O'Donnell's Drug Injury

O'Donnell's Drug Injury, Fifth Edition, presents up-to-date information on adverse events caused by drugs via direct pharmacological action or indirectly through injury caused by impairment or an altered mental state. The impact of drug injury on legal cases is emphasized throughout the book. This book serves as a comprehensive reference for attorneys, pharmacists, physicians, risk managers, nurses, drug manufacturers, and regulators—as well as anyone with an interest in drug use and drug injury. It lays out general pharmacological principles, presents an in-depth discussion of high-risk drugs often implicated in drug injury, details best practices to improve medication safety in clinical pharmacy practice, and discusses a variety of important forensic toxicology concepts such as drug testing.

Key areas covered include:

- Pharmacology and toxicology of high-alert and high-risk drugs often implicated in legal cases.
- Application of pharmacological and toxicological principles to the law.
- Coverage of processes to ensure medication safety, gaps and blind spots in this process, and recommendations on how to enhance drug safety.
- Eight new chapters covering timely topics such as Antineoplastics Therapy, Contrast Media Neurotoxicity, Drug Recognition Evaluation, RxISK Adverse Drug Reaction Reporting Program, Compounding Pharmacy Fraud, Involuntary Intoxication, and Total Parenteral Nutrition Errors and Injuries.
- Contributions by 43 authors with diverse expertise, including pharmacologists; toxicologists; clinical pharmacists; physicians; attorneys; nephrologists, and a neurologist, hepatologist, epidemiologist, addiction expert, and an investigative health reporter.

O'Donnell's Drug Injury
Fifth Edition

Edited by
James J. O'Donnell III, M.S., Ph.D.
James T. O'Donnell, Pharm.D., M.S., FCP, ABCP, FACN
Gourang P. Patel, Pharm.D., M.Sc., BCCCP, FCCP, FCCM
Jennifer Splawski, Pharm.D., M.S., BCPS

CRC Press
Taylor & Francis Group
Boca Raton London New York

CRC Press is an imprint of the
Taylor & Francis Group, an informa business

Fifth edition published 2026
by CRC Press
2385 NW Executive Center Drive, Suite 320, Boca Raton FL 33431

and by CRC Press
4 Park Square, Milton Park, Abingdon, Oxon, OX14 4RN

CRC Press is an imprint of Taylor & Francis Group, LLC

First edition published 2000 by Lawyers & Judges Publishing Company, Inc.
Fourth edition published 2016 by Lawyers & Judges Publishing Company, Inc.

ISBN: 9781041015451 (hbk)
ISBN: 9781041020806 (pbk)
ISBN: 9781003615323 (ebk)

DOI: 10.1201/9781003615323

For Product Safety Concerns and Information please contact our EU representative: GPSR@taylorandfrancis.com
Taylor & Francis Verlag GmbH,
Kaufingerstraße 24,
80331 München, Germany.

To my parents, for their love and support.

James J. O'Donnell, December, 2024

To Michael

James T. O'Donnell, December, 2024

To my family, without their support, sacrifice, and guidance I would not have been able to advance my professional career as far as I have today.

Gourang P. Patel, December, 2024

To my parents, for always loving and supporting me and to James T. O'Donnell for his mentorship and guidance throughout my pharmacy career.

Jennifer Splawski, December, 2024

Contents

PART III Pharmacists, Pharmacy, and Pharmacy Practice

PART IV Forensic and Toxicology Issues

About the Editors

James J. O'Donnell III, M.S., Ph.D., is a chemist and research pharmacologist. He is an associate professor at Rosalind Franklin University of Medicine and Science, where he teaches at the Chicago Medical School and the College of Pharmacy. He is the pharmacology coordinator at the Chicago Medical School, and in the College of Pharmacy he was the founding course director of the core pharmacology courses as well as a forensic toxicology and pharmacology elective. He has also given guest lectures at Rush University on pharmacokinetics and other pharmacology topics. He served as an NIH T32 training grant postdoctoral fellow in respiratory biology at the University of Chicago. He has also held a postdoctoral appointment at the Indiana University School of Medicine at South Bend. His research has primarily focused on inflammatory diseases and pharmacokinetics. He has conducted organometallic chemistry research at the University of Wisconsin–Madison and at Northwestern University in Evanston, IL. He currently serves as President of the American Society for Pharmacology and Experimental Therapeutics—Great Lakes Chapter (ASPET-GLC) and is a member of the American College of Clinical Pharmacology (AACP) and the American Academy of Clinical Toxicology (AACT). He is a co-editor of *O'Donnell's Drug Injury, Fourth Edition*, and the chief editor of *Drug Discovery and Development, Third Edition*. He consults in drug injury, analytical toxicology, and other related matters. Dr. O'Donnell received a Bachelor of Science degree in electrical engineering and computer science from the Massachusetts Institute of Technology (MIT), a Master of Science degree in chemistry from the University of Wisconsin–Madison, and a Doctor of Philosophy in pharmacology from Rush University in Chicago, IL.

James T. O'Donnell, Pharm.D., M.S., FCP, ABCP, FACN, is a pharmacologist, pharmacist, and nutritionist in Barrington Hills, Illinois. He is Associate Professor of Pharmacology at Rush University Medical Center in Chicago, IL, where he served as the course director of the medical pharmacology course. He also held faculty appointments at the University of Illinois Colleges of Medicine and Pharmacy. Dr. O'Donnell is a diplomate of the American Board of Clinical Pharmacology; a fellow of the American College of Clinical Pharmacology; a fellow of the American College of Nutrition; the founding editor-in-chief of the *Journal of Pharmacy Practice*, and the editor of *Drug Injury: Liability, Analysis, and Prevention, First Edition, Second Edition, Third Edition*; a co-editor of *O'Donnell's Drug Injury, Fourth Edition*; a co-editor of *Pharmacy Law: Litigating Pharmaceutical Cases*; and a co-editor of *Drug Discovery and Development, Second and Third Editions.* He consults and testifies in matters involving pharmaceuticals, medication errors, nutritionals, dietary supplements, alcohol and recreational drug toxicity, and drug injuries throughout the United States, for defense and plaintiffs' counsel. Dr. O'Donnell received a Bachelor of Science in pharmacy from the University of Illinois, a Doctor of Pharmacy from the University of Michigan, and a Master of Science in clinical nutrition from Rush University.

Gourang P. Patel, Pharm.D., M.Sc., BCCCP, FCCP, FCCM, is Director of Clinical Pharmacy Services at the University of Chicago Medicine—Chicago, IL. Dr. Patel earned a Bachelor of Chemistry from Truman State University, a Doctor of Pharmacy from the St. Louis College of Pharmacy, and a Master of Clinical Research from the Rush Graduate College. He also reviews medical malpractice cases for both defense and plaintiff sides in the areas of pharmacology, toxicology, and pharmacy practices. Dr. Patel is board certified in critical care (BCCCP) and is a fellow in the American College of Clinical Pharmacy (FCCP) and the Society of Critical Care Medicine (FCCM).

Jennifer Splawski, Pharm.D., M.S., BCPS, is currently a Senior Consultant with Visante's consolidated services centers and pharmacy operations team. Her experience includes clinical pharmacy practice specializing in emergency medicine, operational leadership, and implementing technology within the healthcare space. She also consults and testifies on legal matters for both defense and plaintiff cases related to medication errors and clinical pharmacology/toxicology throughout the United States. Dr. Splawski earned a Bachelor of Science in psychology and Doctor of Pharmacy degree from the University of Illinois at Chicago and a Master of Science degree in pharmacy, focusing on clinical toxicology and a forensic toxicology certificate, from the University of Florida. She served a postgraduate pharmacy residency at the University of California in San Francisco and is a Board-Certified Clinical Pharmacy Specialist (BCPS).

Contributors

Peter D. Anderson, Pharm.D., BCPP, Clinical Pharmacist and Forensic Pharmacologist, Randolph, MA

Frank J. Ascione, Pharm.D., MPH, Ph.D., Professor of Pharmacy, University of Michigan College of Pharmacy, Ann Arbor, MI

Meagan Bailey, M.D., Rush University, Section of Movement Disorders, Chicago, IL

Henry Cohen, B.S., M.S., Pharm.D., FCCM, BCPP, BCGP, Dean and Professor, Touro University, College of Pharmacy, New York, NY

Samantha P. Jellinek-Cohen, Pharm.D., BCPS, CGP, Assistant Clinical Professor, College of Pharmacy and Health Sciences, St. John's University, Queens, NY

Victor Cohen, B.S., Pharm.D., BCPS, CGP, R.Ph., Assistant Vice President, Corporate Clinical Director, Pharmacy Services, Division of Medical and Professional Affairs, NY Health and Hospitals, New York City, NY

Paul N. Danese, Ph.D., Principal, FDAble LLC, Glastonbury, CT

S. Albert Edwards, Pharm.D., RAC, FRAPS, FDA Consultant and Drug Information Expert, Lake Forest, IL

Erica M. Fernandez, Pharm.D., BCCCP, BCPS, Clinical Coordinator, Loyola Medicine—MacNeal Hospital, Berwyn, IL

Todd W. B. Gehr, M.D., Professor of Medicine, Chairman, Division of Nephrology, Medical College of Virginia of Virginia Commonwealth University, Richmond, VA

Fran M. Gengo, Pharm.D., FCP, Associate Professor of Pharmacy and Neurology, University at Buffalo, Dent Neurologic Institute, Amherst, NY

Barry D. Hargan, M.S., MHA, President, Barry Hargan & Associates LLC, Milwaukee, WI

David Healy, MD, FRCPsych, Chief Scientific Officer, Data Based Medicine, Toronto, Canada

Vanessa Juettner, M.S., Ph.D., McCann Health/Caudex, Chicago, IL

Jason M. Kidd, M.D., Associate Professor of Medicine, Division of Nephrology, Virginia Commonwealth University School of Medicine, Richmond, VA

Michael Liu, Pharm.D., MBA, BCCCP, BCNSP, BCPS, Assistant Dean of Clinical & Professional Affairs, and Associate Professor of Pharmacy Practice, Touro College of Pharmacy, New York, NY

Rita Marcoux, R.Ph., MBA, Clinical Professor, University of Rhode Island, College of Pharmacy Kingston, RI

Donald H. Marks, M.D., Ph.D., Morris County, NJ

Anna G. Mattle, Pharm.D., M.S., Division of Neuropharmacology, Dent Neurologic Institute, Amherst, NY

Ned Milenkovich, Pharm.D., J.D., Principal—Much Shelist, Chicago, IL

Heather Minger, Pharm.D., BCPS, Pharmacotherapy Consultant. Lake Forest, IL

Roger N. Morris, R.Ph., J.D., Partner-Chairman Health and Life Science Industry, Quarles & Brady, LLP, Phoenix, AZ

Megan Musselman, Pharm.D., M.S., BCPS, BCCCP, DPLA, FCCP, Clinical Pharmacist Specialist, PGY2 Emergency Medicine Residency Program Director, Emergency Medicine, North Kansas City Hospital, Kansas City, MO

Jadwiga Najib, B.S., Pharm.D., MPH, Professor of Pharmacy Practice, LIU, Arnold and Mary Schwartz College of Pharmacy and Health Sciences, Brooklyn, NY; Clinical Pharmacist, Zucker Hillside Hospital of Northwell, Glen Oaks, NY

James C. Norris, Ph.D., D.A.B.T., ERT, Consulting Pharmacologist and Toxicologist, Searcy, AR

James J. O'Donnell III, M.S., Ph.D., Associate Professor of Pharmacology. Rosalind Franklin University of Medicine and Science, and Pharmaconsultant Inc., Barrington, IL

James T. O'Donnell, Pharm.D., M.S., FCP, Associate Professor of Pharmacology, Rush University Medical Center, IL and Pharmaconsultant Inc., Barrington, IL

Damani Parran, Ph.D., MBA, DABT, Senior Toxicologist, Parran Consulting Group, LLC., Westfield, NJ

Gourang P. Patel, Pharm.D., M.Sc., BCCCP, FCCP, FCCM, Director of Clinical Pharmacy Services, University of Chicago, Chicago, IL

Rodney G. Richmond, MS, PharmD, BCGP, FASCP, Professor and Chair of Pharmacy Practice, Harding University College of Pharmacy, Searcy, AR

Martha Rosenberg, Investigative Journalist/Author, Evanston, IL

Kathryn Schultz, Pharm.D., BCOP, Hematology/Oncology/Cell Therapy Clinical Pharmacy Specialist, Rush University Medical Center; Elmwood Park, IL

Domenic A. Sica, M.D., Professor of Medicine and Pharmacology, Chairman, Section of Clinical Pharmacology and Hypertension, Division of Nephrology, MCV Station, Medical College of Virginia of Virginia Commonwealth University, Richmond, VA

Jennifer Splawski PharmD, MS, BCPS, Senior Consultant, Visante. and ClinPharmRX, Inc. Chicago, IL

William J. Stilling, R.Ph., M.S., J.D., Partner, Stilling & Harrison, Salt Lake City, UT

Stephanie E. Tedford, Ph.D., Director of Clinical and Medical Affairs, LumiThera Inc., Pharmacologist, Pharmacologics, LLC., Seattle, WA

Eris Tollkuci, Pharm.D., BCOP, Hematology/Oncology/Cell Therapy Clinical Pharmacy Specialist, Rush University Medical Center, Assistant Professor of Pharmacotherapy at Rosalind Franklin University of Medicine and Science, River Forest, IL

Willis C. Triplett, Pharm.D., Principal, 503 Quality Matters, LLC., Principal, Compoundium, LLC., Zionsville, IN

William Vaughn, J.D., Vaughn Law, Houston, TX

F. Randy Vogenberg, R.Ph., Ph.D., Principal, Institute for Integrated Healthcare, Greenville, SC, Adjunct Professor of Pharmacy Practice, Department of Pharmacy Practice, University of Rhode Island, College of Pharmacy, Kingston, RI, and Adjunct Professor, Department of Pharmacy Practice, Health Outcomes Policy and Economics Center, Rutgers University, Ernest Mario School of Pharmacy, Piscataway, NJ

Lindsay E. Wagner, Pharm.D., BCPS, CDR, USPHS, Branch Chief, Education and Outreach Branch, Division of Drug Information, Office of Communications, Center for Drug Evaluation and Research, Food and Drug Administration, Silver Spring, MD

Megan Walter, Pharm.D., Pharmacist, Education and Outreach Branch, Division of Drug Information, Office of Communications, Center for Drug Evaluation and Research, Food and Drug Administration, Silver Spring, MD

Jonathan C. Young, Ph.D., M.S., Research Associate, Office of Health Affairs, West Virginia University, Morgantown, WV

Preface to the First Edition

Drug Injury: Liability, Analysis and Prevention is a culmination of my practice, training, consultations, and professional efforts. It follows publication of Pharmacy law (1995). As a pharmacologist, pharmacist, and nutritionist, I have been fortunate to have practiced these three disciplines in a variety of settings. My current professional practice focuses largely on forensics, in which injuries caused by the use of drugs, alcohol, and dietary supplements are examined. My analysis determines what happened, where responsibility lies, and how the injury could have been avoided or prevented.

Pharmacists are trained to be, and are responsible as, drug experts. The public relies on pharmacists to provide the right drug for the right patient, to assure that there are no allergies, contraindications, or interactions from diseases or other drugs, to advise the patients how to safely and effectively use the drugs to the fullest benefit, with a goal of safe and effective drug therapy. The practice of pharmacy has changed dramatically since my entry into practice. What was once a singular and "independent" practice is now largely a corporate practice, consisting of chains of hundreds of units and employing thousands of pharmacists. It remains, however, the individual pharmacist who provides pharmacy services to patients through face-to-face contact, by mail or over the Web. This new corporate focus requires additional layers of control and quality assurance to assure that the individual pharmacists providing service within the corporation are doing so according to the law, the standards of practice, and corporate policy and procedure. The corporate practice of pharmacy has been accompanied by pharmacy litigation which goes beyond the issue of simple negligence, such as a patient who receives the wrong prescription drug, to litigation that addresses inadequate patient monitoring and lack of requisite counseling, and the corporate responsibility for institutional controls to ensure that the corporation's pharmacists are adhering to safe and effective practices.

Drug Injury includes several chapters which describe new and unique specialized pharmacist practices beyond the current chain and traditional retail setting, including long-term care, compounding, home and infusion care, government regulation, and even describe forensic pharmacy practice.

As a pharmacologist, I have conducted clinical research on drugs and devices, and have consulted with and observed how pharmaceutical, medical device, and dietary supplement companies conduct their business. The pharmaceutical industry, especially the segment that is involved with new drug development, is one of the most highly regulated in this country—for good reason! The lives of the public are at stake.

Molzon, a pharmacist-attorney and senior FDA official provides insight into FDA operations, whose mission is to provide risk management for the use of drugs in the United States. Several discussions throughout the book address the role of the FDA in drug development and the regulation of labeling for safety and warnings of toxicity. Since most litigation involving pharmaceutical companies involves inadequate warning, several cases are reviewed to shed light on the controlling regulatory language. The pharmacologists who conduct clinical research to evaluate new drugs, and new uses for old drugs, must address safety and ethical issues to guarantee patient safety. Flawed clinical research practices and inadequate informed consent by subjects may provide grounds for complaints against manufacturers of newly introduced drugs. This subject is well covered in Chapter 4, "Clinical Research," by Tislow, Nesbitt, and Belcher at Gulf Coast Clinical Research. Ron Gottrich of the Illinois Department of Public Health gives us an up-to-date look at regulation in Chapter 20, "Regulation of Pharmacy Practice." Middlekoop addresses the unusual toxicity associated with the powerful acne medication, Accutane, in Chapter 17.

As a nutritionist, I have had the opportunity to work with patients who were unable to eat, did not eat the right nutrients, or just ate too much! I have watched the vitamin craze of the '70s expand to the dietary supplement craze of the '90s. The toxicities associated with various components of substances exempted from FDA enforcement as drugs is covered under a wide umbrella of "non-regulation" under the DSHEA (Dietary Supplement Health Education Act). Molzon's second chapter contribution gives a good history and interpretation of DSHEA, and sets the tone for understanding the regulatory issues of DSHEA and dietary supplements.

As a pharmacist and pharmacologist, I have always been cognizant of safety, and have designed my practice to predict problem areas and focus resources on these areas in the hope of avoiding harm to patients. Adverse drug reactions, drug interactions, allergic reactions, overdoses, and other types of medication errors, are not new to me or to other pharmacists. However, when the Institute of Medicine released its report *To Err is Human* in 1999 on the scope of medical errors, the publicity was astounding. The idea that fifty to one hundred thousand people die each year as a result of medical error was highly disturbing and in fact describes an important new form of disease. The second most frequent type of medical error is the subject of this book. Medication-related errors occur frequently, though most do not result in actual harm. But those that do are costly and sometimes deadly. Almost two percent of hospital admissions experienced an adverse drug effect in spite of underreporting that represents less than twenty percent of the actual unreported totals. A recent *JAMA* article described the enormity of drug related deaths as the equivalent of two 747s crashing every week!

Chapter 5, "Adverse Drug Reaction and Causality Assessment," reviews how causality is assessed in individual adverse reactions. Chapter 27, "Medication Errors," provides dozens of examples of serious medication errors, and analysis and tips for prevention.

It is the intent of this book to go beyond the issue of what went wrong and who did it. Case reports are frequently presented. Analysis of drug injury can help prevent recurrence by educating the entire health care profession. When education and safe pharmacy practice fail, affected patients have a right to investigate and seek damages for their injuries. Many times, that is all that they can do, because their injuries are permanent or fatal.

Described as the largest drug disaster in modern history, the Fen/Phen diet is described from two points of view: by surgeon-attorney Restaino, from a medical legal perspective and; by this author, from the pharmacological and warning perspective. As this book goes to press, a $4 billion plus nationwide settlement is being scrutinized by the court, and an additional 50,000 lawsuits remain to be resolved outside of the nationwide settlement. These two chapters are current and should be quite provocative.

Cohen, an accomplished practitioner who specializes in geriatric pharmacotherapy, and the new Editor-in-Chief of the *Journal of Pharmacy Practice*, has contributed a chapter on antidepressants, describing the complex pharmacology and toxicity issues which apply to this vulnerable population, and compares the pharmacology and toxicology of the agents in use. A large portion of the geriatric population uses medication to treat depression and frequently suffers drug injuries which result in litigation.

Najib, a psychiatric pharmacist from New York, provides a discussion of drug-induced movement disorders associated with antidepressants and with neuroleptics, the drugs used to treat severe mental disorders.

The 1980s had a mass tort involving L-Tryptophan. One of the MDL pharmaceutical torts of the nineties, involved Omniflox, a promising new fluoroquinolone antibiotic. Brian Branch, Esq., an attorney from Albuquerque, New Mexico, has contributed an analysis of this litigation which was quite active in the first half of the '90s. Coincidentally, Margaret and Turner Branch contributed a thorough review of the L-Tryptophan litigation in *Pharmacy Law*, a predecessor to this book. Sheller's chapter is repeated for determining when a physician or hospital may be the subject of litigation in Chapter 9.

We have updated other chapters in the book, including Chapter 28, "Mistakes Pharmacists Make—and Why," by Trinque who brings a unique perspective from a pharmacist in the trenches. The vaccine chapter by Dodd is repeated, because, unfortunately, patients continue to suffer severe and debilitating adverse reactions from vaccine products. The chapter on corticosteroids has been expanded and updated. The misuse of steroids continues, resulting in unnecessary and debilitating injuries, frequently involving destruction of the skeleton and joints. Robinson, a California attorney, presents a legal perspective of steroid-induced avascular necrosis (AVN) of the bone. As an attorney, Ms. Robinson is representing dozens of people throughout the country who have suffered serious steroid induced injuries. Theophylline is included even though it has not been a first-line drug for asthma and chronic obstructive lung disease for at least ten years, because its continued use by physicians often leads to serious toxicity. Ten percent of patients on insulin and hypoglycemics suffer hypoglycemic reactions which results in scores of death each year. Salemi, an athlete and soccer referee, reviews performance-enhancing drugs (athlete doping), including anabolic steroids, involving amateur and professional athletes, which are in the news daily. Several cases involving this wide variety of therapeutic agents are analyzed in individual chapters, which have been contributed by accomplished practitioners in their topic or practice area.

Drug Injury includes chapters addressing specialized pharmacy practice by Klotz, an innovative practitioner from California, and long-term care (nursing home) by Zlotnick of New Jersey, and managed care, by Vogenberg, a recognized academician and researcher from Massachusetts. Allen discusses the specialty pharmacy practice of compounding drugs to prescription order in Chapter 23, "Pharmacy Compounding Regulations." These are new and expanded areas of independent practice, providing new services and new risks.

Peter Anderson's chapter, "The Forensic Pharmacist," discusses alcohol, cocaine, marijuana, and other selected "recreational drugs." It discusses forensic drug testing and its use in litigation. Recreational drugs affect every walk of life. Employers, pharmacists, administrators and attorneys can all benefit from this insightful addition. The chapter addresses the roles and functions of a pharmacist and pharmacologist in forensic matters, with specific case examples. ImObersteg's chapter on drug testing is the companion chapter to the "Forensic Pharmacist." These two chapters can serve any practitioner, since any practitioner can be called upon to serve as an expert in court, a regulatory hearing, or other arena outside clinical practice where scientific and professional issues are examined.

"Pain Medication" covers the use of opiate analgesics for chronic pain and describes how to help a jury assess the amount and type of pain a patient has suffered through the technique of pain equilibration.

Drug Injury is intended to serve as a reference for attorneys, pharmacists, physicians, risk managers, nurses, drug manufacturers, and regulators, as well as anyone with any interest in drug use and drug injury. It summarizes the FDA's responsibility in monitoring drug safety. It reviews drug product related liability issues that focus on the manufacturer's role in providing for drug safety. The book identifies important roles that pharmacists play in enhancing medication safety and effectiveness, and what happens when pharmacists do not function adequately. The medication errors chapter by Iyer focuses on the system of providing safe medications, and addresses the multidisciplinary tasks involved in safe drug delivery. By focusing on the most dangerous drugs, the reader can learn from the tragedies and mistakes of others, look at their own practice setting, and avoid repeating the same or similar mistakes.

James O'Donnell, Pharm.D., M.S., A.B.C.P., C.N.S., F.A.C.N.
Assistant Professor of Pharmacology
Rush Medical College-Chicago
President, Pharmaconsultant Inc.
Palatine, IL and Monarch Beach, CA

Preface to the Fifth Edition

O'Donnell's Drug Injury welcomes two new editors, Gourang P. Patel, Pharm.D., BCCCP, and Jennifer Splawski, Pharm.D., M.S., BCPS, both accomplished clinicians with extensive clinical, academic, publishing, and consulting experience. Their contributions expand the clinical expertise of the editors for *O'Donnell's Drug Injury, Fifth Edition* (*DI V*).

DI V continues the tradition of serving as a reference for attorneys, pharmacists, physicians, risk managers, nurses, drug manufacturers, and regulators—as well as anyone with any interest in drug use and drug injury. It summarizes the FDA's responsibility in monitoring drug development and safety, reviews current drug products that are most frequently the cause of drug injury, and addresses a few drug liability topics. Drug product liability lawsuits have decreased in frequency, hence the lesser coverage in the Fifth Edition. Seven new chapters include Antineoplastic Therapy; Contrast Media Neurotoxicity Following Myelography; Drug Evaluation and Classification Program: An Evidence-Based Analysis; The Safety of Medicines: PharmacoVigilance, PharmacoSurveillance, PharmacoEmpowerment?; Compounding Pharmacy Fraud and Unethical Practices; Involuntary Intoxication; and Parenteral Nutrition Related Errors and Complications. *DI V* identifies important roles that pharmacists play in enhancing medication safety and effectiveness and demonstrates what can happen when pharmacists and other practitioners and healthcare institutions do not meet regulatory standards or operational/clinical duties of a pharmacy and pharmacist. By focusing on the most high-alert and high-risk drugs, the reader can learn from the tragedies and errors of others, evaluate their own practice settings, and avoid making similar errors. The Forensic and Toxicology Issues section has been updated and expanded, reflecting the landscape, and concordant with the editors' consulting practice—a good source for real-life forensic reports.

The Fifth Edition contains forty-two chapters. Forty-three contributors include practicing clinical pharmacists, pharmacologists, toxicologists, nurses, physicians, hepatologists, nephrologists, epidemiologists, attorneys, an investigative health reporter, and an addictionologist. These contributors practice at the FDA, healthcare industry, pharmaceutical industry, academia, regulatory agencies, law firms, medical practices, and hospitals throughout the United States and Canada. Many hold academic appointments and perform clinical research.

The book is divided into four sections:

I. The Pharmaceutical Process: How are drugs developed, regulated, monitored, advertised, and evaluated, and how do they work?
II. High-Risk Drug Therapies Resulting in Injury and Litigation: Which drugs cause the most injury? What types of injuries? Which organ systems are most commonly and seriously injured?
III. Pharmacists, Pharmacy, and Pharmacy Practice: What can pharmacists and health systems do to minimize and mitigate risk while improving medication safety?
IV. Forensic and Toxicology Issues: Recreational drugs, drug testing, involuntary intoxication, and postmortem distribution of drugs.

There are seven new chapters. The remaining chapters have been extensively revised and updated since the publication of *DI IV.* Several chapters with similar topics have been combined and integrated in order to provide a consolidated review of the particular drug class or pathology. A few chapters are re-published, which are either basic topics (Pharmacy Law Review, Regulation of Pharmacists) or there is little or no new information on the topic, but the topic remains relevant, and thus the inclusion. Fourteen (14) chapters have been retired (including Dietary Supplements, Counterfeit Drugs, Legal Consequences of Controlled Substances, HIV Pharmacotherapy, Ketorolac Abuse in Collegiate Athletics, Clinical Research Testing, The Forensic Pharmacist, After-Hours Pharmacy Services, Pain Equipotency, Pharmaceutical Revolution, Nonscientific Uses and Illegal Marketing of Drugs and Dietary Supplements, Institutional Review Boards and Protection of Subjects in Clinical Research, Pharmacogenomics: Using Precision Medicine to Decrease Adverse Drug Reactions, and Forensic Diabetic Drugs), either due to a lack of currency or resolution of some of the necessary problems. Many relevant issues from the retired chapters have been incorporated into other revised, merged, and new chapters. A major focus of the new chapters and revised chapters has been to incorporate expert forensic reports prepared by the editors in litigation consultations. The goal of incorporating forensic reports is to demonstrate the application of forensic sciences content into real drug injury and regulatory scenarios.

We have included updated chapters on all of the specialized pharmacist chapters from the Fourth Edition. We believe that the pharmacist's most important responsibility is to ensure that drugs are used safely and effectively and to do no harm. Everyone in the healthcare system is responsible for medication safety, and pharmacists are the system's safety net.

Because drugs are ubiquitous, and because drugs affect people's lives and practice outside the walls of the hospital and the drugstore, we again include chapters on the most frequently abused drugs (alcohol, marijuana, cocaine), forensic drug testing, and postmortem redistribution. We also significantly updated the "Dangers of Opioids" chapter to include the opioid epidemic, as well as care for patients with opioid use disorder. As stated earlier, a focused audience of *DI V* is attorneys, who usually have no training in FDA, pharmacy, or regulatory law and who certainly have no training in pharmacology or the pathology of drugs. Yet, in a wide spectrum of practices, attorneys must master these complex topics to represent their clients and routinely consult with a clinical pharmacist or pharmacologist to assist. That same expert is frequently called as an expert to provide testimony on drug actions, effects, interactions, causation, and pharmacist standard of care. To assist in the daunting learning curve facing the non-clinician in assessing drug injury matters, we have included an extensive review of the General Principles of Pharmacology (Chapter 9), which details principles applicable to all drugs. The First, Second, Third, and Fourth Editions of *O'Donnell's Drug Injury* were well received by legal, medical, pharmacy, and nursing practitioners and scholars. *O'Donnell's Drug Injury* books have been used as text and reference books in several universities and can be found in numerous medical, pharmacy, manufacturer, and law libraries, the FDA library, and private law offices throughout the United States.

SUMMARY

In closing, *O'Donnell's Drug Injury, Fifth Edition* is intended to serve as a broad and deep reference for anyone with a professional or personal interest in drug use, development, or testing.

James J. O'Donnell III, M.S., Ph.D.
Associate Professor of Pharmacology
Rosalind Franklin University of Medicine and Science, North Chicago, IL, and
Pharmaconsultant Inc. Barrington, Il

James T. O'Donnell, Pharm.D., M.S., FCP, ABCP, FACN
Associate Professor of Pharmacology,
Rush University Medical Center, Chicago, IL and
Pharmaconsultant Inc., Barrington, IL

Gourang P. Patel, Pharm.D., M.Sc., BCCCP, FCCP, FCCM
Director of Clinical Pharmacy Services
University of Chicago Medicine
Chicago, IL

Jennifer Splawski, Pharm.D., M.S., BCPS
Senior Consultant- Visante and
ClinPharmRX Inc., Chicago, IL

Acknowledgements

Gerald Walsh, for diligence and excellence in communications and file maintenance.

Stephanie Tedford Ph.D., for diligence and excellence in technical editing, formatting, and organization.

Part I

The Pharmaceutical Process

1 FDA and Drug Approval Process

Megan Walter and Lindsay E. Wagner

The views are of the authors and should not be construed to represent FDA's views or policies.

SYNOPSIS

DOI: 10.1201/9781003615323-2

1.1 INTRODUCTION

The U.S. Food and Drug Administration (FDA) is charged with protecting the public health by ensuring the safety, effectiveness, quality, and security of human and veterinary drugs, biological products, and medical devices; ensuring the safety of foods, cosmetics, and radiation-emitting products; and regulating tobacco products. Fundamental to the FDA's core mission of promoting and protecting public health is regulatory science. As a science-based agency, the FDA must have access to the best available scientific data to inform regulatory decision-making and improve access to FDA-regulated products that benefit the public health and enhance oversight.[1]

The controlling statute governing the approval of drugs in the U.S. is 21 U.S.C. § 301. The Federal Food Drug and Cosmetic Act (also known as the "FDCA" or "FD&C Act") contains the basic definitions of a drug and a new drug, for purposes of FDA approval. Subsections 201 (g); 21 U.S.C. 321 (g); 21 C.F.R. parts 310 and 314 provide insight into this process.

As defined in FD&C Act 201 (g), a drug is an article recognized by the United States Pharmacopeia, or other officially recognized national formulary. The definition also includes articles intended for use in the diagnosis, cure, mitigation, treatment, or prevention of disease in man or other animals. The statute covers articles other than food that are designed to affect the structure or any function of the body.[2] The classification of a product as a drug is based on the claims or representations made by the manufacturer in the labeling or advertising literature of the product.

Since its beginnings as the United States Department of Agriculture's (USDAs) Bureau of Chemistry, the FDA's institutional organization has changed significantly. Today, the FDA is organized into eight centers with responsibility for regulating specific product areas, as well as a number of administrative and program offices under the Office of the Commissioner. The focus of this chapter is the FDA's largest center, the Center for Drug Evaluation and Research (CDER). CDER's mission is to assure that safe and effective drugs, both prescription and over-the-counter, are available to the American people.

In the United States, medical products are developed and used within a complex system involving players with various goals and responsibilities:

- Manufacturers who develop and test products and submit applications for their approval to the FDA
- The FDA, which has an extensive premarketing review and approval process and which uses a series of post-marketing surveillance programs to gather data on and assess risks[3]
- Healthcare practitioners involved in the healthcare delivery system
- Patients, who rely on this complex system to provide them with the necessary interventions to protect them from injury.

Although medical products are required to be safe, safety does not mean zero risk.[4] A safe product is one that has reasonable risks when balancing the benefits to the American public as a whole.[5] The medical product development and delivery system regulated by the FDA must maintain balance in the risk–benefit ratio by ensuring that medical products are developed, tested, manufactured, labeled, prescribed, dispensed, and used such that risks are known and can be evaluated against alternative treatment options.[6]

The FDA's responsibilities in this system—as laid out in the FDCA—are largely devoted to pre- and post-marketing risk assessment. The FDA's decision to approve or not approve a medical product is the agency's central risk-management action. The FDA must ensure that beneficial medical products are available and labeled with adequate information on their risks and benefits while protecting the public from unsafe products and false claims. The FDA approves a product when it judges the benefits to outweigh the risks for the specified use in the intended population.[7] A major goal of premarket review is to ensure that products are truthfully and adequately labeled. Labeling is given considerable emphasis because it is the chief tool the agency uses to communicate risk and benefit to the healthcare community and patients.[8]

Once medical products are on the market, ensuring continued safety is principally the responsibility of healthcare providers and their patients, as they are the ones making risk–benefit decisions on an individual, rather than on a population, basis. They are expected to use the labeling information to select and use products wisely, thereby minimizing exposure to risks and adverse events. To assist with post-marketing risk management, the agency maintains a system of complex post-marketing surveillance and risk-assessment programs to identify adverse events that are not identified during medical product development and premarket review.[9] The FDA thoroughly evaluates and investigates reported adverse events, therapeutic failures, and medication errors associated with the use of an approved medical product. The agency uses this information to initiate labeling updates and, on rare occasions, to reevaluate the approval decision.[10,11,12]

1.2 THE NEW DRUG DEVELOPMENT PROCESS

American consumers benefit from having access to the safest and most advanced pharmaceutical system in the world.[13] The main consumer watchdog in this system is CDER. CDER ensures that drugs, both brand name and generic, work correctly and that their health benefits outweigh their known risks.[14]

1.2.1 Discovery and Preclinical Research

Researchers test thousands of molecular compounds to find new therapeutics, new uses of old therapeutics, and ways new technology can improve existing knowledge. Only a small fraction of the compounds tested will show promise and progress further.[15]

Before a drug can be tested in humans, information must be gathered to determine its pharmacokinetic properties.[16] It is important to understand how it is absorbed, distributed, metabolized, and excreted. Preclinical research is usually referred to as either *in vivo* or *in vitro*. *In vivo* means "in the body," whereas *in vitro* means "outside the body." Researchers are required to follow the FDA's Good Laboratory Practices (GLPs) set forth in 21 Code of Federal Regulations (CFR) Part 58. These regulations set the minimum basic requirements that lab researchers must follow when conducting preclinical testing.[17]

During a new drug's early preclinical development, the sponsor's primary goal is to determine whether the product is reasonably safe for initial use in humans, as well as whether the compound exhibits pharmacological activity that justifies commercial development. Usually, preclinical studies are not very large. However, these studies must provide detailed information on dosing and toxicity levels. After preclinical testing, researchers review their findings and decide whether the drug should be tested in people.

1.2.2 Clinical Research

While preclinical research answers basic questions about a drug's safety, it is not a substitute for studies of ways the drug will interact with the human body. "Clinical research" refers to studies, or trials, that are done in people (known as subjects in clinical research). When a product is identified as a viable candidate for further development, the sponsor then focuses on collecting the data and information necessary to establish that the product will not expose humans to unreasonable risks when used in limited, early-stage clinical studies. Generally, this includes data and information in three broad areas:

- *Animal pharmacology and toxicology studies.* These include preclinical data to permit an assessment as to whether the product is reasonably safe for initial testing in humans. Also included are any previous experience with the drug in humans (often foreign use).
- *Manufacturing information.* This includes information pertaining to the composition, manufacture, stability, and controls used for manufacturing the drug substance and the drug product. This information is assessed as to whether the company can adequately produce and supply consistent batches of the drug.
- *Clinical protocols and investigator information.* These include detailed protocols for proposed clinical studies to assess whether the initial-phase trials will expose subjects to unnecessary risks. Also included is information on the qualifications of clinical investigators—professionals (generally physicians) who oversee the administration of the experimental compound—to assess whether they are qualified to fulfill their clinical trial duties. Finally, commitments to obtain informed consent from the research subjects, to obtain review of the study by an institutional review board (IRB), and to adhere to the investigational new drug regulations are included.

Clinical trials represent the ultimate premarket testing for unapproved drugs.[18] During these trials, an investigational compound is administered to humans and is evaluated for its safety and effectiveness in treating, preventing, or diagnosing a specific disease or condition. The results of this testing will comprise the single most important factor in deciding whether the new drug receives FDA approval.[19]

Although the goal of clinical trials is to obtain safety and efficacy data to support the drug development plan, the top priority always must be the safety of those in the trials.[20]

The FDA's CDER monitors the study design and conduct of clinical trials to ensure that people in the trials are not exposed to unnecessary risks.

As the developers design clinical studies, they consider what they want to accomplish for each of the different clinical research phases and begin the Investigational New Drug Application (IND), a process they must initiate before clinical research begins.

1.2.3 Investigational New Drug Application

The IND is the vehicle through which a sponsor advances to the next stage of drug development known as clinical trials (human trials).[21] It is not an application for marketing approval. Rather, it is a request for an exemption from the federal statute that prohibits an unapproved drug from being shipped in interstate commerce. Current federal law requires that a drug be the subject of an approved marketing application before it is transported or distributed across state lines. Because a sponsor will probably want to ship the investigational drug to clinical investigators in many states, it must seek an exemption from that legal requirement. The IND is the means through which the sponsor technically obtains this exemption from the FDA; however, its main purpose is to detail the data that provide documentation that it is, indeed, reasonable to proceed with certain human trials with the drug.

In the IND application, developers must include:

- Animal study data and toxicity (side effects that cause great harm) data
- Manufacturing information
- Clinical protocols (study plans) for studies to be conducted
- Data from any prior human research
- Information about the investigator

The FDA offers a wealth of resources to researchers and sponsors to aid in understanding how to submit a complete IND application.[22] For sponsors who are still unsure, the FDA offers pre-IND meetings. These meetings can be very important when the product is intended to treat a serious or life-threatening disease, there is a novel indication, there are no current guidance documents, the sponsor is new to drug development, there are questions from the sponsor, there are pharmacologic or toxicologic signals of concern, or when the drug is a new molecular entity.

Pre-IND meetings are requested through a formal process and require the sponsor submit a pre-IND meeting packet. The packet includes an overall program synopsis, full description of the development plan, along with other information critical to providing input on the research plan. Before requesting a pre-IND meeting, sponsors and researchers must do their due diligence to review all available information from the FDA through the regulations, web information, and guidance documents.

Even though the FDA offers extensive technical assistance, drug developers are in some cases not required to take the FDA's suggestions. As long as clinical trials are thoughtfully designed, reflect what developers know about a product, safeguard participants, and otherwise meet Federal standards, the FDA allows wide latitude in clinical trial design. In fact, the FDA has communicated through guidance on how sponsors can enrich their studies to increase the efficiency of drug development and support precision medicine as well as to share the agency's current thinking related to enhancing the diversity of clinical trial populations.[23,24]

Once an IND is received, the FDA's review team has 30 days to review the submission. FDA responds to IND applications in one of two ways:

1. authorization to begin clinical trials, or
2. clinical hold to delay or stop the investigation.

The FDA can place a clinical hold for specific reasons, including:

- Participants are exposed to unreasonable or significant risk.
- Investigators are not qualified.
- Materials for the volunteer participants are misleading.
- The IND application does not include enough information about the trial's risks.

A clinical hold is rare; instead, the FDA often provides comments intended to improve the quality of a clinical trial. In most cases, if the FDA is satisfied that the trial meets Federal standards, the applicant is allowed to proceed with the proposed study.

The developer is responsible for informing the review team about new protocols, as well as serious side effects seen during the trial. This information ensures that the team can monitor the trials carefully for signs of any problems. After the trial ends, researchers must submit study reports.

This process continues until the developer decides to end clinical trials or files a marketing application. Before filing a marketing application, a developer must generally have adequate data from two large, controlled clinical trials.

1.2.4 Phases of Clinical Studies

The four phases of clinical studies are:

- Phase 1: the initial introduction of an investigational new drug into healthy volunteers to evaluate safety
- Phase 2: small clinical studies conducted with patients to obtain preliminary data on the effectiveness of the drug and further safety data

- Phase 3: large clinical trials to evaluate safety and efficacy in groups of patients with the disease to be treated[25]
- Phase 4: post-marketing commitments and post-market requirements.

1.2.4.1 Phase I

Phase 1 includes the initial introduction of an investigational new drug to human research subjects. These studies are closely monitored and may be conducted in patients but are usually conducted in healthy volunteer subjects. These studies are designed to determine the metabolic and pharmacologic actions of the drug in humans, to determine the side effects associated with increasing doses, and, if possible, to gain early evidence on effectiveness. During Phase 1, sufficient information about the drug's pharmacokinetics and pharmacological effects should be obtained to permit the design of well-controlled, scientifically valid, Phase 2 studies.

Phase 1 studies also evaluate drug metabolism, structure–activity relationships, and the mechanism of action in humans. These studies also determine which investigational drugs are used as research tools to explore biological phenomena or disease processes. The total number of subjects included in Phase I studies varies with the drug but is generally in the range of 20 to 80.

In Phase 1 studies, CDER can impose a clinical hold (i.e., prohibit the study from proceeding or stop a trial that has started) for reasons of safety, or because of a sponsor's failure to accurately disclose the risk of study to investigators. Although CDER routinely provides advice in such cases, investigators may choose to ignore any advice regarding the design of Phase 1 studies in areas other than patient safety.

1.2.4.2 Phase II

Phase 2 includes the early controlled clinical studies conducted to obtain preliminary data on the effectiveness of the drug for a particular indication or indications in patients with the disease or condition. This phase of testing also helps uncover the common short-term side effects and risks associated with the drug. Phase 2 studies are typically well-controlled, closely monitored, and conducted in a relatively small number of subjects (usually several hundred people).

1.2.4.3 Phase III

Phase 3 studies are expanded controlled and uncontrolled trials. They are performed after preliminary evidence suggesting effectiveness of the drug has been obtained in Phase 2 and are intended to gather the additional information about efficacy and safety that is needed to evaluate the overall benefit–risk relationship of the drug. Phase 3 studies also provide an adequate basis for extrapolating the results to the general population and transmitting that information in the prescribing information. Phase 3 studies usually include several hundred to several thousand people.

In both Phases 2 and 3, the CDER can impose a clinical hold if a study is unsafe (as in Phase 1) or if the protocol is clearly deficient in design in meeting its stated objectives. Great care is taken to ensure that this determination is not made in isolation, but that it reflects current scientific knowledge, agency experience with the design of clinical trials, and experience with the therapeutic class of drugs under investigation.

1.2.4.4 Phase IV

Studies are sometimes referred to as Phase IV when they occur after approval, or post-marketing.[26] These are often studies required by the FDA as part of the drug's approval. Post-marketing phase IV studies can be found in a searchable database and in the approval letter for a new drug that is posted on Drugs@FDA.[27,28]

1.2.5 Expanded Access Programs

Sometimes called "compassionate use," expanded access is a potential pathway for a patient with an immediately life-threatening condition or serious disease or condition to gain access to an investigational medical product (drug, biologic, or medical device) for treatment outside of clinical trials when no comparable or satisfactory alternative therapy options are available.[29]

Expanded access may be appropriate when all the following apply:

- Patient has a serious disease or condition, or whose life is immediately threatened by their disease or condition
- There is no comparable or satisfactory alternative therapy to diagnose, monitor, or treat the disease or condition
- Patient enrollment in a clinical trial is not possible
- Potential patient benefit justifies the potential risks of treatment
- Providing the investigational medical product will not interfere with investigational trials that could support a medical product's development or marketing approval for the treatment indication.

Investigational drugs, biologics, or medical devices have not yet been approved or cleared by the FDA, and the FDA has not found these products to be safe and effective for their specific use. Furthermore, the investigational medical product may, or may not, be effective in the treatment of the condition, and use of the product may cause unexpected serious side effects.

An immediately life-threatening disease means a stage of a disease in which there is a reasonable likelihood that death will occur within a matter of months, or in which premature death is likely without early treatment. For example, advanced cases of certain cancers, herpes simplex encephalitis, and subarachnoid hemorrhage are all considered to be immediately life-threatening diseases. Treatment INDs are made available to patients before general marketing begins, typically during Phase 3 studies. Treatment INDs also allow the FDA to obtain additional data on the drug's safety and effectiveness.

Under the FDA's current regulations, there are three categories of expanded access to improve access to investigational drugs: expanded access to investigational drugs for individual patients, including in emergencies, intermediate-size patient populations, and larger populations under a treatment protocol or treatment IND for widespread use.

For many years, the FDA authorized charging for investigational drugs made available under all three categories of expanded access. The regulations set forth the requirements for authorization to charge for an investigational drug in a clinical trial, provide criteria for charging for an investigational drug for the different types of expanded access, and clarify what costs can be recovered.

1.2.6 Right to Try

The Right to Try Act, or the Trickett Wendler, Frank Mongiello, Jordan McLinn, and Matthew Bellina Right to Try Act, was signed into law on May 30, 2018.[30] This law is another way for patients who have been diagnosed with life-threatening diseases or conditions who have tried all approved treatment options and who are unable to participate in a clinical trial to access certain unapproved treatments. The Right to Try Act permits/allows eligible patients to have access to eligible investigational drugs.

An eligible patient is a patient who has:

- Been diagnosed with a life-threatening disease or condition
- Exhausted approved treatment options and is unable to participate in a clinical trial involving the eligible investigational drug (this must be certified by a physician who is in good standing with their licensing organization or board and who will not be compensated directly by the manufacturer for certifying)
- And has provided, or their legally authorized representative has provided, written informed consent regarding the eligible investigational drug to the treating physician

An eligible investigational drug is an investigational drug:

- For which a Phase 1 clinical trial has been completed
- That has not been approved or licensed by the FDA for any use
- For which an application has been filed with the FDA or is under investigation in a clinical trial that is intended to form the primary basis of a claim of effectiveness in support of FDA approval and is the subject of an active investigational new drug application submitted to the FDA
- Whose active development or production is ongoing, and that has not been discontinued by the manufacturer or placed on clinical hold by the FDA

1.3 NEW DRUG AND THERAPEUTIC BIOLOGIC APPLICATION PROCESS

Since 1938, every new drug has been the subject of an approved New Drug Application (NDA) or Biologics License Application (BLA) before U.S. commercialization.[31]

A team of CDER physicians, statisticians, chemists, pharmacologists, and other scientists reviews the company's data and proposed labeling.[14] If this independent and unbiased review establishes that a drug's health benefits outweigh its known risks, the drug is approved for sale. CDER doesn't test drugs itself, although it does conduct limited research in the areas of drug quality, safety, and effectiveness standards.

Until the 20th century, prescribing and taking drugs was a risky business for doctors and patients alike. Little was known about drugs, no scientific standards existed, and sometimes medicines caused illnesses rather than curing or preventing them. The U.S. drug review process assures that drugs are safe and effective.

1.3.1 New Drug Applications and Biologic License Applications

The NDA or BLA is the vehicle through which drug sponsors formally propose that the FDA approve a new pharmaceutical for use in the United States.[32] To obtain this authorization, a drug manufacturer submits an NDA or BLA, which includes nonclinical (animal) and clinical (human) test data and analyses, drug information, and descriptions of manufacturing procedures.

The application submitted must provide sufficient information, data, and analyses to permit FDA reviewers to reach several key decisions, including whether the

- drug (used hereafter to also encompass therapeutic biologics license applications reviewed by CDER) is safe and effective for its proposed uses, and whether the benefits of the drug outweigh its risks;
- drug's proposed labeling is appropriate and, what it should contain; and
- methods used in manufacturing the drug and the conditions used to maintain the drug's quality are adequate to preserve the drug's identity, strength, quality, and purity.

For decades, the regulation and control of new drugs in the United States has been based on the NDA and BLA. Since 1938, every new drug has been the subject of an approved application before U.S. commercialization. Whereas an NDA is used for drugs subject to the drug approval provisions of the FDCA, a BLA is required for biological products subject to licensure under the Public Health Service (PHS) Act.[33]

Applications have evolved considerably over time. When the FDCA was passed in 1938, NDAs were required to contain only information pertaining to the investigational drug's safety. In 1962, the Kefauver–Harris Amendments to the FDCA required NDAs to contain evidence both that a new drug was effective for its intended use and that the established benefits of the drug outweighed its known risks.[34]

The NDA was again the subject of change in 1985, when the FDA completed a comprehensive revision of the regulations pertaining to NDAs.[19] While this revision, commonly called the NDA Rewrite, modified content requirements, it was mainly intended to restructure the ways in which information and data are organized and presented in the NDA to expedite FDA reviews.

Further modification of formatting of the NDA is now required as part of an initiative of the International Council for Harmonisation of Technical Requirements for Pharmaceuticals for Human Use (ICH) (www.ich.org). Through the ICH process, considerable harmonization has been achieved among the three regions (Japan, Europe, and the United States) in the organization of a submission for the registration of pharmaceuticals for human use. The culmination of these efforts is the electronic Common Technical Document (eCTD), a modular presentation of technical documentation acceptable by ICH regulators.[35]

1.3.2 Fundamentals of NDA and BLA Submissions

Although the quantity of information and data submitted in NDAs can vary significantly, the components of the application are fairly uniform. The components of any application are, in part, a function of the nature of the subject drug and the information available to the applicant at the time of submission. As outlined in Form FDA-356h, "Application to Market a New Drug, Biologic or an Antibiotic Drug for Human Use," NDAs or BLAs can consist of a dozen or more different sections.[36]

1.3.3 NDA Classifications

CDER classifies NDAs with a code that reflects both the type of drug being submitted and its intended uses.[37] The numbers one through 10 are used to describe the type of drug:

1 New molecular entity (NME)
2 New active ingredient (new salt, new noncovalent derivative, new ester)
3 New dosage form
4 New combination
5 New formulation or new manufacturer
6 New indication [no longer used]
7 Drug already marketed without an approved NDA
8 OTC switch
9 New indication submitted as distinct NDA, consolidated with original NDA after approval
10 New indication submitted as distinct NDA—not consolidated

The following letter codes describe the review priority of the drug:[38]

S. Standard review for drugs similar to currently available drugs
P. Priority review for drugs that represent significant advances over existing treatments

1.4 FDA Review

1.4.1 Expedited Development and Review Programs

The application review process begins upon receipt of the application. For a high-level illustration of the timeline for NME and original BLAs under PDUFA V, see Figure 1.1.[39]

1.4.1.1 Accelerated Approval

When studying a new drug, it can sometimes take many years to learn whether a drug actually provides a real effect

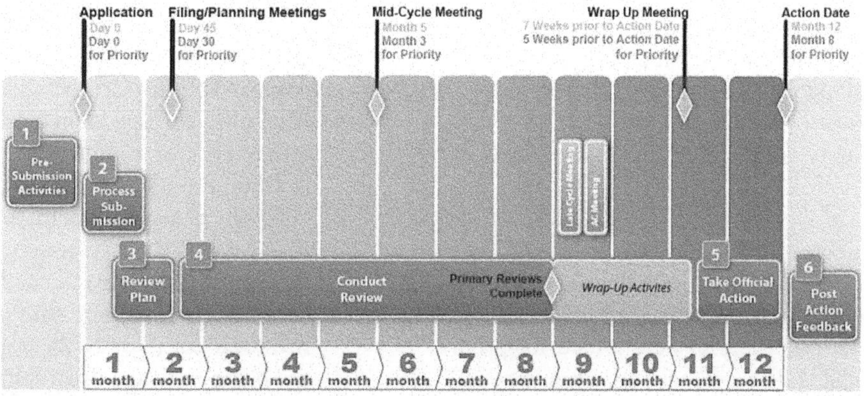

FIGURE 1.1 Application Review Process.

on how a patient survives, feels, or functions.[40] A positive therapeutic effect that is clinically meaningful in the context of a given disease is known as "clinical benefit." Mindful of the fact that it may take an extended period of time to measure a drug's intended clinical benefit, in 1992 the FDA instituted the Accelerated Approval regulations. These regulations allowed drugs for serious conditions that filled an unmet medical need to be approved based on a surrogate endpoint. Using a surrogate endpoint enabled the FDA to approve these drugs faster.

A surrogate endpoint used for accelerated approval is a marker—a laboratory measurement, radiographic image, physical sign, or other measure that is thought to predict clinical benefit—but is not itself a measure of clinical benefit. Likewise, an intermediate clinical endpoint is a measure of a therapeutic effect that is considered reasonably likely to predict the clinical benefit of a drug, such as an effect on irreversible morbidity and mortality (IMM).

Where Phase 4 confirmatory trials verify clinical benefit, the FDA will generally terminate the requirement. Approval of a drug may be withdrawn or the labeled indication of the drug changed if trials fail to verify clinical benefit or do not demonstrate sufficient clinical benefit to justify the risks associated with the drug (e.g., show a significantly smaller magnitude or duration of benefit than was anticipated based on the observed effect on the surrogate).

1.4.1.2 Priority Review

The Prescription Drug User Fee Act of 1992 added a six-month priority review designation for drug applications versus the 10-month standard review. The qualifying criteria is for drugs that treat a serious condition and if approved, would provide a significant improvement in safety or effectiveness, or that proposes a labeling change pursuant to a report on a pediatric study under the Best Pharmaceuticals for Children Act (505A of the FDCA), or that has been designated as a qualified infectious disease product.[41,42]

Significant improvement may be demonstrated by the following examples:

- evidence of increased effectiveness in treatment, prevention, or diagnosis of condition;
- elimination or substantial reduction of a treatment-limiting drug reaction;
- documented enhancement of patient compliance that is expected to lead to an improvement in serious outcomes; or
- evidence of safety and effectiveness in a new subpopulation

Another approach to obtain priority review is through priority review vouchers (PRVs), which give the same benefits of priority review to sponsors of approved product applications that meet certain criteria. PRVs are issued for products that are for a tropical disease, material threat medical countermeasures, or rare pediatric disease.[43,44,45] Once the sponsor obtains a PRV, the voucher can be used to obtain priority review designation for a subsequent application that does not itself qualify for priority review as described in the guidance.

1.4.1.3 Fast Track

Fast track is a process designed to facilitate the development and expedite the review of drugs to treat serious conditions and fill an unmet medical need.[46] The purpose is to get important new drugs to the patient earlier. Fast Track addresses a broad range of serious conditions.

Determining whether a condition is serious is a matter of judgment but generally is based on whether the drug will have an impact on such factors as survival, day-to-day functioning, or the likelihood that the condition, if left untreated, will progress from a less severe condition to a more serious one. Filling an unmet medical need is defined as providing a therapy where none exists or providing a therapy that may be potentially better than the available therapy.

Any drug being developed to treat or prevent a condition with no current therapy obviously is directed at an unmet need. If there are available therapies, a Fast Track drug must show some advantage over available therapy, such as:

- Showing superior effectiveness, effect on serious outcomes or improved effect on serious outcomes
- Avoiding serious side effects of an available therapy
- Improving the diagnosis of a serious condition where early diagnosis results in an improved outcome
- Decreasing a clinically significant toxicity of an available therapy that is common and causes discontinuation of treatment
- Ability to address emerging or anticipated public health need
- A drug that receives Fast Track designation is eligible for some or all of the following:
    - More frequent meetings with the FDA to discuss the drug's development plan and ensure collection of appropriate data needed to support drug approval
    - More frequent written communication from the FDA about such things as the design of the proposed clinical trials and use of biomarkers
    - Eligibility for accelerated approval and priority review, if relevant criteria are met
    - Rolling Review, which means that a drug company can submit completed sections of its BLA or NDA for review by the FDA, rather than waiting until every section of the NDA is completed before the entire application can be reviewed. BLA or NDA review usually does not begin until the drug company has submitted the entire application to the FDA

Fast Track designation must be requested by the drug company. The request can be initiated at any time during the drug development process. The FDA will review the request and make a decision within 60 days based on whether the drug fills an unmet medical need in a serious condition.

Once a drug receives Fast Track designation, early and frequent communication between the FDA and a drug company is encouraged throughout the entire drug development and review process. The frequency of communication assures that questions and issues are resolved quickly, often leading to earlier drug approval and access by patients.

1.4.1.4 Breakthrough Therapy

A drug designated as a breakthrough therapy is intended to treat a serious condition, and preliminary clinical evidence indicates that the drug may demonstrate substantial improvement on a clinically significant endpoint(s) over available therapies.[47]

To determine whether the improvement over available therapy is substantial is a matter of judgment and depends on both the magnitude of the treatment effect, which could include duration of the effect, and the importance of the observed clinical outcome. In general, the preliminary clinical evidence should show a clear advantage over available therapy.

For purposes of breakthrough therapy designation, clinically significant endpoint generally refers to an endpoint that measures an effect on irreversible morbidity or mortality (IMM) or on symptoms that represent serious consequences of the disease. A clinically significant endpoint can also refer to findings that suggest an effect on IMM or serious symptoms, including:

- An effect on an established surrogate endpoint
- An effect on a surrogate endpoint or intermediate clinical endpoint considered reasonably likely to predict a clinical benefit (i.e., the accelerated approval standard)
- An effect on a pharmacodynamic biomarker(s) that does not meet criteria for an acceptable surrogate endpoint, but strongly suggests the potential for a clinically meaningful effect on the underlying disease
- A significantly improved safety profile compared to available therapy (e.g., less dose-limiting toxicity for an oncology agent), with evidence of similar efficacy
- A drug that receives Breakthrough Therapy designation is eligible for the following:
- All Fast Track designation features
- Intensive guidance on an efficient drug development program, beginning as early as Phase 1
- Organizational commitment involving senior managers

Breakthrough Therapy designation is requested by the drug company. If a sponsor has not requested Breakthrough Therapy designation, the FDA may suggest that the sponsor consider submitting a request if (1) after reviewing submitted data and information (including preliminary clinical evidence), the agency thinks the drug development program may meet the criteria for Breakthrough Therapy designation and (2) the remaining drug development program can benefit from the designation.

Ideally, a Breakthrough Therapy designation request should be received by the FDA no later than the end-of-phase-2 meetings if any of the features of the designation are to be obtained. Because the primary intent of Breakthrough Therapy designation is to develop evidence needed to support approval as efficiently as possible, the FDA does not anticipate that Breakthrough Therapy designation requests will be made after the submission of an original BLA or NDA or a supplement. The FDA will respond to Breakthrough Therapy designation requests within sixty days of receipt of the request.

1.4.2 Labeling Review

Each statement proposed for drug labeling must be justified by data and results submitted in the application. The CFR describes labeling requirements in 21 CFR Part 201—Labeling.[48]

The regulations phase in the requirement for drug manufacturers to submit prescription drug labeling, or prescribing information, in a new format.[49] The labeling format contains three main sections, highlights, contents, and full prescribing information. Format changes include consolidating and adding new sections, emphasizing *"Patient Counseling Information,"* which establishes a minimum font size, and encourages adverse event reporting.

When an NDA nears approval, agency reviewers evaluate draft labeling for accuracy and consistency with the regulatory requirements for applicable prescription or over-the-counter drugs. Each element of the proposed labeling—including indications, use instructions, and warnings—is evaluated in terms of conclusions drawn from animal and human testing. All claims, instructions, and precautions must accurately reflect submitted clinical results. The PI, which is directed to the healthcare provider, must: contain a summary of the essential scientific information needed for the safe and effective use of the drug and be informative and accurate and neither promotional in tone nor false or misleading.

If the review division has concerns about the draft labeling, they will contact the sponsor detailing suggested revisions. CDER comments can relate to almost any aspect of the proposed labeling. For example, CDER can comment on drug indications and warnings or suggest general changes in wording and format.

The labeling "negotiation process," through which a drug's final approved labeling is agreed on, can take from a few weeks to many months. The length of the process depends on the number of Agency comments and an applicant's willingness to reach agreement. Sometimes a sponsor will submit several revisions of labeling before agreement with the FDA on the labeling can be reached. New regulations enhance the FDA's ability to make suggested labeling changes when new safety information is identified. Manufacturers are limited to 30 days to respond to these suggestions although the timeline can be shortened if the change is necessary due to a public health threat.

New product labeling is now being cataloged on "DailyMed," an interagency online health information clearinghouse that provides the most up-to-date drug product information to consumers, healthcare providers, and others. Labeling can be accessed through the National Library of Medicine at http://dailymed.nlm.nih.gov.

1.4.2.1 Physician Labeling Rule (PLR)

In 2006, the FDA issued new regulations making labeling easier for healthcare providers to access, read, and use prescribing information, and enhance the safe and effective use of prescription drug products.[50]

Application holders are strongly encouraged to voluntarily convert PI approved in "old" format to PLR format because PLR format labeling enhances the safe and effective use of human prescription drugs, including biological products, and reduces the number of adverse reactions resulting from medication errors due to misunderstood or incorrectly applied drug information.

1.4.2.2 Pregnancy and Lactation Labeling Rule (PLLR)

In December 2014, the FDA published updated regulations, referred to as the "Pregnancy and Lactation Labeling Rule" (PLLR). The final rule creates a consistent format for providing information about the risks and benefits of drug use during pregnancy and lactation and by females and males of reproductive potential. The PLLR removes pregnancy letter categories—A, B, C, D and X.

1.4.2.3 Additional FDA-Approved Patient Labeling

- Patient package inserts: For some prescription medicines, the FDA approves special patient materials to instruct patients about the safe use of the product. These materials may be given to patients by their healthcare provider or pharmacist and are considered part of FDA-regulated product labeling.[51]
- Medication guides: The FDA may require distribution of Medication Guides. Medication Guides are FDA-approved patient information, for selected prescription drugs that pose a serious and significant public-health concern.[52]

1.4.3 Risk Evaluation and Mitigation Strategies

The Food and Drug Administration Amendments Act of 2007 gave the FDA the authority to require a Risk Evaluation and Mitigation Strategy (REMS) from manufacturers to ensure that the benefits of a drug or biological product outweigh its risks.[53] Once the FDA determines a REMS is necessary for a drug, pharmaceutical manufacturers must develop, implement, and assess the specific REMS for their drug product.[54] Without a REMS, these medications would not be approved or would be withdrawn from the market because of known or potential serious risks associated with medication. In 2015, the FDA launched the REMS@FDA Database, where the public can view information on current, historical, and released REMS.[55]

The FDA may release a REMS or remove certain components of a REMS, if, after review of REMS assessments or other information, the FDA determines that the extra measures in a REMS are no longer necessary to ensure a medication's benefits outweigh its risks. In 2011, the FDA published the Guidance on Medication Guides—Distribution Requirements and Inclusion in Risk Evaluation and Mitigation Strategies (REMS).[56] This guidance clarified that the Agency no longer intended to include every Medication Guide as part of a REMS (prior to this date, the Agency had, as a matter of policy, considered any new Medication Guide to be part of a REMS). Depending on the risks involved, the Agency began approving some Medication Guides as part of the approved labeling. Currently, all Medication Guides are approved as part of a drug's labeling, but only a small number of Medication Guides are included as part of REMS.

Medication guides are required if the FDA determines that one or more of the following circumstances exist:

- certain information is necessary to prevent serious adverse effects
- patient decision-making should be informed by information about a known serious side effect with a product, or
- patient adherence to directions for the use of a product are essential to its effectiveness.

For more information about REMS, visit the REMS@FDA Database at www.fda.gov/REMS. To view a Medication Guide, look up the drug's approved labeling in Drugs@FDA at www.fda.gov/drugsatfda, or http://labels.fda.gov, the FDA's Online Label Repository.

1.4.4 Advisory Committee Meetings

Advisory committees provide the FDA with independent opinions and recommendations from outside experts on applications to market new drugs, and on FDA policies.[57]

The FDA generally follows an advisory committee's recommendation, but it is important to note the Agency is not bound to do so. They are a valuable resource and make an important contribution to the agency's decision-making processes.[58]

An advisory committee lends credibility to the product review process and provides a forum for public discussion of certain controversial issues. The process helps air issues that do not have simple answers. For specific products, advisory committees consider the available evidence and provide scientific and medical advice on safety, effectiveness, and appropriate use. Committees might also advise the agency on broader regulatory and scientific issues.[59]

An advisory committee ordinarily consist of nine fixed or "standing" members including the chairperson. Members are selected because they are knowledgeable in expertise specific to the committee's function. Most committees will also have a consumer representative and an industry representative. Additional experts may be added for specific meetings, as needed.

The committee should represent all geographic locations and be balanced as far as gender and minority status. The FDA's advisory committee program is governed by a number of Federal laws and regulations that set forth standards for holding advisory committees and reviewing potential conflicts of interest, among other things. On the FDA's website the public can view the FDA Advisory Committee Calendar.[60] This information includes the date, time, location, webcast information (when available), registration information (when required), presentations, agenda and points of contact for AC meetings.

1.5 THE GENERIC DRUG APPROVAL PROCESS

The FDA requires a generic drug company to produce enough data to demonstrate it can make a drug that can be appropriately substituted for its brand-name counterpart.

1.5.1 Abbreviated New Drug Applications

An abbreviated new drug application (ANDA) contains data which is submitted to the FDA for the review and potential approval of a generic drug product.[61] Generic drug applications are termed "abbreviated" because they are generally not required to include preclinical (animal) and clinical (human) data to establish safety and effectiveness. Instead, generic applicants must scientifically demonstrate that their product is performs in the same manner as the innovator drug. One way applicants demonstrate that a generic product performs in the same way as the innovator drug is to measure the time it takes the generic drug to reach the bloodstream in healthy volunteers. This demonstration of "bioequivalence" gives the rate of absorption, or bioavailability, of the generic drug, which can then be compared to that of the innovator drug. To be approved by the FDA, the generic version must deliver the same amount of active ingredients into a patient's bloodstream in the same amount of time as the innovator drug.

A generic drug product must also demonstrate that it is comparable to an innovator drug product in dosage form, strength, route of administration, quality, performance characteristics, and intended use. All approved products, both innovator and generic, are listed in the FDA's *Approved Drug Products with Therapeutic Equivalence Evaluations* (Orange Book).[62]

While there could be an entire chapter dedicated to the review of generic drug applications, for the purposes of this chapter, we will summarize that a generic drug application submitted to the FDA for approval must show the following:[63]

- The generic drug is pharmaceutically equivalent to the brand.
- The manufacturer is capable of making the drug correctly.
- The manufacturer is capable of making the drug consistently.
- The "active ingredient" is the same as that of the brand.
- The right amount of the active ingredient gets to the place in the body where it has effect.
- The inactive ingredients of the drug are safe.
- The drug does not break down over time.
- The container in which the drug will be shipped and sold is appropriate.
- The labeling is the same as the brand-name drug's labeling.
- Relevant patents or legal exclusivities are expired.

1.5.2 ANDA Approval

After all components of the application are found to be acceptable, an approval letter is issued to the applicant, detailing the conditions of the approval, and providing the company with the ability to market the generic-drug product.[60] If the approval occurs prior to the expiration of any patents or exclusivities accorded to the reference listed drug product, a tentative approval letter is issued to the applicant detailing the tentative approval of the generic-drug product until the patent or exclusivity condition has expired.[64] A tentative approval does not allow the applicant to market the generic drug product.

1.5.3 Generic Drug User Fee Amendments

On July 9, 2012, the Generic Drug User Fee Amendments (GDUFA) was signed into law by the President as part of the Food and Drug Administration Safety and Innovation Act (FDASIA).[65] Up until October 2012, the law only required user fees for firms submitting NDAs. As of October 1, 2012, under GDUFA, all firms that manufacture human generic drug products, and active ingredients for human generic drug products, that are the subject of an application and distributed in U.S. commerce became subject to FDA user fees.[66]

Congress enacted and reauthorized GDUFA in 2017 (known as GDUFA II) to ensure patients have access to safe, high-quality, and affordable generic drugs. The current reauthorization lasts through September 2022. GDUFA is based on an agreement negotiated by the FDA and representatives of the generic drug industry to address a growing number of regulatory challenges and must be reauthorized every five years.[67]

GDUFA and GDUFA II overhauled the generic drug program and aimed to put the FDA's generic drug program on a firm financial footing and ensure timely access to safe, high-quality, affordable generic drugs. GDUFA enables the FDA to assess user fees to fund critical and measurable enhancements to the performance of the FDA's generic drugs program, bringing greater predictability and timeliness to the review of generic drug applications. To learn more, visit www.fda.gov/gdufa.

1.6 BIOSIMILAR PATHWAY

The Patient Protection and Affordable Care Act (Affordable Care Act), signed into law on March 23, 2010, amends the Public Health Service Act (PHS Act) to create an abbreviated licensure pathway for biological products that are demonstrated to be "biosimilar" to or "interchangeable" with an FDA-licensed biological product. This pathway is provided in the part of the law known as the Biologics Price Competition and Innovation Act (BPCI Act). Under the BPCI Act, a biological product may be demonstrated to be "biosimilar" if data show that, among other things, the product is "highly similar" to an already-approved biological product.[68],[69]

The nature of biological products, including the inherent variations that can result from the manufacturing process, can present challenges in characterizing and manufacturing these products that often do not exist in the development of small molecule drugs. Slight differences between manufactured lots of the same biological product (i.e., acceptable within-product variations) are normal and expected within the manufacturing process. As part of its review, the FDA assesses the manufacturing process and the manufacturer's strategy to control within-product variations. These control strategies are put in place to help ensure that manufacturers produce biological products with consistent clinical performance.[70,71]

A biosimilar product is a biological product that is approved based on a showing that it is highly similar to an FDA-approved biological product, known as a reference product, and has no clinically meaningful differences in terms of safety and effectiveness from the reference product. Only minor differences in clinically inactive components are allowable in biosimilar products.[72]

An *interchangeable* biological product is biosimilar to an FDA-approved reference product and meets additional standards for interchangeability. An interchangeable biological product may be substituted for the reference product by a pharmacist without the intervention of the health care provider who prescribed the reference product. Also, for products administered to a patient more than once, the risk in terms of safety and reduced efficacy of switching back and forth between an interchangeable product and a reference product will have been evaluated.[73]

The FDA requires licensed biosimilar and interchangeable biological products to meet the Agency's rigorous standards of safety and efficacy. That means patients and healthcare professionals will be able to rely upon the safety and effectiveness of the biosimilar or interchangeable product, just as they would the reference product.[74]

1.7 OVER-THE-COUNTER DRUG PRODUCTS

Over-the-counter (OTC) drug products are drugs available to consumers without a prescription.[75] There are more than 80 classes (therapeutic categories) of OTC drugs, ranging from acne drug products to weight-control drug products.[76] As with prescription drugs, CDER oversees OTC drugs to ensure that they are properly labeled and that their benefits outweigh their risks.[77]

OTC drugs play an increasingly vital role in America's healthcare system by providing easy access to certain drugs that can be used safely without the help of a healthcare practitioner.[78] This enables consumers to take control of their own health care in many situations. OTC drug products have been marketed for many years. For this reason, the FDA has been evaluating the ingredients and labeling of these products as part of "The OTC Drug Review Program." The goal of this program was to establish OTC drug monographs for each class of products through a three-phase public rulemaking process.[79] OTC drug monographs are a kind of "recipe book" covering acceptable ingredients, doses, formulations, and labeling.[73] Monographs have been continually updated, adding additional ingredients and labeling, as needed. Products conforming to a monograph may be marketed without further FDA clearance, while those that do not must undergo separate review and approval through the New Drug Application (NDA) process. Some OTC products (previously available only by prescription) are first approved through the NDA system, and their "switch" to OTC status is approved via the NDA system.[80]

In March 2020, the President signed the Coronavirus Aid, Relief, and Economic Security Act (CARES Act) to aid response efforts and ease the economic impact of COVID-19. In addition to the COVID-19 response efforts, the CARES Act includes statutory provisions that reform and modernize the way OTC monograph drugs are regulated in the United States.[81] Specifically, the CARES Act replaces the rulemaking process with an administrative order process for issuing, revising, and amending OTC monographs. The CARES Act also provides the FDA the authority to assess and collect user fees dedicated to OTC monograph drug activities.[82] The FDA anticipates that this user fee program will provide additional resources to help the agency conduct these important regulatory activities in a timely manner and ultimately help provide the public with access to innovative OTC monograph drugs. See Table 1.1 OTC Monograph Drug Regulation Before and

TABLE 1.1
OTC Monograph Drug Regulation Before and After Coronavirus Aid, Relief, and Economic Security (CARES) Act.

What stays the same?	What is new?
Ingredient-based review	Administrative order process
Active Ingredients grouped by therapeutic category	OTC monograph order request (OMOR)
GRASE (generally recognized as safe and effective) determination	Clarification of status of existing OTC monograph drugs, including drugs that were previously subject to tentative final monographs (TFM) and advanced notice of proposed rulemakings (ANPR)
Drugs complying with OTC monograph and other applicable requirements may be marketed without FDA approval	Process for minor changes in dosage forms
Process includes public comment period	Exclusivity period for certain OTC monograph drugs
	OTC monograph user fees
	Formal meetings

Source: Michelle, T. M., "Monograph Reform is Here!," Last modified May 29, 2020, https://www.fda.gov/media/139503/download.

After CARES Act below for more information about OTC monograph reform.[83]

1.8 POST-MARKETING SURVEILLANCE

Drug safety is the focus of CDER's Office of Surveillance and Epidemiology.[84] The Office of Surveillance and Epidemiology (OSE) works with the Office of New Drugs (OND) and other programs in CDER to evaluate the safety profiles of drugs available to U.S. consumers using a variety of tools and disciplines throughout the lifespan of drugs. OSE maintains a system of post-marketing surveillance and risk-assessment programs to identify medication errors and adverse events that did not appear during the drug-development process.

Adverse event data is collected through required reporting by companies and through voluntary reports submitted to the FDA's MedWatch program, which, together, total over two million reports per year.[85] Staff in OSE use this information to identify drug-safety concerns and recommend actions to improve product safety and protect the public health.[86] Potential actions include updating drug labeling, providing more information to the community, implementing or revising a risk-management program, and, on rare occasions, removing products from the market. OSE, OND and other CDER offices also evaluate data and initiate appropriate regulatory actions regarding medication errors related to confusing container labels, carton labeling, drug packaging, and drug names that look or sound similar.[87]

The goal of the CDER's post-marketing surveillance system is to monitor the ongoing safety of marketed drugs. This is accomplished by reassessing drug risks based on new data obtained after the drug is marketed and recommending ways to appropriately manage that risk. This is accomplished through a variety of activities and tools that are outlined below.

The FDA maintains a website with post-market drug safety information for patients and providers.[88] This website contains links to post-market drug safety information to improve transparency and communication to patients and healthcare providers.

1.8.1 Adverse Event Reporting

Even the large, well-designed Phase 3 clinical studies that are conducted by drug manufacturers cannot uncover every problem that can come to light once a product is widely used.[89] For this reason, receipt of adverse event reports after a product is FDA approved is critical in order to continuously evaluate product safety over its lifecycle. To capture this critical data, especially serious adverse-event data, CDER receives adverse events from drug manufacturers, who are required by regulation to submit adverse event reports to the FDA.[9] In addition, the FDA has a medical product reporting program called "MedWatch" to promote and facilitate voluntary reporting of serious adverse events, medication errors, and product problems with drugs by healthcare practitioners and patients.[90]

The FDA is especially interested in learning of "serious" events that follow drug use. Serious events are generally defined as those that involve death, a life-threatening condition, hospitalization, disability, a congenital anomaly, or intervention to avoid one of these serious outcomes.[91] Additionally, the FDA is interested in learning of all medication errors regardless of patient outcome. In return, the FDA keeps healthcare professionals informed about new safety concerns and may issue a communication to the public describing the concern. The FDA shares information in the interest of informing doctors, other healthcare providers and patients. It generally includes information about the safety issue, factors to consider when making treatment decisions, and other information that patients need to know in order to safely use the drug. The FDA's information sharing is mainly accomplished through MedWatch Safety Alerts, Drug Safety Communications, Drug Safety-related Labeling Changes, and other FDA safety web postings.[92]

1.8.2 FDA Adverse Event Reporting System

A powerful drug-safety tool is FDA Adverse Event Reporting System (FAERS).[9] This computerized system combines the voluntary adverse drug event and medication error reports from MedWatch and the required reports from manufacturers. These reports often form the basis of "signals" that there may be a potential for serious, unrecognized, drug-associated events and medication errors. When a signal is detected, further testing of the hypothesis is undertaken using various epidemiological and analytic databases, studies, and other instruments and resources.[93] The reports in FAERS are evaluated by clinical reviewers in CDER to detect safety signals and to monitor drug safety. They form the basis for further epidemiological studies when appropriate. As a result, the FDA may take regulatory actions to improve product safety and protect the public health.

The FDA conducts regular screenings of FAERS and posts on the Internet a quarterly report of new safety information or potential signals of a serious risk identified from the FAERS. The appearance of a drug on this list does not mean that the FDA has concluded that the drug has this listed risk. It means that the FDA has identified only a potential safety issue. If after further evaluation the FDA determines that the drug is associated with the risk, it may take a variety of actions including some previously mentioned.

The FAERS Public Dashboard is an interactive search tool that allows the user to count and view adverse event reports sent to the FDA.[94] In addition to being able to search for adverse drug events, users can "drill down" into an individual case and view approximately 60 data fields specific to the record that include non-confidential information such as demographic, drugs, and therapy information.

While the FAERS dashboard offers stakeholders many more ways of searching for and organizing data on adverse events reported to the FDA for many drug and biologic products, there remain limitations to the data. For example, while FAERS contains reports on a particular drug or biologic, this does not mean that the drug or biologic caused the adverse event. Importantly, the FAERS data by themselves are not an indicator of the safety profile of the drug or biologic. A full disclaimer is provided on the FDA's website and upon entering the FAERS Public Dashboard to ensure good stewardship of the data provided.

1.8.3 Post-Marketing Requirements and Commitments

The Food and Drug Administration Amendments Act (FDAAA) was passed in 2007 and gave the FDA new authorities to require manufacturers to conduct necessary post-approval studies and post-approval clinical trials to assess a known serious risk related to the use of a drug, to assess signals of serious risk related to the use of a drug, or to identify an unexpected serious risk when available data indicates the potential for a serious risk. A post-marketing requirement (PMR) is a study or trial that a sponsor is required to conduct post-approval. PMRs are sometimes necessary as a condition of approval and are useful to collect more safety information. In contrast, a post-marketing commitment (PMC) is a study or trial to conduct post-approval that a sponsor agrees to in writing, but not required by law. The FDA tracks and monitors the progress of PMRs and PMCs to ensure that they are completed in a timely manner.

Most recently, in April 2020, CDER released a new policy to describe how CDER collaboratively identifies, evaluates, and resolves *newly identified safety signals* (NISS) associated with marketed drugs.[95]

Using medical and scientific judgment and procedures consistent with established pharmacovigilance practice for identifying safety signals or established review practices for identifying quality signals, CDER staff apply the general criteria to determine if data from a signal source is a NISS. CDER's criteria for a NISS generally includes:

- a serious adverse event; medication error; or an adverse event that suggests therapeutic inequivalence or product quality issue; AND the information indicates a likely safety signal that warrants further investigation into whether there is a causal association or a new aspect of a known association.

OR

- a product quality issue that:
  - could negatively affect public health or the benefit–risk profile of a product; and
  - cannot be resolved through existing routine processes (e.g., drug recalls, adverse inspection findings).

1.8.4 Sentinel Network

In the fall of 2007, Congress passed FDA Amendments Act (FDAAA), mandating the FDA to establish an Active Postmarket Risk Identification and Analysis (ARIA).[96] FDAAA requires the FDA to develop, in collaboration with public, academic, and private entities, methods to obtain access to disparate data sources and validated methods for the establishment of a system to link and analyze safety data from multiple sources. In May 2008, the FDA launched the Sentinel Initiative to create a national electronic system, the Sentinel System, for medical product safety surveillance.[97]

The FDA has long used administrative and insurance claims databases to investigate safety questions about Agency-regulated products, but until Sentinel, the Agency generally was only able to work with one particular healthcare system at a time to evaluate a given safety issue.

Sentinel has the largest multisite distributed database in the world dedicated to medical product safety. This plan is intended to serve as a roadmap to guide the development of the Sentinel System between 2019 and 2023. Specifically, the plan discusses five strategic aims:

- Enhance and expand the Sentinel System's foundation (i.e. data, infrastructure, operations, technology).
- Augment the Sentinel System's safety analysis capabilities by leveraging advances in data sciences and signal detection.
- Leverage the Sentinel System to accelerate access to and broader use of Real-World Data (RWD) for Real-World Evidence (RWE) generation.
- Broaden the Sentinel System's ecosystem of stakeholders to pursue the vision of a national resource.
- Disseminate knowledge and advance regulatory science to encourage innovation and meet Agency scientific needs.

1.8.5 Drug Safety Oversight Board

The Drug Safety Oversight Board (DSB) established since 2005 and mandated by law in the FDA Amendments Act of 2007 continues to provide independent oversight and advice to CDER leadership on the management of important drug safety issues and manage the flow of emerging safety information to healthcare professionals and patients.[98] The DSB is an internal government committee comprised of members from the FDA and medical experts from other Health and Human Services agencies and government departments. The Board discusses drug safety topics that are of potential significant impact in the post-market setting as well as issues concerning matters of internal policy, such as collaboration among agency divisions to enhance drug safety management. An important drug safety issue is one that has the potential to alter the benefit/risk analysis for a drug in such a way as to affect decisions about prescribing or taking the drug.

1.9 APPLICABLE STATUTES AND IMPLEMENTING REGULATIONS

1.9.1 Food and Drug Acts—1906

The passage of the 1906 Pure Food and Drugs Act marked a monumental shift in the use of government powers to enhance consumer protection by requiring that foods and drugs bear truthful labeling statements and meet certain standards for purity and strength.[99] While the 1906 law laid the cornerstone for the modern FDA, as time went on it became clear that it had major shortcomings, which limited the agency's ability to protect consumers. The law offered no way to remove inherently dangerous drugs from the market and set such a high burden of proof for misbranding, i.e., intent to defraud, that the agency was rarely able to take action against a company for fraudulent products. In addition, the law provided no authority over cosmetics, medical devices, or advertising, and imposed no standards for foods.[100]

1.9.2 Food, Drug and Cosmetic Act—1938

By the 1930s it was widely recognized that the Food and Drugs Act of 1906 was obsolete, but bitter disagreement arose as to what should replace it. By 1937 most of the arguments had been resolved but Congressional action was stalled. Then came a shocking development—the deaths of more than 100 people after using a drug that was clearly unsafe.[101] The incident hastened final enactment in 1938 of the Federal Food, Drug, and Cosmetic Act, the statute that today remains the basis for FDA regulation of these products. During September and October 1937 Elixir Sulfanilamide was responsible for the deaths of more than 100 people in 15 states, as far east as Virginia and as far west as California. The drug and the deaths led to the passage of the 1938 Food, Drug, and Cosmetic Act, which increased the FDA's authority to regulate drugs.[102]

1.9.3 Durham-Humphrey Amendment—1951

Within two months of the passage of the act, the FDA began to identify drugs such as the sulfas that simply could not be labeled for safe use directly by the patient—they would require a prescription from a physician.[103] The ensuing debate by the FDA, industry, and health practitioners over what constituted a prescription and an over the counter drug was resolved in this amendment.[104]

1.9.4 Kefauver-Harris Amendment—1962

As with the 1938 act, a therapeutic disaster compelled passage of the new law; in this case the disaster was narrowly averted.[95] Thalidomide, a sedative that was never approved in this country, produced thousands of grossly deformed newborns outside of the United States. The new law mandated efficacy as well as safety before a drug could be marketed, required the FDA to assess the efficacy of all drugs introduced since 1938, instituted stricter agency control over drug trials (including a requirement that patients involved must give their informed consent), transferred from the Federal Trade Commission to the FDA regulation of prescription drug advertising, established good manufacturing practices by the drug industry, and granted the FDA greater powers to access company production and control records to verify those practices. The FDA contracted with the National Academy of Sciences/National Research Council (NAS/NRC) to make an initial evaluation of the effectiveness of more than 3,400 drugs that had been approved only for safety between 1938 and 1962.[105] The agency reviewed and reevaluated the NAS/NRC reports and published its initial findings in Federal Register notices. These amendments also required manufacturers to report serious side effects to the FDA.[106]

1.9.5 Orphan Drug Act—1983

"Orphans" are drugs and other products for treating rare diseases. They may offer little or no profit to the manufacturer, because of the limited market, but may benefit people with the rare disease. To foster orphan product development, this law allows drug companies to take tax deductions for about three-quarters of the costs of their clinical studies.[107] Firms also are given exclusive marketing rights for seven years for any orphan products that are approved.

1.9.6 Drug Price and Competition and Patent Term Restoration Act—1984

This law expands the number of drugs suitable for an Abbreviated New Drug Application, or ANDA.[108] ANDAs make it less costly and time-consuming for generic drugs, which are often sold at lower prices than brand-name drugs, to reach the market. "Patent term restoration" refers to the 17 years of legal protection given a firm for each drug patent. Some of that time allowance is used while the drug goes through the approval process, so this law allows restoration of up to five years of lost patent time.

Though not involving changes in law, the following changes in three of the FDA's drug regulations are noteworthy.

1.9.6.1 Revision of New Drug Application Regulations—1985

These changes provide for safety reports after an application for a new drug is submitted, more focused and better organized data, use of summaries and tables for easier review, earlier problem solving, and allowance of approval on the basis of foreign studies alone. It also strengthens the monitoring of adverse reactions from marketed drugs.[109]

1.9.6.2 Revision of Investigational New Drug Application Regulations—1987

Encourages problem-solving meetings with the FDA, requires deadlines in safety reports, and increases sponsor control over initial human test design, if subjects face no unreasonable, significant risks.[110]

1.9.6.3 Treatment Use of Investigational New Drugs—1987

Patients with serious or immediately life-threatening diseases, such as AIDS, may now get treatment with experimental drugs that show reasonable evidence of potential benefit—provided no satisfactory approved therapy exists. This applies only to drugs already being studied in controlled clinical studies. Also, the drugs cannot expose patients to unreasonable risks.[100]

1.9.7 Prescription Drug User Fee Act (PDUFA)—1992

The Prescription Drug User Fee Act (PDUFA) was created by Congress in 1992 and authorizes the FDA to collect fees from companies that produce certain human drug and biological products.[111] Since the passage of PDUFA, user fees have played an important role in expediting the drug approval process. PDUFA provides the FDA with resources for a period of five years to accelerate the review of applications, without compromising safety and efficacy standards. The goal of PDUFA is to focus on reviewing timeliness. By improving FDA review efficiency, while concurrently improving the quality of submissions by the industry, overall approval times will improve and result in earlier patient access to safe and effective new therapies.

1.9.8 FDA Modernization Act (FDAMA)—1997

The Modernization Act (FDAMA) implemented important provisions regarding patient access to experimental drugs and medical devices, information on clinical trials, pharmacy compounding, food safety and labeling, and other matters.[112]

One provision of the act abolishes a prohibition on manufacturers' dissemination of information about unapproved uses of drugs and devices, permitting them to disseminate peer-reviewed journal articles, provided that they commit to file, within a specified timeframe, an application to establish the safety and effectiveness of the unapproved use for a period of five years. The statute also added a new provision requiring tracking of the status of post-marketing approval studies. One of the most important pieces of the legislation is one that reauthorizes, for another five years, user fees paid by manufacturers for prescription drugs. Since 1992, funding from the fees provided the Agency with resources to reduce the average time for new drug review.

1.9.9 FDA Amendments Act (FDAAA)—2007

The FDA Amendments Act (FDAAA) of 2007 is a combination of six different pieces of prescription drug and medical device legislation reflecting new authorities given to the FDA.[113]

Four sections of the Act are reauthorizations—the Prescription Drug User Fee Act, the Medical Device User Fee and Modernization Act, the Best Pharmaceuticals for Children Act, and the Pediatric Research Equity Act. The fifth legislative amendment expands the authority of the FDA to assess and manage drug risks. The sixth is new legislation to encourage specialized pediatric medical device development and to create a foundation (Reagan-Udall) to modernize product development, accelerate innovation, and enhance product safety.[114] Although www.clinicaltrials.gov was established in 1997 with FDAMA, this clinical trial registry became more useful under FDAAA. FDAAA required the availability of more clinical trials and related information in the registry, including basic results.

1.9.10 Food and Drug Administration Safety and Innovation Act (FDASIA)—2012

The Food and Drug Administration Safety and Innovation Act (FDASIA), expands the FDA's authorities and strengthens the agency's ability to safeguard and advance public health by including the fifth authorization of the Prescription Drug User Fee Act (PDUFA), first enacted in 1992 to collect user fees from industry to fund reviews of innovator drugs. FDASIA also gave the FDA the authority to initiate new user fee programs for the review of generic drugs (Generic Drug User Fee Amendments of 2012 [GDUFA]) and biosimilar biological products (Biosimilar User Fee Act of 2012 [BsUFA]); promote innovation to speed patient access to safe and effective products; increase stakeholder involvement in FDA processes; and enhance the safety of the drug supply chain.[115]

FDASIA-related stakeholder engagement efforts include FDA initiation of a five-year Patient Focused Drug Development (PFDD) program to learn from patients about the impact of their disease on their daily lives.[116] From 2012 to 2017, the FDA conducted 24 disease-specific PFDD meetings to more systematically obtain the patient perspective on specific diseases and their treatments.[117]

FDASIA gave the FDA a new and powerful expedited drug development tool, known as the "breakthrough therapy" designation. This new designation helps the FDA assist drug developers to expedite the development and review of new drugs with preliminary clinical evidence that indicates the drug may offer a substantial improvement over available therapies for patients with serious or life-threatening diseases.

1.9.10.1 FDASIA Supply Chain

With nearly 40 percent of finished drugs being imported, and nearly 80 percent of active ingredients coming from overseas sources, protecting the global drug supply chain and making sure that patients have access to the drugs they need is a priority for the FDA.[118] FDASIA includes a set of provisions which give FDA new authorities to address the challenges posed by an increasingly global drug supply chain.[119] The new authorities include:

- Extending the agency's administrative detention authority to include drugs
- Defining conduct the agency considers delaying, denying, limiting or refusing inspection, resulting in a drug being deemed adulterated
- Higher penalties for adulterated and counterfeit drugs before the U.S. Sentencing Commission
- Protecting the drug supply chain
- Establishing a unique facility identifier (UFI) system for drug establishment registration
- Requiring the FDA to replace the previous two-year drug inspectional frequency requirement with a risk-based inspection schedule for domestic and foreign drug facilities.

Grant FDA authority to protect from disclosure information obtained from a foreign government agency if the information concerns the inspection of a facility, is part of an investigation, alerts the United States to the potential need for an investigation, or concerns a drug that has a reasonable probability of causing serious adverse health consequences or death, and such information is provided voluntarily on the condition that it not be released and is covered by a written agreement.

1.9.11 The Drug Quality and Security Act (DQSA)—2013

The Drug Quality and Security Act (DQSA) signed into law on November 27, 2013, includes the Drug Supply Chain Security Act (DSCSA), to modernize and expand the drug pedigree requirements of the Prescription Drug Marketing Act of 1987. The law outlines critical steps to build an electronic, interoperable system to identify and trace certain prescription drugs as they are distributed in the United States.[120]

DQSA also addresses the compounding of human drugs with the Compounding Quality Act.[121] The new law describes the conditions under which certain compounded human drug products are entitled to exemptions from three sections of the FDCA requiring compliance with current good manufacturing practices (CGMP) labeling with adequate directions for use and FDA approval prior to marketing. The law also creates a new section in the FDCA. Under section 503B, a compounder can become an "outsourcing facility." An outsourcing facility will be able to qualify for exemptions from FDA approval requirements and the requirement to label products with adequate directions for use, but not the exemption from CGMP requirements. In addition, outsourcing facilities will be inspected by the FDA according to a risk-based schedule, and must meet certain other conditions, such as reporting adverse events and providing the FDA with certain information about the products they compound.

The DSCSA outlines critical steps to build an electronic, interoperable system to identify and trace certain prescription drugs as they are distributed in the United States. Ten years after enactment, the system will facilitate the exchange of information at the individual package level about where a drug has been in the supply chain.

1.9.12 21st Century Cures Act—2016

The 21st Century Cures Act (Cures Act), signed into law on December 13, 2016, is designed to help accelerate medical product development and bring new innovations and advances to patients who need them faster and more efficiently.[122]

The law builds on the FDA's ongoing work to incorporate the perspectives of patients into the development of drugs, biological products, and devices in the FDA's decision-making process. Cures enhances our ability to modernize clinical trial designs, including the use of real-world evidence, and clinical outcome assessments, which will speed the development and review of novel medical products, including medical countermeasures.[123]

The Cures Act also directs the FDA to create one or more inter-center institutes to help coordinate activities in major disease areas between the drug, biologics and device centers and improves the regulation of combination products (ex: Oncology Center of Excellence).

1.9.13 Food and Drug Administration Reauthorization Act (FDARA)—2017

The FDA Reauthorization Act of 2017 (FDARA), signed into law on August 18, 2017, amends the FDCA to revise and extend the user fee programs for drugs, medical devices, generic drugs, and biosimilar biological products, and for other purposes.[124]

1.9.14 Coronavirus Aid, Relief, and Economic Security Act (CARES Act)—2020

On March 27, 2020, the President signed the Coronavirus Aid, Relief, and Economic Security Act (CARES Act) to aid response efforts and ease the economic impact of COVID-19. In addition to the COVID-19 response efforts, the CARES Act includes an important legislative initiative that reforms and modernizes the way certain nonprescription, over-the-counter (or OTC) drugs are regulated in the United States. These drugs, known as OTC monograph drugs, may be marketed without an approved drug application under section 505 of the FDCA if they meet the requirements of section 505G of the FDCA, as well as other applicable requirements.

Section 744M of the FDCA, as added by the CARES Act, establishes an OTC monograph drug user fee program, under which the FDA will assess and collect fees from submitters of OTC Monograph Order Requests (OMORs) as well as facility fees from certain manufacturers of OTC monograph drugs, to support the agency's OTC monograph drug activities.[125] As with our other user fee programs, we anticipate that this new user fee program will provide additional resources to help the agency conduct these important regulatory activities in a timely manner and ultimately help provide the public with access to innovative OTC monograph drugs.

OTC Monograph Reform is expected to accomplish the following:

- Improve the process by replacing rulemaking with administrative orders;
- Improve efficiency, timeliness, and predictability;
- Facilitate innovation;
- Establish a process to rapidly address safety issues;
- Finalize pending monographs; and
- Provide the FDA with user fees to support OTC monograph drug activities.

During the first three years of OTC Monograph Reform, essentially all effective review capacity is expected to be consumed by current external mandates, safety activities, and OTC Monograph Reform implementation and infrastructure development activities. Beginning in Years 4 and 5 (and to a limited extent in Year 3), the FDA expects to have built sufficient effective review capacity to begin to have timelines and performance goals for review activities expected to be part of the steady state of a monograph review program.

The FDA will collect two types of user fees under OMUFA: Facility Fees and OTC Monograph Order Request (OMOR) fees.

1.10 SUMMARY AND CONCLUSIONS

In conclusion, the Agency will continue to promote the adoption of safety and quality policies, practices, and standards, both domestically and internationally, aimed at reducing risks in the manufacturing, production, and distribution of FDA-regulated products.

1.11 GLOSSARY OF TERMS

1.11.1 Word and Phrase List for Index

Abbreviated New Drug Application (ANDA). Contains data that, when submitted to the FDA's Center for Drug Evaluation and Research, Office of Generic Drugs, provides for the review and ultimate approval of a generic drug product. Generic drug applications are called "abbreviated" because they are generally not required to include preclinical (animal) and clinical (human) data to establish safety and effectiveness. Instead, a generic applicant must scientifically demonstrate that its product is bioequivalent (i.e., performs in the same manner as the innovator drug). Once approved, an applicant may manufacture and market the generic drug product to provide a safe, effective, low cost alternative to the American public.

Adverse Event. A drug reaction is also known as a side effect, is any undesirable experience associated with the use of a medicine in a patient. Adverse events can range from mild to severe. Serious adverse events are those that can cause disability, are life-threatening, result in hospitalization or death, or are birth defects.

Biologic License Application (BLA). Biological products are approved for marketing under the provisions of the Public Health Service (PHS) Act. The Act requires a firm who manufactures a biologic for sale in interstate commerce to hold a license for the product. A biologics license application is a submission that contains specific information on the manufacturing processes, chemistry, pharmacology, clinical pharmacology and the medical effects of the biologic product. If the information provided meets FDA requirements, the application is approved, and a license is issued allowing the firm to market the product.

Biological Product. Biological products include a wide range of products such as vaccines, blood and blood components, allergenics, somatic cells, gene therapy, tissues, and recombinant therapeutic proteins. Biologics can be composed of sugars, proteins, or nucleic acids or complex combinations of these substances, or may be living entities such as cells and tissues. Biologics are isolated from a variety of natural sources—human, animal, or microorganism—and may be produced by biotechnology methods and other cutting-edge technologies. Gene-based and cellular biologics, for example, often are at the forefront of biomedical research, and may be used to treat a variety of medical conditions for which no other treatments are available. In General, the Term "Drugs" Includes Therapeutic Biological Products.

Code of Federal Regulations. The Code of Federal Regulations (CFR) is the codification of the general and permanent rules published in the Federal Register by the departments and agencies of the Federal Government produced by the Office of the Federal Register (OFR) and the Government Publishing Office. Available from: www.ecfr.gov.

DailyMed. Developed with the National Library of Medicine, DailyMed is a Web site that gives physicians and patients electronic access to FDA-approved drug labels.

Drug. A drug is defined as:

- A substance recognized by an official pharmacopoeia or formulary.
- A substance intended for use in the diagnosis, cure, mitigation, treatment, or prevention of disease.
- A substance (other than food) intended to affect the structure or any function of the body.
- A substance intended for use as a component of a medicine but not a device or a component, part or accessory of a device.
- Biological products are included within this definition and are generally covered by the same laws and regulations, but differences exist regarding their manufacturing processes (chemical process versus biological process.)

Drugs@FDA. Drugs@FDA is a resource allows you to search for information about FDA-approved brand name and generic drugs and therapeutic biological products. These are proteins derived from living material (such as cells or tissues) used to treat or cure disease. You can search in many ways, including by drug name and active ingredient.

Drug Product. The finished dosage form that contains a drug substance, generally, but not necessarily in association with other active or inactive ingredients.

Drug Withdrawal. In rare cases, the FDA may need to reassess and change its approval decision on a drug. A conclusion that a drug should no longer be marketed is based on the nature and frequency of the adverse events and how the drug's benefit and risk balance compares with treatment alternatives. When the FDA believes that a drug's benefits no longer outweigh its risks, the agency will ask the manufacturer to withdraw the drug.

Expanded Access. Also called "compassionate use," provides a pathway for patients to gain access to investigational drugs, biologics and medical devices for serious diseases or conditions. Investigational drugs and devices have not yet been approved by the FDA and they have not been proven to be safe and effective. Therefore, they may be effective in the treatment of a condition, or they may not. It is important to remember that the drug/biologic/medical device may have unexpected serious side effects and that patients need to consider all the possible risks when seeking access to an investigational medical product.

To gain access to an investigational medical product outside of a clinical trial, the sponsors must decide whether to make their experimental medical product available to patients via expanded access. FDA regulations specify two groups of people eligible for expanded access:

- those with life-threatening diseases or conditions for which "there is a reasonable likelihood that death will occur within a matter of months or in which premature death is likely without early treatment"
- those with serious diseases or conditions that have a "substantial impact on day-to-day functioning"

In most cases, patients who seek compassionate use must have exhausted all approved therapies for their condition and be unable to enroll in a clinical trial.

FDA Adverse Event Reporting System (FAERS). A computerized database containing reports of adverse events. It supports the FDA's post-market safety surveillance program for all approved drugs and therapeutic biologics.

Generic Drug. A generic drug is the same as a brand name drug in dosage, safety, strength, how it is taken, quality, performance, and intended use. Before approving a generic drug product, the FDA requires many rigorous tests and procedures to assure that the generic drug can be substituted for the brand name drug. The FDA bases evaluations of substitutability, or "therapeutic equivalence," of generic drugs on scientific evaluations. By law, a generic drug product must contain the identical amounts of the same active ingredient(s) as the brand name product. Drug products evaluated as "therapeutically equivalent" can be expected to have equal effect and no difference when substituted for the brand name product.

In vitro. In glass, as in a test tube. An in vitro test is one that is done in glass or plastic vessels in the laboratory. In vitro is the opposite of in vivo.

In vivo. In the living organism. For example, an experiment that is done in vivo is done in the body of a living organism. In vivo is the opposite of in vitro.

Investigational Drug. This can also be called an experimental drug and is being studied to see if your disease or medical condition improves while taking it. Scientists are trying to prove in clinical trials:

- If the drug is safe and effective.
- How the drug might be used in that disease.
- How much of the drug is needed.
- Information about the potential benefits and risks of taking the drug.
- effect and no difference when substituted for the brand name product.

Label. The FDA-approved label is the official description of a drug product which includes indication (what the drug is used for); who should take it; adverse events (side effects); instructions for uses in pregnancy, children, and other populations; and safety information for the patient. Labels are often found inside drug product packaging.

Medication Guides (Med Guide). These are paper hand-outs/pamphlets that are required to be given to patients with certain medications by the pharmacist. Medication Guides communicate risk information that is specific to particular drugs and drug classes, and they contain FDA-approved information that can help patients avoid serious adverse events.

MedWatch. MedWatch is FDA's safety information and adverse event reporting program. It provides important and timely medical product information to healthcare professionals, including information on prescription and over-the-counter drugs, biologics, medical devices, and special nutritional products. Healthcare professionals and consumers can also report serious problems they suspect are related to certain FDA-regulated products.

New Drug Application (NDA). When the sponsor of a new drug believes that enough evidence on the drug's safety and effectiveness has been obtained to meet the FDA's requirements for marketing approval, the sponsor submits to the FDA a new drug application (NDA). The application must contain data from specific technical viewpoints for review, including chemistry, pharmacology, medical, biopharmaceutics, and statistics. If the NDA is approved, the product may be marketed in the United States. For internal tracking purposes, all NDA's are assigned an NDA number.

New Drug Approval Process. After the animal testing stage, the FDA decides whether it is reasonably safe for the company to move forward with clinical trials—studies that evaluate the safety and effectiveness of a drug in healthy people and in patients. The drug company submits the results of such studies to the FDA for review. The agency conducts a thorough review of the safety and effectiveness data and considers how the benefits compare to the risks when making a decision of whether to approve a drug.

Nonprescription Drug Label ("Drug Facts"). For an over-the-counter (OTC), or nonprescription medicine, information printed on the medication bottle or package under the heading Drug Facts is important for taking care of yourself and your family. The Drug Facts tell you what a medicine is supposed to do, who should or should not take it, and how to use it. Safety information and instructions for use are displayed in a uniform and easy-to-read format.

"Off Label Use." Also called unapproved use of an approved product, is when your healthcare provider uses an FDA-approved medical product for a use that has not been studied yet.

Over-the-Counter Drugs (OTC). The FDA defines OTC drugs as safe and effective for use by the general public without a doctor's prescription.

Patient Package Insert (PPI). A patient package insert contains information for patients' understanding of how to safely use a drug product.

Post-Market Surveillance. This is the process by which a drug's safety is monitored on an ongoing basis after a drug is approved by the FDA. Post-market surveillance looks to identify problems that were not observed or recognized before approval and any problems that may arise because a drug may not be used as described in the drug labeling, or because a drug is being manufactured incorrectly.

Pre-Clinical Data. Before a drug can be tested in people in the United States; sponsors (drug manufacturers, research institutions, and other organizations that develop drugs) must show the FDA results of testing they have done in laboratory animals and what they propose to do for human testing.

Prescription Drug Product. A prescription drug product requires a doctor's authorization to purchase.

Regulatory Agency. This is a public authority or government agency responsible for exercising autonomous authority over some area of human activity in a regulatory or supervisory capacity. An independent regulatory agency is a regulatory agency that is independent from other branches or arms of the government. Regulatory agencies deal in the area of administrative law—regulation or rulemaking (codifying and enforcing rules and regulations and imposing supervision or oversight for the benefit of the public at large).

Review. A review is the basis of the FDA's decision to approve an application. It is a comprehensive analysis of clinical trial data and other information prepared by FDA drug application reviewers. A review is divided into sections on medical analysis, chemistry, clinical pharmacology, biopharmaceutics, pharmacology, statistics, and microbiology.

Reference Listed Drug (RLD). An approved drug product to which new generic versions are compared to show that they are bioequivalent. A drug company seeking approval to market a generic equivalent must refer to the RLD in its ANDA by designating a single reference listed drug as the standard to which all generic versions must be shown to be bioequivalent, the FDA hopes to avoid possible significant variations among generic drugs and their brand name counterpart.

Sponsors. Clinical trials are sponsored or funded by various organizations or individuals, including physicians, foundations, medical institutions, voluntary groups, and pharmaceutical companies, as well as Federal agencies such as NIH, FDA, the Department of Defense, and the Department of Veterans Affairs.

Tentative Approval. If a generic drug product is ready for approval before the expiration of any patents or exclusivities accorded to the reference listed drug product, the FDA issues a tentative approval letter to the applicant. The tentative approval letter details the circumstances associated with the tentative approval. The FDA delays final approval of the generic drug product until all patent or exclusivity issues have been resolved. A tentative approval does not allow the applicant to market the generic drug product.

Therapeutic Biological Product. A protein derived from living material (such as cells or tissues) used to treat or cure disease. The therapeutic biological products include: monoclonal antibodies for in-vivo use; cytokines, growth factors, enzymes, immunomodulators, and thrombolytics; proteins intended for therapeutic use that are extracted from animals or microorganisms, including recombinant versions of these products (except clotting factors); and other non-vaccine therapeutic immunotherapies.

NOTES

1 Office of the Commissioner. (2018, February 1). *History of FDA's Centers and Offices*. U.S. Food and Drug Administration. https://www.fda.gov/about-fda/history-fdas-internal-organization/history-fdas-centers-and-offices

2 Center for Food Safety and Applied Nutrition. (2020, August 24). *Is It a Cosmetic, a Drug, or Both? (Or Is It Soap?)*. U.S. Food and Drug Administration. https://www.fda.gov/cosmetics/cosmetics-laws-regulations/it-cosmetic-drug-or-both-or-it-soap#Intended_use

3 Center for Drug Evaluation and Research. (2020, June 1). *New Drug Development and Review Process*. U.S. Food and Drug Administration. https://www.fda.gov/drugs/cder-small-business-industry-assistance-sbia/new-drug-development-and-review-process

4 Center for Drug Evaluation and Research. (2018, June 18). *Think It Through: Managing the Benefits and Risks of Medicines*. U.S. Food and Drug Administration. https://www.fda.gov/drugs/information-consumers-and-patients-drugs/think-it-through-managing-benefits-and-risks-medicines

5 Office of the Commissioner. (2020, September 30). *FDA-TRACK: Center for Drug Evaluation & Research—Pre-Approval Safety Review*. U.S. Food and Drug Administration. https://www.fda.gov/about-fda/fda-track-agency-wide-program-performance/fda-track-center-drug-evaluation-research-pre-approval-safety-review

6 U.S. Food and Drug Administration. (2018, March 30). *Benefit Risk Assessment in Drug Regulatory Decision Making*. https://www.fda.gov/files/about%20fda/published/Benefit-Risk-Assessment-in-Drug-Regulatory-Decision-Making.pdf

7 Center for Drug Evaluation and Research. (2018, March 20). *Enhancing Benefit-Risk Assessment in Regulatory Decision-Making*. U.S. Food and Drug Administration. https://www.fda.gov/industry/prescription-drug-user-fee-amendments/enhancing-benefit-risk-assessment-regulatory-decision-making

8 Center for Drug Evaluation and Research. (2021, January 7). *Prescription Drug Labeling Resources*. U.S. Food and Drug Administration. https://www.fda.gov/drugs/laws-acts-and-rules/prescription-drug-labeling-resources

9 Center for Drug Evaluation and Research. (2020, April 2). *Postmarketing Surveillance Programs*. U.S. Food and Drug Administration. https://www.fda.gov/drugs/surveillance/postmarketing-surveillance-programs

10 Office of Regulatory Affairs. (2021, January 29). *Recalls, Market Withdrawals, & Safety Alerts*. U.S. Food and Drug Administration. https://www.fda.gov/safety/recalls-market-withdrawals-safety-alerts

11 Center for Drug Evaluation and Research. (2016, February 26). *FDA Drug Approval Process Infographic (Horizontal)*. U.S. Food and Drug Administration.

https://www.fda.gov/drugs/information-consumers-and-patients-drugs/fda-drug-approval-process-infographic-horizontal
12 Center for Drug Evaluation and Research. (2017, November 24). *The FDA's Drug Review Process: Ensuring Drugs Are Safe and Effective*. U.S. Food and Drug Administration. https://www.fda.gov/drugs/information-consumers-and-patients-drugs/fdas-drug-review-process-ensuring-drugs-are-safe-and-effective
13 Center for Drug Evaluation and Research. (2019, October 28). *Development & Approval Process|Drugs*. U.S. Food and Drug Administration. https://www.fda.gov/drugs/development-approval-process-drugs
14 Center for Drug Evaluation and Research. (2016, May 4). *CDER: The Consumer Watchdog for Safe and Effective Drugs*. U.S. Food and Drug Administration. https://www.fda.gov/drugs/information-consumers-and-patients-drugs/cder-consumer-watchdog-safe-and-effective-drugs
15 Office of the Commissioner. (2018, January 4). *Step 1: Discovery and Development*. U.S. Food and Drug Administration. https://www.fda.gov/patients/drug-development-process/step-1-discovery-and-development
16 U.S. Food and Drug Administration. (2006, January). *Guidance for Industry, Investigators, and Reviewers: Exploratory IND Studies*. https://www.fda.gov/regulatory-information/search-fda-guidance-documents/exploratory-ind-studies
17 Office of the Commissioner. (2018, January 4). *Step 2: Preclinical Research*. U.S. Food and Drug Administration. https://www.fda.gov/patients/drug-development-process/step-2-preclinical-research
18 Center for Drug Evaluation and Research. (2015, February 2). *Information for Clinical Investigators (INDs)*. U.S. Food and Drug Administration. https://www.fda.gov/drugs/investigational-new-drug-ind-application/information-clinical-investigators-inds
19 Center for Drug Evaluation and Research. (2015, August 20). *Drug Development and Review Definitions*. U.S. Food and Drug Administration. https://www.fda.gov/drugs/investigational-new-drug-ind-application/drug-development-and-review-definitions
20 Office of the Commissioner. (2018, January 4). *Step 3: Clinical Research*. U.S. Food and Drug Administration. https://www.fda.gov/patients/drug-development-process/step-3-clinical-research
21 Center for Drug Evaluation and Research. (2020, May 12). *Investigational New Drug (IND) Application*. U.S. Food and Drug Administration. https://www.fda.gov/drugs/types-applications/investigational-new-drug-ind-application
22 Center for Drug Evaluation and Research. (2020, February 4). *Small Business and Industry Assistance: Frequently Asked Questions on the Pre-Investigational New Drug (IND) Meeting*. U.S. Food and Drug Administration. https://www.fda.gov/drugs/cder-small-business-industry-assistance-sbia/small-business-and-industry-assistance-frequently-asked-questions-pre-investigational-new-drug-ind
23 U.S. Food and Drug Administration. (2019, March). *Guidance for Industry: Enrichment Strategies for Clinical Trials to Support Approval of Human Drugs and Biological Products*. https://www.fda.gov/regulatory-information/search-fda-guidance-documents/enrichment-strategies-clinical-trials-support-approval-human-drugs-and-biological-products
24 U.S. Food and Drug Administration. (2020, November). *Guidance for Industry: Enhancing the Diversity of Clinical Trial Populations—Eligibility Criteria, Enrollment Practices, and Trial Designs*. https://www.fda.gov/regulatory-information/search-fda-guidance-documents/enhancing-diversity-clinical-trial-populations-eligibility-criteria-enrollment-practices-and-trial
25 Phases of an Investigation, 21 CFR 312.21 (1987).
26 Center for Drug Evaluation and Research. (2016, January 12). *Postmarketing Requirements and Commitments: Introduction*. U.S. Food and Drug Administration. https://www.fda.gov/drugs/guidance-compliance-regulatory-information/postmarket-requirements-and-commitments
27 U.S. Food and Drug Administration. (n.d.). *Postmarket Requirements and Commitments*. FDA. https://www.accessdata.fda.gov/scripts/cder/pmc/index.cfm
28 U.S. Food and Drug Administration. (n.d.). *Drugs@FDA: FDA-Approved Drugs*. FDA. https://www.accessdata.fda.gov/scripts/cder/daf/
29 Office of the Commissioner. (2020, April 27). *Expanded Access*. U.S. Food and Drug Administration. https://www.fda.gov/news-events/public-health-focus/expanded-access
30 Office of the Commissioner. (2020, January 14). *Right to Try*. U.S. Food and Drug Administration. https://www.fda.gov/patients/learn-about-expanded-access-and-other-treatment-options/right-try
31 Center for Drug Evaluation and Research. (2019, June 10). *New Drug Application (NDA)*. U.S. Food and Drug Administration. https://www.fda.gov/drugs/types-applications/new-drug-application-nda
32 Center for Drug Evaluation and Research. (2019, June 10). *New Drug Application (NDA)*. U.S. Food and Drug Administration. https://www.fda.gov/drugs/types-applications/new-drug-application-nda
33 Center for Drug Evaluation and Research. (2015, July 7). *Frequently Asked Questions About Therapeutic Biological Products*. U.S. Food and Drug Administration. https://www.fda.gov/drugs/therapeutic-biologics-applications-bla/frequently-asked-questions-about-therapeutic-biological-products

34 Office of the Commissioner. (2012, September 10). *Kefauver-Harris Amendments Revolutionized Drug Development*. U.S. Food and Drug Administration. https://www.fda.gov/consumers/consumer-updates/kefauver-harris-amendments-revolutionized-drug-development
35 The International Council for Harmonisation of Technical Requirements for Pharmaceuticals for Human Use (ICH). (2003, July). *ICH Official Website: ICH*. M4: The Common Technical Document. https://www.ich.org/page/ctd
36 Center for Drug Evaluation and Research. (2018, May 4). *Forms & Submission Requirements*. U.S. Food and Drug Administration. https://www.fda.gov/drugs/development-approval-process-drugs/forms-submission-requirements
37 Center for Drug Evaluation and Research. (2021, January 22). *Office of Pharmaceutical Quality NDA Classification Codes MAPP 5018.2*. U.S. Food and Drug Administration. https://www.fda.gov/about-fda/center-drug-evaluation-and-research-cder/cder-manual-policies-procedures-mapp
38 Office of the Commissioner. (2018, January 4). *Priority Review*. U.S. Food and Drug Administration. https://www.fda.gov/patients/fast-track-breakthrough-therapy-accelerated-approval-priority-review/priority-review
39 U.S. Food and Drug Administration. (2014, September 26). *CDER 21st Century Review*. FDA. https://www.accessdata.fda.gov/cder/sb-navigate/topic3/topic3/da_01_03_0030.htm
40 Office of the Commissioner. (2018, January 4). *Accelerated Approval*. U.S. Food and Drug Administration. https://www.fda.gov/patients/fast-track-breakthrough-therapy-accelerated-approval-priority-review/accelerated-approval
41 Center for Drug Evaluation and Research. (2014, May). *Expedited Programs for Serious Conditions: Drugs and Biologics*. https://www.fda.gov/regulatory-information/search-fda-guidance-documents/expedited-programs-serious-conditions-drugs-and-biologics
42 Center for Drug Evaluation and Research. (2018, January). *Qualified Infectious Disease Product Designation Questions and Answers*. U.S. Food and Drug Administration. https://www.fda.gov/regulatory-information/search-fda-guidance-documents/qualified-infectious-disease-product-designation-questions-and-answers
43 Center for Drug Evaluation and Research. (2020, July 15). *Tropical Disease Priority Review Voucher Program*. U.S. Food and Drug Administration. https://www.fda.gov/about-fda/center-drug-evaluation-and-research-cder/tropical-disease-priority-review-voucher-program
44 Office of the Commissioner. (2018, January). *Material Threat Medical Countermeasure Priority Review Vouchers: Draft Guidance for Industry*. U.S. Food and Drug Administration. https://www.fda.gov/regulatory-information/search-fda-guidance-documents/material-threat-medical-countermeasure-priority-review-vouchers-draft-guidance-industry
45 Office of the Commissioner. (2020, April 16). *Rare Pediatric Disease Priority Review Vouchers*. U.S. Food and Drug Administration. https://www.fda.gov/regulatory-information/search-fda-guidance-documents/rare-pediatric-disease-priority-review-vouchers
46 Office of the Commissioner. (2018, January 4). *Fast Track*. U.S. Food and Drug Administration. https://www.fda.gov/patients/fast-track-breakthrough-therapy-accelerated-approval-priority-review/fast-track
47 Office of the Commissioner. (2018, January 4). *Breakthrough Therapy*. U.S. Food and Drug Administration. https://www.fda.gov/patients/fast-track-breakthrough-therapy-accelerated-approval-priority-review/breakthrough-therapy
48 Labeling, 21 CFR 201 (2007).
49 Center for Drug Evaluation and Research. (2013, February). *Labeling for Human Prescription Drug and Biological Products: Implementing the PLR Content and Format Requirements*. U.S. Food and Drug Administration. https://www.fda.gov/regulatory-information/search-fda-guidance-documents/labeling-human-prescription-drug-and-biological-products-implementing-plr-content-and-format
50 Federal Register. (2006, January 24). *Requirements on Content and Format of Labeling for Human Prescription Drug and Biological Products*. https://www.federalregister.gov/documents/2006/01/24/06-545/requirements-on-content-and-format-of-labeling-for-human-prescription-drug-and-biological-products
51 Office of the Commissioner. (2018, January 8). *Learn About Your Medicines*. https://www.fda.gov/patients/learn-about-your-medicines
52 Center for Drug Evaluation and Research. (2020, January 3). *Medication Guides*. U.S. Food and Drug Administration. https://www.fda.gov/drugs/drug-safety-and-availability/medication-guides
53 Center for Drug Evaluation and Research. (2019, August 8). *Risk Evaluation and Mitigation Strategies|REMS*. U.S. Food and Drug Administration. https://www.fda.gov/drugs/drug-safety-and-availability/risk-evaluation-and-mitigation-strategies-rems
54 Center for Drug Evaluation and Research. (2018, January 26). *Frequently Asked Questions (FAQs) About REMS*. U.S. Food and Drug Administration. https://www.fda.gov/drugs/risk-evaluation-and-mitigation-strategies-rems/frequently-asked-questions-faqs-about-rems
55 U.S. Food and Drug Administration. (n.d.). *Approved Risk Evaluation and Mitigation Strategies (REMS)*.

FDA. https://www.accessdata.fda.gov/scripts/cder/rems/index.cfm
56 Center for Drug Evaluation and Research. (2011, November). *Medication Guides: Distribution Requirements and Inclusion in Risk Evaluation and Mitigation Strategies (REMS)*. U.S. Food and Drug Administration. https://www.fda.gov/regulatory-information/search-fda-guidance-documents/medication-guides-distribution-requirements-and-inclusion-risk-evaluation-and-mitigation-strategies
57 Center for Drug Evaluation and Research. (2017, October 5). *Human Drug Advisory Committees*. U.S. Food and Drug Administration. https://www.fda.gov/advisory-committees/committees-and-meeting-materials/human-drug-advisory-committees
58 Office of the Commissioner. (2020, October 19). *Learn About FDA Advisory Committees*. U.S. Food and Drug Administration. https://www.fda.gov/patients/about-office-patient-affairs/learn-about-fda-advisory-committees
59 Biopharma/Tech Education—Education—Valhalla. https://forums.ascendedtrading.com/t/biopharma-tech-education/14844
60 Office of the Commissioner. (2020, September 16). *Advisory Committee Calendar*. U.S. Food and Drug Administration. https://www.fda.gov/advisory-committees/advisory-committee-calendar
61 Center for Drug Evaluation and Research. (2019, May 22). *Abbreviated New Drug Application (ANDA)*. U.S. Food and Drug Administration. https://www.fda.gov/drugs/types-applications/abbreviated-new-drug-application-anda
62 U.S. Food and Drug Administration. (n.d.). *Orange Book: Approved Drug Products with Therapeutic Equivalence Evaluations*. FDA. https://www.accessdata.fda.gov/scripts/cder/ob/index.cfm
63 Center for Drug Evaluation and Research. (2017, August 31). *What Is the Approval Process for Generic Drugs?* U.S. Food and Drug Administration. https://www.fda.gov/drugs/generic-drugs/what-approval-process-generic-drugs
64 Center for Drug Evaluation and Research. (2020, September). *ANDA Submissions: Amendments and Requests for Final Approval to Tentatively Approved ANDAs*. U.S. Food and Drug Administration. https://www.fda.gov/regulatory-information/search-fda-guidance-documents/anda-submissions-amendments-and-requests-final-approval-tentatively-approved-andas
65 Office of the Commissioner. (2018, March 28). *Food and Drug Administration Safety and Innovation Act (FDASIA)*. U.S. Food and Drug Administration. https://www.fda.gov/regulatory-information/selected-amendments-fdc-act/food-and-drug-administration-safety-and-innovation-act-fdasia
66 Center for Drug Evaluation and Research. (2021, January 27). *Generic Drug User Fee Amendments*. U.S. Food and Drug Administration. https://www.fda.gov/industry/fda-user-fee-programs/generic-drug-user-fee-amendments
67 Center for Drug Evaluation and Research. (2020, July 20). *Building on Successes of the Generic Drug Program, FDA Sets the Stage for the Next Generic Drug User Fee Amendments (GDUFA) Reauthorization Process*. U.S. Food and Drug Administration. https://www.fda.gov/drugs/news-events-human-drugs/building-successes-generic-drug-program-fda-sets-stage-next-generic-drug-user-fee-amendments-gdufa
68 Center for Drug Evaluation and Research. (2020, February 3). *Biosimilars*. U.S. Food and Drug Administration. https://www.fda.gov/drugs/therapeutic-biologics-applications-bla/biosimilars
69 Biosimilar: K-Message. https://k-message.com/glossary/biosimilar/
70 Office of the Commissioner. (2020, February 20). *Definition of the Term "Biological Product" Final Regulatory Impact Analysis*. U.S. Food and Drug Administration. https://www.fda.gov/about-fda/economic-impact-analyses-fda-regulations/definition-term-biological-product-final-regulatory-impact-analysis
71 Biosimilar: K-Message. https://k-message.com/glossary/biosimilar/
72 Center for Drug Evaluation and Research. (2017, October 23). *Biosimilar and Interchangeable Products*. U.S. Food and Drug Administration. https://www.fda.gov/drugs/biosimilars/biosimilar-and-interchangeable-products
73 Biosimilar: K-Message. https://k-message.com/glossary/biosimilar/
74 Biosimilar: K-Message. https://k-message.com/glossary/biosimilar/
75 Center for Drug Evaluation and Research. (2016, May 4). *Now Available Without a Prescription*. U.S. Food and Drug Administration. https://www.fda.gov/drugs/information-consumers-and-patients-drugs/now-available-without-prescription
76 Center for Drug Evaluation and Research. (2014, October 23). *Types of Applications*. U.S. Food and Drug Administration. https://www.fda.gov/drugs/how-drugs-are-developed-and-approved/types-applications
77 Center for Drug Evaluation and Research. (2019, October 28). *Frequently Asked Questions About CDER*. U.S. Food and Drug Administration. https://www.fda.gov/about-fda/center-drug-evaluation-and-research-cder/frequently-asked-questions-about-cder
78 Center for Drug Evaluation and Research. (2020, March 31). *Drug Applications for Over-the-Counter (OTC) Drugs*. U.S. Food and Drug Administration.

https://www.fda.gov/drugs/types-applications/drug-applications-over-counter-otc-drugs

79 Center for Drug Evaluation and Research. (2020, September 3). *Over-the-Counter (OTC) Drug Monograph Process*. U.S. Food and Drug Administration. https://www.fda.gov/drugs/over-counter-otc-drug-monograph-process

80 Center for Food Safety and Applied Nutrition. (2020, August 24). *Is It a Cosmetic, a Drug, or Both? (Or Is It Soap?)*. U.S. Food and Drug Administration. https://www.fda.gov/cosmetics/cosmetics-laws-regulations/it-cosmetic-drug-or-both-or-it-soap

81 Center for Drug Evaluation and Research. (2020, December 8). *Over-the-Counter (OTC) Drug Review|OTC Monograph Reform in the CARES Act*. U.S. Food and Drug Administration. https://www.fda.gov/drugs/over-counter-otc-nonprescription-drugs/over-counter-otc-drug-review-otc-monograph-reform-cares-act

82 Center for Drug Evaluation and Research. (2021, January 10). *Over-the-Counter Monograph User Fee Program (OMUFA)*. U.S. Food and Drug Administration. https://www.fda.gov/industry/fda-user-fee-programs/over-counter-monograph-user-fee-program-omufa

83 Center for Drug Evaluation and Research. (2020, May 29). *Monograph Reform is Here! Learn What to Expect and How to Prepare*. U.S. Food and Drug Administration. https://www.fda.gov/drugs/news-events-human-drugs/webinar-monograph-reform-here-learn-what-expect-and-how-prepare-05292020-05292020

84 CDER Office of Surveillance and Epidemiology. (2020, March 23). U.S. Food and Drug Administration. https://www.fda.gov/about-fda/center-drug-evaluation-and-research-cder/cder-office-surveillance-and-epidemiology

85 Office of the Commissioner. (2019, October 21). *MedWatch: The FDA Safety Information and Adverse Event Reporting Program*. U.S. Food and Drug Administration. https://www.fda.gov/safety/medwatch-fda-safety-information-and-adverse-event-reporting-program

86 Center for Drug Evaluation and Research. (2018, June 4). *Questions and Answers on FDA's Adverse Event Reporting System (FAERS)*. U.S. Food and Drug Administration. https://www.fda.gov/drugs/surveillance/questions-and-answers-fdas-adverse-event-reporting-system-faers

87 Center for Drug Evaluation and Research. (2020, March 23). *Office of Surveillance and Epidemiology (OSE): Divisions*. U.S. Food and Drug Administration.https://www.fda.gov/about-fda/center-drug-evaluation-and-research-cder/office-surveillance-and-epidemiology-ose-divisions

88 Center for Drug Evaluation and Research. (2020, May 26). *Postmarket Drug Safety Information for Patients and Providers*. U.S. Food and Drug Administration. https://www.fda.gov/drugs/drug-safety-and-availability/postmarket-drug-safety-information-patients-and-providers

89 U.S. Food and Drug Administration. (2017, January). *22 Case Studies Where Phase 2 and Phase 3 Trials Had Divergent Results*. FDA. https://www.fda.gov/about-fda/reports/22-case-studies-where-phase-2-and-phase-3-trials-had-divergent-results

90 Office of the Commissioner. (2018, May 22). *Reporting Serious Problems to FDA*. U.S. Food and Drug Administration. https://www.fda.gov/safety/medwatch-fda-safety-information-and-adverse-event-reporting-program/reporting-serious-problems-fda

91 Office of the Commissioner. (2016, February 1). *What is a Serious Adverse Event?* U.S. Food and Drug Administration. https://www.fda.gov/safety/reporting-serious-problems-fda/what-serious-adverse-event

92 Center for Drug Evaluation and Research. (2020, May 26). *Postmarket Drug Safety Information for Patients and Providers*. U.S. Food and Drug Administration. https://www.fda.gov/drugs/drug-safety-and-availability/postmarket-drug-safety-information-patients-and-providers

93 Center for Drug Evaluation and Research. (2021, January 27). *Potential Signals of Serious Risks/New Safety Information Identified From the FDA Adverse Event Reporting System (FAERS)*. U.S. Food and Drug Administration. https://www.fda.gov/drugs/questions-and-answers-fdas-adverse-event-reporting-system-faers/potential-signals-serious-risksnew-safety-information-identified-fda-adverse-event-reporting-system

94 Center for Drug Evaluation and Research. (2020, October 29). *FDA Adverse Event Reporting System (FAERS) Public Dashboard*. U.S. Food and Drug Administration. https://www.fda.gov/drugs/questions-and-answers-fdas-adverse-event-reporting-system-faers/fda-adverse-event-reporting-system-faers-public-dashboard

95 Center for Drug Evaluation and Research. (2020, April 30). *CDER Manual of Policies & Procedures|MAPP: Collaborative Identification, Evaluation, and Resolution of a Newly Identified Safety Signal (NISS) 4121.3*. U.S. Food and Drug Administration. https://www.fda.gov/about-fda/center-drug-evaluation-and-research-cder/cder-manual-policies-procedures-mapp

96 Office of the Commissioner. (2020, March 9). *FDA's Sentinel Initiative: Background*. U.S. Food and Drug Administration.https://www.fda.gov/safety/fdas-sentinel-initiative/fdas-sentinel-initiative-background

97 FDA. *FDA's Sentinel Initiative: Background.* https://www.fda.gov/safety/fdas-sentinel-initiative/fdas-sentinel-initiative-background
98 Center for Drug Evaluation and Research. (2020, November 24). *Drug Safety Oversight Board.* U.S. Food and Drug Administration. https://www.fda.gov/about-fda/center-drug-evaluation-and-research-cder/drug-safety-oversight-board
99 Office of the Commissioner. (2018, July 11). *80 Years of the Federal Food, Drug, and Cosmetic Act.* U.S. Food and Drug Administration. https://www.fda.gov/about-fda/virtual-exhibits-fda-history/80-years-federal-food-drug-and-cosmetic-act
100 FDA. *80 Years of the Federal Food, Drug, and Cosmetic Act.* https://www.fda.gov/about-fda/fda-history-exhibits/80-years-federal-food-drug-and-cosmetic-act
101 Office of the Commissioner. (2018, January 31). *Sulfanilamide Disaster.* U.S. Food and Drug Administration. https://www.fda.gov/about-fda/histories-product-regulation/sulfanilamide-disaster
102 FDA. *Sulfanilamide Disaster.* https://www.fda.gov/about-fda/histories-product-regulation/sulfanilamide-disaster
103 Office of the Commissioner. (2018, February 1). *Part III: Drugs and Foods Under the 1938 Act and Its Amendments.* U.S. Food and Drug Administration. https://www.fda.gov/about-fda/fdas-evolving-regulatory-powers/part-iii-drugs-and-foods-under-1938-act-and-its-amendments
104 FDA. *Part III: Drugs and Foods Under the 1938 Act and Its Amendments.* https://www.fda.gov/about-fda/changes-science-law-and-regulatory-authorities/part-iii-drugs-and-foods-under-1938-act-and-its-amendments
105 Center for Drug Evaluation and Research. (2020, August 28). *Drug Efficacy Study Implementation (DESI).* U.S. Food and Drug Administration. https://www.fda.gov/drugs/enforcement-activities-fda/drug-efficacy-study-implementation-desi
106 FDA. *Part III: Drugs and Foods Under the 1938 Act and Its Amendments.* https://www.fda.gov/about-fda/changes-science-law-and-regulatory-authorities/part-iii-drugs-and-foods-under-1938-act-and-its-amendments
107 Office of the Commissioner. (2018, March 9). *Orphan Drug Act: Relevant Excerpts.* U.S. Food and Drug Administration. https://www.fda.gov/industry/designating-orphan-product-drugs-and-biological-products/orphan-drug-act-relevant-excerpts
108 Center for Drug Evaluation and Research. (2018, July 19). *Hatch-Waxman Letters.* U.S. Food and Drug Administration. https://www.fda.gov/drugs/abbreviated-new-drug-application-anda/hatch-waxman-letters
109 Office of the Commissioner. (2019, April 24). *New Drug and Antibiotic Regulations.* U.S. Food and Drug Administration. https://www.fda.gov/science-research/clinical-trials-and-human-subject-protection/new-drug-and-antibiotic-regulations
110 Center for Drug Evaluation and Research. (2015, September 22). *New Drug, Antibiotic, and Biologic Drug Product Regulations.* U.S. Food and Drug Administration. https://www.fda.gov/science-research/clinical-trials-and-human-subject-protection/new-drug-antibiotic-and-biologic-drug-product-regulations
111 Center for Drug Evaluation and Research. (2015, December 16). *PDUFA Legislation and Background.* U.S. Food and Drug Administration. https://www.fda.gov/industry/prescription-drug-user-fee-amendments/pdufa-legislation-and-background
112 Office of the Commissioner. (2018, March 28). *FDA Backgrounder on FDAMA.* U.S. Food and Drug Administration. https://www.fda.gov/regulatory-information/food-and-drug-administration-modernization-act-fdama-1997/fda-backgrounder-fdama
113 Office of the Commissioner. (2018, March 29). *Food and Drug Administration Amendments Act (FDAAA) of 2007.* U.S. Food and Drug Administration. https://www.fda.gov/regulatory-information/selected-amendments-fdc-act/food-and-drug-administration-amendments-act-fdaaa-2007
114 Federal Register. (2007, September 27). *Agencies: Reagan-Udall Foundation for the Food and Drug Administration.* https://www.federalregister.gov/agencies/reagan-udall-foundation-for-the-food-and-drug-administration
115 Office of the Commissioner. (2018, March 28). *Food and Drug Administration Safety and Innovation Act (FDASIA).* U.S. Food and Drug Administration. https://www.fda.gov/regulatory-information/selected-amendments-fdc-act/food-and-drug-administration-safety-and-innovation-act-fdasia
116 Center for Drug Evaluation and Research. (2020, December 22). *CDER Patient-Focused Drug Development.* U.S. Food and Drug Administration. https://www.fda.gov/drugs/development-approval-process-drugs/cder-patient-focused-drug-development
117 Center for Drug Evaluation and Research. (2020, November 24). *FDA-Led Patient-Focused Drug Development (PFDD) Public Meetings.* U.S. Food and Drug Administration. https://www.fda.gov/industry/prescription-drug-user-fee-amendments/fda-led-patient-focused-drug-development-pfdd-public-meetings
118 Office of the Commissioner. (2018, March 28). *FDASIA Title VII Overview.* U.S. Food and Drug Administration. https://www.fda.gov/regulatory-information/food-and-drug-administration-safety-and-innovation-act-fdasia/fdasia-title-vii-overview

119 Office of the Commissioner. (2018, March 28). *FDASIA Title VII Drug Supply Chain Provisions*. U.S. Food and Drug Administration. https://www.fda.gov/regulatory-information/food-and-drug-administration-safety-and-innovation-act-fdasia/fdasia-title-vii-drug-supply-chain-provisions

120 *Testimony: Scott Gottlieb on the Compounding Quality Act. 1.30.18*. (2018, January 30). U.S. Food and Drug Administration. https://www.fda.gov/news-events/congressional-testimony/examining-implementation-compounding-quality-act-01292018-01292018

121 Center for Drug Evaluation and Research. (2020, September 10). *Compounding Laws and Policies*. U.S. Food and Drug Administration. https://www.fda.gov/drugs/human-drug-compounding/compounding-laws-and-policies

122 Office of the Commissioner. (2020, January 31). *21st Century Cures Act*. U.S. Food and Drug Administration. https://www.fda.gov/regulatory-information/selected-amendments-fdc-act/21st-century-cures-act

123 FDA. *21st Century Cures Act*. https://www.fda.gov/regulatory-information/selected-amendments-fdc-act/21st-century-cures-act

124 Office of the Commissioner. (2018, June 21). *FDA Reauthorization Act of 2017 (FDARA)*. U.S. Food and Drug Administration. https://www.fda.gov/regulatory-information/selected-amendments-fdc-act/fda-reauthorization-act-2017-fdara

125 Center for Drug Evaluation and Research. (2021, January 10). *Over-the-Counter Monograph User Fee Program(OMUFA)*. U.S. Food and Drug Administration. https://www.fda.gov/industry/fda-user-fee-programs/over-counter-monograph-user-fee-program-omufa

2 The Front Lines of Clinical Research
The Industry and Ethical Considerations

Jonathan C. Young

SYNOPSIS

2.1 INTRODUCTION

Drug development in the United States is both risky and expensive. The cost of developing a drug has increased from approximately $500 million in 1990[1] to more than $2.8 billion in 2016.[2,3,4] At the same time, the research and development (R&D) costs of the pharmaceutical industry have increased from approximately 12% of sales to 21%.[5,6] As of 2019, only about 14% of drugs with clinical trials will be successful, and the drug development process takes at least 10 years. Importantly, only 3.4% of oncology drug trials will be successful.[7,8]

Given the growing number of clinical trials required for FDA approval, opportunities are numerous in the provision of clinical research services. In addition, the FDA is becoming more vigilant in enforcing the ethical conduct of clinical research and the protection of research participants. Lastly, to avoid conflicts of interest or perceived improprieties,

DOI: 10.1201/9781003615323-3

pharmaceutical and device manufacturers frequently outsource all or part of the clinical trial process to niche service providers. For these reasons, the clinical trial industry has become segmented. Each segment or service provider performs a necessary step in the clinical trial value chain. In addition to niche service providers, the growing clinical trial industry has created a need for service organizations, publications, and web sites devoted to the specialized field.

To have a thorough understanding of the industry requires a working knowledge of the freedoms, constraints, and political environments in which each service provider must operate. Perhaps a better way to stress the complexities of the industry is to realize that drug development is characterized by a high rate of failure. It is a disorderly process where very few research efforts ever bear fruit. In fact, the typical pharmaceutical company spends about 40% of its R&D budget on compounds that do not make it to market. As one expert has stated, "Drug innovation is something that is sought but not known in advance .... Only by aiming high can genuine innovation be coaxed into existence .... Innovation must be able to pay the price of failure."[9] Unfortunately, even if the new compound under study is safe and efficacious, failure can occur because of undercapitalization of the pharmaceutical company, poor data quality on the part of the sponsor or investigative site, or disapproval by the FDA.

2.2 CLINICAL TRIAL SERVICE PROVIDERS

Although it is estimated that 102 billion dollars was spent on human drug development (Phases I to III) in 2018, the industry is quite small and very specialized.[10] In fact, most Americans have a limited knowledge of how new medications end up in their pharmacies.[11,12] The service providers challenged with bringing new treatments and cures to the masses include (1) the Food and Drug Administration, (2) the clinical trial sponsor, (3) contract research organizations (CROs), (4) study monitors, (5) the clinical trial site, (6) site management organizations (SMOs), (7) the institutional review board (IRB), and (8) study participants.

2.2.1 Food and Drug Administration

The FDA's very noble mission is "to promote and protect public health by helping safe and effective products reach the market in a timely way, and monitoring products for continued safety after they are in use."[13] The scope of this mission has grown substantially during the past century. In addition to its consumer protection role regarding all prescription and over-the-counter drugs, the FDA establishes and enforces standards for all food (except meat and poultry), all blood products, vaccines and tissues for transplantation, all medical equipment, all devices that emit radiation, all animal drugs and foods, and all cosmetics.

Given the complex and diverse tasks performed by the FDA, it is not surprising that there are critics on both sides of the drug approval fence. Many argue that the FDA has taken away the human right to make an informed choice regarding whether to take an investigational drug. Others argue that the FDA acts too hastily in approving drugs that are later shown to be unsafe. Thus, there is a constant tension between those who want greater consumer protection and those who want greater freedom of choice.

In 1992, Congress passed the Prescription Drug User Fee Act (PDUFA).[14] The purpose was to establish a mechanism for financing the resources that would be needed to speed up the process of reviewing NDAs. PDUFA allows the FDA to collect user fees from pharmaceutical companies to support the review of applications. A recent report by the U.S. General Accounting Office (GAO)[15] concludes that "PDUFA has been successful in providing FDA with the funding necessary to hire additional drug reviewers, thereby making new drugs available in the United States more quickly" (p. 6).

Supporting this conclusion is the fact that approval times have decreased from 27 to 10 months.[16] However, the GAO also reported a small increase in the drug-withdrawal rate since the implementation of PDUFA, although these results seem to have been mitigated in more recent years. Initially, after PDUFA went into effect, a higher percent of approved drugs had been withdrawn from the market because of safety issues. FDA officials argued that the increase is insignificant—from 3.1% in the 8-year period before PDUFA to 3.47% in the 8-year period after. A more recent study showed that from 2001 to 2010, only 1.35% of 222 approved drugs were withdrawn from the market.[17]

This protection–freedom dynamic is even more intensive when it comes to drugs that are being tested for use in patients with terminal illnesses that have no other viable treatment options. In these situations, the FDA receives tremendous pressure to approve these drugs rapidly. The rationale is that the most serious risk of death from an experimental drug is no risk at all compared with the certainty of death in patients with a lethal disease.

2.2.2 Clinical Trial Sponsor

The clinical trial sponsor is an individual, company, institution, or organization that assumes responsibility for the initiation, management, or financing of the clinical trial. The sponsor is required by the FDA to conduct clinical trials to determine the safety and efficacy of the investigational agent. Safety data are usually derived through documented occurrence of adverse pharmacokinetic or pharmacodynamic effects. Alternatively, efficacy data can be evaluated by the prevention of a medical condition or through improvement of specific symptoms of a disease process.[18]

In the conduct of the clinical trial, according to the Code of Federal Regulations (CFR), the study sponsor is responsible for all aspects of the study including, but not limited to, maintaining quality assurance and quality control, medical expertise, trial design, trial management, data handling, record keeping, investigator selection, allocation of duties and functions, determining compensation to subjects and investigators, financing, notification/submission to regulatory authorities, product information, preparing and supplying study medications, monitoring and assuring that all clinical trial sites comply with federal regulatory requirements.[19]

The sponsor bears ultimate responsibility for the success, failure, and safety of the treatment under study, even after FDA approval. In addition, the sponsor is the true innovator in the clinical trial process. Innovation is expensive, causing newly available treatments to be costly to the end user. Thus, because of the escalating price of medications, the innovators are under increased scrutiny by consumers and policymakers. Paradoxically, as the population ages, the consumers are driving the demand for new cures and better treatments.

Given the high rate of "failure" in the drug industry, it is reasonable to hypothesize that drug development would take place in economies characterized by relatively free markets and prices. The ideal environment would provide adequate incentives for investing in high-risk ventures. Such an environment exists in the United States. Although the United States is home to only about 4% of the world's population, roughly 22% of the worldwide pharmaceutical R&D is conducted in the United States on a yearly basis.[20,21]

The United States is the world's quantitative and qualitative leader in drug development,[22] but what is the price of that leadership? Many taxpayers and consumers are outraged at the high cost of prescription drugs compared with those available in nations with price controls, such as Canada, Mexico, and the United Kingdom. In 2018, the White House Ways and Means Committee released a report claiming drug prices in the United States are nearly four times higher than the combined average price of 11 comparator nations. The list of nations included several European nations where price controls exist, Japan, and Australia.[23] Having established this comparison, it was an easy step for the writer to conclude that what was a good deal for these other countries would be a good deal for the United States. The point that escapes the writer is that if such controls were in effect here, many of the sampled drugs would never have been developed and made available to price-controlled countries.

Citizens and policymakers misunderstand that although drug development is expensive, production costs of the pills are comparatively low. It is the formula, not the ingredients, that is costly. In addition, drug expenditure is just part of the overall expense of health care and must not be looked at in a vacuum. For example, it is estimated that, on average, U.S. citizens spend about 29% more per capita on pharmaceutical goods—or about 228 dollars per person per year more—than the most expensive price-controlled nation.[24]

2.2.3 Contract Research Organizations

The daily attendance of the clinical trial process can require time, labor, and training that many sponsors feel do not match their current capabilities. Therefore, sponsors may elect to outsource any or all their trial-related duties to a CRO. Full-service CROs offer provide data monitoring, data management, protocol development, medical writing, statistical analysis, contract management, site selection, and shipping and handling of investigational supplies. Niche CROs may elect to provide only a few of these services, such as data monitoring or medical writing. The CRO should maintain its own system of quality assurance and quality control. However, regardless of the duties assumed by the CRO, the final responsibility for the quality and integrity of the data always resides with the sponsor, and any duties not specifically transferred to a CRO remain the responsibility of the sponsor.

CROs are growing and mutating, making it difficult to identify specific trends. However, one thing is certain, pharmaceutical, biotechnology, and medical devices sponsors expect to increase outsourcing to the several hundred CROs. In fact, pharmaceutical companies have already increased their use of CROs: from 28% of clinical studies in 1993 to 61% in 2017.[25,26] Another study suggests that, as of 2015, 100% of sponsors performed at least some amount of outsourcing to CROs.[27] This reflects increased spending on the CRO services of phases I-IV study monitoring, data management, pharmacoeconomic analysis, and medical writing. Although these specialties remain the most frequently used, CROs are also offering new services to satisfy sponsors demands for faster trials and globalization.

To meet this challenge, CROs seem to be taking one of the two tracks: they are either strategically planning to become mega-CROs or niche providers. Industry observers believe the midsize CROs will disappear, mostly through merger and acquisition activity by larger CROs and by non-CROs with a strategic interest in entering the business. Analysts had forecasted that the midsize CRO will be gone, but niche players with special capabilities (statistical consulting, data management, monitoring) may survive.[28] Indeed, in 2016, merger and acquisition spending in the CRO industry had increased to $24 billion, and only nine CROs possessed 60% of the market share.[29] As the CRO industry consolidates, some large publicly traded CROs are making acquisitions that diversify the breadth of service beyond conducting studies. This move enables sponsors to do one-stop shopping instead of contracting with multiple companies throughout the discovery—development process. In addition, CROs are positioning themselves to gain access to populations in emerging markets such as Israel, Russia, Latin America, China, and India.

2.2.4 Study Monitors

Study monitors or clinical research associates (CRAs) can be employed by the study sponsor, CRO, or independently contracted for a specific study and, according to the International Committee on Harmonisation (ICH) and formalized by FDA in the Guidance for Industry: Good Clinical Practice (GCP), the purpose of a CRA is to:[30]

1. Verify that the rights and well-being of human subjects are protected.
2. Verify that the reported trial data are accurate, complete, and verifiable from source documentation.
3. Verify that the conduct of the trial is in compliance with the currently approved protocol/amendment(s), with GCPs, and with applicable regulatory requirement(s).

CRAs achieve these tasks through frequent visits to the clinical trial site. During these visits, the monitor will verify source data, audit regulatory documents for accuracy and completion, perform drug accountability assessments, and communicate any concerns, problems, or new information with the study staff.

2.3 CLINICAL TRIAL SITE

The front line of clinical trials is the site. It is at the site level that participants are given informed consent, study-related procedures are conducted according to the clinical trial protocol, and data are collected and reported. It is these data, aggregated from all sites, that ultimately determine the fate of the investigational drug or device. With the rigor in which clinical trials must be conducted today, site research personnel usually include the principal investigator (PI), sub-investigators, study coordinators, and regulatory managers. However, depending on the amount of research being conducted at a given location, the study coordinators are often also responsible for the regulatory compliance.

The PI is the individual who is ultimately responsible for the clinical trial at the trial site and the one who verifies that the data reported to the study sponsor are accurate. Although not required by the FDA, the PI is usually a physician. If the PI is not a physician, adequate physician oversight of the trial must be readily evident. As addressed by ICH and GCP guidance, the PI should be qualified through education, training, and experience to assume responsibility for the proper conduct of the trial and should meet all the qualifications specified by the applicable regulatory requirements (Section 4.1.1, p. 18).[31] Not all physicians are well suited for clinical research. A successful PI has distinct characteristics as listed in Table 2.1.

As defined by ICH and GCP guidelines, a sub-investigator is any individual member of the clinical trial team designated and directly supervised by the PI to perform trial-related procedures or make trial-related decisions (Section 1.56, p. 13).[32] Examples of sub-investigators include other physicians, pharmacists, pharmacologists, nurses, physician assistants, and study coordinators.

Clinical research coordinators (CRCs) are the research personnel who assist with patient visits and perform study-related procedures that do not require a physician (phlebotomy, vital signs, adverse event, and concomitant medication discussions, etc.). CRCs provide the PI or physician with data required for interpretation, medical decisions (inclusion/exclusion, dosage adjustment, patient withdrawal, adverse event causality, etc.), and trial oversight. In addition, CRCs are usually responsible for transcribing source documentation (medical records, clinic notes, laboratory reports, etc.) into case report forms (CRF) supplied by the study sponsor.

TABLE 2.1
Qualities Needed by a Successful Principal Investigator.

Not Everyone Makes a Successful Principal Investigator, a Good PI:

- Has an intrinsic interest in science
- Is knowledgeable about the protocol
- Always places patient care above all other priorities
- Is willing to carve out time for the study
- Is very involved in medical oversight
- Knows his or her limitations and when to ask for help
- Is tolerant of the increased need for regulatory scrutiny
- Understands that being a respected clinician does not mean being a good researcher and is open to learning about the conduct of clinical research
- Is prompt in the turnaround on documentation
- Meets participant recruitment and enrollment goals established with the sponsor

Another important function of the CRC is to interact with the sponsor or CRO appointed CRA. Because the CRA is an agent for the sponsor, the CRC–CRA relationship is one that can make or break a study. If a CRC is doing an excellent job, and the documents are available and accurate, the CRA's interactions with the site should be positive and productive. Unfortunately, this does not always happen. There are dynamics on both sides of the CRF. Some common complaints are:

- The CRA assigned to a given study changes frequently. Each CRA communicates different directives to the site, causing the site to redo work.
- The CRA has a condescending attitude toward the site and the investigator.
- The CRA is not well trained.
- The CRC is inexperienced.
- The CRA cannot obtain rapid answers to questions, often creating patient-care issues.
- The CRC cannot obtain rapid answers to queries, often extending timelines for study closure.
- The CRC makes numerous errors in the CRF.
- The CRC does not seem dedicated to the study.

In an industry where there is virtually full employment, it is difficult to find trained CRCs and CRAs, therefore; conflicts can arise from interaction between untrained or inexperienced personnel. Although technology can eliminate some of the need for CRA–CRC interaction, all parties need to understand the roles and pressures on the other person.[33]

For example, many CRAs travel four days per week and see various levels of work quality at different sites. On the other hand, CRCs are often responsible for more than one study and have requests from multiple CRAs on any given day. In addition, the CRA must respond to the needs of the research participant first, which can cause time delays in completing data queries.

Regulatory managers are usually charged with submitting regulatory documents to the IRB and study sponsor and with maintaining a regulatory binder. A regulatory binder should contain a protocol, protocol amendments, IRB approvals and correspondence, all versions of the IRB-approved patient informed consent, investigators' brochure, sponsor correspondence, curriculum vitas and licensures of the PI and sub-investigators, and any safety reports.

2.3.1 Site Management Organizations

As the number of clinical research sites have grown, a new entity, the SMOs, has arisen. SMOs, in the traditional sense, were established to offer the sponsor consolidated services at the site level. SMOs took the CRO business model and brought it to the front lines. For example, CROs offer a variety of services for the sponsor, such as site monitoring, contract administration, shipping and receiving of study supplies, and data management. SMOs offer PI recruitment, patient recruitment, and regulatory and contract management for multiple sites. As sponsors often must recruit 50 to 200 clinical trial sites, SMOs offer a one-stop shop. SMOs can provide the sponsors with multiple PIs and centralized contract and regulatory services, expediting study initiation.

SMO models vary widely in the industry. Some SMOs hire physician investigators as employees of the company. Others subcontract for investigator services. However, few offer turnkey solutions for investigators who wish to be involved in clinical research but lack the specialized training or necessary personnel. Full-service SMOs act as a liaison between the pharmaceutical, device, or biotechnology company (or CRO), and the research patient. Services often include patient and investigator recruitment, regulatory document preparation and compliance, and study coordination.

SMOs provide an interesting entry for investigators into the clinical trial business. Specifically, some SMOs can present new investigators with clinical trial opportunities, essential training, and qualified research personnel. In turn, the investigator assumes ultimate responsibility for the ethical conduct of the study. By alleviating the physician, hospital, and health care staff from time-consuming, nonclinical tasks, SMOs can make research not only feasible but also lucrative for investigators and hospitals. This risk-sharing model can be beneficial to all parties.

2.3.2 Institutional Review Boards

Since the Kefauver–Harris Amendment[34] was adopted in 1962, pharmaceutical manufacturers have been held responsible by the FDA for providing new medications that are both safe and effective. In addition to the Kefauver–Harris Amendment, the Belmont Report (written in 1979),[35] established the ethical principles and guidelines for conducting research. The FDA requires that clinical trials be conducted in compliance with a protocol that has been approved by an IRB or Independent Ethics Committee (IEC). The terms IRB or IEC refer to any board, committee, or other group formally designated by an institution to review, approve initiation, and conduct periodic review of research involving human participants.[36] The FDA expects the IRB to review all research-related documents and activities that pertain directly to the rights and welfare of the participants of proposed research. The IRB has the authority to approve, require modification to, or disapprove all research activities as specified in the federal regulations. The primary purpose of the IRB and this formal review process is to protect the rights and welfare of human participants involved in these clinical trials. It is the federally mandated charge of the IRB to ensure the safety of the research participant.

The FDA is not the only agency governing the function of an IRB. The FDA only oversees clinical trials when they involve an FDA-regulated product (i.e., drug, device, or biologic). The Department of Health and Human Services (HHS), Office for Human Research Protection (OHRP) oversees federally funded research. The Federal Policy for the Protection of Human Subjects,[37] known as the "Common Rule," is the basic HHS policy for protection of human subjects, now codified in the CFR.[38] Even though the FDA regulations are not part of the Common Rule, the basic requirements for IRB's and informed consent are largely congruent. On January 21, 2019 HHS revisions to the Common Rule went into effect.[39] Changes included new requirements for informed consent and changes to the IRB review processes for expedited studies and continuing reviews. Even though the FDA has not yet harmonized with the HHS 2019 Common Rule revisions, the FDA has released guidance that states its intent to harmonize in the future.[40]

The differences between the Common Rule and the FDA regulations are differences in applicability. HHS regulations are based on federal funding, and FDA regulations are based on the use of FDA-regulated products. Examples of some of the differences in the FDA regulations and the Common Rule include the following:

- Differing definitions of a "human subject."
- HHS discusses "research" whereas FDA discusses "clinical investigations."
- FDA makes no provisions for waiving informed consent whereas HHS regulations provide for certain conditions in which an IRB can waive or alter elements of informed consent.
- FDA regulations states that subjects must be informed about FDA inspections.
- FDA requires that subjects sign and date the informed consent.

- FDA allows the sponsor to request a waiver of IRB review; under HHS regulations, certain categories of research are exempt, and department heads can waive regulations.
- HHS and FDA both have adopted additional protections for children, but HHS also has additional protections for fetuses, pregnant women, and prisoners.
- FDA has responsibility and authority over all parties participating in FDA-regulated research and has regulations unique to product review responsibilities.
- The FDA requires annual review for all FDA-regulated research, even if the research is deemed to be approvable under one or more of the expedited IRB review categories; whereas, under the HHS 2019 Common Rule, studies approvable under the expedited review categories may not require annual review.

IRBs should be knowledgeable in both FDA and HHS regulations and should know which regulations to apply when conducting its review. FDA regulations apply when products are regulated by the FDA. The Common Rule applies when the research is federally supported or conducted or when it is being conducted in an institution that has agreed to review all research under the Common Rule. Both rules apply if the research is federally funded and involves FDA-regulated products or if the FDA-regulated research is being conducted in an institution that has agreed to review all research under the Common Rule. As a rule of thumb, no matter which regulations apply, IRB members should use the Belmont Report[41] and its guidelines in all their daily decisions.

2.4 THE EVOLUTION OF ETHICAL PRINCIPLES IN CLINICAL RESEARCH

As the demand to develop new and improved medical treatments has grown so has the need for human participants to test the potential new treatments. The federal government has taken an increasingly prominent role in the oversight of human subject protection. The Belmont Report[42] established the ethical principles and guidelines for conducting research. It describes the three basic ethical principles (respect for persons, beneficence, and justice) that are relevant to clinical research involving humans. These principles dictate to the clinical research industry that it does not have the right to use people for scientific benefit without their permission—no matter how noble the cause may seem. The research must do something good, and it must be fair—people cannot be exploited for research purposes. Applying these ethical principles brings the research industry closer to providing sound, ethical research. The regulations that govern the conduct and oversight of clinical research involving human participants were written to implement these ethical principles.

The history of the development of formal ethical principles of research with humans can be traced to World War II. Physicians in Nazi Germany performed "medical experiments" on thousands of concentration camp prisoners. These experiments included determining how long humans would survive in freezing water and high altitudes, injecting people with viruses, and forcing people to ingest poison. Whereas the German physicians argued that the experiments were medically justified, the Nuremberg Military Tribunal declared them to be "crimes against humanity." Seven of the physicians were sentenced to death. The judges who wrote the verdict in 1947 included a section on medical experiments, which became known as the Nuremberg Code.[43] This code was the first formal set of ethical principles for researchers. The first item in the Nuremberg Code emphasizes obtaining informed consent as a primary responsibility of the researcher:

> "The voluntary consent of the human subject is essential. This means that the person involved should have legal capacity to give consent; should be so situated as to be able to exercise free power of choice, without the intervention of any element of force, fraud, deceit, duress, over-reaching, or other ulterior form of constraint or coercion; and should have sufficient knowledge and comprehension of the elements of the subject matter involved as to enable him to make an understanding and enlightened decision. This latter element requires that, before the acceptance of an affirmative decision by the experimental subject, there should be made known to him the nature, duration, and purpose of the experiment; the method and means by which it is to be conducted; all inconveniences and hazards reasonably to be expected; and the effects upon his health or person, which may possibly come from his participation in the experiment."

The duty and responsibility for ascertaining the quality of the consent rests upon everyone who initiates, directs, or engages in the experiment. It is a personal duty and responsibility, which may not be delegated to another with impunity.[44]

In 1964, the World Medical Association adopted the "Declaration of Helsinki"[45] to guide researchers in the ethical conduct of medical research. This document has been revised several times since originally adopted. These guidelines reinforced the importance of informed consent, although it added a provision to allow for that consent process to be performed with a legal guardian for people unable to provide consent for themselves. The Declaration of Helsinki also delineated the difference between clinical research, defined as "medical research in which the aim is essentially diagnostic or therapeutic for a patient" and non-clinical biomedical research, defined as "medical research, the essential object of which is purely scientific and without implying direct diagnostic or therapeutic value to the person subjected to the research."

At the time of unfolding this history of medical research ethics internationally, a deplorable medical experiment was being conducted in the United States in Tuskegee by the U.S. Public Health Service. The purpose of this research, which began in the 1930s, was to study the natural history of untreated syphilis. More than 400 African Americans with syphilis were recruited into the study without their permission. They were also deceived; they were told that some study tests were "special free treatment." During the course of this study, the researchers learned that the mortality rate was twice as high in subjects with syphilis when compared with controls without syphilis. In the 1940s, penicillin was proven an effective treatment for syphilis. Despite this finding, the research continued. The subjects were not told of the available treatment, and it was not given to them.

Reports of the Tuskegee study began appearing in the media in 1972. Overwhelming and justified public shock and anger resulted in federal action to compensate for the egregious ethical breaches and to prevent them from recurring. The National Commission for the Protection of Human Subjects of Biomedical and Behavioral Research was established in 1974 to identify the basic ethical principles to guide all research with humans. The Commission's work was documented in The Belmont Report—Ethical Principles and Guidelines for the Protection of Human Subjects.[46] That report contained the three ethical principles mentioned above that guide the work of modern researchers and that became the foundation for federal regulations governing research with humans: respect for persons, beneficence, and justice. The principles are described in greater detail below.

2.4.1 Respect for Persons

The first of the ethical principles reflects the emphasis in the Nuremberg Code on informed consent. That is, respect for research participants means treating them as autonomous agents. The Belmont Report defines "autonomous agent" as "an individual capable of deliberation about personal goals and of acting under such deliberation . . . ." This means that the informed consent process is needed so that the potential participants are given all the information they need to determine whether participating in the study is in their best interest. The principle of respect also means that researchers conducting trials with "vulnerable" populations (e.g., children or the cognitively impaired) should ensure that extra provisions are made to protect those participants who have diminished autonomy. Of course, the principle of respect includes the notion that the consent process must be completed with no coercion or pressure by the researchers to participate.

2.4.2 Beneficence

The Belmont Report's principle of beneficence refers to the need to ensure that all aspects of a study are designed to obtain the desired knowledge in a way that maximizes benefits and minimizes risks to the participants. The principle of beneficence also means that a risk–benefit analysis must be performed on every proposed study. In determining if this ratio is ethical, consideration must be given to the impact on both the participants and society.

2.4.3 Justice

The principle of justice refers to the fairness or equity involved in the selection of research participants. The point is to ensure that risks or benefits incurred by research participants are not unfairly concentrated in one segment of the population.

2.4.4 How the Investigator Applies Ethical Principles

An investigator applies these ethical principles daily by ensuring that the informed consent process is performed perfectly with every research participant. This means that all staff involved in the consent process must be well trained, not only in the research protocol in question, but also in the proper elements of informed consent. A good rule of thumb for the people conducting consent discussions is for them to think about what they would want their mother, father, spouse, or friend to know about the study to enable them to make an informed decision. The investigator should never allow this process to be rushed. In addition, to reduce the possibility that the potential participant feels pressured by the power differential that often characterizes the doctor–patient relationship, some ethicists argue that the physician should not be the primary person conducting the consent discussion. This means that, ideally, other individuals should be on the study staff, and they should be charged with carrying out the consent process with prospective subjects.

The researcher complies with the concept of beneficence in two ways. First, the investigator carefully reviews the study protocol to determine whether the design provides a generally favorable ratio between the potential risks to the subjects and the potential benefits to the subject and society. If the researcher decides to conduct the study, the second strategy is to carefully review each potential candidate to ensure that this ratio is favorable for each potential participant. Of course, the investigator also encourages the potential participant to weigh the risks and benefits for themselves through the consent process. Indeed, a central principle of the 1964 Declaration of Helsinki was that "Concern for the interests of the subject must always prevail over the interests of science and society." This means that societal benefits should always carry less weight than individual, subject-level benefits.

Finally, the investigator fulfills the principle of justice by ensuring that his or her subject-recruitment strategies do not systematically discriminate against any specific group. In the Tuskegee study, all the risks were concentrated among African American males. In other cases, the benefits might be concentrated in a particular group. One of the current ethical dilemmas facing research professionals is the conduct of research involving children. Because of the focus on protecting vulnerable populations, drug research in children has been very limited. Thus, the benefits of research were concentrated in adults. The result was that physicians had little scientific basis for prescribing medications in children. To improve the practice of pediatric medicine and to expand the benefits of research beyond adults, the federal government established incentives to pharmaceutical companies to sponsor research with children. This, in turn, led to additional regulations designed to protect the rights of minors who participate in research. This is just one example of the delicate balance of justice in selecting research populations.

2.5 REGULATIONS GOVERNING INSTITUTIONAL REVIEW BOARDS

Investigators embarking on research path might be tempted to focus their energies exclusively on those aspects of the study that involve direct patient care and medical decisions. They might be tempted to skip the remaining portions of this chapter that focus on the regulations governing IRBs. Why, after all, does an investigator need to know about IRBs?

The answer is that the FDA holds investigators responsible for ensuring that the studies they conduct are reviewed by an IRB that meets FDA regulations governing the function of IRBs. More specifically, when an investigator signs FDA Form 1572 the investigator is making the following commitment (among others): "I will ensure that an IRB that complies with the requirements of 21 CFR Part 56 will be responsible for the initial and continuing review and approval of the clinical investigation. I also agree to promptly report to the IRB all changes in the research activity and all unanticipated problems involving risks to human subjects or others. Additionally, I will not make any changes in the research without IRB approval, except where necessary to eliminate apparent immediate hazards to human subjects." Therefore, it is prudent that the investigator contacts their IRB to make sure it complies with all requirements under 21 CFR Part 56, and that the PI maintain contact with the IRB staff to ensure adequate reporting and his or her own compliance with regulations.

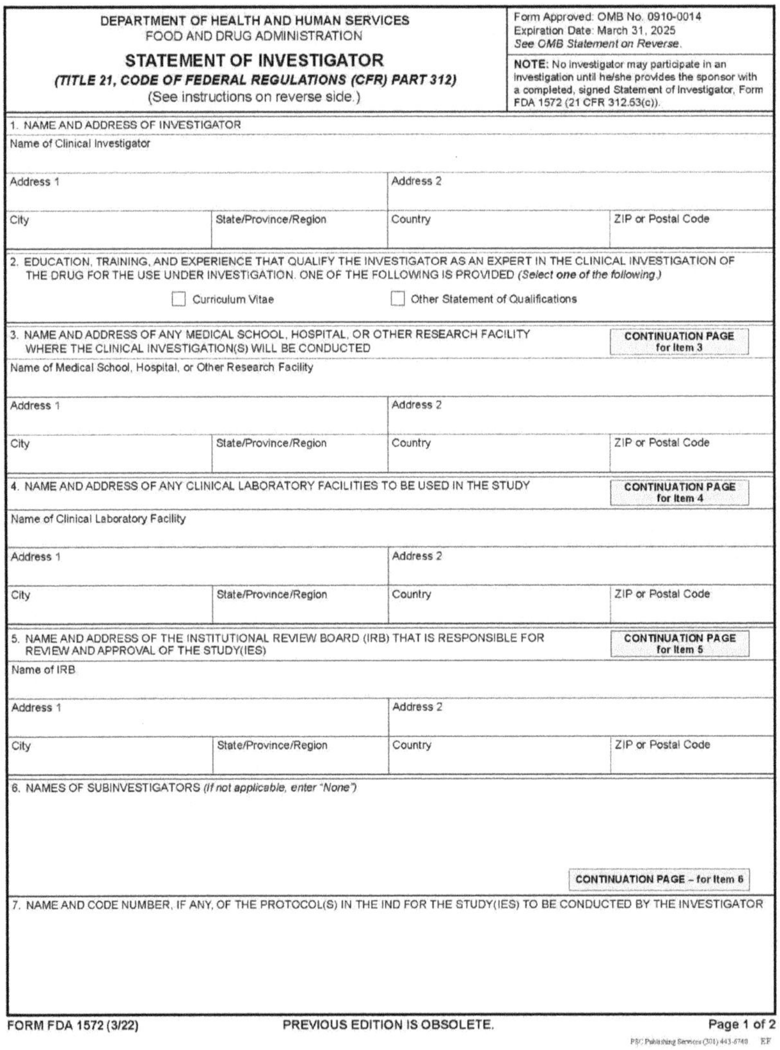

DEPARTMENT OF HEALTH AND HUMAN SERVICES
FOOD AND DRUG ADMINISTRATION

STATEMENT OF INVESTIGATOR
(TITLE 21, CODE OF FEDERAL REGULATIONS (CFR) PART 312)
(See instructions on reverse side.)

Form Approved: OMB No. 0910-0014
Expiration Date: March 31, 2025
See OMB Statement on Reverse.

NOTE: No investigator may participate in an investigation until he/she provides the sponsor with a completed, signed Statement of Investigator, Form FDA 1572 (21 CFR 312.53(c)).

1. NAME AND ADDRESS OF INVESTIGATOR
Name of Clinical Investigator
Address 1 | Address 2
City | State/Province/Region | Country | ZIP or Postal Code

2. EDUCATION, TRAINING, AND EXPERIENCE THAT QUALIFY THE INVESTIGATOR AS AN EXPERT IN THE CLINICAL INVESTIGATION OF THE DRUG FOR THE USE UNDER INVESTIGATION. ONE OF THE FOLLOWING IS PROVIDED *(Select one of the following.)*
☐ Curriculum Vitae ☐ Other Statement of Qualifications

3. NAME AND ADDRESS OF ANY MEDICAL SCHOOL, HOSPITAL, OR OTHER RESEARCH FACILITY WHERE THE CLINICAL INVESTIGATION(S) WILL BE CONDUCTED
CONTINUATION PAGE for Item 3
Name of Medical School, Hospital, or Other Research Facility
Address 1 | Address 2
City | State/Province/Region | Country | ZIP or Postal Code

4. NAME AND ADDRESS OF ANY CLINICAL LABORATORY FACILITIES TO BE USED IN THE STUDY
CONTINUATION PAGE for Item 4
Name of Clinical Laboratory Facility
Address 1 | Address 2
City | State/Province/Region | Country | ZIP or Postal Code

5. NAME AND ADDRESS OF THE INSTITUTIONAL REVIEW BOARD (IRB) THAT IS RESPONSIBLE FOR REVIEW AND APPROVAL OF THE STUDY(IES)
CONTINUATION PAGE for Item 5
Name of IRB
Address 1 | Address 2
City | State/Province/Region | Country | ZIP or Postal Code

6. NAMES OF SUBINVESTIGATORS *(If not applicable, enter "None")*
CONTINUATION PAGE – for Item 6

7. NAME AND CODE NUMBER, IF ANY, OF THE PROTOCOL(S) IN THE IND FOR THE STUDY(IES) TO BE CONDUCTED BY THE INVESTIGATOR

FORM FDA 1572 (3/22) PREVIOUS EDITION IS OBSOLETE. Page 1 of 2
PSC Publishing Services (301) 443-6740 EF

FIGURE 2.1 Statement of Investigator: Form FDA 1572.

2.5.1 What Institutional Review Board Members Should Know About Clinical Research

Although IRB members can and should come from a variety of backgrounds, all board members should know the basic elements of clinical research and should stay focused on their role in the ethical review process. Any board member who does not have a research background should take the time to learn the basics of the industry. Books, such as this one, can introduce the language, regulations, and ethical issues in the conduct of research with humans.

Board members should look carefully at an investigator's qualifications for conducting the research. If a protocol proposes to study the effects of a new treatment for hypertension, the investigator should not be a podiatrist. The investigator is responsible for overseeing the medical care and conduct of the trial and, therefore, must have the proper qualifications to accomplish that task.

Board members should understand the need to avoid conflicts of interest. Any board member with a conflicting interest in a study should not participate in the deliberations or voting on that study. The IRB may ask that member to leave the room during deliberations and voting to avoid a political environment that is not conducive to objective ethical review. The recusal and attendance requirements for IRB members with a conflict of interest mentioned above should be stated in the institution's IRB policies.

Finally, board members should understand that clinical research involves tremendous coordination of systems, staff, and supplies; however, it is not the responsibility of the IRB to plan, facilitate, or verify that the investigator has resolved the logistics of a given study. The logistics are something the investigator works out with the sponsor. The IRB members should stay focused on evaluating the risks and benefits of conducting the study, but sometimes IRB members may find that the study is planned so poorly that it may affect scientific validity. In the case where scientific validity is affected, IRB members can (and should) make the argument that subjecting research participants to the study may not provide any benefit at all and thus should not be conducted. A study in which the PI is subjecting participants to risks while no benefit may be provided is not approvable by the IRB.

2.5.2 What Institutional Review Board Members Should Know About Their Responsibilities

IRB members should be aware that their duties include (but are not limited to) evaluating proposed investigations and approving or disapproving the investigation after considering the medical soundness considering the rights and safety of the human participants involved; determining compliance with acceptable standards of professional conduct and practice; and assessing community, ethical, and moral values. The members also evaluate the qualifications of the PI with emphasis placed on that individual's professional development as it relates to the degree of protocol complexity and the risk to human research participants. Because the primary purpose of an IRB is to ensure—in advance and by periodic review—that appropriate measures are taken to safeguard the rights, safety, and wellbeing of human participants involved in a clinical trial, the board members must determine that the following requirements are satisfied:

- Human participants are protected from ill-advised research or research protocols in light of both ethical and scientific concerns.
- Risks to participants are minimized.
- Risks to participants are reasonable in relation to anticipated benefits and the importance of the knowledge that may be expected to result.
- Selection of participants is equitable.
- Informed consent will be obtained from each prospective participant or the participant's legally authorized representative and will be documented in accordance with IRB, FDA, and ICH informed consent regulations and guidelines.
- Adequate provisions are made for monitoring the data collected to ensure the safety of participants.
- Adequate provisions are made to protect the privacy of participants and maintain confidentiality of data.
- Appropriate additional safeguards have been included to protect the rights and welfare of participants who are members of a particularly vulnerable group,[14] such as persons with acute or severe physical or mental illness, persons with limited capacity to consent, or persons who are economically or educationally disadvantaged.
- Participant selection and exclusion criteria—including justification of the use of special participant populations, such as children, pregnant women, human fetuses, and neonates or the mentally handicapped—are appropriately established.
- The study design includes a discussion of the appropriateness of the research methods.

In addition to the above, the IRB has additional and special review requirements to protect the well-being of children when children are to be involved in the research (Subpart D, Sections 401–409).[47]

2.6 WHAT THE SITE SHOULD KNOW ABOUT INSTITUTIONAL REVIEW BOARDS

When choosing an IRB, the investigator may have the option of using a "local" IRB or a "central" IRB, depending upon the investigator's institutional policies. A local IRB is one that is housed within an institution and has been developed for overseeing research conducted within the institution or by the staff of the institution. For example, many community hospitals and academic medical centers have their own internal IRB, composed largely of clinicians who conduct research at that institution.

A central IRB is an "outside" or "independent" IRB. The central IRB serves to review research for non-IRB institutions, private practices, outpatient clinical trials, NIH studies where a central IRB is mandated, or institutions that allow the investigator to cede IRB review authority to the central IRB. Investigators conducting research in a non-institutional setting often choose to use an established central IRB rather than forming their own. In addition, some smaller hospitals and other institutions are choosing to eliminate their internal IRBs and outsource this function. The benefits of the decision to outsource include:

- Reduced likelihood of conflict of interest or the appearance of bias because the board members reviewing the proposed protocols are unlikely to be friends, colleagues, or acquaintances of the researchers whose work they are reviewing.
- Reduced liability by selecting to outsource to an organization whose sole focus and expertise is in ensuring compliance with the many regulations governing the work of IRBs.
- Potential cost savings by eliminating staff currently dedicated to performing IRB duties by outsourcing to an IRB that achieves economies of scale through higher volumes of reviews.

However, some potential hazards of relying upon a central IRB include:[48]

- The central IRB may be less able to provide a complete and thorough review of the documents included in the IRB submission since local IRBs tend to have a better understanding of local study population norms, values, cultural context, and economic factors. Thus, when local IRB review is used, the consent and recruitment process may be enhanced.
- A local IRB may be better able to promote the Belmont principle of justice in that they can more readily seek input from the local community so that risks and benefits are distributed appropriately. Local IRBs tend to be more accountable and accessible.
- Local IRBs are more willing and better able to communicate with investigators at the site-level, and better able to provide information and training that may be needed.

An investigator must be qualified by education, training, and experience to assume responsibility for the proper conduct of a clinical trial and should meet all qualifications specified by the applicable regulatory requirements. Investigators must agree to abide by the decisions of their selected IRB and should comply with all governing rules and regulations.

2.6.1 What Research Requires Institutional Review Board Approval and Oversight

According to the Belmont Report,[49] items that must go before an IRB for review, for the protection of human participants, include any projects that include any element of research in an activity. The definition of research is described as "a systemic investigation, including research development, testing, and evaluation, designed to develop or contribute to generalizable knowledge."[50] Medical research involving human participants also includes research on identifiable human material and identifiable data.[18] The obvious material requiring submission to, and review by, an IRB would be industry-funded research, which would include biomedical, behavioral, medical devices, and humanitarian-use devices. If there is confusion about whether a project is research, several questions can be asked to help make this determination:

- Is there a hypothesis?
- Does it include research development?
- Will the knowledge be used outside the institution?
- Is there a question to be answered for reasons other than clinical care or routine evaluation?
- Is there an intent to generalize the information?
- Is there a specific intent?
- Is the purpose for the scientific community?
- If it were not going to be published, would you do it anyway?

Investigators should be aware that some research projects may qualify for expedited review. Research that would qualify for this type of review includes certain categories of research that involve no more-than-minimal risk. A list of research categories that qualify was published in the Federal Register in 1998.

2.6.1.1 Categories of Clinical Investigations That Can Go Through an Expedited Review

1. Clinical studies of drugs and medical devices only when condition (a) or (b) is met.
   a. Research on drugs for which an investigational new drug application (21 CFR Part 312) is not required. (Note: Research on marketed drugs that significantly increases the risks or decreases the acceptability of the risks associated with the use of the product is not eligible for expedited review.)
   b. Research on medical devices for which (i) an investigational device exemption application (21 CFR Part 812) is not required; or (ii) the medical device is cleared/approved for marketing and the medical device is being used in accordance with its cleared/approved labeling.

2. Collection of blood samples by finger stick, heel stick, ear stick, or venipuncture as follows:
   a. from healthy, nonpregnant adults who weigh at least 110 pounds. For these subjects, the amounts drawn may not exceed 550 ml in an 8 week period and collection may not occur more frequently than 2 times per week; or
   b. from other adults and children [2], considering the age, weight, and health of the subjects, the collection procedure, the amount of blood to be collected, and the frequency with which it will be collected. For these subjects, the amount drawn may not exceed the lesser of 50 ml or 3 ml per kg in an 8 week period and collection may not occur more frequently than 2 times per week.
3. Prospective collection of biological specimens for research purposes by noninvasive means.
   Examples:
   a. hair and nail clippings in a non-disfiguring manner
   b. deciduous teeth at time of exfoliation or if routine patient care indicates a need for extraction
   c. permanent teeth if routine patient care indicates a need for extraction
   d. excreta and external secretions (including sweat);
   e. un-cannulated saliva collected either in an unstimulated fashion or stimulated by chewing gumbase or wax or by applying a dilute citric solution to the tongue
   f. placenta removed at delivery
   g. amniotic fluid obtained at the time of rupture of the membrane prior to or during labor
   h. supra- and subgingival dental plaque and calculus, provided the collection procedure is not more invasive than routine prophylactic scaling of the teeth and the process is accomplished in accordance with accepted prophylactic techniques
   i. mucosal and skin cells collected by buccal scraping or swab, skin swab, or mouth washings
   j. sputum collected after saline mist nebulization.
4. Collection of data through non-invasive procedures (not involving general anesthesia or sedation) routinely employed in clinical practice, excluding procedures involving x-rays or microwaves. Where medical devices are employed, they must be cleared/approved for marketing. (Studies intended to evaluate the safety and effectiveness of the medical device are not generally eligible for expedited review, including studies of cleared medical devices for new indications).
   Examples:
   a. physical sensors that are applied either to the surface of the body or at a distance and do not involve input of significant amounts of energy into the subject or an invasion of the subjects' privacy
   b. weighing or testing sensory acuity
   c. magnetic resonance imaging
   d. electrocardiography, electroencephalography, thermography, detection of naturally occurring radioactivity, electroretinography, ultrasound, diagnostic infrared imaging, doppler blood flow, and echocardiography
   e. moderate exercise, muscular strength testing, body composition assessment, and flexibility testing where appropriate given the age, weight, and health of the individual.
5. Research involving materials (data, documents, records, or specimens) that have been collected, or will be collected solely for nonresearch purposes (such as medical treatment or diagnosis).
   a. (NOTE: Some research in this category may be exempt from the HHS regulations for the protection of human subjects. 45 CFR 46.101(b)(4). This listing refers only to research that is not exempt.)
6. Collection of data from voice, video, digital, or image recordings made for research purposes.
7. Research on individual or group characteristics or behavior (including, but not limited to, research on perception, cognition, motivation, identity, language, communication, cultural beliefs or practices, and social behavior) or research employing survey, interview, oral history, focus group, program evaluation, human factors evaluation, or quality assurance methodologies.
   a. NOTE: Some research in this category may be exempt from the HHS regulations for the protection of human subjects. 45 CFR 46.101(b)(2) and (b)(3). This listing refers only to research that is not exempt).
8. Continuing review of research previously approved by the convened IRB as follows
   a. where (i) the research is permanently closed to the enrollment of new subjects; (ii) all subjects have completed all research-related interventions; and (iii) the research remains active only for long-term follow-up of subjects; or
   b. where no subjects have been enrolled and no additional risks have been identified; or
   c. where the remaining research activities are limited to data analysis.
9. Continuing review of research, not conducted under an investigational new drug application or investigational device exemption where categories two (2) through eight (8) do not apply but the IRB has determined and documented at a convened meeting that the research involves no greater than minimal risk and no additional risks have been identified.[51]

2.6.2 Requirements of an Investigator for Institutional Review Board Research Approval

For an investigator to obtain IRB approval for a research proposal, required information should be provided to the prospective IRB for review and consideration in a timely manner. PIs should know what their IRBs expect and should ask questions early in the process to avoid any delays. Investigators should remember that an IRB review is based on human-participant concerns and should expect questions. It is very helpful for the investigator to contact the IRB before making a submission to inquire about its document-submission requirements. Incomplete submissions to the IRB will cause the review of the research project to be delayed. When IRBs must request a number of modifications or seek additional information, IRB approval must be deferred, pending subsequent review by the full board upon receipt of the requested information. Providing the IRB with all required documents with the initial submission, however, will help eliminate undue delays and make the IRB review process more expedient. The pertinent information that the investigator will need to provide may vary from IRB to IRB; however, in general, the standard, required information would include the material listed in Table 2.2.

Additional requirements of a PI include the following:

- The investigator should be committed to a trial before the IRB issues its written approval.
- The investigator should not deviate from, or initiate, any changes to the protocol, without prior written approval from the IRB for an appropriate amendment, except when necessary to eliminate immediate hazards to the participants or when changes involve only logistical or administrative aspects of the trial (e.g., a change of the monitor telephone number).

TABLE 2.2
Information that IRBs May Be Required from a Principal Investigator (PI).

- Brief letter, memorandum, or note requesting approval of the research
- Completed, signed original of the IRB application or Information and Site Survey (if required by the IRB)
- Investigational Device Exemption (IDE), Humanitarian Device Exemption (HDE), or Premarket Approval (PMA) numbers for device trials
- Copy of the protocol/amendments; (title of study; purpose, including expected benefits obtained by doing the study; participant selection criteria; participant exclusion criteria; study design, including as needed, a discussion of the appropriateness of research methods; description of methods performed)
- Written informed consent document and consent form updates (which include all of the required elements of an informed consent)
- Completed FDA 1572 form, if applicable (not required for device trials)
- Investigator's brochure (if applicable)
- Curriculum vitae and licensure for the principal investigator and each subinvestigator
- Disclosure of any payments or compensation to a participant for participating in the study
- Participant recruitment procedures, materials, or advertisements
- Provisions for managing adverse reactions
- Written information that will be provided to the participant
- Justification for use of special/vulnerable participant populations; as well as additional safeguards that will be used to protect these participants (i.e., the mentally retarded, children, prisoners, pregnant women, etc.)
- A disclosure of any compensation provided to the participant for participating in the study
- A disclosure of extra costs to the participant because of participation in the study
- Protection of the participant's privacy
- Name of the sponsor
- Results of previous related research (i.e., investigator's brochure)

Additional Items the PI Should Provide:

- Any changes in the study after initiation
- A report of any unexpected serious adverse reactions or information regarding similar reports received from the sponsor as soon as possible and, in no event later than 15 calendar days after the investigator discovers the information
- Progress reports as requested by the IRB, but in any event, no less than on an annual basis, including the number of participants withdrawing from the study and the reasons for each withdrawal
- Any significant protocol deviation that considerably affects the safety of the participant, or the scientific quality of the study
- A final report

- The investigator should promptly report the following to the IRB:
  1. Deviations from, or changes in, the protocol to eliminate immediate hazards to the trial participants.
  2. Changes that increase the risk to participants or significantly affect the conduct of the trial.
  3. All adverse drug reactions that are both serious and unexpected.
  4. New information that may adversely affect the safety of the participants or the conduct of the trial.

The investigator should be aware that the IRB has the authority to suspend or terminate approval of research that is not being conducted in accordance with IRB requirements or FDA regulations or that has been associated with unexpected serious harm to participants.

In cases in which an investigator engages in serious or continuing noncompliance, it is the responsibility of the IRB to report that activity to the sponsor, to the federal Office of Human Research Protections (OHRP), and to the FDA. Noncompliance issues may include, but are not limited to, unreported changes in the protocol, misuse or nonuse of the informed consent document, failure to submit protocols to the IRB in a timely manner and avoiding or ignoring the IRB.

2.7 RISK-BENEFIT ANALYSIS: THE HUMAN ADVOCATE

To ensure that the rights and welfare of human research participants are protected, the IRB takes on the task of performing a risk-benefit analysis. Before a clinical trial can be initiated, foreseeable risks and inconveniences should be weighed against the anticipated benefit for the trial participant and for society.[52] Risks associated with participation in research should be justified by the anticipated benefits; only then, can the trial be initiated. Because this requirement is clearly stated in the federal regulations, it is, therefore, one of the major responsibilities of the IRB to assess the risks and benefits associated with proposed research. Definitions of the terms that the IRB uses to assess risk include the following:

- Benefit—a valued or desired outcome, an advantage.
- Minimal risk—the probability and magnitude of harm or discomfort anticipated in the proposed research are not greater, in and of themselves, than those ordinarily encountered in daily life or during the performance of routine physical or psychological examinations or tests (45 CFR 46.102(j)).[53]
- Risk—the probability of harm or injury (physical, psychological, social, or economic) occurring because of participation in a research study. Both the probability and magnitude of possible harm can vary from minimal to significant.

The IRB must determine whether the anticipated benefit—either of new knowledge or of improved health for a research participant—justifies asking individuals to expose themselves to the potential risks. The IRB's assessment of risks and anticipated benefits involves the following steps:

- Identifying the risks associated with the research in comparison to the risks of treatments the participants would receive if not participating in research.
- Determining that the risks will be minimized to the extent possible.
- Identifying the probable benefits to be derived from the research.
- Determining that the risks are reasonable in relation to the benefits to the participants, if any, and the importance of the knowledge to be gained.
- Assuring those potential participants will be provided with an accurate and fair description of the risks or discomforts and the anticipated benefits.
- Determining intervals of periodic review and, where appropriate, determining that adequate provisions are in place for monitoring the data collected.

In addition, the IRB should determine that the provisions to protect the privacy of participants and to maintain the confidentiality of the data are adequate. When participants are members of a vulnerable population, the IRB should ensure that appropriate additional safeguards are being used to protect the rights and welfare of these participants.[54]

2.7.1 Identifying and Assessing the Risks

In the process of identifying what constitutes a risk, only risks that can result directly from the research should be considered, but before an activity involving participants is eliminated from the risk–benefit analysis as therapy, the IRB should be very sure that the activity is not actually research. IRB member should be aware that the potential risks faced by research participants could be associated with the design mechanisms used to ensure valid results and by the interventions that may be performed during the research. Designs involving randomization to treatment groups have the risk that the participant may not receive a treatment that could be effective. Participants involved in a double-blinded study are at risk of the necessary information for individual treatment not being available to the proper individuals when needed. The added risk of invasion of privacy and violations of confidentiality are also possible within the methods used for gathering information in behavioral, social, and biomedical research.

Risks to which research participants may be exposed have been grouped as physical, psychological, legal, social, and economic harms.[55] The description of each classification is as follows:

- Physical harms: Medical research often involves exposure to minor pain, discomfort, injury from invasive medical procedures, or harm from possible side effects of drugs. All of these should be considered "risks" for purposes of the IRB review.
- Psychological harms: Participation in research may result in undesired changes in the thought processes and emotions. These changes may be temporary, recurrent, or permanent. IRB members should be aware that some research has the potential to cause serious psychological harm. Stress and feelings of guilt or embarrassment may arise from thinking or talking about one's own behavior or attitudes on sensitive topics. These feelings may occur when a participant is being interviewed or filling out a questionnaire. IRBs will confront the possibility of psychological harm when reviewing behavioral research that involves a component of deception, particularly if the deception includes false feedback to the participants about their own performance.
- Legal: Invasion of privacy: Access to a person's body or behavior without consent constitutes an invasion of privacy. The IRB must determine if the invasion of privacy is acceptable considering the participant's reasonable expectations of privacy in the situation under which the study is being performed and if the research questions are of sufficient importance to justify this intrusion. The IRB should determine if the research could be modified so that the study could be conducted without the invasion of the participants' privacy.
- Legal: Breach of confidentiality: Confidentiality of data requires safeguarding information that has been given voluntarily by one person to another. Some research requires access to the participants' hospital, school, or employment records. Such access is generally acceptable if the researcher protects the confidentiality of that information. The IRB should be aware that a breach of confidentiality could result in psychological or social harm.
- Social and economic harms: Some invasions of privacy or breaches of confidentiality could result in embarrassment with one's business or social group, loss of employment, or criminal prosecution. Confidential safeguards must be strong in these instances. Examples of these sensitivities include information about alcohol or drug abuse, mental illness, illegal activities, and sexual behavior. Participation in research may also result in additional costs to the participant.

2.7.2 Minimal Risk versus Greater-than-Minimal Risk

Once the risks have been determined, the IRB must then assess whether the research involves greater-than-minimal risk. Regulations governing the functions of an IRB allow approval through the expedited review process for research projects that contain no more-than-minimal risk and that involve participants only in one or more approved categories.

In research involving more-than-minimal risk, potential participants must be informed of the availability of medical treatment and compensation for a research-related injury, including who will pay for the treatment and the availability of other financial compensation.[56] Institutions are not required to provide care or payment for research injuries; however, some institutions provide hospitalization and necessary medical treatment in an emergency.

2.7.3 Vulnerable Populations and Minimal Risk

When research involves especially vulnerable populations (e.g., fetuses and pregnant women, prisoners, and children) regulations strictly limit research involving more-than-minimal risk. Special limitations are recommended when the research involves individuals who are institutionalized or mentally disabled. For these situations, it is recommended that minimal risk be defined in terms of the risks normally encountered in the daily lives or the routine medical and psychological examination of healthy participants. In these cases, the IRB should determine whether the proposed participant populations would be more sensitive or vulnerable to the risks involved by the research because of their general condition or disabilities. These concerns are also equally applicable to other participants (e.g., taking blood samples from a person with hemophilia, outdoor exercises with asthma patients if the air is polluted, changes in diet for a diabetic, and giving over-the-counter drugs for minor ailments to pregnant women).

2.7.4 Determining Whether Risks Are Minimized

The IRB is responsible for assuring that risks to participants are minimized. In assuring that the risks are minimized, the IRB should obtain and review the protocol, including the investigational design, scientific rationale, and the statistical reason for the structure of the proposed research. Results from previous studies (e.g., the investigator's brochure) should also be reviewed during this process. The expected beneficial and harmful effects within the research, as well as the effects of any treatments that may be ordinarily administered, and those associated with receiving no treatment should also be analyzed. Whether potential harmful effects can be detected, prevented, or treated should be considered. Risks and complications of any underlying disease that may be present should be assessed as well.

The IRB should determine whether the investigators are competent in the area of the proposed research and whether they are serving in more than one role, which may complicate their interactions with participants. Potential investigator conflict-of-interest issues should be identified and resolved before IRB approval.

Deciding whether the research design will produce useful data will assist the IRB in determining whether risks are minimized. Participants may be exposed to risk without sufficient justification when the research design does not contain a sample size large enough to produce valid data or conclusions. Faulty or poor research design means that the risks are not likely to be reasonable in relation to the benefits. Sometimes, procedures that are included for purposes of good research design, but which add disproportionate risks to participants, may be unacceptable. Assuring that adequate safeguards such as data and safety monitoring are incorporated into the research design is a useful method of minimizing the risks.

2.7.5 Assessing Anticipated Benefits

Benefits to participants and to society are considered benefits of research. Research often involves the evaluation of procedures that may benefit the participants by improving their conditions or providing a better understanding of their diseases or disorders. In this type of research, participants undergo treatment for a particular illness or abnormal condition. Patients and healthy volunteers may choose to take part in research that is neither related to any illness or condition they might have nor structured to provide any diagnostic or therapeutic benefit. This type of research is designed to gain knowledge about human behavior and physiology. Research that contains no immediate therapeutic intent may benefit society overall by providing increased knowledge, improved safety, advances in technology, and overall better health. Anticipated benefits to the participant and the expected knowledge to be gained should be clearly stated within the protocol.

2.7.6 Determining Whether Risks Are Reasonable

The IRB must consider many factors when determining of whether the risks are reasonable in relation to the anticipated benefits. The evaluation of the risk–benefit ratio is an ethical judgment that an IRB must make, and each case must be reviewed separately. This judgment often depends on subjective determinations and community standards. When making its decision, the IRB relies on currently available information regarding the risks and benefits of the interventions from previous bench, animal, and human studies (e.g., from the investigator's brochure), and the extent of confidence in the knowledge. However, human responses may differ from those of animals; therefore, although that information may suggest possible risks and benefits to humans, it is not conclusive. Hence, first in human research is often considered riskier and the IRB should more carefully weigh the risks and benefits of such a study. Within its assessment, the IRB should also consider the proposed participants and be sensitive to the different feelings and views individuals may have about risks and benefits.

The risk–benefit assessments depend on whether the research involves the use of interventions that have the intent and reasonable possibility of providing a benefit to the participant, or whether it only involves procedures for research purposes. In research containing interventions expected to provide direct benefit to the participants, a certain amount of risk is justifiable. In research where no direct benefits are anticipated, the IRB should evaluate whether the risks presented by procedures only to obtain generalized knowledge are ethically acceptable.[57]

2.7.7 Continuing Review and Monitoring of Data

Regulations governing the functions of an IRB require that an IRB reevaluate research projects at intervals appropriate to the degree of risk but not less than annually. Note that, under the revised Common Rule effective January 21, 2019, only full board studies require renewal. However, the IRB may determine upon review that expedited studies require renewal if there is an adequate and well-documented reason.[58] The reevaluation is performed to review the entire research project again and to reassess the risk–benefit ratio, which may have changed since the last review. During a study, new information regarding the risks and benefits, unexpected side effects, unanticipated findings involving risks to participants, or knowledge resulting from another research project may become apparent. The IRB should determine whether these situations have occurred and whether there is any additional information regarding risks or benefits that should be revealed to the participants.

The investigator should be aware that the interval for IRB review can be more frequent than once per year. The approval period for a study can be shorter (i.e., less than a year) if the IRB feels that the study is of considerable risk and should be monitored by the IRB more frequently. If an investigator allows an IRB approval date to lapse, the research no longer has IRB approval. No approval means that all aspects of the research must stop. Extensions of approvals do not exist. Investigators should provide the IRB with an adequate detailed report in a timely manner to avoid expiration (and thus stoppage) of their study. Any monitoring reports (e.g., from a formally constituted data safety monitoring board) should be submitted with or before the annual renewal.

2.8 INFORMED CONSENT: NOT JUST A DOCUMENT

One of the most important pieces of a research trial is the informed consent of the research participant. However, a signature on an informed consent document does not constitute the end of the informed consent. It is very important for the research community (the sponsor, the investigator, and the IRB) to remember that informed consent is not just a document, but is, instead, a continuing process that carries through to the end of the individual's participation in the trial.

Informed consent involves the information presented to the participant, comprehension of that information by the participant, and the participant's voluntary and fully, continuously informed agreement to participate in the study. The informed consent process begins with the recruitment of potential participants, whether by radio advertisement, flyer, or initial contact with the PI or the research staff. The initial consent involves explaining to a potential participant the risks, benefits, alternatives, procedures, and purpose of the study; allowing that individual to ask questions and providing satisfactory answers to those questions; sharing new information with the participants as it becomes available during the study because it may change their willingness to continue participation; and for long-term studies, revisiting the consent because of possible capacity changes.

The written informed consent form should be presented to potential participants in a language that they understand and written in terms that they can comprehend. This is one of the important functions of an IRB. The IRB members review every informed consent form to determine if it contains all the required elements and any additional required elements of an informed consent form as set forth in the governing regulations. The informed consent form is also reviewed to determine that complete, accurate, and pertinent study-related information is being provided to the potential participants and that medical terms are clearly defined, in simple language that the study population can understand. A recommended approach is to—after presenting the consent form and study information—ask the participant to recall key facets of the study to assess study procedure comprehension.

The consent process is not simply completed at the initial recruitment visit. The consent process continues throughout the participant's study enrollment. Thus, for example, if during the study there is a newly discovered risk associated with the study drug, all participants who may have received the study drug should be notified of the risk in an appropriate manner. The consent process requires continuous and fully informed consent throughout the study.

Human participant protection is a shared responsibility between the sponsor, the investigator, and the IRB. It is their responsibility as a team to ensure that the participants remain well informed and that their rights and welfare are protected. It is important that all members of the research team understand the informed consent form regulations,[59] their part of the informed consent process, and apply this knowledge to each informed consent form that is reviewed, presented, and distributed to a potential participant.

2.8.1 Elements of an Informed Consent

The investigator is responsible for providing every potential research participant with complete, accurate, and pertinent study-related information while adhering to the applicable governing rules and regulations. The process of providing this information to potential participants is informed consent. Except as provided in the regulations,[60] no investigator may involve a human being as subject in research unless the investigator has obtained the legally effective informed consent for the participant or the participant's legally authorized representative.[61] The exceptions include the participant being in a life-threatening situation that makes it necessary to use the test article; being unable to communicate with the participant to obtain a legally effective consent; insufficient time to obtain the consent from the participant's legally authorized representative; and no available alternative method of approved or generally recognized therapy that provides an equal or greater chance of saving the participants life.[62]

The governing rules and regulations require certain elements (information) be included within every informed consent form that is provided to a potential research participant. These required elements are outlined in Table 2.3.

2.8.2 Additional Required Elements

When appropriate, one or more of the following elements of information should also be provided to each participant. Note that additional required elements are not optional but are required when applicable:

- A statement that the particular treatment or procedure may involve risk to the participant (or to the embryo or fetus if the participant is, or may become, pregnant and to nursing infants) that are currently unforeseeable.
- Anticipated circumstances under which the participant's participation may be terminated by the investigator without regard to the participant's or the legally authorized representative's consent.
- Any additional costs to the participant that may result from participation in the research.
- The consequences of a participant's decision to withdraw from the research and procedures for orderly termination of participation by the participant.
- A statement that significant new findings developed during the course of the research, that may relate to the participant's willingness to continue participation, will be provided to the participant.
- The approximate number of subjects involved in the study.
- A statement that the subject's biospecimens (even if identifiers are removed) may be used for commercial profit and whether the subject will or will not share in this commercial profit.
- A statement regarding whether clinically relevant research results, including individual research results, will be disclosed to subjects, and if so, under what conditions; and
- For research involving biospecimens, whether the research will (if known) or might include whole genome sequencing (i.e., sequencing of a human

TABLE 2.3
Elements Required in an Informed Consent.

- A statement that the study involves research, an explanation of the purposes of the research and the expected duration of the subject's participation, a description of the procedures to be followed, and identification of any procedures that are experimental
- The approximate number of participants involved in the trial and the participant's responsibilities
- A description of any reasonably foreseeable risks or discomforts to the participant
- A description of any benefits to the participant or to others that may reasonably be expected from the research; when there is no intended clinical benefit to the participant, the participant should be made aware of this fact
- A disclosure of appropriate alternative procedures or courses of treatment that might be advantageous to the participant and the alternative procedure's important potential benefits and risks
- A statement describing the extent of confidentiality of records, which notes the possibility that the monitors, auditors, IRB, and the regulatory authorities may inspect the records for verification of clinical trial procedures and data without violating the confidentiality of the participant to the extent permitted by the applicable laws and regulations and that, by signing a written informed consent form, the participant or the participant's legally acceptable representative is authorizing such access; that records identifying the participant will be kept confidential and, to the extent permitted by the applicable laws or regulations, will be made publicly available; and that if the results of the trial are published, the participant's identity will remain confidential
- An explanation of whether compensation or medical treatment is available if injury occurs and, if so, what they consist of, or where further information may be obtained
- The anticipated prorated payment, if any, to the participant for participating in the trial (see 2018 FDA Payment and Reimbursement to Research Subjects Guidance)[64]
- A statement of dosage/frequency and the probability for random assignment to each treatment
- An explanation of whom to contact for answers to pertinent questions about the research and research participants' rights and whom to contact in the event of a research-related injury to the participant
- A statement that participation is voluntary, that refusal to participate will involve no penalty or loss of benefits to which the participant is otherwise entitled, and that the participant may discontinue participation at any time without penalty or loss of benefits to which the participant is otherwise entitled
- One of the following statements about any research that involves the collection of identifiable private information or identifiable biospecimens:
- A statement that identifiers might be removed from the identifiable private information or identifiable biospecimens and that, after such removal, the information or biospecimens could be used for future research studies or distributed to another investigator for future research studies without additional informed consent from the subject or the legally authorized representative, if this might be a possibility
- A statement that the subject's information or biospecimens collected as part of the research, even if identifiers are removed, will not be used or distributed for future research studies.
- A place for signatures by the participant, physician, person obtaining consent, and witness (less signatures may be required); it depends on the policies and procedures of the IRB

germline or somatic specimen with the intent to generate the genome or exome sequence of that specimen).[63]

In addition to the required elements of an informed consent form, an IRB can and may require other standard information or signatures be added to all informed consent forms being reviewed by the board.

2.9 RESEARCH PARTICIPANTS

Research participants are what drive the entire clinical trial process. Without enough volunteers, statistically significant conclusions about new drugs and devices would not be possible. Given that research volunteers have a wide variety of medical knowledge, there are mechanisms in place to ensure subjects can make educated decisions regarding study participation. The informed consent form alleviates the need for specialized knowledge on the part of the volunteer. In lay terms, the informed consent form describes, in detail, potential risks and benefits.

Regulations also exist to protect the confidentiality of the research participant. All information collected throughout the clinical trial remains with the study staff. For the purposes of data capture, each subject is identified by initials or study number only. In addition, the informed consent discusses who will have access to the trial documents.

Research participants are the true pioneers of medicine. Through their participation, novel therapeutic cures and treatments have been made possible. Furthermore, their participation also protects the public from approval of drugs that have a poor benefit-to-risk relationship. Thus, data obtained via research volunteers may be used to provide medical advances or to protect against insidious drugs entering the marketplace.

2.10 INDUSTRY TRADE ORGANIZATIONS AND SUPPORT SERVICES

The pharmaceutical industry must concede to a high failure rate. To minimize failures owing to poor performance on the part of any niche service providers, the need for structured education, training, and communication is clear. The largest trade organizations devoted to the clinical trial industry include the Associates of Clinical Research Professionals (ACRP, www.arcpnet.org), the Drug Information Associates (DIA, www.diahome.org), and the Pharmaceutical Research and Manufacturers Association (PhRMA, www.phrma.org). In addition, the FDA offers many training sessions and hosts a web site for consumers as well as researchers. CenterWatch is the leading publication (and a leading web site, www.centerwatch.com) for clinical trial information and industry news. Publications, such as the Good Clinical Practice Handbook, the Code of Federal Regulations, and the ICH Guidelines outline industry-specific standards and regulations. These publications are also available at no cost online.

2.11 SUMMARY: ETHICAL DILEMMAS IN CLINICAL RESEARCH

The rapid growth in the clinical research industry is met by a similar increase in knowledge, medical innovations, new technologies, and scientific breakthroughs. Yet despite these goods, many ethical dilemmas have also been raised. Such dilemmas as ethical violations, conflicts of interest, coercion, and misrepresentation date back to the 1930s. Ethical breaches include the study of untreated syphilis (commonly referred to as the Tuskegee Syphilis Study) conducted by the United States Public Health Services from 1932 to 1972, in which patients were not told they had syphilis, were not offered effective treatment, and were not allowed to be drafted because then they would receive treatment in the military. Clearly, these human subjects were deceived, coerced, and treated unjustly. In Nuremburg, Germany, 23 doctors were charged with crimes against humanity for performing incredibly egregious medical experiments on concentration camp inmates and others without their consent. In the 1950s' Willowbrook incident, intellectually disabled children were deliberately infected with the hepatitis virus. The parents were coerced when they were told that if their child enrolled into the study, the child could occupy one of the very few beds in the hospital. In 1951, a physician obtained a sample of Henrietta Lacks' cervical cancer without her knowledge or consent and developed the HeLa cell line, creating decades of controversy. In the 1960s, live cancer cells were injected into 22 senile patients at the Jewish Chronic Disease Hospital. These patients were not told and were incapable of understanding the experiment. Between 1986 and 1990, there were as many as 3000 women with high-risk pregnancies were involved in experiments by the University of South Florida and Tampa General Hospital without their consent, a case that was settled for $3.8 million.[29] Other cases in which ethical or regulatory lapses have been sited include the 1999 death of an 18-year-old man participating in a gene therapy trial at the University of Pennsylvania and the death of a healthy 24-year-old woman participating in a clinical trial at Johns Hopkins using hexamethonium, a drug not approved by the FDA, to induce asthma like symptoms in healthy volunteers.

Within these examples are unethical acts, coercion, conflicts of interest, and misrepresentation. Conflicts of interest are not limited to the rewards and stock options of investigators; they involve the entire research endeavor. Recently, financial conflicts of interest in medical research along with widely publicized episodes of scientific misconduct have been brought to the public's attention. In some episodes, researchers have been accused of falsifying or fabricating research data on therapeutic products in which they had substantial financial interests. There have now been many steps taken to keep such actions from occurring.

In April 2000, the American Society of Gene Therapy issued new guidelines controlling conflicts of interest in research. Among the reasons for the guidelines was the discovery that a researcher of a gene therapy trial, which involved the death of an 18-year-old subject, was heavily invested in the company that was funding the research. The American Society of Gene Therapy issued a statement making it clear that financial conflicts are unacceptable. It stated, "All investigators and team members directly involved with patient selection, the informed consent process, or clinical management in a trial must not have equity, stock options, or comparable arrangements in the companies sponsoring the trials."[65]

Because of several highly publicized deaths of patients involved in experimental studies at universities, the impetus for Congress and the federal bureaucracy to proceed with human research rules has become overwhelming. In 2011, HHS issued an advanced notice of proposed rulemaking (ANPRM) affecting subpart A of 45 CFR 46, known as the Common Rule. Commentary on the ANPRM was completed in 2015, and a noted of proposed rulemaking (NPRM) was issued on September 8, 2015. The NPRM to the Common Rule was revised and went into effect on January 21st, 2019. The driving purpose of the Common Rule revisions is to enhance protection of human subjects while also decreasing the administrative burden on investigators and IRB staff. The major burden-reducing provisions included:[66]

- The revised definition of "research," which explicitly deems particular activities not to be research
- The allowance for no annual continuing review for certain categories of research
- The elimination of the requirement that IRBs review grant applications or other funding proposals related to the research

CROs are increasingly conducting drug company research privately. The number of private practice-based investigators has grown almost fourfold within a 5-year span. This change is a response to the pressures of being the first to get a new drug to market. So, managing conflicts of interest outside of academic settings increasingly take place on a national level, as opposed to following guidelines set by an academic center. On the national level, efforts are being made to control this issue. Sponsors now have their investigators as well as any other individuals involved in their trial's complete financial disclosures. They are also requiring statements about which IRB members abstained from voting (for a conflicting interest) on the approval letter from the IRB.

Publicity surrounding these activities is often inflamed rather than informative, showing clinical research in a poor light instead of offering the public the big picture of clinical research, the realities of the present, and the possibilities of the future. Thousands of investigators and their staffs who participate in clinical trials are dedicated to advancing science and developing new therapeutic treatments, and they use the highest professional standards. Reporting the positive side of clinical research along with the negative publicity about events such as those described, the health care consumer would have more complete information to make an educated choice about participating in clinical trials. The clinical research community and federal government have worked hard to create and enforce guidelines and standards of practice for the protection of human subjects. ACRP offers training programs and certifications for CRCs and CRAs and is initiating certification programs for investigators.

The research community is charged with effectively protecting human subjects and ensuring that research is conducted ethically. Ethical violations in research are often caused by lack of awareness rather than malice. However, without clinical research, medical innovations and scientific breakthroughs would not be possible. So, practicing ethical conduct, seeking continued training, and complying with the governing regulations will promote good, sound, ethical research, which will, in turn, benefit society.

We have the many years of research and the hard work of the researchers to thank for providing the treatments that we now have available for the many diseases that plague our society. Keeping the trust, interest, and confidence of the public will allow for continued, successful clinical research with new scientific developments and breakthroughs.

NOTES

1 Orzechowski W and Walker R. Dose of Reality: How Drug Price Controls Would Hurt Americans, Policy Paper No. 25, February 7, 2000.

2 DiMasi JA. *Cost of Developing a New Drug*. Boston, MA: Briefing: Tufts Center for the Study of Drug Development, November 18, 2014. Available at: http://csdd.tufts.edu/news/complete_story/cost_study_press_event_webcast. Accessed October 17, 2018.

3 Pammoli F, Magazzini L and Riccaboni M. The Productivity Crisis in Pharmaceutical R&D. Nature Reviews Drug Discovery, 2011; 10(6) 429–438.

4 DiMasi JA, Grabowski HG and Hansen RW. Innovation in the Pharmaceutical Industry: New Estimates of R&D Costs. Journal of Health Economics, 2016; 47. Available at: https://dukespace.lib.duke.edu/dspace/bitstream/handle/10161/12742/DiMasi-Grabowski-Hansen-RnD-JHE-2016.pdf;jsessionid=5D6800B7C44E6303EFEE76FB7DD9807A?sequence=1.

5 Orzechowski W and Walker R. Dose of Reality: How Drug Price Controls Would Hurt Americans, Policy Paper No. 25, February 7, 2000.

6 McClung T. PhRMA Member Companies R&D Investments Hit Record High in 2017—$71.4 Billion; August 9, 2018. Available at: https://catalyst.phrma.org/phrma-member-companies-rd-investments-hit-record-high-in-2017-71.4-billion-0. Accessed October 17, 2018.

7 McClung T. PhRMA Member Companies R&D Investments Hit Record High in 2017—$71.4 Billion; August 9, 2018. Available at: https://catalyst.phrma.org/phrma-member-companies-rd-investments-hit-record-high-in-2017-71.4-billion-0. Accessed October 17, 2018.

8 Wong CH, Siah KW and Lo AW. Estimation of Clinical Trial Success Rates and Related Parameters, Biostatistics, April 2019; 20(2) 273–286.

9 Orzechowski W and Walker R. Dose of Reality: How Drug Price Controls Would Hurt Americans, Policy Paper No. 25, February 7, 2000.

10 PhRMA. 2020 Profile: Biopharmaceutical Research Industry; 2020. Available at: https://www.phrma.org/-/media/Project/PhRMA/PhRMA-Org/PhRMA-Org/PDF/G-I/Industry-Profile-2020_1.pdf.

11 Orzechowski W and Walker R. Dose of Reality: How Drug Price Controls Would Hurt Americans, Policy Paper No. 25, February 7, 2000.

12 Research!America, U.S. Investments in Medical and Health Research and Development, 2013–2016, Arlington, VA; Fall 2017. Available at: https://www.researchamerica.org/sites/default/files/RA-2017_InvestmentReport.pdf.

13 DiMasi JA. *Cost of Developing a New Drug*. Boston, MA: Briefing: Tufts Center for the Study of Drug Development, November 18, 2014. Available at: http://csdd.tufts.edu/news/complete_story/cost_study_press_event_webcast. Accessed October 17, 2018.

14 Pammoli F, Magazzini L and Riccaboni M. The Productivity Crisis in Pharmaceutical R&D. Nature Reviews Drug Discovery, 2011; 10(6) 429–438.

15 McClung T. PhRMA Member Companies R&D Investments Hit Record High in 2017—$71.4 Billion; August 9, 2018. Available at: https://catalyst.phrma.org/phrma-member-companies-rd-investments-hit-record-high-in-2017-71.4-billion-0. Accessed October 17, 2018.

16 FDA. FY 2017 Performance Report to Congress for the Prescription Drug User Fee Act; September 20, 2017. Available at: https://www.fda.gov/downloads/AboutFDA/ReportsManualsForms/Reports/UserFeeReports/PerformanceReports/UCM606719.pdf.

17 Downing NS, Shah ND, Aminawung JA, Pease AM, Zeitoun JD, Krumholz HM and Ross JS. Postmarket Safety Events Among Novel Therapeutics Approved by the US Food and Drug Administration Between 2001 and 2010. Journal of the American Medical Association, May 9, 2017; 317(18) 1854–1863. Available at: https://jamanetwork.com/journals/jama/fullarticle/2625319.
18 Research!America. U.S. Investments in Medical and Health Research and Development, 2013–2016, Arlington, VA; Fall 2017. Available at: https://www.researchamerica.org/sites/default/files/RA-2017_InvestmentReport.pdf.
19 FDA. Food and Drugs: Additional Safeguards for Children, Code of Federal Regulations, Title 21, Part 50, Subpart D, Rev, April 2003, p. 293.
20 Orzechowski W and Walker R. Dose of Reality: How Drug Price Controls Would Hurt Americans, Policy Paper No. 25, February 7, 2000.
21 PhRMA. 2020 Profile: Biopharmaceutical Research Industry, 2020. Available at: https://www.phrma.org/-/media/Project/PhRMA/PhRMA-Org/PhRMA-Org/PDF/G-I/Industry-Profile-2020_1.pdf.
22 Levine R. *Ethics and Regulation of Clinical Research*, 2nd ed. Baltimore, MD: Urban and Schwarzenberg, 1988, p. 42.
23 White House Ways and Means Committee. A Painful Pill to Swallow: U.S. Vs. International Prescription Drug Prices; September 2019. Available at: https://waysandmeans.house.gov/sites/democrats.waysandmeans.house.gov/files/documents/U.S.%20vs.%20International%20Prescription%20Drug%20Prices_0.pdf.
24 The Commonwealth Fund. National Trends in Per Capita Pharmaceutical Spending, 1980–2015; October 2017. Available at: https://www.commonwealthfund.org/sites/default/files/documents/___media_files_publications_issue_brief_2017_oct_pdf_sarnak_paying_for_rx_exhibits.pdf.
25 ACRP. *Where We Are and Where We Are Going, 2000 White Paper*. Alexandria, VA: Association of Clinical Research Professionals, 2000. Available at: www.acrpnet.org/whitepaper2/html/ii_contract_research_organizations.html.
26 The Avoca Group. Article: Avoca Group's Industry Research Report on Clinical Outsourcing: Spend, Models, and Measures; September 2019. Available at: https://www.theavocagroup.com/news_events/article-avoca-groups-industry-research-report-on-clinical-outsourcing-spend-models-and-measures/.
27 Hennig M, Hundt F, Busta S, Mikus S, Sanden PH, Sörgel A and Ruppert T. Current Practice and Perspectives in CRO Oversight Based on a Survey Performed Among Members of the German Association of Research-Based Pharmaceutical Companies (VFA); January 26, 2017. German Medical Science. Available at: https://www.ncbi.nlm.nih.gov/pmc/articles/PMC5278541/.
28 ACRP. *Where We Are and Where We Are Going, 2000 White Paper*. Alexandria, VA: Association of Clinical Research Professionals, 2000. Available at: www.acrpnet.org/whitepaper2/html/ii_contract_research_organizations.html.
29 ISR Reports. 2017 Edition of the CRO Market Size Projections: 2016–2021. Available at: https://www.isrreports.com/reports/2017-edition-of-the-cro-market-size-projections-2016-2021/.
30 International Conference on Harmonisation of Technical Requirements for Registration of Pharmaceuticals for Human Use. *Guidance for Industry: E6—Good Clinical Practice*. Geneva, Switzerland: Consolidated Guidance, March 2018. Available at: https://www.fda.gov/downloads/Drugs/Guidances/UCM464506.pdf.
31 International Conference on Harmonisation of Technical Requirements for Registration of Pharmaceuticals for Human Use. *Guidance for Industry: E6—Good Clinical Practice*. Geneva, Switzerland: Consolidated Guidance, March 2018. Available at: https://www.fda.gov/downloads/Drugs/Guidances/UCM464506.pdf.
32 International Conference on Harmonisation of Technical Requirements for Registration of Pharmaceuticals for Human Use. *Guidance for Industry: E6—Good Clinical Practice*. Geneva, Switzerland: Consolidated Guidance, March 2018. Available at: https://www.fda.gov/downloads/Drugs/Guidances/UCM464506.pdf.
33 ACRP. *The CRC—CRA Relationship, 2000 White Paper*. Alexandria, VA: Association of Clinical Research Professionals, 2000. Available at: www.acrpnet.org/whitepaper2/html/viii._crc_cra_relatioship.html.
34 Kefauver–Harris Amendment of 1962, PL 87-78, 76 Stat 780, Codified in Section 21 U.S.C. §502(n).
35 The National Commission for the Protection of Human Subjects of Biomedical and Behavioral Research. *The Belmont Report: Ethical Principles and Guidelines for the Protection of Human Subjects of Research*. Washington, DC: Department of Health, Education, and Welfare, April 18, 1979.
36 FDA. *Food and Drugs: Institutional Review Boards, Code of Federal Regulations, Title 21, Part 56*. Rockville, MD: Food and Drug Administration, Rev. April 2003.
37 HHS. *Federal Policy for the Protection of Human Subjects, Federal Register, 56(117)*. Washington, DC: Department of Health and Human Services, 1991, p. 18.
38 HHS. *Public Welfare: Protection of Human Subjects, Code of Federal Regulations, Title 45, Part 46 Subtitle A*. Washington, DC: Department of Health and Human Services, Rev. January 2017, pp. 107–125.
39 HHS. *Public Welfare: Protection of Human Subjects, Code of Federal Regulations, Title 45, Part 46 Subtitle*

A. Washington, DC: Department of Health and Human Services, Rev. January 2017, pp. 107–125.
40 HHS and FDA. Impact of Certain Provisions of the Revised Common Rule on FDA-Regulated Clinical Investigations: Guidance for Sponsors, Investigators, and Institutional Review Boards; October 2018. Available at: https://www.fda.gov/downloads/RegulatoryInformation/Guidances/UCM623211.pdf?utm_campaign=Impact%20Guidance&utm_medium=email&utm_source=Eloqua&elqTrackId=B10F41E07EB29CFEE1F2ED0B62E45601&elq=ea9d7d8ca2c646ecb92fcb56108f3048&elqaid=5431&elqat=1&elqCampaignId=4386.
41 The National Commission for the Protection of Human Subjects of Biomedical and Behavioral Research. *The Belmont Report: Ethical Principles and Guidelines for the Protection of Human Subjects of Research.* Washington, DC: Department of Health, Education, and Welfare, April 18, 1979.
42 The National Commission for the Protection of Human Subjects of Biomedical and Behavioral Research. *The Belmont Report: Ethical Principles and Guidelines for the Protection of Human Subjects of Research.* Washington, DC: Department of Health, Education, and Welfare, April 18, 1979.
43 U.S. Government Printing Office. *Trials of War Criminals Before the Nuremberg Military Tribunals Under Control Council Law No. 10*, Vol. 2. Washington, DC: U.S. Government Printing Office, 1949, pp. 181–182.
44 U.S. Government Printing Office. *Trials of War Criminals Before the Nuremberg Military Tribunals Under Control Council Law No. 10*, Vol. 2. Washington, DC: U.S. Government Printing Office, 1949, pp. 181–182.
45 World Medical Organization. Declaration of Helsinki: Ethical Principles for Medical Research Involving Human Subjects, Adopted by the 18th WMA General Assembly, Helsinki, Finland; June 1964.
46 The National Commission for the Protection of Human Subjects of Biomedical and Behavioral Research. *The Belmont Report: Ethical Principles and Guidelines for the Protection of Human Subjects of Research.* Washington, DC: Department of Health, Education, and Welfare, April 18, 1979.
47 HHS. *Public Welfare: Protection of Human Subjects, Code of Federal Regulations, Title 45, Part 46 Subtitle A.* Washington, DC: Department of Health and Human Services, Rev. January 2017, pp. 107–125.
48 Resnik DB. Centralized Institutional Review Boards: Assessing the Arguments and Evidence. Journal of Clinical Research Best Practices, November 2012; 8(11).
49 The National Commission for the Protection of Human Subjects of Biomedical and Behavioral Research. *The Belmont Report: Ethical Principles and Guidelines for the Protection of Human Subjects of Research.* Washington, DC: Department of Health, Education, and Welfare, April 18, 1979.
50 HHS. *Public Welfare: Protection of Human Subjects, Code of Federal Regulations, Title 45, Part 46 Subtitle A.* Washington, DC: Department of Health and Human Services, Rev. January 2017, pp. 107–125.
51 FDA. Protection of Human Research Subjects; Clinical Investigations Which May Be Reviewed Through Expedited Review Procedure Set forth in FDA Regulations. Federal Register, November 9, 1998; 63(216).
52 International Conference on Harmonisation of Technical Requirements for Registration of Pharmaceuticals for Human Use. *Guidance for Industry: E6—Good Clinical Practice.* Geneva, Switzerland: Consolidated Guidance, March 2018. Available at: https://www.fda.gov/downloads/Drugs/Guidances/UCM464506.pdf.
53 HHS. *Public Welfare: Protection of Human Subjects, Code of Federal Regulations, Title 45, Part 46 Subtitle A.* Washington, DC: Department of Health and Human Services, Rev. January 2017, pp. 107–125.
54 Amdur R and Bankert EA. *Institutional Review Board: Member Handbook*, 3rd ed. Boston, MA: Jones and Bartlett Publishers, 2011.
55 Levine R. *Ethics and Regulation of Clinical Research*, 2nd ed. Baltimore, MD: Urban and Schwarzenberg, 1988, p. 42.
56 HHS. *Public Welfare: Protection of Human Subjects, Code of Federal Regulations, Title 45, Part 46 Subtitle A.* Washington, DC: Department of Health and Human Services, Rev. January 2017, pp. 107–125.
57 Amdur R and Bankert EA. *Institutional Review Board: Member Handbook*, 3rd ed. Boston, MA: Jones and Bartlett Publishers, 2011.
58 HHS. *Public Welfare: Protection of Human Subjects, Code of Federal Regulations, Title 45, Part 46 Subtitle A.* Washington, DC: Department of Health and Human Services, Rev. January 2017, pp. 107–125.
59 FDA. *Institutional Review Boards: IRB Functions and Operations, Code of Federal Regulations, Title 21, Part 56, Section 108.* Rockville, MD: Food and Drug Administration, Rev. April 2004, pp. 325–326.
60 FDA. *Protection of Human Subjects: Exception From General Requirements, Code of Federal Regulations, Title 21, Part 50, Subpart b 50.23*, Rev. April 2004, pp. 310–312.
61 FDA. *Protection of Human Subjects: General Requirements for Informed Consent, Code of Federal Regulations, Title 21,* Part 50, *Subpart b 50.20*, Rev. April 2004, p. 310.
62 FDA. *Protection of Human Subjects: Exception From Informed Consent Requirements for Emergency Research, Code of Federal Regulations, Title 21,* Part 50, *Subpart b 50.24*, Rev. April 2004, pp. 313–314.
63 HHS. *Public Welfare: Protection of Human Subjects, Code of Federal Regulations, Title 45, Part 46 Subtitle A.* Washington, DC: Department of Health and Human Services, Rev. January 2017, pp. 107–125.

64 FDA. Information Sheet: Payment and Reimbursement to Research Subjects, Guidance for Institutional Review Boards and Clinical Investigators; January 2018. Available at: https://www.fda.gov/regulatory-information/search-fda-guidance-documents/payment-and-reimbursement-research-subjects.

65 ASGT. *Policy of the American Society of Gene Therapy Financial Conflict of Interest in Clinical Research*. Milwaukee, WI: American Society of Gene Therapy, adopted April 5, 2000.

66 HHS. HHS and 16 Other Federal Departments and Agencies Issue a Final Rule to Delay for an Additional 6 Months the General Compliance Date of Revisions to the Common Rule While Allowing the Use of Three Burden-Reducing Provisions During the Delay Period; June 18, 2018. Available at: https://www.hhs.gov/ohrp/final-rule-delaying-general-compliance-revised-common-rule.html.

3 Search and Analysis of the Food and Drug Administration's FDA Adverse Event Reporting System (FAERS)

Paul N. Danese

SYNOPSIS

3.1 INTRODUCTION

In the United States, the Food and Drug Administration (FDA) monitors the safety of marketed prescription and non-prescription medications using an electronic database known as the FDA Adverse Event Reporting System (FAERS). The FDA routinely mines FAERS to search for unexpected drug safety issues, and in recent years it has improved the ability of the extramural researchers to mine the database as well. This chapter discusses the FAERS database in depth, with emphasis on how the FDA and others use FAERS to increase drug safety and promote public health.

DOI: 10.1201/9781003615323-4

3.2 BACKGROUND

The FDA approves and regulates the sale of prescription and non-prescription medications in the United States. FDA approval of prescription drugs is usually based on the results of randomized, controlled, Phase 3 clinical trials, which are typically designed to assess both drug safety and efficacy.[1–3]

Although clinical trials do much to assess drug safety, they are inherently limited in their ability to identify all possible drug safety issues. These limitations arise because of the following characteristics of clinical trials:

3.2.1 Small Clinical Trial Populations

First, although clinical trials may recruit thousands of patients for safety and efficacy testing,[1,3] the trial populations are almost always relatively small in comparison to the number of patients who will be exposed to a medication after its approval. As such, clinical trials are often underpowered with respect to their ability to identify rare drug-related adverse events.[4,5]

3.2.2 Narrow Patient Demographics

Second, patients recruited into clinical trials often belong to narrowly defined demographic groups. For example, children rarely participate in clinical trials.[6] However, once approval is granted, the spectrum of patients exposed to a medication typically expands beyond the boundaries of the demographic groups assessed in the clinical trial. Consequently, members of previously untested demographic groups, who are now exposed to the newly approved pharmaceutical, may reveal drug safety issues that were not apparent from the original clinical trials used as the basis for drug approval.[7,8]

3.2.3 Restricted Co-Administration of Medications

Third, clinical trials often impose restrictions on the types of medications that may be co-administered with the pharmaceutical being tested.[1,9] Once a medication is approved for marketing, however, there is less control over the types and quantities of medications that are co-administered with a newly approved medication. As a result, administration of a medication to members of the public can reveal drug-drug interactions that might not have been observed in the more controlled settings of a clinical trial.

Because of the inherent limitations of conventional clinical trials to identify rare or unanticipated drug safety issues, the FDA has established several surveillance systems to identify drug safety issues that arise *after* a drug has been approved for sale.

This chapter focuses on the FDA's primary pharmacovigilance tool, the FAERS, which monitors the safety of approved drug and biologic agents,[10] and briefly discusses other surveillance systems that are used to monitor the safety of approved vaccines and medical devices.

3.3 HISTORY OF THE FDA'S DRUG SAFETY SURVEILLANCE SYSTEMS

From 1968 to 1997, the FDA collected over 1.6 million reports of suspected drug safety issues from manufacturers, healthcare professionals, and the lay public using the Spontaneous Reporting System (SRS).[11,12] SRS reports captured patient demographic information (e.g., age and gender), adverse reaction information, and patient outcomes. In late 1997, the FDA replaced the SRS with the Adverse Event Reporting System (AERS),[12] which differed from the SRS in that it (1) captured a wider array of information and (2) allowed for the electronic submission of adverse event reports, in anticipation of the increasing importance of the internet as a means of information exchange.

The AERS was subsequently upgraded in the fourth quarter of 2012 and renamed *F*AERS (*F*DA *A*dverse *E*vent *R*eporting *S*ystem). FAERS is almost identical in structure and content to the AERS, but it contains a handful of new data fields that were not previously captured by the AERS.

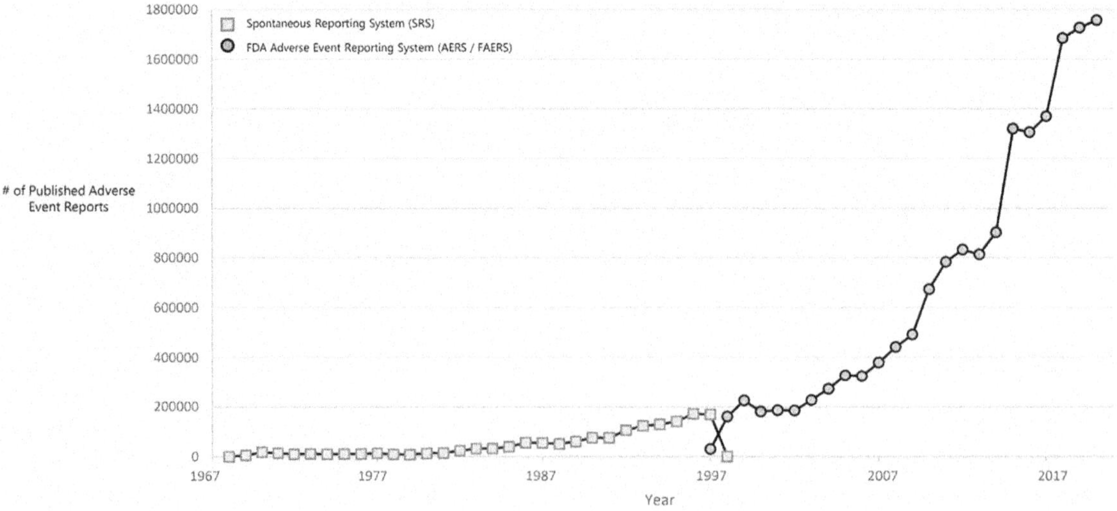

FIGURE 3.1 Number of Drug and Biologic Adverse Event Reports Published by the FDA from 1968 to the fourth quarter of 2020.

Today, FAERS is used to collect and analyze suspected safety issues for all FDA-approved prescription and non-prescription medications. Since its inception in late 1997, the AERS and FAERS databases have documented over 16.6 million adverse event reports, with almost every successive year seeing an increase in the number of submitted reports (Figure 3.1). Remarkably, even though there were more than 430,000 reports submitted to the FDA in the fourth quarter of 2020, only a small minority of suspected drug adverse reactions is reported to the FDA (see Section 8C for a detailed discussion).[13,14]

3.4 SUBMISSION OF ADVERSE EVENT REPORTS TO THE FDA

There are two classes of reports submitted into FAERS: mandatory reports submitted by drug and biologic manufacturers, and voluntary reports submitted by the lay public and their representatives.

3.4.1 Mandatory Reports

The overwhelming majority of adverse event reports (> 94 %) are submitted to the FDA by drug and biologic manufacturers. Manufacturers are legally obligated to submit to the FDA reports of both serious and non-serious adverse events in a timely manner. Specifically, manufacturers must report serious, unexpected adverse events to the FDA within 15 calendar days of their notification of an adverse event. These reports are referred to as Expedited Reports. In addition, manufacturers must also submit quarterly reports that summarize all adverse events (serious and non-serious) associated with their marketed medications for the first three years after approval of a New Drug Application or Biologics License Application. After three years, manufacturers must submit annual summaries of adverse events associated with their marketed medications.[15]

3.4.2 Voluntary Reports

The FDA also receives a small fraction (< 6 %) of its adverse event reports directly from healthcare professionals (physicians, pharmacists, nurses, and other healthcare providers) as well as consumers and consumer representatives (patients, family members, lawyers, and others). These reports are voluntarily submitted to the FDA and are not subject to the reporting deadlines mandated for manufacturers.

3.5 ADVERSE DRUG REACTION INFORMATION CAPTURED BY FAERS

Each adverse event report submitted to the FDA contains an array of information that attempts to provide a clear picture of the patient who suffered the adverse event, the medications taken during the time surrounding the event, the specific adverse events suffered by the patient and the overall patient outcome after the adverse event. Table 3.1 summarizes the information that can be captured within each report. Although each report can contain the information outlined in Table 1, the actual information included in a report varies depending on the extent of information known at the time the report is submitted.

TABLE 3.1
An Abridged List of Information Captured in Individual Safety Reports Submitted into the FDA's Adverse Events Reporting System (FAERS).

Patient Information
- Date Information
- Adverse Event Date
- Date of Death (when applicable)
- Demographic Information
- Age
- Weight
- Gender

Reporter Information
- Date Information
- Date Report Was Submitted
- Manufacturer Notification Date
- FDA Notification Date
- Name of Manufacturer Sending Report (when applicable)
- Manufacturer's Internal Report Identification Code
- Occupation of the Person Submitting the Report
- Whether a reporter requested that his identity not be disclosed to the manufacturer
- Reporter's Country
- Occurring Country*
- Literature Reference*
- Regulatory Authority Number*

(Continued)

TABLE 3.1
Continued

Drug Information
- Drug Name
- Administration Route
- Drug Dose
- Cumulative Dose to First Adverse Reaction*
- Active Pharmaceutical Ingredient*
- Drug's Reported Role (Primary Suspect, Secondary Suspect, Interacting or Concomitant)
- Dechallenge Information (Was the severity of the adverse reaction ameliorated when administration of the drug was stopped?)
- Rechallenge Information (Did the severity of the adverse reaction increase after a medication was re-administered?)
- Drug's Lot Number
- Drug's Expiration Date
- Drug's Start Date
- Drug's End Date
- Duration of Drug Therapy

Adverse Reaction and Outcome Information
- Preferred Term for Adverse Reaction (medical term describing the adverse event using MedDRA, the Medical Dictionary for Regulatory Activities)
- Patient Outcome(s) (Congenital Anomaly, Death, Disability, Life-Threatening, Other, Required Intervention to Prevent Permanent Impairment/ Damage)

Source: * Fields added during the transition from AERS to FAERS

3.6 SEARCHING FAERS DATA TO IDENTIFY POSSIBLE SAFETY PROBLEMS

Given the vast number of existing reports and the rapid pace at which new reports are currently received (an average of over 4,500 reports submitted daily), one may ask how the FDA and other organizations analyze FAERS.

3.6.1 Statistical Methods to Identify Drug Safety Signals

Researchers at the FDA, as well as those in academia and the pharmaceutical industry, chiefly use FAERS to search for drug *safety signals*, unexpected adverse reactions that may be causally linked to the administration of a pharmaceutical.[16]

The methods employed to search for safety signals are statistical in nature, and in general, they attempt to identify adverse reactions that are more frequently, or disproportionately, co-reported with one drug (or class of drugs) than with a comparator drug (or comparator class of drugs).[17] Adverse reactions that are disproportionately associated with a particular drug represent safety signals that may warrant further investigation to assess the possibility of a causal link between the drug and the adverse reaction.

Figure 3.2 shows a safety signal analysis of the intranasal spray, Zicam®, using AERS data from early 2005 and using a statistical method known as the Proportional Reporting Ratio (PRR) that measures reporting disproportionality.[17–19] Interestingly, the strongest safety signals shown in Figure 3.2 are primarily related to dysfunctions in smell and taste (anosmia and dysgeusia). It is noteworthy

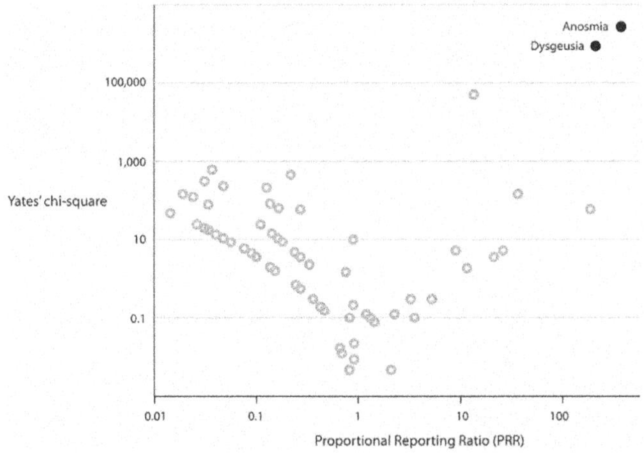

FIGURE 3.2 Safety Signal Analysis of Zicam® using AERS data from 1997 to the first quarter of 2005.

that these signals were present using AERS data available four years before a 2009 FDA public advisory that warned the public of the relationship between intra-nasal Zicam® and anosmia.[20]

FDA researchers have published several peer-reviewed manuscripts describing their analysis of FAERS data. It is clear from these manuscripts that the FDA uses statistical methods that measure reporting disproportionality, including the PRR and the Multi-item Gamma Poisson Shrinker methods to identify safety signals (MGPS).[17–19] However, the FDA's methods in searching for safety signals are opaque in two noteworthy respects. First, it is unclear if FDA researchers systematically use FAERS to search for safety signals of all marketed medications or whether they selectively focus on a subset of medications. Second, it is unclear if the FDA employs additional quantitative or qualitative methods beyond the PRR and MGPS to search for safety signals.

3.6.2 Dechallenge and Rechallenge Data and Causality

Although it is not always possible to definitively demonstrate a causal relationship between a drug and a particular adverse reaction using FAERS data alone, FAERS reports may contain data that help support a causal relationship. Specifically, individual safety reports often include information on whether the severity of an adverse reaction was ameliorated when administration of a drug was discontinued (known as a positive dechallenge) or whether an adverse reaction was exacerbated upon re-administration of a drug (known as a positive rechallenge). When analyzing FAERS data, dechallenge and rechallenge data can provide evidence of a causal link between a drug and a particular adverse reaction.[21,22]

3.6.3 Identifying Drug-Drug Interactions

Recent research has also shown that the FDA's FAERS data can be used to search for previously unexpected drug-drug interactions. Specifically, Tatonetti et al.[23] mined FAERS database to identify medications that were disproportionately associated with adverse reactions involving increased blood glucose levels (hyperglycemia) but *only when co-administered.* This approach identified two medications, paroxetine and pravastatin, that appear to cause hyperglycemia only in combination. Tatonetti et al. subsequently tested the hypothesis that co-administration of paroxetine and pravastatin interfered with blood glucose levels by mining an independent registry of medical records. Their subsequent analysis also supported the link between hyperglycemia and co-administration of these medications.[23]

3.6.4 Timelines and Deadlines of Adverse Event Reporting

FAERS reports also contain a wealth of date-related information, including the date when a manufacturer receives an adverse event report. It is therefore possible to use FAERS to determine when a manufacturer was first notified of a possible link between a medication and a specific adverse reaction. Therefore, it is also possible to use FAERS to determine whether manufacturers have complied with FDA-mandated reporting deadlines for serious adverse reactions.

Specifically, because FAERS reports contain information on when a manufacturer was notified of an adverse event and when the manufacturer subsequently notified the FDA, it is possible to use FAERS to determine whether a manufacturer has forwarded reports of serious and unexpected adverse reactions to the FDA within the mandated 15 calendar day period. For example, in 2013, the FDA indicated that Pfizer and other unnamed organizations had submitted adverse event reports related to the medication varenicline through "improper channels" and had initially submitted adverse event reports to the FDA "in a way that did not allow for [the FDA to conduct] comprehensive evaluation." These improper submissions included reports of varenicline-associated suicides and serious psychiatric episodes that were submitted to the FDA as periodic summaries rather than as expedited, 15-calendar-day, reports.[24]

3.7 THE FOOD AND DRUG ADMINISTRATION'S USE OF FAERS IN REGULATORY DECISIONS

As noted above, the FDA uses FAERS to search for unexpected safety issues associated with marketed medications. The FDA uses this information as part of its strategy to communicate drug safety issues to the public and to guide changes in the regulation of marketed medications. In 2008, the FDA began releasing lists of newly identified "Potential Signals of Serious Risks/New Safety Information Identified from the Adverse Event Reporting System".[25] These lists, which are released quarterly, include three items:

- The name of the drug or class of drugs under investigation
- The potential adverse reaction (safety signal) associated with the drug in question
- Additional information on what steps the FDA has taken or is taking to further its investigation.

From 2008 to the third quarter of 2020, the FDA has published over 600 potential signals of serious risks based on its examination of FAERS. The safety signals identified by the FDA are a remarkable testament to the diverse types of adverse reactions that can be revealed by analyzing FAERS. They include the following:

- Overdoses related to confusion over packaging (for arginine hydrochloride)
- Organ and tissue failure (specifically: liver failure and dronedarone)
- Drug-drug interactions (e.g., ranolazine and simvastatin associated with rhabdomyolysis)
- Age-related adverse reactions (e.g., serious adverse events in neonates associated with lopinavir/ritonavir)

The range of actions taken by the FDA in response to its investigation of these safety signals also covers a wide range, including:

3.7.1 Boxed Warnings

The most serious actions include addition of boxed warnings to the prescribing information of several medications (e.g., extraneal, lapatinib, trastuzumab[25]) and recommendations that prescribers limit the use of high doses of certain medications like simvastatin.[26,27]

3.7.2 Other Changes to a Medication's Prescribing Information

The FDA has also used its investigation of FAERS to orchestrate more moderate changes to the prescribing information of numerous medications (e.g., minocycline, tapentadol, saquinavir).[25] In these cases, prescribing information of an investigated drug was changed to include the newly identified safety signals as part of a list of adverse reactions that have been observed in post-marketing reports.

3.7.3 Determinations That No Action Is Needed and Continuing Investigations

The bulk of the remaining medications under investigation for potential safety issues are either still under investigation, or the FDA has determined that no regulatory action is needed at the time, either because there is insufficient evidence to support the initial safety signal or because the FDA believes that the medication's existing prescribing information adequately addresses the potential safety issue (e.g., mefloquine[28]).

3.8 LIMITATIONS OF FAERS

Although analysis of FAERS can identify rare and unexpected drug safety issues, the FDA notes that FAERS does have certain limitations, including:

3.8.1 Lack of Demonstration of Causality for Individual Reports

For any individual report, the information contained therein does not necessarily demonstrate that a particular medication caused the reported adverse reactions. However, as noted above, dechallenge and rechallenge data, when available, may support causality.

3.8.2 Extensive Under-Reporting

FAERS is a *voluntary* drug safety surveillance system. That is, drug safety reports are either voluntarily submitted directly to the FDA by members of the public or they are voluntarily submitted to manufacturers who are then obligated to submit the reports to the FDA. Because of its voluntary underpinnings, most suspected drug adverse reactions are not reported into FAERS. Several studies have attempted to estimate the degree of underreporting (1) within the AERS and (2) the general degree of under-reporting within all voluntary pharmacovigilance adverse event reporting systems. A 2006 analysis estimates that only 6 % of known, suspected, or expected adverse drug reactions are reported in voluntary pharmacovigilance systems like FAERS (with an interquartile range of 2–18%).[14] Similar conclusions were drawn in a 2008 FDA study, which estimated the degree of under-reporting for the serious adverse reaction, rhabdomyolysis for the class of drugs colloquially known as statins (3-hydroxy-3-methylglutaryl coenzyme A [HMG-CoA] reductase inhibitors). The FDA study estimated that only 5–15% of rhabdomyolysis adverse events were reported for the statins in general. Moreover, even after theh FDA publicized the safety issue by disseminating a "Dear Health Care Provider" letter notifying healthcare practitioners of this potential issue and to submit suspected cases to the FDA, the FDA estimated that the reporting frequency was still only 5–30% for the entire class of statin medications.[13]

3.8.3 Reporting Biases

The voluntary nature of FAERS reporting can make the number of reports filed for a particular medication susceptible to publicity surrounding a particular medication.[10,13]

3.8.4 Lack of Comparator Populations (Lack of a Denominator)

Under ideal conditions, one would be able to determine the frequency at which a particular adverse reaction is associated with a particular drug using the following equation (Equation 3.1).

$$\begin{matrix}\textit{Frequency of} \\ \textit{Association}\end{matrix} = \frac{\begin{matrix}\textit{\# of Cases where Adverse Event X} \\ \textit{occurs when Patients are Exposed to Drug Y}\end{matrix}}{\textit{Total \# of Patients Exposed to Drug Y}} \quad (3.1)$$

One could then compare this frequency to the frequency of occurrence Adverse Event X in the population as a whole (or in another suitable control population). Comparisons of this type would then allow investigators to calculate the strength of association between a particular adverse event and a particular drug. However, it is often difficult to estimate the total number of patients exposed to a particular medication. Therefore, most analyses of FAERS cannot compute an incidence frequency owing to a lack of a denominator in the equation shown above.[29] However, as noted in Section 6A, other statistical methods have been developed to address this issue, primarily by identifying adverse reactions that are disproportionately co-reported with specific medications.[17–19]

3.9 SEARCH AND RETRIEVAL OF ADVERSE EVENT REPORTS FROM THE FDA'S FAERS

There are four general approaches that researchers outside the FDA may use to analyze FAERS data.

3.9.1 Raw Data Files

First, researchers can download FAERS data from the FDA website as raw text files.[30] As one might expect, there are both benefits and drawbacks to this approach. The obvious benefit is that researchers have unfettered access to the underlying data and can therefore filter and analyze FAERS in any way that they find suitable. Conversely, the clear downside is that these files can only be searched using advanced computational methods.

3.9.2 FDA Public Dashboard

Second, the FDA has recently created a publicly accessible search engine for FAERS (termed the FAERS Public Dashboard).[31] Although the search engine is publicly available and free, users are restricted to relatively simple searches, and it is therefore difficult to use the dashboard to conduct nuanced statistical analysis.

3.9.3 FOIA Requests

Third, interested parties may also file a Freedom of Information Act (FOIA) request with the FDA and search FAERS by specifying search parameters (e.g., all cases reporting both ibuprofen and cardiac arrest). Upon receipt of a FOIA request, an FDA liaison will search FAERS using the FDA's internal query system and subsequently return electronic copies of matching case reports. The FDA charges a fee for FOIA requests that is dependent on the complexity of the search. The time required for the FDA to complete these requests varies from a few weeks to longer periods.[32]

3.9.4 Commercial Vendors

Fourth, commercial organizations (including ours)[33,34] have built search engines that allow users to mine and analyze the complete FAERS data set more rapidly than is possible by conventional FOIA request and with greater sophistication than is possible with the FAERS Public Dashboard. Depending on the commercial vendor, search results can provide end-users with both raw data and statistical analysis of their search results, allowing users to search for safety signals (Figure 3.2) and to see statistics like patient outcome distributions and co-reported adverse reactions (Figure 3.3).

3.10 OTHER FDA-ADVERSE EVENT REPORTING SYSTEMS

As noted above, FAERS is not the only post-marketing surveillance system employed by the FDA. The FDA uses other surveillance systems, each of which is designed to monitor adverse events for a specific type of medical treatment.

3.10.1 VAERS

For example, the FDA (in conjunction with the Centers for Disease Control and Prevention) monitors reports of vaccine-associated adverse events using an electronic database known as VAERS. VAERS was launched in 1990 and currently contains over 810,000 reports. The FDA and CDC use VAERS to search for vaccine safety signals in a manner similar to that employed for safety signal analysis of FAERS.[35,36]

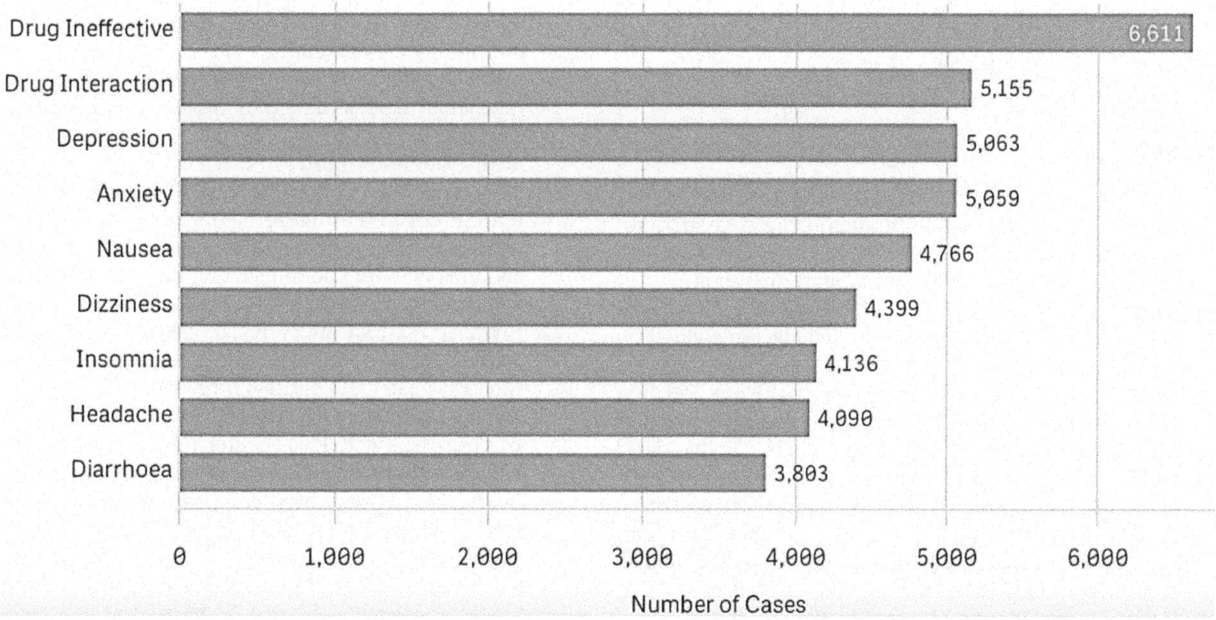

FIGURE 3.3 Most frequently reported adverse reactions for the antidepressant, Zoloft® (sertraline) using FAERS data from 1997 to 2020.

3.10.2 MAUDE

The FDA also maintains a separate database that collects adverse event reports for medical devices and medical facilities. This database is known as MAUDE (Medical Device and User Facility Device Experience). MAUDE reports are available from 1991 to the present and the database currently contains more than 10.9 million reports.[37]

3.10.3 Sentinel Initiative

In May 2008, the FDA announced a new program, termed the Sentinel Initiative, whereby it would track all FDA-approved products by mining electronic health record systems and insurance claims databases from several external organizations. After initial pilot studies, the FDA expanded the Sentinel Initiative in September 2019 to include an array of health insurance providers and public health research institutes distributed across the United States.[38,39]

3.11 SUMMARY AND CONCLUSIONS

This chapter has described the FDA Adverse Event Reporting System (FAERS), the primary tool employed to monitor the safety of marketed medications in the United States. The FDA uses FAERS to identify unexpected drug safety issues and guide regulatory changes based on its findings. The FDA has used FAERS to identify a diverse array of drug safety issues, including unexpected drug-drug interactions, organ failure, overdoses related to confusion over drug packaging and age-related adverse reactions. Although the ability to search FAERS through the FDA's web site is somewhat limited, commercial vendors also provide access to FAERS, allowing interested parties the ability to search for drug safety signals and compile statistical data on medications of interest. Ultimately, expanded access to these data should enhance drug safety efforts and promote greater public health.

REFERENCES

1. Gad SC, ed. *Clinical Trials Handbook* (Wiley, 2009).
2. U.S. Food and Drug Administration. Drug study designs: Information sheet (July 12, 2018). http://www.fda.gov/RegulatoryInformation/Guidances/ucm126501.htm
3. National Institutes of Health. Glossary of clinical trial terms. https://www.nia.nih.gov/research/dgcg/nia-glossary-clinical-research-terms
4. Alsheikh-Ali AA, Ambrose MS, Kuvin JT, Karas RH. The safety of rosuvastatin as used in common clinical practice: A postmarketing analysis. Circulation. 111(23):3051–3057 (2005).
5. Strangfeld A, Listing J. Infection and musculoskeletal conditions: Bacterial and opportunistic infections during anti-TNF therapy. Best Pract. Res. Clin. Rheumatol. 20(6):1181–1195 (2006).
6. U.S. Food and Drug Administration. Would your child benefit from a clinical trial? (March 21, 2017). http://www.fda.gov/ForConsumers/ConsumerUpdates/ucm048699.htm
7. Johann-Liang R, Wyeth J, Chen M, Cope JU. Pediatric drug surveillance and the food and drug administration's adverse event reporting system: An overview of reports, 2003–2007. Pharmacoepidemiol. Drug Saf. 18(1):24–27 (2008).
8. Rivkees S, Szarfman A. Dissimilar hepatotoxicity profiles of propylthiouracil and methimazole in children. J. Clin. Endocrinol. Metable. 95(7):3260–3267 (2010).
9. National Institutes of Health. ClinicalTrials.gov. www.clinicaltrials.gov
10. U.S. Food and Drug Administration. Questions and answers on FDA's Adverse Event Reporting System (FAERS) (June 4, 2018). http://www.fda.gov/Drugs/GuidanceComplianceRegulatoryInformation/Surveillance/AdverseDrugEffects/default.htm
11. Rossi AC, Knapp DE. Discovery of new adverse drug reactions: A review of the food and drug administration's spontaneous reporting system. JAMA. 252(8):1030–1033 (1984).
12. Trontell AE. How the U.S. Food and Drug Administration defines and detects adverse drug events. Curr. Therap. Res. 62(9):641–649 (2001).
13. McAdams M, Staffa J, Dal Pan G. Estimating the extent of reporting to FDA: A case study of statin-associated rhabdomyolysis. Pharmacoepidemiol. Drug Saf. 17(3):229–239 (2008).
14. Hazell L, Shakir SAW. Under-reporting of adverse drug reactions: A systematic review. Drug Saf. 29(5):385–396 (2006).
15. Postmarketing reporting of adverse drug experiences (2010). 21 C.F.R. '314.80'.
16. Edwards IR, Biriell C. Harmonisation in pharmacovigilance. Drug Saf. 10(2):93–102 (1994).
17. Almenoff JS, LaCroix KK, Yuen NA, Fram D, DuMouchel W. Comparative performance of two quantitative safety signalling methods: Implications for use in a pharmacovigilance department. Drug Saf. 29(10):875–887 (2006).
18. DuMouchel W. Bayesian data mining in large frequency tables, with an application to the FDA Spontaneous Reporting System. Am. Stat. 53(3):177–202 (1999).
19. Evans SJ, Waller PC, Davis S. Use of proportional reporting ratios (PRRs) for signal generation from spontaneous adverse drug reaction reports. Pharmacoepidemiol. Drug Saf. 10(6):483–486 (2001).
20. U.S. Food and Drug Administration. Homeopathic product regulation: Evaluating FDA's regulatory framework after a quarter-century (April 20, 2015). https://www.fda.gov/media/91697/download
21. Wysowski DK, Corken A, Gallo-Torres H, Talarico L, Rodriguez EM. Postmarketing reports of QT prolongation and ventricular arrhythmia in association with cisapride and food and drug administration regulatory actions. Am. J. Gastroenterol. 96(6):1698–1703 (2001).
22. Bremner JD, McCaffery P. The neurobiology of retinoic acid in affective disorders. Prog. Neuropsychopharmacol. Biol. Psychiatry. 32(2):315–331 (2008).
23. Tatonetti NP, Denny JC, Murphy SN, Fernald GH, Krishnan G, Castro V, Yue P, Tsau PS, Kohane I, Roden DM, Altman RB. Detecting drug interactions from adverse-event reports: Interaction between paroxetine and pravastatin increases blood glucose levels. Clin. Pharmacol. Ther. 90(1):133–142 (2011).
24. U.S. Food and Drug Administration. Chantix: Quarterwatch article (November 2, 2017). https://wayback.archive-it.org/7993/20171102213606/https:/www.fda.gov/Drugs/DrugSafety/ucm255918.htm

25. U.S. Food and Drug Administration. Potential signals of serious risks/new safety information identified from the FDA Adverse Event Reporting System (FAERS) (February 2, 2021). http://www.fda.gov/Drugs/GuidanceComplianceRegulatoryInformation/Surveillance/AdverseDrugEffects/ucm082196.htm
26. U.S. Food and Drug Administration. Potential signals of serious risks/new safety information identified from the Adverse Event Reporting System (AERS) between April–June 2010 (December 15, 2017). http://www.fda.gov/Drugs/GuidanceComplianceRegulatoryInformation/Surveillance/AdverseDrugEffects/ucm223734.htm
27. U.S. Food and Drug Administration. FDA Drug Safety Communication: New restrictions, contraindications, and dose limitations for Zocor (simvastatin) to reduce the risk of muscle injury (December 15, 2017). http://www.fda.gov/Drugs/DrugSafety/ucm256581.htm
28. U.S. Food and Drug Administration. Potential signals of serious risks/new safety information identified from the Adverse Event Reporting System (AERS) between July–September 2008. Potential signals of serious risks/new safety information identified from the FDA Adverse Event Reporting System (FAERS) (February 2, 2021). https://www.fda.gov/drugs/questions-and-answers-fdas-adverse-event-reporting-system-faers/potential-signals-serious-risksnew-safety-information-identified-fda-adverse-event-reporting-system
29. Burke SP, Stratton K, Baciu A. *The Future of Drug Safety: Promoting and Protecting the Health of the Public* (Institute of Medicine of the National Academies, 2007).
30. U.S. Food and Drug Administration. FDA Adverse Event Reporting System (FAERS) quarterly data extract files. https://fis.fda.gov/extensions/FPD-QDE-FAERS/FPD-QDE-FAERS.html
31. U.S. Food and Drug Administration. FDA Adverse Event Reporting System (FAERS) public dashboard (October 29, 2020). https://www.fda.gov/drugs/questions-and-answers-fdas-adverse-event-reporting-system-faers/fda-adverse-event-reporting-system-faers-public-dashboard
32. U.S. Food and Drug Administration. How to make a FOIA request (March 12, 2020). https://www.fda.gov/regulatory-information/freedom-information/how-make-foia-request
33. FDAble, LLC. www.fdable.com
34. United BioSource Corporation. http://www.unitedbiosource.com/
35. Department of Health and Human Services. Vaccine adverse event reporting system (February 20, 2021). http://vaers.hhs.gov/index
36. Iskander J, Pool V, Zhou W, English-Bullard R. Data mining in the U.S. using the vaccine adverse event reporting system. Drug Saf. 29(5):375–384 (2006).
37. U.S. Food and Drug Administration. Manufacturer and user facility device experience database (MAUDE) (January 22, 2021). http://www.fda.gov/MedicalDevices/DeviceRegulationandGuidance/PostmarketRequirements/ReportingAdverseEvents/ucm127891.htm
38. U.S. Food and Drug Administration. FDA's sentinel initiative (October 18, 2019). https://www.fda.gov/safety/fdas-sentinel-initiative
39. Sentinel Initiative. https://www.sentinelinitiative.org/

4 The Safety of Medicines
PharmacoVigilance, PharmacoSurveillance, PharmacoEmpowerment?

David Healy

SYNOPSIS

4.1 RXISK.ORG

RxISK.org, an adverse event reporting website, opened to the world in 2012. The idea underpinning it took shape in 2010, in the form of an idea about Data Based Medicine. This led to a Data Based Medicine company in 2011.

The contrast between Data Based Medicine (DBM) and Evidence Based Medicine (EBM) was deliberate. EBM implies a clinical practice based on data, primarily from randomized clinical trials (RCT), rather than practice based on clinical opinion, which for over a decade before 2010 had been dismissed as Eminence Based Medicine. Several people had tried to open up other avenues, such as Medicine Based Evidence, in support of the idea that what evidently appeared to be happening the person in front of a clinician was important even if the apparent evidence pointed to the contrary (1).

By 2010, it had become increasingly clear that Evidence Based Medicine was not based on what was evident to a clinician but on evidence, that is statistical outputs, largely published in ghost-written papers without access to the data underlying the claims these papers made.

4.2 ANTIDEPRESSANTS: DATA BASED OR EVIDENCE BASED?

The phrase, the plural of anecdote is data, central to Google now, was coined by Raymond Wolfinger, a polling expert in 1969 (2). Two years later, the CEO of NutraSweet claimed "the plural of anecdotes is not data" when his company's sweetener, aspartame, was linked to cancer. The related phrases "anecdotes are not science" and "harm has not been proven" were also coined at this time and used in media interviews by the Pedophile Information Exchange defending sexual relations between adults and children. They are now the stock in trade of corporate risk management, whether by politicians, companies, or churches.

In February 1990, an American Journal of Psychiatry article outlined 6 cases in which people had become suicidal on Eli Lilly's selective serotonin reuptake inhibiting (SSRI) antidepressant Prozac (fluoxetine) (3). Prozac was then on its way to blockbuster status despite minimal RCT evidence for benefits. The suicidality appeared on treatment, stopped when treatment stopped, and reappeared on restarting. By all canons of causality, Prozac caused suicidality. The US Food and Drug Administration (FDA) were forced into a hearing on Prozac.

In preparation for this FDA Hearing, Eli Lilly submitted its RCT data in an article to the British Medical Journal (BMJ). The editor of BMJ at this time, Richard Smith, was an early fan of Evidence Based Medicine (EBM) as a way to control the pharmaceutical industry. Faced with the Lilly article, Smith saw the company seemingly embracing EBM. He missed the small print in a footnote, which shows a statistically significant increased risk of suicide and suicidal events on Prozac compared to placebo. BMJ ran Lilly's article on Prozac on September 20, the day of the FDA hearings (4).

DOI: 10.1201/9781003615323-5

Although the large print showed an increased number of suicidal events on Prozac these were not statistically significant. The article became a key exhibit in Lilly's media defense that there was no evidence Prozac caused suicide.

This defense had three elements:

- "The plural of anecdote is not data."
- "Who are you going to believe the anecdotes or the data?"
- "It's the disease not the drug"

The FDA was meanwhile sitting on RCT evidence showing older antidepressants were more effective than the SSRIs. There was evidence of induced suicidality and suicides in healthy volunteer trials. There was RCT evidence that the soon to be released Zoloft (sertraline) and Paxil (paroxetine) also increased the risk of suicide. Finally, there was very clear evidence that Eli Lilly, Pfizer and SmithKline had to manipulate their data, on some occasions in breach of FDA regulations, to make the data for their individual drugs not statistically significant, as Lilly had done in the Beasley paper (4). Combining the evidence from all three drugs made the risk of suicide indisputable.

The FDA concealed these details and cleared Prozac, saying the fuss was a public relations issue and that warnings would deter people from seeking treatment (5). Up to 15% of the population in many countries now take SSRIs chronically, a large proportion of whom do so because they are physically dependent. This has happened in part because of the climate created on that day, a key feature of which was that people cannot believe the evidence of their own eyes. This climate has fostered an increasing turn to drugs as the only treatment option where once they were one option because the benefits supposedly outweigh any risks.

Clinical practice changed on September 21, 1991. After this, journals faced a choice between articles reporting RCTs or meta-analyses of RCTs, for which companies would pay handsomely for reprints, or they could publish case reports, which up till then had been the mainstream of medical publishing, but which sold few reprints. Journal lawyers began to advise against publication of articles on treatment hazards when the traditional methods of establishing cause and effect no longer seemed to apply.

Up till 2000, most prescribers had a stream of drugs' bulletins assessing new drugs and detailing their hazards, but these became unprofitable and largely vanished. Instead, clinicians had free access to Guidelines, which list drug benefits but not hazards.

As a result, it can now take 20 or 30 years for most prescribers, who have no training in how to link to link treatments to hazards, in particular doctors, to make a link between significant and common hazards and what patients report to them. And in the absence of adverse event data, just as water will flow down the most minimal of gradients in the absence of bumps, even hints of efficacy will sell drugs. Medical prescribers seem particularly poor at interpreting the evidence from RCTs in respect of benefits (6).

The adverse event literature disappeared just as adverse events became a leading cause of death. Few doctors believe scientific journals and meetings are censored, although many concede it would be politically mature to accommodate to commercial sensitivities. Journals and meetings, however, self-censor. In the 1960s, for instance, professional meetings ran entire symposia on the hazards of lithium or problems like tardive dyskinesia, but adverse events now only appear in healthcare meetings if one company is attacking the product of another and covers any liabilities organizers may be worried about.

Simply stating an RCT has not been done ends most discussions, notwithstanding the fact that once a serious hazard has been identified it would, almost by definition, be unethical to run an RCT. For instance, despite convincing epidemiological and biological evidence SSRIs increase miscarriage rates, cause cardiac and other birth defects, and lead to autistic spectrum disorder (ASD) and neurodevelopmental delay (7, 8), all companies need to do to get clinicians onside is to say no RCTs have proven these conditions are linked to our treatments.

As a result, when patients need clinicians to be able to see them, they have become invisible. The scientific job should be to decide the likeliest cause of a suicidal event, fracture, or cognitive failure, in the person who brings a problem for review. Clinical science is first and foremost judicial. If the conclusion is that treatment probably caused the event, but the academic literature gives no hint of this possibility, a second scientific task is to account for the mismatch. In attempting to do this, however, we are now up against the apparent science in a way we had not been before 1991.

In the case of the SSRIs and suicide, the mismatch stemmed from a lack of access to the data, and ghost-written articles, which documents later revealed in some trials were fraudulent. With access it became clear that the evident clinical events that patients presented with and the RCT data lined up.

4.3 ACCESS TO ADVERSE EVENT DATA

Conflict of interest is the most commonly endorsed explanation for things going wrong in clinical research. While conflict of interest is important in areas such as law and ethics, science generates data and conflicts get resolved by a requirement to account for the data. It is not possible to account for data to which we don't have free and full access.

Access to trial data was lost somewhat by accident (2). The early trials were run by universities or hospitals, often supported by companies, and the data held in a chief investigator's filing cabinet. After 1962, pharmaceuticals had to go through RCTs in order to be licensed.

In the 1960s, the pharmaceutical industry had a flood-tide of new drugs which everyone thought would continue. Management consultants, called in to advise on company structure, suggested outsourcing clinical trials, which had never been a core company activity. Running trials was outsourced to contract research organizations (CROs). Quintiles appeared in 1982, followed by Parexel and Covance. By 2010, the CRO business was worth $30 billion (2).

CROs compete for business on price, access to patients and timely completion of studies. Clinicians are paid per patient, with many patients recruited by advertisement rather than through clinical care. While having a specialized company run trials, the arrangement opens up cracks through which important data can be lost. As early as 1996, Richard Borison and Bruce Diamond from the Medical College of Georgia were jailed for recruiting non-existent patients.

In addition, where trials had previously been approved by independent institutional review boards, CROs set up privatized review systems. As the business grew and competition for patients increased, CROs moved trials out of hospitals to primary care and then to Eastern Europe, Asia, Africa, and American foster homes, jails, and lodging houses.

In these trials, people and their medical records are the raw data. Companies don't own this but claiming copyright on the thousands of pages of trial paperwork is enough. Where once academics interrogated the data, CROs cumulate and code adverse events from this paperwork, missing some events in the process. These tables of coded events are the closest anyone gets to the data.

The original paperwork is held by CROs or offshore. The denial of access to the paperwork is an exercise of force majeure without scientific, legal, or moral support. When trials are systematically reviewed the result is called EBM, but it is not data based medicine. Many assumed academ ics presenting company RCTs had access to the data. They don't. At the very least, we all assume regulators like the FDA have seen the data. They haven't.

A key question is what is data? In a trial of one antipsychotic currently on the market, a man who died had his death coded as burns. Companies are required to submit a serious adverse event (SAE) report in the case of deaths and in this case the SAE form made it possible to establish that the man had doused himself in petrol attempting suicide. He died of his burns 5 days later. Without access to the paperwork and ideally the man's medical records, or an ability to interview his family, no-one can know what happened. If science is about interrogating data, people are the data in clinical trials. Statistical outputs are statistical outputs rather than data that challenge observers to make a judgment about what has happened.

In study 329, an RCT of paroxetine compared to placebo in depressed minors, one 15-year-old boy, and three other minors, all taking paroxetine dropped out of the trial coded as "intercurrent illness." No SAE reports have to be filed for intercurrent illnesses. A few weeks after the boy started paroxetine, he was arrested in a public place, waving a gun and threatening to kill people. Someone may have decided he had a bipolar disorder and coded him appropriately as intercurrent illness, but his behavior is more likely to have been caused by paroxetine. To know what happened we have to be able to interview the individual or his family and make a judgment based on the subsequent course of events.

All pharmaceutical companies had in house medical writing divisions through to 1970. After that, just as with clinical trials, medical writing was also outsourced. By 2000, hundreds of writing agencies were competing for contracts on price per article, stature of the academic "authors," and access to prestigious journals. Many of the original companies have since become subsidiaries of public relations companies, which are in turn branches of global advertising companies such as WPP, Omnicon, and Interpublic.

By 2000, Axis Healthcare Communications offered to "brand the science." Envision Pharma recognized "data generated from clinical trials are the most powerful marketing tools available to a pharmaceutical company." GYMR claimed, "We know how to take the language of science and medicine and transform it into the more understandable language of health. We advise clients of the best dissemination strategy for their news and make sure that the message they deliver is compelling, documented and contributes to other national dialogues in a real and meaningful way" (28). Current Medical Directions delivered "scientifically accurate information strategically developed for specific target audiences". [We] "write up studies, review articles, abstracts, journal supplements, product monographs, expert commentaries and textbook chapters, conduct meta-analyses, organize journal supplements, satellite symposia, and consensus conferences as well as advisory boards for clients."

The ghost writers mostly have PhDs in a science subject. They also have codes of practice and ensure submissions meet a journal's requirement for conflict-of-interest statements and authorship declarations in a way academics often fail to do. Ghosts see themselves as resisting the overt promotion that marketing departments favor, while ensuring an article in line with a business rather than an academic timetable.

Until recently, the editors of prestigious journals regularly attend medical writer meetings and liaise with ghosts. In the 1990s, as RCTs became the currency of academic medicine, leading journals realized their influence depended on the publication of key RCTs. Given medical writers produce articles that tick all the quality boxes, avoid the excesses of the marketers, and turn around a product in a timely fashion, with a paper trail that makes for accountability, why would editors not co-operate?

Up to 2000, distinguished biomedical scientists might have authored 400 articles by their sixties. Today, marketing copy describes opinion leaders as people whose views we can trust because they have 1,000 articles to their name. When choosing names for an authorship line, companies put most store on the potential of names as advocates for the drug. For trials run in India or Africa, the authorship line may be entirely Western.

In the 1950s, ghosted articles were a small part of the literature. Today, over 90% of articles on medicines that are on-patent are written by ghosts. No independent research balances these company articles. An antidepressant will have articles festooned with statistical outputs on its use for anxiety, panic disorder, depression, dysthymia, obsessive-compulsive disorder, for children, the elderly, and women, but no articles exploring its hazards other than on trivial features where it beats its competitors (9).

4.4 RCTS AND ADVERSE EVENTS

Beyond access to RCT data, and how ghost-writers represent trial results, the nature of RCTs is in itself an issue. In legal settings, RCTs are pitched as generating generalizable evidence and knowledge that lies within confidence limits in contrast to the views of clinicians and case reports (27). They are characterized as offering gold-standard evidence, which likely leaves many clinicians thinking they offer real knowledge, even though in clinical practice translating from population or average effects to individual patients often doesn't work out.

RCTs are an operation rather than an evaluation. They were introduced in a Medical Research Council (MRC) trial of streptomycin in 1947 (2). Prior to 1947, clinical trials like a Mayo Clinic trial of streptomycin controlled for known confounders. In 1925, Ronald Fisher proposed that randomization could in principle control for unknown confounders. The MRC trial used randomization as a method for fair allocation, rather than a means of controlling for unknowns. The MRC trial missed the tolerance that develops to streptomycin and the deafness and other problems it causes, which the prior Mayo clinic trial detected (27).

RCTs brought statistical significance in their wake because Fisher argued that the only things that can interfere with expert judgment not being correct every time are unknown confounders and chance. Significance testing could control for chance and randomization for unknown confounders. Fisher's model had an anchor in the real world—an expert whose judgments were invariably correct—such as offering a view that wearing a parachute if you jump from a plane at 5,000 feet will evidently save your life unless some chance event intervenes (27).

For Fisher, experiments were a means to demonstrate that we knew what we were doing rather than a leap into the unknown. They should get the same result every time. The more prescribers know what they are doing, the more they approach Fisher's expert. This is not what RCTs are now. Company trials are assay systems rather than experiments. The results hold for the assay (provided we can access them) but they have an uncertain value for clinical practice.

Jerzy Neyman and Egon Pearson took issue with Fisher's real-world anchor—a semi-infallible expert. They borrowed from Carl Friedrich Gauss' use of confidence intervals to manage the error in astronomical measurements of stars (2, 27). Applied to imprecise measuring instruments and invariant entities like stars, confidence intervals have an anchor in the real world, helping us to decide if our varying measures reflect the presence of one or two stars. Taking successive measurements of a pulse in an individual in two emotional states is similar to determining the precise location of a star; the tighter the confidence interval bounding our measurements the more apparent we can do things reliably and that in these two emotional states pulse rates vary (27).

Confidence intervals could be used in a manner consistent with their use in astronomy to distinguish between a repeated set of pulse measurements before and during (but not after) administration of a drug to one individual (27). The presence of an attractive member of the opposite sex might introduce measurement error that confidence intervals control for. The current use of confidence intervals in RCTs is predicated on the idea that a cohort of patients in standard parallel group trials can be regarded as a single object like a galaxy. When pulses increase in response to a drug in one individual and decrease in a second in response to the same drug, however, this is not measurement error (27).

In cases like this, claiming the true effect of the drug lies near some mean of the effects in a group of individuals, potentially giving us a best estimate of no effect, is wrong (27). A mechanism to decide if we have one or two stars should not turn up the answer there are none. If the gap between Average Treatment Effects (ATE) and Heterogenous Treatment Effects (THE) is too large, the notion of ATE falls apart. In the case of stars, we knew enough about what we were doing to make reasonable inferences from varying measurements (27). We rarely know as much to make comparably reasonable inferences when prescribing medicines.

4.5 RCTS AND PRIMARY ENDPOINTS

The 1938 U.S. Food, Drugs and Cosmetics Act required pharmaceutical companies to establish the safety of their products. The birth defects thalidomide caused triggered a political crisis in 1962, in which safety needed to be seen to be enhanced. Arguing that an ineffective treatment cannot be safe, Louis Lasagna proposed companies should be required to demonstrate treatment effectiveness. The 1962 Amendments to the 1938 Act paired the word Effectiveness with Safety throughout, with two placebo-controlled RCTs as the means of demonstrating effectiveness (27).

These provisions were put in place before it was realized that demonstrating effectiveness rather than a treatment effect was not a realistic gateway to the market. In 1962, it was also assumed that RCTs offered generalizable knowledge and a positive result would invariably be replicated but this has not been borne out (27).

Before 1962, RCTs were not seen as offering gold standard knowledge about what drugs do. As Tony Hill, the person who ran the original MRC trial, put it in a 1965 lecture, RCTs have a place in the study of therapeutic efficacy, but they are only one way of doing so and any belief to the contrary is mad (11, 27). Hill's lecture ties RCTs to the investigation of one effect and places the information they yield within the framework of clinical judgment.

In medical RCTs, a focus on a primary endpoint is key to ensuring that only chance (Fisher) or measurement error (Neyman and Pearson) will get in way of the correct result (27). This means RCTs are not a good way to evaluate a medicine; a recent study of finasteride demonstrated it has over 3,700 effects on gene expression (12).

It is often assumed that the primary endpoint in an RCT is the commonest effect of a drug (27). Heterogeneity of treatment effects (HTE) leading to wider confidence intervals than are ideal can be accommodated against this background as can missing effects assumed to be rare or not appearing within the duration of the trial. But the RCT telescope is often not trained on the commonest thing a drug does. The commonest effect of an SSRI is genital anesthesia, which appears almost universally and within 30 minutes of taking a first pill (13, 27). It should not be possible to miss this when evaluating a drug, but RCTs have missed this effect because of a required focus on a primary endpoint, which in this case is the effect of commercial interest.

The attention given to measuring a primary endpoint creates an act of hypnosis in which common treatment effects can be missed entirely or given an incidental status. Casting RCTs as offering gold standard evidence about a drug, rather than one effect of the drug, therefore, creates an ignorance about the ignorance they generate (27).

RCT evidence should never trump an evident safety effect that appears after treatment. If a person becomes suicidal after taking an antidepressant, the issue of what is happening in that case is a matter of assessing the effects of their condition, circumstances, prior exposure to similar drugs, dose changes on the medication and whether there are other evident effects of treatment consistent with a link between suicidality and treatment (27).

Unless RCTs have been designed specifically to look at the effects of treatment on a possible emergence of an effect like suicidality (and there have been none), RCT evidence is irrelevant. In these circumstances, it becomes pernicious to pitch irrelevant RCTs as science that should count for more than clinical "anecdotes" containing CDR, dose response, and other evidence. The transformation of RCTs from a hurdle industry had to surmount to make gold into gold standard knowledge has made them a gold standard way to hide the hundreds of other effects a drug has (27).

4.6 POST-1962: CONFOUNDING AND CAUSALITY

Discussions of the results of epidemiological studies apparently linking drugs to treatment effects often caution that confounding by indication undercuts any easy assumption of a link. Many clinicians likely think that randomization takes care of confounding by all unknown unknowns, including by indication, with many saying RCTs demonstrate cause and effect where other epidemiological studies produce correlations (27).

Consider scenarios involving the antidepressants imipramine and paroxetine. Imipramine was discovered in 1957 and launched in 1958 without any RCT input. Among other actions, it is a serotonin reuptake inhibitor. In later RCTs, it "beat" SSRI antidepressants in trials involving patients with melancholia (severe depression). Melancholic patients are 80 times more likely to commit suicide than mildly depressed patients (27).

By 1959, clinicians praising imipramine's benefits also noted it could cause agitation and suicidality in some patients that cleared when the drug was stopped and reappeared when restarted. This Challenge-Dechallenge-Rechallenge (CDR) evidence, especially as it was replicated by several clinicians with different patients, offers close to Fisherian expert like certainty that imipramine causes suicide in certain individuals (27).

Despite being able to cause suicide, in RCTs of melancholic patients imipramine seems likely to protect against suicide on average by reducing the risk from melancholia to a greater extent than placebo. In contrast, in the RCTs that brought SSRIs to the market, these drugs doubled the rate of suicidal acts. This was because, weaker than imipramine, SSRIs had to be tested in people with mild depression at little risk of suicide. The low placebo suicidal act rate revealed the risk from the SSRI—as it does for imipramine when put into trials of mild depression. RCTs can, in other words, mislead as regards cause and effect (27).

In any trial where both condition and treatment cause superficially similar problems, RCTs can produce results all the way along a spectrum from "causes" to possible risk, likely protective and "cannot cause". This range of interpretations likely apply to a majority of trials in clinical conditions, which are Treatment Trials rather than Drug Trials (27).

Drug Trials are done on healthy volunteers, and ordinarily do not have a primary endpoint. In these, treatment effects stand out more clearly. SSRI Drug Trials in the 1980s demonstrated sexual effects were common, often debilitating, and might endure after treatment stopped, that agitation up to suicidality was common and that dependence commonly occurred after exposures of two weeks. The choice of primary endpoint in later Treatment Trials almost eliminated these effects (27).

Paroxetine was later put into Treatment Trials of patients with Major Depressive Disorder (MDD) and patients with Intermittent Brief Depressive Disorders (IBDD). IBDD patients are repeated self-harmers who can readily meet criteria for borderline personality disorder or MDD (1, 27).

In April 2006, GlaxoSmithKline (GSK) released RCT data showing an increase in suicidal events in MDD patients on paroxetine (Table). The data from IBDD RCTs in the GSK release were better. We can add 16 suicidal events to the paroxetine IBDD column below and still get an apparently protective rather than problematic result for paroxetine when MDD and IBDD data are added together (27).

This effect has been noted as a hazard of meta-analyses but it must apply to some extent in every trial that recruits patients who have a superficially similar but in fact heterogenous conditions such as depression, pain, breast cancer,

TABLE 4.1
Suicidal Events in MDD and IBDD Trials (27).

	Paroxetine	Placebo	Relative Risk
MDD Trials Acts/Patients	11/2943	0/1671	Inf (1.3, inf)
IBDD Trials Acts/Patients	32/147	35/151	0.9
Combined Acts/Patients	43/3090	35/1822	0.7

Parkinson's disease, diabetes or almost any medical disorder. Every time there is a mixture of more than one patient group in a trial, randomization will ensure some patients hide some treatment effects—good and bad. Trials of standard treatments for back pain, for instance, mask the beneficial treatment effects of an antibiotic on back pains linked to infections (up to 10% of back pains) (27).

This is Heterogeneity of Treatment Conditions (HTC) rather than HTE. In epidemiological studies confounding by indication is commonly taken to mean that we should not for example interpret results apparently associating a treatment like an antidepressant with suicidality given the possibility that depression can cause suicidality, but this effect almost certainly more commonly hides the adverse effects of treatment (27). As the example shows, it is even possible to design Treatment Trials to hide adverse effects.

A quantitative approach to data generated by algorithm rather than an approach based on judgment also increases the risk that minor events in a placebo arm will be offset against significant events in an "active" treatment arm creating an opportunity to claim that nothing specific has happened, when it has.

In 1947, treatment with medicines was viewed as therapeutic poisoning (27). In 1951, the FDA made most new medicines prescription-only on the basis that they are unavoidably risky. But from the mid-1990s, regulators have licensed drugs on the basis of a favorable risk-benefit profile. This implies a balance, in which benefits and risks can be weighed (27). There is no balance on which this can be done. One statistically significant effect is taken to count for more than all other effects, even serious effects that occur more frequently and can include death, but which by design are not significant. Poisons have been transformed into sacraments (agents from which only good can come) (27).

The statistical outputs from RCTs act like GDP (Gross Domestic Product) figures. They don't capture all the data, and in particular don't capture the data for clean air, pure water, trees, and many other things that we might think contribute more to "true" national wealth than accidents like the Exxon Valdez oil spill.

Like GDP, RCTs and EBM create an arms race where the answer to the efficacy of guns is more guns rather than a mindset that appreciates efficacy provided it is embedded in safety. An over-emphasis on efficacy means many prescribers of an antidepressant facing a patient reporting worsening depression, agitation or suicidality on treatment appear to think there is no option but to increase the dose of treatment or switch to another antidepressant, often of the same class, as nothing else is licensed to help in this situation.

Combined with an increased degree of medical specialism, another consequence of RCTs has been a loss of a sense for forensic pharmacology (toxicology). Specialists in neurology or dermatology, faced with patients who have multi-system or atypical effects following an anticonvulsant or isotretinoin, and unequipped to manage changes in other systems, are likely to diagnose these patients as having functional neurological or other disorders. There is a loss of a sense that effects not confined to one body system are a feature of drug effects, especially when a treatment is having toxic effects.

4.7 PHARMACOVIGILANCE

Pharmacovigilance came into being in the late 1960s, with the first efforts to establish adverse event reporting systems and definitions for adverse events. RCTs by then were on their way to creating the belief that they had evaluated the important effect of a drug and all other effects were rare or idiosyncratic (2).

The labels of drugs evolved to list effects noted in RCTs, most of which were deemed non-significant. Another set of other effects were included on the label under Other Effects reported to the company outside of clinical trials. The wording surrounding these is designed to suggest to readers that there may be no link to treatment.

4.8 RxISK.ORG AND PHARMACOVIGILANCE 1.0

Aware that RCTs were failing to collect the bulk of the data stemming from drug use, such as the effect of antidepressants on hair and skin, and that RCTs discarding much of the data they did collect, the focus of Data Based Medicine, when it was created, was to bring the missing data into view. Over 90% of the data was going missing and much of it like clear air, pure water, and trees might be of greater importance to the takers of medicine than the effects they were being told about.

RxISK.org, an adverse event reporting site, was created. Visitors to RxISK.org were invited to list their drugs and report events linked to their treatment, after which they were taken through a set of questions derived from the Naranjo algorithm designed to give them a score as to whether the effect they reported was likely linked to their drug or not.

Sample RxISK Summary Report (29):

RxISK report ID: R16-8dcddf

Thank you for completing a RxISK report. This report includes a causality assessment in the form of a RxISK score together with details of how it was calculated. See the attached PDF file for the full report.

Suspect drug: SSRI not sure which

You describe the primary side effect as: I took fluoxetine for a 1.5 years. Zoloft 7 days and lexapro 1 month and I had side effects on all of them that were very mild. Then I took citalopram for 8 days and then stopped taking it and 1 week later after stopping I got blunted emotions and sexual dysfunction.

You link the primary side effect to: Stopping the drug

RxISK score

Your RxISK score is: 9

RxISK score guide:

0–4—Not enough information to confirm a link

5–8—Likely link between medicine and side effect

9 +—Strong possibility of a link between medication and side effect

This report is designed to be used in conversation with your doctor or pharmacist on the possible linkage between the suspect drug and the primary side effect. You can also invite them to add to your RxISK report to indicate whether they agree that there is a linkage: http://rxisk.org/hcp-comment/(they will need the RxISK report ID from the top of this report).

Thank you for helping make medicines safer for all of us.

Dr. David Healy & Dr. Dee Mangin

Data Based Medicine Americas Ltd.

David Braley Health Sciences Centre

McMaster University

Hamilton, ON

Canada L8P 1H6

Armed with a report from a respectable site, we hoped people with an adverse effect would feel able to raise problems with their prescriber, as clearly many were nervous about doing so. Levelling the playing field might help get a problem managed early. If the prescriber took up the patient's invitation to submit a report also, this process might enable RxISK to map out prescribers who listen and offer a quality mark for those who did. We envisaged offering this system to pharmacist, nurse, clinical psychology as well as medical prescribers.

However, even armed with a RxISK report, most patients find doctors too intimidating to approach. Many patients with conditions like Post-SSRI Sexual Dysfunction (PSSD) who are desperate and commonly contemplating drastic measures like suicide or medical assistance in dying, have faced ridicule from doctors (14). Presenting a RxISK report and peer-reviewed articles about the condition has in a few instances led to a more sympathetic response but rarely to an endorsement of the validity of what the patient is saying.

In addition to producing a causality index, the RxISK form has a section from which the economic cost of an adverse event can be calculated, along with sections on impact on a life and trip-advisor options—would you recommend this medicine to others?

TABLE 4.2
RxISK Causality Questions (29).

Question	Answer	Score
Did the side effect start before or after REDUCING the dose of the drug?	Side effect started after reducing the dose	3
Was the side effect different from the original condition for which the drug was prescribed?	Different from the original condition	2
Did the side effect start after STOPPING the drug?	Side effect started or got worse after stopping	2
Did the side effect improve or clear up if the person RESTARTED the drug?	Didn't restart	0
Did the side effect improve if the person INCREASED the dose of the drug?	Didn't increase the dose	0
How soon after RESTARTING the drug or INCREASING the dose did the problem improve?	Didn't restart the drug or increase the dose	0
Did the problem improve on a related drug?	Didn't try a related drug	0
Has the person ever experienced the SAME side effect on STOPPING another drug? (If the experience was different in any way answer "No.")	No	.0
Has the person ever experienced any OTHER side effects on STOPPING another drug?	No	0
Could anything else be causing this side effect?	Don't know	0
Are there previous reports of side effects on STOPPING the drug in the RxISK database or in a drug regulator database (e.g., FDA, Health Canada, Yellow Card) or elsewhere?	Yes	2
Total:		9

Unlike other pharmacovigilance systems, RxISK doesn't shrink from making causal connections. It has helped put Post-SSRI Sexual Dysfunction (PSSD) on the map and linked this to similar problems following finasteride and isotretinoin and a mirror image condition Persistent Genital Arousal Disorder (PGAD) (14). In 2019, following representations from RxISK, the European Medicines Agency (EMA) requested companies to add a mention of persistent sexual dysfunction to their labels. Health Canada followed suit.

RxISK has also raised the profile of antidepressant induced alcoholism as well as increased blood alcohol levels on treatment (15, 16). A further paper reports on unrecognized visual effects of antidepressant treatment (17).

As RxISK developed, we became aware that pharmaceutical companies were outsourcing their pharmacovigilance divisions. There are a number of reasons for this.

Since the 1950s, pharmacovigilance has been a legal requirement for pharmaceutical companies, just as autovigilance is for motor manufactures. If an automobile maker becomes aware of a potential hazard, they recall the vehicle and repair any defect. In the case of a pharmaceutical company, remedying the problem means adding anything thought to be causally linked to their treatment to the drug's label. Establishing causality means companies are obliged to track down anyone who reports an adverse event to them.

While concerned about adverse events from the 1950s, the FDA only created MedWatch, an Adverse Event Reporting System in 1993. This was initially aimed at doctors and companies. It was revamped in 2004, and in 2010 the public were also encouraged to report. In 2014, the FDA created a public facing website that allows everyone to see the reports sent to them. The bulk of reports come from companies to whom patients or clinicians have reported problems. In other countries, reports are more likely to come from doctors. But no country does anything with enthusiasm. The FDA state that little more than 1% of serious adverse events are reported to them.

All regulators categorize these reports as anecdotes or hearsay and caution against inferring causality. A prime reason for the inability to establish causality is that regulators remove any names of patients from reports and do not track the patients down or attempt to establish causality. Nameless subjects cannot be invited into court to be cross-examined about any event. Rather than being good evidence, reports with names removed are no longer evidence, they have become hearsay.

Reporting to regulators is at present meaningless. The failure of their reports to make a difference, rather than any remiss behavior on the part of doctors or other prescribers, may explain why there is such a low rate of reporting of even serious events.

In 2007, company prepared prescription drug package inserts and company websites began encouraging prescribers and others to report adverse events to the FDA's MedWatch scheme. Companies find Direct-to-Company communication from patients is awkward. It can force a company to add a warning to their label, if the company decides their drug has caused an adverse event. The judgment that there is a causal link becomes more likely if the event is followed up to see what happened when treatment stops, or on re-exposure.

Manufacturers are obliged to follow up reports that come to them. They commonly decide there is a causal link, and at that point, they add a mention of the problem to the drug label, in the section for Other Effects. Most prescribers and patients have the impression that reports in this section, placed as it is below the adverse effects noted in RCTs, are from Flat Earthers or others hostile to medicines and pay little heed to them, when in fact little gets included here unless companies have not been able to find another way to explain it away.

The FDA, in contrast, is unable to follow events because reports to them are anonymized. Encouraging patients and prescribers to report directly to MedWatch sounds as though companies are avoiding a conflict of interest, but it makes the recognition of a causal link between a hazard and a drug less likely. People get paid to notice how to game the system in ways prescribers and patients are unlikely to spot.

Although anonymized, reports to the FDA are useful. They are like the data exhaust we leave behind on social media. They can be analyzed using a number of functions developed to exploit the idea of proportional reporting ratios. Does Drug X have more reports of a particular problem, as a proportion of all reports on it, compared with this problem reported as a function of all reports on all other drugs. Reporting ratios generated in this way can offer a useful signal of problems.

Reporting ratios can also offer a possible business model for companies offering to undertake a parent company's pharmacovigilance. Analyzing data exhaust streams, like MedWatch data, enables pharmacovigilance companies to let pharmaceutical companies know what the profile of their drug looks like compared to comparators.

Companies like Advera and eHealthMe, supported by adverts, have made a business of this, while the Institute for Safe Medication Practices issues quarterly bulletins on new treatments or new problems based on analyzing these reports.

Another group of companies like PatientsLikeMe and Sermo have pitched the conversations that happen on their sites about the treatment of various conditions as offering important insights on medicines that might inform pharmaceutical companies, ostensibly for pharmacovigilance purposes but in practice more likely for marketing purposes.

We presented the RxISK model to health insurers like United HealthCare, offering the evidence that nipping treatment induced problems in the bud could reduce outpatient and inpatient costs. But there was no uptake.

We presented the model to generic pharmaceutical companies making the case that RxISK might enable generic companies to produce not only less expensive but also better drugs. The argument is that given a drug is a chemical with information on how to use it to best advantage, an instrument like RxISK could help produce more and better information, and in so doing make the generic a better drug than the branded one. But there was no uptake.

We presented the model to pharmaceutical companies, once termed branded but now rebranded as research intensive, as enabling them to discover new drugs. But there was no uptake.

We prepared versions of RxISK's offer for nurse and pharmacist prescribers but to date have had no uptake (available on request).

Around 2015, it seemed to make sense to go in a somewhat different direction and this led to TaperMD outlined below.

4.9 PHARMACOSURVEILLANCE

In addition to pharmacovigilance, pharmaceutical companies are supposed to engage in post-marketing surveillance of their drugs. This commonly means setting up phase IV trials. These are widely seen as offering opportunities to market products rather than the safety exercises they are supposed to be.

The creation of health apps in recent years has opened up new possibilities for surveillance. These apps track their users vital and not so vital functions, from the number of steps taken, to sleep duration and quality, heart rate, and flickers of emotions or moods. While data like this might shed light on hazards, if generated by companies at one remove from parent pharmaceutical companies, the risks to the pharmaceutical company can be managed, while companies can also dismiss such adverse events as not generated in controlled trials.

All data however open up market opportunities, and drugs in particular can be pitched as the answer to aberrant health data.

It looks likely that psychedelics when marketed will come with Apps (MyDelica for example), purporting to make their use safer. The problem with psychedelics for pharmaceutical companies is that these drugs are old and require minimal daily intake. The need is to find a model that can be used to add value to the product, allowing an extra charge, which in this case would have the added benefit of yielding data potentially supporting further use of mainstream medicines.

It seems possible that vaccines could follow suit, especially a suite of vaccines being developed for behavioral purposes, such as managing drug addiction. No App, no Jab, no Job may be the future.

4.10 TAPERMD AND PHARMACOVIGILANCE 2.0

First generation pharmacovigilance was based on case reports and case series, supplemented with epidemiological studies. It focused on dramatic but relatively uncommon events and brought problems like treatment-induced hepatic failure, severe skin reactions, neuroleptic malignant syndrome, blood dyscrasias, and hypersensitivity reactions into focus (18).

Important although these adverse effects are, falls leading to fractures, confusion, fatigue, and hemorrhages are more common and more important in terms of disability and mortality than idiosyncratic adverse events.

Falls, confusion, and bleeding events, however, occur more commonly against a background of multiple medications. In these circumstances, traditional pharmacovigilance, which works best where there is one treatment and one event, breaks down.

Traditional pharmacovigilance linked events to treatment, which companies included in drug labels. Second generation pharmacovigilance is a safety matter for health systems. Heavy medication burdens almost certainly lead to more hospitalizations and premature deaths than the conditions for which the individual medicines in a treatment cocktail are given.

Polypharmacy became a systemic problem in the 1980s when companies discovered risk prevention, often called chronic disease, or non-communicable disease, management. This discovery offered companies a chance to promote the treatment of relatively minor changes in risk factors such as blood pressure, blood sugar, bone density, peak flow rates, or variations on behavioral rating scales. With the creation of guidelines for disease management, based on a ghost-written literature with no access to trial data, which advocated treatment with medicines, there was a dramatic increase in the number of medicines people took. We moved from being on less that one medicine per day, in the early eighties, to over 40% of those over forty-five now being on three medicines every day, and over 40% of those over sixty-five being on five medicines per day (2).

These increases in medication do not happen just with age. They are growing on a cohort basis; younger people today are on vastly more medicines than people of the comparable age were several decades ago. Some of these medicines are psychotropics and will be difficult to stop.

Polypharmacy was noted as a hazard in its own right in the late 1990s. The first suggestion that it might be appropriate to reduce medication burdens, to deprescribe, came in 2003 (19). In 2010, Garfinkel and Mangin demonstrated that it was feasible to reduce medication burdens from 10 or more drugs toward 5 and that this appeared to reduce hospitalizations, extend life, and improve quality of life (20).

The efficacy of treatments came into the frame in 1962 for the contribution it might make to safety. Since 1990, however, with the primacy of RCTs and a focus on efficacy endpoints, safety has been displaced. The evidence on reducing medication burdens now reintroduces safety for the contribution it might make to efficacy. As with the arms race, when it comes to medication, efficacy has its limits. To get the greatest benefit from medicines, we may need to be on less rather than more and it makes sense for patient values to shape the choice of what is retained.

In 2015, based primarily on Dee Mangin's research, this thinking led data-based medicine to develop TaperMD, a clinical decision support tool.

TaperMD was envisaged as an app that could be free-standing or incorporated in an Electronic Medical Record (EMR). Its public facing dashboard shows all the medicines a person is on, and a set of the most significant treatment hazards linked to polypharmacy such as falls, confusion, anticholinergic burden, or serotonergic burden. Sample patient data from TaperMD is shown in Figure 4.1. Once a person's drugs are entered the dashboard automatically shows whether they are on two, three, four or more drugs that might increase any of these risks such as falls or anti-cholinergic burden.

Since 2015, there has been a growing amount of talk about deprescribing. Very little of this talk has any effect. Medication burdens are growing rapidly, particularly in younger people. There are a number of platforms—the University of British Columbia linked MedStopper, Optum Health's ScriptSwitch, and others aiming to feed into this.

In an era of EMRs, talk about deprescribing doesn't lead to deprescribing unless built into an EMR or a medication review process. TaperMD is the only clinical decision support tool at present that is evidence based with preliminary

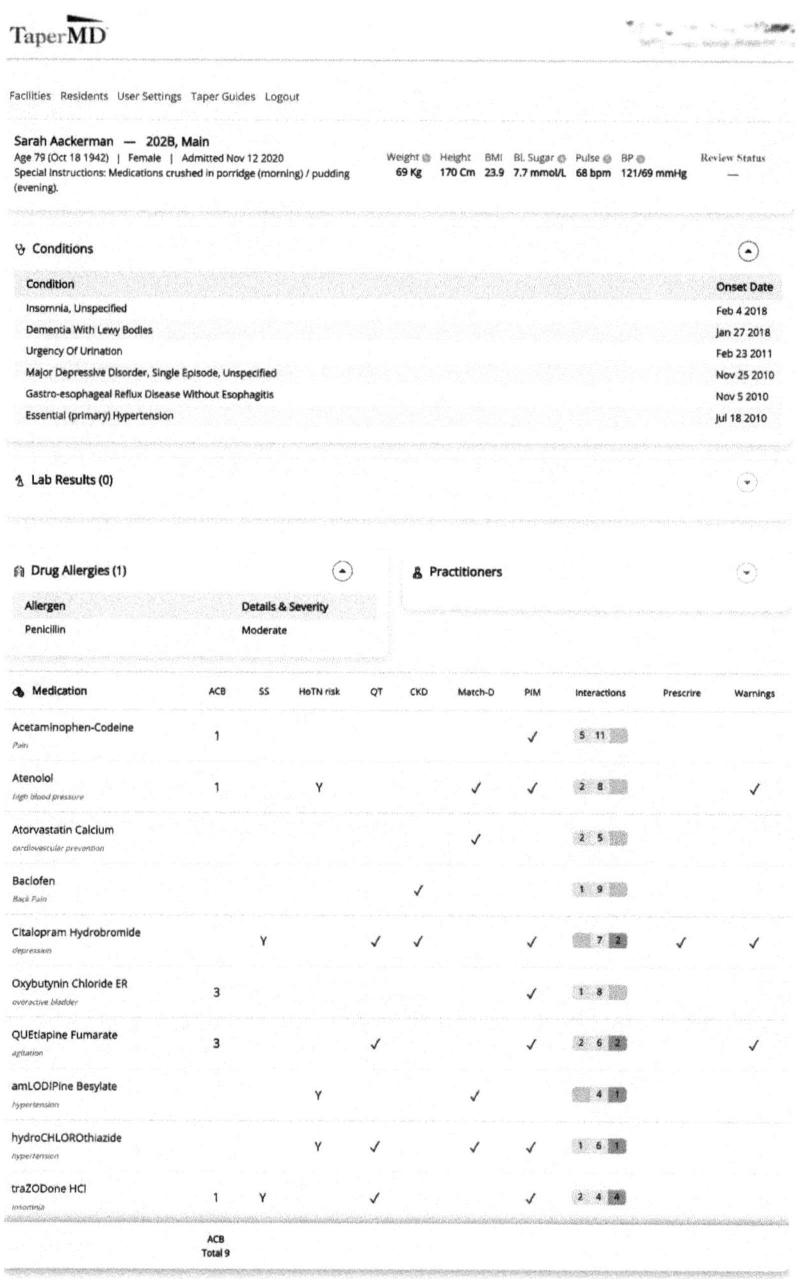

FIGURE 4.1 TaperMD Sample Patient Data.

trial results (21, 22) and several RCTs in progress in Canada and Australia due to complete data collection in 2021.

There are a growing number of studies aimed at reducing inappropriate medicines in older subjects, which in general show that a reduction in hospital admissions accompanies reducing medication burden but not dramatically so, suggesting more work is needed to identify the patient groups most likely to benefit (23). Of note also are several studies indicating that a greater medication burden is linked to increased rates of death from Covid (24, 25).

TaperMD made contact with a large Canadian EMR company in 2018 and has since developed links to other EMR companies. It has also established contact with Canadian pharmacy chains and Canadian Health Insurers.

Pharmacists are the profession most engaged in medication review. TaperMD established links with the American Society of Consultant Pharmacists in 2018 and has collaborated with them in developing lists of Potentially Inappropriate Medicines (PIMS) (25).

At present, medication burdens are primarily an older person's issue, and long-term care (LTC) facilities are arguably the best place to test whether medication review actually makes a difference. TaperMD is actively engaged with partners in pilot schemes in Canada LTC facilities as well as in New Zealand and Australia.

In an ideal world, pharmacists, who in many jurisdictions can get paid for medication reviews, would use TaperMD to reduce medication burdens in the elderly. Everyone needs data on the feasibility of reducing medication burdens, which medicines can be reduced, what strategies work best, and whether reductions make a substantial difference. Use of TaperMD can generate such data en passant.

Demonstrations of this sort do not necessarily map onto the priorities of pharmacy chains, unless the arrangements with LTC facilities hinge on the quality of pharmacy services rather than the amount of medicines provided, or other benefits. Similarly, having more alert patients may not be in the interest of LTC facilities, who may also prefer cheaper medicines rather than quality services.

Pharmacy chains similarly may be more interested to use clinical decision support tools to standardize pharmacist input, make review processes more efficient, or switch from branded medicines to generics, than in actually achieving a reduction of medication burdens or improved quality of life. TaperMD's pharmacist review and recommendations to prescribers segue into a discussion between prescriber and patient module, which can lead to medication reductions on a pause-and-monitor basis.

It is not yet clear how this will play out with older patients and even less so with younger patients where medical consumerism is still an incoming tide.

While TaperMD aims at facilitating conversations between patient, family, pharmacist, and prescriber, it seems useful also to build a degree of artificial intelligence (AI) into the process. This may reveal that we know less about deprescribing than we might think, about both the values of different stakeholders and the process itself. With AI, Taper would offer an opportunity to build a system based on data. This comes with a risk that a data-driven, algorithmic system might supplant the original intention to foster conversations based on shared values.

There are other options for decision support tools like TaperMD. The Covid pandemic has opened up clinical consults by video. One option for a tool providing decision support in respect of medication burdens is to link with one of the increasing number of platforms providing clinical services.

Finally at present, the TaperMD dashboard refers to anticholinergic, serotonergic, and other burdens. This speaks to professionals. It could be turned around to focus on the commonest patient complaints, from falls to confusion, fatigue, weight gain and others. This could be public facing and lead to a much greater awareness among the public of the deleterious impacts heavy medication burdens may be having on their lives, prompting consults with pharmacists in the first instance and then prescribers.

A public facing version of TaperMD would draw wider attention to the ways in which medication burdens can compromise a person's quality of life. It incentivizes people to seek out consult with pharmacists or doctors in person, or through online services, about how these burdens might be lessened.

This would be a people driven medication reduction, aimed at changing the climate of healthcare over time, in contrast to an expert driven approach, which has led to a relentless increase in the consumption of both medicines and tests. The footfall on the TaperMD site that leads to further development would be quite different in both instances.

4.11 SUMMARY AND CONCLUSIONS

Technological platforms, like RxISK or TaperMD, are inherently unidimensional, whereas living with conditions and on medicines is multidimensional. The technology can be optimized. However, just as one of the 100 things a drug does can be optimized but not all of them, technology platforms can be optimized with respect to one function such as standardizing pharmacist medication reviews or making the process more efficient or more likely to support patient safety.

REFERENCES

1. Healy D, Mangin D, Antonuccio D. Data based medicine & clinical judgement. Int J Risk Saf Med. 2013;25:111–121. With commentary by Edwards R. Data and evidence, there is a difference. Int J Risk Saf Med. 2013;25:123–129.
2. Healy D. *The Shipwreck of the Singular: Healthcare's Castaways*. Toronto: Samizdat-Health, 2019.
3. Teicher MH, Glod C, Cole JO. Emergence of intense suicidal preoccupation during fluoxetine treatment. Am J Psychiatry. 1990;147(2):207–210.
4. Beasley CM, Dornseif BE, Bosomworth JC, Sayler ME, Rampey AH, Heiligenstein JH, Thomson VL, Murphy DJ, Masica DN. Fluoxetine and suicide: A meta-analysis of controlled trials of treatment for depression. Br Med J. 1991;303:685–692.

5. Healy D, Le Noury J, Wood J. *Children of the Cure*. Toronto: Samizdat-Health, 2020.
6. Morgan DJ, Pineles L, Owczarzak J, Magder L, Scherer L, Brown JP, Pfeiffer C, Terndrup C, Leykum L, Feldstein D, Foy A. Clinician conceptualization of the benefits of treatments for individual patients. JAMA Netw Open. 2021;4:e2119747.
7. Healy D, Mangin D, Mintzes B. The ethics of randomized placebo controlled trials of antidepressants with pregnant women. Int J Risk Saf Med. 2010;22:7–16. doi:10.3233/JRS-2010-0487.
8. Healy D, Le Noury J, Mangin D. Links between serotonin reuptake inhibition pregnancy & neurodevelopmental delay spectrum disorders: A review of epidemiological and physiological evidence. Int J Risk Saf Med. 2016;28:125–141. doi:10.3233/JRS-160726.
9. Healy D, Cattell D. The interface between authorship, industry and science in the domain of therapeutics. Br J Psychiatry. 2003;182:22–27.
10. Howell S, Song W, Pastuszak A, Khera M. Differential gene expression in post-finasteride syndrome patients. J Sex Med. 2021;18:1479–1490.
11. Healy D. Antidepressants and sexual dysfunction, a history. J R Soc Med. 2020;113:133–135.
12. Healy D, Le Noury J, Mangin D. Post-SSRI sexual dysfunction: Patient experiences of engagement with healthcare professionals. Int J Risk Saf Med. 2019;31:1–7. doi:10.3233/JRS-191005.
13. Healy D, Le Noury J, Mangin D. Enduring sexual dysfunction after treatment with antidepressants, 5α-reductase inhibitors and isotretinoin: 300 cases. Int J Risk Saf Med. 2019;30:167–178.
14. Healy D, Atigari OV, Kelly AM, Jabeen Q. New onset alcohol dependence linked to treatment with selective serotonin reuptake inhibitors. Int J Risk Saf Med. 2013;25:105–109.
15. Healy D, Brookwell L, Hogan C, Mangin D. Ninety-three cases of alcohol dependence following SSRI treatment. Int J Risk Saf Med. 2014;26:99–107.
16. Healy D, Mangin D, Lochead J. Development and persistence of patient reported visual problems associated with serotonin reuptake inhibiting antidepressants. Int J Risk Saf Med. 2022;33(1):37–47.
17. Laporte J-R. Fifty years of pharmacovigilance: Medicines safety and public health. Pharmacoepidemiol Drug Saf. 2016;25:725–732.
18. Woodward MC. Deprescribing: Achieving better health outcomes for older people through reducing medicines. J Pharm Pract Res. 2003;33:323–328.
19. Garfinkel D, Mangin D. Feasibility study of a systematic approach for discontinuation of multiple medications in older adults. Arch Intern Med. 2010;170:1648–1654.
20. Parkinson L, Magin P, Etherton-Beer C, Naganathan V, Mangin D. Engaging general practice and patients with AusTAPER, a pharmacist facilitated web-based deprescribing tool. J Pharm Pract Res. 2021;51:154–159.
21. Blum MR, Sallevelt BT, Spinewine A, O'Mahony D, Moutzouri E, Feller M, Baumgartner C, Roumet M, Jungo KT, Schwab N, Bretagne L. Optimizing therapy to prevent avoidable hospital admissions in multi-morbid older adults. BMJ. 2021;374:n1585.
22. Wu H, Kouladjian O'Donnell L, Fujita K, Masnoon N, Hilmer SN. Deprescribing in the older patient. Int J Geriatr Med. 2021;14:3793–3807.
23. Ottenhoff MC, Ramos LA, Potters W, Janssen ML, Hubers D, Hu S, Fridgeirsson EA, Piña-Fuentes D, Thomas R, van der Horst IC, Herff C. Predicting mortality of individual patients with Covid-19. BMJ Open. 2021;11:e047347.
24. McKeigue PM, Kennedy S, Weir A, Bishop J, McGurnaghan SJ, McAllister D, Robertson C, Wood R, Lone N, Murray J, Caparrotta TM. Associations of severe Covid-19 with polypharmacy and the prescribing of psychotropic drugs in the REACT-SCOT case control study. BMC Med. 2021;19:51.
25. Healy D. The fault lies in our stars. https://davidhealy.org/the-fault-lies-in-our-stars/
26. Healy D. Manufacturing consensus. Cult Med Psychiatry. 2006;30(2):135–156. doi:10.1007/s11013-006-9013-3.
27. Complete a RxISK report. https://rxisk.org/complete-a-rxisk-report/

5 Important Code of Federal Regulations Applicable to Drug Product Liability Suits

S. Albert Edwards

SYNOPSIS

5.1 §20.61 TRADE SECRETS AND COMMERCIAL OR FINANCIAL INFORMATION WHICH IS PRIVILEGED OR CONFIDENTIAL

(a) A trade secret may consist of any commercially valuable plan, formula, process, or device that is used for the making, preparing, compounding, or processing of trade commodities and that can be said to be the end product of either innovation or substantial effort. There must be a direct relationship between the trade secret and the productive process.

(b) Commercial or financial information that is privileged or confidential means valuable data or information which is used in one's business and is of a type customarily held in strict confidence or regarded as privileged and not disclosed to any member of the public by the person to whom it belongs.

(c) Data and information submitted or divulged to the Food and Drug Administration which fall within the definitions of a trade secret or confidential commercial or financial information are not available for public disclosure.

(d) A person who submits records to the Government may designate part or all of the information in such records as exempt from disclosure under exemption 4 of the Freedom of Information Act.

DOI: 10.1201/9781003615323-6

TABLE 5.1
Topics and Associated Code of Federal Regulation Citations

Adverse event reporting	310.305, 312.32, & 314.80
Approved drug, adverse event reports	314.80
Confidential, trade secret information	20.61
Investigational drug, adverse event reports	312.32
Informed consent, elements required	50.25
Informed consent, required documents	50.27
Institutional Review Boards, IRBs	56.109
Labeling, approved drug	201.56 & 201.57
Labeling, changes prior to FDA approval	314.70(c)(6)(iii)
Labeling, changes to promotional labeling	314.70(a)(4)
Labeling, older drugs, approved before June 30, 2006	201.80
Mailing important information on drugs	200.5
Marketed drug, adverse events reports	310.305
National Drug Code, requested vs required	201.2
OTC drug, identity statement	201.61
OTC drug, labeling format/content req.	201.66
OTC drug, meeting monograph standards	330.1
OTC drug, net contents declaration	201.62
OTC drug, pregnancy, breast feeding	201.63
OTC drug, sodium labeling	201.64
Pregnancy, breast feeding, OTC drug	201.63
Pregnancy, lactation, breast feeding, labor, and delivery, prescription drug labeling	201.57(i)
Review of research, IRB duties	56.109
Side effect reporting, approved drugs	314.80
Side effect reporting, investigational drugs	312.32
Side effect reporting, marketed drug	310.305
Side effect reporting, unapproved drug	310.305
Trade secret, confidential information	20.61
Unapproved drugs, side effect reporting	310.305

The person may make this designation either at the time the records are submitted to the Government or within a reasonable time thereafter. The designation must be in writing. Where a legend is required by a request for proposals or request for quotations, pursuant to 48 CFR 352.215-12, then that legend is necessary for this purpose. Any such designation will expire 10 years after the records were submitted to the Government.

(e) The procedures in this paragraph apply to records on which the submitter has designated information as provided in paragraph (d) of this section. These procedures also apply to records that were submitted to the Food and Drug Administration when the agency has substantial reason to believe that information in the records could reasonably be considered exempt under exemption 4 of the Freedom of Information Act. Certain exceptions to these procedures are set forth in paragraph (f) of this section.

(1) When the Food and Drug Administration receives a request for such records and determines that disclosure may be required, the Food and Drug Administration will make reasonable efforts to notify the submitter about these facts. The notice will include a copy of the request, and it will inform the submitter about the procedures and time limits for submission and consideration of objections to disclosure. If the Food and Drug Administration must notify a large number of submitters, notification may be done by posting or publishing a notice in a place where the submitters are reasonably likely to become aware of it.

(2) The submitter has 10 working days from the date of the notice to object to disclosure of any part of the records and to state all bases for its objections. The Division of Freedom of Information may extend this period as appropriate and necessary.

(3) The Food and Drug Administration will give consideration to all bases that have been stated in a timely manner by the submitter. If the Food and Drug Administration decides to disclose the records, the Food and Drug Administration will notify the submitter in writing. This notice will briefly explain why the agency did not sustain the submitter's objections. The Food and Drug Administration will include with the notice a copy of the records about which the submitter objected, as the agency proposes to disclose them. The notice will state that the Food and Drug Administration intends to disclose the records 5 working days after the submitter receives the notice unless a U.S. District Court orders the agency not to release them.

(4) If a requester files suit under the Freedom of Information Act to obtain records covered by this paragraph, the Food and Drug Administration will promptly notify the submitter.

(5) Whenever the Food and Drug Administration sends a notice to a submitter under paragraph (e)(1) of this section, the Food and Drug Administration will notify the requester that the Food and Drug Administration is giving the submitter a notice and an opportunity to object. Whenever the Food and Drug Administration sends a notice to a submitter under paragraph (e)(3) of this section, the Food and Drug Administration will notify the requester of this fact.

(f) The notice requirements in paragraph (e) of this section do not apply in the following situations:

(1) The Food and Drug Administration decided not to disclose the records;

(2) The information has previously been published or made generally available;
(3) Disclosure is required by a regulation issued after notice and opportunity for public comment, that specifies narrow categories of records that are to be disclosed under the Freedom of Information Act, but in this case a submitter may still designate records as described in paragraph (d) of this section, and in exceptional cases, the Food and Drug Administration may, at its discretion, follow the notice procedures in paragraph (e) of this section;
(4) The information requested has not been designated by the submitter as exempt from disclosure when the submitter had an opportunity to do so at the time of submission of the information or within a reasonable time thereafter, unless the Food and Drug Administration has substantial reason to believe that disclosure of the information would result in competitive harm; or
(5) The designation appears to be obviously frivolous, but in this case the Food and Drug Administration will still give the submitter the written notice required by paragraph (e)(3) of this section (although this notice need not explain our decision or include a copy of the records), and the Food and Drug Administration will notify the requester as described in paragraph (e)(5) of this section.

5.2 §50.25 ELEMENTS OF INFORMED CONSENT

(a) *Basic elements of informed consent.* In seeking informed consent, the following information shall be provided to each subject:
(1) A statement that the study involves research, an explanation of the purposes of the research and the expected duration of the subject's participation, a description of the procedures to be followed, and identification of any procedures which are experimental.
(2) A description of any reasonably foreseeable risks or discomforts to the subject.
(3) A description of any benefits to the subject or to others which may reasonably be expected from the research.
(4) A disclosure of appropriate alternative procedures or courses of treatment, if any, that might be advantageous to the subject.
(5) A statement describing the extent, if any, to which confidentiality of records identifying the subject will be maintained and that notes the possibility that the Food and Drug Administration may inspect the records.
(6) For research involving more than minimal risk, an explanation as to whether any compensation and an explanation as to whether any medical treatments are available if injury occurs and, if so, what they consist of, or where further information may be obtained.
(7) An explanation of whom to contact for answers to pertinent questions about the research and research subjects' rights, and whom to contact in the event of a research-related injury to the subject.
(8) A statement that participation is voluntary, that refusal to participate will involve no penalty or loss of benefits to which the subject is otherwise entitled, and that the subject may discontinue participation at any time without penalty or loss of benefits to which the subject is otherwise entitled.

(b) *Additional elements of informed consent.* When appropriate, one or more of the following elements of information shall also be provided to each subject:
(1) A statement that the particular treatment or procedure may involve risks to the subject (or to the embryo or fetus, if the subject is or may become pregnant) which are currently unforeseeable.
(2) Anticipated circumstances under which the subject's participation may be terminated by the investigator without regard to the subject's consent.
(3) Any additional costs to the subject that may result from participation in the research.
(4) The consequences of a subject's decision to withdraw from the research and procedures for orderly termination of participation by the subject.
(5) A statement that significant new findings developed during the course of the research which may relate to the subject's willingness to continue participation will be provided to the subject.
(6) The approximate number of subjects involved in the study.

(c) When seeking informed consent for applicable clinical trials, as defined in 42 U.S.C. 282(j)(1)(A), the following statement shall be provided to each clinical trial subject in informed consent documents and processes. This will notify the clinical trial subject that clinical trial information has been or will be submitted for inclusion in the clinical trial registry databank under paragraph (j) of section 402 of the Public Health Service Act. The statement is: "A description of this clinical trial will be available on http://www.ClinicalTrials.gov, as required by U.S. Law. This Web site will not include information that can identify you. At most, the Web site will include a summary of the results. You can search this Web site at any time."

(d) The informed consent requirements in these regulations are not intended to preempt any applicable Federal, State, or local laws which require additional information to be disclosed for informed consent to be legally effective.

(e) Nothing in these regulations is intended to limit the authority of a physician to provide emergency medical care to the extent the physician is permitted to do so under applicable Federal, State, or local law.

5.3 §50.27 DOCUMENTATION OF INFORMED CONSENT

(a) Except as provided in §56.109(c), informed consent shall be documented by the use of a written consent form approved by the IRB and signed and dated by the subject or the subject's legally authorized representative at the time of consent. A copy shall be given to the person signing the form.

(b) Except as provided in §56.109(c), the consent form may be either of the following:

  (1) A written consent document that embodies the elements of informed consent required by §50.25. This form may be read to the subject or the subject's legally authorized representative, but, in any event, the investigator shall give either the subject or the representative adequate opportunity to read it before it is signed.

  (2) A *short form* written consent document stating that the elements of informed consent required by §50.25 have been presented orally to the subject or the subject's legally authorized representative. When this method is used, there shall be a witness to the oral presentation. Also, the IRB shall approve a written summary of what is to be said to the subject or the representative. Only the short form itself is to be signed by the subject or the representative. However, the witness shall sign both the short form and a copy of the summary, and the person actually obtaining the consent shall sign a copy of the summary. A copy of the summary shall be given to the subject or the representative in addition to a copy of the short form.

5.4 §56.109 IRB REVIEW OF RESEARCH

(a) An IRB shall review and have authority to approve, require modifications in (to secure approval), or disapprove all research activities covered by these regulations.

(b) An IRB shall require that information given to subjects as part of informed consent is in accordance with §50.25. The IRB may require that information, in addition to that specifically mentioned in §50.25, be given to the subjects when in the IRB's judgment the information would meaningfully add to the protection of the rights and welfare of subjects.

(c) An IRB shall require documentation of informed consent in accordance with §50.27 of this chapter, except as follows:

  (1) The IRB may, for some or all subjects, waive the requirement that the subject, or the subject's legally authorized representative, sign a written consent form if it finds that the research presents no more than minimal risk of harm to subjects and involves no procedures for which written consent is normally required outside the research context; or

  (2) The IRB may, for some or all subjects, find that the requirements in §50.24 of this chapter for an exception from informed consent for emergency research are met.

(d) In cases where the documentation requirement is waived under paragraph (c)(1) of this section, the IRB may require the investigator to provide subjects with a written statement regarding the research.

(e) An IRB shall notify investigators and the institution in writing of its decision to approve or disapprove the proposed research activity, or of modifications required to secure IRB approval of the research activity. If the IRB decides to disapprove a research activity, it shall include in its written notification a statement of the reasons for its decision and give the investigator an opportunity to respond in person or in writing. For investigations involving an exception to informed consent under §50.24 of this chapter, an IRB shall promptly notify in writing the investigator and the sponsor of the research when an IRB determines that it cannot approve the research because it does not meet the criteria in the exception provided under §50.24(a) of this chapter or because of other relevant ethical concerns. The written notification shall include a statement of the reasons for the IRB's determination.

(f) An IRB shall conduct continuing review of research covered by these regulations at intervals appropriate to the degree of risk, but not less than once per year, and shall have authority to observe or have a third party observe the consent process and the research.

(g) An IRB shall provide in writing to the sponsor of research involving an exception to informed consent under §50.24 of this chapter a copy of information that has been publicly disclosed under

§50.24(a)(7)(ii) and (a)(7)(iii) of this chapter. The IRB shall provide this information to the sponsor promptly so that the sponsor is aware that such disclosure has occurred. Upon receipt, the sponsor shall provide copies of the information disclosed to FDA.

(h) When some or all of the subjects in a study are children, an IRB must determine that the research study is in compliance with part 50, subpart D of this chapter, at the time of its initial review of the research. When some or all of the subjects in a study that was ongoing on April 30, 2001, are children, an IRB must conduct a review of the research to determine compliance with part 50, subpart D of this chapter, either at the time of continuing review or, at the discretion of the IRB, at an earlier date.

5.5 §200.5 MAILING OF IMPORTANT INFORMATION ABOUT DRUGS

Manufacturers and distributors of drugs and the Food and Drug Administration occasionally are required to mail important information about drugs to physicians and others responsible for patient care. In the public interest, such mail should be distinctive in appearance so that it will be promptly recognized and read. The Food and Drug Administration will make such mailings in accordance with the specifications set forth in this section. Manufacturers and distributors of drugs are asked to make such mailings as prescribed by this section and not to use the distinctive envelopes for ordinary mail.

(a) Use first class mail and No. 10 white envelopes.

(b) The name and address of the agency or the drug manufacturer or distributor is to appear in the upper left corner of the envelope.

(c) The following statements are to appear in the far left third of the envelope front, in the type and size indicated, centered in a rectangular space approximately 3 inches wide and $2\frac{1}{4}$ inches high with an approximately $\frac{3}{8}$ inch-wide border in the color indicated:

(1) When the information concerns a significant hazard to health, the statement:
IMPORTANT
DRUG
WARNING
The statement shall be in three lines, all capitals, and centered. "Important" shall be in 36 point Gothic Bold type. "Drug" and "Warning" shall be in 36 point Gothic Condensed type. The rectangle's border and the statement therein shall be red.

(2) When the information concerns important changes in drug package labeling, the statement:
IMPORTANT
PRESCRIBING
INFORMATION
The statement shall be in three lines, all capitals, and centered. "Important" shall be in 36 point Gothic Bold type. "Prescribing" and "Information" shall be in 36 point Gothic Condensed type. The rectangle's border and the statement therein shall be blue.

(3) When the information concerns a correction of prescription drug advertising or labeling, the statement:
IMPORTANT
CORRECTION
OF DRUG
INFORMATION
The statement shall be in four lines, all capitals, and centered. "Important" shall be in 36 point Gothic Bold type. "Correction," "Of Drug," and "Information" shall be in 36 point Gothic Condensed type. The rectangle's border and the statement therein shall be brown.

5.6 §201.2 DRUGS AND DEVICES; NATIONAL DRUG CODE NUMBERS

The National Drug Code (NDC) number is requested but not required to appear on all drug labels and in all drug labeling, including the label of any prescription drug container furnished to a consumer.

5.7 §201.56 REQUIREMENTS ON CONTENT AND FORMAT OF LABELING FOR HUMAN PRESCRIPTION DRUG AND BIOLOGICAL PRODUCTS

(a) *General requirements.* Prescription drug labeling described in §201.100(d) must meet the following general requirements:

(1) The labeling must contain a summary of the essential scientific information needed for the safe and effective use of the drug.

(2) The labeling must be informative and accurate and neither promotional in tone nor false or misleading in any particular. In accordance with §§314.70 and 601.12 of this chapter, the labeling must be updated when new information becomes available that causes the labeling to become inaccurate, false, or misleading.

(3) The labeling must be based whenever possible on data derived from human experience. No implied claims or suggestions of drug use

may be made if there is inadequate evidence of safety or a lack of substantial evidence of effectiveness. Conclusions based on animal data but necessary for safe and effective use of the drug in humans must be identified as such and included with human data in the appropriate section of the labeling.

(b) *Categories of prescription drugs subject to the labeling content and format requirements in §§201.56(d) and 201.57.* (1) The following categories of prescription drug products are subject to the labeling requirements in paragraph (d) of this section and §201.57 in accordance with the implementation schedule in paragraph (c) of this section:
   (i) Prescription drug products for which a new drug application (NDA), biologics license application (BLA), or efficacy supplement was approved by the Food and Drug Administration (FDA) between June 30, 2001 and June 30, 2006;
   (ii) Prescription drug products for which an NDA, BLA, or efficacy supplement is pending on June 30, 2006; or
   (iii) Prescription drug products for which an NDA, BLA, or efficacy supplement is submitted anytime on or after June 30, 2006.
   (2) Prescription drug products not described in paragraph (b)(1) of this section are subject to the labeling requirements in paragraph (e) of this section and §201.80.

(c) *Schedule for implementing the labeling content and format requirements in §§201.56(d) and 201.57.* For products described in paragraph (b)(1) of this section, labeling conforming to the requirements in paragraph (d) of this section and §201.57 must be submitted according to the following schedule:
   (1) For products for which an NDA, BLA, or efficacy supplement is submitted for approval on or after June 30, 2006, proposed conforming labeling must be submitted as part of the application.
   (2) For products for which an NDA, BLA, or efficacy supplement is pending on June 30, 2006, or that has been approved any time from June 30, 2005, up to and including June 30, 2006, a supplement with proposed conforming labeling must be submitted no later than June 30, 2009.
   (3) For products for which an NDA, BLA, or efficacy supplement has been approved anytime from June 30, 2004, up to and including June 29, 2005, a supplement with proposed conforming labeling must be submitted no later than June 30, 2010.
   (4) For products for which an NDA, BLA, or efficacy supplement has been approved anytime from June 30, 2003, up to and including June 29, 2004, a supplement with proposed conforming labeling must be submitted no later than June 30, 2011.
   (5) For products for which an NDA, BLA, or efficacy supplement has been approved anytime from June 30, 2002, up to and including June 29, 2003, a supplement with proposed conforming labeling must be submitted no later than June 30, 2012.
   (6) For products for which an NDA, BLA, or efficacy supplement has been approved anytime from June 30, 2001, up to and including June 29, 2002, a supplement with proposed conforming labeling must be submitted no later than June 30, 2013.

(d) *Labeling requirements for new and more recently approved prescription drug products.* This paragraph applies only to prescription drug products described in paragraph (b)(1) of this section and must be implemented according to the schedule specified in paragraph (c) of this section.
   (1) Prescription drug labeling described in §201.100(d) must contain the specific information required under §201.57(a), (b), and (c) under the following headings and subheadings and in the following order:
   Highlights of Prescribing Information
   Product Names, Other Required Information
   Boxed Warning
   Recent Major Changes
   Indications and Usage
   Dosage and Administration
   Dosage Forms and Strengths
   Contraindications
   Warnings and Precautions
   Adverse Reactions
   Drug Interactions
   Use in Specific Populations
   Full Prescribing Information: Contents
   Full Prescribing Information
   Boxed Warning
   1 Indications and Usage
   2 Dosage and Administration
   3 Dosage Forms and Strengths
   4 Contraindications
   5 Warnings and Precautions
   6 Adverse Reactions
   7 Drug Interactions
   8 Use in Specific Populations
      8.1 Pregnancy
      8.2 Lactation
      8.3 Females and Males of Reproductive Potential
      8.4 Pediatric use
      8.5 Geriatric use

9 Drug Abuse and Dependence
  9.1 Controlled substance
  9.2 Abuse
  9.3 Dependence
10 Overdosage
11 Description
12 Clinical Pharmacology
  12.1 Mechanism of action
  12.2 Pharmacodynamics
  12.3 Pharmacokinetics
13 Nonclinical Toxicology
  13.1 Carcinogenesis, mutagenesis, impairment of fertility
  13.2 Animal toxicology and/or pharmacology
14 Clinical Studies
15 References
16 How Supplied/Storage and Handling
17 Patient Counseling Information

(2) Additional nonstandard subheadings that are used to enhance labeling organization, presentation, or ease of use (e.g., for individual warnings or precautions, or for each drug interaction) must be assigned a decimal number that corresponds to their placement in labeling. The decimal numbers must be consistent with the standardized identifying numbers listed in paragraph (d)(1) of this section (e.g., subheadings added to the "Warnings and Precautions" section must be numbered 5.1, 5.2, and so on).
(3) Any reference in Highlights to information appearing in the full prescribing information must be accompanied by the identifying number (in parentheses) corresponding to the location of the information in the full prescribing information.
(4) Omit clearly inapplicable sections, subsections, or specific information. If sections or subsections required under paragraph (d)(1) of this section are omitted from the full prescribing information, the heading "Full Prescribing Information: Contents" must be followed by an asterisk and the following statement must appear at the end of Contents: "*Sections or subsections omitted from the full prescribing information are not listed."
(5) Any risk information that is required under §201.57(c)(9)(iv) is considered "appropriate pediatric contraindications, warnings, or precautions" within the meaning of section 505A(l)(2) of the Federal Food, Drug, and Cosmetic Act (the act) (21 U.S.C. 355A(l)(2)), whether such information appears in the "Contraindications," "Warnings and Precautions," or "Use in Specific Populations" section of labeling.

(e) *Labeling requirements for older prescription drug products.* This paragraph applies only to approved prescription drug products not described in paragraph (b)(1) of this section.
(1) Prescription drug labeling described in §201.100(d) must contain the specific information required under §201.80 under the following section headings and in the following order:
Description
Clinical Pharmacology
Indications and Usage
Contraindications
Warnings
Precautions
Adverse Reactions
Drug Abuse and Dependence
Overdosage
Dosage and Administration
How Supplied
(2) The labeling may contain the following additional section headings if appropriate and if in compliance with §201.80(l) and (m):
Animal Pharmacology and/or Animal Toxicology
Clinical Studies
References
(3) Omit clearly inapplicable sections, subsections, or specific information.
(4) The labeling may contain a "Product Title" section preceding the "Description" section and containing only the information required by §201.80(a)(1)(i), (a)(1)(ii), (a)(1)(iii), and (a)(1)(iv) and §201.100(e). The information required by §201.80(a)(1)(i) through (a)(1)(iv) must appear in the "Description" section of the labeling, whether or not it also appears in a "Product Title."
(5) The labeling must contain the date of the most recent revision of the labeling, identified as such, placed prominently immediately after the last section of the labeling.
(6) The requirement in §201.80(f)(2) to reprint any FDA-approved patient labeling at the end of prescription drug labeling or accompany the prescription drug labeling must be implemented no later than June 30, 2007.

5.8 §201.57 SPECIFIC REQUIREMENTS ON CONTENT AND FORMAT OF LABELING FOR HUMAN PRESCRIPTION DRUG AND BIOLOGICAL PRODUCTS DESCRIBED IN §201.56(B)(1)

The requirements in this section apply only to prescription drug products described in §201.56(b)(1) and must be implemented according to the schedule specified in §201.56(c), except for the requirement in paragraph (c)(18) of this section to reprint any FDA-approved patient labeling at the end of prescription drug labeling or accompany the prescription drug labeling, which must be implemented no later than June 30, 2007.

(a) *Highlights of prescribing information.* The following information must appear in all prescription drug labeling:

(1) *Highlights limitation statement.* The verbatim statement "These highlights do not include all the information needed to use (*insert name of drug product*) safely and effectively. See full prescribing information for (insert name of drug product)."

(2) *Drug names, dosage form, route of administration, and controlled substance symbol.* The proprietary name and the established name of the drug, if any, as defined in section 502(e)(3) of the Federal Food, Drug, and Cosmetic Act (the act) or, for biological products, the proper name (as defined in §600.3 of this chapter) including any appropriate descriptors. This information must be followed by the drug's dosage form and route of administration. For controlled substances, the controlled substance symbol designating the schedule in which the controlled substance is listed must be included as required by §1302.04 of this chapter.

(3) *Initial U.S. approval.* The verbatim statement "Initial U.S. Approval" followed by the four-digit year in which FDA initially approved a new molecular entity, new biological product, or new combination of active ingredients. The statement must be placed on the line immediately beneath the established name or, for biological products, proper name of the product.

(4) *Boxed warning.* A concise summary of any boxed warning required by paragraph (c)(1) of this section, not to exceed a length of 20 lines. The summary must be preceded by a heading, in upper-case letters, containing the word "WARNING" and other words that are appropriate to identify the subject of the warning. The heading and the summary must be contained within a box and bolded. The following verbatim statement must be placed immediately following the heading of the boxed warning: "See full prescribing information for complete boxed warning."

(5) *Recent major changes.* A list of the section(s) of the full prescribing information, limited to the labeling sections described in paragraphs (c)(1), (c)(2), (c)(3), (c)(5), and (c)(6) of this section, that contain(s) substantive labeling changes that have been approved by FDA or authorized under §314.70(c)(6) or (d)(2), or §601.12(f)(1) through (f)(3) of this chapter. The heading(s) and, if appropriate, the subheading(s) of the labeling section(s) affected by the change must be listed together with each section's identifying number and the date (month/year) on which the change was incorporated in labeling. These labeling sections must be listed in the order in which they appear in the full prescribing information. A changed section must be listed under this heading in Highlights for at least 1 year after the date of the labeling change and must be removed at the first printing subsequent to the 1 year period.

(6) *Indications and usage.* A concise statement of each of the product's indications, as required under paragraph (c)(2) of this section, with any appropriate subheadings. Major limitations of use (e.g., lack of effect in particular subsets of the population, or second line therapy status) must be briefly noted. If the product is a member of an established pharmacologic class, the concise statement under this heading in Highlights must identify the class in the following manner: "(Drug) is a (name of class) indicated for (indication(s))."

(7) *Dosage and administration.* A concise summary of the information required under paragraph (c)(3) of this section, with any appropriate subheadings, including the recommended dosage regimen, starting dose, dose range, critical differences among population subsets, monitoring recommendations, and other clinically significant clinical pharmacologic information.

(8) *Dosage forms and strengths.* A concise summary of the information required under paragraph (c)(4) of this section, with any appropriate subheadings (e.g., tablets, capsules, injectable, suspension), including the strength or potency of the dosage form in metric system (e.g., 10-milligram tablets) and whether the product is scored.

(9) *Contraindications.* A concise statement of each of the product's contraindications, as required under paragraph (c)(5) of this section, with any appropriate subheadings.

(10) *Warnings and precautions.* A concise summary of the most clinically significant information required under paragraph (c)(6) of this section, with any appropriate subheadings, including information that would affect decisions about whether to prescribe a drug, recommendations for patient monitoring that are critical to safe use of the drug, and measures that can be taken to prevent or mitigate harm.

(11) *Adverse reactions.*

(i) A list of the most frequently occurring adverse reactions, as described in paragraph (c)(7) of this section, along with the criteria used to determine inclusion (e.g., incidence rate). Adverse reactions important for other reasons (e.g., because they are serious or frequently lead to discontinuation or dosage adjustment) must not be repeated under this heading in Highlights if they are included elsewhere in Highlights (e.g., Warnings and Precautions, Contraindications).

(ii) For drug products other than vaccines, the verbatim statement "To report SUSPECTED ADVERSE REACTIONS, contact (*insert name of manufacturer*) at (*insert manufacturer's phone number*) or FDA at (*insert current FDA phone number and Web address for voluntary reporting of adverse reactions*)."

(iii) For vaccines, the verbatim statement "To report SUSPECTED ADVERSE REACTIONS, contact (insert name of manufacturer) at (insert manufacturer's phone number) or VAERS at (insert the current VAERS phone number and Web address for voluntary reporting of adverse reactions)."

(iv) For manufacturers with a Web site for voluntary reporting of adverse reactions, the Web address of the direct link to the site.

(12) *Drug interactions.* A concise summary of the information required under paragraph (c)(8) of this section, with any appropriate subheadings.

(13) *Use in specific populations.* A concise summary of the information required under paragraph (c)(9) of this section, with any appropriate subheadings.

(14) *Patient counseling information statement.* The verbatim statement "See 17 for Patient Counseling Information" or, if the product has FDA-approved patient labeling, the verbatim statement "See 17 for Patient Counseling Information and (insert either FDA-approved patient labeling or Medication Guide)."

(15) *Revision date.* The date of the most recent revision of the labeling, identified as such, placed at the end of Highlights.

(b) *Full prescribing information: Contents.* Contents must contain a list of each heading and subheading required in the full prescribing information under §201.56(d)(1), if not omitted under §201.56(d)(4), preceded by the identifying number required under §201.56(d)(1). Contents must also contain any additional subheading(s) included in the full prescribing information preceded by the identifying number assigned in accordance with §201.56(d)(2).

(c) *Full prescribing information.* The full prescribing information must contain the information in the order required under paragraphs (c)(1) through (c)(18) of this section, together with the headings, subheadings, and identifying numbers required under §201.56(d)(1), unless omitted under §201.56(d)(4). If additional subheadings are used within a labeling section, they must be preceded by the identifying number assigned in accordance with §201.56(d)(2).

(1) *Boxed warning.* Certain contraindications or serious warnings, particularly those that may lead to death or serious injury, may be required by the FDA to be presented in a box. The boxed warning ordinarily must be based on clinical data, but serious animal toxicity may also be the basis of a boxed warning in the absence of clinical data. The box must contain, in uppercase letters, a heading inside the box that includes the word "WARNING" and conveys the general focus of the information in the box. The box must briefly explain the risk and refer to more detailed information in the "Contraindications" or "Warnings and Precautions" section, accompanied by the identifying number for the section or subsection containing the detailed information.

(2) *lIndications and usage.* This section must state that the drug is indicated for the treatment, prevention, mitigation, cure, or diagnosis of a recognized disease or condition, or of a manifestation of a recognized disease or condition, or for the relief of symptoms associated with a recognized disease or condition.

(i) This section must include the following information when the conditions listed are applicable:

(A) If the drug is used for an indication only in conjunction with a primary mode of therapy (e.g., diet, surgery, behavior changes, or some other drug), a statement that the drug is indicated as an adjunct to that mode of therapy.

(B) If evidence is available to support the safety and effectiveness of the drug or biological product only in selected subgroups of the larger population (e.g., patients with mild disease or patients in a special age group), or if the indication is approved based on a surrogate endpoint under §314.510 or §601.41 of this chapter, a succinct description of the limitations of usefulness of the drug and any uncertainty about anticipated clinical benefits, with reference to the "Clinical

Studies" section for a discussion of the available evidence.

(C) If specific tests are necessary for selection or monitoring of the patients who need the drug (e.g., microbe susceptibility tests), the identity of such tests.

(D) If information on limitations of use or uncertainty about anticipated clinical benefits is relevant to the recommended intervals between doses, to the appropriate duration of treatment when such treatment should be limited, or to any modification of dosage, a concise description of the information with reference to the more detailed information in the "Dosage and Administration" section.

(E) If safety considerations are such that the drug should be reserved for specific situations (e.g., cases refractory to other drugs), a statement of the information.

(F) If there are specific conditions that should be met before the drug is used on a long term basis (e.g., demonstration of responsiveness to the drug in a short term trial in a given patient), a statement of the conditions; or, if the indications for long term use are different from those for short term use, a statement of the specific indications for each use.

(ii) If there is a common belief that the drug may be effective for a certain use or if there is a common use of the drug for a condition, but the preponderance of evidence related to the use or condition shows that the drug is ineffective or that the therapeutic benefits of the product do not generally outweigh its risks, FDA may require that this section state that there is a lack of evidence that the drug is effective or safe for that use or condition.

(iii) Any statements comparing the safety or effectiveness of the drug with other agents for the same indication must, except for biological products, be supported by substantial evidence derived from adequate and well-controlled studies as defined in §314.126(b) of this chapter unless this requirement is waived under §201.58 or §314.126(c) of this chapter. For biological products, such statements must be supported by substantial evidence.

(iv) For drug products other than biological products, all indications listed in this section must be supported by substantial evidence of effectiveness based on adequate and well-controlled studies as defined in §314.126(b) of this chapter unless the requirement is waived under §201.58 or §314.126(c) of this chapter. Indications or uses must not be implied or suggested in other sections of the labeling if not included in this section.

(v) For biological products, all indications listed in this section must be supported by substantial evidence of effectiveness. Indications or uses must not be implied or suggested in other sections of the labeling if not included in this section.

(3) *2 Dosage and administration.*

(i) This section must state the recommended dose and, as appropriate:

(A) The dosage range,

(B) An upper limit beyond which safety and effectiveness have not been established, or beyond which increasing the dose does not result in increasing effectiveness,

(C) Dosages for each indication and subpopulation,

(D) The intervals recommended between doses,

(E) The optimal method of titrating dosage,

(F) The usual duration of treatment when treatment duration should be limited,

(G) Dosing recommendations based on clinical pharmacologic data (e.g., clinically significant food effects),

(H) Modification of dosage needed because of drug interactions or in special patient populations (e.g., in children, in geriatric age groups, in groups defined by genetic characteristics, or in patients with renal or hepatic disease),

(I) Important considerations concerning compliance with the dosage regimen,

(J) Efficacious or toxic concentration ranges and therapeutic concentration windows of the drug or its metabolites, if established and clinically significant. Information on therapeutic drug concentration monitoring (TDM) must also be included in this section when TDM is necessary.

(ii) Dosing regimens must not be implied or suggested in other sections of the labeling if not included in this section.

(iii) Radiation dosimetry information must be stated for both the patient receiving a radioactive drug and the person administering it.

(iv) This section must also contain specific direction on dilution, preparation (including the strength of the final dosage solution, when prepared according to instructions, in terms of milligrams of active ingredient per milliliter of reconstituted solution, unless another measure of the strength is more appropriate), and administration of the dosage form, if needed (e.g., the rate of administration of parenteral drug in milligrams per minute; storage conditions for stability of the reconstituted drug, when important; essential information on drug incompatibilities if the drug is mixed in vitro with other drugs or diluents; and the following verbatim statement for parenterals: "Parenteral drug products should be inspected visually for particulate matter and discoloration prior to administration, whenever solution and container permit.")

(4) *3 Dosage forms and strengths.* This section must contain information on the available dosage forms to which the labeling applies and for which the manufacturer or distributor is responsible, including:
 (i) The strength or potency of the dosage form in metric system (e.g., 10 milligram tablets), and, if the apothecary system is used, a statement of the strength in parentheses after the metric designation; and
 (ii) A description of the identifying characteristics of the dosage forms, including shape, color, coating, scoring, and imprinting, when applicable. The National Drug Code number(s) for the drug product must not be included in this section.

(5) *4 Contraindications.* This section must describe any situations in which the drug should not be used because the risk of use (e.g., certain potentially fatal adverse reactions) clearly outweighs any possible therapeutic benefit. Those situations include use of the drug in patients who, because of their particular age, sex, concomitant therapy, disease state, or other condition, have a substantial risk of being harmed by the drug and for whom no potential benefit makes the risk acceptable. Known hazards and not theoretical possibilities must be listed (e.g., if severe hypersensitivity to the drug has not been demonstrated, it should not be listed as a contraindication). If no contraindications are known, this section must state "None."

(6) *5 Warnings and precautions.*
 (i) *General.* This section must describe clinically significant adverse reactions (including any that are potentially fatal, are serious even if infrequent, or can be prevented or mitigated through appropriate use of the drug), other potential safety hazards (including those that are expected for the pharmacological class or those resulting from drug/drug interactions), limitations in use imposed by them (e.g., avoiding certain concomitant therapy), and steps that should be taken if they occur (e.g., dosage modification). The frequency of all clinically significant adverse reactions and the approximate mortality and morbidity rates for patients experiencing the reaction, if known and necessary for the safe and effective use of the drug, must be expressed as provided under paragraph (c)(7) of this section. In accordance with §§314.70 and 601.12 of this chapter, the labeling must be revised to include a warning about a clinically significant hazard as soon as there is reasonable evidence of a causal association with a drug; a causal relationship need not have been definitely established. A specific warning relating to a use not provided for under the "Indications and Usage" section may be required by FDA in accordance with sections 201(n) and 502(a) of the act if the drug is commonly prescribed for a disease or condition and such usage is associated with a clinically significant risk or hazard.
 (ii) *Other special care precautions.* This section must contain information regarding any special care to be exercised by the practitioner for safe and effective use of the drug (e.g., precautions not required under any other specific section or subsection).
 (iii) *Monitoring: Laboratory tests.* This section must identify any laboratory tests helpful in following the patient's response or in identifying possible adverse reactions. If appropriate, information must be provided on such factors as the range of normal and abnormal values expected in the particular situation and the recommended frequency with which tests should be performed before, during, and after therapy.
 (iv) *Interference with laboratory tests.* This section must briefly note information on any known interference by the product with laboratory tests and reference the section where the detailed information is presented (e.g., "Drug Interactions" section).

(7) *6 Adverse reactions.* This section must describe the overall adverse reaction profile of the drug based on the entire safety database. For purposes of prescription drug labeling, an adverse reaction is an undesirable effect,

reasonably associated with use of a drug, that may occur as part of the pharmacological action of the drug or may be unpredictable in its occurrence. This definition does not include all adverse events observed during use of a drug, only those adverse events for which there is some basis to believe there is a causal relationship between the drug and the occurrence of the adverse event.

(i) *Listing of adverse reactions.* This section must list the adverse reactions that occur with the drug and with drugs in the same pharmacologically active and chemically related class, if applicable. The list or lists must be preceded by the information necessary to interpret the adverse reactions (e.g., for clinical trials, total number exposed, extent and nature of exposure).

(ii) *Categorization of adverse reactions.* Within a listing, adverse reactions must be categorized by body system, by severity of the reaction, or in order of decreasing frequency, or by a combination of these, as appropriate. Within a category, adverse reactions must be listed in decreasing order of frequency. If frequency information cannot be reliably determined, adverse reactions must be listed in decreasing order of severity.

(A) *Clinical trials experience.* This section must list the adverse reactions identified in clinical trials that occurred at or above a specified rate appropriate to the safety database. The rate of occurrence of an adverse reaction for the drug and comparators (e.g., placebo) must be presented, unless such data cannot be determined or presentation of comparator rates would be misleading. If adverse reactions that occurred below the specified rate are included, they must be included in a separate listing. If comparative rates of occurrence cannot be reliably determined (e.g., adverse reactions were observed only in the uncontrolled trial portion of the overall safety database), adverse reactions must be grouped within specified frequency ranges as appropriate to the safety database for the drug (e.g., adverse reactions occurring at a rate of less than 1/100, adverse reactions occurring at a rate of less than 1/500) or descriptively identified, if frequency ranges cannot be determined. For adverse reactions with significant clinical implications, the listings must be supplemented with additional detail about the nature, frequency, and severity of the adverse reaction and the relationship of the adverse reaction to drug dose and demographic characteristics, if data are available and important.

(B) *Postmarketing experience.* This section of the labeling must list the adverse reactions, as defined in paragraph (c)(7) of this section, that are identified from domestic and foreign spontaneous reports. This listing must be separate from the listing of adverse reactions identified in clinical trials.

(iii) *Comparisons of adverse reactions between drugs.* For drug products other than biological products, any claim comparing the drug to which the labeling applies with other drugs in terms of frequency, severity, or character of adverse reactions must be based on adequate and well-controlled studies as defined in §314.126(b) of this chapter unless this requirement is waived under §201.58 or §314.126(c) of this chapter. For biological products, any such claim must be based on substantial evidence.

(8) *7 Drug interactions.*

(i) This section must contain a description of clinically significant interactions, either observed or predicted, with other prescription or over-the-counter drugs, classes of drugs, or foods (e.g., dietary supplements, grapefruit juice), and specific practical instructions for preventing or managing them. The mechanism(s) of the interaction, if known, must be briefly described. Interactions that are described in the "Contraindications" or "Warnings and Precautions" sections must be discussed in more detail under this section. Details of drug interaction pharmacokinetic studies that are included in the "Clinical Pharmacology" section that are pertinent to clinical use of the drug must not be repeated in this section.

(ii) This section must also contain practical guidance on known interference of the drug with laboratory tests.

(9) *8 Use in specific populations.* This section must contain the following subsections:

(i) *8.1 Pregnancy.* This subsection of the labeling must contain the fol lowing information in the following order under the subheadings "Pregnancy Exposure Registry," "Risk Summary," "Clinical Considerations," and "Data":

(A) *Pregnancy exposure registry.* If there is a scientifically acceptable pregnancy exposure registry for the drug, contact information needed to enroll in the registry or to obtain information about the registry must be provided following the statement: "There is a pregnancy exposure registry that monitors pregnancy outcomes in women exposed to (*name of drug*) during pregnancy."

(B) *Risk summary.* The Risk Summary must contain risk statement(s) based on data from all relevant sources (human, animal, and/or pharmacologic) that describe, for the drug, the risk of adverse developmental outcomes (*i.e.,* structural abnormalities, embryo-fetal and/or infant mortality, functional impairment, alterations to growth). When multiple data sources are available, the statements must be presented in the following order: Human, animal, pharmacologic. The source(s) of the data must be stated. The labeling must state the percentage range of live births in the United States with a major birth defect and the percentage range of pregnancies in the United States that end in miscarriage, regardless of drug exposure. If such information is available for the population(s) for which the drug is labeled, it must also be included. When use of a drug is contraindicated during pregnancy, this information must be stated first in the Risk Summary. When applicable, risk statements as described in paragraphs (c)(9)(i)(B)(*1*) and (*2*) of this section must include a cross-reference to additional details in the relevant portion of the "Data" subheading in the "Pregnancy" subsection of the labeling. If data demonstrate that a drug is not systemically absorbed following a particular route of administration, the Risk Summary must contain only the following statement: "(*Name of drug*) is not absorbed systemically following (route of administration), and maternal use is not expected to result in fetal exposure to the drug."

(1) *Risk statement based on human data.* When human data are available that establish the presence or absence of any adverse developmental outcome(s) associated with maternal use of the drug, the Risk Summary must summarize the specific developmental outcome(s); their incidence; and the effects of dose, duration of exposure, and gestational timing of exposure. If human data indicate that there is an increased risk for a specific adverse developmental outcome in infants born to women exposed to the drug during pregnancy, this risk must be quantitatively compared to the risk for the same outcome in infants born to women who were not exposed to the drug but who have the disease or condition for which the drug is indicated to be used. When risk information is not available for women with the disease or condition for which the drug is indicated, the risk for the specific outcome must be compared to the rate at which the outcome occurs in the general population. The Risk Summary must state when there are no human data or when available human data do not establish the presence or absence of drug-associated risk.

(2) *Risk statement based on animal data.* When animal data are available, the Risk Summary must summarize the findings in animals and based on these findings, describe, for the drug, the potential risk of any adverse developmental outcome(s) in humans. This statement must include: The number and type(s) of species affected, timing of exposure, animal doses expressed in terms of human dose or exposure equivalents, and outcomes for pregnant animals and offspring. When animal studies do not meet current standards for nonclinical developmental toxicity studies, the Risk Summary must so state. When there are no animal data, the Risk Summary must so state.

(3) *Risk statement based on pharmacology.* When the drug has a well-understood mechanism of action that may result in adverse developmental outcome(s), the Risk Summary must explain the mechanism of action and the potential associated risks.

(C) *Clinical considerations.* Under the subheading "Clinical Considerations," the labeling must provide relevant information, to the extent it is available, under the headings "Disease-associated maternal and/or embryo/fetal risk," "Dose adjustments during pregnancy and the postpartum period," "Maternal adverse reactions," "Fetal/Neonatal adverse reactions," and "Labor or delivery":

(1) *Disease-associated maternal and/or embryo/fetal risk.* If there is a serious known or potential risk to the pregnant woman and/or the embryo/fetus associated with the disease or condition for which the drug is indicated to be used, the labeling must describe the risk.

(2) *Dose adjustments during pregnancy and the postpartum period.* If there are pharmacokinetic data that support dose adjustment(s) during pregnancy and the postpartum period, a summary of this information must be provided.

(3) *Maternal adverse reactions.* If use of the drug is associated with a maternal adverse reaction that is unique to pregnancy or if a known adverse reaction occurs with increased frequency or severity in pregnant women, the labeling must describe the adverse reaction and available intervention(s) for monitoring or mitigating the reaction. The labeling must describe, if known, the effect of dose, timing, and duration of exposure on the risk to the pregnant woman of experiencing the adverse reaction.

(4) *Fetal/Neonatal adverse reactions.* If it is known or anticipated that treatment of the pregnant woman increases or may increase the risk of an adverse reaction in the fetus or neonate, the labeling must describe the adverse reaction, the potential severity and reversibility of the adverse reaction, and available intervention(s) for monitoring or mitigating the reaction. The labeling must describe, if known, the effect of dose, timing, and duration of exposure on the risk.

(5) *Labor or delivery.* If the drug is expected to affect labor or delivery, the labeling must provide information about the effect of the drug on the pregnant woman and the fetus or neonate; the effect of the drug on the duration of labor and delivery; any increased risk of adverse reactions, including their potential severity and reversibility; and must provide information about available intervention(s) that can mitigate these effects and/or adverse reactions. The information described under this heading is not required for drugs approved for use only during labor and delivery.

(D) *Data—(1) "Data" subheading.* Under the subheading "Data," the labeling must describe the data that are the basis for the Risk Summary and Clinical Considerations.

(2) *Human and animal data headings.* Human and animal data must be presented separately, beneath the headings "Human Data" and "Animal Data," and human data must be presented first.

(3) *Description of human data.* For human data, the labeling must describe adverse developmental outcomes, adverse reactions, and other adverse effects. To the extent applicable, the labeling must describe the types of studies or reports, number of subjects and the duration of each study, exposure information, and limitations of the data. Both positive and negative study findings must be included.

(4) *Description of animal data.* For animal data, the labeling must describe the following: Types of studies, animal species, dose, duration and timing of exposure, study findings, presence or absence of maternal toxicity, and limitations of the data. Description of maternal and offspring findings must include dose-response and severity of adverse developmental outcomes. Animal doses or exposures must be described in terms of human dose or exposure equivalents and the basis for those calculations must be included.

(ii) *8.2 Lactation.* This subsection of the labeling must contain the following information in the following order under the subheadings "Risk Summary," "Clinical Considerations," and "Data":

(A) *Risk summary.* When relevant human and/or animal lactation data are available, the Risk Summary must include a cross-reference to the "Data" subheading in the "Lactation" subsection of the labeling. When human data are available, animal data must not be included unless the animal model is specifically known to be predictive for humans. When use of a drug is contraindicated during breastfeeding, this information must be stated first in the Risk Summary.

(1) *Drug not absorbed systemically.* If data demonstrate that the drug is not systemically absorbed by the mother, the Risk Summary must contain only the following statement: "(*Name of drug*) is not absorbed systemically by the mother following (route of administration), and breastfeeding is not expected to result in exposure of the child to (*name of drug*)."

(2) *Drug absorbed systemically.* If the drug is absorbed systemically, the Risk

Summary must describe the following to the extent relevant information is available:

(*i*) *Presence of drug in human milk.* The Risk Summary must state whether the drug and/or its active metabolite(s) are present in human milk. If there are no data to assess this, the Risk Summary must so state. If studies demonstrate that the drug and/or its active metabolite(s) *are* not detectable in human milk, the Risk Summary must state the limits of the assay used. If studies demonstrate the presence of the drug and/or its active metabolite(s) in human milk, the Risk Summary must state the concentration of the drug and/or its active metabolite(s) in human milk and the actual or estimated daily dose for an infant fed exclusively with human milk. The actual or estimated amount of the drug and/or its active metabolite(s) ingested by the infant must be compared to the labeled infant or pediatric dose, if available, or to the maternal dose. If studies demonstrate the presence of the drug and/or its active metabolite(s) in human milk but the drug and/or its active metabolite(s) are not expected to be systemically bioavailable to the breast-fed child, the Risk Summary must describe the disposition of the drug and/or its active metabolite(s). If only animal lactation data are available, the Risk Summary must state only whether or not the drug and/or its active metabolite(s) were detected in animal milk and specify the animal species.

(*ii*) *Effects of drug on the breast-fed child.* The Risk Summary must include information, on the known or predicted effects on the child from exposure to the drug and/or its active metabolite(s) through human milk or from contact with breast or nipple skin (for topical products). The Risk Summary also must include information on systemic and/or local adverse reactions. If there are no data to assess the effects of the drug and/or its active metabolite(s) on the breast-fed child, the Risk Summary must so state.

(*iii*) *Effects of drug on milk production.* The Risk Summary must describe the effects of the drug and/or its active metabolite(s) on milk production. If there are no data to assess the effects of the drug and/or its active metabolite(s) on milk production, the Risk Summary must so state.

(3) *Risk and benefit statement.* For drugs absorbed systemically, unless breastfeeding is contraindicated during drug therapy, the following risk and benefit statement must appear at the end of the Risk Summary: "The developmental and health benefits of breastfeeding should be considered along with the mother's clinical need for (*name of drug*) and any potential adverse effects on the breast-fed child from (*name of drug*) or from the underlying maternal condition."

(B) *Clinical considerations.* Under "Clinical Considerations," the following information must be provided to the extent it is available and relevant:

(1) *Minimizing exposure.* The labeling must describe ways to minimize exposure in the breast-fed child if: The drug and/or its active metabolite(s) are present in human milk in clinically relevant concentrations; the drug does not have an established safety profile in infants; and the drug is used either intermittently, in single doses, or for short courses of therapy. When applicable, the labeling must also describe ways to minimize a breast-fed child's oral intake of topical drugs applied to the breast or nipple skin.

(2) *Monitoring for adverse reactions.* The labeling must describe available intervention(s) for monitoring or mitigating the adverse reaction(s) presented in the Risk Summary.

(C) *Data.* Under the subheading "Data," the labeling must describe the data that are the basis for the Risk Summary and Clinical Considerations.

(iii) *8.3 Females and males of reproductive potential.* When pregnancy testing and/or contraception are required or recommended before, during, or after drug therapy and/or when there are human and/or animal data that suggest drug-associated fertility effects, this subsection of labeling must contain this information under the subheadings "Pregnancy Testing," "Contraception," and "Infertility," in that order.

(iv) *8.4 Pediatric use.*

(A) Pediatric population(s)/pediatric patient(s): For the purposes of paragraphs (c)(9)(iv)(B) through (c)(9)(iv)(H) of this section, the terms *pediatric population(s)* and *pediatric patient(s)* are defined as the pediatric age group, from birth to 16 years, including age groups often called neonates, infants, children, and adolescents.

(B) If there is a specific pediatric indication different from those approved for adults that is supported by adequate and well-controlled studies in the pediatric population, it must be described under the "Indications and Usage" section, and appropriate pediatric dosage information must be given under the "Dosage and Administration" section. The "Pediatric use" subsection must cite any limitations on the pediatric indication, need for specific monitoring, specific hazards associated with use of the drug in any subsets of the pediatric population (e.g., neonates), differences between pediatric and adult responses to the drug, and other information related to the safe and effective pediatric use of the drug. Data summarized in this subsection should be discussed in more detail, if appropriate, under the "Clinical Pharmacology" or "Clinical Studies" section. As appropriate, this information must also be contained in the "Contraindications" and/or "Warnings and Precautions" section(s).

(C) If there are specific statements on pediatric use of the drug for an indication also approved for adults that are based on adequate and well-controlled studies in the pediatric population, they must be summarized in the "Pediatric use" subsection and discussed in more detail, if appropriate, under the "Clinical Pharmacology" and "Clinical Studies" sections. Appropriate pediatric dosage must be given under the "Dosage and Administration" section. The "Pediatric use" subsection of the labeling must also cite any limitations on the pediatric use statement, need for specific monitoring, specific hazards associated with use of the drug in any subsets of the pediatric population (e.g., neonates), differences between pediatric and adult responses to the drug, and other information related to the safe and effective pediatric use of the drug. As appropriate, this information must also be contained in the "Contraindications" and/or "Warnings and Precautions" section(s).

(D) (1) When a drug is approved for pediatric use based on adequate and well-controlled studies in adults with other information supporting pediatric use, the "Pediatric use" subsection of the labeling must contain either the following statement or a reasonable alternative:

The safety and effectiveness of (*drug name*) have been established in the age groups ___ to ___ (note any limitations, e.g., no data for pediatric patients under 2, or only applicable to certain indications approved in adults). Use of (*drug name*) in these age groups is supported by evidence from adequate and well-controlled studies of (*drug name*) in adults with additional data (*insert wording that accurately describes the data submitted to support a finding of substantial evidence of effectiveness in the pediatric population*).

(2) Data summarized in the preceding prescribed statement in this subsection must be discussed in more detail, if appropriate, under the "Clinical Pharmacology" or the "Clinical Studies" section. For example, pediatric pharmacokinetic or pharmacodynamic studies and dose response information should be described in the "Clinical Pharmacology" section. Pediatric dosing instructions must be included in the "Dosage and Administration" section. Any differences between pediatric and adult responses, need for specific monitoring, dosing adjustments, and any other information related to safe and effective use of the drug in pediatric patients must be cited briefly in the "Pediatric use" subsection and, as appropriate, in the "Contraindications," "Warnings and Precautions," and "Dosage and Administration" sections.

(E) If the requirements for a finding of substantial evidence to support a pediatric indication or a pediatric use statement have not been met for a particular pediatric population, the "Pediatric use" subsection must contain an appropriate statement such as "Safety and effectiveness in pediatric patients below the age of (__) have not been established." If use of the drug in this pediatric population is associated with a specific hazard, the hazard must be described in this subsection, or, if appropriate, the hazard must be stated in the "Contraindications" or "Warnings and Precautions" section and this subsection must refer to it.

(F) If the requirements for a finding of substantial evidence to support a pediatric indication or a pediatric use statement have not been met for any pediatric population, this subsection must contain the following statement: "Safety and effectiveness in pediatric patients have not been established." If use of the drug in premature or neonatal infants, or other pediatric subgroups, is associated with a specific hazard, the hazard must be described in this subsection, or, if appropriate, the hazard must be stated in the "Contraindications" or "Warnings and Precautions" section and this subsection must refer to it.

(G) If the sponsor believes that none of the statements described in paragraphs (c)(9)(iv)(B) through (c)(9)(iv)(F) of this section are appropriate or relevant to the labeling of a particular drug, the sponsor must provide reasons for omission of the statements and may propose alternative statement(s). FDA may permit use of an alternative statement if FDA determines that no statement described in those paragraphs is appropriate or relevant to the drug's labeling and that the alternative statement is accurate and appropriate.

(H) If the drug product contains one or more inactive ingredients that present an increased risk of toxic effects to neonates or other pediatric subgroups, a special note of this risk must be made, generally in the "Contraindications" or "Warnings and Precautions" section.

(v) *8.5 Geriatric use.*

(A) A specific geriatric indication, if any, that is supported by adequate and well-controlled studies in the geriatric population must be described under the "Indications and Usage" section, and appropriate geriatric dosage must be stated under the "Dosage and Administration" section. The "Geriatric use" subsection must cite any limitations on the geriatric indication, need for specific monitoring, specific hazards associated with the geriatric indication, and other information related to the safe and effective use of the drug in the geriatric population. Unless otherwise noted, information contained in the "Geriatric use" subsection must pertain to use of the drug in persons 65 years of age and older. Data summarized in this subsection must be discussed in more detail, if appropriate, under "Clinical Pharmacology" or the "Clinical Studies" section. As appropriate, this information must also be contained in the "Warnings and Precautions" and/or "Contraindications" section(s).

(B) Specific statements on geriatric use of the drug for an indication approved for adults generally, as distinguished from a specific geriatric indication, must be contained in the "Geriatric use" subsection and must reflect all information available to the sponsor that is relevant to the appropriate use of the drug in elderly patients. This information includes detailed results from controlled studies that are available to the sponsor and pertinent information from well-documented studies obtained from a literature search. Controlled studies include those that are part of the marketing application and other relevant studies available to the sponsor that have not been previously submitted in the investigational new drug application, new drug application, biologics license application, or a supplement or amendment to one of these applications (e.g., postmarketing studies or adverse drug reaction reports). The "Geriatric use" subsection must contain the following statement(s) or reasonable alternative, as applicable, taking into account available information:

(1) If clinical studies did not include sufficient numbers of subjects aged 65 and over to determine whether elderly subjects respond differently from younger subjects, and other reported clinical experience has not identified such differences, the "Geriatric use" subsection must include the following statement:
Clinical studies of (*name of drug*) did not include sufficient numbers of subjects aged 65 and over to determine whether they respond differently from younger subjects. Other reported clinical experience has not identified differences in responses between the elderly and younger patients. In general, dose selection for an elderly patient should be cautious, usually starting at the low end of the dosing range, reflecting the greater frequency of decreased hepatic, renal, or cardiac function, and of concomitant disease or other drug therapy.

(2) If clinical studies (including studies that are part of marketing applications and other relevant studies available to the sponsor that have not been submitted in the sponsor's applications) included enough elderly subjects to make it likely that differences in safety or effectiveness between elderly and younger subjects would have been detected, but no such differences (in safety or effectiveness) were observed, and other reported clinical experience has not identified

such differences, the "Geriatric use" subsection must contain the following statement:

Of the total number of subjects in clinical studies of (*name of drug*), __ percent were 65 and over, while __ percent were 75 and over. (Alternatively, the labeling may state the total number of subjects included in the studies who were 65 and over and 75 and over.) No overall differences in safety or effectiveness were observed between these subjects and younger subjects, and other reported clinical experience has not identified differences in responses between the elderly and younger patients, but greater sensitivity of some older individuals cannot be ruled out.

(3) If evidence from clinical studies and other reported clinical experience available to the sponsor indicates that use of the drug in elderly patients is associated with differences in safety or effectiveness, or requires specific monitoring or dosage adjustment, the "Geriatric use" subsection must contain a brief description of observed differences or specific monitoring or dosage requirements and, as appropriate, must refer to more detailed discussions in the "Contraindications," "Warnings and Precautions," "Dosage and Administration," or other sections.

(C) (1) If specific pharmacokinetic or pharmacodynamic studies have been carried out in the elderly, they must be described briefly in the "Geriatric use" subsection and in detail under the "Clinical Pharmacology" section. The "Clinical Pharmacology" and "Drug Interactions" sections ordinarily contain information on drug/disease and drug/drug interactions that is particularly relevant to the elderly, who are more likely to have concomitant illness and to use concomitant drugs.

(2) If a drug is known to be substantially excreted by the kidney, the "Geriatric use" subsection must include the statement:

This drug is known to be substantially excreted by the kidney, and the risk of adverse reactions to this drug may be greater in patients with impaired renal function. Because elderly patients are more likely to have decreased renal function, care should be taken in dose selection, and it may be useful to monitor renal function.

(D) If use of the drug in the elderly appears to cause a specific hazard, the hazard must be described in the "Geriatric use" subsection, or, if appropriate, the hazard must be stated in the "Contraindications" or "Warnings and Precautions" section, and the "Geriatric use" subsection must refer to those sections.

(E) Labeling under paragraphs (c)(9)(v)(A) through (c)(9)(v)(C) of this section may include statements, if they are necessary for safe and effective use of the drug, and reflect good clinical practice or past experience in a particular situation, e.g., for a sedating drug, it could be stated that:

Sedating drugs may cause confusion and over-sedation in the elderly; elderly patients generally should be started on low doses of (*name of drug*) and observed closely.

(F) If the sponsor believes that none of the requirements described in paragraphs (c)(9)(v)(A) through (c)(9)(v)(E) of this section are appropriate or relevant to the labeling of a particular drug, the sponsor must provide reasons for omission of the statements and may propose an alternative statement. FDA may permit omission of the statements if FDA determines that no statement described in those paragraphs is appropriate or relevant to the drug's labeling. FDA may permit use of an alternative statement if the agency determines that such statement is accurate and appropriate.

(vi) *Additional subsections.* Additional subsections may be included, as appropriate, if sufficient data are available concerning the use of the drug in other specified subpopulations (e.g., renal or hepatic impairment).

(10) *9 Drug abuse and dependence.* This section must contain the following information, as appropriate:

(i) *9.1 Controlled substance.* If the drug is controlled by the Drug Enforcement Administration, the schedule in which it is controlled must be stated.

(ii) *9.2 Abuse.* This subsection must state the types of abuse that can occur with the drug and the adverse reactions pertinent to them, and must identify particularly susceptible patient populations. This subsection must be based primarily on human data and human experience, but pertinent animal data may also be used.

(iii) *9.3 Dependence.* This subsection must describe characteristic effects resulting from both psychological and physical dependence that occur with the drug and must identify the quantity of the drug over a period of time that may lead to tolerance or dependence, or both. Details must be provided on the adverse effects of chronic abuse and the effects of abrupt withdrawal. Procedures necessary to diagnose the dependent state and the principles of treating the effects of abrupt withdrawal must be described.

(11) *10 Overdosage*. This section must be based on human data. If human data are unavailable, appropriate animal and in vitro data may be used. The following specific information must be provided:

(i) Signs, symptoms, and laboratory findings associated with an overdosage of the drug;

(ii) Complications that can occur with the drug (for example, organ toxicity or delayed acidosis);

(iii) Concentrations of the drug in biologic fluids associated with toxicity or death; physiologic variables influencing excretion of the drug, such as urine pH; and factors that influence the dose response relationship of the drug, such as tolerance. The pharmacokinetic data given in the "Clinical Pharmacology" section also may be referenced here, if applicable to overdoses;

(iv) The amount of the drug in a single dose that is ordinarily associated with symptoms of overdosage and the amount of the drug in a single dose that is likely to be life threatening;

(v) Whether the drug is dialyzable; and

(vi) Recommended general treatment procedures and specific measures for support of vital functions (e.g., proven antidotes, gastric lavage, forced diuresis, or as per Poison Control Center). Such recommendations must be based on data available for the specific drug or experience with pharmacologically related drugs. Unqualified recommendations for which data are lacking for the specific drug or class of drugs must not be stated.

(12) *11 Description*.

(i) This section must contain:

(A) The proprietary name and the established name, if any, as defined in section 502(e)(2) of the act, of the drug or, for biological products, the proper name (as defined in §600.3 of this chapter) and any appropriate descriptors;

(B) The type of dosage form(s) and the route(s) of administration to which the labeling applies;

(C) The same qualitative and/or quantitative ingredient information as required under §201.100(b) for drug labels or §§610.60 and 610.61 of this chapter for biological product labels;

(D) If the product is sterile, a statement of that fact;

(E) The pharmacological or therapeutic class of the drug;

(F) For drug products other than biological products, the chemical name and structural formula of the drug; and

(G) If the product is radioactive, a statement of the important nuclear physical characteristics, such as the principal radiation emission data, external radiation, and physical decay characteristics.

(ii) If appropriate, other important chemical or physical information, such as physical constants or pH, must be stated.

(13) *12 Clinical pharmacology*.

(i) This section must contain information relating to the human clinical pharmacology and actions of the drug in humans. Pharmacologic information based on in vitro data using human biomaterials or pharmacologic animal models, or relevant details about in vivo study designs or results (e.g., drug interaction studies), may be included in this section if essential to understand dosing or drug interaction information presented in other sections of the labeling. This section must include the following subsections:

(A) *12.1 Mechanism of action*. This subsection must summarize what is known about the established mechanism(s) of the drug's action in humans at various levels (e.g., receptor, membrane, tissue, organ, whole body). If the mechanism of action is not known, this subsection must contain a statement about the lack of information.

(B) *12.2 Pharmacodynamics*. This subsection must include a description of any biochemical or physiologic pharmacologic effects of the drug or active metabolites related to the drug's clinical effect in preventing, diagnosing, mitigating, curing, or treating disease, or those related to adverse effects or toxicity. Exposure-response relationships (e.g., concentration-response, dose-response) and time course of pharmacodynamic response (including short-term clinical response) must be included if known. If this information is unknown, this subsection must contain a statement about the lack of information. Detailed dosing or monitoring recommendations based on pharmacodynamic information that appear in other sections (e.g., "Warnings and Precautions" or "Dosage and Administration") must not be repeated in this subsection, but the location of such recommendations must be referenced.

(C) *12.3 Pharmacokinetics.* This subsection must describe the clinically significant pharmacokinetics of a drug or active metabolites, (i.e., pertinent absorption, distribution, metabolism, and excretion parameters). Information regarding bioavailability, the effect of food, minimum concentration (C_{min}), maximum concentration (C_{max}), time to maximum concentration (T_{max}), area under the curve (AUC), pertinent half-lives ($t_{1/2}$), time to reach steady state, extent of accumulation, route(s) of elimination, clearance (renal, hepatic, total), mechanisms of clearance (e.g., specific enzyme systems), drug/drug and drug/food (e.g., dietary supplements, grapefruit juice) pharmacokinetic interactions (including inhibition, induction, and genetic characteristics), and volume of distribution (V_d) must be presented if clinically significant. Information regarding nonlinearity in pharmacokinetic parameters, changes in pharmacokinetics over time, and binding (plasma protein, erythrocyte) parameters must also be presented if clinically significant. This section must also include the results of pharmacokinetic studies (e.g., of metabolism or interaction) that establish the absence of an effect, including pertinent human studies and in vitro data. Dosing recommendations based on clinically significant factors that change the product's pharmacokinetics (e.g., age, gender, race, hepatic or renal dysfunction, concomitant therapy) that appear in other sections (e.g., "Warnings and Precautions," "Dosage and Administration" or "Use in Specific Populations") must not be repeated in this subsection, but the location of such recommendations must be referenced.

(ii) Data that demonstrate activity or effectiveness in in vitro or animal tests and that have not been shown by adequate and well-controlled clinical studies to be pertinent to clinical use may be included under this section only under the following circumstances:

(A) In vitro data for anti-infective drugs may be included if the data are immediately preceded by the statement "The following in vitro data are available but their clinical significance is unknown."

(B) For other classes of drugs, in vitro and animal data that have not been shown by adequate and well-controlled studies, as defined in §314.126(b) of this chapter, to be necessary for the safe and effective use may be included in this section only if a waiver is granted under §201.58 or §314.126(c) of this chapter.

(14) *13 Nonclinical toxicology.* This section must contain the following subsections as appropriate:

(i) *13.1 Carcinogenesis, mutagenesis, impairment of fertility.* This subsection must state whether long term studies in animals have been performed to evaluate carcinogenic potential and, if so, the species and results. If results from reproduction studies or other data in animals raise concern about mutagenesis or impairment of fertility in either males or females, this must be described. Any precautionary statement on these topics must include practical, relevant advice to the prescriber on the significance of these animal findings. Human data suggesting that the drug may be carcinogenic or mutagenic, or suggesting that it impairs fertility, as described in the

"Warnings and Precautions" section, must not be included in this subsection of the labeling.

(ii) *13.2 Animal toxicology and/or pharmacology.* Significant animal data necessary for safe and effective use of the drug in humans that is not incorporated in other sections of labeling must be included in this section (e.g., specifics about studies used to support approval under §314.600 or §601.90 of this chapter, the absence of chronic animal toxicity data for a drug that is administered over prolonged periods or is implanted in the body).

(15) *14 Clinical studies.* This section must discuss those clinical studies that facilitate an understanding of how to use the drug safely and effectively. Ordinarily, this section will describe the studies that support effectiveness for the labeled indication(s), including discussion of study design, population, endpoints, and results, but must not include an encyclopedic listing of all, or even most, studies performed as part of the product's clinical development program. If a specific important clinical study is mentioned in any section of the labeling required under §§201.56 and 201.57 because the study is essential to an understandable presentation of the information in that section of the labeling, any detailed discussion of the study must appear in this section.

(i) For drug products other than biological products, any clinical study that is discussed in prescription drug labeling that relates to an indication for or use of the drug must be adequate and well-controlled as described in §314.126(b) of this chapter and must not imply or suggest indications or uses or dosing regimens not stated in the "Indications and Usage" or "Dosage and Administration" section. For biological products, any clinical study that is discussed that relates to an indication for or use of the biological product must constitute or contribute to substantial evidence and must not imply or suggest indications or uses or dosing regimens not stated in the "Indications and Usage" or "Dosage and Administration" section.

(ii) Any discussion of a clinical study that relates to a risk from the use of the drug must also refer to the other sections of the labeling where the risk is identified or discussed.

(16) *15 References.* When prescription drug labeling must summarize or otherwise rely on a recommendation by an authoritative scientific body, or on a standardized methodology, scale, or technique, because the information is important to prescribing decisions, the labeling may include a reference to the source of the information.

(17) *16 How supplied/storage and handling.* This section must contain information on the available dosage forms to which the labeling applies and for which the manufacturer or distributor is responsible. The information must include, as appropriate:

(i) The strength or potency of the dosage form in metric system (e.g., 10 milligram tablets) and, if the apothecary system is used, a statement of the strength in parentheses after the metric designation;

(ii) The units in which the dosage form is ordinarily available for prescribing by practitioners (e.g., bottles of 100);

(iii) Appropriate information to facilitate identification of the dosage forms, such as shape, color, coating, scoring, imprinting, and National Drug Code number; and

(iv) Special handling and storage conditions.

(18) *17 Patient counseling information.* This section must contain information necessary for patients to use the drug safely and effectively (e.g., precautions concerning driving or the concomitant use of other substances that may have harmful additive effects). Any FDA-approved patient labeling must be referenced in this section and the full text of such patient labeling must be reprinted immediately following this section or, alternatively, accompany the prescription drug labeling. Any FDA-approved patient labeling printed immediately following this section or accompanying the labeling is subject to the type size requirements in paragraph (d)(6) of this section, except for a Medication Guide to be detached and distributed to patients in compliance with §208.24 of this chapter. Medication Guides for distribution to patients are subject to the type size requirements set forth in §208.20 of this chapter.

(d) *Format requirements.* All labeling information required under paragraphs (a), (b), and (c) of this section must be printed in accordance with the following specifications:

(1) All headings and subheadings required by paragraphs (a) and (c) of this section must be highlighted by bold type that prominently distinguishes the headings and subheadings from other labeling information. Reverse type is not permitted as a form of highlighting.

(2) A horizontal line must separate the information required by paragraphs (a), (b), and (c) of this section.
(3) The headings listed in paragraphs (a)(5) through (a)(13) of this section must be presented in the center of a horizontal line.
(4) If there are multiple subheadings listed under paragraphs (a)(4) through (a)(13) of this section, each subheading must be preceded by a bullet point.
(5) The labeling information required by paragraphs (a)(1) through (a)(4), (a)(11)(ii) through (a)(11)(iv), and (a)(14) of this section must be in bold print.
(6) The letter height or type size for all labeling information, headings, and subheadings set forth in paragraphs (a), (b), and (c) of this section must be a minimum of 8 points, except for labeling information that is on or within the package from which the drug is to be dispensed, which must be a minimum of 6 points.
(7) The identifying numbers required by §201.56(d) and paragraphs (c)(1) through (c)(18) of this section must be presented in bold print and must precede the heading or subheading by at least two square m's (i.e., two squares of the size of the letter "m" in 8 point type).
(8) The information required by paragraph (a) of this section, not including the information required under paragraph (a)(4) of this section, must be limited in length to an amount that, if printed in 2 columns on a standard sized piece of typing paper ($8^1/_2$ by 11 inches), single spaced, in 8 point type with $^1/_2$ -inch margins on all sides and between columns, would fit on one-half of the page.
(9) Sections or subsections of labeling that are identified as containing recent major changes under paragraph (a)(5) of this section must be highlighted in the full prescribing information by the inclusion of a vertical line on the left edge of the new or modified text.
(10) For the information required by paragraph (b) of this section, each section heading must be in bold print. Each subheading within a section must be indented and not bolded.

5.8.1 §201.57(i) Specific Requirements on Content and Format of Labeling for Human Prescription Drug and Biological Products With Emphasis on Pregnancy, Lactation, Breast Feeding, Labor, and Delivery

(i) *8.1 Pregnancy.* This subsection of the labeling must contain the following information in the following order under the subheadings "Pregnancy Exposure Registry," "Risk Summary," "Clinical Considerations," and "Data":

(A) *Pregnancy exposure registry.* If there is a scientifically acceptable pregnancy exposure registry for the drug, contact information needed to enroll in the registry or to obtain information about the registry must be provided following the statement: "There is a pregnancy exposure registry that monitors pregnancy outcomes in women exposed to (*name of drug*) during pregnancy."

(B) *Risk summary.* The Risk Summary must contain risk statement(s) based on data from all relevant sources (human, animal, and/or pharmacologic) that describe, for the drug, the risk of adverse developmental outcomes (*i.e.,* structural abnormalities, embryo-fetal and/or infant mortality, functional impairment, alterations to growth). When multiple data sources are available, the statements must be presented in the following order: Human, animal, pharmacologic. The source(s) of the data must be stated. The labeling must state the percentage range of live births in the United States with a major birth defect and the percentage range of pregnancies in the United States that end in miscarriage, regardless of drug exposure. If such information is available for the population(s) for which the drug is labeled, it must also be included. When use of a drug is contraindicated during pregnancy, this information must be stated first in the Risk Summary. When applicable, risk statements as described in paragraphs (c)(9)(i)(B)(*1*) and (*2*) of this section must include a cross-reference to additional details in the relevant portion of the "Data" subheading in the "Pregnancy" subsection of the labeling. If data demonstrate that a drug is not systemically absorbed following a particular route of administration, the Risk Summary must contain only the following statement: "(*Name of drug*) is not absorbed systemically following (route of administration), and maternal use is not expected to result in fetal exposure to the drug."

(*1*) *Risk statement based on human data.* When human data are available that establish the presence or absence of any adverse developmental outcome(s) associated with maternal use of the drug, the Risk Summary must summarize the specific developmental outcome(s); their incidence; and the effects of dose, duration of exposure, and gestational timing of exposure. If human data indicate that there is an increased risk for a specific adverse developmental outcome in infants born to women exposed to the drug during pregnancy, this risk must be quantitatively compared to the risk for the same outcome in infants born to women who were not exposed to the drug but who have the disease or condition for which the drug is indicated to be used. When risk information is not available for women with the disease or condition for which the drug is indicated, the risk for the specific outcome must be compared to the rate at which the outcome occurs in the general population. The Risk Summary must state when there are no human data or when available human data do not establish the presence or absence of drug-associated risk.

(*2*) *Risk statement based on animal data.* When animal data are available, the Risk Summary must summarize the findings in animals and based on these findings, describe, for the drug, the potential risk of any adverse developmental outcome(s) in humans. This statement must include: The number and type(s) of species affected, timing of exposure, animal doses expressed in terms of human dose or exposure equivalents, and outcomes for pregnant animals and offspring. When animal studies do not meet current standards for nonclinical developmental toxicity studies, the Risk Summary must so state. When there are no animal data, the Risk Summary must so state.

(*3*) *Risk statement based on pharmacology.* When the drug has a well-understood mechanism of action that may result in adverse developmental outcome(s), the Risk Summary must explain the mechanism of action and the potential associated risks.

(C) *Clinical considerations.* Under the subheading "Clinical Considerations," the labeling must provide relevant information, to the extent it is available, under the headings "Disease-associated maternal and/or embryo/fetal risk," "Dose adjustments during pregnancy and the postpartum period," "Maternal adverse reactions," "Fetal/Neonatal adverse reactions," and "Labor or delivery":

(*1*) *Disease-associated maternal and/or embryo/fetal risk.* If there is a serious known or potential risk to the pregnant woman and/or the embryo/fetus associated with the disease or condition for which the drug is indicated to be used, the labeling must describe the risk.

(*2*) *Dose adjustments during pregnancy and the postpartum period.* If there are pharmacokinetic data that support dose adjustment(s) during pregnancy and the postpartum period, a summary of this information must be provided.

(*3*) *Maternal adverse reactions.* If use of the drug is associated with a maternal adverse reaction that is unique to pregnancy or if a known adverse reaction occurs with increased frequency or severity in pregnant women, the labeling must describe the adverse reaction and available intervention(s) for monitoring or mitigating the reaction. The labeling must describe, if known, the effect of dose, timing, and duration of exposure on the risk to the pregnant woman of experiencing the adverse reaction.

(*4*) *Fetal/Neonatal adverse reactions.* If it is known or anticipated that treatment of the pregnant woman increases or may increase the risk of an adverse reaction in the fetus or neonate, the labeling must describe the adverse reaction, the potential severity and reversibility of the adverse reaction, and available intervention(s) for monitoring or mitigating the reaction. The labeling must describe, if known, the effect of dose, timing, and duration of exposure on the risk.

(*5*) *Labor or delivery.* If the drug is expected to affect labor or delivery, the labeling must provide information about the effect of the drug on the pregnant woman and the fetus or neonate; the effect of the drug on the duration of labor and delivery; any increased risk of adverse reactions, including their potential severity and reversibility; and must provide information about available intervention(s) that can mitigate these effects and/or adverse reactions. The information described under this heading is not required for drugs approved for use only during labor and delivery.

(D) *Data—(1) "Data" subheading.* Under the subheading "Data," the labeling must describe the data that are the basis for the Risk Summary and Clinical Considerations.

(2) *Human and animal data headings.* Human and animal data must be

presented separately, beneath the headings "Human Data" and "Animal Data," and human data must be presented first.

(*3*) *Description of human data.* For human data, the labeling must describe adverse developmental outcomes, adverse reactions, and other adverse effects. To the extent applicable, the labeling must describe the types of studies or reports, number of subjects and the duration of each study, exposure information, and limitations of the data. Both positive and negative study findings must be included.

(*4*) *Description of animal data.* For animal data, the labeling must describe the following: Types of studies, animal species, dose, duration and timing of exposure, study findings, presence or absence of maternal toxicity, and limitations of the data. Description of maternal and offspring findings must include dose-response and severity of adverse developmental outcomes. Animal doses or exposures must be described in terms of human dose or exposure equivalents and the basis for those calculations must be included.

(ii) *8.2 Lactation.* This subsection of the labeling must contain the following information in the following order under the subheadings "Risk Summary," "Clinical Considerations," and "Data":

(A) *Risk summary.* When relevant human and/or animal lactation data are available, the Risk Summary must include a cross-reference to the "Data" subheading in the "Lactation" subsection of the labeling. When human data are available, animal data must not be included unless the animal model is specifically known to be predictive for humans. When use of a drug is contraindicated during breastfeeding, this information must be stated first in the Risk Summary.

(*1*) *Drug not absorbed systemically.* If data demonstrate that the drug is not systemically absorbed by the mother, the Risk Summary must contain only the following statement: "(*Name of drug*) is not absorbed systemically by the mother following (route of administration), and breastfeeding is not expected to result in exposure of the child to (*name of drug*)."

(*2*) *Drug absorbed systemically.* If the drug is absorbed systemically, the Risk Summary must describe the following to the extent relevant information is available:

(*i*) *Presence of drug in human milk.* The Risk Summary must state whether the drug and/or its active metabolite(s) are present in human milk. If there are no data to assess this, the Risk Summary must so state. If studies demonstrate that the drug and/or its active metabolite(s) *are* not detectable in human milk, the Risk Summary must state the limits of the assay used. If studies demonstrate the presence of the drug and/or its active metabolite(s) in human milk, the Risk Summary must state the concentration of the drug and/or its active metabolite(s) in human milk and the actual or estimated daily dose for an infant fed exclusively with human milk. The actual or estimated amount of the drug and/or its active metabolite(s) ingested by the infant must be compared to the labeled infant or pediatric dose, if available, or to the maternal dose. If studies demonstrate the presence of the drug and/or its active metabolite(s) in human milk but the drug and/or its active metabolite(s) are not expected to be systemically bioavailable to the breast-fed child, the Risk Summary must describe the disposition of the drug and/or its active metabolite(s). If only animal lactation data are available, the Risk Summary must state only whether or not the drug and/or its active metabolite(s) were detected in animal milk and specify the animal species.

(*ii*) *Effects of drug on the breast-fed child.* The Risk Summary must include information, on the known or predicted effects on the child from exposure to the drug and/or its active metabolite(s) through human milk or from contact with breast or nipple skin (for topical products). The Risk Summary also must include information on systemic and/or local adverse reactions. If there are no data to assess the effects of the drug and/or its active metabolite(s) on the breast-fed child, the Risk Summary must so state.

(*iii*) *Effects of drug on milk production.* The Risk Summary must describe the effects of the drug and/or its active metabolite(s) on milk production. If there are no data to assess the effects of the drug and/or its active metabolite(s) on milk production, the Risk Summary must so state.

(*3*) *Risk and benefit statement.* For drugs absorbed systemically, unless breastfeeding is contraindicated during drug therapy, the following risk and benefit statement must appear at the end of the Risk Summary: "The developmental and health benefits of breastfeeding should be considered along with the mother's clinical need for (*name of drug*) and any potential adverse effects on the breastfed child from (*name of drug*) or from the underlying maternal condition."

(B) *Clinical considerations.* Under "Clinical Considerations," the following information must be provided to the extent it is available and relevant:

(*1*) *Minimizing exposure.* The labeling must describe ways to minimize exposure in the breast-fed child if: The drug and/or its active metabolite(s) are present in human milk in clinically relevant concentrations; the drug does not have an established safety profile in infants; and the drug is used either intermittently, in single doses, or for short courses of therapy. When applicable, the labeling must also describe ways to minimize a breastfed child's oral intake of topical drugs applied to the breast or nipple skin.

(*2*) *Monitoring for adverse reactions.* The labeling must describe available intervention(s) for monitoring or mitigating the adverse reaction(s) presented in the Risk Summary.

(C) *Data.* Under the subheading "Data," the labeling must describe the data that are the basis for the Risk Summary and Clinical Considerations.

(iii) *8.3 Females and males of reproductive potential.* When pregnancy testing and/or contraception are required or recommended before, during, or after drug therapy and/or when there are human and/or animal data that suggest drug-associated fertility effects, this subsection of labeling must contain this information under the subheadings "Pregnancy Testing," "Contraception," and "Infertility," in that order.

5.9 §201.61 STATEMENT OF IDENTITY

(a) The principal display panel of an over-the-counter drug in package form shall bear as one of its principal features a statement of the identity of the commodity.

(b) Such statement of identity shall be in terms of the established name of the drug, if any there be, followed by an accurate statement of the general pharmacological category(ies) of the drug or the principal intended action(s) of the drug. In the case of an over-the-counter drug that is a mixture and that has no established name, this requirement shall be deemed to be satisfied by a prominent and conspicuous statement of the general pharmacological action(s) of the mixture or of its principal intended action(s) in terms that are meaningful to the layman. Such statements shall be placed in direct conjunction with the most prominent display of the proprietary name or designation and shall employ terms descriptive of general pharmacological category(ies) or principal intended action(s); for example, "antacid," "analgesic," "decongestant," "antihistaminic," etc. The indications for use shall be included in the directions for use of the drug, as required by section 502(f)(1) of the act and by the regulations in this part.

(c) The statement of identity shall be presented in bold face type on the principal display panel, shall be in a size reasonably related to the most prominent printed matter on such panel, and shall be in lines generally parallel to the base on which the package rests as it is designed to be displayed.

5.10 §201.62 DECLARATION OF NET QUANTITY OF CONTENTS

(a) The label of an over-the-counter drug in package form shall bear a declaration of the net quantity of contents. This shall be expressed in the terms of weight, measure, numerical count, or a combination or numerical count and weight, measure, or size. The statement of quantity of drugs in tablet, capsule, ampule, or other unit form and the quantity of devices shall be expressed in terms of numerical count; the statement of quantity for drugs in other dosage forms shall be in terms of weight if the drug is solid, semisolid, or viscous, or in terms of fluid measure if the drug is liquid. The drug quantity statement shall be augmented when necessary to give accurate information as to the strength of such drug in the package; for example, to differentiate between several strengths of the same drug "100 tablets, 5 grains each" or "100 capsules, 125 milligrams each" or "100 capsules, 250 milligrams each": *Provided,* That:

(1) In the case of a firmly established, general consumer usage and trade custom of declaring the quantity of a drug in terms of linear measure

or measure of area, such respective term may be used. Such term shall be augmented when necessary for accuracy of information by a statement of the weight, measure, or size of the individual units or of the entire drug; for example, the net quantity of adhesive tape in package form shall be expressed in terms of linear measure augmented by a statement of its width.

(2) Whenever the Commissioner determines for a specific packaged drug that an existing practice of declaring net quantity of contents by weight, measure, numerical count, or a combination of these does not facilitate value comparisons by consumers, he shall by regulation designate the appropriate term or terms to be used for such article.

(b) Statements of weight of the contents shall be expressed in terms of avoirdupois pound and ounce. A statement of liquid measure of the contents shall be expressed in terms of the U.S. gallon of 231 cubic inches and quart, pint, and fluid-ounce subdivisions thereof, and shall express the volume at 68 °F (20 °C). See also paragraph (p) of this section.

(c) The declaration may contain common or decimal fractions. A common fraction shall be in terms of halves, quarters, eights, sixteenths, or thirty-seconds; except that if there exists a firmly established, general consumer usage and trade custom of employing different common fractions in the net quantity declaration of a particular commodity, they may be employed. A common fraction shall be reduced to its lowest terms; a decimal fraction shall not be carried out to more than two places. A statement that includes small fractions of an ounce shall be deemed to permit smaller variations than one which does not include such fractions.

(d) The declaration shall be located on the principal display panel of the label, and with respect to packages bearing alternate principal panels it shall be duplicated on each principal display panel.

(e) The declaration shall appear as a distinct item on the principal display panel, shall be separated, by at least a space equal to the height of the lettering used in the declaration, from other printed label information appearing above or below the declaration and, by at least a space equal to twice the width of the letter "N" of the style of type used in the quantity of contents statement, from other printed label information appearing to the left or right of the declaration. It shall not include any term qualifying a unit of weight, measure, or count, such as "giant pint" and "full quart", that tends to exaggerate the amount of the drug in the container. It shall be placed on the principal display panel within the bottom 30 percent of the area of the label panel in lines generally parallel to the base on which the package rests as it is designed to be displayed: *Provided,* That:

(1) On packages having a principal display panel of 5 square inches or less the requirement for placement within the bottom 30 percent of the area of the label panel shall not apply when the declaration of net quantity of contents meets the other requirements of this part; and

(2) In the case of a drug that is marketed with both outer and inner retail containers bearing the mandatory label information required by this part and the inner container is not intended to be sold separately, the net quantity of contents placement requirement of this section applicable to such inner container is waived.

(3) The principal display panel of a drug marketed on a display card to which the immediate container is affixed may be considered to be the display panel of the card, and the type size of the net quantity of contents statement is governed by the dimensions of the display card.

(f) The declaration shall accurately reveal the quantity of drug or device in the package exclusive of wrappers and other material packed therewith: *Provided,* That in the case of drugs packed in containers designed to deliver the drug under pressure, the declaration shall state the net quantity of the contents that will be expelled when the instructions for use as shown on the container are followed. The propellant is included in the net quantity declaration.

(g) The declaration shall appear in conspicuous and easily legible boldface print or type in distinct contrast (by typography, layout, color, embossing, or molding) to other matter on the package; except that a declaration of net quantity blown, embossed, or molded on a glass or plastic surface is permissible when all label information is so formed on the surface. Requirements of conspicuousness and legibility shall include the specifications that:

(1) The ratio of height to width of the letter shall not exceed a differential of 3 units to 1 unit, i.e., no more than 3 times as high as it is wide.

(2) Letter heights pertain to upper case or capital letters. When upper and lower case or all lower case letters are used, it is the lower case letter "o" or its equivalent that shall meet the minimum standards.

(3) When fractions are used, each component numeral shall meet one-half the minimum height standards.

(h) The declaration shall be in letters and numerals in a type size established in relationship to the area of the principal display panel of the package and shall be uniform for all packages of substantially the same size by complying with the following type specifications:

(1) Not less than one-sixteenth inch in height on packages the principal display panel of which has an area of 5 square inches or less.

(2) Not less than one-eighth inch in height on packages the principal display panel of which has an area of more than five but not more than 25 square inches.

(3) Not less than three-sixteenths inch in height on packages the principal display panel of which has an area of more than 25 but not more than 100 square inches.

(4) Not less than one-fourth inch in height on packages the principal display panel of which has an area of more than 100 square inches, except not less than one-half inch in height if the area is more than 400 square inches.

Where the declaration is blown, embossed, or molded on a glass or plastic surface rather than by printing, typing, or coloring, the lettering sizes specified in paragraphs (h) (1) through (4) of this section shall be increased by one-sixteenth of an inch.

(i) On packages containing less than 4 pounds or 1 gallon and labeled in terms of weight or fluid measure:

(1) The declaration shall be expressed both in ounces, with identification by weight or by liquid measure and, if applicable (1 pound or 1 pint or more) followed in parentheses by a declaration in pounds for weight units, with any remainder in terms of ounces or common or decimal fractions of the pound (see examples set forth in paragraphs (k) (1) and (2) of this section), or in the case of liquid measure, in the largest whole units (quarts, quarts and pints, or pints, as appropriate) with any remainder in terms of fluid ounces or common or decimal fractions of the pint or quart (see examples set forth in paragraphs (k) (3) and (4) of this section). If the net weight of the package is less than 1 ounce avoirdupois or the net fluid measure is less than 1 fluid ounce, the declaration shall be in terms of common or decimal fractions of the respective ounce and not in terms of drams.

(2) The declaration may appear in more than one line. The term *net weight* shall be used when stating the net quantity of contents in terms of weight. Use of the terms *net* or *net contents* in terms of fluid measure or numerical count is optional. It is sufficient to distinguish avoirdupois ounce from fluid ounce through association of terms; for example, "Net wt. 6 oz" or "6 oz net wt.," and "6 fl oz" or "net contents 6 fl oz".

(j) On packages containing 4 pounds or 1 gallon or more and labeled in terms of weight or fluid measure, the declaration shall be expressed in pounds for weight units with any remainder in terms of ounces or common or decimal fractions of the pound; in the case of fluid measure, it shall be expressed in the largest whole unit (gallons, followed by common or decimal fractions of a gallon or by the next smaller whole unit or units (quarts or quarts and pints)) with any remainder in terms of fluid ounces or common or decimal fractions of the pint or quart; see paragraph (k)(5) of this section.

(k) Examples:

(1) A declaration of $1\frac{1}{2}$ pounds weight shall be expressed as "Net wt. 24 oz (1 lb 8 oz)," or "Net wt. 24 oz ($1\frac{1}{2}$ lb)" or "Net wt. 24 oz (1.5 lb)".

(2) A declaration of three-fourths pound avoirdupois weight shall be expressed as "Net wt. 12 oz".

(3) A declaration of 1 quart liquid measure shall be expressed as "Net contents 32 fl oz (1 qt)" or "32 fl oz (1 qt)".

(4) A declaration of $1\frac{3}{4}$ quarts liquid measure shall be expressed as "Net contents 56 fl oz (1 qt 1 pt 8 oz)" or "Net contents 56 fl oz (1 qt 1.5 pt)," but not in terms of quart and ounce such as "Net 56 fl oz (1 qt 24 oz)."

(5) A declaration of $2\frac{1}{2}$ gallons liquid measure shall be expressed as "Net contents 2 gal 2 qt," "Net contents 2.5 gallons," or "Net contents $2\frac{1}{2}$ gal" but not as "2 gal 4 pt".

(l) For quantities, the following abbreviations and none other may be employed. Periods and plural forms are optional:

Gallon gal
milliliter ml
quart qt
cubic centimeter cc
pint pt
yard yd
ounce oz
feet or foot ft
pound lb
inch in
grain gr
meter m
kilogram kg
centimeter cm
gram g
millimeter mm
milligram mg
fluid fl
microgram mcg
square sq
liter l
weight wt

(m) On packages labeled in terms of linear measure, the declaration shall be expressed both in terms of inches and, if applicable (1 foot or more), the largest whole units (yards, yards and feet, feet). The declaration in terms of the largest whole units shall be in parentheses following the declaration in terms of inches and any remainder shall be in terms of inches or common or decimal fractions of the foot or yard; if applicable, as in the case of adhesive tape, the initial declaration in linear inches shall be preceded by a statement of the width. Examples of linear measure are "86 inches (2 yd 1 ft 2 in)," "90 inches ($2\frac{1}{2}$ yd)," "30 inches (2.5 ft)," " $\frac{3}{4}$ inch by 36 in (1 yd)," etc.

(n) On packages labeled in terms of area measure, the declaration shall be expressed both in terms of square inches and, if applicable (1 square foot or more), the largest whole square unit (square yards, square yards and square feet, square feet). The declaration in terms of the largest whole units shall be in parentheses following the declaration in terms of square inches and any remainder shall be in terms of square inches or common or decimal fractions of the square foot or square yard; for example, "158 sq inches (1 sq ft 14 sq in)."

(o) Nothing in this section shall prohibit supplemental statements at locations other than the principal display panel(s) describing in nondeceptive terms the net quantity of contents, provided that such supplemental statements of net quantity of contents shall not include any term qualifying a unit of weight, measure, or count that tends to exaggerate the amount of the drug contained in the package; for example, "giant pint" and "full quart." Dual or combination declarations of net quantity of contents as provided for in paragraphs (a) and (i) of this section are not regarded as supplemental net quantity statements and shall be located on the principal display panel.

(p) A separate statement of net quantity of contents in terms of the metric system of weight or measure is not regarded as a supplemental statement and an accurate statement of the net quantity of contents in terms of the metric system of weight or measure may also appear on the principal display panel or on other panels.

(q) The declaration of net quantity of contents shall express an accurate statement of the quantity of contents of the package. Reasonable variations caused by loss or gain of moisture during the course of good distribution practice or by unavoidable deviations in good manufacturing practice will be recognized. Variations from stated quantity of contents shall not be unreasonably large.

(r) A drug shall be exempt from compliance with the net quantity declaration required by this section if it is an ointment labeled "sample," "physician's sample," or a substantially similar statement and the contents of the package do not exceed 8 grams.

5.11 §201.63 PREGNANCY/BREAST-FEEDING WARNING

(a) The labeling for all over-the-counter (OTC) drug products that are intended for systemic absorption, unless specifically exempted, shall contain a general warning under the heading "Warning" (or "Warnings" if it appears with additional warning statements) as follows: "If pregnant or breast-feeding, ask a health professional before use." [first four words of this statement in bold type] In addition to the written warning, a symbol that conveys the intent of the warning may be used in labeling.

(b) Where a specific warning relating to use during pregnancy or while nursing has been established for a particular drug product in a new drug application (NDA) or for a product covered by an OTC drug final monograph in part 330 of this chapter, the specific warning shall be used in place of the warning in paragraph (a) of this section, unless otherwise stated in the NDA or in the final OTC drug monograph.

(c) The following OTC drugs are exempt from the provisions of paragraph (a) of this section:
  (1) Drugs that are intended to benefit the fetus or nursing infant during the period of pregnancy or nursing.
  (2) Drugs that are labeled exclusively for pediatric use.

(d) The Food and Drug Administration will grant an exemption from paragraph (a) of this section where appropriate upon petition under the provisions of §10.30 of this chapter. Decisions with respect to requests for exemptions shall be maintained in a permanent file for public review by the Division of Dockets Management (HFA-305), Food and Drug Administration, 5630 Fishers Lane, rm. 1061, Rockville, MD 20852.

(e) The labeling of orally or rectally administered OTC aspirin and aspirin-containing drug products must bear a warning that immediately follows the general warning identified in paragraph (a) of this section. The warning shall be as follows:
"It is especially important not to use" (select "aspirin" or "carbaspirin calcium," as appropriate) "during the last 3 months of pregnancy unless definitely directed to do so by a doctor because it may cause problems in the unborn child or complications during delivery."

5.12 §201.64 SODIUM LABELING

(a) The labeling of over-the-counter (OTC) drug products intended for oral ingestion shall contain the sodium content per dosage unit (e.g., tablet, teaspoonful) if the sodium content of a single maximum recommended dose of the product (which may be one or more dosage units) is 5 milligrams or more. OTC drug products intended for oral ingestion include gum and lozenge dosage forms, but do not include dentifrices, mouthwashes, or mouth rinses.

(b) The sodium content shall be expressed in milligrams per dosage unit and shall include the total amount of sodium regardless of the source, i.e., from both active and inactive ingredients. The sodium content shall be rounded-off to the nearest whole number. The sodium content per dosage unit shall follow the heading "Other information" as stated in §201.66(c)(7).

(c) The labeling of OTC drug products intended for oral ingestion shall contain the following statement under the heading "Warning" (or "Warnings" if it appears with additional warning statements) if the amount of sodium present in the labeled maximum daily dose of the product is more than 140 milligrams: "Ask a doctor before use if you have [in bold type] [bullet] a sodium-restricted diet". The warnings in §§201.64(c), 201.70(c), 201.71(c), and 201.72(c) may be combined, if applicable, provided the ingredients are listed in alphabetical order, e g., a calcium or sodium restricted diet.

(d) The term sodium free may be used in the labeling of OTC drug products intended for oral ingestion if the amount of sodium in the labeled maximum daily dose is 5 milligrams or less and the amount of sodium per dosage unit is 0 milligram (when rounded-off in accord with paragraph (b) of this section).

(e) The term very low sodium may be used in the labeling of OTC drug products intended for oral ingestion if the amount of sodium in the labeled maximum daily dose is 35 milligrams or less.

(f) The term low sodium may be used in the labeling of OTC drug products intended for oral ingestion if the amount of sodium in the labeled maximum daily dose is 140 milligrams or less.

(g) The term salt is not synonymous with the term sodium and shall not be used interchangeably or substituted for the term sodium.

(h) The terms sodium free, very low sodium, and low sodium shall be in print size and style no larger than the product's statement of identity and shall not be unduly prominent in print size or style compared to the statement of identity.

(i) Any product subject to this paragraph that contains sodium bicarbonate, sodium phosphate, or sodium biphosphate as an active ingredient for oral ingestion and that is not labeled as required by this paragraph and that is initially introduced or initially delivered for introduction into interstate commerce after April 22, 1997, is misbranded under sections 201(n) and 502 (a) and (f) of the Federal Food, Drug, and Cosmetic Act (the act).

(j) Any product subject to paragraphs (a) through (h) of this section that is not labeled as required and that is initially introduced or initially delivered for introduction into interstate commerce after the following dates is misbranded under sections 201(n) and 502(a) and (f) of the Federal Food, Drug, and Cosmetic Act.

  (1) As of the date of approval of the application for any single entity and combination products subject to drug marketing applications approved on or after April 23, 2004.

  (2) September 24, 2005, for all OTC drug products subject to any OTC drug monograph, not yet the subject of any OTC drug monograph, or subject to drug marketing applications approved before April 23, 2004.

(k) The labeling of OTC drug products intended for rectal administration containing dibasic sodium phosphate and/or monobasic sodium phosphate shall contain the sodium content per delivered dose if the sodium content is 5 milligrams or more. The sodium content shall be expressed in milligrams or grams. If less than 1 gram, milligrams should be used. The sodium content shall be rounded-off to the nearest whole number if expressed in milligrams (or nearest tenth of a gram if expressed in grams). The sodium content per delivered dose shall follow the heading "Other information" as stated in §201.66(c)(7). Any product subject to this paragraph that contains dibasic sodium phosphate and/or monobasic sodium phosphate as an active ingredient intended for rectal administration and that is not labeled as required by this paragraph and that is initially introduced or initially delivered for introduction into interstate commerce after November 29, 2005, is misbranded under sections 201(n) and 502(a) and (f) of the act.

5.13 §201.66 FORMAT AND CONTENT REQUIREMENTS FOR OVER-THE-COUNTER (OTC) DRUG PRODUCT LABELING

(a) *Scope.* This section sets forth the content and format requirements for the labeling of all OTC drug products. Where an OTC drug product is the subject of an applicable monograph or regulation that contains content and format requirements that conflict with this section, the content and format requirements in this section must be followed unless otherwise specifically provided in the applicable monograph or regulation.

(b) *Definitions.* The following definitions apply to this section:

(1) *Act* means the Federal Food, Drug, and Cosmetic Act (secs. 201 *et seq.* (21 U.S.C. 321 *et seq.*)).
(2) *Active ingredient* means any component that is intended to furnish pharmacological activity or other direct effect in the diagnosis, cure, mitigation, treatment, or prevention of disease, or to affect the structure or any function of the body of humans. The term includes those components that may undergo chemical change in the manufacture of the drug product and be present in the drug product in a modified form intended to furnish the specified activity or effect.
(3) *Approved drug application* means a new drug (NDA) or abbreviated new drug (ANDA) application approved under section 505 of the act (21 U.S.C. 355).
(4) *Bullet* means a geometric symbol that precedes each statement in a list of statements. For purposes of this section, the bullet style is limited to solid squares or solid circles, in the format set forth in paragraph (d)(4) of this section.
(5) *Established name* of a drug or ingredient thereof means the applicable official name designated under section 508 of the act (21 U.S.C. 358), or, if there is no designated official name and the drug or ingredient is recognized in an official compendium, the official title of the drug or ingredient in such compendium, or, if there is no designated official name and the drug or ingredient is not recognized in an official compendium, the common or usual name of the drug or ingredient.
(6) *FDA* means the Food and Drug Administration.
(7) *Heading* means the required statements in quotation marks listed in paragraphs (c)(2) through (c)(9) of this section, excluding subheadings (as defined in paragraph (a)(9) of this section).
(8) *Inactive ingredient* means any component other than an active ingredient.
(9) *Subheading* means the required statements in quotation marks listed in paragraphs (c)(5)(ii) through (c)(5)(vii) of this section.
(10) *Drug facts labeling* means the title, headings, subheadings, and information required under or otherwise described in paragraph (c) of this section.
(11) *Title* means the heading listed at the top of the required OTC drug product labeling, as set forth in paragraph (c)(1) of this section.
(12) *Total surface area available to bear labeling* means all surfaces of the outside container of the retail package or, if there is no such outside container, all surfaces of the immediate container or container wrapper except for the flanges at the tops and bottoms of cans and the shoulders and necks of bottles and jars.

(c) *Content requirements.* The outside container or wrapper of the retail package, or the immediate container label if there is no outside container or wrapper, shall contain the title, headings, subheadings, and information set forth in paragraphs (c)(1) through (c)(8) of this section, and may contain the information under the heading in paragraph (c)(9) of this section, in the order listed.
(1) (Title) "Drug Facts". If the drug facts labeling appears on more than one panel, the title "Drug Facts (continued)" shall appear at the top of each subsequent panel containing such information.
(2) "Active ingredient" or "Active ingredients" "(in each [insert the dosage unit stated in the directions for use (e.g., tablet, 5 mL teaspoonful) or in each gram as stated in §§333.110 and 333.120 of this chapter])", followed by the established name of each active ingredient and the quantity of each active ingredient per dosage unit. Unless otherwise provided in an applicable OTC drug monograph or approved drug application, products marketed without discrete dosage units (e.g., topicals) shall state the proportion (rather than the quantity) of each active ingredient.
(3) "Purpose" or "Purposes", followed by the general pharmacological category(ies) or the principal intended action(s) of the drug or, where the drug consists of more than one ingredient, the general pharmacological categories or the principal intended actions of each active ingredient. When an OTC drug monograph contains a statement of identity, the pharmacological action described in the statement of identity shall also be stated as the purpose of the active ingredient.
(4) "Use" or "Uses", followed by the indication(s) for the specific drug product.
(5) "Warning" or "Warnings", followed by one or more of the following, if applicable:
  (i) "For external use only" [in bold type] for topical drug products not intended for ingestion, or "For" (select one of the following, as appropriate: "rectal" or "vaginal") "use only" [in bold type].
  (ii) All applicable warnings listed in paragraphs (c)(5)(ii)(A) through (c)(5)(ii)(G) of this section with the appropriate subheadings highlighted in bold type:
    (A) Reye's syndrome warning for drug products containing salicylates set forth in §201.314(h)(1). This warning shall follow the subheading "Reye's syndrome:"

(B) *Allergic reaction and asthma alert warnings.* Allergic reaction warnings set forth in any applicable OTC drug monograph or approved drug application for any product that requires a separate allergy warning. This warning shall follow the subheading "Allergy alert:" The asthma alert warning set forth in §§341.76(c)(5) and 341.76(c)(6) of this chapter. This warning shall follow the subheading "Asthma alert:"

(C) Flammability warning, with appropriate flammability signal word(s) (e.g., §§341.74(c)(5)(iii), 344.52(c), 358.150(c), and 358.550(c) of this chapter). This warning shall follow a subheading containing the appropriate flammability signal word(s) described in an applicable OTC drug monograph or approved drug application.

(D) Water soluble gums warning set forth in §201.319. This warning shall follow the subheading "Choking:"

(E) Liver warning set forth in §201.326(a)(1)(iii) and/or stomach bleeding warning set forth in §201.326(a)(2)(iii). The liver warning shall follow the subheading "Liver warning:" and the stomach bleeding warning shall follow the subheading "Stomach bleeding warning:"

(F) Sore throat warning set forth in §201.315. This warning shall follow the subheading "Sore throat warning:"

(G) Warning for drug products containing sodium phosphates set forth in §201.307(b)(2)(i) or (b)(2)(ii). This warning shall follow the subheading "Dosage warning:"

(H) Sexually transmitted diseases (STDs) warning for vaginal contraceptive and spermicide drug products containing nonoxynol 9 set forth in §201.325(b)(2). This warning shall follow the subheading "Sexually transmitted diseases (STDs) alert:"

(iii) "Do not use" [in bold type], followed by all contraindications for use with the product. These contraindications are absolute and are intended for situations in which consumers should not use the product unless a prior diagnosis has been established by a doctor or for situations in which certain consumers should not use the product under any circumstances regardless of whether a doctor or health professional is consulted.

(iv) "Ask a doctor before use if you have" [in bold type] or, for products labeled only for use in children under 12 years of age, "Ask a doctor before use if the child has" [in bold type], followed by all warnings for persons with certain preexisting conditions (excluding pregnancy) and all warnings for persons experiencing certain symptoms. The warnings under this heading are those intended only for situations in which consumers should not use the product until a doctor is consulted.

(v) "Ask a doctor or pharmacist before use if you are" [in bold type] or, for products labeled only for use in children under 12 years of age, "Ask a doctor or pharmacist before use if the child is" [in bold type], followed by all drug-drug and drug-food interaction warnings.

(vi) "When using this product" [in bold type], followed by the side effects that the consumer may experience, and the substances (e.g., alcohol) or activities (e.g., operating machinery, driving a car, warnings set forth in §369.21 of this chapter for drugs in dispensers pressurized by gaseous propellants) to avoid while using the product.

(vii) "Stop use and ask a doctor if" [in bold type], followed by any signs of toxicity or other reactions that would necessitate immediately discontinuing use of the product. For all OTC drug products under an approved drug application whose packaging does not include a toll-free number through which consumers can report complaints to the manufacturer or distributor of the drug product, the following text shall immediately follow the subheading: "[Bullet] side effects occur. You may report side effects to FDA at 1–800-FDA-1088." The telephone number must appear in a minimum 6-point bold letter height or type size.

(viii) Any required warnings in an applicable OTC drug monograph, other OTC drug regulations, or approved drug application that do not fit within one of the categories listed in paragraphs (c)(5)(i) through (c)(5)(vii), (c)(5)(ix), and (c)(5)(x) of this section.

(ix) The pregnancy/breast-feeding warning set forth in §201.63(a); the third trimester warning set forth in §201.63(e) for products containing aspirin or carbaspirin calcium; the third trimester warning set forth in approved drug applications for products containing ketoprofen, naproxen sodium, and ibuprofen (not intended exclusively for use in children).

(x) The "Keep out of reach of children" warning and the accidental overdose/ingestion warning set forth in §330.1(g) of this chapter.

(6) "Directions", followed by the directions for use described in an applicable OTC drug monograph or approved drug application.

(7) "Other information", followed by additional information that is not included under paragraphs (c)(2) through (c)(6), (c)(8), and (c)(9) of this section, but which is required by or is made optional under an applicable OTC drug monograph, other OTC drug regulation, or is included in the labeling of an approved drug application.

(i) Required information about certain ingredients in OTC drug products (e.g., sodium in §201.64(b), calcium in §201.70(b), magnesium in §201.71(b), and potassium in §201.72(b)) shall appear as follows: "each (insert appropriate dosage unit) contains:" [in bold type (insert name(s) of ingredient(s) (in alphabetical order) and the quantity of each ingredient). This information shall be the first statement under this heading.

(ii) The phenylalanine/aspartame content required by §201.21(b), if applicable, shall appear as the next item of information.

(iii) Additional information that is authorized to appear under this heading shall appear as the next item(s) of information. There is no required order for this subsequent information.

(8) "Inactive ingredients", followed by a listing of the established name of each inactive ingredient. If the product is an OTC drug product that is not also a cosmetic product, then the inactive ingredients shall be listed in alphabetical order. If the product is an OTC drug product that is also a cosmetic product, then the inactive ingredients shall be listed as set forth in §701.3(a) or (f) of this chapter, the names of cosmetic ingredients shall be determined in accordance with §701.3(c) of this chapter, and the provisions in §701.3(e), (g), (h), (l), (m), (n), and (o) of this chapter and §720.8 of this chapter may also apply, as appropriate. If there is a difference in the labeling provisions in this §201.66 and §§701.3 and 720.8 of this chapter, the labeling provisions in this §201.66 shall be used.

(9) "Questions?" or "Questions or comments?", followed by the telephone number of a source to answer questions about the product. It is recommended that the days of the week and times of the day when a person is available to respond to questions also be included. A graphic of a telephone or telephone receiver may appear before the heading. The telephone number must appear in a minimum 6-point bold type.

(d) *Format requirements.* The title, headings, subheadings, and information set forth in paragraphs (c)(1) through (c)(9) of this section shall be presented on OTC drug products in accordance with the following specifications. In the interest of uniformity of presentation, FDA strongly recommends that the Drug Facts labeling be presented using the graphic specifications set forth in appendix A to part 201.

(1) The title "Drug Facts" or "Drug Facts (continued)" shall use uppercase letters for the first letter of the words "Drug" and "Facts." All headings and subheadings in paragraphs (c)(2) through (c)(9) of this section shall use an uppercase letter for the first letter in the first word and lowercase letters for all other words. The title, headings, and subheadings in paragraphs (c)(1), (c)(2), and (c)(4) through (c)(9) of this section shall be left justified.

(2) The letter height or type size for the title "Drug Facts" shall appear in a type size larger than the largest type size used in the Drug Facts labeling. The letter height or type size for the title "Drug Facts (continued)" shall be no smaller than 8-point type. The letter height or type size for the headings in paragraphs (c)(2) through (c)(9) of this section shall be the larger of either 8-point or greater type, or 2-point sizes greater than the point size of the text. The letter height or type size for the subheadings and all other information described in paragraphs (c)(2) through (c)(9) of this section shall be no smaller than 6-point type.

(3) The title, heading, subheadings, and information in paragraphs (c)(1) through (c)(9) of this section shall be legible and clearly presented, shall have at least 0.5-point leading (i.e., space between two lines of text), and shall not have letters that touch. The type style for the title, headings, subheadings, and all other required information described in paragraphs (c)(2) through (c)(9) of this section shall be any single, clear, easy-to-read type style, with no

more than 39 characters per inch. The title and headings shall be in bold italic, and the subheadings shall be in bold type, except that the word "(continued)" in the title "Drug Facts (continued)" shall be regular type. The type shall be all black or one color printed on a white or other contrasting background, except that the title and the headings may be presented in a single, alternative, contrasting color unless otherwise provided in an approved drug application, OTC drug monograph (e.g., current requirements for bold print in §§341.76 and 341.80 of this chapter), or other OTC drug regulation (e.g., the requirement for a box and red letters in §201.308(c)(1)).

(4) When there is more than one statement, each individual statement listed under the headings and subheadings in paragraphs (c)(4) through (c)(7) of this section shall be preceded by a solid square or solid circle bullet of 5-point type size. Bullets shall be presented in the same shape and color throughout the labeling. The first bulleted statement on each horizontal line of text shall be either left justified or separated from an appropriate heading or subheading by at least two square "ems" (i.e., two squares of the size of the letter "M"). If more than one bulleted statement is placed on the same horizontal line, the end of one bulleted statement shall be separated from the beginning of the next bulleted statement by at least two square "ems" and the complete additional bulleted statement(s) shall not continue to the next line of text. Additional bulleted statements appearing on each subsequent horizontal line of text under a heading or subheading shall be vertically aligned with the bulleted statements appearing on the previous line.

(5) The title, headings, subheadings, and information set forth in paragraphs (c)(1) through (c)(9) of this section may appear on more than one panel on the outside container of the retail package, or the immediate container label if there is no outside container or wrapper. The continuation of the required content and format onto multiple panels must retain the required order and flow of headings, subheadings, and information. A visual graphic (e.g., an arrow) shall be used to signal the continuation of the Drug Facts labeling to the next adjacent panel.

(6) The heading and information required under paragraph (c)(2) of this section shall appear immediately adjacent and to the left of the heading and information required under paragraph (c)(3) of this section. The active ingredients and purposes shall be aligned under the appropriate headings such that the heading and information required under paragraph (c)(2) of this section shall be left justified and the heading and information required under paragraph (c)(3) of this section shall be right justified. If the OTC drug product contains more than one active ingredient, the active ingredients shall be listed in alphabetical order. If more than one active ingredient has the same purpose, the purpose need not be repeated for each active ingredient, provided the information is presented in a manner that readily associates each active ingredient with its purpose (i.e., through the use of brackets, dot leaders, or other graphical features). The information described in paragraphs (c)(4) and (c)(6) through (c)(9) of this section may start on the same line as the required headings. None of the information described in paragraph (c)(5) of this section shall appear on the same line as the "Warning" or "Warnings" heading.

(7) Graphical images (e.g., the UPC symbol) and information not described in paragraphs (c)(1) through (c)(9) of this section shall not appear in or in any way interrupt the required title, headings, subheadings, and information in paragraphs (c)(1) through (c)(9) of this section. Hyphens shall not be used except to punctuate compound words.

(8) The information described in paragraphs (c)(1) through (c)(9) of this section shall be set off in a box or similar enclosure by the use of a barline. A distinctive horizontal barline extending to each end of the "Drug Facts" box or similar enclosure shall provide separation between each of the headings listed in paragraphs (c)(2) through (c)(9) of this section. When a heading listed in paragraphs (c)(2) through (c)(9) of this section appears on a subsequent panel immediately after the "Drug Facts (continued)" title, a horizontal hairline shall follow the title and immediately precede the heading. A horizontal hairline extending within two spaces on either side of the "Drug Facts" box or similar enclosure shall immediately follow the title and shall immediately precede each of the subheadings set forth in paragraph (c)(5) of this section, except the subheadings in paragraphs (c)(5)(ii)(A) through (c)(5)(ii)(G) of this section.

(9) The information set forth in paragraph (c)(6) of this section under the heading "Directions" shall appear in a table format when dosage directions are provided for three or more age groups or populations. The last line of the table may be the horizontal barline immediately preceding the heading of the next section of the labeling.

(10) If the title, headings, subheadings, and information in paragraphs (c)(1) through (c)(9) of this section, printed in accordance with the specifications in paragraphs (d)(1) through (d)(9) of this section, and any other FDA required information for drug products, and, as appropriate, cosmetic products, other than information required to appear on a principle display panel, requires more than 60 percent of the total surface area available to bear labeling, then the Drug Facts labeling shall be printed in accordance with the specifications set forth in paragraphs (d)(10)(i) through (d)(10)(v) of this section. In determining whether more than 60 percent of the total surface area available to bear labeling is required, the indications for use listed under the "Use(s)" heading, as set forth in paragraph (c)(4) of this section, shall be limited to the minimum required uses reflected in the applicable monograph, as provided in §330.1(c)(2) of this chapter.
   (i) Paragraphs (d)(1), (d)(5), (d)(6), and (d)(7) of this section shall apply.
   (ii) Paragraph (d)(2) of this section shall apply except that the letter height or type size for the title "Drug Facts (continued)" shall be no smaller than 7-point type and the headings in paragraphs (c)(2) through (c)(9) of this section shall be the larger of either 7-point or greater type, or 1-point size greater than the point size of the text.
   (iii) Paragraph (d)(3) of this section shall apply except that less than 0.5-point leading may be used, provided the ascenders and descenders do not touch.
   (iv) Paragraph (d)(4) of this section shall apply except that if more than one bulleted statement is placed on the same horizontal line, the additional bulleted statements may continue to the next line of text, and except that the bullets under each heading or subheading need not be vertically aligned.
   (v) Paragraph (d)(8) of this section shall apply except that the box or similar enclosure required in paragraph (d)(8) of this section may be omitted if the Drug Facts labeling is set off from the rest of the labeling by use of color contrast.

(11) (i) The following labeling outlines the various provisions in paragraphs (c) and (d) of this section:

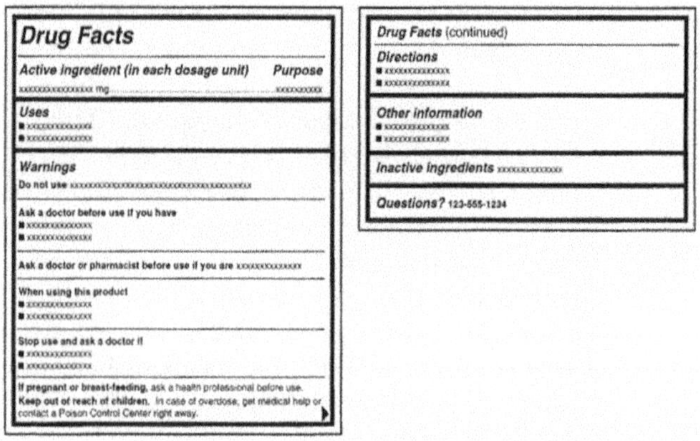

FIGURE 5.1 Over-The-Counter Drug Product Labeling Outline.

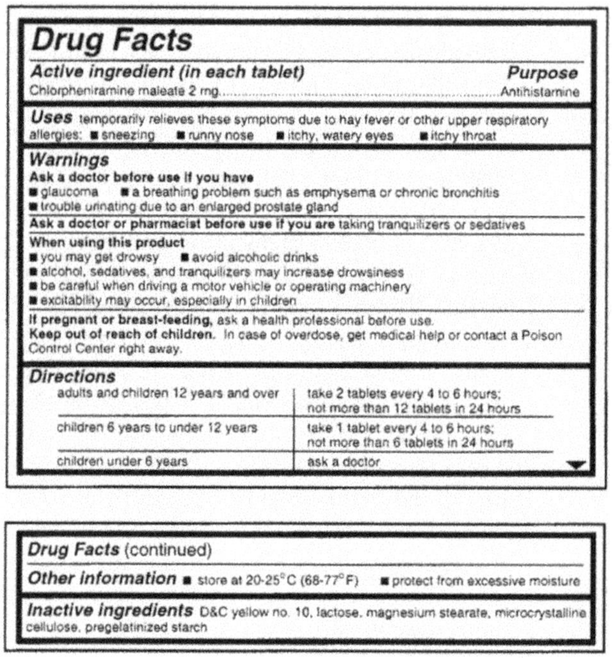

FIGURE 5.2 Sample Label Illustration Example 1.

(e) *Exemptions and deferrals.* FDA on its own initiative or in response to a written request from any manufacturer, packer, or distributor, may exempt or defer, based on the circumstances presented, one or more specific requirements set forth in this section on the basis that the requirement is inapplicable, impracticable, or contrary to public health or safety. Requests for exemptions shall be submitted in three copies in the form of an "Application for Exemption" to the Food and Drug Administration, 5630 Fishers Lane, rm. 1061, Rockville, MD 20852. The request shall be clearly identified on the envelope as a "Request for Exemption from 21 CFR 201.66 (OTC Labeling Format)" and shall be directed to Docket No. 98N-0337. A separate request shall be submitted for each OTC drug product. Sponsors of a product marketed under an approved drug application shall also submit a single copy of the exemption request to their application. Decisions on exemptions and deferrals will be maintained in a permanent file in this docket for public review. Exemption and deferral requests shall:

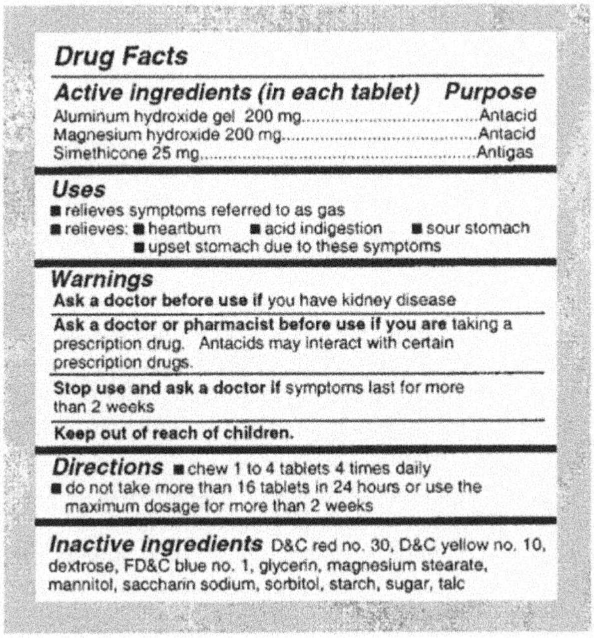

FIGURE 5.3 Sample Label Illustration Example 2.

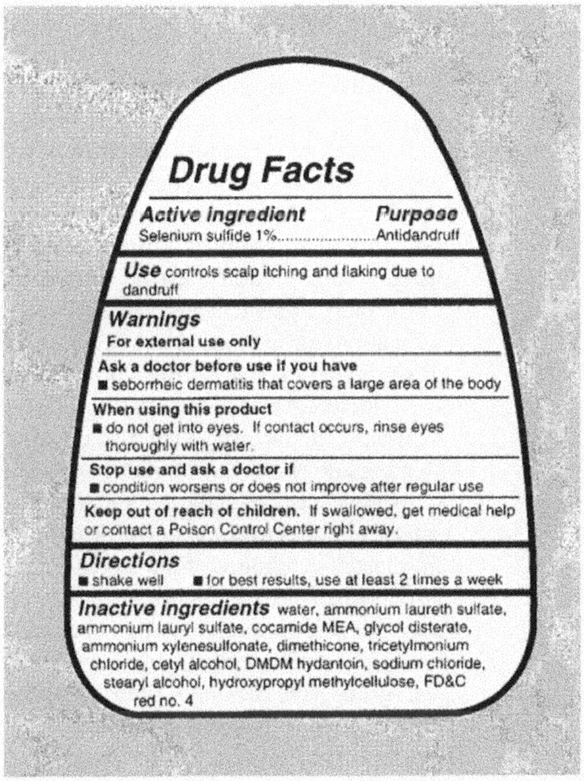

FIGURE 5.4 Sample Label Illustration Example 3.

(1) Document why a particular requirement is inapplicable, impracticable, or is contrary to public health or safety; and
(2) Include a representation of the proposed labeling, including any outserts, panel extensions, or other graphical or packaging techniques intended to be used with the product.

(f) *Interchangeable terms and connecting terms.* The terms listed in §330.1(i) of this chapter may be used interchangeably in the labeling of OTC drug products, provided such use does not alter the meaning of the labeling that has been established and identified in an applicable OTC drug monograph or by regulation. The terms listed in §330.1(j) of this chapter may be deleted from the labeling of OTC drug products when the labeling is revised to comply with this section, provided such deletion does not alter the meaning of the labeling that has been established and identified in an applicable OTC drug monograph or by regulation. The terms listed in §330.1(i) and (j) of this chapter shall not be used to change in any way the specific title, headings, and subheadings required under paragraphs (c)(1) through (c)(9) of this section.
(g) *Regulatory action.* An OTC drug product that is not in compliance with the format and content requirements in this section is subject to regulatory action.

5.14 §201.80 SPECIFIC REQUIREMENTS ON CONTENT AND FORMAT OF LABELING FOR HUMAN PRESCRIPTION DRUG AND BIOLOGICAL PRODUCTS; OLDER DRUGS NOT DESCRIBED IN §201.56(B)(1)

Each section heading listed in §201.56(d), if not omitted under §201.56(d)(3), shall contain the following information in the following order:

(a) *Description.*
  (1) Under this section heading, the labeling shall contain:
    (i) The proprietary name and the established name, if any, as defined in section 502(e)(2) of the act, of the drug;
    (ii) The type of dosage form and the route of administration to which the labeling applies;
    (iii) The same qualitative and/or quantitative ingredient information as required under §201.100(b) for labels;
    (iv) If the product is sterile, a statement of that fact;
    (v) The pharmacological or therapeutic class of the drug;
    (vi) The chemical name and structural formula of the drug;
    (vii) If the product is radioactive, a statement of the important nuclear physical characteristics, such as the principal radiation

emission data, external radiation, and physical decay characteristics.

(2) If appropriate, other important chemical or physical information, such as physical constants, or pH, shall be stated.

(b) *Clinical Pharmacology.*

(1) Under this section heading, the labeling shall contain a concise factual summary of the clinical pharmacology and actions of the drug in humans. The summary may include information based on in vitro and/or animal data if the information is essential to a description of the biochemical and/or physiological mode of action of the drug or is otherwise pertinent to human therapeutics. Pharmacokinetic information that is important to safe and effective use of the drug is required, if known, e.g., degree and rate of absorption, pathways of biotransformation, percentage of dose as unchanged drug and metabolites, rate or half-time of elimination, concentration in body fluids associated with therapeutic and/or toxic effects, degree of binding to plasma proteins, degree of uptake by a particular organ or in the fetus, and passage across the blood brain barrier. Inclusion of pharmacokinetic information is restricted to that which relates to clinical use of the drug. If the pharmacological mode of action of the drug is unknown or if important metabolic or pharmacokinetic data in humans are unavailable, the labeling shall contain a statement about the lack of information.

(2) Data that demonstrate activity or effectiveness in in vitro or animal tests and that have not been shown by adequate and well-controlled clinical studies to be pertinent to clinical use may be included under this section of the labeling only under the following circumstances:

(i) In vitro data for anti-infective drugs may be included if the data are immediately preceded by the statement "The following in vitro data are available but their clinical significance is unknown."

(ii) For other classes of drugs, in vitro and animal data that have not been shown by adequate and well-controlled clinical studies, as defined in §314.126(b) of this chapter, to be pertinent to clinical use may be used only if a waiver is granted under §201.58 or §314.126(c) of this chapter.

(c) *Indications and Usage.*

(1) Under this section heading, the labeling shall state that:

(i) The drug is indicated in the treatment, prevention, or diagnosis of a recognized disease or condition, e.g., penicillin is indicated for the treatment of pneumonia due to susceptible pneumococci; and/or

(ii) The drug is indicated for the treatment, prevention, or diagnosis of an important manifestation of a disease or condition, e.g., chlorothiazide is indicated for the treatment of edema in patients with congestive heart failure; and/or

(iii) The drug is indicated for the relief of symptoms associated with a disease or syndrome, e.g., chlorpheniramine is indicated for the symptomatic relief of nasal congestion in patients with vasomotor rhinitis; and/or

(iv) The drug, if used for a particular indication only in conjunction with a primary mode of therapy, e.g., diet, surgery, or some other drug, is an adjunct to the mode of therapy.

(2) (i) For drug products other than biological products, all indications listed in this section must be supported by substantial evidence of effectiveness based on adequate and well-controlled studies as defined in §314.126(b) of this chapter unless the requirement is waived under §201.58 or §314.126(c) of this chapter. Indications or uses must not be implied or suggested in other sections of labeling if not included in this section.

(ii) For biological products, all indications listed in this section must be supported by substantial evidence of effectiveness. Indications or uses must not be implied or suggested in other sections of labeling if not included in this section.

(3) This section of the labeling shall also contain the following additional information:

(i) If evidence is available to support the safety and effectiveness of the drug only in selected subgroups of the larger population with a disease, syndrome, or symptom under consideration, e.g., patients with mild disease or patients in a special age group, the labeling shall describe the available evidence and state the limitations of usefulness of the drug. The labeling shall also identify specific tests needed for selection or monitoring of the patients who need the drug, e.g., microbe susceptibility tests. Information on the approximate kind, degree, and duration of improvement to be anticipated shall be stated if available and shall be based on substantial evidence derived from adequate and well-controlled studies as defined in §314.126(b) of this chapter unless the requirement is waived under §201.58 or §314.126(c) of this chapter. If the information is relevant to the recommended intervals between doses, the usual duration of treatment, or any modification of dosage, it shall be stated in the "Dosage and Administration" section of the labeling and referenced in this section.

(ii) If safety considerations are such that the drug should be reserved for certain situations, e.g., cases refractory to other drugs, this information shall be stated in this section.

(iii) If there are specific conditions that should be met before the drug is used on a long-term basis, e.g., demonstration of responsiveness to the drug in a short-term trial, the labeling shall identify the conditions; or, if the indications for long-term use are different from those for short-term use, the labeling shall identify the specific indications for each use.

(iv) If there is a common belief that the drug may be effective for a certain use or if there is a common use of the drug for a condition, but the preponderance of evidence related to the use or condition shows that the drug is ineffective, the Food and Drug Administration may require that the labeling state that there is a lack of evidence that the drug is effective for that use or condition.

(v) Any statements comparing the safety or effectiveness, either greater or less, of the drug with other agents for the same indication shall be supported by adequate and well-controlled studies as defined in §314.126(b) of this chapter unless this requirement is waived under §201.58 or §314.126(c) of this chapter.

(d) *Contraindications.* Under this section heading, the labeling shall describe those situations in which the drug should not be used because the risk of use clearly outweighs any possible benefit. These situations include administration of the drug to patients known to have a hypersensitivity to it; use of the drug in patients who, because of their particular age, sex, concomitant therapy, disease state, or other condition, have a substantial risk of being harmed by it; or continued use of the drug in the face of an unacceptably hazardous adverse reaction. Known hazards and not theoretical possibilities shall be listed, e.g., if hypersensitivity to the drug has not been demonstrated, it should not be listed as a contraindication. If no contraindications are known, this section of the labeling shall state "None known."

(e) *Warnings.* Under this section heading, the labeling shall describe serious adverse reactions and potential safety hazards, limitations in use imposed by them, and steps that should be taken if they occur. The labeling shall be revised to include a warning as soon as there is reasonable evidence of an association of a serious hazard with a drug; a causal relationship need not have been proved. A specific warning relating to a use not provided for under the "Indications and Usage" section of the labeling may be required by the Food and Drug Administration if the drug is commonly prescribed for a disease or condition, and there is lack of substantial evidence of effectiveness for that disease or condition, and such usage is associated with serious risk or hazard. Special problems, particularly those that may lead to death or serious injury, may be required by the Food and Drug Administration to be placed in a prominently displayed box. The boxed warning ordinarily shall be based on clinical data, but serious animal toxicity may also be the basis of a boxed warning in the absence of clinical data. If a boxed warning is required, its location will be specified by the Food and Drug Administration. The frequency of these serious adverse reactions and, if known, the approximate mortality and morbidity rates for patients sustaining the reaction, which are important to safe and effective use of the drug, shall be expressed as provided under the "Adverse Reactions" section of the labeling.

(f) *Precautions.* Under this section heading, the labeling shall contain the following subsections as appropriate for the drug:

(1) *General.* This subsection of the labeling shall contain information regarding any special care to be exercised by the practitioner for safe and effective use of the drug, e.g., precautions not required under any other specific section or subsection of the labeling.

(2) *Information for patients.* This subsection must contain information necessary for patients to use the drug safely and effectively (e.g., precautions concerning driving or the concomitant use of other substances that may have harmful additive effects). Any FDA-approved patient labeling must be referenced in this section and the full text of such patient labeling must be reprinted immediately following the last section of labeling or, alternatively, accompany the prescription drug labeling. The type size requirement for the Medication Guide set forth in §208.20 of this chapter does not apply to the Medication Guide that is reprinted in or accompanying the prescription

drug labeling unless such Medication Guide is to be detached and distributed to patients in compliance with §208.24 of this chapter.

(3) *Laboratory tests.* This subsection of the labeling shall identify any laboratory tests that may be helpful in following the patient's response or in identifying possible adverse reactions. If appropriate, information shall be provided on such factors as the range of normal and abnormal values expected in the particular situation and the recommended frequency with which tests should be done before, during, and after therapy.

(4) (i) *Drug interactions.* This subsection of the labeling shall contain specific practical guidance for the physician on preventing clinically significant drug/drug and drug/food interactions that may occur in vivo in patients taking the drug. Specific drugs or classes of drugs with which the drug to which the labeling applies may interact in vivo shall be identified, and the mechanism(s) of the interaction shall be briefly described. Information in this subsection of the labeling shall be limited to that pertaining to clinical use of the drug in patients. Drug interactions supported only by animal or in vitro experiments may not ordinarily be included, but animal or in vitro data may be used if shown to be clinically relevant. Drug incompatibilities, i.e., drug interactions that may occur when drugs are mixed in vitro, as in a solution for intravenous administration, shall be discussed under the "Dosage and Administration" section of the labeling rather than under this subsection of the labeling.

(ii) *Drug/laboratory test interactions.* This subsection of the labeling shall contain practical guidance on known interference of the drug with laboratory tests.

(5) *Carcinogenesis, mutagenesis, impairment of fertility.* This subsection of the labeling shall state whether long-term studies in animals have been performed to evaluate carcinogenic potential and, if so, the species and results. If reproduction studies or other data in animals reveal a problem or potential problem concerning mutagenesis or impairment of fertility in either males or females, the information shall be described. Any precautionary statement on these topics shall include practical, relevant advice to the physician on the significance of these animal findings. If there is evidence from human data that the drug may be carcinogenic or mutagenic or that it impairs fertility, this information shall be included under the "Warnings" section of the labeling. Also, under "Precautions," the labeling shall state: "See 'Warnings' section for information on carcinogenesis, mutagenesis, and impairment of fertility."

(6) *Pregnancy.* This subsection of the labeling may be omitted only if the drug is not absorbed systemically and the drug is not known to have a potential for indirect harm to the fetus. For all other drugs, this subsection of the labeling shall contain the following information:

(i) *Teratogenic effects.* Under this heading the labeling shall identify one of the following categories that applies to the drug, and the labeling shall bear the statement required under the category:

(*a*) If adequate and well-controlled studies in pregnant women have failed to demonstrate a risk to the fetus in the first trimester of pregnancy (and there is no evidence of a risk in later trimesters), the labeling shall state: "Studies in pregnant women have not shown that (*name of drug*) increases the risk of fetal abnormalities if administered during the first (*second, third, or all*) trimester(*s*) of pregnancy. If this drug is used during pregnancy, the possibility of fetal harm appears remote. Because studies cannot rule out the possibility of harm, however, (*name of drug*) should be used during pregnancy only if clearly needed." The labeling shall also contain a description of the human studies. If animal reproduction studies are available and they fail to demonstrate a risk to the fetus, the labeling shall also state: "Reproduction studies have been performed in (*kinds of animal*(*s*)) at doses up to (*x*) times the human dose and have revealed no evidence of impaired fertility or harm to the fetus due to (*name of drug*)." The labeling shall also contain a description of available data on the effect of the drug on the later growth, development, and functional maturation of the child.

(*b*) If animal reproduction studies have failed to demonstrate a risk to the fetus and there are no adequate and well-controlled studies in pregnant women, the labeling shall state:

"Reproduction studies have been performed in (*kind(s) of animal(s)*) at doses up to (*x*) times the human dose and have revealed no evidence of impaired fertility or harm to the fetus due to (*name of drug*). There are, however, no adequate and well-controlled studies in pregnant women. Because animal reproduction studies are not always predictive of human response, this drug should be used during pregnancy only if clearly needed." If animal reproduction studies have shown an adverse effect (other than decrease in fertility), but adequate and well-controlled studies in pregnant women have failed to demonstrate a risk to the fetus during the first trimester of pregnancy (and there is no evidence of a risk in later trimesters), the labeling shall state: "Pregnancy Category B. Reproduction studies in (*kind(s) of animal(s)*) have shown (*describe findings*) at (*x*) times the human dose. Studies in pregnant women, however, have not shown that (*name of drug*) increases the risk of abnormalities when administered during the first (*second, third, or all*) trimester(*s*) of pregnancy. Despite the animal findings, it would appear that the possibility of fetal harm is remote, if the drug is used during pregnancy. Nevertheless, because the studies in humans cannot rule out the possibility of harm, (*name of drug*) should be used during pregnancy only if clearly needed." The labeling shall also contain a description of the human studies and a description of available data on the effect of the drug on the later growth, development, and functional maturation of the child.

(*c*) If animal reproduction studies have shown an adverse effect on the fetus, if there are no adequate and well-controlled studies in humans, and if the benefits from the use of the drug in pregnant women may be acceptable despite its potential risks, the labeling shall state: " (*Name of drug*) has been shown to be teratogenic (or to have an embryocidal effect or other adverse effect) in (*name(s) of species*) when given in doses (*x*) times the human dose. There are no adequate and well-controlled studies in pregnant women. (*Name of drug*) should be used during pregnancy only if the potential benefit justifies the potential risk to the fetus." The labeling shall contain a description of the animal studies. If there are no animal reproduction studies and no adequate and well-controlled studies in humans, the labeling shall state: "Pregnancy Category C. Animal reproduction studies have not been conducted with (*name of drug*). It is also not known whether (*name of drug*) can cause fetal harm when administered to a pregnant woman or can affect reproduction capacity. (*Name of drug*) should be given to a pregnant woman only if clearly needed." The labeling shall contain a description of any available data on the effect of the drug on the later growth, development, and functional maturation of the child.

(*d*) If there is positive evidence of human fetal risk based on adverse reaction data from investigational or marketing experience or studies in humans, but the potential benefits from the use of the drug in pregnant women may be acceptable despite its potential risks (for example, if the drug is needed in a life-threatening situation or serious disease for which safer drugs cannot be used or are ineffective), the labeling shall state: "See 'Warnings' section." Under the "Warnings" section, the labeling states: "(*Name of drug*) can cause fetal harm when administered to a pregnant woman. (*Describe the human data and any pertinent animal data.*) If this drug is used during pregnancy, or if the patient becomes pregnant while taking this drug, the patient should be apprised of the potential hazard to the fetus."

(*e*) If studies in animals or humans have demonstrated fetal abnormalities or if there is positive evidence of fetal risk based on adverse reaction reports from investigational or marketing experience, or both, and the risk of the use of the drug in a pregnant woman clearly outweighs any possible benefit (for example, safer drugs or other forms of therapy are available), the labeling shall state: "See 'Contraindications' section." Under "Contraindications," the labeling shall state: *"(Name of drug)* may *(can)* cause fetal harm when administered to a pregnant woman. *(Describe the human data and any pertinent animal data.)* *(Name of drug)* is contraindicated in women who are or may become pregnant. If this drug is used during pregnancy, or if the patient becomes pregnant while taking this drug, the patient should be apprised of the potential hazard to the fetus."

(ii) *Nonteratogenic effects.* Under this heading the labeling shall contain other information on the drug's effects on reproduction and the drug's use during pregnancy that is not required specifically by one of the pregnancy categories, if the information is relevant to the safe and effective use of the drug. Information required under this heading shall include nonteratogenic effects in the fetus or newborn infant (for example, withdrawal symptoms or hypoglycemia) that may occur because of a pregnant woman's chronic use of the drug for a preexisting condition or disease.

(7) *Labor and delivery.* If the drug has a recognized use during labor or delivery (vaginal or abdominal delivery), whether or not the use is stated in the indications section of the labeling, this subsection of the labeling shall describe the available information about the effect of the drug on the mother and the fetus, on the duration of labor or delivery, on the possibility that forceps delivery or other intervention or resuscitation of the newborn will be necessary, and the effect of the drug on the later growth, development, and functional maturation of the child. If any information required under this subsection is unknown, this subsection of the labeling shall state that the information is unknown.

(8) *Nursing mothers.*

(i) If a drug is absorbed systemically, this subsection of the labeling shall contain, if known, information about excretion of the drug in human milk and effects on the nursing infant. Pertinent adverse effects observed in animal offspring shall be described.

(ii) If a drug is absorbed systemically and is known to be excreted in human milk, this subsection of the labeling shall contain one of the following statements, as appropriate. If the drug is associated with serious adverse reactions or if the drug has a known tumorigenic potential, the labeling shall state: "Because of the potential for serious adverse reactions in nursing infants from *(name of drug)* (or, "Because of the potential for tumorigenicity shown for *(name of drug)* in *(animal or human)* studies), a decision should be made whether to discontinue nursing or to discontinue the drug, taking into account the importance of the drug to the mother." If the drug is not associated with serious adverse reactions and does not have a known tumorigenic potential, the labeling shall state: "Caution should be exercised when *(name of drug)* is administered to a nursing woman."

(iii) If a drug is absorbed systemically and information on excretion in human milk is unknown, this subsection of the labeling shall contain one of the following statements, as appropriate. If the drug is associated with serious adverse reactions or has a known tumorigenic potential, the labeling shall state: "It is not known whether this drug is excreted in human milk. Because many drugs are excreted in human milk and because of the potential for serious adverse reactions in nursing infants from *(name of drug)* (or, "Because of the potential for tumorigenicity shown for *(name of drug)* in *(animal or human)* studies), a decision should be made whether to discontinue nursing or to discontinue the drug, taking into account the importance of the drug to the mother." If the drug is not associated with serious adverse reactions and does not have a known tumorigenic potential, the labeling shall state: "It is not known whether this drug is excreted in human milk. Because many drugs are excreted in human milk, caution should be exercised when *(name of drug)* is administered to a nursing woman."

(9) *Pediatric use.*

(i) Pediatric population(s)/pediatric patient(s): For the purposes of paragraphs (f)(9)(ii) through (f)(9)(viii) of this section, the terms *pediatric population(s)* and *pediatric patient(s)* are defined as the pediatric age group, from birth to 16 years, including age groups often called neonates, infants, children, and adolescents.

(ii) If there is a specific pediatric indication (i.e., an indication different from those approved for adults) that is supported by adequate and well-controlled studies in the pediatric population, it shall be described under the "Indications and Usage" section of the labeling, and appropriate pediatric dosage information shall be given under the "Dosage and Administration" section of the labeling. The "Pediatric use" subsection shall cite any limitations on the pediatric indication, need for specific monitoring, specific hazards associated with use of the drug in any subsets of the pediatric population (e.g., neonates), differences between pediatric and adult responses to the drug, and other information related to the safe and effective pediatric use of the drug. Data summarized in this subsection of the labeling should be discussed in more detail, if appropriate, under the "Clinical Pharmacology" or "Clinical Studies" section. As appropriate, this information shall also be contained in the "Contraindications," "Warnings," and elsewhere in the "Precautions" sections.

(iii) If there are specific statements on pediatric use of the drug for an indication also approved for adults that are based on adequate and well-controlled studies in the pediatric population, they shall be summarized in the "Pediatric use" subsection of the labeling and discussed in more detail, if appropriate, under the "Clinical Pharmacology" and "Clinical Studies" sections. Appropriate pediatric dosage shall be given under the "Dosage and Administration" section of the labeling. The "Pediatric use" subsection of the labeling shall also cite any limitations on the pediatric use statement, need for specific monitoring, specific hazards associated with use of the drug in any subsets of the pediatric population (e.g., neonates), differences between pediatric and adult responses to the drug, and other information related to the safe and effective pediatric use of the drug. As appropriate, this information shall also be contained in the "Contraindications," "Warnings," and elsewhere in the "Precautions" sections.

(iv) FDA may approve a drug for pediatric use based on adequate and well-controlled studies in adults, with other information supporting pediatric use. In such cases, the agency will have concluded that the course of the disease and the effects of the drug, both beneficial and adverse, are sufficiently similar in the pediatric and adult populations to permit extrapolation from the adult efficacy data to pediatric patients. The additional information supporting pediatric use must ordinarily include data on the pharmacokinetics of the drug in the pediatric population for determination of appropriate dosage. Other information, such as data from pharmacodynamic studies of the drug in the pediatric population, data from other studies supporting the safety or effectiveness of the drug in pediatric patients, pertinent premarketing or postmarketing studies or experience, may be necessary to show that the drug can be used safely and effectively in pediatric patients. When a drug is approved for pediatric use based on adequate and well-controlled studies in adults with other information supporting pediatric use, the "Pediatric use" subsection of the labeling shall contain either the following statement, or a reasonable alternative: "The safety and effectiveness of (*drug name*) have been established in the age groups _ to _ (note any limitations, e.g., no data for pediatric patients under 2, or only applicable to certain indications approved in adults). Use of (*drug name*) in these age groups is supported by evidence from adequate and well-controlled studies of (*drug name*) in adults with additional data (insert wording that accurately describes the data submitted to support a finding of substantial evidence of effectiveness in the pediatric population)." Data summarized in the preceding prescribed statement in this subsection of the labeling shall be discussed in more detail, if appropriate, under the "Clinical Pharmacology" or the "Clinical Studies" section. For example, pediatric pharmacokinetic or pharmacodynamic studies and dose-response information should be described in the "Clinical Pharmacology" section. Pediatric dosing instructions shall be included in the "Dosage and Administration" section of the labeling. Any differences between pediatric and adult responses, need for specific monitoring, dosing adjustments, and any other information related to safe and effective use of the drug in pediatric patients shall be cited briefly in the "Pediatric use" subsection and, as appropriate, in the "Contraindications," "Warnings," "Precautions," and "Dosage and Administration" sections.

(v) If the requirements for a finding of substantial evidence to support a pediatric indication or a pediatric use statement have not been met for a particular pediatric population, the "Pediatric use" subsection of the labeling shall contain an appropriate statement such as "Safety and effectiveness in pediatric patients below the age of (_) have not been established." If use of the drug in this pediatric population is associated with a specific hazard, the hazard shall be described in this subsection of the labeling, or, if appropriate, the hazard shall be stated in the "Contraindications" or "Warnings" section of the labeling and this subsection shall refer to it.

(vi) If the requirements for a finding of substantial evidence to support a pediatric indication or a pediatric use statement have not been met for any pediatric population, this subsection of the labeling shall contain the following statement: "Safety and effectiveness in pediatric patients have not been established." If use of the drug in premature or neonatal infants, or other pediatric subgroups, is associated with a specific hazard, the hazard shall be described in this subsection of the labeling, or, if appropriate, the hazard shall be stated in the "Contraindications" or "Warnings" section of the labeling and this subsection shall refer to it.

(vii) If the sponsor believes that none of the statements described in paragraphs (f)(9)(ii) through (f)(9)(vi) of this section is appropriate or relevant to the labeling of a particular drug, the sponsor shall provide reasons for omission of the statements and may propose alternative statement(s). FDA may permit use of an alternative statement if FDA determines that no statement described in those paragraphs is appropriate or relevant to the drug's labeling and that the alternative statement is accurate and appropriate.

(viii) If the drug product contains one or more inactive ingredients that present an increased risk of toxic effects to neonates or other pediatric subgroups, a special note of this risk shall be made, generally in the "Contraindications," "Warnings," or "Precautions" section.

(10) *Geriatric use.*

(i) A specific geriatric indication, if any, that is supported by adequate and well-controlled studies in the geriatric population shall be described under the "Indications and Usage" section of the labeling, and appropriate geriatric dosage shall be stated under the "Dosage and Administration" section of the labeling. The "Geriatric use" subsection shall cite any limitations on the geriatric indication, need for specific monitoring, specific hazards associated with the geriatric indication, and other information related to the safe and effective use of the drug in the geriatric population. Unless otherwise noted, information contained in the "Geriatric use" subsection of the labeling shall pertain to use of the drug in persons 65 years of age and older. Data summarized in this subsection of the labeling shall be discussed in more detail, if appropriate, under "Clinical Pharmacology" or the "Clinical Studies" section. As appropriate, this information shall also be contained in "Contraindications," "Warnings," and elsewhere in "Precautions."

(ii) Specific statements on geriatric use of the drug for an indication approved for adults generally, as distinguished from a specific geriatric indication, shall be contained in the "Geriatric use" subsection and shall reflect all information available to the sponsor that is relevant to the appropriate use of the drug in elderly patients. This information includes detailed results from controlled studies that are available to the sponsor and pertinent information from well-documented studies obtained from a literature search. Controlled studies include those that are part of the marketing application and other relevant studies available to the sponsor that have not been previously submitted in the investigational new drug application, new drug application, biological license application, or a supplement or amendment to one of these applications (e.g., postmarketing studies or adverse drug reaction reports). The "Geriatric use" subsection shall contain the following statement(s) or reasonable alternative, as applicable, taking into account available information:

(A) If clinical studies did not include sufficient numbers of subjects aged 65 and over to determine whether elderly subjects respond differently from younger subjects, and other reported clinical experience has not identified such differences, the "Geriatric use" subsection shall include the following statement:
"Clinical studies of (name of drug) did not include sufficient numbers of subjects aged 65 and over to determine whether they respond differently from younger subjects. Other reported clinical experience has not identified differences in responses between the elderly and younger patients. In general, dose selection for an elderly patient should be cautious, usually starting at the low end of the dosing range, reflecting the greater frequency of decreased hepatic, renal, or cardiac function, and of concomitant disease or other drug therapy."

(B) If clinical studies (including studies that are part of marketing applications and other relevant studies available to the sponsor that have not been submitted in the sponsor's applications) included enough elderly subjects to make it likely that differences in safety or effectiveness between elderly and younger subjects would have been detected, but no such differences (in safety or effectiveness) were observed, and other reported clinical experience has not identified such differences, the "Geriatric use" subsection shall contain the following statement:
Of the total number of subjects in clinical studies of (name of drug), _ percent were 65 and over, while _ percent were 75 and over. (Alternatively, the labeling may state the total number of subjects included in the studies who were 65 and over and 75 and over.) No overall differences in safety or effectiveness were observed between these subjects and younger subjects, and other reported clinical experience has not identified differences in responses between the elderly and younger patients, but greater sensitivity of some older individuals cannot be ruled out.

(C) If evidence from clinical studies and other reported clinical experience available to the sponsor indicates that use of the drug in elderly patients is associated with differences in safety or effectiveness, or requires specific monitoring or dosage adjustment, the "Geriatric use" subsection of the labeling shall contain a brief description of observed differences or specific monitoring or dosage requirements and, as appropriate, shall refer to more detailed discussions in the "Contraindications," "Warnings," "Dosage and Administration," or other sections of the labeling.

(iii) (A) If specific pharmacokinetic or pharmacodynamic studies have been carried out in the elderly, they shall be described briefly in the "Geriatric use" subsection of the labeling and in detail under the "Clinical Pharmacology" section. The "Clinical Pharmacology" section and "Drug interactions" subsection of the "Precautions" section ordinarily contain information on drug-disease and drug-drug interactions that is particularly relevant to the elderly, who are more likely to have concomitant illness and to utilize concomitant drugs.

(B) If a drug is known to be substantially excreted by the kidney, the "Geriatric use" subsection shall include the statement:
"This drug is known to be substantially excreted by the kidney, and the risk of toxic reactions to this drug may be greater in patients with impaired renal function. Because elderly patients are more likely to have decreased renal function, care should be taken in dose selection, and it may be useful to monitor renal function."

(iv) If use of the drug in the elderly appears to cause a specific hazard, the hazard shall be described in the "Geriatric use" subsection of the labeling, or, if appropriate, the hazard shall be stated in the "Contraindications," "Warnings," or

"Precautions" section of the labeling, and the "Geriatric use" subsection shall refer to those sections.

(v) Labeling under paragraphs (f)(10)(i) through (f)(10)(iii) of this section may include statements, if they would be useful in enhancing safe use of the drug, that reflect good clinical practice or past experience in a particular situation, e.g., for a sedating drug, it could be stated that:
"Sedating drugs may cause confusion and over-sedation in the elderly; elderly patients generally should be started on low doses of (name of drug) and observed closely."

(vi) If the sponsor believes that none of the requirements described in paragraphs (f)(10)(i) through (f)(10)(v) of this section is appropriate or relevant to the labeling of a particular drug, the sponsor shall provide reasons for omission of the statements and may propose an alternative statement. FDA may permit omission of the statements if FDA determines that no statement described in those paragraphs is appropriate or relevant to the drug's labeling. FDA may permit use of an alternative statement if the agency determines that such statement is accurate and appropriate.

(g) *Adverse Reactions.* An adverse reaction is an undesirable effect, reasonably associated with the use of the drug that may occur as part of the pharmacological action of the drug or may be unpredictable in its occurrence.

(1) This section of the labeling shall list the adverse reactions that occur with the drug and with drugs in the same pharmacologically active and chemically related class, if applicable.

(2) In this listing, adverse reactions may be categorized by organ system, by severity of the reaction, by frequency, or by toxicological mechanism, or by a combination of these, as appropriate. If frequency information from adequate clinical studies is available, the categories and the adverse reactions within each category shall be listed in decreasing order of frequency. An adverse reaction that is significantly more severe than the other reactions listed in a category, however, shall be listed before those reactions, regardless of its frequency. If frequency information from adequate clinical studies is not available, the categories and adverse reactions within each category shall be listed in decreasing order of severity. The approximate frequency of each adverse reaction shall be expressed in rough estimates or orders of magnitude essentially as follows: "The most frequent adverse reaction(s) to (*name of drug*) is (are) (*list reactions*). This (these) occur(s) in about (e.g., one-third of patients; one in 30 patients; less than one-tenth of patients). Less frequent adverse reactions are (*list reactions*), which occur in approximately (e.g., one in 100 patients). Other adverse reactions, which occur rarely, in approximately (e.g., one in 1,000 patients), are (*list reactions*)." Percent figures may not ordinarily be used unless they are documented by adequate and well-controlled studies as defined in §314.126(b) of this chapter, they are shown to reflect general experience, and they do not falsely imply a greater degree of accuracy than actually exists.

(3) The "Warnings" section of the labeling or, if appropriate, the "Contraindications" section of the labeling shall identify any potentially fatal adverse reaction.

(4) Any claim comparing the drug to which the labeling applies with other drugs in terms of frequency, severity, or character of adverse reactions shall be based on adequate and well-controlled studies as defined in §314.126(b) of this chapter unless this requirement is waived under §201.58 or §314.126(c) of this chapter.

(h) *Drug Abuse and Dependence.* Under this section heading, the labeling shall contain the following subsections, as appropriate for the drug:

(1) *Controlled Substance.* If the drug is controlled by the Drug Enforcement Administration, the schedule in which it is controlled shall be stated.

(2) *Abuse.* This subsection of the labeling shall be based primarily on human data and human experience, but pertinent animal data may also be used. This subsection shall state the types of abuse that can occur with the drug and the adverse reactions pertinent to them. Particularly susceptible patient populations shall be identified.

(3) *Dependence.* This subsection of the labeling shall describe characteristic effects resulting from both psychological and physical dependence that occur with the drug and shall identify the quantity of the drug over a period of time that may lead to tolerance or dependence, or both. Details shall be provided on the adverse effects of chronic abuse and the effects of abrupt withdrawal. Procedures necessary to diagnose the dependent state

shall be provided, and the principles of treating the effects of abrupt withdrawal shall be described.

(i) *Overdosage.* Under this section heading, the labeling shall describe the signs, symptoms, and laboratory findings of acute overdosage and the general principles of treatment. This section shall be based on human data, when available. If human data are unavailable, appropriate animal and in vitro data may be used. Specific information shall be provided about the following:

(1) Signs, symptoms, and laboratory findings associated with an overdosage of the drug.

(2) Complications that can occur with the drug (for example, organ toxicity or delayed acidosis).

(3) Oral LD_{50} of the drug in animals; concentrations of the drug in biologic fluids associated with toxicity and/or death; physiologic variables influencing excretion of the drug, such as urine pH; and factors that influence the dose response relationship of the drug, such as tolerance. The pharmacokinetic data given in the "Clinical Pharmacology" section also may be referenced here, if applicable to overdoses.

(4) The amount of the drug in a single dose that is ordinarily associated with symptoms of overdosage and the amount of the drug in a single dose that is likely to be life-threatening.

(5) Whether the drug is dialyzable.

(6) Recommended general treatment procedures and specific measures for support of vital functions, such as proven antidotes, gastric lavage, and forced diuresis. Unqualified recommendations for which data are lacking with the specific drug or class of drugs, especially treatment using another drug (for example, central nervous system stimulants, and respiratory stimulants) may not be stated unless specific data or scientific rationale exists to support safe and effective use.

(j) *Dosage and Administration.* This section of the labeling shall state the recommended usual dose, the usual dosage range, and, if appropriate, an upper limit beyond which safety and effectiveness have not been established; dosages shall be stated for each indication when appropriate. Dosing regimens must not be implied or suggested in other sections of labeling if not included in this section. This section shall also state the intervals recommended between doses, the optimal method of titrating dosage, the usual duration of treatment, and any modification of dosage needed in special patient populations, e.g., in children, in geriatric age groups, or in patients with renal or hepatic disease. Specific tables or monographs may be included to clarify dosage schedules. Radiation dosimetry information shall be stated for both the patient receiving a radioactive drug and the person administering it. This section shall also contain specific direction on dilution, preparation (including the strength of the final dosage solution, when prepared according to instructions, in terms of milligrams active ingredient per milliliter of reconstituted solution, unless another measure of the strength is more appropriate), and administration of the dosage form, if needed, e.g., the rate of administration of parenteral drug in milligrams per minute; storage conditions for stability of the drug or reconstituted drug, when important; essential information on drug incompatibilities if the drug is mixed in vitro with other drugs; and the following statement for parenterals: "Parenteral drug products should be inspected visually for particulate matter and discoloration prior to administration, whenever solution and container permit."

(k) *How Supplied.* This section of the labeling shall contain information on the available dosage forms to which the labeling applies and for which the manufacturer or distributor is responsible. The information shall ordinarily include:

(1) The strength of the dosage form, e.g., 10-milligram tablets, in metric system and, if the apothecary system is used, a statement of the strength is placed in parentheses after the metric designation;

(2) The units in which the dosage form is ordinarily available for prescribing by practitioners, e.g., bottles of 100;

(3) Appropriate information to facilitate identification of the dosage forms, such as shape, color, coating, scoring, and National Drug Code; and

(4) Special handling and storage conditions.

(l) *Animal Pharmacology and/or Animal Toxicology.* In most cases, the labeling need not include this section. Significant animal data necessary for safe and effective use of the drug in humans shall ordinarily be included in one or more of the other sections of the labeling, as appropriate. Commonly for a drug that has been marketed for a long time, and in rare cases for a new drug, chronic animal toxicity studies have not been performed or completed for a drug that is administered over prolonged periods or is implanted in the body. The unavailability of such data shall be stated in the appropriate section of the labeling for the drug. If the pertinent animal data cannot be appropriately incorporated into other sections of the labeling, this section may be used.

(m) *"Clinical Studies" and "References".* These sections may appear in labeling in the place of a detailed discussion of a subject that is of limited interest but nonetheless important. A reference to a specific important clinical study may be made in any section of the format required under §§201.56 and 201.57 if the study is essential to an understandable presentation of the available information. References may appear in sections of the labeling format, other than the "Clinical Studies" or "References" section, in rare circumstances only. A clinical study or reference may be cited in prescription drug labeling only under the following conditions:

(1) (i) If the clinical study is cited in the labeling in place of a detailed discussion of data and information concerning an indication for use of the drug, the clinical study must constitute an adequate and well-controlled study as described in §314.126(b) of this chapter, except for biological products, and must not imply or suggest indications or uses or dosing regimens not stated in the "Indications and Usage" or "Dosage and Administration" section.

(ii) When prescription drug labeling must summarize or otherwise rely on a recommendation by an authoritative scientific body, or on a standardized methodology, scale, or technique, because the information is important to prescribing decisions, the labeling may include a reference to the source of the information.

(2) If the clinical study or reference is cited in the labeling in the place of a detailed discussion of data and information concerning a risk or risks from the use of the drug, the risk or risks shall also be identified or discussed in the appropriate section of the labeling for the drug.

5.15 §310.305 RECORDS AND REPORTS CONCERNING ADVERSE DRUG EXPERIENCES ON MARKETED PRESCRIPTION DRUGS FOR HUMAN USE WITHOUT APPROVED NEW DRUG APPLICATIONS

(a) *Scope.* FDA is requiring manufacturers, packers, and distributors of marketed prescription drug products that are not the subject of an approved new drug or abbreviated new drug application to establish and maintain records and make reports to FDA of all serious, unexpected adverse drug experiences associated with the use of their drug products. Any person subject to the reporting requirements of paragraph (c) of this section must also develop written procedures for the surveillance, receipt, evaluation, and reporting of postmarketing adverse drug experiences to FDA.

(b) *Definitions.* The following definitions of terms apply to this section:

Adverse drug experience. Any adverse event associated with the use of a drug in humans, whether or not considered drug related, including the following: An adverse event occurring in the course of the use of a drug product in professional practice; an adverse event occurring from drug overdose whether accidental or intentional; an adverse event occurring from drug abuse; an adverse event occurring from drug withdrawal; and any failure of expected pharmacological action.

Disability. A substantial disruption of a person's ability to conduct normal life functions.

Individual case safety report (ICSR). A description of an adverse drug experience related to an individual patient or subject.

ICSR attachments. Documents related to the adverse drug experience described in an ICSR, such as medical records, hospital discharge summaries, or other documentation.

Life-threatening adverse drug experience. Any adverse drug experience that places the patient, in the view of the initial reporter, at *immediate* risk of death from the adverse drug experience as it occurred, *i.e.*, it does not include an adverse drug experience that, had it occurred in a more severe form, might have caused death.

Serious adverse drug experience. Any adverse drug experience occurring at any dose that results in any of the following outcomes: Death, a life-threatening adverse drug experience, inpatient hospitalization or prolongation of existing hospitalization, a persistent or significant disability/incapacity, or a congenital anomaly/birth defect. Important medical events that may not result in death, be life-threatening, or require hospitalization may be considered a serious adverse drug experience when, based upon appropriate medical judgment, they may jeopardize the patient or subject and may require medical or surgical intervention to prevent one of the outcomes listed in this definition. Examples of such medical events include allergic bronchospasm requiring intensive treatment in an emergency room or at home, blood dyscrasias or convulsions that do not result in inpatient hospitalization, or the development of drug dependency or drug abuse.

Unexpected adverse drug experience. Any adverse drug experience that is not listed in the current labeling for the drug product. This includes events that may be symptomatically and pathophysiologically related to an event listed in the labeling, but differ from the event because of greater severity or specificity. For example, under this definition, hepatic necrosis would be unexpected (by virtue of greater severity) if the labeling only referred to elevated hepatic enzymes or hepatitis. Similarly, cerebral thromboembolism and cerebral vasculitis would be unexpected (by virtue of greater specificity) if the labeling only listed cerebral vascular accidents. "Unexpected," as used in this definition, refers to an adverse drug experience that has not been previously observed (*i.e.*, included in the labeling) rather than from the perspective of such experience not being anticipated from the pharmacological properties of the pharmaceutical product.

(c) *Reporting requirements.* Each person identified in paragraph (c)(1)(i) of this section must submit to FDA adverse drug experience information as described in this section. Except as provided in paragraph (e)(2) of this section, 15-day "Alert reports" and follow-up reports, including ICSRs and any ICSR attachments, must be submitted to the Agency in electronic format as described in paragraph (e)(1) of this section.

(1) *Postmarketing 15-day "Alert reports".*

(i) Any person whose name appears on the label of a marketed prescription drug product as its manufacturer, packer, or distributor must report to FDA each adverse drug experience received or otherwise obtained that is both serious and unexpected as soon as possible, but no later than 15 calendar days from initial receipt of the information by the person whose name appears on the label. Each report must be accompanied by the current content of labeling in electronic format as an ICSR attachment unless it is already on file at FDA.

(ii) A person identified in paragraph (c)(1)(i) of this section is not required to submit a 15-day "Alert report" for an adverse drug experience obtained from a postmarketing study (whether or not conducted under an investigational new drug application) unless the applicant concludes that there is a reasonable possibility that the drug caused the adverse experience.

(2) *Postmarketing 15-day "Alert reports"—follow-up.* Each person identified in paragraph (c)(1)(i) of this section must promptly investigate all serious, unexpected adverse drug experiences that are the subject of these postmarketing 15-day Alert reports and must submit follow-up reports within 15 calendar days of receipt of new information or as requested by FDA. If additional information is not obtainable, records should be maintained of the unsuccessful steps taken to seek additional information.

(3) *Submission of reports.* To avoid unnecessary duplication in the submission of, and follow-up to, reports required in this section, a packer's or distributor's obligations may be met by submission of all reports of serious adverse drug experiences to the manufacturer of the drug product. If a packer or distributor elects to submit these adverse drug experience reports to the manufacturer rather than to FDA, it must submit, by any appropriate means, each report to the manufacturer within 5 calendar days of its receipt by the packer or distributor, and the manufacturer must then comply with the requirements of this section even if its name does not appear on the label of the drug product. Under this circumstance, the packer or distributor must maintain a record of this action which must include:

(i) A copy of each adverse drug experience report;

(ii) The date the report was received by the packer or distributor;

(iii) The date the report was submitted to the manufacturer; and

(iv) The name and address of the manufacturer.

(4) [Reserved]

(5) A person identified in paragraph (c)(1)(i) of this section is not required to resubmit to FDA adverse drug experience reports forwarded to that person by FDA; however, the person must submit all *follow-up* information on such reports to FDA.

(d) *Information reported on ICSRs.* ICSRs include the following information:

(1) *Patient information.*

(i) Patient identification code;

(ii) Patient age at the time of adverse drug experience, or date of birth;

(iii) Patient gender; and

(iv) Patient weight.

(2) *Adverse drug experience.*

(i) Outcome attributed to adverse drug experience;

(ii) Date of adverse drug experience;

(iii) Date of ICSR submission;

(iv) Description of adverse drug experience (including a concise medical narrative);

(v) Adverse drug experience term(s);

(vi) Description of relevant tests, including dates and laboratory data; and

(vii) Other relevant patient history, including preexisting medical conditions.

(3) *Suspect medical product(s).*

(i) Name;

(ii) Dose, frequency, and route of administration used;

(iii) Therapy dates;
(iv) Diagnosis for use (indication);
(v) Whether the product is a combination product as defined in §3.2(e) of this chapter;
(vi) Whether the product is a prescription or nonprescription product;
(vii) Whether adverse drug experience abated after drug use stopped or dose reduced;
(viii) Whether adverse drug experience reappeared after reintroduction of drug;
(ix) Lot number;
(x) Expiration date;
(xi) National Drug Code (NDC) number; and
(xii) Concomitant medical products and therapy dates.

(4) *Initial reporter information.*
(i) Name, address, and telephone number;
(ii) Whether the initial reporter is a healthcare professionals; and
(iii) Occupation, if a healthcare professional.

(5) *Manufacturer, packer, or distributor information.*
(i) Manufacturer, packer, or distributor name and contact office address;
(ii) Telephone number;
(iii) Report source, such as spontaneous, literature, or study;
(iv) Date the report was received by manufacturer, packer, or distributor;
(v) Whether the ICSR is a 15-day "Alert report";
(vi) Whether the ICSR is an initial report or follow-up report; and
(vii) Unique case identification number, which must be the same in the initial report and any subsequent follow-up report(s).

(e) *Electronic format for submissions.*
(1) Each report required to be submitted to FDA under this section, including the ICSR and any ICSR attachments, must be submitted in an electronic format that FDA can process, review, and archive. FDA will issue guidance on how to provide the electronic submission (e.g., method of transmission, media, file formats, preparation and organization of files).
(2)Each person identified in paragraph (c)(1)(i) of this section may request, in writing, a temporary waiver of the requirements in paragraph (e)(1) of this section. These waivers will be granted on a limited basis for good cause shown. FDA will issue guidance on requesting a waiver of the requirements in paragraph (e)(1) of this section.

(f) *Patient privacy.* Manufacturers, packers, and distributors should not include in reports under this section the names and addresses of individual patients; instead, the manufacturer, packer, and distributor should assign a unique code for identification of the patient. The manufacturer, packer, and distributor should include the name of the reporter from whom the information was received as part of the initial reporter information, even when the reporter is the patient. The names of patients, individual reporters, healthcare professionals, hospitals, and geographical identifiers in adverse drug experience reports are not releasable to the public under FDA's public information regulations in part 20 of this chapter.

(g) *Recordkeeping.*
(1) Each manufacturer, packer, and distributor must maintain for a period of 10 years records of all adverse drug experiences required under this section to be reported, including raw data and any correspondence relating to the adverse drug experiences, and the records required to be maintained under paragraph (c)(3) of this section.
(2) Manufacturers and packers may retain the records required in paragraph (f)(1) of this section as part of its complaint files maintained under §211.198 of this chapter.
(3) Manufacturers, packers, and distributors must permit any authorized FDA employee, at all reasonable times, to have access to and copy and verify the records established and maintained under this section.

(h) *Disclaimer.* A report or information submitted by a manufacturer, packer, or distributor under this section (and any release by FDA of that report or information) does not necessarily reflect a conclusion by the manufacturer, packer, or distributor, or by FDA, that the report or information constitutes an admission that the drug caused or contributed to an adverse effect. The manufacturer, packer, or distributor need not admit, and may deny, that the report or information submitted under this section constitutes an admission that the drug caused or contributed to an adverse effect.

5.16 §312.32 IND SAFETY REPORTING

(a) *Definitions.* The following definitions of terms apply to this section:
Adverse event means any untoward medical occurrence associated with the use of a drug in humans, whether or not considered drug related.
Life-threatening adverse event or *life-threatening suspected adverse reaction.* An adverse event or suspected adverse reaction is considered "life-threatening" if, in the view of either the investigator or sponsor, its occurrence places the patient or subject at immediate risk of death. It does not include an adverse event or suspected adverse

reaction that, had it occurred in a more severe form, might have caused death.

Serious adverse event or *serious suspected adverse reaction*. An adverse event or suspected adverse reaction is considered "serious" if, in the view of either the investigator or sponsor, it results in any of the following outcomes: Death, a life-threatening adverse event, inpatient hospitalization or prolongation of existing hospitalization, a persistent or significant incapacity or substantial disruption of the ability to conduct normal life functions, or a congenital anomaly/birth defect. Important medical events that may not result in death, be life-threatening, or require hospitalization may be considered serious when, based upon appropriate medical judgment, they may jeopardize the patient or subject and may require medical or surgical intervention to prevent one of the outcomes listed in this definition. Examples of such medical events include allergic bronchospasm requiring intensive treatment in an emergency room or at home, blood dyscrasias or convulsions that do not result in inpatient hospitalization, or the development of drug dependency or drug abuse.

Suspected adverse reaction means any adverse event for which there is a reasonable possibility that the drug caused the adverse event. For the purposes of IND safety reporting, "reasonable possibility" means there is evidence to suggest a causal relationship between the drug and the adverse event. Suspected adverse reaction implies a lesser degree of certainty about causality than adverse reaction, which means any adverse event caused by a drug.

Unexpected adverse event or *unexpected suspected adverse reaction*. An adverse event or suspected adverse reaction is considered "unexpected" if it is not listed in the investigator brochure or is not listed at the specificity or severity that has been observed; or, if an investigator brochure is not required or available, is not consistent with the risk information described in the general investigational plan or elsewhere in the current application, as amended. For example, under this definition, hepatic necrosis would be unexpected (by virtue of greater severity) if the investigator brochure referred only to elevated hepatic enzymes or hepatitis. Similarly, cerebral thromboembolism and cerebral vasculitis would be unexpected (by virtue of greater specificity) if the investigator brochure listed only cerebral vascular accidents. "Unexpected," as used in this definition, also refers to adverse events or suspected adverse reactions that are mentioned in the investigator brochure as occurring with a class of drugs or as anticipated from the pharmacological properties of the drug, but are not specifically mentioned as occurring with the particular drug under investigation.

(b) *Review of safety information*. The sponsor must promptly review all information relevant to the safety of the drug obtained or otherwise received by the sponsor from foreign or domestic sources, including information derived from any clinical or epidemiological investigations, animal or in vitro studies, reports in the scientific literature, and unpublished scientific papers, as well as reports from foreign regulatory authorities and reports of foreign commercial marketing experience for drugs that are not marketed in the United States.

(c) (1) *IND safety reports*. The sponsor must notify FDA and all participating investigators (i.e., all investigators to whom the sponsor is providing drug under its INDs or under any investigator's IND) in an IND safety report of potential serious risks, from clinical trials or any other source, as soon as possible, but in no case later than 15 calendar days after the sponsor determines that the information qualifies for reporting under paragraph (c)(1)(i), (c)(1)(ii), (c)(1)(iii), or (c)(1)(iv) of this section. In each IND safety report, the sponsor must identify all IND safety reports previously submitted to FDA concerning a similar suspected adverse reaction, and must analyze the significance of the suspected adverse reaction in light of previous, similar reports or any other relevant information.

(i) *Serious and unexpected suspected adverse reaction*. The sponsor must report any suspected adverse reaction that is both serious and unexpected. The sponsor must report an adverse event as a suspected adverse reaction only if there is evidence to suggest a causal relationship between the drug and the adverse event, such as:

(A) A single occurrence of an event that is uncommon and known to be strongly associated with drug exposure (e.g., angioedema, hepatic injury, Stevens-Johnson Syndrome);

(B) One or more occurrences of an event that is not commonly associated with drug exposure, but is otherwise uncommon in the population exposed to the drug (e.g., tendon rupture);

(C) An aggregate analysis of specific events observed in a clinical trial (such as known consequences of the underlying disease or condition under investigation or other events that commonly occur in the study population independent of drug therapy) that indicates those events occur more frequently in the drug treatment group than in a concurrent or historical control group.

(ii) *Findings from other studies.* The sponsor must report any findings from epidemiological studies, pooled analysis of multiple studies, or clinical studies (other than those reported under paragraph (c)(1)(i) of this section), whether or not conducted under an IND, and whether or not conducted by the sponsor, that suggest a significant risk in humans exposed to the drug. Ordinarily, such a finding would result in a safety-related change in the protocol, informed consent, investigator brochure (excluding routine updates of these documents), or other aspects of the overall conduct of the clinical investigation.

(iii) *Findings from animal or in vitro testing.* The sponsor must report any findings from animal or in vitro testing, whether or not conducted by the sponsor, that suggest a significant risk in humans exposed to the drug, such as reports of mutagenicity, teratogenicity, or carcinogenicity, or reports of significant organ toxicity at or near the expected human exposure. Ordinarily, any such findings would result in a safety-related change in the protocol, informed consent, investigator brochure (excluding routine updates of these documents), or other aspects of the overall conduct of the clinical investigation.

(iv) *Increased rate of occurrence of serious suspected adverse reactions.* The sponsor must report any clinically important increase in the rate of a serious suspected adverse reaction over that listed in the protocol or investigator brochure.

(v) *Submission of IND safety reports.* The sponsor must submit each IND safety report in a narrative format or on FDA Form 3500A or in an electronic format that FDA can process, review, and archive. FDA will periodically issue guidance on how to provide the electronic submission (e.g., method of transmission, media, file formats, preparation and organization of files). The sponsor may submit foreign suspected adverse reactions on a Council for International Organizations of Medical Sciences (CIOMS) I Form instead of a FDA Form 3500A. Reports of overall findings or pooled analyses from published and unpublished in vitro, animal, epidemiological, or clinical studies must be submitted in a narrative format. Each notification to FDA must bear prominent identification of its contents, i.e., "IND Safety Report," and must be transmitted to the review division in the Center for Drug Evaluation and Research or in the Center for Biologics Evaluation and Research that has responsibility for review of the IND. Upon request from FDA, the sponsor must submit to FDA any additional data or information that the agency deems necessary, as soon as possible, but in no case later than 15 calendar days after receiving the request.

(2) *Unexpected fatal or life-threatening suspected adverse reaction reports.* The sponsor must also notify FDA of any unexpected fatal or life-threatening suspected adverse reaction as soon as possible but in no case later than 7 calendar days after the sponsor's initial receipt of the information.

(3) *Reporting format or frequency.* FDA may require a sponsor to submit IND safety reports in a format or at a frequency different than that required under this paragraph. The sponsor may also propose and adopt a different reporting format or frequency if the change is agreed to in advance by the director of the FDA review division that has responsibility for review of the IND.

(4) *Investigations of marketed drugs.* A sponsor of a clinical study of a drug marketed or approved in the United States that is conducted under an IND is required to submit IND safety reports for suspected adverse reactions that are observed in the clinical study, at domestic or foreign study sites. The sponsor must also submit safety information from the clinical study as prescribed by the postmarketing safety reporting requirements (e.g., §§310.305, 314.80, and 600.80 of this chapter).

(5) *Reporting study endpoints.* Study endpoints (e.g., mortality or major morbidity) must be reported to FDA by the sponsor as described in the protocol and ordinarily would not be reported under paragraph (c) of this section. However, if a serious and unexpected adverse event occurs for which there is evidence suggesting a causal relationship between the drug and the event (e.g., death from anaphylaxis), the event must be reported under §312.32(c)(1)(i) as a serious and unexpected suspected adverse reaction even if it is a component of the study endpoint (e.g., all-cause mortality).

(d) *Follow-up.*
(1) The sponsor must promptly investigate all safety information it receives.
(2) Relevant follow-up information to an IND safety report must be submitted as soon as the information is available and must be identified as such, i.e., "Follow-up IND Safety Report."
(3) If the results of a sponsor's investigation show that an adverse event not initially determined to be reportable under paragraph (c) of this section is so reportable, the sponsor must report such suspected adverse reaction in an IND safety report as soon as possible, but in no case later than 15 calendar days after the determination is made.

(e) *Disclaimer.* A safety report or other information submitted by a sponsor under this part (and any release by FDA of that report or information) does not necessarily reflect a conclusion by the sponsor or FDA that the report or information constitutes an admission that the drug caused or contributed to an adverse event. A sponsor need not admit, and may deny, that the report or information submitted by the sponsor constitutes an admission that the drug caused or contributed to an adverse event.

5.17 §314.70(A)(4) SUPPLEMENTS AND OTHER CHANGES TO AN APPROVED APPLICATION, PROMOTIONAL LABELING

(4) The applicant must promptly revise all promotional labeling and advertising to make it consistent with any labeling change implemented in accordance with paragraphs (b) and (c) of this section.

5.18 §314.70(C)(6)(III) SUPPLEMENTS AND OTHER CHANGES TO AN APPROVED APPLICATION, LABELING, CHANGES BEING EFFECTED

(c) *Changes requiring supplement submission at least 30 days prior to distribution of the drug product made using the change (moderate changes).* (1) A supplement must be submitted for any change . . . *If the supplement provides for a labeling change under paragraph* (c)(6)(iii) of this section, 12 copies of the final printed labeling must be included.

(6) The agency may designate a category of changes for the purpose of providing that, in the case of a change in such category, the holder of an approved application may commence distribution of the drug product involved upon receipt by the agency of a supplement for the change. These changes include, but are not limited to:

(iii) *Changes in the labeling to reflect newly acquired information,* except for changes to the information required in §201.57(a) of this chapter (which must be made under paragraph (b)(2)(v)(C) of this section), to accomplish any of the following:
(A) To add or strengthen a contraindication, warning, precaution, or adverse reaction for which the evidence of a causal association satisfies the standard for inclusion in the labeling under §201.57(c) of this chapter;
(B) To add or strengthen a statement about drug abuse, dependence, psychological effect, or overdosage;
(C) To add or strengthen an instruction about dosage and administration that is intended to increase the safe use of the drug product;
(D) To delete false, misleading, or unsupported indications for use or claims for effectiveness; or
(E) Any labeling change normally requiring a supplement submission and approval prior to distribution of the drug product that FDA specifically requests be submitted under this provision.

5.19 §314.80 POSTMARKETING REPORTING OF ADVERSE DRUG EXPERIENCES

(a) *Definitions.* The following definitions of terms apply to this section:
Adverse drug experience. Any adverse event associated with the use of a drug in humans, whether or not considered drug related, including the following: An adverse event occurring in the course of the use of a drug product in professional practice; an adverse event occurring from drug overdose whether accidental or intentional; an adverse event occurring from drug abuse; an adverse event occurring from drug withdrawal; and any failure of expected pharmacological action.
Individual case safety report (ICSR). A description of an adverse drug experience related to an individual patient or subject.
ICSR attachments. Documents related to the adverse drug experience described in an ICSR, such as medical records, hospital discharge summaries, or other documentation.
Disability. A substantial disruption of a person's ability to conduct normal life functions.
Life-threatening adverse drug experience. Any adverse drug experience that places the patient, in the view of the initial reporter, at *immediate* risk of death from the adverse drug experience as it occurred, *i.e.*, it does not include an adverse drug experience that, had it occurred in a more severe form, might have caused death.
Serious adverse drug experience. Any adverse drug experience occurring at any dose that results in any of the following outcomes: Death, a life-threatening adverse drug experience, inpatient

hospitalization or prolongation of existing hospitalization, a persistent or significant disability/incapacity, or a congenital anomaly/birth defect. Important medical events that may not result in death, be life-threatening, or require hospitalization may be considered a serious adverse drug experience when, based upon appropriate medical judgment, they may jeopardize the patient or subject and may require medical or surgical intervention to prevent one of the outcomes listed in this definition. Examples of such medical events include allergic bronchospasm requiring intensive treatment in an emergency room or at home, blood dyscrasias or convulsions that do not result in inpatient hospitalization, or the development of drug dependency or drug abuse.

Unexpected adverse drug experience. Any adverse drug experience that is not listed in the current labeling for the drug product. This includes events that may be symptomatically and pathophysiologically related to an event listed in the labeling, but differ from the event because of greater severity or specificity. For example, under this definition, hepatic necrosis would be unexpected (by virtue of greater severity) if the labeling only referred to elevated hepatic enzymes or hepatitis. Similarly, cerebral thromboembolism and cerebral vasculitis would be unexpected (by virtue of greater specificity) if the labeling only listed cerebral vascular accidents. "Unexpected," as used in this definition, refers to an adverse drug experience that has not been previously observed (*i.e.*, included in the labeling) rather than from the perspective of such experience not being anticipated from the pharmacological properties of the pharmaceutical product.

(b) *Review of adverse drug experiences.* Each applicant having an approved application under §314.50 or, in the case of a 505(b)(2) application, an effective approved application, must promptly review all adverse drug experience information obtained or otherwise received by the applicant from any source, foreign or domestic, including information derived from commercial marketing experience, postmarketing clinical investigations, postmarketing epidemiological/surveillance studies, reports in the scientific literature, and unpublished scientific papers. Applicants are not required to resubmit to FDA adverse drug experience reports forwarded to the applicant by FDA; however, applicants must submit all follow-up information on such reports to FDA. Any person subject to the reporting requirements under paragraph (c) of this section must also develop written procedures for the surveillance, receipt, evaluation, and reporting of postmarketing adverse drug experiences to FDA.

(c) *Reporting requirements.* The applicant must submit to FDA adverse drug experience information as described in this section. Except as provided in paragraph (g)(2) of this section, these reports must be submitted to the Agency in electronic format as described in paragraph (g)(1) of this section.

(1) (i) *Postmarketing 15-day "Alert reports".* The applicant must report each adverse drug experience that is both serious and unexpected, whether foreign or domestic, as soon as possible but no later than 15 calendar days from initial receipt of the information by the applicant.

(ii) *Postmarketing 15-day "Alert reports"—follow-up.* The applicant must promptly investigate all adverse drug experiences that are the subject of these postmarketing 15-day Alert reports and must submit follow-up reports within 15 calendar days of receipt of new information or as requested by FDA. If additional information is not obtainable, records should be maintained of the unsuccessful steps taken to seek additional information.

(iii) *Submission of reports.* The requirements of paragraphs (c)(1)(i) and (c)(1)(ii) of this section, concerning the submission of postmarketing 15-day Alert reports, also apply to any person other than the applicant whose name appears on the label of an approved drug product as a manufacturer, packer, or distributor (nonapplicant). To avoid unnecessary duplication in the submission to FDA of reports required by paragraphs (c)(1)(i) and (c)(1)(ii) of this section, obligations of a nonapplicant may be met by submission of all reports of serious adverse drug experiences to the applicant. If a nonapplicant elects to submit adverse drug experience reports to the applicant rather than to FDA, the nonapplicant must submit, by any appropriate means, each report to the applicant within 5 calendar days of initial receipt of the information by the nonapplicant, and the applicant must then comply with the requirements of this section. Under this circumstance, the nonapplicant must maintain a record of this action which must include:

(A) A copy of each adverse drug experience report;

(B) The date the report was received by the nonapplicant;

(C) The date the report was submitted to the applicant; and

(D) The name and address of the applicant.

(2) *Periodic adverse drug experience reports.*

(i) The applicant must report each adverse drug experience not reported under paragraph (c)(1)(i) of this section at quarterly intervals, for 3 years from the date of approval of the application, and then at annual intervals. The applicant must submit each quarterly report within 30 days of the close of the quarter (the first quarter beginning on the date of approval of the application) and each annual report within 60 days of the anniversary date of approval of the application. Upon written notice, FDA may extend or reestablish the requirement that an applicant submit quarterly reports, or require that the applicant submit reports under this section at different times than those stated. For example, the agency may reestablish a quarterly reporting requirement following the approval of a major supplement. Follow-up information to adverse drug experiences submitted in a periodic report may be submitted in the next periodic report.

(ii) Each periodic report is required to contain:

(A) *Descriptive information.*

(*1*) A narrative summary and analysis of the information in the report;

(*2*) An analysis of the 15-day Alert reports submitted during the reporting interval (all 15-day Alert reports being appropriately referenced by the applicant's patient identification code, adverse reaction term(s), and date of submission to FDA);

(*3*) A history of actions taken since the last report because of adverse drug experiences (for example, labeling changes or studies initiated); and

(*4*) An index consisting of a line listing of the applicant's patient identification code, and adverse reaction term(s) for all ICSRs submitted under paragraph (c)(2)(ii)(B) of this section.

(B) *ICSRs for serious, expected, and nonserious adverse drug experiences.* An ICSR for each adverse drug experience not reported under paragraph (c)(1)(i) of this section (all serious, expected and nonserious adverse drug experiences). All such ICSRs must be submitted to FDA (either individually or in one or more batches) within the timeframe specified in paragraph (c)(2)(i) of this section. ICSRs must only be submitted to FDA once.

(iii) Periodic reporting, except for information regarding 15-day Alert reports, does not apply to adverse drug experience information obtained from postmarketing studies (whether or not conducted under an investigational new drug application), from reports in the scientific literature, and from foreign marketing experience.

(d) *Scientific literature.* A 15-day Alert report based on information in the scientific literature must be accompanied by a copy of the published article. The 15-day reporting requirements in paragraph (c)(1)(i) of this section (*i.e.*, serious, unexpected adverse drug experiences) apply only to reports found in scientific and medical journals either as case reports or as the result of a formal clinical trial.

(e) *Postmarketing studies.* An applicant is not required to submit a 15-day Alert report under paragraph (c) of this section for an adverse drug experience obtained from a postmarketing study (whether or not conducted under an investigational new drug application) unless the applicant concludes that there is a reasonable possibility that the drug caused the adverse experience.

(f) *Information reported on ICSRs.* ICSRs include the following information:

(1) *Patient information.*

(i) Patient identification code;

(ii) Patient age at the time of adverse drug experience, or date of birth;

(iii) Patient gender; and

(iv) Patient weight.

(2) *Adverse drug experience.*

(i) Outcome attributed to adverse drug experience;

(ii) Date of adverse drug experience;

(iii) Date of ICSR submission;

(iv) Description of adverse drug experience (including a concise medical narrative);

(v) Adverse drug experience term(s);

(vi) Description of relevant tests, including dates and laboratory data; and

(vii) Other relevant patient history, including preexisting medical conditions.

(3) *Suspect medical product(s).*

(i) Name;

(ii) Dose, frequency, and route of administration used;

(iii) Therapy dates;

(iv) Diagnosis for use (indication);

(v) Whether the product is a prescription or nonprescription product;

(vi) Whether the product is a combination product as defined in §3.2(e) of this chapter;

(vii) Whether adverse drug experience abated after drug use stopped or dose reduced;

(viii) Whether adverse drug experience reappeared after reintroduction of drug;
(ix) Lot number;
(x) Expiration date;
(xi) National Drug Code (NDC) number; and
(xii) Concomitant medical products and therapy dates.

(4) *Initial reporter information.*
(i) Name, address, and telephone number;
(ii) Whether the initial reporter is a health care professional; and
(iii) Occupation, if a healthcare professional.

(5) *Applicant information.*
(i) Applicant name and contact office address;
(ii) Telephone number;
(iii) Report source, such as spontaneous, literature, or study;
(iv) Date the report was received by applicant;
(v) Application number and type;
(vi) Whether the ICSR is a 15-day "Alert report";
(vii) Whether the ICSR is an initial report or follow-up report; and
(viii) Unique case identification number, which must be the same in the initial report and any subsequent follow-up report(s).

(g) *Electronic format for submissions.*
(1) Safety report submissions, including ICSRs, ICSR attachments, and the descriptive information in periodic reports, must be in an electronic format that FDA can process, review, and archive. FDA will issue guidance on how to provide the electronic submission (e.g., method of transmission, media, file formats, preparation and organization of files).
(2) An applicant or nonapplicant may request, in writing, a temporary waiver of the requirements in paragraph (g)(1) of this section. These waivers will be granted on a limited basis for good cause shown. FDA will issue guidance on requesting a waiver of the requirements in paragraph (g)(1) of this section.

(h) *Multiple reports.* An applicant should not include in reports under this section any adverse drug experiences that occurred in clinical trials if they were previously submitted as part of the approved application. If a report applies to a drug for which an applicant holds more than one approved application, the applicant should submit the report to the application that was first approved. If a report refers to more than one drug marketed by an applicant, the applicant should submit the report to the application for the drug listed first in the report.

(i) *Patient privacy.* An applicant should not include in reports under this section the names and addresses of individual patients; instead, the applicant should assign a unique code for identification of the patient. The applicant should include the name of the reporter from whom the information was received as part of the initial reporter information, even when the reporter is the patient. The names of patients, healthcare professionals, hospitals, and geographical identifiers in adverse drug experience reports are not releasable to the public under FDA's public information regulations in part 20 of this chapter.

(j) *Recordkeeping.* The applicant must maintain for a period of 10 years records of all adverse drug experiences known to the applicant, including raw data and any correspondence relating to adverse drug experiences.

(k) *Withdrawal of approval.* If an applicant fails to establish and maintain records and make reports required under this section, FDA may withdraw approval of the application and, thus, prohibit continued marketing of the drug product that is the subject of the application.

(l) *Disclaimer.* A report or information submitted by an applicant under this section (and any release by FDA of that report or information) does not necessarily reflect a conclusion by the applicant or FDA that the report or information constitutes an admission that the drug caused or contributed to an adverse effect. An applicant need not admit, and may deny, that the report or information submitted under this section constitutes an admission that the drug caused or contributed to an adverse effect. For purposes of this provision, the term "applicant" also includes any person reporting under paragraph (c)(1)(iii) of this section.

5.20 §330.1 GENERAL CONDITIONS FOR GENERAL RECOGNITION AS SAFE, EFFECTIVE AND NOT MISBRANDED

An over-the-counter (OTC) drug listed in this subchapter is generally recognized as safe and effective and is not misbranded if it meets each of the conditions contained in this part and each of the conditions contained in any applicable monograph. Any product which fails to conform to each of the conditions contained in this part and in an applicable monograph is liable to regulatory action.

(a) The product is manufactured in compliance with current good manufacturing practices, as established by parts 210 and 211 of this chapter.

(b) The establishment(s) in which the drug product is manufactured is registered, and the drug product is listed, in compliance with part 207 of this chapter. It is requested but not required that the number assigned to the product pursuant to part 207 of this chapter appear on all drug labels and in all drug labeling. If this number is used, it shall be placed in the manner set forth in part 207 of this chapter.

(c) (1) The product is labeled in compliance with chapter V of the Federal Food, Drug, and Cosmetic Act (the act) and subchapter C *et seq.* of this chapter, including the format and content requirements in 201.66 of this chapter. An OTC drug product that is not in compliance with chapter V and subchapter C, including 201.66 of this chapter, is subject to regulatory action. For purposes of 201.61(b) of this chapter, the statement of identity of the product shall be the term or phrase used in the applicable OTC drug monograph established in this part.

(2) The "Uses" section of the label and labeling of the product shall contain the labeling describing the "Indications" that have been established in an applicable OTC drug monograph or alternative truthful and nonmisleading statements describing only those indications for use that have been established in an applicable monograph, subject to the provisions of section 502 of the act relating to misbranding and the prohibition in section 301(d) of the act against the introduction or delivery for introduction into interstate commerce of unapproved new drugs in violation of section 505(a) of the act. Any other labeling under this subchapter and subchapter C *et seq.* of this chapter shall be stated in the exact language where exact language has been established and identified by quotation marks in an applicable OTC drug monograph or by regulation (e.g., 201.63 of this chapter), except as provided in paragraphs (i) and (j) of this section.

(d) The advertising for the product prescribes, recommends, or suggests its use only under the conditions stated in the labeling.

(e) The product contains only suitable inactive ingredients which are safe in the amounts administered and do not interfere with the effectiveness of the preparation or with suitable tests or assays to determine if the product meets its professed standards of identity, strength, quality, and purity. Color additives may be used only in accordance with section 721 of the act and subchapter A of this chapter.

(f) The product container and container components meet the requirements of 211.94 of this chapter.

(g) The labeling for all drugs contains the general warning: "Keep out of reach of children." [Highlighted in bold type]. The labeling of drugs shall also state as follows: For drugs used by oral administration, "In case of overdose, get medical help or contact a Poison Control Center right away"; for drugs used topically, rectally, or vaginally and not intended for oral ingestion, "If swallowed, get medical help or contact a Poison Control Center right away"; and for drugs used topically and intended for oral use, "If more than used for" (insert intended use, e.g., pain) "is accidentally swallowed, get medical help or contact a Poison Control Center right away." The Food and Drug Administration will grant an exemption from these general warnings where appropriate upon petition, which shall be maintained in a permanent file for public review by the Division of Dockets Management, Food and Drug Administration, 5630 Fishers Lane, rm. 1061, Rockville, MD 20852.

(h) Where no maximum daily dosage limit for an active ingredient is established in this part, it is used in a product at a level that does not exceed the amount reasonably required to achieve its intended effect.

(i) The following terms may be used interchangeably in the labeling of OTC drug products, provided such use does not alter the meaning of the labeling that has been established and identified in an applicable monograph or by regulation. The following terms shall not be used to change in any way the title, headings, and subheadings required under 201.66(c)(1) through (c)(9) of this chapter:

(1) "Abdominal" or "stomach" (in context only).
(2) "Administer" or "give".
(3) "Aggravate(s)" or "make(s) worse".
(4) "Application of this product" or "applying".
(5) "Are uncertain" or "do not know".
(6) "Ask" or "consult" or "contact".
(7) "Asking" or "consulting".
(8) "Assistance" or "help" or "aid".
(9) "Associated with" or "due to" or "caused by".
(10) "Avoid contact with eyes" or "do not get into eyes".
(11) "Avoid inhaling" or "do not inhale".
(12) "Before a doctor is consulted" or "without first consulting your doctor" or "consult your doctor before".
(13) "Beverages" or "drinks".
(14) "Clean" or "cleanse".
(15) "Consulting" or "advising".
(16) "Continue(s)" or "persist(s)" or "is persistent" or "do(es) not go away" or "last(s)".
(17) "Daily" or "every day".
(18) "Develop(s)" or "begin(s)" or "occur(s)".
(19) "Difficulty" or "trouble".
(20) "Difficulty in urination" or "trouble urinating".
(21) "Discard" or "throw away".
(22) "Discontinue" or "stop" or "quit".
(23) "Doctor" or "physician".
(24) "Drowsiness" or "the drowsiness effect".
(25) "Drowsiness may occur" or "you may get drowsy".
(26) "Enlargement of the" or "an enlarged".

(27) "Especially in children" or especially children".
(28) "Exceed" or "use more than" or "go beyond".
(29) "Exceed recommended dosage" or "use more than directed".
(30) "Excessive" or "too much".
(31) "Excitability may occur" or "you may get excited".
(32) "Experience" or "feel".
(33) "For relief of" or "relieves".
(34) "For temporary reduction of" or "temporarily reduces".
(35) "For the temporary relief of" or "temporarily relieves".
(36) "For the treatment of" or "treats".
(37) "Frequently" or "often".
(38) "Give to" or "use in".
(39) "Immediately" or "right away" or "directly".
(40) "Immediately" or "as soon as".
(41) "Immediately following" or "right after".
(42) "Improve(s)" or "get(s) better" or "make(s) better".
(43) "Increased" or "more".
(44) "Increase your risk of" or "cause".
(45) "Indication(s)" or "Use(s)".
(46) "Inhalation" or "puff".
(47) "In persons who" or "if you" or "if the child".
(48) "Instill" or "put".
(49) "Is (are) accompanied by" or "you also have" (in context only) or "(optional: that) occur(s) with".
(50) "Longer" or "more".
(51) "Lung" or "pulmonary".
(52) "Medication(s)" or "medicine(s)" or "drug(s)".
(53) "Nervousness, dizziness, or sleeplessness occurs" or "you get nervous, dizzy, or sleepless".
(54) "Not to exceed" or "do not exceed" or "not more than".
(55) "Obtain(s)" or "get(s)".
(56) "Passages" or "passageways" or "tubes".
(57) "Perforation of" or "hole in".
(58) "Persistent" or "that does not go away" or "that continues" or "that lasts".
(59) "Per day" or "daily".
(60) "Presently" or "now".
(61) "Produce(s)" or "cause(s)".
(62) "Prompt(ly)" or "quick(ly)" or "right away".
(63) "Reduce" or "minimize".
(64) "Referred to as" or "of".
(65) "Sensation" or "feeling".
(66) "Solution" or "liquid".
(67) "Specifically" or "definitely".
(68) "Take" or "use" or "give".
(69) "Tend(s) to recur" or "reoccur(s)" or "return(s)" or "come(s) back".
(70) "To avoid contamination" or "avoid contamination" or "do not contaminate".
(71) "To help" or "helps".
(72) "Unless directed by a doctor" or "except under the advice of a doctor" or "unless told to do so by a doctor".
(73) "Use caution" or "be careful".
(74) "Usually" or "generally" (in context only).
(75) "You" ("Your") or "the child" ("the child's").
(76) "You also have" or "occurs with".
(77) "When practical" or "if possible".
(78) "Whether" or "if".
(79) "Worsen(s)" or "get(s) worse" or "make(s) worse".

(j) The following connecting terms may be deleted from the labeling of OTC drug products, provided such deletion does not alter the meaning of the labeling that has been established and identified in an applicable monograph or by regulation. The following terms shall not be used to change in any way the specific title, headings, and subheadings required under 201.66(c)(1) through (c)(9) of this chapter:
(1) "And".
(2) "As may occur with".
(3) "Associated" or "to be associated".
(4) "Consult a doctor".
(5) "Discontinue use".
(6) "Drug Interaction Precaution".
(7) "Due to".
(8) "Except under the advice and supervision of a physician".
(9) "If this occurs".
(10) "In case of".
(11) "Notice".
(12) "Or".
(13) "Occurring with".
(14) "Or as directed by a doctor".
(15) "Such as".
(16) "Such as occurs with".
(17) "Tends to".
(18) "This product".
(19) "Unless directed by a doctor".
(20) "While taking this product" or "before taking this product".
(21) "Within".

6 The Regulation of Drug Product Information to Consumers

Frank J. Ascione

SYNOPSIS

6.1 THE HISTORICAL DEVELOPMENT OF FOOD AND DRUG ADMINISTRATION'S REGULATORY ROLE

One of the major roles of the Food and Drug Administration (FDA) is to ensure that information about drug products is accurate and aids patients in minimizing risks. Specifically, the FDA's role is "to minimize risks through education, regulation, and enforcement and it must do this by communicating frequently and clearly about risks and benefits and what organizations and individuals can do to minimize risk."[1]

This approach has evolved along with the elucidation of the role of the government in health and consumer protection. Figure 6.1 illustrates this role.

As indicated in the figure, the role of the FDA is to ensure that information about the drug product is sufficient to ensure safe and effective use. This role is influenced by the science that exists (e.g., human behavior and decision-making) and the technological changes that occur in the delivery of information to the public (e.g., the shift from solely written information sources to multimedia platforms). The "contract" between society and the FDA is the assurance that the public will be properly informed about how to use medications safely and effectively.

6.1.1 Early Phase (Prior to 1906): No Significant Government Intervention

Prior to 1906, federal involvement in ensuring appropriate use of drug products was very limited. The absence of regulations was due to the lack of science about drug products and a public emphasis on citizen self-responsibility for their decisions (caveat emptor or "let the buyer beware").

Although federal efforts were limited, a variety of state laws existed that focused on trade issues related to food quality and purity. In addition, private efforts were extensive regarding the purity of the drug product. The United States Pharmacopoeia (USP) was created in 1825 by a group of physicians to provide drug product ingredient standards. The National Formulary was created by the American Pharmaceutical Association to address products not listed in the USP.[2]

DOI: 10.1201/9781003615323-7

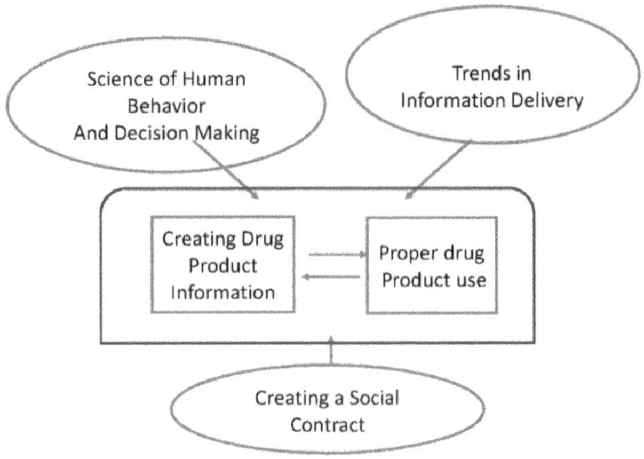

FIGURE 6.1 Illustration of the Social Contract between the FDA and the US Public.

The first real attempt at addressing drug product quality issues started with the creation of US customs laboratories to administer the Import Drugs Act of 1848. The 1848 act was an ambitious federal regulatory program that originally enjoyed overwhelming support in Congress and the medical community because it addressed a growing issue of counterfeit drugs prevalent in the US, especially those used by US soldiers in the Mexican-American War. Support, however, dwindled, and the program gradually disappeared.

The result of the laissez-faire approach to drug regulation was a relatively unsupervised marketplace for drug products. Dangerous drugs such as opium and morphine were sold without any restrictions. In addition, product labels usually contain fraudulent information. Innocuous or inert preparations were labeled as a panacea. Product ingredients and warnings against misuse were not labeled.

A good example of misleading information was the ad for Lydia Pinkham's Vegetable Compound. An 1886 ad is shown in Figure 6.2.

This preparation, which was the result of Mrs. Pinkham's efforts to market her home remedies, was the highest-selling product of its time. A major reason was her effort to address women's health issues (e.g., poor menstruation), which were commonly neglected during that era. The claims were very broad and not supported by any scientific evidence. One ad stated that the compound: "will cure entirely the worst form of Female complaints, all ovarian troubles . . . faintness, flatuancy . . . feeling of bearing down, backache." Analysis of the original formula revealed five herbs with broad medicinal properties (e.g., pleurisy root, life root, fenugreek, unicorn root, and black cohosh), but it also contained drinking alcohol and ethanol derivatives.

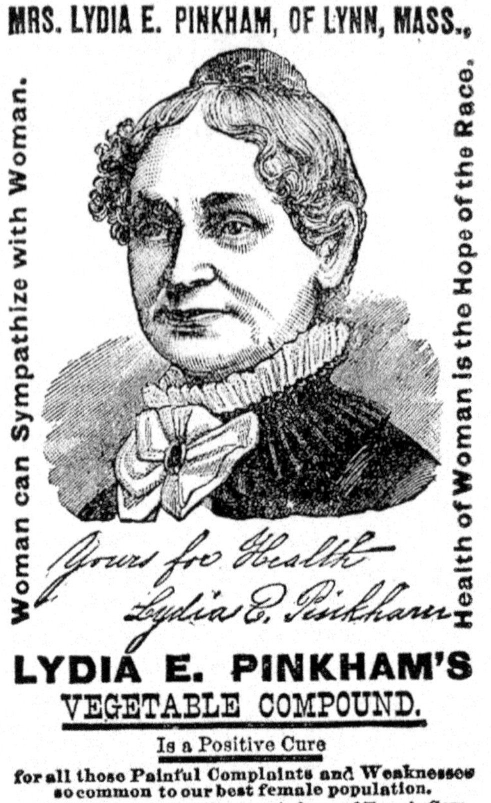

FIGURE 6.2 Example of a print ad for Lydia Pinkham's Vegetable Compound.

Source: http://www.mum.org/mrspink3.htm.

6.1.2 Early Regulatory Phase (1906–1938): Minimal Government Control

Widespread falsifying claims and undisclosed product ingredients became untenable and less acceptable when medical science became more advanced and when economic interest in abolishing drug adulteration became stronger. The movement for greater regulation of drug products began in earnest in the late 1800s although opposition to any federal involvement in policing citizen behavior remained strong. Nevertheless, after a series of scandals, Congress was finally pushed into action. The key legislation was the 1906 Federal Food and Drug Act that was created to prohibit interstate commerce of adulterated and misbranded food and drugs.[3]

The original agency charged with administering the act was the Bureau of Chemistry. Although the act addressed both food and drug product standards, the bureau originally focused on the enforcement of food standards, which was perceived at the time to pose a greater health problem. Drug product quality was addressed, but the enforcement of misbranding of drug products was difficult to prove. While the act required that a drug had to be labeled accurately regarding its ingredients, misleading advertising was difficult to enforce. Manufacturers only had to prove that they believed their remedy to be effective, regardless of the existing scientific evidence. Fortunately, legislation passed in 1912 (Shirley Amendment) improved the legal basis for the outlawing of therapeutic claims intended to defraud the purchaser. Although several clearly fraudulent products were removed from the market through legal action, the government still lost several key cases during that period.

An example of misleading advertising at this time was for the drug Urodonal, which was being promoted for a range of disorders such as rheumatism, gout, acidity, and obesity (Figure 6.3).

The active ingredients were methenamine (an antibiotic), lithium (now used specifically for bipolar disorders), and piperazine (an anthelmintic used primarily for worm

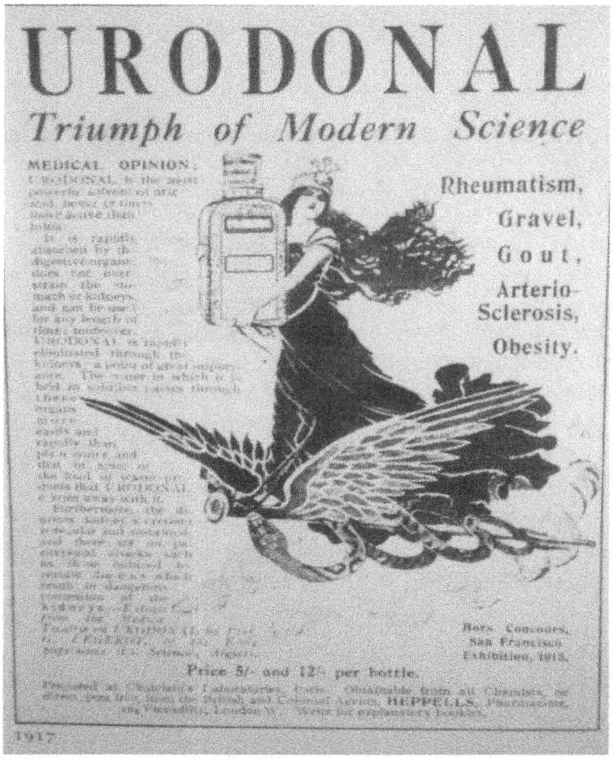

FIGURE 6.3 Ad for Urodonal in 1917.

Source: https://www.bing.com/images/search?q=urodonal+ad&qpvt=urodonal+ad&form=IGRE&first=1&tsc=ImageHoverTitle.

infections). While the safety of the product was assured, the therapeutic claims did not match the known effects of the ingredients.

The Bureau of Chemistry's expanded work eventually led to the creation of the FDA in 1931, which is considered the oldest comprehensive consumer protection agency in the federal government. While the responsibilities of the FDA have expanded greatly since 1906, it continues to remain focused on ensuring public health safety for food and drugs distributed in the US.

6.1.3 Greater Government Control (1938–1961)

The weaknesses of the 1906 law and the increased availability of new potent drugs created pressure for more federal regulation in the 1930s. Finally, deaths due to ingestion of a misbranded sulfanilamide elixir in 1937 convinced Congress to be more concerned about ensuring drug safety for the public. The Federal Food, Drug, and Cosmetic Act (FDCA) of 1938 was enacted to improve drug product regulation and represented a significant change in the public's view of the government's role in monitoring medication use in the US. While many aspects of the law focused on food and drug quality, the act also enhanced the regulation of drug product information. Proof of fraud was no longer required to prevent false drug claims. Although the act was clear in its prohibition of false therapeutic claims for drug products, jurisdiction of drug advertising was given to the Federal Trade Commission (FTC).[3]

Despite the new law, the upsurge in the availability of the number of new drugs created concern about an increased danger to the public. For example, in 1938, the FDA issued a letter warning manufacturers to avoid mislabeling of drug products containing aminopyrine because of numerous deaths from agranulocytosis. The aminopyrine and sulfanilamide cases highlighted concerns about whether the newly created drug products could be handled safely through improved labeling for consumers. An alternative approach was to legislate that some of these products should be prescribed only by physicians. The idea of prescription drugs was not a new regulatory concept (narcotics were restricted under the 1914 Harrison Act) but was first formally addressed through section 503b of the 1938 act. However, the categorizations and enforcement of which drugs would be classified as prescription versus non-prescription was very limited.

The issue was comprehensively addressed with the passage of the Durham-Humphrey Amendment in 1951.[4] For the first time, it required that certain drugs (besides narcotics) be dispensed only through a prescription. It also clearly identified a long-needed statutory definition of what kinds of drugs must be labeled for prescription use. The eligible drugs were divided into those that were habit forming and those that could be safely used only with professional supervision. The Amendment required drugs that were unsafe to use without medical supervision to be labeled with a statement: "Caution: Federal law prohibits dispensing without prescription." "Professional supervision" was viewed as management by a "learned intermediary," often defined by the practice acts of each state. Thus, the typical professionals designated to prescribe were physicians and dentists, while pharmacists were the most typical healthcare professionals authorized to dispense the product.

In addition to its restriction on public accessibility of drug products, the Durham-Humphrey Amendment provided the FDA with legal authority to require the inclusion of health professional information in prescription drug packages. Under the law, the FDA began to require professional information packages for injectable drugs. However, the FDA was still reluctant to require this labeling regulation for all prescription medications because of its apprehension that such information would inadvertently get into the hands of the lay public. The agency emphasized the need to keep prescription drug information primarily disseminated through professional channels. The premise was that practitioners could better obtain complete information from "readily available" sources such as textbooks and journals.

While this system effectively managed harm associated with dangerous drug products, it also inadvertently restricted the availability of information to the public. The question as to whether a drug was available with or without a prescription was still often left to drug manufacturers to decide. Many manufacturers targeted their product distribution to health professionals and labeled their drug products accordingly. Thus, no consumer labeling was available, although some of these drug products could be used safely and effectively without medical supervision. When the number of drugs entering the market dramatically increased, this inadvertent result became more noticeable. The FDA was soon concerned that the current regulations might hamper the government's desire to ensure the public received the information they needed to use the drug product safely and effectively.

The large increase in new innovative drug therapies in the 1950s added to this concern. The information provided by the manufacturer to the physician tended to understate the real risks associated with using the drug product. Because the public almost entirely relied on their physician's judgment regarding drug therapy, it was likely that consumers would not be fully aware of the side effects associated with the drug.

A typical ad of the period was for the drug Mornidine. The ad was directed toward physicians and a sample is shown in Figure 6.4.

Mornidine contained pipamazine, which is a drug of the phenothiazine class that has negligible antipsychotic activity and produces few extrapyramidal (movement disorder) side effects. It was introduced in 1959 and was advertised for morning sickness and postoperative nausea and vomiting. The manufacturer also claimed to reduce the need for postoperative analgesia. The drug was eventually withdrawn from the US market in 1969, after reports of hepatotoxicity (liver injury).

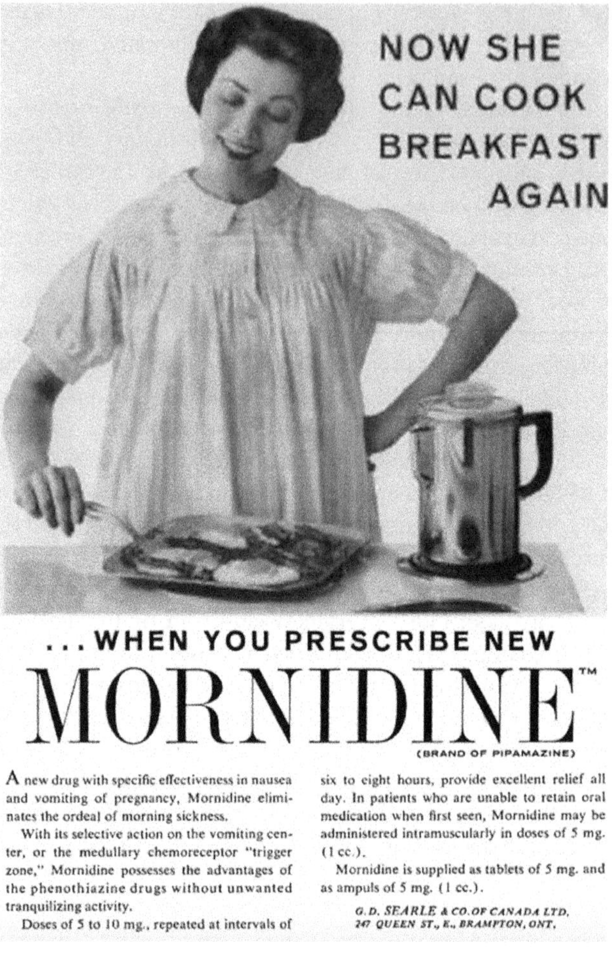

FIGURE 6.4 Mornidine Ad.

Source: http://www.bonkersinstitute.org/medshow/mornidine.html.

6.1.4 Debating Increased Consumer Access to Drug Product Information (1961–1983)

The concerns about the unavailability of drug product information to consumers began a gradual effort in the 1960s within the federal government to more comprehensively address this issue. At the same time, a significant social movement, often referred to as the Consumer Health Information Movement, was emerging. This movement was the result of several social shifts in American society that focused on the individual's right to control important aspects of their life. A key purpose of the movement was to explore ways to enable patients and consumers to gain power to control her/his own health and well-being by obtaining relevant knowledge.[3–6]

The FDA and other parts of the federal government recognized these trends and slowly began to develop regulations to better provide consumers with accessible, accurate, and unbiased drug product information. In 1961, the FDA issued a "full disclosure" regulation for all prescription drug package inserts and promotional literature distributed to physicians. The regulation required package inserts to include complete drug information regarding hazards, side effects, and precautions to assure complete information to health professionals. The "full disclosure" concept was extended the following year to prescription drug advertising directed to medical professionals.

In addition to expanding the information available to the public, the FDA remained concerned about the quality of the information that would be provided. A big boost to its ability to control and regulate that information occurred with the 1962 Kefauver–Harris Amendments to the FDCA. Prior to 1962, there was no effective control of advertisements directed to the medical profession or the public. Under the 1938 FDCA, the responsibility for direct regulation of advertising of all domestic commodities in interstate commerce was granted to the FTC. However, this effort was ineffective largely due to the lack of scientific expertise within the FTC and its limited legal power to hold manufacturers responsible. While legislative change had been suggested prior to 1962, the Thalidomide tragedy and other allegations of misleading and uninformative promotions to physicians led Congress to amend the FDC Act to include extensive drug approval procedures for both safety and efficacy. [6]

The authority to regulate prescription drug advertising was transferred from the FTC to the FDA. All promotional materials were required to be thoroughly reviewed by the FDA and were expected to disclose accurate information about the side effects and efficacy of treatments. A specific requirement implemented by the FDA was to mandate that ads must contain a "brief summary" statement describing full information on possible side effects, contraindications, and effectiveness of the drug being promoted. For prescription drugs, the focus was on promotional material directed toward healthcare professionals because the regulatory view at the time was that patients lacked the knowledge to act independently in managing these medications. Non-prescription drug ("over-the-counter") advertising was allowed, but the manufacturers were eventually required to justify their claims of efficacy and safety or remove the product from the market. While the regulation of over-the-counter quality, safety, and labeling was subject to FDA regulation, the responsibility for how the drug was advertised remained with the FTC.

The Kefauver–Harris Amendment enhanced the FDA's role in ensuring accurate information about drug products. Because of the original focus on the health professional and not the patient, consumer groups began demonstrating a need for more information about prescription drug products. These demands expanded with the "self-care" movements in the 1970s, which encouraged consumers to seek more information to take better control over their health and achieve better lifestyles. During that period, "do-it-yourself" books, newspaper columns, and television programs regarding health inquiry became widespread. In the late 1970s and early 1980s, the Physicians' Desk References became available in consumer bookstores and became very popular as a source of prescription information. Various health professional groups responded by urging their constituents to better educate their patients about the drug products they were taking. Many were effective in improving patient knowledge, although the impact on medication side effects and adherence was unclear. Thus, public pressure increased on the federal government to provide leadership in better informing the public better informed about the medications they were taking.

Congress responded to this public pressure by proposing a system in which all patients would receive FDA-approved information about their prescription drugs. This federal effort became known as the "patient package insert" (PPI) initiative.[7,8] The main regulatory objective was to ensure that individual patients comprehended their illnesses and treatment regimens—especially an understanding of the proper and safe use of medications they used. PPIs were defined as "standardized monographs of information about a drug or drug class intended for users of prescription medicines." The purpose was to promote the safe and effective use of drugs by patients and to ensure that they can be informed of the risk–benefit information of their medications. The first PPI was required for isoproterenol inhalators in 1968. In 1970, the FDA required a PPI for oral contraceptives and extended this provision to other drugs in the following years. In the late 1970s, the FDA instituted a series of regulatory policies to require PPIs for all prescription drugs. The FDA's initial intent was that PPIs would be available through the physician. However, since the FDA has no jurisdiction over medical practice, it interpreted PPIs as labeling that needed to accompany the drug product at the time of dispensing. Although most stated support for providing more drug information to patients, healthcare professionals and pharmaceutical companies strongly opposed the regulation. Stated reasons for this opposition included lack of evidence that it would improve efficacy and safety, potential increased liability to health professionals if they do not faithfully adhere to the mandate, and the increased costs associated with the preparation and distribution of the leaflets to every patient.

Nevertheless, the mandate was moving toward implementation during the last months of the Carter Administration. However, in the Regan administration, the PPI regulation was deemed unnecessary and not to be enforced. The FDA officially rescinded the PPI regulation in 1982 in favor of a plan under which pharmaceutical companies, and the various health professions would voluntarily make more information about their products available to consumers. [8]

6.1.5 Expanding Information Available to Consumers (1983–Present)

Despite the legislative failure of the PPI initiative, the need to bridge the gap between what patients wanted to know about their medications and what they learned from existing communications with health professionals remained a high priority at the FDA.[9,10] The FDA encouraged the private sector to develop its own initiatives. The pharmaceutical industry managed their initiative by sponsoring the formation of the National Center for Patient Information and Education, which continues today as a leading non-profit coalition that focuses on the communication of information on the appropriate use of medications to consumers and healthcare professionals. The pharmaceutical manufacturers also joined other organizations such as the American Medical Association, the American Pharmacists Association, the USP, and other related organizations to encourage their membership to provide more written drug product information to the public. Their efforts, combined with increased activity from pharmaceutical manufacturers, resulted in the development of more than 1000 instructional sheets covering the major classes of drugs.

Legislative activity also increased. In 1990, Congress strengthened the requirement for appropriate patient information through the Omnibus Budget Reconciliation Act (OBRA 90), which mandated pharmacists to offer counseling to all Medicaid recipients who have prescriptions filled. Most states responded with statutes or regulations that expanded the requirement to all patients. The regulations varied by state; some only required it for new prescriptions; others believed that counseling should be required for all prescription drugs. Face-to-face counseling was required in almost all states. Although the regulatory requirement was followed inconsistently among pharmacists and rarely enforced, the act spurred more efforts toward patient information provided both orally and in writing by pharmacists.

At the same time, the FDA re-examined the issue of PPIs through its MedGuide Project. The goal was to develop computer-generated medication guides that would come with selected medications. Unlike the PPI initiative, the objective was not to mandate leaflets for all prescription medications approved by the FDA. Rather, the guides were intended to address issues that were specific to particular drugs and drug classes and would contain FDA-approved information that would help patients avoid serious adverse events. The MedGuide Project at the FDA has been very successful. The guides are necessary for specific prescription drugs and biological products when the agency determines the following: certain information is necessary to prevent serious adverse effects; patient decision-making should be informed by information about a known serious side effect with a product; or patient adherence to directions for the use of a product is essential to its effectiveness. The FDA now recommends that medication guides be considered a key part of any Risk Evaluation and Mitigation Strategy (REMS) submitted by manufacturers for new drug approvals. [11]

6.2 CURRENT STATE OF PRESCRIPTION DRUG PRODUCT-RELATED INFORMATION PROVIDED TO CONSUMERS[12–28]

Federal efforts have created almost universal public access to FDA-approved information about drug products. The current agency's focus has been to ensure that the drug product information provided to patients is accessible, accurate, balanced, and understandable.

6.2.1 Written Information Dispensed With the Prescription

The most frequent source of prescription drug information is provided through the written material that is typically distributed with the drug product.[12] There are generally three types of information provided to patients when a prescription is dispensed: Medication Guides (also referred to MedGuides), PPIs, and Consumer Medication Information (CMI). Medication guides are based on product labeling and are required if the FDA believes that specific labeling information is needed to minimize risks and ensure important adherence to directions. Distribution of medication guides is considered necessary for those drug products that need to have a REMS to be safely used. [13]

The PPI is another type of written information distributed with the dispensing of the prescription. PPIs are developed by the manufacturer, approved by the FDA, and are required to be given with specific products or classes of products (e.g., oral contraceptives and estrogen-containing products). Other PPIs are submitted to the FDA voluntarily by the manufacturer and approved by the FDA, but their distribution is not required.[14,15]

CMI is the most commonly distributed information with the prescription drug product. This information is developed by third-party sources and is not officially part of FDA-approved labeling and not reviewed by the agency. However, the FDA has published guidelines to assist the third-party developers in developing this written information. A CMI is considered useful when the information presented is consistent with the most recent version of the manufacturer's professional labeling or PI, which includes the necessary information components suggested by the FDA and substantially conforms to the formatting recommendations made by the agency. Specifically, written CMIs should be scientifically accurate; be unbiased in content and tone; be sufficiently specific and comprehensive; be presented in an understandable and legible format that is readily comprehensible to consumers; be timely/up to date; and contain information that is needed for the safe use of the medication.[14,15]

6.2.2 Electronic Sources of Medication Information

Written information given at the time of dispensing has been the primary source of drug product information, but technological advances offer the opportunity to transition to more digital platforms.[16,17] Thus, there has been an increased public effort to move from paper to the more versatile electronic patient information leaflets, often known as e-PILs. The main value of this approach is its dynamic nature.[18] The product information can be easily updated and individualized as new information is produced, especially about emerging side effects. In addition, electronic information portals have the potential to enable real-time interaction with health professionals and other sources such as the FDA or the product manufacturer. However, despite the value of transmitting drug product information electronically, patients still appear to prefer the written information form.[19]

6.2.3 Sources of Information on the Internet

The internet has evolved vastly as a drug information source for consumers. Since much of the internet is unregulated, the drug information available needs to be scrutinized. A key characteristic to assessing the quality of the drug product information on the internet is the source of the content. Two reliable sources on the internet are the FDA and the drug product's manufacturer.[20,21] The FDA Drug Labeling Program contains drug labeling information on every drug product, although it may be difficult to understand. The manufacturer of the product is also a highly reliable source of product information, and its medical information department will answer patient inquiries even though its focus is on health professionals. Other respected sources include healthcare professionals organizations such as the Mayo Clinic, DailyMed, and others.[22] An evolving source is the collection of patient experiences about a drug on the internet.[23,24] These sites solicit ratings from patients about their experiences with the drug and comments about those experiences. These comments may be helpful, but they are based on spontaneous responses and may represent only those individuals who have a unique perspective rather than the experiences of the general user population.

6.2.4 Value of Written Product Information

Research suggests that consumers, especially for information about side effects, value written product information.[25,26] However, the use is limited by the readability of the written information, its format, and the relevance of the information provided.[27,28] Consumers are likely to read the written product information when they receive it with the prescription but less likely to refer to it later. They tend to seek further information through internet sources or their health professional. Perception of the information seems to be affected by individual characteristics. In one study, older adults were more concerned about the risks associated with taking prescription drug products than younger adults. Despite the widespread availability of prescription drug product information, they are best used in conjunction with counseling provided by a health professional, typically a physician, physician assistant, nurse, or pharmacist.

All health professional organizations, particularly the federal government, involved in the provision of drug information to patients are now actively trying to determine the best approaches to ensuring that the information is accurate, balanced, and useful.[28] The result of these efforts has been the creation of general guidelines about providing this information, especially about risks. The guidelines include the following general recommendations: [28]

- Information should be provided so that the patient can properly understand both the benefits and risks of taking the medication.
- Consumer-friendly language ought to be used and jargon or technical terms should be avoided.
- Words that are understandable to an audience with various levels of literacy skills need to be used.
- The information should be presented visually in a manner designed for ease of use by consumers. Brief summary formats that organize information in an understandable manner such as a "Drug Fact Box" or a "Question/Answer" format are preferred.

6.3 EVOLUTION OF DRUG ADVERTISING TO US CONSUMERS (DTCA)

During the late 1970s to the early 1980s, drug companies were uncertain if they should communicate directly to consumers regarding their products because they feared doctors would never accept programs that bypassed them. In addition, it was not clear whether the FDA would sanction such practices. Thus, many drug companies used limited advertising campaigns promoting their organizational name rather than promoting their individual drug products. A classic example was Pfizer's "Partners in Health Care" series, which used both television and print media for patient education. The campaign covered topics such as diabetes, arthritis, and hypertension, and new choices of treatment. The campaign also highlighted the dedication of the company and its employees to improve public health. Around this time, Ayerst launched a print ad encouraging women to seek treatment for osteoporosis, while Merrell-Dow used television and print media for a "quit" campaign to make consumers aware of a product available to help with nicotine withdrawal symptoms. Institution-orientated campaigns were used by many firms such as Upjohn, DuPont, Ciba-Geigy, and Eli-Lilly to increase consumers' awareness of the firm and its reputation. Although the campaigns used the company's name, they did not mention the name of specific drug products.

6.3.1 Emergence of DTCA (1981–1982)

Drug product advertising directed at consumers first began when Naprosyn® was introduced in England.[29–31] At that time, Naprosyn (naproxen) was a new drug used in the treatment of arthritis and had soon become the subject of broadcast talk shows where its risks and benefits were discussed. Syntex, Naprosyn's manufacturer, soon realized that merely brief exposure of Naprosyn messages to the public had dramatically reduced the length of its introductory stage. Although Naprosyn was introduced into a saturated non-steroidal anti-inflammatory drug market, product sales substantially increased in only a few short months after its introduction. Presumably, patients independently learned of Naprosyn early and their requests for the drug accelerated its use by physicians.

The Naprosyn phenomenon did not go unnoticed in the US. In 1981, a few drug companies began direct advertising. The most notable of these pioneers were Merck, Sharpe, & Dohme and Boots Pharmaceuticals, who launched the first two product-specific advertisements: Pneumovax® (a pneumonia vaccine) and Rufen® (a brand name for ibuprofen, which was approved for the treatment of arthritis), respectively.

Pneumovax vaccine advertising was very distinctive because it targeted the healthy elderly who were potential users of the product (Figure 6.5). The vaccine was advertised in consumer magazines, where readers were encouraged to take a tear-off coupon to their physicians for an examination of whether they were candidates for Pneumovax therapy. The advertisement caused little controversy for the FDA for two reasons. First, it contained a public health benefit by increasing consumers' awareness of the existence of a preventive health measure, and, second, Merck, Sharpe, & Dohme also surveyed physicians to determine whether they would be offended by such advertisements.

At the same time, Rufen (which was another brand name for ibuprofen) was the subject of talk shows, commercial spots, magazines, and a newspaper in the Tampa, Florida, area. The Rufen advertisement was basically price advertising, making no claims. The primary message to consumers was that "Rufen® was the same as Motrin® but cost less." Boots also had a nationwide rebate coupon program for Rufen purchasers. Besides price information, Rufen advertising was interpreted as conveying comparative effectiveness claims with Motrin® without providing adequate risk information or directions of use. This ad created substantial internal discussions in the FDA, which eventually prompted the FDA to order Boots to stop the Rufen ad.

Although consumers' awareness of the Rufen advertisement doubled during the six-week period of the campaign and the Pneumovax advertisements were viewed to be beneficial to the public, neither the Boots nor Merck campaigns reported a significant increase in product sales. Even so, several pharmaceutical companies expressed their interest in advertising their products directly to the public.

6.3.2 Voluntary Moratorium Period of DTCA (1983–1985)

Witnessing trends in consumer demand for prescription drug information and a dramatic increase of sources of health care information, the FDA predicted that

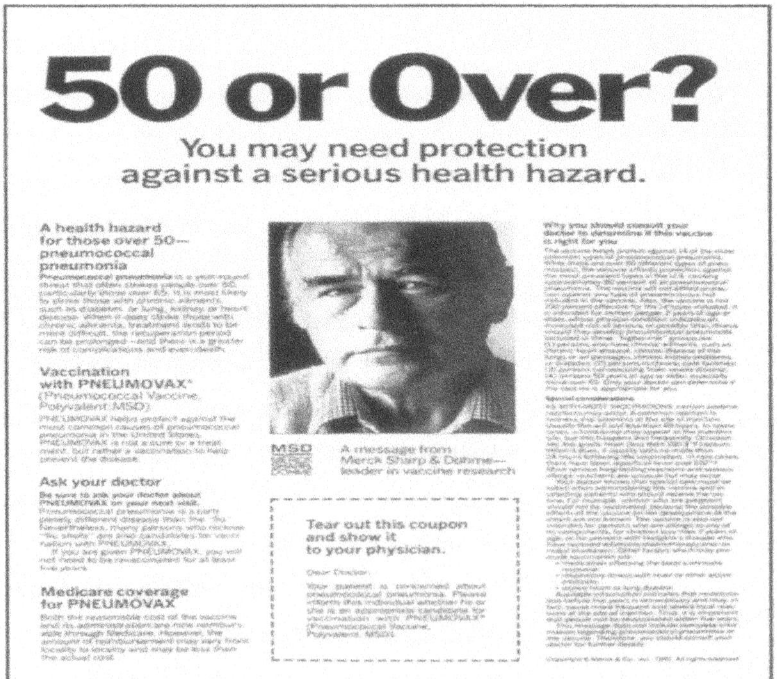

FIGURE 6.5 Pneumovax ad, the first DTC ad appeared in Readers Digest in 1981.

Source: https://www.knowpneumonia.com/about-pneumococcal-pneumonia?cmp=eee20a03-84c7-4038-b27b-5e36a5b7bf9e&gclid=1f84d4406ea31a9e9a06b4c5c94631bd&gclsrc=3p.ds&

"exponential growth" of DTCA would follow. In 1982, FDA Commissioner Arthur Hull Hayes made a speech to the Pharmaceutical Advertising Council with the intent of simply summarizing the state of DTCA from his perspective. However, Hayes' remarks had the unintended impact of creating misconceptions for the drug industry about the FDA's position, which resulted in a very large number of DTC ads being submitted to the FDA's Division of Drug Advertising and Labeling. In the middle of his speech, Hayes predicted "exponential growth" in advertising directly to consumers. The statement was not an indication of FDA support or passive approval of DTCA. However, the drug industry interpreted this statement as a change in FDA policy regarding this new form of advertising. Responding to this confusion, the FDA in September 1983 issued a formal request to the drug industry to voluntarily stop prescription drug advertising directly to consumers. The request was made to allow the FDA to develop appropriate guidelines for future DTCA regulations. During the moratorium period, several groups, including the FDA, conducted DTCA research varying in design and rigor.[29–34]

Overall, consumers expressed interest in receiving information and positively viewed the concept of DTCA. Thus, in 1983, the FDA commissioned research to investigate the appropriateness of applying a "brief summary" requirement to DTCA. Overall results revealed that DTCA could communicate information regarding risk and benefits, although benefit information (rather than risk information) tended to be more frequently recalled. Compared to those who examined general risk ads, subjects who viewed specific information ads reported a more negative evaluation of the drug product and ad. In addition, interaction relationships were discovered. For example, opinions toward the ad appeared to be a function of how specific risk information and emphasis of risk information were presented.[32,35–37]

A different study revealed that the presence of risk information was positively associated with the believability of the ad. Additionally, the relationship between subjects' evaluation of the ad and the disclosure of risk information appeared to depend on the type of drug. Disclosing risk information for anti-acne drugs was viewed as overemphasizing risk information, while that for a pain-reliever drug increased the perceived value of the information.[38] These studies and other research provided insight to the FDA regarding what would be appropriate prescription drug product advertising to consumers. The key goal would be to provide a balance between medication benefits and risks. While there was no standardized definition, it appeared that the "fair balance" goal could be reached by advertising directly to the consumer and patient.

6.3.3 Establishment of DTCA Regulations (1985–1999)

After gathering information and evaluating study results, the moratorium was lifted in September 1985, but no specific policy was announced. The agency concluded that existing regulations could "provide sufficient safeguards to protect consumers." The FDA applied the same standards as those for physician-directed prescription drug advertising to regulate DTCA. There was no differentiation of DTCA regulations by type of media. Both print and broadcast advertisements were regulated using the same "fair balance" requirements. Product-specific ads were required to include the "brief summary" statement describing full information on possible side effects, contraindications, and effectiveness of the drug being promoted.[35–39]

After the FDA lifted its moratorium, drug companies began advertising their products. For the print media, product-specific DTCA posed no problem because the brief summary could be included as part of the advertisement. In contrast, the use of product-specific DTCA in broadcast media was more challenging because the brief summary could not easily fit into the limited broadcast timeframe (usually 30–60 seconds). Thus, drug companies had to use two other kinds of advertisements: a help-seeking ad or a reminder notice ad. Help-seeking ads could describe diseases or symptoms without mentioning the product name. This basic message is to encourage consumers to see a doctor. A classic example of help-seeking ads was Rogaine® (a hair-restorer) by the Upjohn Company. This ad encouraged consumers who had premature baldness to see their doctors or to call a toll-free number for additional information. Reminder ads merely mentioned the product name without describing its uses. A typical example was Claritin® (a non-sedating antihistamine) by Schering-Plough, which showed a hot-air balloon floating across the sky with a voice "Blue skies smiling at me, nothing but blue skies I do see . . . See your doctor about Claritin® . . . (because a) clear answer is out there."[40–42]

Given that DTCA was a relatively new phenomenon at that time, consumers could not tell from the help-seeking or reminder ads the product's indication was for or its prescription drug status. The FDA realized that messages in these types of commercials were not sufficiently communicative and could create confusion rather than benefit consumers. Thus, in 1995, the FDA held a public hearing on the appropriateness of elements in the current DTCA regulations and the role of fair balance for disclosure of risk in broadcast media.[40–42]

In 1997, the FDA established a new provision, "The Draft Guidance for Industry: Consumer-Directed Broadcast Advertisements," that applied to broadcast DTCA. The FDA's rationale was to ensure that consumers receive adequate communication about risk information needed for an informed decision and to facilitate the process used by drug sponsors to disseminate drug product information to consumers. The guidance did not introduce a dramatic change in the principle of DTCA regulations but rather clarified the FDA's interpretation of the "adequate provision" requirement for broadcast DTCA structure so that broadcast advertisements can comply with regulatory objectives. According to the guidance, broadcast DTCA could present the product's name and its indications, but important risk information (or the major statement) must always be included. Additionally, the broadcast DTCA must provide a toll-free telephone number, an internet address, a reference to print advertisements, and a statement that additional information about the product is available from a doctor or pharmacist.

The 1997 guidance was in draft form and the FDA evaluated the policy after two years. To revise and finalize the guidance, the FDA requested feedback on new guidelines regarding the effects of DTCA on public health, the degree to which consumers were taking advantage of the mechanisms for obtaining approved package labeling in connection with broadcast advertisements, and how risk information can be best integrated into broadcast advertisements.[43,44]

In August 1999, the FDA issued a final guidance on DTCA broadcasts.[45] The final guidance did not differ substantially from the draft guidance but elucidated and supplemented the existing adequate provision requirements. Revisions required, for example, (1) reference to an internet site that provides access to more extensive drug product information, (2) an explicit address where health care providers other than physicians and pharmacists can be sources of drug product information, (3) a toll-free number that provides access to additional information via mail or fax or by being read to on the phone, and (4) print material associated with widely broadcasted DTCA to be "comparably broadly disseminated in terms of the target audiences" (i.e., reference to a magazine that has a high circulation).

6.4 CURRENT STATE OF DIRECT-TO-CONSUMER ADVERTISING[46–60]

After the final guidance was published in 1999 regarding DTCA, efforts by manufacturers increased substantially. The venues used to promote prescription drug products have also expanded significantly, especially with the rapid increase in the use of the internet. The growth is due to an apparent increase in sales attributed to DTCA of specific new drug products, especially during the "launch" phase when a product is first entering a crowded market. An additional reason is the significant growth of all forms of DTCA beyond drug products. This growth is enabled by the newer technology that allows consumers direct access to product selection choices without significant assistance from an intermediary.

While the 1999 guidance provides the basic framework for appropriate DTCA, the FDA has published several draft or final guidances that clarify or address new activities by the manufacturers. These guidances include ones that address the use of ads on television, social media, and the specific use of risk information.[46–51]

The general responsibility for overseeing these activities currently rests with the FDA's Center for Drug Evaluation and Research (CDER). Within CDER, the Office of Prescription Drug Promotion (OPDP) is assigned the specific responsibility of watching over prescription drug ad activities. OPDP is focused on three major activities: (1) reviewing existing advertisements to identify those that may violate the law; (2) educating industry and others about the specifics of the law; and (3) working with consumers and health professions to encourage enlightened use of such promotional information.[52,53]

While federal law requires that all drug product risks need to be communicated, it does not mandate that pharmaceutical manufacturers submit their ads for approval prior to their use. Although many do, the FDA often views ads after they are used publicly. If the agency believes that an ad violates the law, it will send a warning letter to request a stoppage immediately. Court action may follow, but the warning letter is usually a sufficient deterrent.

Based on past practices, the FDA organizes its regulatory guidance by dividing DTCA into three broad categories: product claims, reminders, and help-seeking. Although the requirements for these types of ads had been used prior to the publication of the guidance, their content is now formally described. The categories are shown in Table 6.1.[54,55]

Since DTCA is largely self-regulated, efforts have been made within the pharmaceutical industry to ensure that manufacturers adhere to best practices and to avoid unnecessary conflict with the FDA. An example is the "Guiding Principles for the DTCA about Prescription Medicines" published by PhRMA, the Pharmaceutical Research and Manufacturers of America, which represents the country's leading biopharmaceutical researchers and biotechnology companies.

These principles are summarized here:[56–60]

1. DTCA is based on the recognition that DTC advertising of prescription medicines can benefit public health.
2. DTCA should be accurate, not misleading, and be consistent with FDA-approved labeling.
3. DTCA should balance its marketing efforts with a similar effort to responsibly educate the consumer about that medicine and, where appropriate, the condition for which it may be prescribed. The educational impact should be assessed through planned solicitations of consumer and health professional feedback.
4. DTCA should clearly indicate that the medicine is a prescription drug to distinguish such advertising from other advertising for non-prescription products.
5. DTCA should foster responsible communications between patients and healthcare professionals to help patients achieve better health and understand the benefits and risks of the medicine being advertised.
6. Companies should spend an appropriate amount of time educating healthcare professionals about a new medicine or a new therapeutic indication and alert them to the upcoming advertising campaign

TABLE 6.1
Categories of Ads Supervised by the FDA

Types of Advertisement	Purpose	Specific Regulatory Requirements: Print	Specific Regulatory Requirements: Broadcast
Product-claim ads	Name a drug and discuss its benefits and risks	Fair balance between benefits/risks Brief summary of the drug including all risks noted in approval documents Statement that "You are encouraged to report negative side effects of prescription drugs to the FDA. Visit MedWatch or call 1-800-FDA-1088."	Fair balance between benefits/risks Fulfillment of the "adequate provision" requirement for the drug risk information: Most important risks (i.e., "Major Statement") presented in the audio portion Either all the risks listed in the drug's prescribing information or a variety of sources for viewers to find the prescribing information for the drug Appropriate sources for finding additional drug information (e.g., health care providers, toll-free manufacturer number, website address)
Reminder ads	Give the name of a drug but not the drug's uses. These ads assume that the audience already knows the drug's use. Excluded from promoting high-risk drug products	No product-specific information allowed	No product-specific information allowed
Help-seeking ads	Describe a disease or condition but do not recommend or suggest a specific drug treatment. Excluded from promoting high-risk drug products	No product-specific information allowed	No product-specific information allowed

before commencing the first DTC advertising campaign.

7. Companies should continue to responsibly alter or discontinue a DTC advertising campaign if new and reliable information indicates a serious previously unknown safety risk.
8. Companies should submit all new DTC television advertisements to the FDA before releasing these advertisements for broadcast.
9. DTCA for prescription medicines should include the FDA's toll-free MedWatch telephone number and website for reporting potential adverse events.
10. Companies that choose to feature actors in the roles of healthcare professionals or actual health professionals in DTCA should acknowledge the advertisement that is being used.
11. DTCA that features a celebrity endorser should ensure that endorsements accurately reflect the opinions, findings, beliefs, or experiences of the endorser.
12. DTCA should include information about the availability of other options such as diet and lifestyle changes where appropriate for the advertised condition.
13. DTCA that identifies a product by name should clearly state the health conditions for which the medicine is approved and the major risks associated with the medicine being advertised.
14. DTCA should be designed to achieve a balanced presentation of both the benefits and the risks associated with the advertised prescription medicine. DTCA should direct patients to healthcare professionals as well as print advertisements and/or websites where additional benefit and risk information are available.
15. DTCA should respect the seriousness of the health conditions and the medicine being advertised.
16. DTC television and print advertisements should be targeted to avoid audiences that are not age appropriate for the messages involved, especially children.
17. Companies are encouraged to promote health and disease awareness as part of their DTCA.
18. Companies should include information in all DTC advertising, where practical and appropriate, directing patients to company resources that may help them with the cost of their medicine.

19. All DTC television advertising that identifies a prescription medicine by name should include directions as to where patients can find information about the cost of the medicine, such as a company-developed website, including the list price and average, estimated or typical patient out-of-pocket costs, or other context about the potential cost of the medicine.

6.4.1 Advantages and Disadvantages of DTCA[61–66]

6.4.1.1 Advantages

One of the key advantages of DTCA is the empowerment of patients by providing them with relevant information about their disease that focuses on the available treatment options (emphasizing new drugs). DTCA is viewed by some groups as a highly visible source of health information that complements the advice of the patient's physician and other health professionals.[61,62] Several organizations suggest that DTCA offers patients significant amounts of relevant health information that may encourage them to be more active in seeking the advice of health professionals.[63,64] In particular, DTCA may reduce the under-diagnosis or under-treatment of certain conditions with social stigma (e.g., mental health or erectile dysfunction) by encouraging patients to seek health professional advice. Other bodies have suggested that DTCA encourages consumers to seek appropriate care or pursue screening for a condition that they did not previously deem relevant to their health. Another reported advantage is a possible enhancement of the patient–physician relationship. Various surveys suggest that DTCA has initiated more thoughtful questions from patients and may make them more involved in their treatment choices.

6.4.1.2 Disadvantages

A major criticism of DTCA is how the ads convey risk information. Although the FDA guidance does not clearly define what the "fair balance" of benefit-to-risk drug information is, research suggests that the quantity of the benefit information is usually higher than the facts about the risks, with significant variation by drug product. Ad imagery is also distorted toward the benefits of the drug product, even when risk information is provided. In addition, the language often used to describe the risks seems to be more complicated than information describing the drug's benefits.[65–66]

Another criticism is that DTCA provides consumers with biased, incomplete, and misleading drug product information that may generate unneeded visits and inappropriate requests for medications. In addition, these ads may encourage drug products over healthier (and safer) lifestyle choices. The DTCA may also lead to the "medicalization" of nonmedical conditions, ultimately promoting the needs of the pharmaceutical industry rather than the public's health. Finally, the ads have historically not discussed the cost of the advertised drug, which is likely to be much higher than the existing treatment.

The existing research shows that the value of DTCA in health care and medical use is controversial. Manufacturers view it as a successful tool for marketing their products and fulfilling their role as public educators. They have attempted to address the criticisms of DTCA through the PhRMA Principles, especially the emphasis on the key role of the physician, promoting a balanced approach to providing both the drug benefits and the risks and including a discussion about drug costs. Health professionals, especially physicians, have historically opposed such advertising because they believe that it is inherently misleading and interferes with their relationships with patients. However, they have begun to accept it as an important source of drug information. Consumer groups generally endorse DTCA as a readily accessible source of approved drug product information. The federal government, especially the FDA, views DTCA as a legitimate means of providing approved product information to the public, endorsed by the First Amendment. Thus, the FDA focuses on ensuring that information is accurate and balanced between the drug product's benefits and risks and that the role of the physician in prescribing the drug product is emphasized. While the various groups disagree on certain aspects of DTCA, these manufacturer-initiated efforts will continue and remain an important source of prescription drug product information in the future.

6.5 CONCLUSION

The history of drug product regulation in the US is long and complicated. However, some basic principles do appear. As indicated in Figure 6.1, the regulations represent a "social contract" between the US government (represented primarily by the FDA) and the citizens it serves to ensure that only safe and effective drug products are available. This contract, though clear, represents a tension between the citizens and their government in reaching the optimal goal of promoting health but protecting against unnecessary risks. Societal trends such as belief in individual rights and technological advances such as the internet have minimized the ability of the FDA to control access to product information. Rather, its role has evolved into ensuring that drug product information remains accurate and balanced.

It has been stated by unknown pundits that, if the FDA did not exist, we would have to create it. Its role is necessary for a society where access to drug products is great, and the information about the drugs is massive, occasionally misleading, and often overwhelming.

REFERENCES

1. US Food and Drug Administration. *FDA's Strategic Plan for Risk Communication.* Department of Health and Human Services Food and Drug Administration Center for Drug Evaluation and Research (CDER); Fall 2009.
2. Ascione FJ, Kirking DM, Gaither CA, Welage LS. Historical overview of generic medication policy. *Journal of the American Pharmaceutical Association.* 2001;41:567–577.

3. Janssen W. Outline of the history of U.S. drug regulation and labeling. *Food Drug Cosmetic Law Journal.* 1981;36:420–441.
4. Swann J. FDA and the practice of pharmacy: Prescription drug regulation before the Durham-Humphrey Amendment of 1951. *Pharmacy History.* 1994;36(2):55–70.
5. Huber J, Gillaspy M. Knowledge/power transforming the social landscape: The case of the Consumer Health Information Movement. *The Library Quarterly: Information, Community, Policy.* 2011;81(4):405–430.
6. Hamburg M. 50 Years after thalidomide: Why regulation matters. *FDA Voice*, February 7, 2012.
7. Symposium on patient package inserts. *Drug Information Journal.* 1977 (Jan. supp).
8. Prescription drug products; revocation of patient package insert requirements—Food and Drug Administration. Final rule. *Federal Register.* 1982;47(Sep 7):39147–39155.
9. Kessler D. Communicating with patients about their medications. *New England Journal of Medicine.* 1991; 325:1650–1652.
10. Vivian J, Fink J. OBRA'90 at sweet sixteen: A retrospective review. *U.S. Pharmacist.* 2008;33(3):59–65.
11. US Food and Drug Administration. *Guidance on Medication Guides Distribution Requirements and Inclusion in Risk Evaluation and Mitigation Strategies (REMS).* U.S. Department of Health and Human Services Food and Drug Administration Center for Drug Evaluation and Research (CDER); November 2011.
12. Food and Drug Administration. *Title 21-Food and Drugs. Part 310-New Drugs, Subpart E-Requirements for a Specific New Drugs or Devices, Sec. 310.501 Patient Package Inserts for Oral Contraceptives.* U.S. Department of Health and Human Services Food and Drug Administration Center for Drug Evaluation and Research (CDER); April 2020.
13. Brodsky E. *Consistency in Labeling and Methods to Optimize Communication in Labeling.* Prescription Drug Labeling Conference, U.S. Department of Health and Human Services Food and Drug Administration Center for Drug Evaluation and Research (CDER); November 2017.
14. Walker M. *Instructions for Use (IFU) Content and Format Draft Guidance for Industry.* CDER Prescription Drug Labeling Conference U.S. Department of Health and Human Services Food and Drug Administration Center for Drug Evaluation and Research (CDER); December 4–5, 2019.
15. US Food and Drug Administration. *Guidance on Useful Written Consumer Medication Information FDA (CMI).* U.S. Department of Health and Human Services Food and Drug Administration Center for Drug Evaluation and Research (CDER); July 2006.
16. Bolislis WR, Mortazavi C, Riccioni R, Schaeffer PE, Kühler TC. From print to screen: Regulatory considerations to adopting innovative approaches for patient information and safety. *Therapeutic Innovation & Regulatory Science.* 2020;54:831–838. https://doi.org/10.1007/s43441-019-00018-0.
17. Murrell D. Electronic patient information leaflets: The future. *Archives of Disease in Childhood.* 2020;105(Suppl 1): A84–A85.
18. Smith-Gick J, Barnes N, Barone R, Bedford J, James JR, Reisner SF, Stephenson M. The near-term viability and benefits of eLabels for patients, clinical sites, and sponsors. *Therapeutic Innovation & Regulatory Science.* 2018;52:537–545. https://doi.org/10.1177/2168479018765463tirs.sagepub.com.
19. Hammer T, Nilsson A, Hovstadius B. Patients' views on electronic patient information leaflets. *Pharmacy Practice.* 2016;14(2):702.
20. US Food and Drug Administration. *FDA Label: Full-Text Search of Drug Product Labeling.* U.S. Department of Health and Human Services Food and Drug Administration Center for Drug Evaluation and Research (CDER); April 2021.
21. First Data Bank. Drug database and medical device leader. https://www.fdbhealth.com/. Last Accessed April 2021.
22. Paquette-Lemieux E, Hays S, Gaspo R. US Medical Information websites benchmarking: How is the industry fairing in usability? *Therapeutic Innovation & Regulatory Science.* 2019;53(3):340–348. https://doi.org/10.1177/2168479018786481.
23. Brunetti L, Desantis E. The internet as a drug information resource. *US Pharm*, 2010;35.
24. Candelario DM, Vazquez V, Jackson W, Reilly T. Completeness, accuracy, and readability of Wikipedia as a reference for patient medication information. *Journal of the American Pharmacists Association.* 2017;57:197–200.
25. Balog-Way H, Lofstedt R. Pharmaceutical benefit-risk perception and older age: A pilot study. *Therapeutic Innovation & Regulatory Science.* 2020;54(3):645–657. https://doi.org/10.1007/s43441-019-00099.
26. Munsour EE, Awaisu A, Hassali MA, Abdoun E, Dabbous Z, Zahran N, Ali H. The effect of tailored consumer medicine information on patients with type 2 diabetes mellitus: A randomised controlled interventional study. *International Journal of Clinical Practice.* 2020;74(8):1357. https://doi.org/10.1111/ijcp.13527.
27. Sharp ML, Hall L, Eleftherion A, Simpson K, Neuhauser L. Comparison of brief summary formats through a health literacy lens. *Therapeutic Innovation & Regulatory Science.* 2019;53(1):100–109. https://doi.org/10.1177/2168479018769291 tirs.sagepub.com.
28. Yiu A, Ng KK, Lee VW, Bajorek BV. Evaluating the understandability and actionability of web-based education materials for patients taking non-vitamin K oral anticoagulants. *Therapeutic Innovation & Regulatory Science.* 2020;54(2):476–483. https://doi.org/10.1007/s43441-019-00079-1.
29. Morris LA, Brinberg D, Klimberg R, Rivera C, Millstein LG. The attitudes of consumers toward direct advertising of prescription drugs. *Public Health Reports.* 1986;101:82–89.
30. Perri M III, Shinde S, Banavali R. The past, present, and future of direct-to-consumer prescription drug advertising. *Clinical Therapeutics.* 1999;21:1798–1811.
31. Perri M, Nelson AA Jr. An exploratory analysis of consumer recognition of direct-to-consumer advertising of prescription medications. *Journal of Health Care Marketing.* 1987;7:9–17.
32. Christensen T. Effect of direct-to-consumer advertising of prescription medications in an elderly population. *Dissertation Abstracts.* Ann Arbor, MI: University of Michigan; 1995.
33. Feisullin S, Sause R. Update on direct-to-consumer advertising of prescription drugs. *American Pharmacy.* 1991;NS31:47–52.
34. Anonymous. Rx-to-consumer advertising debate starts up again. *Drug Topics.* 1985;129:20–21.
35. Pines W. A history and perspective on direct-to-consumer promotion. *Food Drug Law Journal.* 1999;54:489–518.

36. Murphy D. Direct to consumer advertising of prescription drugs. *American Pharmacy.* 1984;NS24:20–22.
37. Morris LA, Ruffner M, Klimberg R. Warning disclosures for prescription drugs. *Journal of Advertising Research.* 1985;25:25–32.
38. Morris LA, Brinberg D, Plimpton L. Prescription drug information for consumers: An experiment of source and format. *Current Issues and Research in Advertising.* 1984;7:65–78.
39. US Food and Drug Administration. Withdrawal of moratorium on direct-to-consumer advertising of prescription drugs. *Federal Register.* 1985;50:36677.
40. Gilgore L. A consideration of direct-to-consumer advertising of prescription drugs and potential legal problems with the brief summary requirement: Is the FDA's regulatory authority illusory? *Food and Drug Law Journal.* 1991;46:849–859.
41. Schwartz T. Consumer-directed prescription drug advertising and the learned intermediary doctrine. *Food and Drug Law Journal.* 1991;46:829–848.
42. US Food and Drug Administration. Direct-to-consumer promotion public hearing announced. *Federal Register.* 1995;60:42581.
43. US Food and Drug Administration. Consumer-directed broadcast advertisements (draft guidance). *Federal Register.* 1997;62:43171.
44. Nordenberg T. Direct to you: TV drug ads that make sense. *FDA Consumer*, January–February 1998:7–10.
45. US Food and Drug Administration. *Guidance for Industry: Consumer-Directed Broadcast Advertisements.* U.S. Department of Health and Human Services Food and Drug Administration Center for Drug Evaluation and Research (CDER); August 1999.
46. US Food and Drug Administration. *Internet/Social Media Platforms: Correcting Independent Third-Party Misinformation About Prescription Drugs and Medical Devices Draft Guidance for Industry.* U.S. Department of Health and Human Services Food and Drug Administration Center for Drug Evaluation and Research (CDER); June 2014.
47. US Food and Drug Administration. *Guidance on Distributing Scientific and Medical Publications on Risk Information for Approved Prescription Drugs and Biological Products: Recommended Practices.* U.S. Department of Health and Human Services Food and Drug Administration Center for Drug Evaluation and Research (CDER); June 2014.
48. US Food and Drug Administration. *Guidance on Distributing Scientific and Medical Publications on Unapproved New Uses: Recommended Practices.* U.S. Department of Health and Human Services Food and Drug Administration Center for Drug Evaluation and Research (CDER); February 2014.
49. US Food and Drug Administration. *Guidance on Fulfilling Regulatory Requirements for Postmarketing Submissions of Interactive Promotional Media for Prescription Human and Animal Drugs and Biologics.* U.S. Department of Health and Human Services Food and Drug Administration Center for Drug Evaluation and Research (CDER); January 2014.
50. US Food and Drug Administration. *Guidance on Presenting Risk Information in Prescription Drug and Medical Device Promotion.* U.S. Department of Health and Human Services Food and Drug Administration Center for Drug Evaluation and Research (CDER); May 2009.
51. US Food and Drug Administration. *Guidance on Product Name Placement, Size, and Prominence in Advertising and Promotional Labeling.* U.S. Department of Health and Human Services Food and Drug Administration Center for Drug Evaluation and Research (CDER); December 2017.
52. Kenton W. What is direct to consumer advertising. *Investopedia*, April 2020.
53. Lee B. How is consumer drug advertising regulated in the United States? *GoodRx*, June 17, 2019.
54. Matthews M. Direct-to-consumer drug advertising benefits. *Orange County Register*, December 19, 2019.
55. Mialki S. Direct-to-consumer advertising: What sets it apart & what are the 3 primary benefits for brands? *Advertising*, June 13, 2019.
56. PhRMA. PhRMA members take a new approach direct to consumer advertising, October 15, 2018.
57. PhRMA. PhRMA guiding principles on direct to consumer advertisements about prescription medicines, October 2018.
58. PhRMA. Direct to consumer advertising survey results, 2017.
59. PhRMA. Report of the PhRMA member signatory companies to the PhRMA guiding principles on direct to consumer advertisements about prescription medicines, 2019.
60. Shmerling R. What you should know about direct-to-consumer ads. *Harvard Health AD Watch*, September 2019.
61. Sullivan H. Direct-to-consumer prescription drug advertising and patient-provider interactions. *Journal of the American Board of Family Medicine.* 2020;33:279–283.
62. Fahim G, Toscani M, Barone JA, Wang C, Gandhi S. Evaluation of risk versus benefit information in direct-to-consumer (DTC) prescription drug television advertisements. *Therapeutic Innovation & Regulatory Science.* 2018;52(1):114–117.
63. US Food and Drug Administration. *The Impact of Direct-to-Consumer Advertising.* U.S. Department of Health and Human Services Food and Drug Administration Center for Drug Evaluation and Research (CDER); October 2015.
64. Hwang M, Young H. Enhancing the educational value of direct-to-consumer advertising of prescription drugs. *Journal of the American Pharmacists Association.* 2017;57:571–578.
65. Parekh N, Shrank W. Dangers and opportunities of direct-to-consumer advertising. *Journal of General Internal Medicine.* 2018;33(5):586–587.
66. Weinmeyer R. Direct-to-consumer advertising of drugs. *American Medical Association Journal of Ethics.* 2013;15(11):954–959.

7 The Role of Investigative Journalism in Improving Drug Safety

Martha Rosenberg

SYNOPSIS

DOI: 10.1201/9781003615323-8

7.1 INTRODUCTION

Direct-to-consumer (DTC) advertising began in the 1980s and became increasingly common in the 1990s and beyond, including for prescription drugs. The gap in time between the dawn of DTC drug advertising in the 1980s and the passage of the Physician Financial Transparency Reports (Sunshine Act) in 2010 represented a kind of "Wild West" for the pharmaceutical industry.[1]

Hollywood-handsome drug reps saturated hospitals and medical centers with lunch, gifts and free drug samples for doctors and their staff. Statins, proton pump inhibitors (PPIs), asthma drugs, antipsychotics and ADHD meds became blockbusters. But the "Wild West" was not to last for drug makers.

For one thing, the public was becoming aware of––and infuriated by––drug maker price gouging. In 2016 Martin Shkreli, founder of Turing Pharmaceuticals, refused to justify the company's price hike of the anti-parasitic drug Daraprim from $13.50 to $750[2] on Capitol Hill and took the "fifth."[3] Months later, the drug giant Mylan raised the price of EpiPen, the emergency allergy injection, to $600 from $100 with no warning.[4]

Also, many top-selling drugs went off patent, lucrative psychiatric drug franchises peaked and financial incentives to doctors like "speakers fees" were frowned upon. Still, greater awareness of conflicts of interest between medical leaders and drug makers did not mean those financial relationships stopped. In 2018, ProPublica reported:[5]

> Top researchers at Memorial Sloan Kettering Cancer Center have filed at least seven corrections with medical journals recently, divulging financial relationships with health care companies that they did not previously disclose.
>
> The hospital's chief executive, Dr. Craig B. Thompson, disclosed his relationship with companies including the drugmaker Merck, and Dr. Jedd Wolchok, a noted pioneer in cancer immunotherapy, listed his affiliations with 31 companies.
>
> The corrections followed the resignation in September of Dr. José Baselga . . . the cancer center's chief medical officer, who had failed to disclose his company ties in dozens of articles in medical journals . . . totaling millions of dollars.

CEO Thompson sat on the boards of Merck and Charles River Laboratories and actually founded a cancer start-up, said news reports.[6]

In response to the developments, drug makers launched a love affair with biologics––larger proteins, peptides, nucleic acids and cells administered parenterally replaced the huge revenues[7] drug makers had enjoyed for orally administered "small molecules."[8] Monoclonal antibodies, man-made proteins that behave like human antibodies, were used to create blockbuster TNF blockers such as AbbVie's Humira, which became the best-selling medication in the U.S. year after year.[9] But the medications' costs and safety profiles were alarming.

In addition to the TNF blockers, drug makers launched expensive, specialty and disease-specific biologic drugs, some priced so high and without clear benefit that the House Committee on Oversight and Reform conducted continual investigations.[10] In fact, according to a 2019 article in *JAMA Internal Medicine*, only 19 of 93 cancer drugs approved since 1992 were shown to increase survival.[11]

Other noteworthy biologics that emerged once small molecules began to disappoint were hepatitis C virus (HCV) medications like Harvoni (ledipasvir/sofosbuvir) and Sovaldi (sofosbuvir), which we discuss later in this chapter. Their prices ranged from $78,000 to $87,000 per round of treatment.[12]

Before the COVID-19 pandemic put a halo on drug makers' heads in 2020 as the world craved a vaccine, revelations had emerged that opioid makers deliberately created the opioid addiction and overdose epidemic for profit.

In 2020, OxyContin-manufacturer Purdue Pharma pled guilty to three counts of a felony charge, with resulting penalties including a criminal fine of $3.544 billion and $2 billion in criminal forfeiture.[13,14] Other popular and widely used medications were also beset with new safety concerns though the COVID-19 pandemic tended to eclipse other pharmaceutical news.

7.2 DIRECT-TO-CONSUMER ADVERTISING INCREASED WITH COVID

DTC advertising debuted at the same time as the World Wide Web, and both had the immediate effect of giving patients more information about diseases, symptoms and drugs than they ever had before, fostering "cyberchondria." DTC drug advertising enriched drug makers and media outlets, and for some magazines and TV shows, DTC ads were the primary revenue drivers, explaining the lack of coverage about safety concerns.

While some people say they enjoy ads, other TV viewers have their guard up. They know the butterflies, sunsets and puppies in the ads are designed to distract them from the listing of alarming side effects that could be reasons to not "ask your doctor" about the advertised drug. Since only brand drugs are advertised, DTC marketing also sells expensive drugs when cheaper drugs would work just as well.

It was no surprise to media or industry watchers that drug advertising increased during the COVID pandemic with a greater potential audience of millions now isolated at home. A month after the COVID pandemic was declared, drug makers' TV ad expenditures for the top 10 prescription drugs increased to $183 million from $156 million in March according to FiercePharma.[15] Overall spending on prescription drug ads rose 123%.[16] In the first six months of 2020, Pfizer's digital advertising was up 532% while Amgen's was up 216% and GlaxoSmithKline was up 151%.[17]

7.2.1 Unbranded DTC Advertising

Another kind of popular marketing from drug makers which persisted during COVID is called "unbranded" advertising. Its purpose is to "raise awareness" about a disease or condition, and the drug that is really being promoted is never mentioned.

The hallmark of unbranded advertising is fear. It implies that even though someone may feel healthy, they may be ill or even have a "silent killer" disease. Unbranded advertising often sends people to online "symptom checkers," which then circuitously lead a person to the drug being sold. Risks of diseases are also peddled though patients are symptom-free, and clearly if patients take the med, they can't know if the drug is working or if they ever even needed it.

Unbranded advertising can fly under the public's radar because it appears to be official information from the CDC or the government. Even radio and TV stations have been known to wave unbranded ads through to run free as "public service announcements" because producers do not see drug makers' fingerprints on them but rather "altruistic" ads. Unbranded advertising has sold everything from depression and bipolar disorder to obscure conditions like exocrine pancreatic insufficiency and non-24-hour sleep-wake disorder.

7.2.2 Industry-Funded Disease Awareness Groups

Unbranded ads can also carry the name of the patient and the imprimatur of groups that have been organized to "raise awareness" about certain diseases and fight them. What the public does not usually realize (and nor do even members of these groups, sometimes) is that they are generally bankrolled by drug makers.

One of the biggest and most aggressive of such patient groups is the National Alliance on Mental Illness or NAMI, which gets most of its donations from drug makers.[18] To create a market for high-priced psychiatric drugs, groups like NAMI actually "sell" mental illness by enlarging its definition to include everyday blue moods or anxiety and claiming that one in four people has a mental illness. When the drugs failed to treat a condition, possibly because it was not "mental illness" to begin with, a lucrative "add-on" drug market emerged.

While patient "front groups" are connected to many diseases and specialties, they are especially prevalent in the psychiatric field not only because psychoactive drugs are among the most expensive but also because psychiatric conditions usually lack blood and diagnostic tests to confirm them and boil down to judgment calls.

Several psychiatric-oriented patient groups have been investigated by Congress for undisclosed drug company funding including Children and Adults with Attention Deficit/Hyperactivity Disorder, Depression and Bipolar Support Alliance, Mental Health America, National Alliance for Research on Schizophrenia and Depression and Screening for Mental Health.[19]

"When insurers balk at reimbursing patients for new prescription medications, these groups typically swing into action, rallying sufferers to appear before public and consumer panels [and] contact lawmakers," wrote the Los Angeles Times.[20]

Pulling at lawmakers' heartstrings, such groups testify at FDA meetings and lobby state health officials over the need for high-priced drugs. For example, in 2014, NAMI helped defeat a White House proposal that would have limited Medicare coverage of expensive psychiatric drugs such as Wellbutrin, Paxil, Prozac, Abilify and Seroquel.[21] "The proposal undermines a key protection for some of the sickest, most vulnerable Medicare beneficiaries," said Andrew Sperling, a NAMI lobbyist using the image of pathetic, elderly victims to funnel billions of taxpayer dollars to drug makers.[22]

7.2.3 Encouraging Victim Politics

In the past few years, public figures are increasingly cancelled, disenfranchised and shamed for straying from "Woke" orthodoxy, which deifies "victims." As a health reporter, I see the roots of "cancel culture" in DTC advertising.

Long before cancel culture made general reporters afraid, health reporters received vehement patient backlashes when we dared to report that some drugs have a downside (opioids) or some "diseases" are hyped by drug makers ("adult ADHD," "Exocrine Pancreatic Insufficiency").

"How dare you suggest I/my son is not sick?" "How dare you suggest my medication has risks?" "You're not taking my drugs!" the outraged patients would write us or Tweet.

Before DTC advertising, people did not derive their identities from aggressively advertised conditions that they might happen to have like bipolar disorder, adult ADHD, seasonal allergies, insomnia, gastroesophageal reflux disease (GERD) and osteopenia. They did not begin sentences with "As a migraine (depression or fibromyalgia) sufferer" and baste in self-pity. They did not chastise health reporters.

Today's victim culture owes a lot to DTC advertising which told the public that health conditions and concerns are somehow "good" and bestow a ready-made identity that wins sympathy.

Before DTC advertising, there were no Internet "disease clubs" for someone to have fellow "sufferers," an Internet identity from a celebrated disease and a monthly marketing newsletter. Drug makers have capitalized on "disease clubs" and identity marketing because it creates loyal customers and patient-to-patient selling and sells products.

The "victim" mentalities that DTC advertising has conferred on those with health conditions—or "at risk" of health conditions—fan the flames of current victim politics. They are not good for healthcare or today's argumentative, polarized times. They only benefit drug makers.

7.3 THE OPIOID EPIDEMIC

The U.S. opioid epidemic began in the 1990s and by 2017 the Department of Health and Human Services (HHS) declared a public health emergency.[23] The epidemic encompassed prescription drugs like oxycodone, hydrocodone, fentanyl, hydromorphone, morphine and methadone; and street drugs like heroin, which people who were addicted to prescription drugs turned to when they couldn't procure legal drugs.

According to the Centers for Disease Control and Prevention, 128 people die daily in the U.S. from an opioid overdose.[24]

7.3.1 Growing an Untapped Market

The opioid epidemic did not "just happen"—it was facilitated by drug makers. Sensing an untapped market, OxyContin-maker Purdue Pharma and other drug makers began to aggressively market opioids for almost every pain condition in the late 1990s, promising practitioners that the drugs were not addictive.

Doctors soon began prescribing opioids for all "causes of human suffering," said a Bloomberg analysis, "be it back pain, fibromyalgia, toothaches, cancer, depression, divorce, boredom, mental illness, unemployment, hip replacement, or withdrawal symptoms" from opioids.[25]

It had been decades since narcotics had been a social scourge that required tight controls. With the heroin abuse of U.S. servicemen in the Vietnam War, the opiate addictions of the middle of the 20th century[26] and the notorious opium dens of early America fading from memory, the pharmaceutical industry questioned why these drugs should be so highly restricted. Relying on the short memory of the U.S., Pharma pushed for opioid use to be expanded beyond short-term surgical pain, accidents and treatment of cancer and terminal pain conditions.[27]

Between 1996 and 2002, Purdue "funded more than 20,000 pain-related 'educational programs' through direct sponsorship or financial grants and launched a multifaceted campaign to encourage long-term use of [opioid painkillers] for chronic non-cancer pain," reported Vox Media.[28]

Promotional swag distributed by Purdue sales reps to prescribers included OxyContin-branded fishing hats and stuffed plush toys as well as compact discs with songs such as "Get in the Swing With Oxycontin." This type of shameless promotion was "unprecedented for a schedule II opioid," said a paper in the *American Journal of Public Health*.[29,30] Purdue also funded authoritative societies and other groups with influence on opioid prescribing such as the American Pain Society, the American Academy of Pain Medicine, the Federation of State Medical Boards, the Joint Commission and pain patient groups.[31,32] As a result, these groups then "advocated for more aggressive identification and treatment of pain, especially use of [opioid painkillers]."[33,34] The University of Pain & Policy Studies group advocated for fewer opioid restrictions while taking $2.5 million in support from opioid-producing companies, a clear conflict of interest.

Additionally, financial ties to individual members of a society may influence the acts of that body. For example, half of the panel at the American Geriatric Society responsible for changing the pain guidelines to encourage opioid use had financial ties to opioid manufacturers.[35] These financial relationships included serving as "a paid speaker, consultant, or an adviser at the time the guidelines were issued."[36,37] Based on these guidelines, a pain guide called Finding Relief: Pain Management for Older Adults concluded that opioids "allow people with chronic pain to get back to work, run, and play sports." The guide was unsurprisingly endorsed by the American Geriatric Society, but in another conflict of interest, the guide itself was funded by Jannsen, the producers of opioids such as Duragesic, Nucynta ER and Ultram ER.[38] In truth, study after study shows patients became less active on opioids and their return to work is delayed.[39] The guide defends the safety of long-term opioid use though studies show no value in long-term opioid use and serious harm.

7.3.2 Aggressive Opioid Marketing

More influence peddling was seen with IMMPACT,[40] a lobbying group funded by 11 drug makers including makers of narcotic painkillers. Federal regulators and Pharma executives held private meetings at expensive hotels under IMMPACT auspices.[41]

IMMPACT's goal of "improving the design, execution, and interpretation of clinical trials of treatments for pain" through "enriched enrollment" allowed the elimination of poor responders from trials. This increases the chance of a drug being approved, streamlines approval and lowers drug maker costs say experts. Both Purdue and Janssen have acknowledged the value of IMMPACT's efforts in "improving" clinical trial procedures.[42]

As early as 2003, National Institutes of Health (NIH) official Raymond Dionne raised ethical concerns about the influence of industry at meetings on the NIH campus. He suggested meetings in which federal officials and industry were present should be open and further stated in his correspondence to IMMPACT that federal officials should not accept expensive dinners from the pharmaceutical industry.[43] In response, one IMMPACT co-founder, Robert Dworkin, mocked these concerns in an email, suggesting that they would provide "inexpensive sandwiches" to Dionne if he insisted. He continued derisively, "The rest of us undoubtedly will feel guilty, but we will probably resist the temptation to have tuna fish in respect for your plight." Dworkin is a pain expert who is a professor at the University of Rochester Medical Center.[44,45]

7.3.3 Fostering Opioid Addiction

Initially, long-acting opioids like OxyContin seemed to solve a problem associated with *short-acting* opioid drugs. Most short acting opioids were combined with acetamino phen, putting patients at risk for liver damage if they needed a "rescue" dose. Long-acting opioids lacked acetaminophen. Short-acting opioids were seen to encourage "reward-seeking," addictive behavior by making patients focus on their pain, a phenomenon that long-acting opioids, taken on a time-contingent basis, seemed to obviate.

But of course there was one problem, and it was a big one. Recreational drug users soon discovered they could crush and snort long-acting opioids or even inject them intravenously like heroin.[46]

Manufacturers moved to create abuse-deterrent pills that would lose their effectiveness when crushed in compliance with FDA directives. But, in some ways, the FDA seemed to be playing both sides of the street when it came to the opioid epidemic.

In 2013, days after the FDA tightened opioid labels and indications, it approved a new, long-acting drug called Zohydro ER that contained a similar ingredient, hydrocodone bitartrate, and was easy to crush and abuse.[47] In 2015 the FDA even approved opioids for children as young as 11.[48]

In 2016, the government also looked like it was abetting the epidemic. A law was passed that year that curtailed the power of the Drug Enforcement Agency to pursue pharmacies and drug wholesalers whose misconduct was fanning the flames of the opioid epidemic.[49,50]

Meanwhile, Purdue emails, memos, meeting minutes, sales reports, FDA records, patient records and journal articles collected by the *Los Angeles Times*[51] found the company deliberately marketed OxyContin as a 12-hour med knowing the drug only provided *eight hours* of pain relief. Consequently, patients were subject to the re-emergence of pain and withdrawal symptoms in the four hours preceding each subsequent dose.[52,53]

In a letter to the FDA, Purdue claimed a 12-hour dose was more convenient for patients, but it also made more money for the company, reported the *Times*—even though higher doses are more likely to cause death.[54]

7.3.4 Pill Mills and Addiction Medicine

Not surprisingly, as opioids received an image makeover, "pill mills" erupted dispensing the drugs to almost anyone who walked in the door. Physicians could earn $37,500 a week, said media reports.[55] On their heels, "opioid addiction" treatment clinics boomed, dispensing narcotic agonists like Suboxone, a combination of buprenorphine and naloxone, which produced its own high—and addictions.[56] "Subs" and "Bupes" became popular on the street.

Moreover, "At least 1,350 of 12,780 buprenorphine doctors have been sanctioned for offenses that include excessive narcotics prescribing, insurance fraud, sexual misconduct and practicing medicine while impaired," reported the *New York Times*.[57] "Some have been suspended or arrested, leaving patients in the lurch."

The new opioid addiction treatment clinics, unlike traditional "rehabs," which de-emphasized prescription drugs and promoted abstinence, were predicated on medication. Industry lobbying helped recast addiction as a *psychiatric condition* requiring life-long medication.

Psychiatrist and *Psychiatryland* author Phil Sinaikin explained, "The insurance companies told the rehabs they would no longer pay for inpatient rehab for heroin, cocaine or alcohol unless there was also another Axis 1 psychiatric disorder like bipolar disorder or major depression." He continued,

> I was working in a drug treatment facility when the change happened. Since addicts typically complain of anxiety and depression, a completely understandable emotional response to their toxic lifestyles, it was no problem to add a new label and throw a few psychiatric drugs at their now relabeled "dual diagnosis."[58,59]

Soon drug makers groups promoted "awareness."

The American Society of Addiction Medicine (ASAM), a big player in opioid addiction treatment efforts, cited support "by an unrestricted educational grant to ASAM from Reckitt-Benckiser Pharmaceutics Inc., manufacturer of Subutex and Suboxone," in a 2011 Consensus Panel statement.[60] The taxpayer-supported National Institute on Drug Abuse (NIDA)[61] worked with and embraced ASAM.[62]

The marketing of buprenorphine is supported by its own advocacy group called the National Alliance of Advocates for Buprenorphine Treatment (NAABT), which admits to having taken money from pharmaceutical companies. NAABT's stated mission is to

> educate the public about the disease of opioid addiction and the buprenorphine treatment option; help reduce the stigma and discrimination associated with patients with addiction disorders; and serve as a conduit connecting patients in need of treatment to buprenorphine treatment providers.[63]

Treating addictions that drug makers helped to cause and "playing both sides of the street" proved another significant revenue stream. In fact, in 2018, Richard Sackler, the past president of Purdue, was granted a patent for a formulation of buprenorphine.[64]

In 2018, the biopharma company Alkermes combined buprenorphine with samidorphan, an opioid blocker, in a drug candidate to counteract the abuse potential of buprenorphine. An FDA advisory group advised against approving it.[65]

7.3.5 Opioid Lawsuits Surface

As opioid addiction became something that could not be ignored, law enforcement agencies became involved. In 2014, the former director of pharmacy services for Beth Israel Medical Center in New York City was arrested and charged with stealing and illegally possessing oxycodone with a street value of almost $5.6 million.[66]

The same year, Santa Clara County in California sued the drug companies Purdue Pharma, Cephalon, Janssen Pharmaceuticals, Endo Health Solutions and Actavis for allegedly addicting Californians to prescription opioids for profit.[67] "Defendants' deceptive marketing campaign deprived California patients and their doctors of the ability to make informed medical decisions and, instead, caused important, sometimes life-or-death decisions to be made based not on science, but hype," the lawsuit alleged. Assistant Santa Clara County Counsel Danny Chou accused the drug companies of a "decades-long marketing plan . . . to create a market for these drugs that never should have existed" which "spawned a new generation of addicts and abusers."

Also, in 2014, federal prosecutors filed an indictment against FedEx that included charges of money laundering and knowingly shipping illegal prescription drugs from two online pharmacies. Opioid users had died soon after receiving shipments of illegal prescription drugs sent by FedEx said the prosecutors.[68]

That year it also became apparent that the opioid epidemic had reached the sports world when the Drug Enforcement Administration launched an investigation into opioid misuse within the National Football League.[69] Attorneys representing about 1300 NFL retirees filed a class-action lawsuit that the league illegally provided prescription painkillers to keep players on the field without informing them of the long-term risks.[70]

7.3.6 Lack of Opioid Efficacy and Serious Side Effects

The automatic administering of opioids for pain care substitutes short-term savings at the price of long-term results, wrote Barry Meier, a *New York Times* reporter.[71] "In the short run, treating a patient with an opioid like OxyContin, which costs about $6000 a year, is less expensive than putting a patient through a pain-treatment program that emphasizes physical therapy and behavior modification," but over time multidisciplinary programs "might yield far lower costs," he observed.[72]

An average worker compensation claim without opioids, for example, is $13,000 but leaps to $39,000 when short-acting opioids are added and $117,000 when long-acting opioids are added, wrote Meier in a related *New York Times* article, in 2013.[73] According to a study by the California Workers' Compensation Institute, workers who received high opioid doses stayed out of work three times longer than those who took lower doses. "What we see is an association between the greater use of opioids and delayed recovery from workplace injuries," explained Alex Swedlow, head of research at the Institute.[74]

A 2008 study in the journal *Spine* concluded patients taking opioids for more than seven days during the first six weeks following an injury were more than twice as likely to be disabled or unemployed a year later. In an earlier study in the same journal, workers receiving opioids early in recovery of amounts exceeding a morphine equivalent amount of 450 mg "were, on average, disabled 69 days longer than those who received no early opioids" and their "risk for surgery was three times greater."[75] The use of opioids for acute lower back pain "may be counterproductive to recovery," the study concludes.[76]

There is little evidence that opioids are even effective after six weeks, and there is a concerning dearth of long-term studies.[77] A study of 300,000 Workers' Compensation claims by the Workers Compensation Research Institute found that pain and day-to-day function were not substantially improved in workers when they remained on opioids.[78]

In addition to tolerance progressing toward physical dependence and addiction, opioids cause hormonal changes (decreases in testosterone), constipation and a decrease in immune responses.[79] According to Responsible Opioid Prescribing, other opioid side effects include "heightened fracture risk related to effects and bone metabolism and from falls," with at-risk groups including the elderly and those with impaired renal or hepatic function; individuals with cardiopulmonary disorders, such as chronic obstructive pulmonary disease (COPD); congestive heart failure (CHF), sleep apnea, or mental illness; and in patients who combine opioids with other respiratory depressants such as alcohol, sedative-hypnotics, benzodiazepines, or barbiturates.[80,81]

Moreover, many are not fully aware of the phenomenon of opioid-induced hyperalgesia (OIH)––a paradoxical heightened pain sensitization in people who use opioids to treat pain.[82] I have interviewed both patients and practitioners who say, in some cases, when the opioids were terminated pain was markedly reduced.

7.3.7 Paying for the Opioid Epidemic

The costs of the opioid epidemic to society and taxpayers have been astounding. In addition to the healthcare expenses posed by overdoses, hospitalizations, complications and addiction treatment, law enforcement and criminal justice continue to incur huge costs. According to the Centers for Disease Control and Prevention, the estimated economic burden of the opioid epidemic is $78.5 billion a year.[83,84] Yet in 2017, the government announced it was giving tens of millions of dollars to opioid makers to address the epidemic in a public–private partnership between the NIH and opioid makers including Purdue.[85]

Drug makers liked the reward. Purdue Pharma Vice President for Policy J. David Haddox said he liked the idea of "converting" the opioid market to abuse-deterrent drugs. Craig Landau, CEO of Purdue, wrote in a letter to the *Times* that he appreciated the "regulatory framework to incentivize" the pharmaceutical companies to develop post-opioid crisis drugs and that the industry cannot "abandon" pain patients.[86]

Drug industry critics asked, as they did in 2020 when billions were given to drug makers to develop vaccines, why taxpayers, not industry, should fund the efforts, especially when profits went to industry.

Soon, the tides began turning against opioid makers. In October of 2020, Purdue, according to CNN:[87]

> *agreed to plead guilty to three federal criminal charges for its role in creating the nation's opioid crisis and will pay more than $8 billion and close down the company.*
>
> *The money will go to opioid treatment and abatement programs. The privately held company has agreed to pay a $3.5 billion fine as well as forfeit an additional $2 billion in past profits, in addition to the $2.8 billion it agreed to pay in civil liability . . .*
>
> *The company doesn't have $8 billion in cash available to pay the fines. So Purdue will be dissolved as part of the settlement, and its assets will be used to create a new "public benefit company" controlled by a trust or similar entity designed for the benefit of the American public. The Justice Department said it will function entirely in the public interest rather than to maximize profits. Its future earnings will go to paying the fines and penalties, which in turn will be used to combat the opioid crisis.*

In November 2020, media outlets reported that four companies that manufactured or distributed opioids had reached a tentative settlement with counties and cities suing them for $26 billion.[88] The companies were Johnson & Johnson and McKesson, Cardinal Health and AmerisourceBergen, considered the top three opioid distributors. Monies from the settlement would be earmarked for communities harmed by the opioid addiction crisis if the announced settlement was approved by judges handling the litigation in federal and state courts.

7.4 EFFECTIVE HEPATITIS C DRUGS DEBUT

In 2013, the Centers for Disease Control and Prevention estimated that 2.7 million Americans suffered from hepatitis C (Hep C), a liver-attacking virus that can lead to cancer, cirrhosis and the necessity of having a transplant.

So when Gilead Science launched Sovaldi, the first drug that could effectively cure hepatitis C, that year the nation stood up. The older, interferon-based regimens that were used before Sovaldi and similar drugs that followed "were complex and toxic and required 6–12 months of therapy, with cure rates averaging around 40–45% for HCV genotype 1," according to *Therapeutic Advances in Gastroenterology*.[89]

The nation stood up for the hepatitis C drugs until it saw the initial price––$1000 a pill or $84,000 for a course of treatment.[90] Sovaldi earned Gilead $10.28 billion in sales in 2014, and Harvoni, a more expensive hepatitis C drug Gilead launched the next year, made the company $13.86 billion in 2015.[91]

7.4.1 Lawmakers Investigate Hepatitis C Prices

Since many who have hepatitis C are poor, on Medicare and in prison, the implications for state Medicaid programs were immediately clear to lawmakers and public health policy makers. "If Gilead's approach is the future of how blockbuster drugs are launched in America, it's going to cost billions and billions of dollars to treat just a fraction of patients in America," said Oregon Senator Ron Wyden.[92] Makers of hepatitis C treatments initially attempted to reframe the outrageous prices as recouping research and development costs, but this was even rejected by mainstream business reporters. Why would the same hepatitis C drug that costs only $900 a year in Egypt cost almost 100 times more in the U.S., asked Avid Roy in *Forbes* magazine.[93] "Hepatitis C patients in the U.S. are mostly uninsured, underinsured and/or incarcerated. Medicaid, the VA and our prison system bear the brunt of the cost impact, and by extension so do all of us as taxpayers."[94]

Roy was right. Two years after the release of the drugs, 33 states had already given more than $1 billion to Gilead reported National Public Radio.[95]

A case study released in 2018 by Senate Finance Committee Ranking Minority Member Ron Wyden and Republican member Charles Grassley found that Gilead's pricing and marketing strategy for Solvaldi and Harvoni were "designed to maximize revenue with little concern for access or affordability."[96] The 18-month investigation based on 20,000 internal documents and data from state Medicaid programs found that creating "broad, affordable success was not a key consideration in the process of setting the wholesale prices" and that "Gilead justified Sovaldi's high price point based on price-per-cure."

According to *Policy & Medicine*, Gilead was aware[97]

> *that it was in a position to create clear savings for payers, but instead chose to pursue a "regimen neutral" price that was justified by "cost-per-cure" calculations. Such a pricing structure resulted in "greater revenue per treatment than previous direct acting anti-virals." Gilead felt they were more than justified in using the cost-per-cure pricing model given the increased efficiency of Sovaldi . . .*
>
> *By raising the price for the new standard of care set by Sovaldi, Gilead wanted to raise the price floor for all future Hepatitis C treatments, including its follow-on drugs and those of its competitors.*

In 2014 alone, Medicare and Medicaid spent over $5 billion on Sovaldi and Harvoni, reported *Policy & Medicine*, and, "despite significant apparent access restrictions, Gilead refused to lower the net price by much"[98]—causing financial stress to already strapped states.

According to Sen. Wyden, the prices that Gilead set for the two drugs did not reflect "basic financial matters such as R&D costs or the multi-billion dollar acquisition of Pharmasset, the drug's first developer" and were opportunistic. "Gilead knew these prices would put treatment out of the reach of millions and cause extraordinary problems for Medicare and Medicaid, but still the company went ahead," he asserted. " Ireject the idea that America has to choose between soaring, out-of-reach drug prices and one-size-fits-all government policies."[99]

7.4.2 Aggressive Hepatitis C Marketing

According to Stat News, about 3.5 million Americans have hepatitis C versus the much greater numbers of people with erectile dysfunction or psoriasis, but the advertising campaign for Gilead's Harvoni was over the top in spending and reach.[100]

By 2016, 11,000 ads for Harvoni had aired on TV channels, representing a spend of between $60 and $80 million.[101]

Gildead's print buy for Harvoni in magazines like *People* and *Better Homes and Gardens* totaled $30 million, and the drug makers spent $5 million on online ads. Since hepatitis C is more common in men, Gilead ran ads on ESPN, the *Golf Channel* and in *Sports Illustrated* and *Men's Journal*.[102] It also targeted baby boomers and African-American baby boomers in its media buy, groups that are more likely to have hepatitis C.

To sell Harvoni, Gilead also used the unbranded advertising discussed early in this chapter. Its magazine and TV spots urged viewers to go to a website for hepatitis C information and––presto––the viewers found themselves on the Harvoni website.[103]

7.4.3 Screening as a Hepatitis C Sales Tool

There is an old saying that if you keep going to a barbershop, eventually you will get a haircut. Drug makers often use the same logic, urging the public to get tested, screened or checked for depression, ADHD, bipolar disorder, bone thinning, obscure conditions like exocrine pancreatic insufficiency and of course cancers.

Screening can be a sales tool. A blog on the *Scientific American* website reported that the now-defunct TeenScreen, which screened for early signs of mental illness and risk of suicide in young people, had "ties to the pharmaceutical industry."[104,105] It can also be dangerous. Over-screening can detect cancers that "grow so slowly (or even not at all) that if they went undetected, they wouldn't cause any problems," reported Cancer Research UK.[106] "Even if left untreated, a person wouldn't be harmed by their cancer," said the group's website.

Screening has been a huge tool in selling bone drugs. In 2018, Jane Brody, a columnist in the *New York Times* science section, urged women to get their "bone density checked." There is "solid evidence that treatment with a bone-preserving or bone-building drug is beneficial when a bone density test reveals a level of bone loss defined as osteoporosis in the spine or a hip," she wrote.[107]

Brody omitted the fact that bone density machines were planted in doctor's offices by drug makers[108] to sell drugs and that the "bone-preserving or bone-building drug[s]" themselves, known as bisphosphonates, that she extols are associated with fractures[109] and osteonecrosis of the jaw.[110] In fact, Merck knew about the osteonecrosis of the jaw links since 1977 because of its own rat studies but proceeded to develop and market a bisphosphonate anyway.[111]

In 2017, Harvoni advertisements on TV, broadcast and posters along train commuter lines unabashedly promoted screening. They warned people born between 1945 and 1965 could have hepatitis C and not even know it, so they should get tested.[112] Even if you have no symptoms, you might silently be at risk and need these drugs, said the Pharma messaging, often called "disease mongering" because it employs fear of diseases to grow customers. Ads telling baby boomers to get screened were not limited to the U.S. In British Columbia, a campaign called Generation Hep was formed.[113]

The move to scare tactics and promotion of screening was not just a coincidence. According to FiercePharma, Gilead's blockbuster hepatitis drugs at that time were

> in freefall, and its pool of eligible patients has shrunk dramatically thanks to the success of its meds. If all baby boomers got tested for the virus, though? That could help stem the tide —and it's exactly the move the company is recommending with its latest awareness push.[114,115]

Some of the ads included a CDC logo, which increased credibility but raised questions about what Gilead donations to the CDC foundation netted.[116] Many are unaware of the CDC Foundation, which lists Abbott, AbbVie, Bayer, AstraZeneca, Merck, Pfizer, GlaxoSmithKline Biologicals, Eli Lilly, Amgen, Genentech and other drug makers as donors in addition to Gilead.

The Gilead VP of U.S. sales and marketing for liver diseases, David Johnson, admitted to intentionally promoting "disease awareness" so its products could reach more customers. "This has been a planned evolution of our disease awareness efforts, to reach a much broader audience once the pool of already-diagnosed patients, who often had advanced disease and were in need of curative therapy, had been treated," he said.

> This staged approach was also important to ensure healthcare providers were equipped to support patients asking to be tested, as even for primary care providers, this disease was not something that was high on their radar due to the lack of scientific advances in the past to treat the disease.[117]

In a 2017 piece on the Pharma Marketing Network, the wisdom of mass marketing for hepatitis C screening was questioned. The writer, who calls himself "Pharma Guy," said:

> *Disease awareness ads are scaring a large portion of the population to get tested for a medical condition they most likely do not have. A case in point is a new Hepatitis C disease awareness ad by Gilead Sciences focused on "Baby Boomers."*[118]
>
> *Let's look at the numbers and do some math.*
>
> *The Centers for Disease Control and Prevention (CDC) estimates that 2.7–3.9 million people in the United States have chronic hepatitis C. According to Google, there are 76.4 million baby boomers—people born from 1945–1965—in the U.S.*
>
> *The CDC says that 75% of people with Hep C are baby boomers. That means 2–3 million baby boomers have Hep C. Now that's a big number, especially if Gilead can sell its Hep C cures (Sovaldi and Harvoni) to all those people! However, is it necessary to scare 76 million people into getting tested for Hep C when only 3–4% (the Gilead ad says 1 in 30) of them have it?*

7.4.4 Hepatitis C Safety Signals Emerge

Before new drugs and treatments are released to the public, they are tested on a relatively small group of people for a relatively short period of time while post-marketing studies are relied upon to detect safety signals.

As many objected to the price of the hepatitis C drugs and some objected to marketing them to patients with no symptoms, a surprising safety signal surfaced in 2017 when the drugs were already in wide use. The American Pharmacists Association website quotes the *New York Times* reporting:[119]

> *A new report from the Institute for Safe Medication Practices suggest[s] that drugs approved in recent years that can cure hepatitis C may have severe adverse effects, including liver failure. The number of adverse events appears relatively small, and the findings are not conclusive, but observers say the report is a warning that should not be ignored.*
>
> *It involves nine widely used antiviral drugs that were heralded as a huge advance because they greatly increased cure rates, seemingly with few adverse events. The report's findings are based on an analysis of FDA's database of reports from doctors around the world of adverse events that might be related to medications.*
>
> *About 250,000 people took the newer drugs in 2015, the report said. In those treated during the year ending June 30, 2016, the report identified 524 with liver failure, 165 of whom died. Of those with liver failure, 386 were from outside the United States. An additional 1,058 had severe liver injury, and in 761 the drugs appeared not to work.*

The *New York Times* report was not the first safety signal that regulators received about the new hepatitis C drugs. In 2016, the FDA found that, while effective at eliminating hepatitis C, these antiviral drugs reactivated pre-existing, dormant hepatitis B infections in 24 patients.[120] As a result of this reactivation, two patients died and another one required a liver transplant. In response, the FDA added black box warnings on the hepatitis C drug labels about the possible reactivation of hepatitis B infections.

Thomas Moore of the Institute for Safe Medication Practices asked whether these hepatitis C drugs may have been approved too quickly in the rush to bring a new drug to market, resulting in safety risks to patients.[121]

7.5 ASTHMA DRUG SAFETY SIGNALS

Asthma is big business for drug makers. In 2012, Advair was the third best-selling drug in the world, and in 2013[122] the asthma drugs Singulair[123] and Symbicort[124] were also blockbusters.

Yet the safety of asthma drugs as well as their development and testing has been questioned by media. A few years ago, Robert Davidson, M.D., a former clinical research subinvestigator at Vivra, a major allergy and respiratory management company in Tucson, Arizona,[125] reported clinical trial irregularities. Trials of Singular (montelukast), Serevent (salmeterol), Foradil (formoterol), Flovent (fluticasone propionate), Xolair (omalizumab), Accolate (zafirlukast) and Xopenex (levosalbutamol) were corrupted by protocol violations and outright falsifications said Davidson.[126]

Because investigators earned as much as $10,000 per subject, they were prescreened for trials without their knowledge, enrolled when they had important risk factors that would have disqualified them, serially enrolled in studies despite health and data risks and even plucked from the parking lot charged Davidson.[127] He stated that staff were observed entering rooms where placebo and experimental drugs were prepared, thereby unblinding and thus invalidating entire studies used in new drug applications (NDAs) to the FDA.[128,129]

Tipped off about the irregularities, the FDA inspected the facility and corroborated Davidson's charges. "Three study coordinators stated that they saw diary card blank prior to subject entering exam room with PI for visit 2," reads a report from an inspection over two months in 1999. "Five to ten minutes after, the diary had approximately two weeks of diary symptoms and peak flow entered."[130,131]

According to Davidson, Vivra staff made the charge that pulmonary function tests, required before subject enrollment, were performed on all facility patients to prepare them for possible participation and billed to insurers. Despite the revelations, acknowledged by the FDA, clinical trials at the Vivra Tucson facility were not stopped and the research was cited and not retracted in the *Annals of Internal Medicine* and trials[132]

Vivra Asthma & Allergy was taken over by Gambro in 1997 and DaVita in 2005.[133] In 2004, Gambro agreed to pay $350 million in criminal fines and civil penalties regarding healthcare fraud in the Medicare, Medicaid and TRICARE programs.[134]

7.5.1 Xolair Leaves a Trail of Questions

Because of the large and profitable market for asthma drugs, the prospect of a new drug that reduces the frequency of allergic responses characteristic of asthma made drug makers sit up and take notice. Such a biologic sounded so lucrative that Novartis actually sued Genentech, which was developing a similar drug to its own for "trade secret violations" until the drug giants decided to team up and sell omalizumab, marketed as Xolair, together.[135]

Xolair, developed from humanized rodent cells, soon became part of the push by drug makers to replace the small-molecule drugs, which were not as lucrative or had increasingly gone off patent with biologics.[136] Novartis and Genetech ambitiously applied for FDA approval of this drug for four conditions in 2001, including pediatric and adult asthma and pediatric and adult seasonal allergic rhinitis symptoms (SARS). However, the FDA approved only one indication in 2013: "moderate to severe persistent asthma" in patients over 12 years old whose symptoms are "not adequately controlled on inhaled corticosteroids" and who have allergic asthma as demonstrated by a positive skin test or reactivity to an allergen."[137] The narrowly defined indication limited the number of patients who could be prescribed Xolair, making it a disappointment[138] in terms of marketing and a black box warning for anaphylaxis work on the drug did not help.[139,140]

Novartis and Genentech were faced with the prospect of trying to sell a SARS drug that was too risky for children and cost as much as $24,000 a year.[141] Moreover, the drug could be used only after corticosteroids had failed and an IgE serum test had been conducted. And Xolair was so linked to anaphylaxis it could only be administered in a medical setting where patients could remain for observation.[142]

According to whistleblowers who detailed Xolair at Novartis and Genentech to prescribers, sales of this drug were boosted by kickbacks, bribes, misrepresentations of Xolair's approved uses and side effects and insurance fraud.[143]

The companies marketing Xolair, which included Novartis, Genentech and Roche, "determined as early as 2003 that they would never succeed in transforming Xolair into a blockbuster or near-blockbuster drug unless they broke the law," said a legal complaint the whistleblowers filed.[144]

> And that is exactly what they have knowingly done, by aggressively and illegally marketing Xolair, on a national basis, to induce HCPs [health care providers] to prescribe Xolair for wide-ranging use—despite the drug's very limited efficacy and proven threats to patient safety.[145,146]

Heading the list of Novartis/Genentech's wrongdoing, said the whistleblowers,[147] was off-label marketing, which reps flagrantly conducted at the clear behest of their sales managers and drug company officials. Almost from the start, according to sales training modules included in a complaint, Xolair reps were instructed to use the invented term "active asthma" when soliciting physicians instead of "moderate to severe persistent asthma," which would have more limited sales.[148,149]

This worked. Though Xolair was not approved, effective or safe for mild asthma, many patients with only mild asthma which was not persistent were prescribed Xolair, thanks to the contrived term "active asthma" said the reps.[150]

According to the whistleblower, sales reps were told to assure physicians that the two-hour wait to monitor for an anaphylactic reaction was unnecessary and that patients could self-administer the injectable Xolair drug at home in some cases. Further, reps were even told to contact physicians and assert that Xolair was safe for children under 12 years old, which blatantly contradicts Xolair's indications and safety profile listed on its label.[151,152]

Reps said on sales calls they were also told to show "studies" compiled by doctors paid by Novartis and Genentech that suggested non-FDA uses of Xolair.[153] One suggestion was using "rush immunotherapy"—accelerated exposure of patients to their allergen via injection to shorten treatment—simultaneously with Xolair.[154] Rush immunotherapy is also linked to anaphylaxis putting patients at double risk.[155]

According to the complaint, physicians and medical staff who were successful in boosting prescriptions of Xolair unethically were unethically compensated with rewards such as American Express travelers checks, expensive tickets to entertainment events, expensive dinners and even a vacation to a tropical island. Often payments were disguised as compensation for bogus studies, "advisory board" service, "speaker" programs in lavish settings, unrestricted research grants and thousands of dollars in honoraria for no work.[156,157]

Nor were monetary gifts the only inducements. Xolair reps also provided free computers, refrigerators for offices, pulmonary function machines, IgE test kits and drug swirlers/spinners to make the use of Xolair easier. Since Xolair was a cumbersome drug to prepare, reps said they would volunteer to do the preparation for office nurses or staff.[158]

To help doctors get around Medicare and Medicaid restrictions, the reps recommended "Buy and Bill" arrangements from the specialty pharmacies that provided Xolair, which amounted to kickbacks if a patient were denied coverage or didn't show up for treatment. Reps also delivered Xolair to patients' homes according to the complaint.[159]

7.5.2 More Improper Xolair Marketing

Reps assisted medical staff in coding and reimbursement, some of which was illegal, say complaints.[160] At up to $24,000 a year, Xolair's original cost was prohibitive, so physicians had to sign a statement of medical necessity to secure reimbursement. To circumvent this and the potential inhibition of Xolair prescription numbers, sales reps "instructed and nudged" medical office staff to submit insurance claims for this drug "at improper rates."[161] The alleged fraud included "upcoding"—calling patients at levels 1–2, 4–5 and other falsifications of Current Procedural Terminology ("CPT") and Diagnosis Codes ("ICD-9s").[162]

Reps were advised to pursue Medicare and Medicaid sales, which were called "soft targets," and $412 million tax dollars from such public insurance programs were estimated to be spent on Xolair from 2004 through 2011. Reps were even told to seek to work in medical settings in poor neighborhoods such as Queens and the Bronx in New York City, where patients were more likely to be on Medicaid, said complaints.[163]

In other unsavory marketing, Novartis and Genentech hired and trained well-regarded doctors to extol Xolair because they were considered to be "Key Opinion Leaders" who are thought to influence other doctors, said whistleblowers. William Busse, M.D. with the Allergy, Asthma & Immunology Clinic, Adult & Pediatric at the University of Wisconsin School of Medicine & Public Health, was one of the most visible Xolair cheerleaders and received $100,000 between 2002 and 2003, said legal filings.[164]

Additionally, "Patient Experience Programs" (PEPs) run by Novartis and Genentech compensated patients for not only participation but also positive feedback about Xolair. Specifically, PEP participants were awarded a waiver of the copayment for Xolair and "paid cash or reimbursed to speak favorably about Xolair." According to the complaint PEP participants:[165]

> *were flown to Arizona, with all expenses paid and payment of a stipend, for Defendants to train these patients to speak favorably about their Xolair experiences at future patient speaker events, and to study how to further maximize their experiences for marketing purposes. The patient speakers are then also paid for their future speaking events (speaking to HCPs and prospective Xolair patients), with the speakers' travel, hotel, food, and other expenses paid by Defendants—as well as that of many of the HCPs in attendance.*

7.5.3 Safety Signals Surface With Xolair and a Lawsuit Is Dismissed

The improper marketing cited by whistleblowers was all the more concerning because of Xolair's safety profile. At 2012 FDA panel hearings, safety reports were presented that described 81 serious pediatric cases and five deaths.[166] Three of the fatal outcomes were in utero, and two were pediatric patients.[167] Of 169 pregnancies, according to researchers,[168] there are "156 live births, 1 fetal death/stillbirth [and] 11 spontaneous abortions." Overall, "20 infants had congenital anomalies confirmed," reported researchers.[169]

In 2014, the FDA announced additional safety signals that were arising with Xolair:[170]

> *A U.S. Food and Drug Administration (FDA) review of safety studies suggests a slightly increased risk of problems involving the heart and blood vessels supplying the brain among patients being treated with the asthma drug Xolair (omalizumab) than in those who were not treated with Xolair. As a result, we have added information about these potential risks to the drug label . . .*
>
> *The heart and brain blood vessel problems included mini-strokes known as transient ischemic attacks or TIAs; heart attacks; sudden, unexpected chest pain; high blood pressure in the arteries of the lungs called pulmonary hypertension; and blood clots in the lungs and veins.*

While the FDA termed the risk of the side effects only "slightly increased," the effects themselves such as heart attack, stroke and blood clots were, and continue to be, alarming.

Despite an extensive legal journey involving deposing and even "wiring" pharmaceutical sales reps to collect evidence, Judge William Young of Boston dismissed the Xolair claims.[171,172] He ruled that although "fraud was probable," the whistleblowers and the U.S. Department of Justice (DOJ), which joined the suit, failed to prove that the improper marketing had led to false claims being filed in government health programs.[173]

In 2020, the U.S. DOJ announced that a settlement with Novartis for ten of the company's drugs, including the antihypertension drug Lotrel, had been reached.[174] According to the DOJ, the $678 million settlement was "for operating sham speaker programs through which it paid over $100 million to doctors to unlawfully induce them to prescribe Novartis drugs."[175] Novartis admitted to "certain conduct" and said it would curtail its unlawful inducements. The settlement was believed to be the biggest under the federal anti-kickback law to date.[176]

Since the settlement[177] did not include Xolair or name the original whistleblowers yet retained many of their charges, they suspected there was "horse-trading" between Novartis, the DOJ and a new whistleblower[178] who suddenly surfaced. Protecting the sales of Novartis's new drug,

Cosentyx (secukinumab), launched after Xolair and molecularly similar, was a possible factor for the omissions in the settlement, whistleblowers further said.

7.6 LONG-ACTING BETA AGONISTS

As we noted earlier in this chapter, asthma has been big business for drug makers and drugs that contain long-acting beta agonists (LABAs) like Symbicort, Advair Diskus, Serevent Diskus, Dulera and Foradil have led the way. While inhaled corticosteroids reduce the airway inflammation correlated with the frequency and severity of asthma, LABAs are said to expand constricted airways and protect against bronchospasm.[179] Both inhaled corticosteroids and LABAs are prescribed as maintenance therapy for asthma.[180]

According to published reports, the success of LABAs did not just happen––it grew from financial links between their drug makers and medical associations that promoted them.[181] For example, 15 members of an 18-member National Heart, Lung and Blood Institute panel that revised guidelines in 2007 to promote LABAs had financial ties to Advair maker GlaxoSmithKline or other LABA makers reported the *Journal Sentinel*/MedPage Today.[182] Compensation to physicians on the panel by LABA makers totaled more than $400,000 over a two-year period.[183,184]

Yet despite paid cheerleaders, LABA makers had a tough row to hoe. While they were valued for their bronchoprotective actions, studies showed that the effects had a downside: they could "mask" worsening asthma[185] and produce desensitization or "down regulation."[186] The loss of bronchoprotection that has been seen and studied is attributed to the inhibition of farnesylation,[187] a process of modification of proteins.[188]

LABAs are especially risky for children and African-Americans, a *Journal Sentinel*/MedPage Today investigation found.[189] In fact, between 1994 and 2007, LABAs contributed to a possible 14,000 asthma deaths according to an FDA researcher.[190]

The Salmeterol Multi-center Asthma Research Trial, or SMART trial, had to be terminated in 2003 after 16 deaths and adverse results resulting in 44 intubations and 369 hospitalizations. Most of those affected were African-American.[191,192] As a result, a huge safety cloud hung over LABAs. Black box warnings were added to their labels much to the chagrin of their manufacturers who have continued to fight back.[193]

In 2010, the FDA strengthened LABA warnings by adding that the drugs should be discontinued if possible after the achievement of asthma control.[194] An article in the *New England Journal of Medicine* (*NEJM*) by Badrul Chowdhury, M.D., then director of the FDA's Division of Pulmonary, Allergy, and Rheumatology Products,[195] and Gerald Dal Pan, M.D., then Director of the FDA's Office of Surveillance and Epidemiology Center for Drug Evaluation and Research,[196] noted that the studies on which the recommendation of long-term LABA use were based "have several limitations."[197]

But LABA promoters pushed back. In a 2011 *NEJM* letter, William Busse, M.D., and Stanley Szefler, M.D., bristled at the idea of further LABA safety trials. They wrote:

> Labeling these trials as safety studies suggests that LABAs have some direct toxicity that causes death or leads to hospitalization. Many experts believe that the adverse outcomes in the Salmeterol Multicenter Asthma Research Trial were due to a failure of efficacy.

Busse, who led the National Heart, Lung and Blood Institute guidelines panel that promoted LABAs, disclosed that at the time he worked as a speaker and adviser for LABA maker GlaxoSmithKline and other drug companies.[198] Dr. Szefler, also on the panel, was forced to disclose financial relationships to several asthma drug companies, including GlaxoSmithKline.[199,200]

7.6.1 GlaxoSmithKline Settlement Included a LABA

As we saw with Xolair, brisk sales of expensive drugs can signal improper marketing. In what the Department of Justice characterized as the largest healthcare fraud settlement in U.S. history, asthma drug maker GlaxoSmithKline pled guilty and paid $3 billion to resolve criminal and civil liability related to its unlawful promotion of Advair and other drugs.[201,202] Reporter John Fauber wrote:

> The company paid kickbacks to doctors to induce them to prescribe and recommend Advair and other drugs, according to the settlement. The payments included speaking and consulting fees; gifts, travel and entertainment costs; payments for serving on "sham advisory boards"; and continuing medical education programs.

Nonetheless, the government's 2007 asthma guidelines, which were chaired by Dr. Busse and are still online,[203] promote the "established beneficial effects of LABA for the great majority of patients who require more therapy than low-dose ICS alone to control asthma" and refer to LABAs as a "preferred option" that "improves lung function, decreases symptoms [and] reduces exacerbations." Busse also said to have received stipends to promote Xolair in the whistleblower complaint[204] and lists financial links to GlaxoSmithKline, Merck, Novartis, Pfizer Genentech/Novartis, Schering and five other drug makers in the government guidelines.[205]

In 2011, the Department of Justice stated Advair marketing resulted in "significant safety risks" to patients and noted "scores of lawsuits" from people "whose relatives have died while taking Advair."[206,207] As LABA safety signals continued to surface, the FDA asked LABA makers to conduct studies on LABA safety.[208] To drug safety advocates that seemed like asking the fox to guard the hen-house. In 2017 on the basis of industry studies, the FDA repealed the LABA black box warnings.[209] Busse led the analysis by LABA makers that led to the repeal.[210]

7.7 SAFETY QUESTIONS ABOUT LEUKOTRIENE RECEPTOR ANTAGONISTS

Merck's Singulair (montelukast), a leukotriene receptor antagonist or LTRA, has been another blockbuster asthma drug. In 2019–2020, it was among the top ten asthma drugs in the world and made 0.708 billion for Merck.[211] Singulair was heavily marketed to children for allergies, and, according to Fox News in 2010, both Scholastic Press and the American Academy of Pediatrics accepted money from Merck to promote it.[212]

In a statement prompted by Fox's revelations, the American Academy of Pediatrics said it had received "an educational grant to provide funding" for $651,530 from Merck but that "the content is determined solely by the AAP using guidelines from the NHLBI. It is not a conflict of interest. By accepting external grants like this, the AAP is able to disseminate its educational messages to mass audiences."[213]

In addition to problematical marketing to children, Singulair posed disturbing side effects. Fox News reported that parents were seeing behavioral problems in their children such as aggression, hostility, hallucinations, night terrors, tremors, irritability, anxiety, depression and even suicide.[214,215]

In 2009, 15-year-old Cody Miller of Queensbury, N.Y., took his own life 17 days after being given Singulair.[216] "Cody was never mentally ill nor did he have ongoing problems," his mother, Kate Miller, told me. "I would not have given my son a drug that causes depression for a simple allergy. Who would? But my choice was taken away by a company that buried the risks."[217]

The first week Cody, who played high school football, took Singulair and experienced cramps in his legs, said his mother. The second week he "was sweating profusely and couldn't calm down. He was very agitated, anxious, really having a hard time."[218]

On the last day of his life, Cody's eyes appeared sleep deprived, recounted Miller, and he said, "Sometimes you feel like you can't take it." After taking a nap on the porch while the family ordered pizza for dinner, Cody went upstairs to shower but instead took his own life. Cody was the Millers' only child.[219]

Also in 2009, the FDA announced an update to the precautions section of the prescribing information for Singulair and other drugs "to include information about neuropsychiatric events reported in patients using these products."[220]

7.7.1 Parents Report LTRA Side Effects

On the drug-rating website *askapatient.com*, parents echoed the behavioral side effects produced in their children who had been given the drug cited by Fox. "Singulair caused hyperactivity, tantrums, depression, crying, school trouble, facial tics, strange eye movements and self-harm in their children, some as young as one," wrote parents over the years.[221]

One parent wrote in 2020:[222]

> *My son has been taking this drug since he was 4 years old. He stopped taking it by 11 years old. This drug gave him nightmares, depression, suicidal thoughts headaches, and anxiety. He doesn't want to be around people or go outside. My son likes to stay inside play his video games and text in the phone with family.*

Another parent wrote of Singulair:[223]

> *My 7/8 year old daughter took this and experienced severe night terrors, anxiety, fear of death, INSANE aggressive behavior, kicking, hitting, etc., After discontinuing the medication she returned back to her normal, kind self although she still has some residual fear/night terrors . . .*
>
> *the pulmonologist basically said it wasn't even needed. And he was right. She's gotten better in her behavior and asthma since stopping it.*

7.7.2 LTRA Safety Signals Emerged Early

Shortly after the FDA approval of Singulair, FDA reviewers began to warn that adult studies of the drug "may not be predictive of the response" in children.[224,225]

Singulair's approval documents added to the red flags, especially about the drug's effects on children.[226] Reviewers noted differences in drug concentrations between adolescents and adults, and the forced euthanization of an infant monkey after adverse drug reactions caused them to speculate that "infants may be more sensitive to the toxicity."[227,228,229]

In Singulair's new drug approval documents, one study showed that beclamethasone [qVar] was more efficacious than montelukast, suggesting that it may be better to leave patients on beclomethasone.[230,231,232]

Additionally, there were ten pages left blank and marked, "This section was determined NOT to be releasable."[233,234]

Dr. William Busse, who chaired the National Heart, Lung and Blood Institute LABA guidelines panel, the expert panel that wrote the government's 2007 National Asthma Education and Prevention Program Guidelines, the industry studies that led to the repeal of LABA black boxes in 2017 and promoted Xolair, was also an investigator in Singulair approval trials.[235] He was issued an FDA warning letter after a facility inspection uncovered improper consent forms, patient enrollments and errors in drug inventory and labeling.[236,237]

7.7.3 Patients and Parents Fight Back

Since the Singulair and generic montelukast labels only warned against "neuropsychiatric events," patients and especially parents began to fight back, forming advocacy groups.[238]

A 2016 Vigibase report found that suicidal ideation "and completed suicide appear to be more frequently reported than previously thought in practice."[239] A couple of years later, a study in the journal *Drug Safety* reported, "Ten pharmacovigilance studies using different global databases detected the signals" of neuropsychiatric events.[240,241]

In 2019, amid growing reports concerning the side effects of Singulair, the FDA held a Joint Meeting of the Pediatric and Drug Safety and Risk Management Advisory Committees.[242] Parents of children who had committed suicide or experienced severe adverse events after taking the drug testified at the meeting.[243,244]

According to the activist parents, the briefing documents released by the FDA for the hearings contained disturbing new pharmacological information.[245] Though the Singulair prescribing information had indicated that the drug acts on the CysLT1 receptor, Singulair's action on the brain as a competitive antagonist of GPR17 was revealed for the first time in the FDA documents.[246] The parents felt that the new information was relevant to the neuropsychiatric side effects under investigation and stated so at the hearing.[247,248]

Much of the hearings centered on the question of whether greater warnings should be added to Singulair.

Steven Meisel, PharmD, FDA committee member and Director of Medication Safety Fairview Health Services, agreed that a black box warning was necessary, citing FAERS data that showed "between six and 800 neuropsychiatric events have been reported every year." In light of this and the 35 million prescriptions of montelukast per year, Meisel concluded that this drug was "being prescribed in a cavalier manner."[249] Internist and pediatrician Christy Turer, also a committee member, agreed that a black box warning was warranted. "In thinking about risk-benefit, I think the black box would send a message and would decrease prescribing," she said. "We as a country, our physicians, our prescribers, we over-prescribe."[250]

However, others on the FDA advisory committee disagreed. Allergist and associate professor Jim Tracy said a boxed warning would cause patients to become "terrified" and "without supervision . . . just stop their drug," thus creating "obstacles to care," UCLA child psychiatrist and committee member James McGough agreed, reasoning that the black box warning about suicide risk on selective serotonin reuptake inhibitor (SSRI) antidepressant labels in 2004 backfired. He explained, "There's a clear association between declining antidepressant use and increased suicide among youth." However, it is worth noting that both antidepressant use[251] and the suicide rate have never been higher.[252] This implies that describing prescriptions of antidepressants due to the boxed warning is not a causal factor in rising suicides.[253]

7.7.4 Black Box Added to Singulair

Following the 2019 Joint Meeting of the Pediatric and Drug Safety and Risk Management Advisory Committees, in March 2020, the FDA announced that it was adding a boxed warning to Singulair.[254,255]

> *We are taking this action after a review of available information led us to reevaluate the benefits and risks of montelukast use. Montelukast prescribing information already includes warnings about mental health side effects, including suicidal thoughts or actions; however, many healthcare professionals and patients/caregivers are not aware of the risk. We decided a stronger warning is needed after conducting an extensive review of available information and convening a panel of outside experts, and therefore determined that a Boxed Warning was appropriate.*
>
> *Because of the risk of mental health side effects, the benefits of montelukast may not outweigh the risks in some patients, particularly when the symptoms of disease may be mild and adequately treated with other medicines. For allergic rhinitis, also known as hay fever, we have determined that montelukast should be reserved for those who are not treated effectively with or cannot tolerate other allergy medicines. For patients with asthma, we recommend that healthcare professionals consider the benefits and risks of mental health side effects before prescribing montelukast.*

While parent groups were pleased with the outcome, industry watchers asked why the serious risks were acknowledged only after the Singulair drug had gone off patent, as is the case with many and possibly most prescription medications.

While it is certainly true that the complete safety profiles of prescription drugs cannot be established before millions of patients use them and the post-marketing data are analyzed, it is *also* true that both drug makers and the government often only acknowledge major risks when all profit has been taken. Risks to statins, SSRI antidepressants, PPIs, non-steroidal anti-inflammatory drugs (NSAIDs), diabetes drugs, sleeping pills and drugs in other popular classes have often only been acknowledged after patents have expired.[256]

7.8 BALDNESS TREATMENTS BECOME POPULAR AND CONTROVERSIAL

According to an article in the journal *Pharmacy and Therapeutics*,[257] DTC pharmaceutical advertising often downplays drug risks as it promotes benefits as we have seen with other drugs covered in this chapter. The journal says that between 1997 and 2006[258]

> *nearly 84% of the regulatory letters for DTCPA ads for either minimizing risks (e.g., omitting information about side effects) or exaggerating a drug's effectiveness (e.g., portraying the indication too broadly or making unsubstantiated claims of superiority over other drugs), or both.*

One of the clearest examples of pharmaceutical marketing that downplayed risks is the drug Propecia (finasteride), an antiandrogen and 5α-reductase inhibitor,[259] approved by the FDA in 1997.[260] Medically indicated for symptomatic benign prostatic hyperplasia, the drug was also found useful in the treatment of male pattern hair loss.[261] Because two-thirds of American men have some hair loss by age 35,[262] and 85% by age 50, Propecia had the potential to become a blockbuster drug like Lipitor or Viagra.[263]

Merck spent $100 million[264] marketing Propecia directly to consumers in 1999 alone. This was during a time period in which when DTC advertising on TV was just beginning.[265] One estimate said Propecia was marketed in 120 countries—half the world.[266] In 2017, it was still popular and the 86th-most commonly prescribed medication in the U.S. with more than nine million prescriptions written.[267]

Early ads addressed the stigma of hair loss and sought to make Propecia a "man's" drug. "You'd be surprised who's treated their HAIR LOSS," said one print ad, depicting athletic-looking, 20-something men.[268] Some ads likened men's thinning scalps to crop circles.[269] Some ads compared twins, one of whom had used the product and one of whom had not.[270,271]

7.8.1 Finasteride Side Effects Create Concern

At the onset, the Propecia label warned that "a small number of men experienced certain sexual side effects, such as less desire for sex, difficulty in achieving an erection, or a decrease in the amount of semen"[272] but assured users the symptoms would go away.

But, increasingly, users and some doctors reported that the symptoms sometimes did not "go away" when men stopped taking Propecia and that their lives were being changed permanently. Symptoms that were irreversible in some included impotence, decreased sexual desire, depression, suicidal ideation and even a reduction in penis or testicle size.[273,274]

According to surgeon and head of the Irish Family Planning Association, Dr. Andrew Rynne, Propecia-maker Merck knew that the disturbing symptoms were sometimes irreversible.

> They know it is not true because I and hundreds of other doctors and thousands of patients have told them that these side effects do not always go away when you stop taking Propecia. We continue to be ignored of course.[275]

Dr. Rynne also stated that finasteride use for even a few months can "condemn" men "to a lifetime of Sexual Anhedonia." Sexual anhedonia is a condition in which an individual cannot feel pleasure from orgasm.[276]

Sarah Temori, a relative of one man disabled by the drug, launched a Change.org petition to have finasteride taken off the market.[277] She wrote,

> Many who have taken Propecia have lost their marriages, jobs and some have committed suicide due to the damage this drug has done to their bodies . . . One of my loved ones is a victim of this drug. It's painful to see how much he has to struggle just to make it through each day and do all the daily things that we take for granted. No doctors have been able to help him and he is struggling to pay for medical bills. He is only 23.[278]

7.8.2 Medical Literature Confirms Finasteride Side Effects

The medical literature has addressed such side effects. A study in the *Journal of Sexual Medicine* from 2011 reported that in finasteride-associated cases of "new-onset persistent sexual dysfunction" in otherwise healthy men aged 21–46 years, "94% developed low libido, 92% developed erectile dysfunction, 92% developed decreased arousal and 69% developed problems with orgasm."[279]

The following year the Journal published a study entitled "Persistent Sexual Side Effects of Finasteride: Could They Be Permanent?"[280] which speculated that changes in cognition, ejaculate quality and genital sensation seen with Propecia might be permanent. The article warned that "prescribers of finasteride and men contemplating its use should be made aware of the potential adverse medication effects."

In 2014, a study in the *Journal of Steroid Biochemistry and Molecular Biology* reported lasting psychological and cognitive changes with the drug. "Altered levels of neuroactive steroids, associated with depression symptoms, are present in androgenic alopecia patients even after discontinuation of the finasteride treatment," the study read.[281]

"Persistent SD [sexual dysfunction] might be a potential risk of low-dose finasteride for androgenic alopecia therapy in young men, and this risk might contribute to SI [suicidal ideation]," read a 2015 study in *Pharmacotherapy*.[282]

Lastly, a 2020 study in the journal *Translational Andrology and Urology* reported organic changes in patients who had taken finasteride,[283] declaring "there may be persistent genitourinary, physical, psycho-cognitive, anti-androgenic and penile vascular changes after 5ARI discontinuation."

7.8.3 FDA Adds Warnings to Finasteride

FDA warnings followed the revelation of side effects and the term "post finasteride syndrome" was coined. In 2003, the FDA posted a warning about Propecia's link to high-grade prostate cancers.[284] In 2011, depression[285] was added to the drug label as a side effect. Also, patients were notified that finasteride could interfere with prostate-specific antigen tests used to detect prostate cancer.[286,287] The risk of "male breast cancer" was also added.[288]

By 2013, Merck conceded that[289] a Propecia-caused decrease in sex drive and Propecia-caused problems with ejaculation could continue "after stopping the medication."

In 2014, the risk of angioedema was added to the warning label.[290]

Propecia approval documents also raised red flags.[291] Finasteride induced such harm to animal fetuses that it is now contraindicated in women when they are or may potentially be pregnant. In fact, women were warned not to even "handle crushed or broken PROPECIA tablets when they are pregnant."[292]

In spite of the observed side effects in animal studies, clinical trials focused on efficacy in slowing hair loss rather than side effects.[293] Absent from surveys of patient subjects in clinical studies were questions about depression, mental health and, notably, sexual function. One FDA reviewer reports that Merck did not list the use of other drugs used by subjects in Propecia clinical studies, suggesting depression may have been a known side effect of the drug.[294,295]

Elsewhere an FDA reviewer cautioned that "low figures" in terms of side effects may be misleading because the time period of the study was "relatively short" and those with sexual adverse events may have already withdrawn from the study.[296] Another FDA reviewer noted that "long term cancer effects are unknown" and that breast cancer was noted as an observed adverse event in clinical trials.[297,298]

7.8.4 Finasteride User Speaks Out

One well-known sufferer of post finasteride syndrome is Paule Innes of the UK. Previously healthy and active, Innes was so debilitated by Propecia's use that he founded a website decrying its use.[299,300]

He appeared on the television show *This Morning* in 2013 to warn others about the serious side effects he experienced after using it on two occasions for a three-month and three-week period, respectively. His side effects included depression, leading to suicidal ideation and hospitalization, sexual dysfunction and the shrinking of his reproductive anatomy. Ironically, the TV segment was sponsored by a UK drug chain which had aggressively advertised hair loss clinics from which Innes himself had ordered Propecia. "With very little effort my pills arrived to my home address in the post," he wrote.[301,302]

A year after his TV appearance, Innes wrote me in an email after our initial interview,

> My health is just the same if not worse since 2013. I am still impotent with a shrunken penis and still have very dark thoughts and currently having to take antidepressants just to get through every day. Prior to Propecia I was a very healthy guy but now I'm a shadow of my former self. I have only just managed to return to work in my role as a police officer since taking Propecia in March 2013!

His website declares forcefully, "PROPECIA IS LETHAL—DO NOT EVEN CONSIDER TAKING IT!!!"[303,304]

7.8.5 No Satisfying End for Finasteride Users

By 2020, the medical literature was almost unwavering on Propecia's risks. A case-control study in *Translational Andrology and Urology* reported penile vascular abnormalities in patients who had used the drug and discontinued it.[305] Research in *JAMA Dermatology* in 2020 found 2,926 reports of psychological adverse events such as depression and anxiety in 3,200 users of finasteride—which amounted to a four-time increase.[306] There were also 356 reports of suicidality including suicidal ideation and attempted suicide, reported the journal—a four-time increase.[307]

Meanwhile, hundreds of lawsuits pertaining to finasteride had been filed and Merck agreed to pay a lump sum of $4.3 million, according to Reuters.[308] While Merck told Reuters that it "stands behind the safety and efficacy of Propecia," confidential court documents suggest that the company "understated the number of men who experienced sexual symptoms in clinical trials, and how long those symptoms lasted," and that "Merck knew roughly 20 years ago that sales of the drug would suffer if the public became aware of Propecia's possible long-term effects on men's sexual health," reported Reuters.[309] Meanwhile, the market for Propecia and finasteride will surpass $130 million by 2026, according to Global Market Insights Inc.[310]

7.9 BIOLOGIC DRUGS

As we noted in the introduction to this chapter, the new profit center for drug makers has been biologics. Serum, antitoxin and antibody therapies, interleukins and vaccines made of proteins, peptides and nucleic acids, and cells, administered parenterally, have largely replaced "small-molecule" drugs as Wall Street-pleasing therapies.[311]

The dramatic shift from small-molecule products to biologics allows much higher drug prices. Not only are the biologically derived drugs more expensive to produce than those that are chemically derived, but they can be classified as advanced therapy medicinal products or "cures," which allows drug makers to charge even higher prices.[312] Deloitte estimates that biologics will soon represent a quarter of the pharmaceutical market.[313]

According to a review article in the *Indian Journal of Medical Research*:[314]

> *The biologicals acting as "targeted therapy" have not only changed the natural history of a large number of incurable/uncontrollable diseases but have also transformed the whole approach towards drug development. From the classical empirical process, there is now a complete shift towards understanding the disease pathobiology focusing on the dysregulated molecule(s) . . .*
>
> *Seminal advances in understanding the disease mechanism, development of remarkably effective new technologies, greater knowledge of the human genome and genetic medicine have all made it possible to reach the stage where artificially developed "targeted" drugs are now therapeutically used in routine clinical medicine.*

7.9.1 Tumor Necrosis Factor Blockers

As biologics became a drug maker profit center, tumor necrosis factor (TNF)-blocking drugs usually made from monoclonal antibodies (mAbs) became blockbusters. The drugs such as Remicade (infliximab), Humira (adalimumab), Cimzia (certolizumab pegol), Simponi (golimumab) and Enbrel (etanercept) suppress the inflammatory response to TNF and target and bind to disease-specific molecules.

Approved for a variety of autoimmune and immune-mediated disorders, the medications brought drug maker profits to a whole new level. Diseases indicated for these TNF blockers include rheumatoid arthritis, ankylosing spondylitis, inflammatory bowel disease, psoriasis, hidradenitis suppurativa, refractory asthma, juvenile idiopathic arthritis and Crohn's disease. Ubiquitous ads raising "awareness" of the conditions they treat were seen on TV and in print.[315]

In 2020, it was reported that Humira cost between $1,800 and $2,400 per month, Enbrel more than $4,000 per month and a single dose of Remicade from $1,250 to $2,500.[316] Humira became the U.S.'s best-selling medicine[317] and was projected to make $103.95 billion between 2019 and 2024, according to Biospace.[318]

One of the leading TNF blockers, Humira, allowed Abbott Labs to spin off the company called AbbVie primarily to market the drug.[319] Abbott enlisted the public relations giant Edelman[320] and the pharmaceutical ad agency Harrison and Star[321] to create initial buzz. Then it announced that it would "provide its recently approved rheumatoid arthritis drug free to Medicare patients without drug coverage until the government agrees to pay for the medicine," according to the *Chicago Tribune*,[322] while simultaneously lobbying Congress to get Medicare coverage for the drug.[323] This maneuver worked.[324,325]

Other questionable tactics were also used to make Humira the blockbuster it became and has continued to be. According to the *Journal Sentinel*,[326] in 2012, AbbVie launched a "nurse ambassador" program through which nurse clinicians allegedly "got kickbacks in the form of cash, meals, drinks, gifts, trips, even patient referrals." The lawsuit alleges that these nurses were told to avoid answering questions from patients about the serious side effects of Humira when making home visits to patients taking this drug.[327,328]

California Insurance Commissioner Ricardo Lara said private insurers in California likely "paid out $1.2 billion in Humira claims from 2013 to 2018, making it potentially the largest insurance fraud case in the department's history."[329,330] In the summer of 2020 AbbVie agreed to pay $24 million to settle a California lawsuit charging Humira-related kickbacks.[331] The difference between billions made in profits and millions paid in fines should escape no one.

7.9.2 TNF Blocker Risks

Clearly, any medication that suppresses the immune system poses serious side effects. In addition to their unprecedented costs, TNF blockers increase the risk of opportunistic infections.[332]

The Enbrel label warns about an "increased risk of serious infections leading to hospitalization or death, including tuberculosis (TB), bacterial sepsis, invasive fungal infections (such as histoplasmosis), and infections due to other opportunistic pathogens" including "Legionella and Listeria."[333] The Humira label warns of "serious, possibly lethal infections, melanoma, lymphoma and unusual cancers in children and teenagers."[334] Other reported side effects according to research published in *Current Neurology and Neuroscience Reports* include congestive heart failure, lupus-like autoimmune diseases, autoimmune hepatitis, vasculitis, uveitis, diabetes mellitus, psoriasis, interstitial lung diseases, sarcoidosis, antiphospholipid syndrome, myositis and myasthenia gravis.[335]

According to the *Journal Sentinel*, since 2000, the FDA has issued more than "25 warnings and safety communications" for Humira and similar biologic drugs—all after the drugs were approved for use in patients.[336] A review by this journal found warnings for various infections due to suppression of the immune system by the drug.[337] Other warnings include the risk of acquiring neurological conditions, liver failure or heart failure in addition to the known cancer risks.[338,339]

In fact, in 2019, the *Journal Sentinel* reported that the drug class was linked to 1 million reported adverse events since 2004, more than 500,000 of which were "deemed serious."[340]

In 2020, the *Journal Sentinel* reported that biologic medications for arthritis and psoriasis had "been linked to 34,000 deaths,"[341] with 13,000 deaths being attributed to Humira use, 8,000 to Embrel and 6,000 to Remicade.[342] The drugs were also correlated with depression and suicide.[343,344]

7.10 OTHER POPULAR MEDICATIONS COME UNDER NEW SCRUTINY

There is an inherent tension between drug sales and drug safety. Drug makers understandably want their products on the market as soon as possible—the impulse behind the Prescription Drug User Fee Act (PDUFA)—but drug safety advocates have been known to tell consumers to wait five years before taking a new drug.

Sadly, accelerated drug approvals can result in safety signals only identified in post-marketing studies, after many have used and are using the medication. In recent years as examples in this chapter have and will show, PPIs, statins, bisphosphonates, histamine receptor antagonists, birth control pills, blood thinners, antibiotics, asthma drugs, psychiatric drugs, NSAIDs, testosterone supplements, hair restoration medications, diabetes drugs and diet preparations have all received new safety scrutiny.

Often this leads to stricter warnings on drug labels, but it can also lead to the removal of the drug from the market.

Sometimes patient advocates and legal entities claim that the drug makers knew about the safety signals during drug development and marketed the product anyway. Other times the drug makers say they did not realize the risks.

Some of the newly identified and publicized risks with popular drugs follow.

7.10.1 *N*-Nitrosodimethylamine Found in Medicines

7.10.1.1 Zantac Taken Off Shelves

In April of 2020, after an investigation of *N*-Nitrosodimethylamine (NDMA) found in Zantac (ranitidine), the FDA requested that manufacturers withdraw all prescription and over-the-counter (OTC) versions of drugs containing ranitidine from the market immediately.[345] Zantac, an H2 histamine receptor antagonist that reduces stomach acid secretion, was used in treating peptic ulcers, gastroesophageal reflux disease and other conditions in which the stomach produces too much acid.[346,347] It was taken by mouth or injection into a muscle or vein.[348]

While ranitidine was associated with headaches and pain or burning when injected and an increased risk of liver problems, pneumonia, a slow heart rate and *Clostridium difficile* colitis, the identification of NDMA in drug preparations caught many by surprise.[349]

According to the FDA:[350]

> *NDMA is a common contaminant found in water and foods including cured and grilled meats, dairy products and vegetables. Everyone is exposed to some level of NDMA. The FDA and the international scientific community do not expect it to cause harm when ingested at low levels. The acceptable daily intake limit for NDMA in the U.S. is 96 nanograms. Genotoxic substances such as NDMA may increase the risk of cancer if people are exposed to them above acceptable levels and over long periods of time, but a person taking a drug that contains NDMA at-or-below the acceptable daily intake limit every day for 70 years is not expected to have an increased risk of cancer.*

The FDA said it first learned of NDMA in ranitidine during the summer of 2019 when it warned the public of the "potential risks and to consider alternative OTC and prescription treatments."[351] The FDA soon strengthened its warning when it learned:[352]

> *that the impurity in some ranitidine products increases over time and when stored at higher than room temperatures and may result in consumer exposure to unacceptable levels of this impurity. As a result of this immediate market withdrawal request, ranitidine products will not be available for new or existing prescriptions or OTC use in the U.S.*

Ranitidine sales were also suspended in the European Union and in Australia.[353] Prior to the FDA's move, drug makers Sandoz, Sanofi, Dr. Reddy's, Perrigo, Apotex and Novitium Pharma withdrew their products containing ranitidine.[354]

Janet Woodcock, director of the FDA's Center for Drug Evaluation and Research, stated,

> We didn't observe unacceptable levels of NDMA in many of the samples that we tested. However, since we don't know how or for how long the product might have been stored, we decided that it should not be available to consumers and patients unless its quality can be assured.[355]

The FDA said it did not find NDMA in Pepcid (famotidine), Tagamet (cimetidine) Nexium (esomeprazole), Prevacid (lansoprazole) or Prilosec (omeprazole) and that

> patients taking prescription ranitidine should speak with their healthcare professionals about other treatment options before stopping the medicine, as there are multiple drugs approved for the same or similar uses as ranitidine that do not carry the same risks from NDMA.[356]

As thousands filed Zantac lawsuits, claiming their cancer was caused by the heartburn drug,[357] the U.S. Department of Justice announced an investigation in 2010 to determine whether the drug makers GlaxoSmithKline (GSK) and Sanofi violated federal law in selling Zantac.[358]

As early as 1981, research in the Lancet addressed whether the nitroso derivatives in ranitidine and another drug were mutagenic.[359] The research was followed by a response by the Glaxo Group Research titled "Safety of Ranitidine,"[360] which questioned the validity of the research but also acknowledged a cancer-causing material in the drug.[361]

A Sanofi spokeswoman, addressing litigation, said the company stands "by the long-standing science that supports the safety of Zantac OTC products, which have been used by consumers for over two decades."[362]

Both GlaxoSmithKline and Sanofi are also the targets of a Zantac-related lawsuit from the New Mexico Attorney General, claiming false advertising, public nuisance and negligence and violations of the state's unfair practices act.[363]

7.10.1.2 NDMA Also Found in Metformin

During the same time period that NDMA was found in Zantac, the FDA also identified dangerous levels of the substance in metformin, which is the first-line drug to treat type 2 diabetes.[364,365] By September 2020, at least seven drug makers had recalled their metformin products after finding high levels of NDMA.[366]

While the FDA admitted the risks as it did with Zantac, it also noted fewer patient options since there are "no alternative medications that treat this condition [diabetes] in the same way":[367]

> *Patients should continue taking metformin to keep their diabetes under control. It could be dangerous for patients with this serious condition to stop taking their metformin*

without first talking to their healthcare professionals. The FDA recommends prescribers continue to use metformin when clinically appropriate, as the FDA investigation is still ongoing.

7.11 POPULAR STIMULANT DRUGS REVEAL RISKS

When the stimulant Provigil (modafinil), made by Cephalon, was approved for U.S. sales in 1998, many hailed it as an alternative to dangerous amphetamines. And, even though it was meant to treat sleepiness due to narcolepsy, shift work sleep disorder or obstructive sleep apnea, it gained widespread off-label use just like amphetamines had done and continue to do. "Modafinil is a memory-improving and mood-brightening psycho stimulant that enhances wakefulness—not unlike cocaine or amphetamines," wrote ABC News in 2007, and the drug not surprisingly gained popularity in the general population.[368]

Sleep-deprived groups ranging from truck drivers to the military have experimented with modafinil, marketed for nearly a decade by Cephalon under what Plotz calls the "creepy, pharma-Orwellian" name Provigil.

Military officials have found it so effective that some now refer to it as a "super drug." But its off-label uses have created a rich debate on how far to push the limits of the human body . . . .

A seemingly perfect stimulant, clinical trials found modafinil to be less likely than amphetamines to cause jitteriness or anxiety or have a "rebound" or "crash" effect.

By 2006, annual modafinil sales were almost $600 million, reported ABC News, and as much as 90% of sales were for off-label use.[369]

In 2008, modafinil maker Cephalon, which was acquired by Teva, paid $425 million to settle charges of off-label marketing of modafinil, Actiq (Fentanyl) and Gabitril (tiagabine). In 2014, a lawsuit was filed claiming Cephalon had a scheme for marketing modafinil and Nuvigil (armodafinil), the R-enantiomer of racemic modafinil approved in 2007,[370] "falsely and misleadingly promoting its drugs for off-label, non-medically accepted uses."[371]

7.11.1 Risks Seen With Modafinil

In addition to off-label charges, the safety profile of modafinil raised serious questions. After an all-day FDA hearings in 2006 about whether to allow the drug to be used for children with ADHD, an advisory committee voted against the usage.[372] Dr. Glen Manheim, a scientist with the FDA, had testified that a young user of modafinil had come down with a case of Stevens-Johnson syndrome, characterized by "peeling and blistering over the entire body, with lips and urinary tract involvement. The drug was stopped, but the rash progressed to involve peeling, blistering, mucosal involvement, over days."[373]

Dr. Manheim and Dr. Paul Andreason presented data showing two cases of Stevens-Johnson syndrome in a group of modafinil-treated subjects at the FDA hearing.[374]

Over time, awareness of the risk of Stevens-Johnson syndrome and the related toxic epidermal necrolysis and drug rashes with eosinophilia grew, especially as popular off-label uses ballooned.[375]

The *Indian Journal of Pharmacology* wrote, presently modafinil:[376]

is being used as a lifestyle medicine; in India, it has been misused as an "over the counter" drug. Modafinil is known to have several cutaneous side effects. Fixed drug eruption (FDE) is a distinctive drug induced reaction pattern characterized by recurrence of eruption at the same site of the skin or mucous membrane with repeated systemic administration . . .

The increasing use of this class of drug amongst the medical personnel might be posing a threat to the proper use and encouraging subsequent abuse. There might be a considerable population using these drugs unaware of the possible adverse effects. Authorities should be more alert regarding the sale and distribution of such medicines.

A Stevens-Johnson case was also reported by the journal *Sleep*.[377]

7.11.2 Fetal Risks Seen With Modafinil and Armodafinil

In 2020, new risks associated with modafinil and Nuvigil (armodafinil) became known—congenital fetal malformations. According to MedPage Today, the Provigil/Nuvigil increased the prevalence of major congenital malformations by more than a factor of four (13% of 102 prospective live births in the Provigil/Nuvigil Pregnancy Registry).[378],[379]

Four of the newborns with malformations were diagnosed with congenital torticollis; two were diagnosed with hypospadias, and three with congenital heart defects, making the cardiac malformation prevalence 3%, compared with about 1% in the general population.

Before the safety signal, "intrauterine growth restrictions and spontaneous abortions" and fetal structural abnormalities in animals had already been identified with the drugs, earning them pregnancy category C on labels.[380]

Neda Ghaffari, MD and Patricia A. Robertson, MD, who wrote an accompanying commentary[381] to the *JAMA Internal Medicine* article that cited the deformities,[382] told MedPage Today:[383]

Given the risks of these medications and the high rate of unintended pregnancy, we recommend that pregnancy be considered a possibility in all individuals of reproductive age who may be prescribed a potential teratogen. . . . To avoid major congenital malformations associated with modafinil and armodafinil, these medications should be avoided or offered along with a reliable contraceptive to individuals who could become pregnant.[384]

7.11.3 European Union SUES Provigil Makers

In addition to the concerning risks, there were pricing questions about Provigil. In 2020, the European Union fined Cephalon and Teva Pharmaceuticals, which Cephalon had acquired, for delaying a generic version of Provigil to receive financial side deals and payments.[385]

The EU antitrust commissioner, Margrethe Vestager, said "Teva's and Cephalon's pay-for-delay agreement harmed patients and national health systems, depriving them of more affordable medicines." Cephalon was ordered to pay 60.5 million euros or $72 million U.S. dollars for the lucrative delaying scheme.[386]

7.12 FETAL RISK SEEN WITH NSAIDS

Fetal risks were also identified with another drug class in 2020—NSAIDS. The use of aspirin, ibuprofen, naproxen, diclofenac and celecoxib after 20 weeks of pregnancy could cause fetal harm, said the FDA.[387]

> *The U.S. Food and Drug Administration (FDA) is warning that use of nonsteroidal anti-inflammatory drugs (NSAIDs) around 20 weeks or later in pregnancy may cause rare but serious kidney problems in an unborn baby. This can lead to low levels of amniotic fluid surrounding the baby and possible complications . . .*
>
> *After around 20 weeks of pregnancy, the unborn babies' kidneys produce most of the amniotic fluid, so kidney problems can lead to low levels of this fluid. Amniotic fluid provides a protective cushion and helps the unborn babies' lungs, digestive system, and muscles develop . . .*
>
> *This issue affects all NSAIDs that are available by prescription and those that can be bought over-the-counter (OTC) without a prescription.*

According to the FDA, there are other NSAID concerns. Between 20 and 30 weeks of pregnancy, NSAIDs can cause heart issues in a fetus, it warned, and NSAIDs should be limited to the lowest dose and duration. If NSAIDs must be used beyond 48 hours, ultrasound monitoring of amniotic fluid was recommended said the FDA.[388]

Though low amniotic fluid levels tend to return to normal when NSAIDs are discontinued, consequences of low amniotic fluid levels are serious, said the FDA in new warnings. Data submitted to the FDA that newborn deaths coincided with kidney failure and/or low amniotic fluid when the mothers took NSAIDs during pregnancy.[389] The correlation of low amniotic fluid with NSAID use is confirmed in the medical literatures, wrote the FDA.[390]

7.13 BISPHOSPHONATES CONTINUE TO PRESENT RISKS

Merck's Fosamax (alendronate), the first bisphosphonate approved for osteoporosis, flew out of the FDA, receiving only a six-month review.[391] Early side effects like acid regurgitation, dyspepsia, dysphagia, erosive esophagitis, esophageal hemorrhage and esophageal perforation were identified after the drug was approved.[392]

Thanks to the esophageal side effects, patients were required to stay upright for a full hour after taking Fosamax. One woman who took Fosamax but remained upright for 30 minutes developed "severe ulcerative esophagitis affecting the entire length of the esophagus."[393,394]

Six months after Fosamax was approved, Merck had received 1,213 adverse effect reports including 32 hospitalizations.[395]

By 2003, dentists and oral surgeons were noting jaw osteonecrosis after simple tooth extractions and other in-office dental work.[396] The condition resembled "phossy jaw," an occupational disease of the 1800s that workers got from working with phosphorus.[397] As Merck added warnings to the Fosamax label,[398] jaw removal, bone grafts and even tracheostomies were seen.[399] In fact, Merck animal studies revealed jaw osteonecrosis in rats given bisphosphonates as early as 1977 Merck bone scientist Don Kimmel, who conducted the research, was admitted under oath in 2008.[400]

Sadly, jaw osteonecrosis was not the only side effect to emerge with Fosamax and the bisphosphonate drug class—patients also faced an increased risk of developing atrial fibrillation.[401] Bisphosphonates were also linked to severe bone, joint or muscle pain, said the FDA in a 2008 press release.[402] The pain could be so severe the FDA cautioned clinicians to "consider whether musculoskeletal pain in patients on bisphosphonates might be caused by the drug, and consider discontinuing it either temporarily or permanently."[403]

Then, in 2009, Diane Wysowski, an epidemiologist with the FDA, reported 23 incidences of Fosamax-associated esophageal cancer in the U.S., which included 8 deaths and 27 incidences of cancer in Europe and Japan with six deaths.[404]

Still, the nail in the bisphosphonate coffin probably came in 2010 when its indication, prevention of fractures, was discredited. Studies revealed that the drugs sometimes caused fractures. "Long-term use of osteoporosis drugs linked to hip breaks," said *USA Today*.[405] "Increased risk of fracture with bisphosphonates," said the Associated Press.[406] "Possible increased risk of thigh bone fracture with bisphosphonates," said the FDA in a 2010 warning.[407]

A *New York Times* article titled "Drugs to Build Bones May Weaken Them" recounts that bisphosphonate users experienced sudden femur breaks doing nothing more than walking or standing. This was reportedly preceded by "weeks or months of unexplained aching."[408,409]

How common was degraded bone from bisphosphonates? Half the doctors at a presentation the *Los Angeles Times* report that half of the doctors at a presentation at the annual meeting of the 2010 American Academy of Orthopaedic Surgeons reported that their patients experienced the effects of bisphosphonate-compromised bone.[410,411]

There was plenty of warning in the medical literature that the action of bisphosphonates—reducing the life span of osteoclasts and so increasing the action of osteoblasts—would result in fracture-prone bone. As early as 2004 Susan M. Ott, M.D., in the *Annals of Internal Medicine*[412] and others warned that the actions of bisphosphonates could paradoxically make bones brittle and cause fractures.

Reports in the *Journal of Clinical Endocrinology & Metabolism*,[413] *Journal of Orthopaedic Trauma*[414] and *Injury*[415] followed. In 2008, Phuli Cohan, M.D., appeared on CBS TV in Boston with X-rays of a woman whose hip had shattered after years on Fosamax. "There is actually bone death occurring," and her worst fears—"that we'd be seeing spontaneous fractures"—had been realized.[416]

As fracture fears cut into sales, pro-bisphosphonate messaging increased. "Currently, many people at risk of a fracture—and often their doctors—are failing to properly weigh the benefits of treating fragile bones against the very rare but widely publicized hazards of bone-preserving drugs, experts say," read a 2018 article in the *New York Times* science section lamenting that Medicare reimbursements for bone density tests are falling.[417] Bone density–measuring machines were widely placed in in medical offices across the country by a Merck contractor according to National Public Radio to foster Merck's bone drug sales.[418] The *New York Times* article quotes a doctor who lamented bad buzz about the drugs had made it so that "Doctors who did them [density tests] in private offices could no longer afford to [do them] which limited patient access and diagnosis and treatment of serious bone loss."[419]

In 2020, a new bisphosphonate "benefit" was floated. According to the *New York Times*, "Osteoporosis drugs such as Fosamax and Actonel may have an additional benefit: A new study suggests they are associated with a reduced risk for pneumonia."[420]

"In the entire [New York Times] story there was only discussion of benefits from bisphosphonates and not one mention of side effects or potential harms," wrote Gary Schwitzer, founder and publisher of HealthNewsReview.org.[421] Schwitzer quoted a *BMJ* article titled "Overdiagnosis of bone fragility in the quest to prevent hip fracture," which stated that drug therapy "can achieve at best a marginal reduction in hip fractures at the cost of unnecessary psychological harms, serious medical adverse events, and forgone opportunities to have greater impacts on the health of older people."[422]

7.14 SSRI ANTIDEPRESSANTS LINKED TO NEW RISKS

Sales of SSRI antidepressants continue to rise. Between 2015 and 2019, their use in the U.S. rose by 15% and prescriptions for antidepressants, along with anti-anxiety medications and sleeping pills had already increased by 21% within two weeks of the COVID pandemic.[423]

SSRI antidepressants have been linked to sexual dysfunction, birth defects, suicidal ideation and other serious side effects.[424] Yet another side effect has been identified—negative effects on bone.

7.14.1 SSRI Bone Thinning

According to 2012 research in *Innovations in Clinical Neuroscience*, "Our examination of 19 studies, one review, and one meta-analysis indicates that these unique antidepressants appear to have negative effects on bone, particularly with regard to bone mineral density and fracture risk."[425] Since then, several studies have confirmed the bone actions from SSRIs such as "impaired fracture healing" and negative effects on jawbones.[426] Though osteoporosis is more common among women than men, bone impairments from SSRIs have also been seen in men in scientific studies.[427]

Some SSRI makers fought the bad buzz about bone mineral density. One employee of antidepressant-maker Janssen asserted in the journal *Translational Psychiatry* that SSRI treatment augmented "bone formation" in animal studies and that these effects were "long-lasting."[428] He continued the findings in these studies "may be relevant to the understanding and treatment of osteoporosis, a condition of increasing prevalence due to the aging population."[429,430]

7.14.2 SSRI Addictive Potential

In 2018, the *New York Times* reported something that many patients had suspected: SSRI antidepressants can be very difficult to quit.[431] In fact, the withdrawal from them—which drug makers call a "discontinuation syndrome"—is similar to that of addictive drugs. The *Times* reported that patients were angry that they were not warned by their doctors; they may be "parked" on the drugs indefinitely due to lingering side effects associated with drug discontinuation such as dizziness, nausea, headache and brain "zaps." One young man who was on SSRI antidepressant explained, "Every time I try to stop, I get something that feels like an electrical current in my head and I can't do it." As a result, he kept taking the SSRI for years.[432]

The *New York Times* article drew a backlash from psychiatrists, many of whom were with medical schools that received drug maker funding.[433] A joint statement by 39 psychiatrists asserts, "By amplifying the social media echo chamber, the article creates the unfortunate impression that most patients are forced to continue antidepressants out of fear of withdrawal rather than out of prevention of recurrence." They insisted that depression was a "chronic" disease that was "undertreated."[434]

At least 35 of the letter signers who were defending the reputation of SSRIs were affiliated with Columbia University's College of Physicians and Surgeons, which received $250 million from former Merck CEO Roy Vagelos and his wife Diana in 2019.[435]

According to Peter Breggin, M.D., a Harvard-trained psychiatrist who served as a full-time consultant to the National Institute of Mental Health, the effects of discontinuing psychoactive drugs are often misdiagnosed.

Too often these mental reactions are termed a 'relapse' of the condition the drugs were prescribed for—when they are actually a result of the process of going through withdrawal. This is obvious because when the withdrawing person is returned to a higher dosage level, the symptoms quickly disappear, sometimes in an hour or two. These risks are why the involvement of the family and caregivers is so important.[436]

7.15 BELVIQ, A DIET DRUG WITHDRAWN FROM MARKET

In 2020, the FDA requested the withdrawal of Belviq (lorcaserin),[437] a weight-loss medication approved in 2012 and made by Eisai.[438,439] According to a 2013 article in *Pharmacy and Therapeutics*, lorcaserin is a "small-molecule agonist of the serotonin 2C (5-HT2C) receptor" thought to avoid the "cardiovascular effects that occurred in previous non-selective serotonergic weight-loss medications."[440] The journal notes that "previous weight-loss medications with a serotonin agonist mechanism of action, such as dexfenfluramine and fenfluramine, also stimulated 5-HT2B receptors, which led to pulmonary hypertension and heart-valve problems."[441] The drugs were withdrawn from the market in 1997.[442]

Citing questions about the potential risks of neoplasms and valvular heart disease, the FDA Endocrinologic and Metabolic Drugs Advisory Committee rejected the NDA of lorcaserin in 2010.[443,444]

The FDA wrote that "diagnostic uncertainty in the classification of mammary masses in female rats, unresolved exposure-response relationship for lorcaserin-emergent mammary adenocarcinoma and unidentified mode of action and unclear safety margin for lorcaserin-emergent brain astrocytoma" caused the rejection.[445]

Though the drug was approved two years later, in 2020, the FDA says it has since identified serious safety signals.[446]

> *When FDA approved lorcaserin in 2012, we required the drug manufacturer to conduct a randomized, double-blind, placebo-controlled clinical trial to evaluate the risk of cardiovascular problems, which found that more patients taking lorcaserin (n = 462; 7.7 percent) were diagnosed with cancer compared to those taking a placebo, which is an inactive treatment (n = 423; 7.1 percent). The trial was conducted in 12,000 patients over 5 years. A range of cancer types was reported, with several different types of cancers occurring more frequently in the lorcaserin group, including pancreatic, colorectal, and lung.*

Late in 2020, New York resident Barbara Zottola filed a class-action lawsuit against Eisai, claiming it knew the negative health effects of Belviq but continued to manufacture and market the drug.[447] Zottola sought certification of a nationwide class of patients who took the drug, amounting to hundreds of thousands of people.[448,449,450] Eisai, also called Arena Pharmaceuticals, subsequently urged a New York federal court to throw any class suit out stating that the plaintiff's "conclusory assertions" of deception fall short of stating any plausible claim.[451]

7.16 SLEEPING PILLS GIVEN BOXED WARNINGS

An estimated 4% of U.S. adults use sleeping pills, but, in 2019, the FDA mandated black box warnings on some of the most popular, called "Z drugs"[452]—Lunesta (eszopiclone), Sonata (zaleplon) and Ambien (zolpidem) citing the danger of associated "sleepwalking, sleep driving, and engaging in other activities while not fully awake." According to the FDA.[453]

> *We identified 66 cases of complex sleep behaviors occurring with these medicines over the past 26 years that resulted in serious injuries, including death... These cases included accidental overdoses, falls, burns, near drowning, exposure to extreme cold temperatures leading to loss of limb, carbon monoxide poisoning, drowning, hypothermia, motor vehicle collisions with the patient driving, and self-injuries such as gunshot wounds and apparent suicide attempts. Patients usually did not remember these events.*

One of the reasons the sale of sleeping pills has accelerated over the past 20 years is aggressive advertising on TV.[454] Drug makers have created numerous subcategories of insomnia to promote more "personalized" sales—treating someone's exact kind of insomnia. Such subcategories of insomnia include chronic, acute, transient, initial, delayed-onset, middle-of-the-night, early-morning and non-restful sleep.[455]

Yet, as the FDA's 2019 warning flags, there has been a dark underside to sleeping pills. In addition to sleepwalking, sleep-driving, sleep-eating and blackout behaviors, the risk of associated falls increased.

Mayo Clinic researchers found that the fall rate on Ambien among 16,000 hospitalized patients was more than four times of those not on the sleeping pill.[456] Ambien posed a greater fall risk and was correlated with more falls overall compared to age and other fall-associated factors.[457] In consideration of this, Mayo's chief patient safety officer stated on behalf of the Mayo Clinic, "As a result of our study, we are now phasing out [Ambien] and moving toward sleep enhancement techniques that are not based on drugs and which we believe are safer and probably as effective."[458,459]

7.16.1 Public Figures on Sleeping Pills Make the News

Some sleeping drugs like Ambien have become household words thanks to their use and apparent abuse by public figures. In 2006, under the influence of the Ambien, former congressman Patrick Kennedy drove to Capitol Hill in the middle of the night because he thought he was "late for a vote" and crashed his car.[460] The vote was actually six hours earlier. Following this incident, Kennedy entered rehab.[461,462]

In 2009, Ambien was again in the news when golf giant Tiger Woods reportedly used it to enhance sex with his mistresses but then crashed his car while under the influence, leading to a national scandal and separation from his wife.[463,464]

Another member of the Kennedy clan encountered Ambien-related legal trouble in 2014. After reportedly weaving in traffic for miles, she swerved into and struck a tractor-trailer and continued driving. She reported to police that she may have confused Ambien with her thyroid medication but later in court attributed her crash to a seizure.[465]

7.16.2 Other Sleeping Pill Risks

There are other risks associated with sleeping pills, also called hypnotics. According to 2012 research in the journal *Pharmacology and Therapeutics Research*:[466]

> *As predicted, patients prescribed any hypnotic had substantially elevated hazards of dying compared to those prescribed no hypnotics. For groups prescribed 0.4–18, 18–132 and >132 doses/year, HRs (95% CIs) were 3.60 (2.92 to 4.44), 4.43 (3.67 to 5.36) and 5.32 (4.50 to 6.30), respectively, demonstrating a dose–response association.*
>
> *HRs were elevated in separate analyses for several common hypnotics, including zolpidem, temazepam, eszopiclone, zaleplon, other benzodiazepines, barbiturates and sedative antihistamines. Hypnotic use in the upper third was associated with a significant elevation of incident cancer.*

According to the authors, "Control of selective prescription of hypnotics for patients in poor health did not explain the observed excess mortality."[467]

Research published on the open-access publishing platform f1000research in 2018 added many concerns.[468]

> *The most important risks of hypnotics include excess mortality (especially overdose deaths, quiet deaths at night, and suicides), infections, cancer, depression, automobile crashes, falls, other accidents, and hypnotic-withdrawal insomnia. Short-term use of one-two prescriptions is associated with even greater risk per dose than long-term use.*
>
> *Hypnotics have usually been prescribed without approved indication, most often with specific contraindications, but even when indicated, there is little or no benefit. The recommended doses objectively increase sleep little if at all, daytime performance is often made worse (not better) and the lack of general health benefits is commonly misrepresented in advertising. Treatments such as the cognitive behavioral treatment of insomnia and bright light treatment of circadian rhythm disorders offer safer and more effective alternative approaches to insomnia.*

7.17 RISKS ASSOCIATED WITH FLUOROQUINOLONE ANTIBIOTICS

Many first became aware of the fluoroquinolone class of antibiotics after an anthrax scare that followed the 9/11 terrorist attacks in the U.S. Cipro, a fluoroquinolone, was the drug of choice to treat and prevent anthrax infections.[469] Other fluoroquinolones include Levaquin, Avelox, Noroxin and Floxin.[470]

Seen in both human and veterinary medicine, fluoroquinolones are often used for genitourinary infections and for hospital-acquired infections connected to urinary catheters.[471] However, a string of dangerous side effects and FDA warnings have shed a negative light on the antibiotic class.

In 2008, the FDA added a boxed warning to fluoroquinolones about an increased risk of tendinitis and tendon rupture.[472]

According to the FDA's Dr. Renata Albrecht fluoroquinolone drugs increased the risk of an Achilles tendon rupture or tendinitis by three to four times.[473] The rupture could also occur suddenly, said Dr. Albrecht. "Sometimes it's been reported on the first day of taking a fluoroquinolone . . . a sudden snap or popping sound that is tendon rupture with no preceding warning." The risks are higher in people older than 60 and recipients of organ transplants, she added.[474]

7.17.1 Fluoroquinolone Warnings Continue

Warnings related to fluoroquinolones continued. In 2013, the FDA added a warning about the potential side effect of "permanent nerve damage."[475] In 2016, the FDA advised that fluoroquinolones should only be used for "certain uncomplicated infections" because of their "disabling side effects," which could involve the musculoskeletal system or nervous system.[476] In 2018, the FDA added warnings about hypoglycemia and mental health side effects.[477]

The risks were also recognized in the European Union. In 2018 an EU-wide review found fluoroquinolone-linked neuropathies associated with paraesthesia, pain in extremities, gait disturbance, depression, fatigue, memory impairment, sleep disorders and even impaired hearing, vision, taste and smell.[478]

Finally, in 2019, the FDA issued a new warning that could further limit fluoroquinolone usage. The agency found[479]

> *that fluoroquinolone antibiotics can increase the occurrence of rare but serious events of ruptures or tears in the main artery of the body, called the aorta. These tears, called aortic dissections, or ruptures of an aortic aneurysm can lead to dangerous bleeding or even death. They can occur with fluoroquinolones for systemic use given by mouth or through an injection . . .*
>
> *People at increased risk include those with a history of blockages or aneurysms (abnormal bulges) of the aorta or other blood vessels, high blood pressure, certain genetic disorders that involve blood vessel changes, and the elderly.*

7.17.2 Hormone Therapy Still Linked to Risks

It is a fluke of the news cycle that when a product's risks aren't communicated frequently, the product can be "forgiven" and thought safe again. In contrast to other toxic products such as cigarettes or toxins like lead or mercury, public opinion has softened on the dangers of hormone replacement therapy (HRT). HRT is a treatment for menopause. So it was noteworthy that follow-up of subjects in the federal Women's Health Initiative completed in 2019[480] revealed that "breast cancer risk from menopause hormones may last decades."[481,482] The Women's Health Initiative had previously established in 2002 that HRT increased the risk of breast cancer by 26% and cardiovascular events such as heart attacks, strokes and blood clots to an even greater degree. It was also linked to a greater risk of ovarian and endometrial cancers as well as lung cancer mortality.[483] HRT was also linked to increased risk in women of dementia,[484] hearing loss,[485] gallbladder disease,[486] urinary incontinence,[487] asthma,[488] melanoma[489] and joint replacement.[490] They were at greater risk of ovarian and endometrial cancers and dying from lung cancers.[491,492]

HRT also complicates cancer detection. In 1995, a publication in the journal *Radiology* noted that continuous combined HRT treatment led to "an increase in mammographic density."[493] HRT's deleterious effects on cancer risk and detection were so dramatic that the incidence of breast cancer fell 7% the year after millions of women stopped HRT (2003).[494] The rate fell 15% in women with estrogen-dependent cancers.[495,496]

In the opinion of this author, the myriad of HRT-induced health outcomes should have been embarrassing to the medical community because HRT's role in causing cancer should have been recognized much earlier. Unfortunately, this was not an isolated incident.

In 1979, research in the *New England Journal of Medicine* said:[497]

> *From July, 1975, to July, 1977, there was a sharp downward trend in the incidence of endometrial cancer that paralleled a substantial reduction in prescriptions for replacement estrogens. Incidence rates were estimated for estrogen users and nonusers among women 50 to 64 years of age with intact uteri; current long-term users had an annual risk for endometrial cancer between 1 and 3 per cent, whereas nonusers had a risk less than 1/10th as great. These incidence rates remained fairly constant over time among users and nonusers; the drop in overall incidence soon after estrogen use declined suggests that the increased risk associated with estrogens falls quickly after discontinuation. The reduction in incidence of endometrial cancer in this group practice was part of a general decline in the United States after 1975.*

7.17.3 Beware of Testosterone Marketing

There has been a lot more media coverage about hormone replacement for women than testosterone replacement for men, yet some of the same issues are at play. A 2015 paper in the *Journal of the American Geriatrics Society* noted that

> a combination of direct-to-consumer product advertising (DTCPA) and lax consensus guidelines for testosterone prescribing have, over the past decade, led to 10 and 40-fold increases in testosterone prescriptions in the United States and Canada, respectively, with Internet pharmacies playing a major role in the latter's increase.[498]

The journal authors, Thomas Perls, M.D., and David J. Handelsman, PhD, further wrote:

> *We join others who characterize the mass marketing of testosterone coupled with the permissive prescribing of testosterone for common, nonspecific, aging-related symptoms as disease mongering of declines in testosterone with advancing age. Disease mongering is defined as "the selling of sickness that widens the boundaries of illness and grows the markets for those who sell and deliver treatments." The prescribing of growth hormone for "antiaging" or "age management" is another example of disease mongering.*

As we noted earlier in this chapter, DTC advertising does less for consumers and patients than it does for drug makers and media outlets. The authors wrote that "when sophisticated mass marketing is directed toward people lacking the technical expertise to critically evaluate the deceptively simplified medical science claims" not only mongers disease but can "effectively pit patients against their doctors, pressuring them for compliant prescribing on demand and distorting clinical judgment."

There are at least two reasons that aggressive testosterone marketing is harmful, Dr. Perls told me in an interview.[499] First, less than one-half of 1% of men have true testosterone deficiency, which would require supplementation. Many other men are just pursuing body-building and acting out of the advertising message that testosterone is an anti-aging elixir. Second, side effects from testosterone administration can include cardiac rhythm disturbances like atrial fibrillation, low levels of good (HDL) cholesterol, symptoms of coronary artery disease and even psychiatric effects, he said.[500]

In summation, Dr. Perls told me, the testosterone supplementation craze resulted from aggressive marketing by drug makers, irresponsible prescribing and a lack of testosterone guidelines with teeth in them.

Learning from marketers of female hormones, marketers "invented the term 'andropause' for a condition that numerous endocrinology experts state does not exist and began selling testosterone," said Dr. Perls.

7.17.4 New PPI Questions

As many as 116 million prescriptions are written for GERD each year in the U.S., often PPIs according to data from the government's Medical Expenditure Panel Survey.[501] The PPI Prilosec was the eighth-most prescribed drug in the

U.S. and, along with other PPIs, has now become an over-the-counter drug.[502]

However, as many of 70% of patients overuse PPIs, according to David Jacobs, PharmD, PhD, assistant professor of pharmacy practice at the University at Buffalo School of Pharmacy and Pharmaceutical Sciences. He further asserts that PPIs should only be used on a short-term basis. There are serious risks to popular drugs if they are used long term.

According to 2017 research in *PLOS One*, "In patients with CAD [coronary artery disease], PPI use is independently associated with an increased incidence of HF [heart failure] and death."[503]

According to Kidney International,[504] PPI use is linked to an increased risk of acute kidney injury and incident chronic kidney disease, which can progress to end-stage renal disease.[505] PPI use is also correlated with osteoporosis in femur research, as reported in the *International Journal of Rheumatic Diseases* reported in 2016.[506]

Research in the *BMJ* Journal *Gut* found that PPIs were associated with the worsening of gastric atrophy, especially in patients infected with *Helicobacter pylori* (HP) and associated gastric cancer.[507] And a 2019 study in the journal *Nature Communications* even suggested that PPI users may be twice as likely to develop allergies than non-users.[508]

The medical literature has even questioned the actual value of PPIs in treating or preventing GERD. Research published in *Gastroenterology* in 2009 found that after taking the medications for eight weeks, healthy adults developed acid reflux symptoms, possibly from a rebound effect.[509]

The media continue to expose dangerous and ineffective drugs and fraudulent marketing of prescription drugs, and sometimes the offending drug makers are brought to justice with penalties and fines. Sadly, the media awareness of risky drugs and "bad actor" drug makers does not seem to be a deterrent to future wrongdoing.

NOTES

1. Pharma Bro' Shkreli is in prison. But Daraprim's price is still high. https://kffhealthnews.org/news/for-shame-pharma-bro-shkreli-is-in-prison-but-daraprims-price-is-still-high/
2. Luthra S. 'Pharma Bro' Shkreli is in prison, but Daraprim's price is still high. *KHN*, May 4, 2018. https://khn.org/news/for-shame-pharma-bro-shkreli-is-in-prison-but-daraprims-price-is-still-high/
3. Zarroli J. Martin Shkreli takes the fifth, but can't resist firing back. *NPR*, February 4, 2016. https://www.npr.org/sections/thetwo-way/2016/02/04/465596177/martin-shkreli-takes-the-fifth-but-cant-resist-firing-back
4. What's being done about EpiPen price hike, from $100 to $600? *Fox 9*, August 24, 2016. https://www.fox9.com/news/whats-being-done-about-epipen-price-hike-from-100-to-600
5. Ornstein C and Thomas K. Sloan Kettering cancer researchers correct the record by revealing company ties. *ProPublica*, October 12, 2018. https://www.propublica.org/article/sloan-ketting-researchers-reveal-company-ties
6. Ornstein C and Thomas K. Sloan Kettering cancer researchers correct the record by revealing company ties. *ProPublica*, October 12, 2018. https://www.propublica.org/article/sloan-ketting-researchers-reveal-company-ties
7. Oxtoby K. How biologics have changed the rules for Pharma. *Chemistry World*, May 7, 2019. https://www.chemistryworld.com/molecule-to-market/how-biologics-have-changed-the-rules-for-pharma/3010301.article
8. Biologics vs small molecule drugs: What's the difference? *Admescope*, November 19, 2018. https://www.admescope.com/whats-new/blog/2018/biologics-vs-small-molecule-drugs-whats-the-difference.html
9. Herman B. The top-selling drugs in the U.S. in 2019. *Axios*, August 12, 2020. https://www.axios.com/top-selling-drugs-america-2019-f32a8818-a37c-4581-a805-bcf73942c1de.html
10. House Committee on Oversight and Reform. Investigation of skyrocketing prescription drug prices, 2011. *Oversight House*. https://oversight.house.gov/investigations/investigation-of-skyrocketing-prescription-drug-prices
11. Gyawali B, Hey SP and Kesselheim AS. Assessment of the clinical benefit of cancer drugs receiving accelerated approval. *JAMA*, May 28, 2019. https://jamanetwork.com/journals/jamainternalmedicine/fullarticle/2733561
12. Hand S. The top 4 most expensive drugs in the US are hepatitis C treatments. *X Talks*, July 31, 2017. https://xtalks.com/expensive-drugs-in-the-us-hepatitis-c-treatments/
13. A drug maker halo for a covid vaccine? Not with this poor track record. *NewsBlaze News*. https://newsblaze.com/usnews/health/a-drug-maker-halo-for-a-covid-vaccine-not-with-this-track-record_171990/
14. U.S. Department of Justice. Justice Department announces global resolution of criminal and civil investigations with opioid manufacturer Purdue Pharma and civil settlement with members of the Sackler family. *U.S. DOJ*, October 21, 2020. https://www.justice.gov/opa/pr/justice-department-announces-global-resolution-criminal-and-civil-investigations-opioid
15. Bulik B. Pharma ups April TV spending for stuck-at-home viewers with AbbVie leading the way. *Fierce Pharma*, May 27, 2020. https://www.fiercepharma.com/marketing/ispot-pharma-tv-spending-for-april-jumps-abbvie-and-regeneron-sanofi-brands-top-list
16. Bulik B. Pharma ups April TV spending for stuck-at-home viewers with AbbVie leading the way. *Fierce Pharma*, May 27, 2020. https://www.fiercepharma.

com/marketing/ispot-pharma-tv-spending-for-april-jumps-abbvie-and-regeneron-sanofi-brands-top-list
17 Bulik B. Pharma ups April TV spending for stuck-at-home viewers with AbbVie leading the way. *Fierce Pharma*, May 27, 2020. https://www.fiercepharma.com/marketing/ispot-pharma-tv-spending-for-april-jumps-abbvie-and-regeneron-sanofi-brands-top-list
18 Harris G. Drug makers are advocacy group's biggest donors. *New York Times*, October 21, 2009. http://www.nytimes.com/2009/10/22/health/22nami.html?_r=0
19 Rosenberg M. Pharma funding advocacy groups. *Center for Health Journalism*, October 15, 2014. https://centerforhealthjournalism.org/2014/10/15/discredited-patient-group-fights-mental-illness
20 Healy M. Sold on drugs. *Los Angeles Times*, August 6, 2007. http://articles.latimes.com/2007/aug/06/health/he-sellingthepatient6/3
21 A drug maker halo for a covid vaccine? Not with this poor track record. *NewsBlaze News*. https://newsblaze.com/usnews/health/a-drug-maker-halo-for-a-covid-vaccine-not-with-this-track-record_171990/
22 Thomas K. and Pear R. Plan to limit some drugs in Medicare is criticized. *New York Times*, February 21, 2014. http://www.nytimes.com/2014/02/22/business/plan-to-alter-medicare-drug-coverage-draws-strong-opposition.html?_r=0
23 U.S. Department of Health and Human Services. What is the U.S. opioid epidemic? *HHS*, September 4, 2019. https://www.hhs.gov/opioids/about-the-epidemic/index.html
24 CDC. Understanding the epidemic. *CDC*, March 19, 2020. https://www.cdc.gov/drugoverdose/epidemic/index.html
25 Gillette F. American pain: Largest U.S. pill mill's rise and fall. *Bloomberg*, June 6, 2012. https://www.bloomberg.com/news/articles/2012-06-06/american-pain-the-largest-u-dot-s-dot-pill-mills-rise-and-fall
26 Frontline. A social history of America's most popular drugs. *PBS*, 2014. http://www.pbs.org/wgbh/pages/frontline/shows/drugs/buyers/socialhistory.html
27 What big pharma does not want you to know about the opioid epidemic. *Truthdig*. https://www.truthdig.com/articles/what-big-pharma-does-not-want-you-to-know-about-the-opioid-epidemic/
28 Lopez G. How big pharma got people hooked on dangerous opioids: And made tons of money off it. *Vox*, September 22, 2016. https://www.vox.com/2016/2/5/10919360/opioid-epidemic-chart
29 What big pharma does not want you to know about the opioid epidemic. *Truthdig*. https://www.truthdig.com/articles/what-big-pharma-does-not-want-you-to-know-about-the-opioid-epidemic/
30 Zee A. Promotion and marketing of OxyContin: Commercial triumph, public health tragedy. *American Journal of Public Health*, February 2009. https://www.ncbi.nlm.nih.gov/pmc/articles/PMC2622774/
31 Abuse and misuse of prescription drugs. ATrain education. https://www.atrainceu.com/content/1-abuse-and-misuse-prescription-drugs
32 Lopez G. How big pharma got people hooked on dangerous opioids: And made tons of money off it. *Vox*, September 22, 2016. https://www.vox.com/2016/2/5/10919360/opioid-epidemic-chart
33 What big pharma does not want you to know about the opioid epidemic. *Truthdig*. https://www.truthdig.com/articles/what-big-pharma-does-not-want-you-to-know-about-the-opioid-epidemic/
34 Lopez G. How big pharma got people hooked on dangerous opioids: And made tons of money off it. *Vox*, September 22, 2016. https://www.vox.com/2016/2/5/10919360/opioid-epidemic-chart
35 Fauber J. Narcotic painkiller use booming among elderly. *MedPage Today*, May 30, 2012. https://www.medpagetoday.com/geriatrics/painmanagement/32967
36 What big pharma does not want you to know about the opioid epidemic. *Truthdig*. https://www.truthdig.com/articles/what-big-pharma-does-not-want-you-to-know-about-the-opioid-epidemic/
37 Fauber J. Narcotic painkiller use booming among elderly. *MedPage Today*, May 30, 2012. https://www.medpagetoday.com/geriatrics/painmanagement/32967
38 What big pharma does not want you to know about the opioid epidemic. *Truthdig*. https://www.truthdig.com/articles/what-big-pharma-does-not-want-you-to-know-about-the-opioid-epidemic/
39 Vasudevan S. *Multidisciplinary Management of Chronic Pain: A Practical Guide for Clinicians*. Springer, 2012. https://www.amazon.com/Multidisciplinary-Management-Chronic-Pain-Clinicians/dp/3319203215
40 IMMPACT. Initiative on methods, measurement, and pain assessment in clinical trials. http://www.immpact.org
41 Rosenberg M. How big pharma and the FDA drive the opioid addiction epidemic. *Center for Health Journalism*, May 15, 2014. https://centerforhealthjournalism.org/2014/05/15/how-big-pharma-and-fda-drive-opioid-addiction-epidemic
42 Fauber J. Emails point to 'troubling' relationship between drug firms, regulators. *Journal Sentinel*, October 6, 2013. https://archive.jsonline.com/watchdog/watchdogreports/emails-point-to-troubling-relationship-between-drug-firms-regulators-b99113286z1-226692641.html/
43 Fauber J. Emails point to 'troubling' relationship between drug firms, regulators. *Journal Sentinel*, October 6, 2013. https://archive.jsonline.com/watchdog/watchdogreports/emails-point-to-troubling-relationship-between-drug-firms-regulators-b99113286z1-226692641.html/

44 How big pharma stoked the opioid epidemic. *OpEd News*. https://www.opednews.com/articles/How-Big-Pharma-Stoked-the-by-Martha-Rosenberg-Addiction_Drugs_Drugs_FDA-140514-303.html
45 University of Rochester Medical Center Robert H. Dworkin, Ph.D. https://www.urmc.rochester.edu/people/23059177-robert-h-dworkin
46 What big pharma does not want you to know about the opioid epidemic. *Truthdig*. https://www.truthdig.com/articles/what-big-pharma-does-not-want-you-to-know-about-the-opioid-epidemic/
47 FDA OKs new hydrocodone painkiller. *Health Day*, October 25, 2013. http://consumer.healthday.com/bone-and-joint-information-4/pain-health-news-520/fda-oks-new-hydrocodone-painkiller-681512.html
48 Johnson A. FDA approves OxyContin for children as young as 11. *NBC News*, August 14, 2015. https://www.nbcnews.com/health/health-news/fda-approves-oxycontin-children-young-11-n409621http:/www.nbcnews.com/health/health-news/fda-approves-oxycontin-children-young-11-n409621
49 What big pharma does not want you to know about the opioid epidemic. *Truthdig*. https://www.truthdig.com/articles/what-big-pharma-does-not-want-you-to-know-about-the-opioid-epidemic/
50 Harris G. Actions by congress on opioids haven't included limiting them. *New York Times*, May 19, 2016. https://www.nytimes.com/2016/05/19/us/politics/opioid-dea-addiction.html
51 Harriet Ryan, Lisa Girion and Scott Glover You want a description of hell? *Los Angeles Times*, May 5, 2016. https://www.latimes.com/projects/oxycontin-part1/
52 What big pharma does not want you to know about the opioid epidemic. *Truthdig*. https://www.truthdig.com/articles/what-big-pharma-does-not-want-you-to-know-about-the-opioid-epidemic/
53 Ryan H., et al. You want a description of hell? *Los Angeles Times*, May 5, 2016. https://www.latimes.com/projects/oxycontin-part1/
54 Ryan H. Full coverage: Oxycontin investigation. *Los Angeles Times*, May 27, 2016. https://www.latimes.com/projects/la-me-oxycontin-full-coverage/
55 Gillette F. American pain: Largest U.S. pill mill's rise and fall. *Bloomberg*, June 6, 2012. https://www.bloomberg.com/news/articles/2012-06-06/american-pain-the-largest-u-dot-s-dot-pill-mills-rise-and-fall
56 Sontag D. Addiction treatment with a dark side. *New York Times*, November 11, 2017. https://www.nytimes.com/2013/11/17/health/in-demand-in-clinics-and-on-the-street-bupe-can-be-savior-or-menace.html
57 Sontag D. Addiction treatment with a dark side. *New York Times*, November 11, 2017. https://www.nytimes.com/2013/11/17/health/in-demand-in-clinics-and-on-the-street-bupe-can-be-savior-or-menace.html
58 How big pharma is cashing in on addiction to alcohol and drugs. "Global possibilities." https://globalpossibilities.org/how-big-pharma-is-cashing-in-on-addiction-to-alcohol-and-drugs/
59 Rosenberg M and Pringle E. How big pharma is cashing in on addiction to alcohol and illicit drugs. *AlterNet*, March 18, 2016. https://www.alternet.org/2016/03/how-big-pharma-cashing-addiction-alcohol-and-illicit-drugs/
60 Kraus M. Statement of the American Society of Addiction Medicine Consensus Panel on the use of buprenorphine in office-based treatment of opioid addiction. *Journal of Addiction Medicine* 5(4), December 2011. https://www.asam.org/docs/advocacy/use-of-buprenorphine-in-office-based-treatment-of-opioid-addiction.pdf
61 National Institute on Drug Abuse (NIDA) Mission. *NIDA*, November 28, 2018. https://www.nih.gov/about-nih/what-we-do/nih-almanac/national-institute-drug-abuse-nida; https://www.nih.gov/news-events/news-releases/nida-experts-discuss-latest-science-stimulant-abuse-asam-annual-scientific-meeting-addiction-specialists-learn-about-newest-treatments-development
62 NIDA experts to discuss latest science on stimulant abuse at asam annual scientific meeting addiction specialists to learn about newest treatments in development. *NIH*, April 25, 2007. https://www.nih.gov/news-events/news-releases/nida-experts-discuss-latest-science-stimulant-abuse-asam-annual-scientific-meeting-addiction-specialists-learn-about-newest-treatments-development
63 About us. *The National Alliance of Advocates for Buprenorphine Treatment*, September 23, 2016. https://www.naabt.org/about_us.cfm
64 Joseph A. Richard Sackler, member of family behind OxyContin, was granted patent for addiction treatment. *Stat News*, September 7, 2018. https://www.statnews.com/2018/09/07/richard-sackler-member-of-family-behind-oxycontin-was-granted-patent-for-addiction-treatment/
65 Idrus A. Biotech FDA panel slams Alkermes' opioid-based depression drug. *Fierce Biotech*, November 2, 2018. https://www.fiercebiotech.com/biotech/fda-panel-slams-alkermes-opioid-based-depression-drug#:~:text=It%20has%20been%20a%20long,a%20likely%20rejection%20come%20January
66 Case of large-scale opioid diversion puts hospitals on alert. *Pain Medicine News*, April 2014. https://www.painmedicinenews.com/Policy-Management/Article/09-14/Case-of-Large-Scale-Opioid-Diversion-Puts-Hospitals-on-Alert/28093/ses=ogst
67 Mintz H. Santa Clara County sues drug makers for hyping painkillers. *San Jose Mercury News*, May 22, 2014. https://www.mercurynews.com/2014/05/22/

santa-clara-county-sues-drug-makers-for-hyping-painkillers/
68 Elias P. Money laundering charge added to FedEx drug case. *Associated Press*, August 15, 2014. https://www.memphisdailynews.com/news/2014/aug/15/money-laundering-charge-added-to-fedex-drug-case/
69 O'Keefe M. Feds quietly investigating prescription drug abuse in NFL locker. *New York Daily News*, July 12, 2014. https://www.nydailynews.com/sports/i-team/feds-probe-prescription-drug-abuse-nfl-locker-rooms-sources-article-1.1864651
70 O'Keefe M. Feds quietly investigating prescription drug abuse in NFL locker. *New York Daily News*, July 12, 2014. https://www.nydailynews.com/sports/i-team/feds-probe-prescription-drug-abuse-nfl-locker-rooms-sources-article-1.1864651
71 Meier B. Profiting from pain. *New York Times*, June 23, 2012. https://www.nytimes.com/2013/06/23/sunday-review/profiting-from-pain.html
72 Meier B. Profiting from pain. *New York Times*, June 23, 2012. https://www.nytimes.com/2013/06/23/sunday-review/profiting-from-pain.html
73 Meier B. Pain pills add cost and delays to job injuries. *New York Times*, June 2, 2013. https://www.nytimes.com/2012/06/03/health/painkillers-add-costs-and-delays-to-workplace-injuries.html
74 Meier B. Pain pills add cost and delays to job injuries. *New York Times*, June 2, 2013. https://www.nytimes.com/2012/06/03/health/painkillers-add-costs-and-delays-to-workplace-injuries.html
75 Webster BS, Verma SK and Gatchel RJ. Relationship between early opioid prescribing for acute occupational low back pain and disability duration, medical costs, subsequent surgery and late opioid use. *Spine* 32(19), 2007. https://pubmed.ncbi.nlm.nih.gov/17762815/
76 TrueValueMetrics . . . impact accounting for the 21st century. https://www.truevaluemetrics.org/DBadmin/DBtxt001.php?vv1=txt00011475
77 Fauber J. Studies find little evidence of benefit from long-term opioid use: Most clinical trials haven't gone beyond 6 weeks. *Milwaukee Journal Sentinel*, January 12, 2015. http://archive.jsonline.com/watchdog/watchdogreports/studies-find-little-evidence-of-benefit-from-long-term-opioid-use-b99421747z1-288307521.html
78 Fauber J. Many injured workers remain on opioids, study finds. *Milwaukee Journal Sentinel*, October 2, 2012. http://archive.jsonline.com/features/health/many-injured-workers-remain-on-opioids-study-finds-km72v1g-172331511.html
79 Fishman S. *Responsible Opioid Prescribing.* Washington, DC: Waterford Life Sciences, 2012.
80 OpEd News. A doctor talks about the opioid addiction epidemic. https://www.opednews.com/populum/page.php?f=A-Doctor-Talks-About-the-O-by-Sridhar-Vasudevan-Addictions_Doctors_Drugs_Patients-160327-625.html
81 Fishman S. *Responsible Opioid Prescribing.* Washington, DC: Waterford Life Sciences, 2012.
82 McAnally H. Opioid-induced hyperalgesia: It's a thing. *MedPage Today*, January 27, 2020. https://www.medpagetoday.com/blogs/pain-points/84551
83 Opioids maker purdue facing $2.2 trillion suit. https://www.medicaldaily.com/purdue-sued-role-opioid-epidemic-455515
84 Opioid overdose crisis. *National Institute on Drug Abuse*, May 27, 2020. https://www.drugabuse.gov/drug-topics/opioids/opioid-overdose-crisis
85 The insanity of taxpayer-funded addiction. *New York Times*, November 10, 2017. https://books.google.com/books?id=O7DXDwAAQBAJ&pg=PA165&lpg=PA165&dq=NIH++" nonaddictive+painkiller and+new+treatment for+addiction+and+overdoses."&source=bl&ots=kUdFtdHN9t&sig=ACfU3U3cF6vni1hE9lprxmFG1rtC9QDd4w&hl=en&sa=X&ved=2ahUKEwj-0IPujfHsAhWaZM0KHdGZA_QQ6AEwA3oECAEQAg#v=onepage&q&f=false
86 Pain management and the opioid crisis. *New York Times*, November 19, 2017. https://www.nytimes.com/2017/11/19/opinion/drug-makers-opioids.html
87 Isidore C. OxyContin maker to plead guilty to federal criminal charges, pay $8 billion, and will close the company. *CNN*, October 27, 2020. https://www.cnn.com/2020/10/21/business/purdue-pharma-guilty-plea/index.html
88 Achenbach J. 4 Drug companies agree to $26 billion opioid settlement. *Washington Post*, November 5, 2020. https://www.washingtonpost.com/health/opioid-settlement-drug-distributors/2020/11/05/6a8da214-1fc7-11eb-b532-05c751cd5dc2_story.html
89 Lam B. The changing landscape of hepatitis C virus therapy: Focus on interferon-free treatment. *Therapeutic Advances in Gastroenterology* 8(5), 2015. https://www.ncbi.nlm.nih.gov/pmc/articles/PMC4530432/
90 Kodjak A. Hepatitis drug among the most costly for Medicaid. *NPR*, December 15, 2015. https://www.npr.org/sections/health-shots/2015/12/15/459873815/hepatitis-drug-among-the-most-costly-for-medicaid
91 Special feature: First year after launch. *Pharma Live.* undated. https://www.pharmalive.com/special-feature-first-year-after-launch-2/#:~:text=Launched%20in%20October%202014%2C%20Harvoni,%2410.28%20billion%20the%20year%20before
92 Robbins R. Inside the $100 million ad blitz for a $1,100-a-pill drug for hepatitis C. *Stat News*, March 8, 2016. https://www.statnews.com/2016/03/08/harvoni-hepatitisc-ads/
93 Roy A. The Sovaldi tax: Gilead can't justify the price it's asking for hepatitis C therapy. *Forbes*, June 17, 2014. https://www.forbes.com/sites/theapothecary/2014/06/17/the-sovaldi-tax-gilead-cant-justify-the-price-its-asking-americans-to-pay/?sh=38eb39a25670

94 Roy A. The Sovaldi tax: Gilead can't justify the price it's asking for hepatitis C therapy. *Forbes*, June 17, 2014. https://www.forbes.com/sites/theapothecary/2014/06/17/the-sovaldi-tax-gilead-cant-justify-the-price-its-asking-americans-to-pay/?sh=38eb39a25670
95 Kodjak A. Hepatitis drug among the most costly for Medicaid. *NPR*, December 15, 2015. https://www.npr.org/sections/health-shots/2015/12/15/459873815/hepatitis-drug-among-the-most-costly-for-medicaid
96 Senate Finance Committee releases results of investigation into Gilead's pricing strategy for hepatitis-C drugs. *Policy Med*, May 5, 2018. https://www.policymed.com/2015/12/senate-finance-committee-releases-results-of-investigation-into-gileads-pricing-strategy-for-hepatitis-c-drugs.html
97 Senate Finance Committee releases results of investigation into Gilead's pricing strategy for hepatitis-C drugs. *Policy Med*, May 5, 2018. https://www.policymed.com/2015/12/senate-finance-committee-releases-results-of-investigation-into-gileads-pricing-strategy-for-hepatitis-c-drugs.html
98 Senate Finance Committee releases results of investigation into Gilead's pricing strategy for hepatitis-C drugs. *Policy Med*, May 5, 2018. https://www.policymed.com/2015/12/senate-finance-committee-releases-results-of-investigation-into-gileads-pricing-strategy-for-hepatitis-c-drugs.html
99 Senate Finance Committee releases results of investigation into Gilead's pricing strategy for hepatitis-C drugs. *Policy Med*, May 5, 2018. https://www.policymed.com/2015/12/senate-finance-committee-releases-results-of-investigation-into-gileads-pricing-strategy-for-hepatitis-c-drugs.html
100 Robbins R. Inside the $100 million ad blitz for a $1,100-a-pill drug for hepatitis C. *Stat News*, March 8, 2016.https://www.statnews.com/2016/03/08/harvoni-hepatitisc-ads/
101 Robbins R. Inside the $100 million ad blitz for a $1,100-a-pill drug for hepatitis C. *Stat News*, March 8, 2016.https://www.statnews.com/2016/03/08/harvoni-hepatitisc-ads/
102 Robbins R. Inside the $100 million ad blitz for a $1,100-a-pill drug for hepatitis C. *Stat News*, March 8, 2016.https://www.statnews.com/2016/03/08/harvoni-hepatitisc-ads/
103 Robbins R. Inside the $100 million ad blitz for a $1,100-a-pill drug for hepatitis C. *Stat News*, March 8, 2016.https://www.statnews.com/2016/03/08/harvoni-hepatitisc-ads/
104 Pharma 'screening' is a ploy to seize more patients. *Intrepid Report.com.* http://www.intrepidreport.com/archives/24640
105 Horgan J. Why screening teens for mental illness is a terrible idea. *Scientific American*, September 2, 2011. https://blogs.scientificamerican.com/cross-check/why-screening-teens-for-mental-illness-is-a-terrible-idea/
106 Just J. Overdiagnosis: When finding cancer can do more harm than good. *Science Blog*, March 6, 2018. https://scienceblog.cancerresearchuk.org/2018/03/06/overdiagnosis-when-finding-cancer-can-do-more-harm-than-good/
107 Brody J. When to get your bone density tested. *New York Times*, July 16, 2018. https://www.nytimes.com/2018/07/16/well/when-to-get-your-bone-density-tested.html
108 Spiegel A. How a bone disease grew to fit the prescription. *National Public Radio*, December 21, 2009. https://www.npr.org/2009/12/21/121609815/how-a-bone- disease-grew-to-fit-the-prescription
109 Erviti J. Oral bisphosphonates are associated with increased risk of subtrochanteric and diaphyseal fractures in elderly women: A nested case–control study. https://bmjopen.bmj.com/content/3/1/e002091
110 Heng C. Bisphosphonate-related osteonecrosis of the jaw in patients with osteoporosis. *American Family Physician*, July 15, 2012. https://www.aafp.org/afp/2012/0615/p1134.html
111 Rosenberg M. Internal Merck emails revealed. *Center for Health Journalism*, December 3, 2012. https://centerforhealthjournalism.org/2012/12/03/internal-merck-emails-revealed
112 Drug prices and fast approvals can harm patients. https://www.kevinmd.com/2023/11/drug-prices-and-fast-approvals-can-harm-patients.html
113 July 28th is World Hepatitis Day. *Generation Hep*, January 24, 2017. https://generationhep.com/#block-views-news_and_events_blog-block_1
114 Big Pharma. *Big Food, Big Lies.* Prometheus: Martha Rosenberg, 2023.
115 To boost sales, Gilead's hep C awareness ad focuses on baby boomers. *Fierce Pharma*, February 23, 2017. https://www.fiercepharma.com/marketing/baby-boomers-targeted-gilead-hepatitis-c-awareness-campaign-even-as-drug-s-fortunes-drop
116 Our partners: Corporations. *CDC Foundation*, 2020. https://www.cdcfoundation.org/partner-list/corporations
117 Our partners: Corporations. *CDC Foundation*, 2020. https://www.cdcfoundation.org/partner-list/corporations
118 Pharma Guy. Gilead pushes hep C testing in baby boomers as its blockbusters plummet. *Pharma Marketing*, February 23, 2017. https://www.pharma-mkting.com/blog/to-boost-sales-gileads-hep-c-awareness/
119 Grady D. Are new drugs for HCV safe? A report raises concerns. *New York Times*, January 25, 2017. https://www.nytimes.com/2017/01/24/health/hepatitis-c-antiviral-drug-study.html
120 FDA Drug Safety Communication. FDA warns about the risk of hepatitis B reactivating in some patients treated with direct-acting antivirals for hepatitis C. *FDA*, October 4, 2016. https://www.fda.gov/drugs/drug-safety-and-availability/

fda-drug-safety-communication-fda-warns-about-risk-hepatitis-b-reactivating-some-patients-treated
121 Grady D. Are new drugs for hepatitis C safe? A report raises concerns. *New York Times*, January 24, 2017. https://www.nytimes.com/2017/01/24/health/hepatitis-c-antiviral-drug-study.html
122 Williams S. The 3 best-selling drugs in the world. *Motley Fool*, October 20, 2013. https://www.fool.com/investing/general/2013/10/20/the-3-best-selling-drugs-in-the-world.aspx
123 King S. The best selling drugs since 1996: Why Abbvie's Humira is set to eclipse Pfizer's Lipitor. *Forbes*, July 15, 2013. https://www.forbes.com/sites/simonking/2013/07/15/the-best-selling-drugs-since-1996-why-abbvies-humira-is-set-to-eclipse-pfizers-lipitor/?sh=7a9f2be66a8d
124 Simon M. 100 Best-selling, most prescribed branded drugs through June. *Medscape*, August 13, 2015. https://www.medscape.com/viewarticle/849457
125 Rosenberg M. FDA waved through asthma drugs despite falsified trials. *opednews.com*, May 27, 2009. http://www.opednews.com/articles/FDA-Waved-Through-Asthma-D-by-Martha-Rosenberg-090527-1.html
126 Rosenberg M. FDA waved through asthma drugs despite falsified trials. *opednews.com*, May 27, 2009. http://www.opednews.com/articles/FDA-Waved-Through-Asthma-D-by-Martha-Rosenberg-090527-1.html
127 Rosenberg M. FDA waved through asthma drugs despite falsified trials. *opednews.com*, May 27, 2009. http://www.opednews.com/articles/FDA-Waved-Through-Asthma-D-by-Martha-Rosenberg-090527-1.html
128 Dissident Voice. Fraudulent trials behind asthma drugs cited. https://dissidentvoice.org/2009/05/fraudulent-trials-behind-asthma-drugs-cited/
129 Rosenberg M. FDA waved through asthma drugs despite falsified trials. *opednews.com*, May 27, 2009. http://www.opednews.com/articles/FDA-Waved-Through-Asthma-D-by-Martha-Rosenberg-090527-1.html
130 Dissident Voice. Fraudulent trials behind asthma drugs cited. https://dissidentvoice.org/2009/05/fraudulent-trials-behind-asthma-drugs-cited/
131 FDA. FDA establishment inspection report, February 20, 2001. https://jimedwardsnrx.files.wordpress.com/2009/06/may-5-1999-tucson-eir.pdf
132 Grossman J, Smith LJ, Wilson AM and Thyrum PT. Long-term safety and efficacy of zafirlukast in the treatment of asthma: Interim results of an open-label extension trial. *Annals of Allergy, Asthma & Immunology* 82(4), 1999. https://pubmed.ncbi.nlm.nih.gov/10227334/
133 Edwards J. FDA's asthma drug warning comes after complaints about testing facility. *CBS News*, June 15, 2009. https://www.cbsnews.com/news/fdas-asthma-drug-warning-comes-after-complaints-about-testing-facility/
134 Gambro Healthcare to pay more than $350 million in Medicare fraud case. *HC Pro*, December 8, 2004. http://www.hcpro.com/CCP-44084-862/Gambro-Healthcare-to-pay-more-than-350-million-in-Medicare-fraud-case.html
135 Wikipedia Omalizumab. https://en.wikipedia.org/wiki/Omalizumab
136 Wikipedia Omalizumab. https://en.wikipedia.org/wiki/Omalizumab
137 Rosenberg M. Novartis and Genentech whistleblowers charge illegal asthma drug sales. *Center For Health Journalism*, March 12, 2016. https://centerforhealthjournalism.org/fellowships/projects/novartis-and-genentech-whistleblowers-charge-illegal-asthma-drug-sales
138 Rosenberg M. Novartis and Genentech whistleblowers charge illegal asthma drug sales. *Center For Health Journalism*, March 12, 2016. https://centerforhealthjournalism.org/fellowships/projects/novartis-and-genentech-whistleblowers-charge-illegal-asthma-drug-sales
139 Did Novartis and Genentech get away with this big marketing scam? *OpEd News*. https://www.opednews.com/populum/page.php?f=Did-Novartis-and-Genentech-by-Martha-Rosenberg-Asthma_Children_Complaint_Doctors-160310-950.html
140 Xolair. Prescribing information. *Genetech and Novartis*, 2020. https://www.gene.com/download/pdf/xolair_prescribing.pdf
141 Xolair. Prescribing information. *Genetech and Novartis*, 2020. https://www.gene.com/download/pdf/xolair_prescribing.pdf
142 Xolair. Prescribing information. *Genetech and Novartis*, 2020. https://www.gene.com/download/pdf/xolair_prescribing.pdf
143 Xolair. Prescribing information. *Genetech and Novartis*, 2020. https://www.gene.com/download/pdf/xolair_prescribing.pdf
144 *United States of America v Novartis*. Civil Action No. 12-CV-10962-JLT. Corporate Crime Reporter, March 17, 2015. https://www.corporatecrimereporter.com/wp-content/uploads/2016/01/Xolair.KellyComplaint.MOSTCURRENT.100912.245pm.p
145 Did Novartis and Genentech get away with this big marketing scam? *OpEd News*. https://www.opednews.com/populum/page.php?f=Did-Novartis-and-Genentech-by-Martha-Rosenberg-Asthma_Children_Complaint_Doctors-160310-950.html
146 Did Novartis and Genentech get away with this big marketing scam? *OpEd News*. https://www.opednews.com/populum/page.php?f=Did-Novartis-and-Genentech-by-Martha-Rosenberg-Asthma_Children_Complaint_Doctors-160310-950.html
147 Rosenberg M. Novartis and Genentech whistleblowers charge illegal asthma drug sales. *Center For*

Health Journalism, March 12, 2016. https://centerforhealthjournalism.org/fellowships/projects/novartis-and-genentech-whistleblowers-charge-illegal-asthma-drug-sales
148 Did Novartis and Genentech get away with this big marketing scam? *OpEd News*. https://www.opednews.com/populum/page.php?f=Did-Novartis-and-Genentech-by-Martha-Rosenberg-Asthma_Children_Complaint_Doctors-160310-950.html
149 *United States of America v Novartis*. Civil Action No. 12-CV-10962-JLT. Corporate Crime Reporter, March 17, 2015. https://www.corporatecrimereporter.com/wp-content/uploads/2016/01/Xolair.KellyComplaint.MOSTCURRENT.100912.245pm.p
150 Rosenberg M. Novartis and Genentech whistleblowers charge illegal asthma drug sales. *Center for Health Journalism*, March 12, 2016. https://centerforhealthjournalism.org/fellowships/projects/novartis-and-genentech-whistleblowers-charge-illegal-asthma-drug-sales
151 Did Novartis and Genentech get away with this big marketing scam? *OpEd News*. https://www.opednews.com/populum/page.php?f=Did-Novartis-and-Genentech-by-Martha-Rosenberg-Asthma_Children_Complaint_Doctors-160310-950.html
152 *United States of America v Novartis*. Civil Action No. 12-CV-10962-JLT. Corporate Crime Reporter, March 17, 2015. https://www.corporatecrimereporter.com/wp-content/uploads/2016/01/Xolair.KellyComplaint.MOSTCURRENT.100912.245pm.p
153 *United States of America v Novartis*. Civil Action No. 12-CV-10962-JLT. Corporate Crime Reporter, March 17, 2015. https://www.corporatecrimereporter.com/wp-content/uploads/2016/01/Xolair.KellyComplaint.MOSTCURRENT.100912.245pm.p
154 *United States of America v Novartis*. Civil Action No. 12-CV-10962-JLT. Corporate Crime Reporter, March 17, 2015. https://www.corporatecrimereporter.com/wp-content/uploads/2016/01/Xolair.KellyComplaint.MOSTCURRENT.100912.245pm.p
155 Lieberman P. The risk and management of anaphylaxis in the setting of immunotherapy. *American Journal of Rhinology & Allergy* 26(6), November–December 2012. https://www.ncbi.nlm.nih.gov/pmc/articles/PMC3903104/
156 Did Novartis and Genentech get away with this big marketing scam? *OpEd News*. https://www.opednews.com/populum/page.php?f=Did-Novartis-and-Genentech-by-Martha-Rosenberg-Asthma_Children_Complaint_Doctors-160310-950.html
157 *United States of America v Novartis*. Civil Action No. 12-CV-10962-JLT. Corporate Crime Reporter, March 17, 2015. https://www.corporatecrimereporter.com/wp-content/uploads/2016/01/Xolair.KellyComplaint.MOSTCURRENT.100912.245pm.pdf
158 *United States of America v Novartis*. Civil Action No. 12-CV-10962-JLT. Corporate Crime Reporter, March 17, 2015. https://www.corporatecrimereporter.com/wp-content/uploads/2016/01/Xolair.KellyComplaint.MOSTCURRENT.100912.245pm.pdf
159 *United States of America v Novartis*. Civil Action No. 12-CV-10962-JLT. Corporate Crime Reporter, March 17, 2015. https://www.corporatecrimereporter.com/wp-content/uploads/2016/01/Xolair.KellyComplaint.MOSTCURRENT.100912.245pm.pdf
160 *United States of America v Novartis*. Civil Action No. 12-CV-10962-JLT. Corporate Crime Reporter, March 17, 2015. https://www.corporatecrimereporter.com/wp-content/uploads/2016/01/Xolair.KellyComplaint.MOSTCURRENT.100912.245pm.pdf
161 Did Novartis and Genentech get away with this big marketing scam? *OpEd News*. https://www.opednews.com/populum/page.php?f=Did-Novartis-and-Genentech-by-Martha-Rosenberg-Asthma_Children_Complaint_Doctors-160310-950.html
162 *United States of America v Novartis*. Civil Action No. 12-CV-10962-JLT. Corporate Crime Reporter, March 17, 2015. https://www.corporatecrimereporter.com/wp-content/uploads/2016/01/Xolair.KellyComplaint.MOSTCURRENT.100912.245pm.pdf
163 *United States of America v Novartis*. Civil Action No. 12-CV-10962-JLT. Corporate Crime Reporter, March 17, 2015. https://www.corporatecrimereporter.com/wp-content/uploads/2016/01/Xolair.KellyComplaint.MOSTCURRENT.100912.245pm.pdf
164 *United States of America v Novartis*. Civil Action No. 12-CV-10962-JLT. Corporate Crime Reporter, March 17, 2015. https://www.corporatecrimereporter.com/wp-content/uploads/2016/01/Xolair.KellyComplaint.MOSTCURRENT.100912.245pm.pdf
165 *United States of America v Novartis*. Civil Action No. 12-CV-10962-JLT. Corporate Crime Reporter, March 17, 2015. https://www.corporatecrimereporter.com/wp-content/uploads/2016/01/Xolair.KellyComplaint.MOSTCURRENT.100912.245pm.pdf
166 Hitt E. FDA panel says omalizumab safe in pediatric patients. *Medscape*, January 31, 2012. https://www.medscape.com/viewarticle/757825?pa=AX12T26%2FIqKidJpJe%2FekuM1Kx7q9JNfnO7mZsYmL3bWnoZ8NN4BvzGYgmZI36SX3VrJxKJt4DRD8mxYr6kYfOw%3D%3D
167 Hitt E. FDA panel says omalizumab safe in pediatric patients. *Medscape*, January 31, 2012. https://www.medscape.com/viewarticle/757825?pa=AX12T26%2FIqKidJpJe%2FekuM1Kx7q9JNfnO7mZsYmL3bWnoZ8NN4BvzGYgmZI36SX3VrJxKJt4DRD8mxYr6kYfOw%3D%3D
168 Namazy J. The Xolair Pregnancy Registry (EXPECT): The safety of omalizumab use during pregnancy. *Journal of Allergy and Clinical Immunology* 135(2), February 2015: 407–412. https://pubmed.ncbi.nlm.nih.gov/25441639/
169 Namazy J. The Xolair Pregnancy Registry (EXPECT): The safety of omalizumab use during pregnancy.

Journal of Allergy and Clinical Immunology 135(2), February 2015: 407–412. https://pubmed.ncbi.nlm.nih.gov/25441639/
170 FDA Drug Safety Communication. FDA approves label changes for asthma drug Xolair (omalizumab), including describing slightly higher risk of heart and brain adverse events. *FDA*, September 26, 2014. https://www.fda.gov/drugs/drug-safety-and-availability/fda-drug-safety-communication-fda-approves-label-changes-asthma-drug-xolair-omalizumab-including
171 Did Novartis and Genentech get away with this big marketing scam? *OpEd News*. https://www.opednews.com/populum/page.php?f=Did-Novartis-and-Genentech-by-Martha-Rosenberg-Asthma_Children_Complaint_Doctors-160310-950.html
172 Staton T. Judge tosses Xolair kickback suit against Novartis, Genentech. *Fierce Pharma*, March 18, 2015. https://www.fiercepharma.com/regulatory/judge-tosses-xolair-kickback-suit-against-novartis-genentech
173 Staton T. Judge tosses Xolair kickback suit against Novartis, Genentech. *Fierce Pharma*, March 18, 2015. https://www.fiercepharma.com/regulatory/judge-tosses-xolair-kickback-suit-against-novartis-genentech
174 Morgenson G. It was his dream job. *NBC News*, July 7, 2020. https://www.nbcnews.com/news/amp/ncna1232971
175 Acting Manhattan U.S. attorney announces $678 million settlement of fraud lawsuit against Novartis Pharmaceuticals for operating sham speaker programs through which it paid over $100 million to doctors to unlawfully induce them to prescribe Novartis drugs. *U.S. Department of Justice*, July 1, 2020. https://www.justice.gov/usao-sdny/pr/acting-manhattan-us-attorney-announces-678-million-settlement-fraud-lawsuit-against
176 Acting Manhattan U.S. attorney announces $678 million settlement of fraud lawsuit against Novartis Pharmaceuticals for operating sham speaker programs through which it paid over $100 million to doctors to unlawfully induce them to prescribe Novartis drugs. *U.S. Department of Justice*, July 1, 2020. https://www.justice.gov/usao-sdny/pr/acting-manhattan-us-attorney-announces-678-million-settlement-fraud-lawsuit-against
177 *United States of America v. Novartis Pharmaceuticals Corp.* 11 Civ. 0071 (PGG). https://www.justice.gov/usao-sdny/press-release/file/1291316/download
178 Morgenson G. It was his dream job. *NBC News*, July 7, 2020. https://www.nbcnews.com/news/amp/ncna1232971
179 Advair: How safe is this drug? *MedPage Today*. https://www.medpagetoday.com/allergyimmunology/asthma/36000
180 Advair: How safe is this drug? *MedPage Today*. https://www.medpagetoday.com/allergyimmunology/asthma/36000
181 Fauber J. Advair boomed amid health risks. *Seacoast Online*, November 25, 2012. https://www.seacoastonline.com/article/20121125/LIFE/211250312
182 Fauber J. Advair boomed amid health risks. *Seacoast Online*, November 25, 2012. https://www.seacoastonline.com/article/20121125/LIFE/211250312
183 Advair: How safe is this drug? *MedPage Today*. https://www.medpagetoday.com/allergyimmunology/asthma/36000
184 Fauber J. Advair boomed amid health risks. *Seacoast Online*, November 25, 2012. https://www.seacoastonline.com/article/20121125/LIFE/211250312
185 Andrew Mcivor R, Pizzichini E, Turner MO, Hussack P, Hargreave FE and Sears MR. Potential masking effects of salmeterol on airway inflammation in asthma. *American Journal of Respiratory and Critical Care Medicine*. https://pubmed.ncbi.nlm.nih.gov/9731027/
186 Cardet JC, Jiang X, Lu Q, Gerard N, McIntire K, Boushey HA, Castro M, Chinchilli VM, Codispoti CD, Dyer AM and Holguin F. Loss of bronchoprotection with ICS plus LABA treatment, β-receptor dynamics, and the effect of alendronate. *Journal of Allergy and Clinical Immunology* 144(2), August 2019. https://pubmed.ncbi.nlm.nih.gov/30872116/
187 Cardet JC, Jiang X, Lu Q, Gerard N, McIntire K, Boushey HA, Castro M, Chinchilli VM, Codispoti CD, Dyer AM and Holguin F. Loss of bronchoprotection with ICS plus LABA treatment, β-receptor dynamics, and the effect of alendronate. *Journal of Allergy and Clinical Immunology* 144(2), August 2019. https://pubmed.ncbi.nlm.nih.gov/30872116/
188 Wikipedia prenylation. https://en.wikipedia.org/wiki/Prenylation#:~:text=Farnesylation%20is%20a%20type%20of,interactions%20and%20protein%E2%80%93membrane%20interactions
189 Fauber J. Advair boomed amid health risks. *Seacoast Online*, November 25, 2012. https://www.seacoastonline.com/article/20121125/LIFE/211250312
190 Fauber J. Advair boomed amid health risks. *Seacoast Online*, November 25, 2012. https://www.seacoastonline.com/article/20121125/LIFE/211250312
191 Black boxes: Health warning or profit warning? *Intrepid Report.com*. http://www.intrepidreport.com/archives/29205
192 Sears M. The FDA-mandated trial of safety of long-acting beta-agonists in asthma: Finality or futility? *Thorax*, July 12, 2012. https://thorax.bmj.com/content/thoraxjnl/early/2012/08/01/thoraxjnl-2012-202414.full.pdf
193 Hitti M. New warnings for 3 asthma drugs. *Web MD*, November 18, 2005. https://www.webmd.com/asthma/news/20051118/new-warnings-for-3-asthma-drugs

194 Chowdhury B and Dal Pan G. The FDA and safe use of long-acting beta-agonists in the treatment of asthma. *New England Journal of Medicine*, April 1, 2010. https://www.nejm.org/doi/full/10.1056/NEJMp1002074
195 Badrul Chowdhury. Director, division of pulmonary, allergy, and rheumatology products, CDER. *Linked In*, 2020. https://www.linkedin.com/in/badrul-chowdhury-md-phd-2461a5151/
196 Adverse event reporting related to antiretroviral agents at FDA. *FDA*, June 11, 2010. https://forumresearch.org/storage/documents/PV/4%2006112010_ii1_dal%20pan.pdf
197 Adverse event reporting related to antiretroviral agents at FDA. *FDA*, June 11, 2010. https://forumresearch.org/storage/documents/PV/4%2006112010_ii1_dal%20pan.pdf
198 Fauber J. Advair boomed amid health risks. *Seacoast Online*, November 25, 2012. https://www.seacoastonline.com/article/20121125/LIFE/211250312
199 Fauber J. Advair boomed amid health risks. *Seacoast Online*, November 25, 2012. https://www.seacoastonline.com/article/20121125/LIFE/211250312
200 Advair: How safe is this drug? *MedPage Today*. https://www.medpagetoday.com/allergyimmunology/asthma/36000
201 Fauber J. Advair boomed amid health risks. *Seacoast Online*, November 25, 2012. https://www.seacoastonline.com/article/20121125/LIFE/211250312
202 https://www.justice.gov/opa/pr/glaxosmithkline-plead-guilty-and-pay-3-billion-resolve-fraud-allegations-and-failure-report
203 Guidelines for the diagnosis and management of asthma. *National Asthma Education and Prevention Program Expert Panel Report 3*. 2007. https://www.nhlbi.nih.gov/sites/default/files/media/docs/asthsumm.pdf
204 *United States of America v Novartis*. Civil Action No. 12-CV-10962-JLT. *Corporate Crime Reporter*, March 17, 2015. https://www.corporatecrimereporter.com/wp-content/uploads/2016/01/Xolair.KellyComplaint.MOSTCURRENT.100912.245pm.pdf
205 Are you taking these asthma drugs? https://www.huffpost.com/entry/asthma-drugs-research_b_1119163
206 Gerth J. Overuse, safety questions cloud Advair's ascent to asthma blockbuster. *Pro Publica*, May 19, 2015. https://www.propublica.org/article/overuse-safety-questions-cloud-advair-ascent-to-asthma-blockbuster
207 Black boxes: Health warning or profit warning. *Intrepid Report.com*. http://www.intrepidreport.com/archives/29205
208 FDA Drug Safety Communication. FDA requires post-market safety trials for long-acting beta-agonists (LABAs). *FDA*, April 15, 2011. https://www.fda.gov/drugs/drug-safety-and-availability/fda-drug-safety-communication-fda-requires-post-market-safety-trials-long-acting-beta-agonists-labas
209 Sullivan M. FDA reverses warning on LABA-containing asthma medications. *Chest Physician*, July 2, 2018. https://www.mdedge.com/chestphysician/article/169302/asthma/fda-reverses-warning-laba-containing-asthma-medications
210 Sullivan M. FDA reverses warning on LABA-containing asthma medications. *Chest Physician*, July 2, 2018. https://www.mdedge.com/chestphysician/article/169302/asthma/fda-reverses-warning-laba-containing-asthma-medications
211 Top 10 asthma drugs in the world. *Market Research Reports*, September 7, 2019. https://www.marketresearchreports.com/blog/2019/09/07/top-10-asthma-drugs-world#:~:text=9.-,Singulair,12months%20of%20age%20and%20older
212 Drug Safety Developments. FOX 5 investigates: Singulair. *Drug Injury*, November 10, 2010. https://www.drug-injury.com/drug_injury/2010/11/fox-5-investigates-singulair.html
213 Drug Safety Developments. FOX 5 investigates: Singulair. *Drug Injury*, November 10, 2010. https://www.drug-injury.com/drug_injury/2010/11/fox-5-investigates-singulair.html
214 Drug Safety Developments. FOX 5 investigates: Singulair. *Drug Injury*, November 10, 2010. https://www.drug-injury.com/drug_injury/2010/11/fox-5-investigates-singulair.html
215 Black boxes: Health warning or profit warning? *Intrepid Report.com*. http://www.intrepidreport.com/archives/29205
216 Rosenberg M. Popular asthma drug's deadly side-effects revealed (once Merck stopped making money from it). *Organic Consumers Association*, October 15, 2014. https://www.organicconsumers.org/news/popular-asthma-drugs-deadly-side-effects-revealed-once-merck-stopped-making-money-it
217 Rosenberg M. Popular asthma drug's deadly side-effects revealed (once Merck stopped making money from it). *Organic Consumers Association*, October 15, 2014. https://www.organicconsumers.org/news/popular-asthma-drugs-deadly-side-effects-revealed-once-merck-stopped-making-money-it
218 Rosenberg M. Popular asthma drug's deadly side-effects revealed (once Merck stopped making money from it). *Organic Consumers Association*, October 15, 2014. https://www.organicconsumers.org/news/popular-asthma-drugs-deadly-side-effects-revealed-once-merck-stopped-making-money-it
219 Rosenberg M. Popular asthma drug's deadly side-effects revealed (once Merck stopped making money from it). *Organic Consumers Association*, October 15, 2014. https://www.organicconsumers.org/news/popular-asthma-drugs-deadly-side-effects-revealed-once-merck-stopped-making-money-it
220 Updated information on leukotriene inhibitors: Montelukast, zafirlukast and zileuton. *FDA*,

August 28, 2009. https://wayback.archive-it.org/7993/20171114124744/https://www.fda.gov/Drugs/DrugSafety/PostmarketDrugSafetyInformationforPatientsandProviders/DrugSafetyInformation-forHeathcareProfessionals/ucm165489.htm
221 Patients remarks about singulair. *Askapatient.* https://www.askapatient.com/viewrating.asp?drug=20829&name=SINGULAIR
222 Patients remarks about singulair. *Askapatient.* https://www.askapatient.com/viewrating.asp?drug=20829&name=SINGULAIR
223 Patients remarks about singulair. *Askapatient.* https://www.askapatient.com/viewrating.asp?drug=20829&name=SINGULAIR
224 Letters. Exercise-induced asthma. *New England Journal of Medcine*, December 10, 1998. https://www.nejm.org/doi/full/10.1056/NEJM199812103392412
225 Black boxes: Health warning or profit warning? *Intrepid Report.com.* http://www.intrepidreport.com/archives/29205
226 Application 20-829. Center For Drug Evaluation and Research. *FDA*, January 28, 1998. https://www.accessdata.fda.gov/drugsatfda_docs/nda/98/020829s000_Singular_Pharma.pdf
227 Application 20-829. Center For Drug Evaluation and Research. *FDA*, January 28, 1998. https://www.accessdata.fda.gov/drugsatfda_docs/nda/98/020829s000_Singular_Pharma.pdf
228 Why were they approved? *Dissident Voice.* https://dissidentvoice.org/2011/11/why-were-they-approved/
229 Are You Taking These Asthma Drugs? *Huffington Post.* https://www.huffpost.com/entry/asthma-drugs-research_b_1119163
230 Application 20-829. Center for Drug Evaluation and Research. FDA, January 28, 1998. https://www.accessdata.fda.gov/drugsatfda_docs/nda/98/020829s000_Singular_Pharma.pdf
231 Are You Taking These Asthma Drugs? *Huffington Post.* https://www.huffpost.com/entry/asthma-drugs-research_b_1119163
232 Why were they approved? Dissident Voice. https://dissidentvoice.org/2011/11/why-were-they-approved/
233 Application 20-829. Center for Drug Evaluation and Research. *FDA*, January 28, 1998. https://www.accessdata.fda.gov/drugsatfda_docs/nda/98/020829s000_Singular_Pharma.pdf
234 Another wonder drug isn't so great once it goes off patent. *Dissident Voice.* https://dissidentvoice.org/2014/11/another-wonder-drug-isnt-so-great-once-it-goes-off-patent/
235 Application 20-829. Center for Drug Evaluation and Research. *FDA*, January 28, 1998, p. 98. https://www.accessdata.fda.gov/drugsatfda_docs/nda/98/020829s000_Singular_Pharma.pdf
236 Application 20-829. Center for Drug Evaluation and Research. *FDA*, January 28, 1998, p. 98. https://www.accessdata.fda.gov/drugsatfda_docs/nda/98/020829s000_Singular_Pharma.pdf
237 Another wonder drug isn't so great once it goes off patent. *Dissident Voice.* https://dissidentvoice.org/2014/11/another-wonder-drug-isnt-so-great-once-it-goes-off-patent/
238 Rosenberg M. Black boxes: Health warning or profit warning? *Kevin MD*, February 1, 2020. https://www.kevinmd.com/blog/2020/02/black-boxes-health-warning-or-profit-warning.html; https://www.kevinmd.com/blog/2020/02/black-boxes-health-warning-or-profit-warning.html
239 Aldea Perona A, García-Sáiz M and Sanz Álvarez E. Psychiatric disorders and montelukast in children: A disproportionality analysis of the vigibase®. *Drug Safety* 39(1), January 2016: 69–78. https://pubmed.ncbi.nlm.nih.gov/26620206/
240 Law SW, Wong AY, Anand S, Wong IC and Chan EW. Neuropsychiatric events associated with leukotriene-modifying agents: A systematic review. *Drug Safety* 41(3), March 2018: 253–265. https://pubmed.ncbi.nlm.nih.gov/29076063/
241 Black boxes: Health warning or profit warning? *Intrepid Report.com.* http://www.intrepidreport.com/archives/29205
242 Food and Drug Administration joint meeting of the pediatric advisory committee & drug safety and risk management advisory committee. *FDA*, September 27, 2019. https://www.fda.gov/media/132560/download
243 Food and Drug Administration joint meeting of the pediatric advisory committee & drug safety and risk management advisory committee. *FDA*, September 27, 2019. https://www.fda.gov/media/132560/download
244 Children's Health Defense. Experts urge caution as American academy of pediatrics calls for mental health screenings for newborns to 21-year-olds. https://childrenshealthdefense.org/defender/american-academy-pediatrics-mental-health-screenings-depression-children/
245 Rosenberg M. Black boxes: Health warning or profit warning? *Kevin MD*, February 1, 2020. https://www.kevinmd.com/blog/2020/02/black-boxes-health-warning-or-profit-warning.html; https://www.kevinmd.com/blog/2020/02/black-boxes-health-warning-or-profit-warning.html
246 Rosenberg M. Black boxes: Health warning or profit warning? *Kevin MD*, February 1, 2020. https://www.kevinmd.com/blog/2020/02/black-boxes-health-warning-or-profit-warning.html; https://www.kevinmd.com/blog/2020/02/black-boxes-health-warning-or-profit-warning.html
247 Rosenberg M. Black boxes: Health warning or profit warning? *Kevin MD*, February 1, 2020. https://www.kevinmd.com/blog/2020/02/black-boxes-health-warning-or-profit-warning.html; https://www.

kevinmd.com/blog/2020/02/black-boxes-health-warning-or-profit-warning.html

248 Black boxes: Health warning or profit warning? *Intrepid Report.com.* http://www.intrepidreport.com/archives/29205

249 Rosenberg M. Black boxes: Health warning or profit warning? *Kevin MD*, February 1, 2020. https://www.kevinmd.com/blog/2020/02/black-boxes-health-warning-or-profit-warning.html; https://www.kevinmd.com/blog/2020/02/black-boxes-health-warning-or-profit-warning.html

250 Black boxes: Health warning or profit warning? *Intrepid Report.com.* http://www.intrepidreport.com/archives/29205

251 Mundell E. Antidepressant use in U.S. soars by 65 percent in 15 years. *CBS News*, August 16, 2017. https://www.cbsnews.com/news/antidepressant-use-soars-65-percent-in-15-years/

252 Ducharme J. U.S. suicide rates are the highest they've been since world war II. *Time*, June 20, 2019. https://time.com/5609124/us-suicide-rate-increase/

253 Black boxes: Health warning or profit warning? *Intrepid Report.com.* http://www.intrepidreport.com/archives/29205

254 FDA requires boxed warning about serious mental health side effects for asthma and allergy drug montelukast (Singulair); advises restricting use for allergic rhinitis. *FDA*, March 4, 2020. https://www.fda.gov/drugs/drug-safety-and-availability/fda-requires-boxed-warning-about-serious-mental-health-side-effects-asthma-and-allergy-drug

255 FDA briefing materials for the September 27, 2019 joint meeting of the pediatric and drug safety and risk management advisory committees. FDA. https://www.fda.gov/advisory-committees/pediatric-advisory-committee/fda-briefing-materials-september-27-2019-joint-meeting-pediatric-and-drug-safety-and-risk-management

256 Rosenberg M. 7 Drugs whose risks emerged when they went off patent, January 18, 2014. https://centerforhealthjournalism.org/2014/01/18/7-drugs-whose-risks-emerged-when-they-went-patent

257 Ventola C. Direct-to-consumer pharmaceutical advertising-therapeutic or toxic? *Pharmacy and Therapeutics* 36(10), October 2011. https://www.ncbi.nlm.nih.gov/pmc/articles/PMC3278148/

258 Ventola C. Direct-to-consumer pharmaceutical advertising-therapeutic or toxic? *Pharmacy and Therapeutics* 36(10), October 2011. https://www.ncbi.nlm.nih.gov/pmc/articles/PMC3278148/

259 Zito PM, Bistas KG, Patel P, et al. Finasteride. [Updated 2024 Feb 28]. In: StatPearls [Internet]. Treasure Island (FL): StatPearls Publishing; 2025 Jan-. Available from: https://www.ncbi.nlm.nih.gov/books/NBK513329/

260 Zito PM, Bistas KG, Patel P, et al. Finasteride. [Updated 2024 Feb 28]. In: StatPearls [Internet]. Treasure Island (FL): StatPearls Publishing; 2025 Jan-. Available from: https://www.ncbi.nlm.nih.gov/books/NBK513329/

261 Zito PM, Bistas KG, Patel P, et al. Finasteride. [Updated 2024 Feb 28]. In: StatPearls [Internet]. Treasure Island (FL): StatPearls Publishing; 2025 Jan-. Available from: https://www.ncbi.nlm.nih.gov/books/NBK513329/

262 Male pattern baldness. *WebMD*, March 1, 2010. https://www.webmd.com/skin-problems-and-treatments/hair-loss/hair-loss-introduction-mens

263 Commonly used drug can make men stop enjoying sex: Irreversibly. *Alternet.org.* https://www.alternet.org/2014/07/commonly-used-drug-can-make-men-stop-enjoying-sex-irreversibly

264 Direct to consumer advertising: Finasteride for male pattern hair loss. *Therapeutics Initiative*, April 30, 2001. https://www.ti.ubc.ca/2001/04/30/direct-to-consumer-advertising-finasteride-for-male-pattern-hair-loss/

265 Direct to consumer advertising: Finasteride for male pattern hair loss. *Therapeutics Initiative*, April 30, 2001. https://www.ti.ubc.ca/2001/04/30/direct-to-consumer-advertising-finasteride-for-male-pattern-hair-loss/

266 Number of nations logging onto PFSFoundation.org rose 29% in 2013. *PFSFoundation.org*, January 6, 2014. https://www.pfsfoundation.org/news/nations-logging-onto-post-finasteride-syndrome-foundation-website-29-2013/

267 Commonly used drug can make men stop enjoying sex: Irreversibly. *Alternet.org.* https://www.alternet.org/2014/07/commonly-used-drug-can-make-men-stop-enjoying-sex-irreversibly

268 Finasteride print ad, undated. https://i.pinimg.com/originals/f4/63/6d/f4636dae9dd7af93de040ade3302b0a1.jpg

269 Propecia ProHair Circles campaign. *Dentsu*, September 1, 2009. https://www.adsoftheworld.com/media/print/propecia_prohair_circles_1

270 Propecia twins 4 years later. *Insight Health & Wellness.* https://www.youtube.com/watch?v=X9JMAgRfppw

271 Commonly used drug can make men stop enjoying sex: Irreversibly. *Alternet.org.* https://www.alternet.org/2014/07/commonly-used-drug-can-make-men-stop-enjoying-sex-irreversibly

272 Propecia side effects. *Drug Reporter.* http://drugreporter.com/propecia/side-effects/

273 Propecia help. https://forum.propeciahelp.com/t/change-in-penis-size/4090

274 Commonly used drug can make men stop enjoying sex: Irreversibly. *Alternet.org.* https://www.alternet.org/2014/07/commonly-used-drug-can-make-men-stop-enjoying-sex-irreversibly

275 McCasker T. Negative side effects of Propecia. *Ask Men.* https://in.askmen.com/health-issues/1097313/article/negative-propecia-side-effects

276 Commonly used drug can make men stop enjoying sex: Irreversibly. *Alternet.org*. https://www.alternet.org/2014/07/commonly-used-drug-can-make-men-stop-enjoying-sex-irreversibly
277 McCasker T. Negative side effects of Propecia. *Ask Men*. https://in.askmen.com/health-issues/1097313/article/negative-propecia-side-effects
278 Commonly used drug can make men stop enjoying sex: Irreversibly. *Alternet.org*. https://www.alternet.org/2014/07/commonly-used-drug-can-make-men-stop-enjoying-sex-irreversibly
279 Irwig M. Persistent sexual side effects of finasteride: Could they be permanent? *The Journal of Sexual Medicine* 9(11), November 2012: 2927–2932. https://pubmed.ncbi.nlm.nih.gov/22789024/
280 Irwig M. Persistent sexual side effects of finasteride: Could they be permanent? *The Journal of Sexual Medicine* 9(11), November 2012: 2927–2932. https://pubmed.ncbi.nlm.nih.gov/22789024/
281 Caruso D, Abbiati F, Giatti S, Romano S, Fusco L, Cavaletti G and Melcangi RC. Patients treated for male pattern hair with finasteride show, after discontinuation of the drug, altered levels of neuroactive steroids in cerebrospinal fluid and plasma. *The Journal of Steroid Biochemistry and Molecular Biology* 146, February 2015: 74–79. https://pubmed.ncbi.nlm.nih.gov/24717976/
282 Ali A et al. Persistent sexual dysfunction and suicidal ideation in young men treated with low-dose finasteride: A pharmacovigilance study. *Pharmacotherapy* 35(7), July 2015: 687–695. https://pubmed.ncbi.nlm.nih.gov/26133534/
283 Khera M. Penile vascular abnormalities in young men with persistent side effects after finasteride use for the treatment of androgenic alopecia. *Translational Andrology and Urology*, 2020. https://files.constantcontact.com/dcf09377601/ffc37595-15ab-4cfa-826e-17dd3fff06c8.pdf
284 Hair loss drug finasteride may reduce risk of prostate cancer. *Healthline*, January 28, 2019. https://www.healthline.com/health-news/prostate-cancer-drug-effective-in-clinical-trial#Years-of-data
285 Center for Drug Evaluation and Research. Approval package for Propecia. *FDA*, April 11, 2013. https://www.accessdata.fda.gov/drugsatfda_docs/nda/2011/020788Orig1s018.pdf
286 Center for Drug Evaluation and Research. Approval package for Propecia. *FDA*, April 11, 2013. https://www.accessdata.fda.gov/drugsatfda_docs/nda/2011/020788Orig1s018.pdf
287 Commonly used drug can make men stop enjoying sex: Irreversibly. *Alternet.org*. https://www.alternet.org/2014/07/commonly-used-drug-can-make-men-stop-enjoying-sex-irreversibly
288 Center for Drug Evaluation and Research. Approval package for Propecia. *FDA*, April 11, 2013. https://www.accessdata.fda.gov/drugsatfda_docs/nda/2011/020788Orig1s018.pdf
289 Patient information PROPECIA. *Merck*. September 2013. https://www.merck.com/product/usa/pi_circulars/p/propecia/propecia_ppi.pdf
290 Propecia. Highlights of prescribing information. *Merck & Co*, January 2014. https://www.accessdata.fda.gov/drugsatfda_docs/label/2014/020788s024lbl.pdf
291 Propecia drug approval package. *FDA*, December 19, 1997. https://www.accessdata.fda.gov/drugsatfda_docs/nda/97/020788_propecia_toc.cfm
292 Commonly used drug can make men stop enjoying sex: Irreversibly. *Alternet.org*. https://www.alternet.org/2014/07/commonly-used-drug-can-make-men-stop-enjoying-sex-irreversibly
293 Propecia tablets, 1 mg medical review part 3. *FDA*. https://www.accessdata.fda.gov/drugsatfda_docs/nda/97/20788_PROPECIA%20TABLETS,%201MG_MEDR_P3.PDF
294 Propecia tablets, 1 mg medical review part 3. *FDA*. https://www.accessdata.fda.gov/drugsatfda_docs/nda/97/20788_PROPECIA%20TABLETS,%201MG_MEDR_P3.PDF
295 Commonly used drug can make men stop enjoying sex: Irreversibly. *Alternet.org*. https://www.alternet.org/2014/07/commonly-used-drug-can-make-men-stop-enjoying-sex-irreversibly
296 Propecia tablets, 1 mg medical review part 3. *FDA*. https://www.accessdata.fda.gov/drugsatfda_docs/nda/97/20788_PROPECIA%20TABLETS,%201MG_MEDR_P3.PDF
297 Propecia tablets, 1 mg medical review part 3. *FDA*. https://www.accessdata.fda.gov/drugsatfda_docs/nda/97/20788_PROPECIA%20TABLETS,%201MG_MEDR_P3.PDF
298 Commonly used drug can make men stop enjoying sex: Irreversibly. *Alternet.org*. https://www.alternet.org/2014/07/commonly-used-drug-can-make-men-stop-enjoying-sex-irreversibly
299 Propecia side effects UK. *Propecia Victims United*, 2014. http://www.propeciasideeffects.co.uk/my-propecia-side-effects-story.html; http://www.propeciasideeffects.co.uk/my-propecia-side-effects-story.html
300 Commonly used drug can make men stop enjoying sex: Irreversibly. *Alternet.org*. https://www.alternet.org/2014/07/commonly-used-drug-can-make-men-stop-enjoying-sex-irreversibly
301 Rosenberg M. Commonly used drug can make men stop enjoying sex: Irreversibly. *AlterNet*, July 9, 2014. https://www.alternet.org/2014/07/commonly-used-drug-can-make-men-stop-enjoying-sex-irreversibly/
302 Controversial baldness treatment still sold. *Dissident Voice*. https://dissidentvoice.org/2014/09/controversial-baldness-treatment-still-sold/
303 Propecia side effects UK. *Propecia Victims United*, 2014. http://www.propeciasideeffects.co.uk/my-propecia-side-effects-story.html

304 Controversial baldness treatment still sold. *Dissident Voice*. https://dissidentvoice.org/2014/09/controversial-baldness-treatment-still-sold/
305 Khera M, Than JK, Anaissie J, Antar A, Song W, Losso B, Pastuszak A, Kohn T and Mirabal JR. Penile vascular abnormalities in young men with persistent side effects after finasteride use for the treatment of androgenic alopecia. *Translational Andrology and Urology* 9(3), June 2020. https://www.ncbi.nlm.nih.gov/pmc/articles/PMC7354335/
306 Nguyen DD, Marchese M, Cone EB, Paciotti M, Basaria S, Bhojani N and Trinh QD. Investigation of suicidality and psychological adverse events in patients treated with finasteride. *JAMA Dermatology*, November 11, 2020. https://jamanetwork.com/journals/jamadermatology/article-abstract/2772818
307 Nguyen DD, Marchese M, Cone EB, Paciotti M, Basaria S, Bhojani N and Trinh QD. Investigation of suicidality and psychological adverse events in patients treated with finasteride. *JAMA Dermatology*, November 11, 2020. https://jamanetwork.com/journals/jamadermatology/article-abstract/2772818
308 Levine D. Court let Merck hide secrets about a popular drug's risks. *Reuters*, September 11, 2019. https://www.reuters.com/investigates/special-report/usa-courts-secrecy-propecia/
309 https://www.reuters.com/investigates/special-report/usa-courts-secrecy-propecia/
310 Finasteride market is slated to surpass $130 million by 2026, says Global Market Insights Inc. *Global Market Insights*, March 9, 2020. https://www.globenewswire.com/news-release/2020/03/09/1996989/0/en/Finasteride-Market-is-slated-to-surpass-130-million-by-2026-Says-Global-Market-Insights-Inc.html
311 How biologics have changed the rules for pharma. *Chemistry World*, May 7, 2019. https://www.chemistryworld.com/molecule-to-market/how-biologics-have-changed-the-rules-for-pharma/3010301.article
312 How biologics have changed the rules for pharma. *Chemistry World*, May 7, 2019. https://www.chemistryworld.com/molecule-to-market/how-biologics-have-changed-the-rules-for-pharma/3010301.article
313 2018 Global life sciences outlook. *Deloitte*, p. 5. https://www2.deloitte.com/content/dam/Deloitte/global/Documents/Life-Sciences-Health-Care/gx-lshc-ls-outlook-2018.pdf
314 Malaviya A and Mehra N. fascinating story of the discovery & development of biologicals for use in clinical medicine. *Indian Journal of Medical Research* 148(3), September 2018. https://www.ncbi.nlm.nih.gov/pmc/articles/PMC6251261/
315 Monaco C. Anti-TNF therapy: Past, present and future. *International Immunology* 27(1), January 2015. https://academic.oup.com/intimm/article/27/1/55/2950852 (graph under subhead what are the other indications for anti-TNF therapy?)
316 Eustice C. How are Enbrel, Remicade, and Humira different? *Very Well Health*, February 5, 2020. https://www.verywellhealth.com/comparing-enbrel-remicade-and-humira-drugs-189233#:~:text=Humira%20cost%20between%20%241%2C800%20and,four%20weeks%20or%20eight%20weeks
317 Herman B. The top-selling drugs in the U.S. in 2019. *Axios*, August 12, 2020. https://www.axios.com/top-selling-drugs-america-2019-f32a8818-a37c-4581-a805-bcf73942c1de.html
318 Terry M. Report: Projected sales of 10 top-selling drugs through 2024. *Biospace*, August 16, 2019. https://www.biospace.com/article/top-10-drug-sales-projected-through-2024/
319 AbbVie spins off from Abbott. *Gen*, January 2, 2013. https://www.genengnews.com/news/abbvie-spins-off-from-abbott/
320 Abbott's HUMIRA® approved in the European Union for treatment of moderate-to-severe plaque psoriasis. *Newswire Today*, December 20, 2007. https://www.newswiretoday.com/news/27630/Abbotts-HUMIRA-Approved-in-the-European-Union-for-Treatment-of-Moderate-to-Severe-Plaque-Psoriasis/
321 Accounts in review. *Media Post*, March 9, 2009. https://www.mediapost.com/publications/article/101614/humira.html
322 Japsen B. Abbott says arthritis drug will be free for seniors. *Chicago Tribune*, January 7, 2003. https://www.chicagotribune.com/news/ct-xpm-2003-01-07-0301070320-story.html
323 Pharma tries to cash in on covid shutdowns with its best-selling drug. *CounterPunch.org*. https://www.counterpunch.org/2020/07/20/pharma-tries-to-cash-in-on-covid-shutdowns-with-its-best-selling-drug/
324 Japsen B. Abbott says arthritis drug will be free for seniors. *Chicago Tribune*, January 7, 2003. https://www.chicagotribune.com/news/ct-xpm-2003-01-07-0301070320-story.html
325 Pharma tries to cash in on covid shutdowns with its best-selling drug. *CounterPunch.org*. https://www.counterpunch.org/2020/07/20/pharma-tries-to-cash-in-on-covid-shutdowns-with-its-best-selling-drug/
326 Fauber J. What's behind the surge of prescriptions for risky, expensive medications? Millions from drugmakers. *Milwaukee Journal Sentinel*, August 7, 2019. https://www.jsonline.com/story/news/investigations/2019/08/07/biologic- drug-makers-pay-doctors-prescribe-risky-pricey-medications/1901753001/
327 Fauber J. What's behind the surge of prescriptions for risky, expensive medications? Millions from drugmakers. *Milwaukee Journal Sentinel*, August 7, 2019. https://www.jsonline.com/story/news/investigations/2019/08/07/biologic- drug-makers-pay-doctors-prescribe-risky-pricey-medications/1901753001/
328 Costly drugs with Bizarre origins raise questions. *Best Case Leads*. https://bestcaseleads.com/costly-drugs-with-bizarre-origins-raise-questions/

329 Fauber J. What's behind the surge of prescriptions for risky, expensive medications? Millions from drugmakers. *Milwaukee Journal Sentinel*, August 7, 2019. https://www.jsonline.com/story/news/investigations/2019/08/07/biologic- drug-makers-pay-doctors-prescribe-risky-pricey-medications/1901753001/
330 Pharma tries to cash in on covid shutdowns with its best-selling drug. *CounterPunch.org*. https://www.counterpunch.org/2020/07/20/pharma-tries-to-cash-in-on-covid-shutdowns-with-its-best-selling-drug/
331 Silverman E. AbbVie pays $24 million to settle lawsuit over using 'nurse ambassadors' to boost Humira sales. *Stat News*, August 7, 2020. https://www.statnews.com/pharmalot/2020/08/07/abbvie-humira-california-nurse-ambassadors-kickbacks/
332 Lis K. Tumor necrosis factor inhibitors: State of knowledge. *Archives of Medical Science*, December 22, 2014. https://www.ncbi.nlm.nih.gov/pmc/articles/PMC4296073/#:~:text=For%20TNF%20inhibitors%2C%20three%20warnings,other%20malignancies%2C%20some% 20fatal%2C%20in
333 Enbrel. Highlights of prescribing information, March 2020. https://www.pi.amgen.com/~/media/amgen/repositorysites/pi-amgen-com/enbrel/enbrel_pi.ashx
334 Humira. Highlights of prescribing information, December 2020. https://www.rxabbvie.com/pdf/humira.pdf
335 Kemanetzoglou E and Andreadou E. CNS demyelination with TNF-α blockers. *Current Neurology and Neuroscience Reports*, March 21, 2017. https://www.ncbi.nlm.nih.gov/pmc/articles/PMC5364240/
336 Crowe K and Fauber J. Biologic medications for arthritis and psoriasis have flooded the market: And been linked to 34,000 deaths. *Milwaukee Journal Sentinel*, May 30, 2019. https://www.jsonline.com/story/news/investigations/2019/05/30/arthritis-psoriasis-drugs-darker-aspect-34-000-reports-deaths/1206103001/
337 Crowe K and Fauber J. Biologic medications for arthritis and psoriasis have flooded the market: And been linked to 34,000 deaths. *Milwaukee Journal Sentinel*, May 30, 2019. https://www.jsonline.com/story/news/investigations/2019/05/30/arthritis-psoriasis-drugs-darker-aspect-34-000-reports-deaths/1206103001/
338 Crowe K and Fauber J. Biologic medications for arthritis and psoriasis have flooded the market: And been linked to 34,000 deaths. *Milwaukee Journal Sentinel*, May 30, 2019. https://www.jsonline.com/story/news/investigations/2019/05/30/arthritis-psoriasis-drugs-darker-aspect-34-000-reports-deaths/1206103001/
339 Pharma tries to cash in on covid shutdowns with its best-selling drug. *CounterPunch.org*. https://www.counterpunch.org/2020/07/20/pharma-tries-to-cash-in-on-covid-shutdowns-with-its-best-selling-drug/
340 Fauber J. What's behind the surge of prescriptions for risky, expensive medications? Millions from drugmakers. *Milwaukee Journal Sentinel*, August 7, 2019. https://www.jsonline.com/story/news/investigations/2019/08/07/biologic- drug-makers-pay-doctors-prescribe-risky-pricey-medications/1901753001/
341 Fauber J. What's behind the surge of prescriptions for risky, expensive medications? Millions from drugmakers. *Milwaukee Journal Sentinel*, August 7, 2019. https://www.jsonline.com/story/news/investigations/2019/08/07/biologic- drug-makers-pay-doctors-prescribe-risky-pricey-medications/1901753001/
342 Fauber J. What's behind the surge of prescriptions for risky, expensive medications? Millions from drugmakers. *Milwaukee Journal Sentinel*, August 7, 2019. https://www.jsonline.com/story/news/investigations/2019/08/07/biologic- drug-makers-pay-doctors-prescribe-risky-pricey-medications/1901753001/
343 Fauber J. What's behind the surge of prescriptions for risky, expensive medications? Millions from drugmakers. *Milwaukee Journal Sentinel*, August 7, 2019. https://www.jsonline.com/story/news/investigations/2019/08/07/biologic- drug-makers-pay-doctors-prescribe-risky-pricey-medications/1901753001/
344 Pharma tries to cash in on covid shutdowns with its best-selling drug. *CounterPunch.org*. https://www.counterpunch.org/2020/07/20/pharma-tries-to-cash-in-on-covid-shutdowns-with-its-best-selling-drug/
345 FDA requests removal of all ranitidine products (Zantac) from the market. *FDA*, April 1, 2020. https://www.fda.gov/news-events/press-announcements/fda-requests-removal-all-ranitidine-products-zantac-market
346 Wikipedia ranitidine. https://en.wikipedia.org/wiki/Ranitidine
347 San Diego Zantac Lawsuit: crot4d. https://helbocklaw.com/services/san-diego-zantac-lawsuit/
348 Wikipedia ranitidine. https://en.wikipedia.org/wiki/Ranitidine
349 Ranitidine. Oral tablet. *Healthline*, May 17, 2018. https://www.healthline.com/health/ranitidine-oral-tablet#side-effects
350 Statement from Janet Woodcock, M.D., director of FDA's Center for Drug Evaluation and Research, on impurities found in diabetes drugs outside the U.S. *FDA*, December 5, 2019. https://www.fda.gov/news-events/press-announcements/statement-janet-woodcock-md-director-fdas-center-drug-evaluation-and-research-impurities-found
351 FDA requests removal of all ranitidine products (Zantac) from the market. *FDA*, April 1, 2020. https://www.fda.gov/news-events/press-announcements/fda-requests-removal-all-ranitidine-products-zantac-market
352 FDA requests removal of all ranitidine products (Zantac) from the market. *FDA*, April 1, 2020. https://www.fda.gov/news-events/press-announcements/fda-requests-removal-all-ranitidine-products-zantac-market

353 Wikipedia Ranitidine. https://en.wikipedia.org/wiki/Ranitidine
354 Wikipedia Ranitidine. https://en.wikipedia.org/wiki/Ranitidine
355 FDA requests removal of all ranitidine products (Zantac) from the market. *FDA*, April 1, 2020. https://www.fda.gov/news-events/press-announcements/fda-requests-removal-all-ranitidine-products-zantac-market
356 FDA requests removal of all ranitidine products (Zantac) from the market. *FDA*, April 1, 2020. https://www.fda.gov/news-events/press-announcements/fda-requests-removal-all-ranitidine-products-zantac-market
357 Papantonio M. Zantac lawsuit. *Consumer Safety*, December 6, 2020. https://www.consumersafety.org/zantac/lawsuit/
358 Moncivais K. Zantac manufacturers under investigation by the Department of Justice. *Consumer Safety*, October 29, 2020. https://www.consumersafety.org/news/doj-zantac-investigation/
359 Flora S. Cimetidine, ranitidine, and their mutagenic nitroso derivatives. *Lancet* 2(8253), October 31, 1981: 993–994. https://pubmed.ncbi.nlm.nih.gov/6117765/
360 Tsuji G, Yokoo H, Demizu Y, Abe Y, Masada S, Uchiyama N, Tsutsumi T and Yamamoto E. Safety of ranitidine. *Lancet* 2(8255), November 14, 1981: 1119. https://pubmed.ncbi.nlm.nih.gov/6118570/
361 https://www.consumersafety.org/news/doj-zantac-investigation/
362 Sagonowsky E. Sanofi, GlaxoSmithKline disclose DOJ investigation into Zantac after recalls. *Fierce Pharma*, August 4, 2020. https://www.fiercepharma.com/pharma/sanofi-glaxosmithkline-disclose-doj-probe-into-zantac-disclosures
363 Sagonowsky E. Sanofi, GlaxoSmithKline disclose DOJ investigation into Zantac after recalls. *Fierce Pharma*, August 4, 2020. https://www.fiercepharma.com/pharma/sanofi-glaxosmithkline-disclose-doj-probe-into-zantac-disclosures
364 Blankenship K. Sun Pharma the latest to recall metformin after carcinogen tests come up positive. *Fierce Pharma*, September 23, 2020. https://www.fiercepharma.com/manufacturing/sun-pharma-latest-to-recall-common-diabetes-drug-after-carcinogen-tests-come-back
365 Look at Pharma's recent record before bestowing a crown: Peace. https://www.pea.cx/2021/02/19/look-at-pharmas-recent-record-before-bestowing-a-crown/
366 Blankenship K. Sun Pharma the latest to recall metformin after carcinogen tests come up positive. *Fierce Pharma*, September 23, 2020. https://www.fiercepharma.com/manufacturing/sun-pharma-latest-to-recall-common-diabetes-drug-after-carcinogen-tests-come-back
367 Statement from Janet Woodcock, M.D., director of FDA's Center for Drug Evaluation and Research, on impurities found in diabetes drugs outside the U.S. *FDA*, December 5, 2019. https://www.fda.gov/news-events/press-announcements/statement-janet-woodcock-md-director-fdas-center-drug-evaluation-and-research-impurities-found
368 James S. Super soldiers? Military drug is rage among students, young professionals. *ABC News*, July 24, 2007. https://abcnews.go.com/Technology/Health/story?id=3408266&page=1
369 Pharmaceutical company Cephalon to pay $425 million for off-label drug marketing. *U.S. Department of Justice*, September 29, 2008. https://www.justice.gov/sites/default/files/civil/legacy/2014/01/09/Cephalon%20Press%20Release.pdf
370 Nuvigil (armodafinil) profile. *Center Watch*, June 1, 2007.https://www.centerwatch.com/directories/1067-fda-approved-drugs/listing/3924-nuvigil-armodafinil
371 *United States of America v. Cephalon*, Case 2:08-cv-00287-TON Document 69, March 4, 2014. https://ffj-online.org/wp-content/uploads/2015/04/INSY-CephQuitTam.pdf
372 Hamilton J. FDA committee rejects ADHD use for modafinil. *NPR*, March 24, 2006. https://www.npr.org/templates/story/story.php?storyId=5298885
373 Hamilton J. FDA committee rejects ADHD use for modafinil. *NPR*, March 24, 2006. https://www.npr.org/templates/story/story.php?storyId=5298885
374 McNeil D. Clinical review. *FDA*, December 21, 2005. https://www.fda.gov/media/88501/download
375 Ghoshal L. and Sinha M. Fixed drug eruptions with modafinil. *Indian Journal of Pharmacology* 47(2), March–April 2015. PMC4386138. https://www.ncbi.nlm.nih.gov/pmc/articles/PMC4386138/
376 Holfinger S. 1230 Stevens-Johnsons syndrome after armodafinil use. *Sleep* 40, April 28, 2017. https://academic.oup.com/sleep/article/40/suppl_1/A458/3782478
377 George J. Narcolepsy drugs linked to fetal malformations. *MedPage Today*, October 19, 2020. https://www.medpagetoday.com/neurology/sleepdisorders/89190
378 George J. Narcolepsy drugs linked to fetal malformations. *MedPage Today*, October 19, 2020. https://www.medpagetoday.com/neurology/sleepdisorders/89190
379 Look at Pharma's recent record before bestowing a crown: Peace. https://www.pea.cx/2021/02/19/look-at-pharmas-recent-record-before-bestowing-a-crown/
380 George J. Narcolepsy drugs linked to fetal malformations. *MedPage Today*, October 19, 2020. https://www.medpagetoday.com/neurology/sleepdisorders/89190
381 Ghaffari N. Caution in prescribing modafinil and armodafinil to individuals who could become pregnant. *JAMA Internal Medicine*, October 19, 2020. https://jamanetwork.com/journals/jamainternalmedicine/article-abstract/2771814
382 Kaplan S, Braverman DL, Frishman I and Bartov N. Pregnancy and fetal outcomes following exposure to

modafinil and armodafinil during pregnancy. *JAMA Internal Medicine*, October 19, 2020.
383 George J. Narcolepsy drugs linked to fetal malformations. *MedPage Today*, October 19, 2020. https://www.medpagetoday.com/neurology/sleepdisorders/89190
384 George J. Narcolepsy drugs linked to fetal malformations. *MedPage Today*, October 19, 2020. https://www.medpagetoday.com/neurology/sleepdisorders/89190
385 EU fines drug makers for keeping cheap medicine off market. *US News*, November 26, 2020. https://www.usnews.com/news/business/articles/2020-11-26/eu-fines-drug-makers-for-keeping-cheap-medicine-off-market
386 EU fines drug makers for keeping cheap medicine off market. *US News*, November 26, 2020. https://www.usnews.com/news/business/articles/2020-11-26/eu-fines-drug-makers-for-keeping-cheap-medicine-off-market
387 FDA recommends avoiding use of NSAIDs in pregnancy at 20 weeks or later because they can result in low amniotic fluid. *FDA*, October 15, 2020. https://www.fda.gov/media/142967/download
388 FDA recommends avoiding use of NSAIDs in pregnancy at 20 weeks or later because they can result in low amniotic fluid. *FDA*, October 15, 2020. https://www.fda.gov/media/142967/download
389 Avoid use of NSAID in pregnancy, even before 30 weeks, warns FDA. https://medicaldialogues.in/obstetrics-gynaecology/news/avoid-use-of-nsaid-in-pregnancy-even-before-30-weeks-warns-fda-70600
390 FDA recommends avoiding use of NSAIDs in pregnancy at 20 weeks or later because they can result in low amniotic fluid. *FDA*, October 15, 2020. https://www.fda.gov/media/142967/download
391 New drug for bone disorders: Fosamax approved as treatment for osteoporosis and Paget's disease of bone. *FDA Consumer*, December 1995. http://the-medical-dictionary.com/paget_s_disease_of_bone_article_8.htm
392 De Groen PC, Lubbe DF, Hirsch LJ, Daifotis A, Stephenson W, Freedholm D, Pryor-Tillotson S, Seleznick MJ, Pinkas H and Wang KK. Esophagitis associated with the use of alendronate. *New England Journal of Medicine*, October 3, 1996. https://pubmed.ncbi.nlm.nih.gov/8793925/
393 De Groen PC, Lubbe DF, Hirsch LJ, Daifotis A, Stephenson W, Freedholm D, Pryor-Tillotson S, Seleznick MJ, Pinkas H and Wang KK. Esophagitis associated with the use of alendronate. *New England Journal of Medicine*, October 3, 1996. https://pubmed.ncbi.nlm.nih.gov/8793925/
394 Big pharma still tries to push dangerous drug class. *CounterPunch.org*. https://www.counterpunch.org/2018/02/16/big-pharma-still-tries-to-push-dangerous-drug-class/
395 Murphy C. Side effect reported with osteoporosis drug Fosamax. *Washington Post*, October 15, 1996. https://www.washingtonpost.com/archive/lifestyle/wellness/1996/10/15/side-effect-reported-with-osteoporosis-drug-fosamax/351bfcc3-d242-4b58-90d8-2f6645623f52/
396 Ruggiero SL, Mehrotra B, Rosenberg TJ and Engroff SL. Osteonecrosis of the jaws associated with the use of bisphosphonates: A review of 63 cases. *Journal of Oral and Maxillofacial Surgery* 62(5), May 2004: 527–534. https://pubmed.ncbi.nlm.nih.gov/15122554/
397 Donoghue A. Bisphosphonates and osteonecrosis: Analogy to phossy jaw. *Medical Journal of Australia* 183(3), 2005: 163–164. https://pubmed.ncbi.nlm.nih.gov/16053423/
398 Harasi P. Osteoporosis drugs could have devastating effect on dental work. *Review Journal*, November 13, 2005.
399 Start M. Naples woman files suit against Merck. *News-Press*, April 14, 2006.
400 Rosenberg M. Internal Merck emails revealed. *Center for Health Journalism*, December 3, 2012. https://centerforhealthjournalism.org/2012/12/03/internal-merck-emails-revealed
401 Heckbert SR, Li G, Cummings SR, Smith NL and Psaty BM. Use of alendronate and risk of incident atrial fibrillation in women. *Archives of Internal Medicine* 168(8), 2008: 826–831. https://pubmed.ncbi.nlm.nih.gov/18443257/
402 Warning: Severe pain can occur with osteoporosis, osteopenia drugs. *Bone Density Blog*, 2008. https://bonedensityblog.com/news/severe-pain-with-osteoporosis-drugs-fda-alert-on-bisphosphonates/
403 Warning: Severe pain can occur with osteoporosis, osteopenia drugs. *Bone Density Blog*, 2008. https://bonedensityblog.com/news/severe-pain-with-osteoporosis-drugs-fda-alert-on-bisphosphonates/
404 Wysowski D. Reports of esophageal cancer with oral bisphosphonate use. *New England Journal of Medicine*, January 1, 2009. https://pubmed.ncbi.nlm.nih.gov/19118315/
405 Lloyd J. Long-term use of osteoporosis drugs linked to hip breaks. *USA Today*, March 11, 2010.
406 Increased risk of fracture with bisphosphonates. *Drug Discovery & Development*, October 14, 2010.
407 Possible increased risk of thigh bone fracture with bisphosphonates. *FDA*, October 2, 2010. http://wayback.archive-it.org/7993/20170112215607; http:/www.fda.gov/NewsEvents/Newsroom/PressAnnouncements/2010/ucm229171.htm
408 Parker-Pope T. Drugs to build bones may weaken them. *New York Times*, July 15, 2008. https://www.nytimes.com/2008/07/15/health/15well.html
409 Why did the medical establishment allow Pharma's 12-year bone scam? http://www.niemanwatchdog.org/index.cfm?fuseaction=ask_this.view&askthisid=551&fontsize=up

410 Adams J. Take bisphosphonates, break a leg? *Los Angeles Times*, March 22, 2010. https://www.latimes.com/archives/la-xpm-2010-mar-22-la-he-closer-20100322-story.html
411 Big pharma still tries to push dangerous drug class. *CounterPunch.org*. https://www.counterpunch.org/2018/02/16/big-pharma-still-tries-to-push-dangerous-drug-class/
412 Ott S. New treatments for brittle bones. *Annals of Internal Medicine*, September 7, 2004. https://www.acpjournals.org/doi/10.7326/0003-4819-141-5-200409070-00023
413 Visekruna M, Wilson D and McKiernan FE. Severely suppressed bone turnover and atypical skeletal fragility. *Journal of Clinical Endocrinology & Metabolism* 93(8), 2008. https://pubmed.ncbi.nlm.nih.gov/18522980/
414 Neviaser AS, Lane JM, Lenart BA, Edobor-Osula F and Lorich DG. Low-energy femoral shaft fractures associated with alendronate use. *Journal of Orthopaedic Trauma*, May–June 2008. https://pubmed.ncbi.nlm.nih.gov/18448990/
415 Kwek EB, Goh SK, Koh JS, Png MA and Howe TS. An emerging pattern of subtrochanteric stress fractures: A long-term complication of alendronate therapy. *Injury*, February 2008. https://pubmed.ncbi.nlm.nih.gov/18222447/
416 Marshall M. Patients feel painful side effects of bone drugs. *CBS News*, May 19, 2008.
417 Brody J. A perfect storm for broken bones. *New York Times*, February 12, 2018. https://www.nytimes.com/2018/02/12/well/bone-fractures-broken-hip-osteoporosis-drugs-treatment-diagnosis.html
418 Spiegel A. How a bone disease grew to fit the prescription. *National Public Radio*, December 21, 2009. https://www.npr.org/2009/12/21/121609815/how-a-bone-disease-grew-to-fit-the-prescription
419 Brody J. A perfect storm for broken bones. *New York Times*, February 12, 2018. https://www.nytimes.com/2018/02/12/well/bone-fractures-broken-hip-osteoporosis-drugs-treatment-diagnosis.html
420 Schwitzer G. Same old, same old, with NY Times Well column: Bisphosphonates for pneumonia this time. *Health News Review*, June 12, 2020. https://www.healthnewsreview.org/2020/06/same-old-same-old-with-ny-times-well-column-bisphosphonates-for-pneumonia-this-time/
421 Schwitzer G. Same old, same old, with NY Times Well column: Bisphosphonates for pneumonia this time. *Health News Review*, June 12, 2020. https://www.healthnewsreview.org/2020/06/same-old-same-old-with-ny-times-well-column-bisphosphonates-for-pneumonia-this-time/
422 Schwitzer G. Same old, same old, with NY Times Well column: Bisphosphonates for pneumonia this time. *Health News Review*, June 12, 2020. https://www.healthnewsreview.org/2020/06/same-old-same-old-with-ny-times-well-column-bisphosphonates-for-pneumonia-this-time/
423 Roy S. Insomnia medication prescriptions increase with spread of coronavirus. *Sleep Review*, April 21, 2020. https://www.sleepreviewmag.com/sleep-treatments/pharmaceuticals/prescription-drugs/insomnia-medication-prescriptions-coronavirus/
424 Causes sexual dysfunction, suicide and birth defects? *RxISK*, March 3, 2020. https://rxisk.org/causes-sexual-dysfunction-suicide-and-birth-defects/
425 Sansone R and Sansone L. SSRIs: Bad to the bone? *Innovations in Clinical Neuroscience* 9(7–8), July–August 2012: 42–47. https://www.ncbi.nlm.nih.gov/pmc/articles/PMC3442753/
426 Gupta B, Acharya A, Singh S, Brazzoli S, Ghorab M, Malik S, Pelekos G and Rossouw E. Evaluation of jawbone morphology and bone density indices in panoramic radiographs of selective serotonin reuptake inhibitor users: A preliminary study. *Dentomaxillofacial Radiology*, January 2019. https://pubmed.ncbi.nlm.nih.gov/30004255/
427 Agacayak KS, Guler R and Ilyasov B. Evaluation of the effect of long-term use of antidepressants in the SSRI group on bone density with dental volumetric tomography. *Drug Design, Development and Therapy*, October 3, 2019. https://www.ncbi.nlm.nih.gov/pmc/articles/PMC6781739/
428 Lee SH, Mastronardi CA, Li RW, Paz-Filho G, Dutcher EG, Lewis MD, Vincent AD, Smith PN, Bornstein SR, Licinio J and Wong ML. Short-term antidepressant treatment has long-lasting effects, and reverses stress-induced decreases in bone features in rats. *Translation Psychiatry*, January 16, 2019. https://www.nature.com/articles/s41398-018-0351-z
429 Lee SH, Mastronardi CA, Li RW, Paz-Filho G, Dutcher EG, Lewis MD, Vincent AD, Smith PN, Bornstein SR, Licinio J and Wong ML. Short-term antidepressant treatment has long-lasting effects, and reverses stress-induced decreases in bone features in rats. *Translation Psychiatry*, January 16, 2019. https://www.nature.com/articles/s41398-018-0351-z
430 Is pharma our covid savior? *Freepress.org*. https://freepress.org/article/pharma-our-covid-savior
431 Carey B and Gebeloff R. Many people taking antidepressants discover they cannot quit. *New York Times*, April 7, 2018. https://www.nytimes.com/2018/04/07/health/antidepressants-withdrawal-prozac-cymbalta.html
432 Article: One in 8 takes antidepressants—Are they working? Are they safe? *OpEd News*. https://www.opednews.com/articles/One-in-8-Takes-Antidepress-by-Martha-Rosenberg-Antidepressant_Depression_Depression_Doctors-180706-122.html
433 Opinion. Withdrawing from antidepressants. *New York Times*, April 9, 2018. https://www.nytimes.com/2018/04/09/opinion/antidepressants.html

434 Article: One in 8 takes antidepressants—Are they working? Are they safe? *OpEd News*. https://www.opednews.com/articles/One-in-8-Takes-Antidepress-by-Martha-Rosenberg-Antidepressant_Depression_Depression_Doctors-180706-122.html
435 Cain A. A former big pharma CEO donated $250 million to Columbia Medical School to help eliminate student loans. *Business Insider*, December 28, 2017. http://www.businessinsider.com/ex-merck-ceo-roy-vagelos-donated-250-million-to-columbia-medical-school-2017-12
436 Rosenberg M. An interview with Dr. Peter Breggin. *Center for Health Journalism*, December 23, 2014. https://centerforhealthjournalism.org/2014/12/23/interview-dr-peter-breggin
437 FDA requests the withdrawal of the weight-loss drug Belviq, Belviq XR (lorcaserin) from the market. *FDA*, February 13, 2020. https://www.fda.gov/drugs/drug-safety-and-availability/fda-requests-withdrawal-weight-loss-drug-belviq-belviq-xr-lorcaserin-market
438 Safety clinical trial shows possible increased risk of cancer with weight-loss medicine Belviq, Belviq XR (lorcaserin). *FDA*, January 14, 2020. https://www.fda.gov/drugs/drug-safety-and-availability/safety-clinical-trial-shows-possible-increased-risk-cancer-weight-loss-medicine-belviq-belviq-xr
439 New Yorker files class-action lawsuit against manufacturers of weight loss drug. *Fingerlakes1.com*. https://www.fingerlakes1.com/2020/11/02/new-yorker-files-class-action-lawsuit-against-manufacturers-of-weight-loss-drug/
440 Gustafson A, King C and Rey JA. Lorcaserin (Belviq) A Selective serotonin 5-HT2C agonist in the treatment of obesity. *Pharmacy and Therapeutics*, September 2013. https://www.ncbi.nlm.nih.gov/pmc/articles/PMC3828930/
441 FDA rejects lorcaserin for weight-loss therapy. *Healio*, November 25, 2010. https://www.healio.com/news/hematology-oncology/20120325/fda-rejects-lorcaserin-for-weight-loss-therapy
442 https://www.cdc.gov/mmwr/preview/mmwrhtml/00049815.htm
443 FDA rejects lorcaserin for weight-loss therapy. *Healio*, November 25, 2010. https://www.healio.com/news/hematology-oncology/20120325/fda-rejects-lorcaserin-for-weight-loss-therapy
444 With 1 in 5 kids now obese, Pharma sets sights on $50B market for weight-loss drugs. https://www.medicalextremism.com/2022-08-14-kids-obese-pharma-sets-sights-on-50b-market.html
445 New Yorker files class-action lawsuit against manufacturers of weight loss drug. *Fingerlakes1*, November 2, 2020. https://fingerlakes1.com/2020/11/02/new-yorker-files-class-action-lawsuit-against-manufacturers-of-weight-loss-drug/
446 FDA requests the withdrawal of the weight-loss drug Belviq, Belviq XR (lorcaserin) from the market. *FDA*, February 13, 2020. https://www.fda.gov/drugs/drug-safety-and-availability/fda-requests-withdrawal-weight-loss-drug-belviq-belviq-xr-lorcaserin-market
447 New Yorker files class-action lawsuit against manufacturers of weight loss drug. *Fingerlakes1*, November 2, 2020. https://fingerlakes1.com/2020/11/02/new-yorker-files-class-action-lawsuit-against-manufacturers-of-weight-loss-drug/
448 New Yorker files class-action lawsuit against manufacturers of weight loss drug. *Fingerlakes1*, November 2, 2020. https://fingerlakes1.com/2020/11/02/new-yorker-files-class-action-lawsuit-against-manufacturers-of-weight-loss-drug/
449 New Yorker files class-action lawsuit against manufacturers of weight loss drug. *Fingerlakes1.com*. https://www.fingerlakes1.com/2020/11/02/new-yorker-files-class-action-lawsuit-against-manufacturers-of-weight-loss-drug/
450 https://casetext.com/case/zottola-v-eisai-inc-1
451 Steinberg S. Eisai, CVS Say Belviq class suit plaintiffs weren't harmed. *Bloomberg Law*, September 10, 2020. https://news.bloomberglaw.com/class-action/eisai-cvs-say-belviq-class-suit-plaintiffs-werent-harmed
452 Taking Z-drugs for insomnia? Know the risks. *FDA*, April 30, 2019. https://www.fda.gov/consumers/consumer-updates/taking-z-drugs-insomnia-know-risks
453 FDA adds boxed warning for risk of serious injuries caused by sleepwalking with certain prescription insomnia medicines. *FDA*, April 30, 2019. https://www.fda.gov/drugs/drug-safety-and-availability/fda-adds-boxed-warning-risk-serious-injuries-caused-sleepwalking-certain-prescription-insomnia
454 No, Ambien does not make you a racist but it does a lot of other concerning things. *CounterPunch.org*. https://www.counterpunch.org/2018/06/01/no-ambien-does-not-make-you-a-racist-but-it-does-a-lot-of-other-concerning-things/
455 The Ambien made me do it, says Roseanne Barr. *Intrepid Report.com*. http://www.intrepidreport.com/archives/24198
456 Sleeping pill linked to hospital falls, researchers say. *MedicineNet*, November 19, 2012. https://www.medicinenet.com/script/main/art.asp?articlekey=165199
457 No, Ambien does not make you a racist but it does a lot of other concerning things. *CounterPunch.org*. https://www.counterpunch.org/2018/06/01/no-ambien-does-not-make-you-a-racist-but-it-does-a-lot-of-other-concerning-things/
458 Sleeping pill linked to hospital falls, researchers say. *MedicineNet*, November 19, 2012. https://www.medicinenet.com/script/main/art.asp?articlekey=165199
459 Wood river mattress: Hailey, Sun Valley, Ketchum, Idaho—Sleeping pill linked to hospital falls. https://woodrivermattress.com/sleeping-pill-linked-to-hospital-falls

460 Wikipedia Patrick J. Kennedy. https://en.wikipedia.org/wiki/Patrick_J._Kennedy

461 Ducharme J. Are sleeping pills safe? Here's what research says. *Time*, May 7, 2019. https://time.com/5584937/sleeping-pills-safe/

462 No, Ambien does not make you a racist but it does a lot of other concerning things. *CounterPunch.org*. https://www.counterpunch.org/2018/06/01/no-ambien-does-not-make-you-a-racist-but-it-does-a-lot-of-other-concerning-things/

463 Gardner D. Tiger woods 'took sleeping pills to spice up sex with mistress.' *Daily Mail*, December 5, 2009. https://www.dailymail.co.uk/news/article-1233303/Tiger-Woods-took-prescription-drugs-boost-sex-mistress.html

464 No, Ambien does not make you a racist but it does a lot of other concerning things. *CounterPunch.org*. https://www.counterpunch.org/2018/06/01/no-ambien-does-not-make-you-a-racist-but-it-does-a-lot-of-other-concerning-things/

465 No, Ambien does not make you a racist but it does a lot of other concerning things. *CounterPunch.org*. https://www.counterpunch.org/2018/06/01/no-ambien-does-not-make-you-a-racist-but-it-does-a-lot-of-other-concerning-things/

466 Kripke DF, Langer RD and Kline LE. Hypnotics' association with mortality or cancer: A matched cohort study. *Pharmacology and Therapeutics*, February 27, 2012. https://bmjopen.bmj.com/content/2/1/e000850.full?sid=f0956753-511d-4e70-9230-c1e8aa5df0d3

467 Gregorian D and Siemaszko C. Kerry Kennedy claims she was accidental Ambien zombie—found not guilty of drugged driving by Westchester County jury, March 1, 2014. https://www.nydailynews.com/news/crime/kerry-kennedy-acquitted-drugged-driving-article-1.1706141

468 Kripke D. Hypnotic drug risks of mortality, infection, depression, and cancer: But lack of benefit. *F1000research*, November 12, 2018. https://www.ncbi.nlm.nih.gov/pmc/articles/PMC4890308/

469 Anthrax emergency: How to take ciprofloxacin to prevent anthrax. *CDC*, November 20, 2020. https://www.cdc.gov/anthrax/medical-care/cipro-eui-recipients.html

470 FDA orders 'black box' label on some antibiotics. *CNN*, July 8, 2008. https://www.cnn.com/2008/HEALTH/07/08/antibiotics.risk/index.html

471 Wikipedia Quinolone antibiotic. https://en.wikipedia.org/wiki/Quinolone_antibiotic

472 Information for healthcare professionals: Fluoroquinolone antimicrobial drugs [ciprofloxacin, ciprofloxacin extended-release, gemifloxacin, levofloxacin, moxifloxacin, norfloxacin, and ofloxacin. *FDA*, July 8, 2008. http://wayback.archive-it.org/7993/20161022101528/http:/www.fda.gov/Drugs/DrugSafety/PostmarketDrugSafetyInformationforPatientsandProviders/ucm126085.htm

473 FDA orders 'black box' label on some antibiotics. *CNN*, July 8, 2008. https://www.cnn.com/2008/HEALTH/07/08/antibiotics.risk/index.html

474 Kripke DF, Langer RD and Kline LE. Hypnotics' association with mortality or cancer: A matched cohort study. *Pharmacology and Therapeutics*, February 27, 2012. https://bmjopen.bmj.com/content/2/1/e000850.full?sid=f0956753-511d-4e70-9230-c1e8aa5df0d3

475 FDA Drug Safety Communication. FDA requires label changes to warn of risk for possibly permanent nerve damage from antibacterial fluoroquinolone drugs taken by mouth or by injection. *FDA*, August 15, 2013. http://wayback.archive-it.org/7993/20161022101530/http:/www.fda.gov/Drugs/DrugSafety/ucm365050.htm

476 FDA Drug Safety Communication. FDA advises restricting fluoroquinolone antibiotic use for certain uncomplicated infections; warns about disabling side effects that can occur together. *FDA*, May 12, 2016. https://www.fda.gov/drugs/drug-safety-and-availability/fda-drug-safety-communication-fda-advises-restricting-fluoroquinolone-antibiotic-use-certain

477 FDA reinforces safety information about serious low blood sugar levels and mental health side effects with fluoroquinolone antibiotics; requires label changes. *FDA*, July 10, 2018. https://www.fda.gov/drugs/drug-safety-and-availability/fda-reinforces-safety-information-about-serious-low-blood-sugar-levels-and-mental-health-side

478 Disabling and potentially permanent side effects lead to suspension or restrictions of quinolone and fluoroquinolone antibiotics. *European Medicines Agency*, November 16, 2018. https://www.ema.europa.eu/en/news/disabling-potentially-permanent-side-effects-lead-suspension-restrictions-quinolone-fluoroquinolone

479 FDA warns about increased risk of ruptures or tears in the aorta blood vessel with fluoroquinolone antibiotics in certain patients. *FDA*, December 20, 2018. https://www.fda.gov/drugs/drug-safety-and-availability/fda-warns-about-increased-risk-ruptures-or-tears-aorta-blood-vessel-fluoroquinolone-antibiotics

480 Marchione M. Breast cancer risk from menopause hormones may last decades. *Associated Press*, December 13, 2019. https://apnews.com/article/a73f6e7c1e77711f3b620caffe8fbcd1

481 Marchione M. Breast cancer risk from menopause hormones may last decades. *Associated Press*, December 13, 2019. https://apnews.com/article/a73f6e7c1e77711f3b620caffe8fbcd1

482 Hormone replacement therapy is still linked to cancer. *Intrepid Report.com*. http://www.intrepidreport.com/archives/28949

483 American Cancer Society. Menopausal hormone therapy and cancer risk, 2020. https://www.cancer.org/cancer/cancer-causes/medical-treatments/

menopausal-hormone-replacement-therapy-and-cancer-risk.html
484 Shumaker SA, Legault C, Rapp SR, Thal L, Wallace RB, Ockene JK, Hendrix SL, Jones III BN, Assaf AR, Jackson RD and Kotchen JM. Estrogen plus progestin and the incidence of dementia and mild cognitive impairment in postmenopausal women: The Women's Health Initiative Memory Study: A randomized controlled trial. *JAMA* 289(20), 28 May 2003: 2651–2662. https://pubmed.ncbi.nlm.nih.gov/12771112/
485 Hormone-replacement therapy hurts hearing, study finds. *AAAS*, September 5, 2006. https://www.eurekalert.org/pub_releases/2006-09/uorm-hth090506.php
486 Biggs W. Oral estrogen not gallbladder-friendly; transdermal seems better. *New England Journal of Medicine*, June 10, 2008. https://www.jwatch.org/wh200807140000001/2008/07/14/oral-estrogen-not-gallbladder-friendly
487 Steinauer JE, Waetjen LE, Vittinghoff E, Subak LL, Hulley SB, Grady D, Lin F and Brown JS. Postmenopausal hormone therapy: Does it cause incontinence? *Obstetrics & Gynecology*, 106(5 Pt 1), November 2005: 940–945. https://pubmed.ncbi.nlm.nih.gov/16260510/
488 Real FG, Svanes C, Björnsson EH, Franklin K, Gislason D, Gislason T, Gulsvik A, Janson C, Jögi R, Kiserud T and Norbäck D. Hormone replacement therapy, body mass index and asthma in perimenopausal women: A cross sectional survey. *Thorax*, January 2006. https://www.ncbi.nlm.nih.gov/pmc/articles/PMC2080706/
489 Koomen ER, Joosse A, Herings RM, Casparie MK, Guchelaar HJ and Nijsten T. Estrogens, oral contraceptives and hormonal replacement therapy increase the incidence of cutaneous melanoma: A population-based case-control study. *Annals of Oncology*, September 2008. https://www.researchgate.net/publication/23192172_Estrogens_oral_contraceptives_and_hormonal_replacement_therapy_increase_the_incidence_of_cutaneous_melanoma_A_population-based_case-control_study
490 Liu B, Balkwill A, Cooper C, Roddam A, Brown A and Beral V. Reproductive history, hormonal factors and the incidence of hip and knee replacement for osteoarthritis in middle-aged women. *Annals of the Rheumatic Diseases* 68(7), 2009: 1165–1170 https://www.researchgate.net/publication/23425177_Reproductive_history_hormonal_factors_and_the_incidence_of_hip_and_knee_replacement_for_osteoarthritis_in_middle-aged_women
491 American Cancer Society. Menopausal hormone therapy and cancer risk, 2020. https://www.cancer.org/cancer/cancer-causes/medical-treatments/menopausal-hormone-replacement-therapy-and-cancer-risk.html
492 Hormone replacement therapy is still linked to cancer. *Intrepid Report.com.* http://www.intrepidreport.com/archives/28949
493 Laya M. Effect of postmenopausal hormonal replacement therapy on mammographic density and parenchymal pattern. *Radiology* 196(2), August 1995: 433–437. https://pubmed.ncbi.nlm.nih.gov/7617857/
494 Kolata G. Breast cancer news brings a range of reactions. *New York Times*, December 18, 2006. https://www.nytimes.com/2006/12/18/health/breast-cancer-news-brings-a-range-of-reactions.html?mtrref=www.google.com&gwh=9D3C82B365B68E1E9E7782D116FCE82C&gwt=pay&assetType=REGIWALL
495 Kolata G. Breast cancer news brings a range of reactions. *New York Times*, December 18, 2006. https://www.nytimes.com/2006/12/18/health/breast-cancer-news-brings-a-range-of-reactions.html?mtrref=www.google.com&gwh=9D3C82B365B68E1E9E7782D116FCE82C&gwt=pay&assetType=REGIWALL
496 Hormone replacement therapy is still linked to cancer. *Intrepid Report.com.* http://www.intrepidreport.com/archives/28949
497 Jick H, Watkins RN, Hunter JR, Dinan BJ, Madsen S, Rothman KJ and Walker AM. Replacement estrogens and endometrial cancer. *New England Journal of Medicine*, February 1, 1979. https://pubmed.ncbi.nlm.nih.gov/759868/
498 Perls T and Handelsman D. Disease mongering of age-associated declines in testosterone and growth hormone levels. *Journal of the American Geriatrics Society*, March 24, 2015. https://onlinelibrary.wiley.com/doi/full/10.1111/jgs.13391
499 Perls T and Handelsman D. Disease mongering of age-associated declines in testosterone and growth hormone levels. *Journal of the American Geriatrics Society*, March 24, 2015. https://onlinelibrary.wiley.com/doi/full/10.1111/jgs.13391
500 Perls T and Handelsman D. Disease mongering of age-associated declines in testosterone and growth hormone levels. *Journal of the American Geriatrics Society*, March 24, 2015. https://onlinelibrary.wiley.com/doi/full/10.1111/jgs.13391
501 Fennessey G. Are GERD drugs worth the risks? *Med Shadow*, March 16, 2020. https://medshadow.org/avoiding-gerd-meds-side-effects/
502 Fennessey G. Are GERD drugs worth the risks? *Med Shadow*, March 16, 2020. https://medshadow.org/avoiding-gerd-meds-side-effects/
503 Pello Lázaro AM, Cristóbal C, Franco-Peláez JA, Tarín N, Aceña Á, Carda R, Huelmos A, Martín-Mariscal ML, Fuentes-Antras J, Martínez-Millá J and Alonso J. Use of proton-pump inhibitors predicts heart failure and death in patients with coronary artery disease. *PLoS*, January 19, 2017. https://journals.plos.org/plosone/article?id=10.1371/journal.pone.0169826

504 Xie Y, Bowe B, Li T, Xian H, Yan Y and Al-Aly Z. Long-term kidney outcomes among users of proton pump inhibitors without intervening acute kidney injury. *Kidney International* 91, 2017: 1482–1494. https://www.kidney-international.org/article/S0085-2538(17)30005-4/pdf

505 Xie Y, Bowe B, Li T, Xian H, Yan Y and Al-Aly Z. Long-term kidney outcomes among users of proton pump inhibitors without intervening acute kidney injury. *Kidney International* 91, 2017: 1482–1494. https://www.kidney-international.org/article/S0085-2538(17)30005-4/pdf

506 Arj A, Razavi Zade M, Yavari M, Akbari H, Zamani B and Asemi Z. Proton pump inhibitors use and change in bone mineral density. *International Journal of Rheumatic Diseases* 19(9), September 2016: 864–868. https://pubmed.ncbi.nlm.nih.gov/27242025/

507 Cheung KS, Chan EW, Wong AY, Chen L, Wong IC and Leung WK. Long-term proton pump inhibitors and risk of gastric cancer development after treatment for *Helicobacter pylori*: A population-based study. *Gut* 67(1), 2018. https://gut.bmj.com/content/67/1/28

508 Jordakieva G, Kundi M, Untersmayr E, Pali-Schöll I, Reichardt B and Jensen-Jarolim E. Country-wide medical records infer increased allergy risk of gastric acid inhibition. *Nature Communications* 10, 2019: 3298. https://www.ncbi.nlm.nih.gov/pmc/articles/PMC6667461/

509 Reimer C, Søndergaard B, Hilsted L and Bytzer P. Proton-pump inhibitor therapy induces acid-related symptoms in healthy volunteers after withdrawal of therapy. *Gastroenterology*, April 13, 2009. https://www.gastrojournal.org/article/S0016-5085(09)00522-8/fulltext

8 Evaluation of Causation in Drug Injury Cases

Donald H. Marks and James T. O'Donnell

SYNOPSIS

8.1 WHAT IS CAUSATION?

Medical causation is the determination of whether an adverse effect (AE) was caused by the use of a medication, biological product, vaccine, device, or procedure, all of which are generally referred to as "treatments." An adverse event refers to an untoward physical sign; symptom; abnormal assessment (lab value, vital sign, ECG, etc.); or a cluster of signs, symptoms, and abnormal assessments within the definition of FDA reg 21 CFR.[1] Physical signs can include fever, hypertension, weight loss, or other physical findings. Symptoms can include any complaint from a patient, including nausea, headache, abdominal pain, or others. A medication can refer to any FDA-approved prescription drug or to an over-the-counter preparation. Biologicals refer to prepared synthetic materials of living origin. Vaccines are preparations designed to induce a protective or therapeutic immune response. Medical devices include both large units (e.g., magnetic resonance imaging (MRI) machines) and miniature units (e.g., intravascular stents).

When determining whether there is causal relatedness between a treatment and an AE, one must follow standard, consistent, and universally accepted rules of causation. It must always be kept in mind that correlation does not imply nor prove causation. Recent examples of faulty correlation include the supposed relatedness between hormone replacement therapy (HRT) and coronary heart disease (*Hormone Therapy and Heart Disease, American College Obstetrics* Gynecology). Also note that even if the logical basis for supporting causation is not reasonable, the causation still may exist.

DOI: 10.1201/9781003615323-9

8.2 IMPORTANCE OF ESTABLISHING CAUSATION

Patients who receive a treatment for an illness generally can be expected to have, as a result of their illness, physical signs and symptoms as manifestations of their illness. As a general statement, all treatments also can cause their own array of physical signs and symptoms separate from the underlying illness being treated, and these new signs and symptoms are referred to as adverse effects. This illustrates the crux of medical causation's difficulty—distinguishing AEs of treatments from signs or symptoms of the underlying illness for which they are being treated.

This problem is illustrated by the medication Lotronex (alosetron, Glaxo Wellcome), an antagonist of the 5-HT3 (serotonin) receptor. Lotronex was indicated for the treatment of severe, chronic, diarrhea-predominant irritable bowel syndrome (IBS) in women for which conventional therapy had failed. IBS patients can typically present with a wide range of gastrointestinal (GI) symptoms and signs. Unfortunately, Lotronex can act both as a serotonergic drug and as a Serotonin Reuptake Inhibitor (SRI). Serotonin is a potent neurotransmitter (NT) which activates a muscle at the neuromuscular (NM) endplate. The intensity and duration of the muscle activation are directly related to the concentration of serotonin at the NM endplate. Lotronex mimics serotonin at the active receptor and blocks serotonin resorption, thereby causing an inordinately high level of serotonin activity in the GI NM endplate. This high serotonin level can be associated with severe vasoconstriction and ischemia.[2]

Elevated serotonin levels are known and accepted causes of many of the serious side effects of Lotronex, including obstruction, perforation, impaction, toxic megacolon, and secondary ischemia. This led to the quandary that the signs and symptoms of an adverse effect[3] from the medication Lotronex, which could have warned of an AE and led to the drug's discontinuation, were similar to the not unexpected signs and symptoms of the underlying disease (IBS) being treated. Ultimately this difficulty of use, not uncommon for a number of medications, led to the removal of Lotronex from the market.

Another significant causation determination of a serotoninergic AE is the development of depression leading to suicidal ideation from the use of metoclopramide, a drug used to treat GI symptoms such as acid reflux and nausea.[4] This drug has both central (nausea) and peripheral (gastric motility) actions, is an antagonist of dopamine, and sensitizes gastric smooth muscle to the effects of acetylcholine stimulation. Metoclopramide (Reglan) has a varied central nervous system (CNS) effect, including drowsiness, extra pyramidal syndrome (dystonias, akathisia), depression, dizziness, and insomnia. It should not be surprising that a drug with antipsychotic efficacy, and which can cause akathisia, may cause an increased risk of suicide, as is pointed out in the prescribing information for Reglan. The establishment of the causation risk led to a significantly decreased clinical use.

8.3 DEFINITIONS

In general, both the pharmaceutical industry and the regulatory bodies use the same definitions for AEs and adverse effects. The FDA's definitions for these terms are included in 21CFR.[5] Providers who observe a potential AE and patients who experience an AE can use different definitions or meanings of commonly used terms such as causation, probable, possible, severe, and serious. The potential for imprecise use of terms can lead to some confusion when AEs are reported to regulatory agencies. Variations in description are just one of several reasons why primary MedWatch reports need to be thoroughly evaluated, rather than simply tabulated. MedWatch reports can supply critical information on unsuspected, previously unreported adverse events (e.g., heart valve thickening and pulmonary hypertension after Fen-Phen) or an incidence rate which is greater than previously known (rhabdomyolysis with statins). The following are definitions of some commonly used terms, which are found in 21CFR 312.32 (revised as of April 1, 2015):

1. Adverse events: "Any untoward medical occurrence associated with the use of a drug in humans, whether or not considered drug-related."
2. Life-threatening adverse events or suspected life-threatening adverse reactions: "An adverse event or suspected adverse reaction is considered 'life-threatening' if, in the view of either the investigator or sponsor, its occurrence places the patient or subject at immediate risk of death. It does not include an adverse event or suspected adverse reaction that, had it occurred in a more severe form, might have caused death."
3. Serious adverse event: As per the FDA, "An adverse event or suspected adverse reaction is considered 'serious' if, in the view of either the investigator or sponsor, it results in any of the following outcomes: Death, a life-threatening adverse event, inpatient hospitalization or prolongation of existing hospitalization, a persistent or significant incapacity or substantial disruption of the ability to conduct normal life functions, or a congenital anomaly/birth defect. Important medical events that may not result in death, be life-threatening, or require hospitalization may be considered serious when, based upon appropriate medical judgment, they may jeopardize the patient or subject and may require medical or surgical intervention to prevent one of the outcomes listed in this definition. Examples of such medical events include allergic bronchospasm requiring intensive treatment in an emergency room or at home, blood dyscrasias or

convulsions that do not result in inpatient hospitalization, or the development of drug dependency or drug abuse."

8.4 DEGREE OF ADVERSE EFFECTS RELATED TO INTERVENTION

Causation—causal relatedness of a drug to an AE—can be rated as: Definitely, probably, possibly, or unrelated to the treatment. Each of the degrees of relatedness has definite meanings, and their structured and consistent application is important for patients receiving the medication and for prescribing physicians. These terms are mentioned in 21CFR,[6] and their use is consistent throughout the pharmaceutical industry, the FDA, CDC, ICH, and WHO. Under the revised reporting FDA requirements *(21CFR 312.32)* for AEs which occur in an investigational new drug application (IND), the definition of "suspected adverse reaction" imposes a greater burden on sponsors to determine whether the drug caused the event, which would transform the temporally related adverse reaction from being an adverse event to an adverse effect. A wider application to these revised rules and definitions should be anticipated by the sponsor when reporting.

In an ideal world, it would be helpful if all observed potential adverse events were reported to the drug manufacturer, or to the FDA, via MedWatch forms, and through established reporting channels to the FDA. This would include all suspected adverse reactions seen as part of clinical use and also within clinical research protocols. In actual practice, less than 10% and possibly as few as less than 1% of all suspected adverse reactions are reported. Those of low seriousness and those well-known are probably reported the least, whereas those of high potential seriousness, new, or different could be expected to be reported. There are strict expectations on the part of the regulatory agencies for reporting of AE by drug manufacturers, but, in practice, these are not always followed.[7] Further, manufacturers maintain their own adverse event reports database, which is not available for inspection to the public and in general not to the regulatory agencies.

The determination of a degree of causation must occur within structured guidelines,[8] such as those of Koch,[9] Hill[10,11], or Riddell.[12] Some degree of flexibility is required, as circumstances demand. A practical definition scheme for assessing the degree of causality is as follows:

Unrelated: The AE is clearly due to extraneous causes (e.g., underlying disease, environment).

Unlikely (must have two):
The AE:

1) Does not have temporal relationship with intervention,
2) Could readily have been produced by the subject's clinical state,
3) Could have been due to environmental or other interventions,
4) Does not follow a known pattern of response to intervention,
5) Does not reappear or worsen with the reintroduction of intervention.

Possible (must have two):
The AE:

1) Has a reasonable temporal relationship with intervention,[13]
2) Could not readily have been produced by the subject's clinical state,
3) Could not readily have been due to environmental or other interventions,
4) Follows a known pattern of response to intervention.

Probable (must have three):
The AE:

1) Has a reasonable temporal relationship with intervention,
2) Could not readily have been produced by the subject's clinical state or have been due to environmental or other interventions,
3) Follows a known pattern of response to intervention,
4) Disappears or decreases with a reduction in dose or cessation of intervention.

Definite (must have all four):
The AE:

1) Has a reasonable temporal relationship with intervention,
2) Could not readily have been produced by the subject's clinical state or have been due to environmental or other interventions,
3) Follows a known pattern of response to intervention,
4) Disappears or decreases with reduction in dose or cessation of intervention and recurs with re-exposure.

For the purposes of 21CFR312.32, a Definite AE is equivalent to an (known) Adverse Reaction. A Probable or Possible AE falls within the FDA definition of Suspected Adverse Reaction until causation can be established:

> Any AE for which there is a reasonable possibility that the drug caused the AE. For the purposes of IND safety reporting, "reasonable possibility" means there is evidence to suggest a causal relationship between the drug and the AE. Suspected adverse reaction implies a lesser degree of certainty about causality than adverse reaction, which means any adverse event caused by a drug.

Under the revised reporting FDA requirements (21CFR 312.32) for AEs which occur in an IND, the relationship of "unknown" is not an option for the causality of SAEs. This creates a greater burden to establish a causal relatedness.

8.5 METHODOLOGY TO INVESTIGATE CAUSATION

Signs or symptoms associated with both regulated treatments can be observed in any phase of development ranging from clinical trial (before a drug is on the market), through initial marketing, up to many years thereafter. Clinical studies beyond the initial and characteristically small Phase I study are designed primarily to demonstrate efficacy—safety data beyond phase I studies is then collected as a secondary parameter. Clinical studies, which can be conducted in a randomized, blinded or non-randomized, non-blinded setting, are varied in their design and strongly influenced by the disease studied, the drug, and the types of information sought (safety, dosing, efficacy, disease-specific). It is for these reasons that referring to the Randomized Clinical Trial (RCT) as the gold standard for demonstrating causation is overly simplistic and deceptive. Important safety data which has allowed the discovery of new counter indications for already-licensed drugs, and caused the removal from market of others, has even come from a few cases presented in collected case series.[14,15,16]

Many clinical trial designs compare newer therapies against placebo. Several advances in clinical trial design have the potential to increase the relevance of trial results to real-world settings. Head-to-head comparisons may incorporate non-inferiority, factorial, and crossover designs. The meta-analysis of multiple studies can yield important conclusions not available via single studies, because of limitations on sample sizes, not completely comparable study designs (such as differences in the patient populations), and other features.

Some of the structured settings in which adverse effects can be evaluated include:

- Randomized Clinical Trial-—in an RCT, efficacy is almost always the primary parameter in which case safety is collected as a secondary parameter. An example would be AEs which are collected during the efficacy trial of an antihypertensive medication. Data can be collected actively (e.g., actively questioned for and data collected in case report forms) or passively collected (as when patients volunteer information on adverse effects about which they are not actively questioned).
- Epidemiologic studies—non-randomized, non-blinded studies that can collect incidence and prevalence data on adverse events in a specific population.
- Case-controlled studies—patients who exhibit an adverse event are matched with multiple demographically similar but nonexposed patients.[17],[18],[19]
- Individual case reports[20] or series—physicians (used here as a general term to include other healthcare providers) publish their observations of novel, unreported adverse effects in individual patients (cases) or groups of patients (series).
- Network meta-analysis—network meta-analysis[21] can combine direct and indirect evidence together and can enable one to compare multiple treatments with each other. Observational data may include disease registries, administrative claims data, and electronic medical records. These varied data can be pooled and linked across these data sources, and newer epidemiologic and analytic methods can provide more valid inferences regarding optimal treatment regimens.

8.6 STRUCTURED ALGORITHMS FOR THE DETERMINATION OF CAUSATION

Koch was perhaps the first to set down rules of causation, albeit not for adverse events.[22] The famous Koch postulates were designed to demonstrate whether a disease was caused by an infectious organism. Some have attempted to adapt Koch's postulates from infectious disease to drug AE causation, but this has generally been unsatisfactory.

8.6.1 Koch's Postulates

1) The suspected agent must be isolated from a patient with the disease in question.
2) The agent must be grown in the laboratory in pure culture.
3) The isolated agent, grown in pure culture, when infected into a healthy host produces exactly the same clinical disease.
4) One is able to isolate the same infective organism from the newly diseased person.[23]

Not only are Koch's postulates not useful for determining AE causation for medications, they are also not practical for many diseases, including HIV (intentional application of the third postulate). In contrast, other criteria, such as those defined by Hill and Riddell, are well-suited for drug adverse causation.

With a set of eight or nine rules, Hill[24] and also Riddell[25] established systematic methods for evaluating potential drug adverse effect causation. Not all of their rules need to be met for causation to be established, and some are more important than others. One of the first rules to meet is temporality, for it is obvious that symptoms of a putative adverse event which occur before the introduction of a treatment could not have been caused by the treatment. However, the symptom or symptom complex, even if preexisting, can be exacerbated by the introduction of the

TABLE 8.1
Criteria for Causation

Hill Criteria[26]	Riddell Criteria[27]
Strength of association	Temporal eligibility
Consistency of results	Latent period
Specificity	Exclusion
Temporal relationship	De-challenge
Dose response	Re-challenge[21,22]
Biologic plausibility	Singularity of the drug
Biologic coherence	Pattern
Experimentation	Drug identification
Analogy	

medication. Hill criteria (537) and Riddell criteria (538) are provided in Table 8.1.

8.6.2 Hill Criteria—Expanded Discussion

(See Section 8.7 for more details.)

1. **Strength of Association**
   A strong association gives support to a causal hypothesis. A weak association requires other information but can be equally as important.
2. **Consistency of Results**
   Repeated findings in different populations and different settings.
3. **Specificity**
   Strengthens confidence in association. Lack of specificity does not rule out causation.
4. **Temporal Relationship**
   Required: Exposure must come before disease.
5. **Dose Response**
   Increased dose = Increased risk. This holds true for both drugs and for vaccines.
6. **Biological Plausibility**
   Known mechanism not required. For example:
   Cigarettes and lung cancer
   Asbestos and lung cancer
   Fen-Phen and valvular heart disease and PPH
7. **Biological Coherence**
   Does not conflict with what is known.
8. **Experimentation**
   RCT is close to experimentation. Removal or reduction of exposure reduces the intensity of disease. Challenge—de-challenge—re-challenge.
9. **Analogy**
   Similarities with other like exposure. For example:
   Aminorex and PPH
   Ergot drugs and VHD

All of these systems for determination can be simplified in an algorithm-based analysis:

1. Temporal relatedness
2. Known or reported AE of medication
3. Presence of concurrent illnesses or medications which could present similarly
4. Challenge—de-challenge—re-challenge

8.7 COMMENTS ON THE INDIVIDUAL RIDDELL CRITERIA FOR CAUSATION[28,29]

Temporal Eligibility: As previously discussed, an effect must occur after a treatment in order to establish causation. The effect should not occur *too* long after the treatment. Inevitably, the question becomes: How long is too long? Regardless of the context, this question, asked without accompanying details, can only have one answer: It depends. Some drugs, such as PCP and Lariam, are known to have neuropsychiatric adverse effects that can last for years after the drug was last taken. Gynecomastia develops only after months of repeated use of risperidone. Autoimmune or neurologic adverse effects of vaccines can be delayed months after administration.[30,31]

Latent Period: Although the closer the interval between the introduction of the treatment and the adverse effect the better, a long latent period can still be consistent with a causal relatedness. Some AEs can have immediate action or a latent period in seconds such as immediate hypersensitivity reactions. Other AEs are more subtle, although equally lethal, and with a longer time delay between exposure and AE, such as liver toxicity from acetaminophen.

Exclusion: It is important to rule out the effect of concurrent medications or underlying medical conditions such as an alternative hypothesis. Liver enzyme elevations in a diabetic patient with underlying fatty liver, and simultaneously taking a statin for hyperlipidemia, can be a challenge for the determination of causation. Regardless, with careful attention to the timeline and details, even in such cases, a determination can be made.

Challenge: The disappearance or improvement of an adverse event after the withdrawal of the treatment is a positive indication of relatedness. Adverse events can however persist after the treatment is withdrawn, which indicates either that there was no relatedness, or that the adverse effect causes persistent injury.

Re-challenge: Reintroduction of a treatment which is again associated with the same or similar adverse event is a good indication of causation. If the AE does not reappear, this can be a sign of lack of causation but may also indicate the development of tolerance. Of course, since the potential association in the first place may prevent the reintroduction of the suspect treatment, this is not always possible to see.

Singularity of the Drug: It is important to determine whether there is something unique about the adverse reaction experience that is not consistent with any other drug taken or any existing disease condition. Even when a supposed unique adverse reaction is noted (e.g., heart valve thickening and pulmonary hypertension with Fen-Phen), careful investigation can show that a pharmacologically similar medication is known to cause similar adverse effects.

Pattern: It is important to determine whether similar AEs have been described in the literature with the treatment in question or by another medication in the same therapeutic class. A characteristic morphologic pattern in a target organ may suggest an association with a particular drug or group of drugs. For example, "Pseudo-tumor cerebri with hypervitaminosis" provides a literature precedent and a biological plausibility for similar neurologic injury with Accutane.

Drug Identification: Identification of the causative agent is of major utility in toxicity and overdose cases. In some cases, such as over-the-counter ephedra associated with intracranial hemorrhage, there may be neither a package insert nor an established laboratory procedure for measuring blood level concentration. It is important to take into account drug metabolism, as it may affect the drug level detected. In some cases, for example with vaccines and biologicals, quantitative determination is not possible, and the demonstration of an immune response will suffice.

8.8 DAUBERT AND THE EVOLUTION OF CAUSATION[32,33]

The accurate determination of causation is a crucial part of every investigation of an adverse effect. Causation can determine whether a treatment receives a marketing authorization, whether a treatment is withdrawn from market, and if the AE frequency will be reported in the accompanying labeling (which has a great influence on the competitive market position). The *Daubert* ruling (*Daubert v. Merrell Dow Pharmaceuticals, Inc.,* 509 U.S. 579, 113 S.Ct. 2786, 125 L.Ed.2d 469, 1993) set the stage for the Federal Rules of Evidence,[34] which is the standard for admitting testimony about scientific evidence. Many, if not most, expert reports concerning causation can expect to have a *Daubert* challenge over scientific validity. The United States Supreme Court upheld the trial court's exclusion of evidence in the *Daubert* case, giving, as part of its opinion, four criteria that the trial judge should consider in determining if evidence should be admitted:

1. The theory's testability,
2. Whether it "has been a subject of peer review or publication,"
3. The "known or potential rate of error," and
4. The "degree of acceptance" within the relevant scientific community.

The Court stressed that this analysis was intended to be flexible, with the trial judge determining how and whether the factors applied in a given case. Although not comparable to the Hill or Riddell criteria, they are just as important, and determinations of causation, while not needing to address all criteria, need to be consistent with them. Any inconsistencies should have a logical and factual basis.

Daubert v. Merrell Dow Pharmaceuticals, Inc., 43 F.3d 1311, 1317 [9th Cir., 1995] expanded on these rules, listing the following as important considerations:

1. The cases versus controls must have a relative risk or odds ratio of ≥ 2.0.
2. The data must be from double or triple-blind clinical trials.
3. The evidence cited should be from relevant peer-reviewed scientific journals.
4. Challenge/de-challenge/re-challenge studies are useful in suggesting causation.
5. Perform or cite epidemiological studies with adequate samples, controls, and appropriate statistical analyses.
6. Theories or methods utilized should be generally accepted in the relevant scientific community or discipline.
7. The investigator must make every effort to account for or rule out alternative explanations of the outcome.
8. Testimony by scientific experts should be non-litigation driven.
9. Purported outcome effects should be from similar purported causes.

Each of these criteria is briefly commented on and explained as follows:

1. Cases versus controls with a relative risk or odds ratio of ≥ 2.0 is a relative and arbitrary standard and not applicable to all conditions, such as idiosyncratic reactions.
2. Blind, randomized, clinical trials are in general supported by drug companies, to demonstrate efficacy as a means to achieving licensure. Safety data is collected as a secondary parameter.
3. Even evidence cited from relevant peer-reviewed scientific journals can be questionable. Ghost writing is a common practice in research supported by the pharmaceutical industry. There also have been a number of recent examples of scientific falsification of data, questionable methods, and conflict of interest in several prominent peer-reviewed medical journals.

4. Challenge/de-challenge/re-challenge studies are useful in suggesting causation.
5. Citing epidemiological studies with adequate samples, controls, and appropriate statistical analyses. There are many instances where the RCT is not appropriate to evaluate a causal relatedness, including:
   a. the difficulties in definition of the population to be studied,
   b. the large sample size needed to detect an event of low incidence (such as suicide, suicide ideation, or homicide), and
   c. the bias introduced by employing multiple investigators in order to generate a large sample size.[28]

   In these cases, an alternative study design, such as challenge-rechallenge, has the potential to better determine whether or not a drug effect is present. These alternative study designs do employ components of the RCT but can remove bias inherent in epidemiologic studies; view patients at higher risk from a wide variety of sources; and employ objective experimental measures to clarify patient selection, diagnostic, and response parameters.
6. Theories or methods utilized should be generally accepted in the relevant scientific community or discipline. This is always important, but not all physicians in all cultures and localities agree on the existence, importance, or cause of some diseases.
7. The investigator must make every effort to account for or rule out alternative explanations of the out come. However, a drug may be a proximate cause without being *the* proximal cause and still be causal. A drug may be a necessary condition for the outcome without being a sufficient (the only) condition. That is, the outcome may not have occurred without the drug, but the outcome may also require some other contributing factor. "Ruling out" is not always possible. Further, alternative explanations can still exist.
8. Testimony by scientific experts should be non-litigation driven. This is important as a demonstration of honesty and objectivity; however, many, if not most, experts have ties to one side of the issue or another and are compensated for their expert opinions. Applying these criteria to FDA Advisory Committee membership, very few experts would be able to serve.
9. Purported outcome effects should be from similar purported causes. No comment is necessary.

8.9 DOES CAUSATION NEED TO BE ESTABLISHED BEFORE A WARNING IS GIVEN?

This is an area of concern for the pharmaceutical industry, for the prescribing clinician, and for the patient. The FDA gives guidance on this issue in 21CFR 201.57. This section provides specific requirements on the content and format (warnings) for human prescription drugs. Section (e) states:

> Warnings: Under this section heading, the labeling shall describe SAE and potential safety hazards, limitations in use imposed by them, and steps that should be taken if they occur. The labeling should be revised to include a warning as soon as there is reasonable evidence of an association of a serious hazard with a drug, and a causal connection need not have been shown.

Key points that can be taken from 21CFR 201.57 are:

1. The FDA regulations provide a broad duty to warn: "All serious and potential." The FDA threshold is not proven causation, but it is as soon as an "association" is detected. This explains why it state that, "a causal connection need not have been shown."
2. The duty to warn is also a continuing duty to amend and revise: "As soon as there is reasonable evidence of a causal association with a drug." The duty to warn is placed on the manufacturer and not on the FDA: Warnings for prescription drugs are typically directed to prescribing physicians, but there are also occasions where warnings must be made directly to the consumer.

8.10 WHAT ARE THE QUALIFICATIONS NEEDED TO GIVE EXPERT CAUSATION OPINIONS?

Thames and Martin address the topic, Pharmacologist as an Expert Witness, in the context of Daubert applications in pharmaceutical cases.[35] They write,

> It is commonplace for an expert pharmacologist to educate a jury by explaining a chemical's or a drug's properties and how it works. Expert pharmacologists are sometimes also used to demonstrate that the information available to a pharmaceutical company should have resulted in an additional or heightened warning. A number of courts have allowed pharmacologists to offer expert opinions related to causation wherever the opinion is based on reliable data and methodology.

They go on to state, "In federal court, expert testimony is admissible if offered by a proffered witness qualified as an expert by knowledge, skill, experience, training, or education" (Fed.R.Civ.Proc. 702). Provided this standard is satisfied, the expert need not hold an advanced degree in pharmacology to offer an expert opinion on an aspect of pharmacology. Interestingly, the article highlights the Daubert challenges to the admissibility of James T. O'Donnell PharmD's testimony.

> One man has almost single-handedly been involved in the decisions constituting the case law in this area. Courts in at least 11 cited cases now have considered whether James O'Donnell Pharm.D., is qualified to testify that either (1) a given warning was inadequate; or (2) a drug is pharmacologically capable of causing a particular effect.

Issues raised in opposition have been that O'Donnell is neither an M.D. nor does he possess a graduate degree in pharmacology. It is noted, however, that O'Donnell is a Diplomate of the American Board of Clinical Pharmacology.[36] The authors note that a few courts have found O'Donnell not qualified, other courts (a majority) have allowed O'Donnell to offer both causation and adequacy of warning expert opinions, finding that his qualifications and background do not, in and of themselves, prevent him from offering admissible expert testimony at trial.[37] One opinion (Ashman) stated, "A person with a doctorate in pharmacy can be qualified as a medical expert."

With reference to the standards and qualifications for a physician serving as a medical expert for medical malpractice cases, the AAFP (2004) provides the following guidelines.[38]

> It is the responsibility of the physician expert witness in a medical liability case to present complete and unbiased information with which the trier of fact can ascertain whether the defendant was medically negligent and whether, as a result, the plaintiff suffered compensable injury and/or damages. The physician expert witness should be aware that transcripts of depositions and courtroom testimony are public records.
>
> The physician expert witness should not become an advocate or a partisan during the trial and, to the extent possible, the testimony presented should reflect the generally accepted standards within the specialty or area of practice about which the expert witness is testifying. When there is no generally accepted standard of practice or when the expert witness presents testimony that is contrary to the generally accepted standard, the expert witness should clearly identify that fact, as well as the basis for the opinions expressed. Ideally, both the defense and the plaintiff should have at least one witness in the same specialty as the defendant physician.
>
> Prior to testifying, the physician expert witness should become familiar with the facts of the case and the medical standard at issue and should review and understand both the current concepts and practices related to that standard as well as the concepts and practices related to that standard at the time of the occurrence which led to the lawsuit.
>
> Compensation to physicians who testify as expert witnesses should be reasonable and commensurate with the time and effort involved in fulfilling the physician's responsibilities as an expert witness. The acceptance of fees that are disproportionately high relative to the time and effort involved may be interpreted as influencing testimony and should be avoided. Under no circumstances should a physician accept compensation for serving as an expert witness when payment of the compensation or the amount of the compensation are contingent upon the outcome of the case.

The AAFP also comments on what should be the minimal qualifications of medical experts for medical malpractice cases:

1. The physician expert witness must have a current, unrestricted license to practice.
2. The physician expert witness should be fully trained in the medical specialty or area of practice about which he or she is testifying.
3. The physician expert witness must have current clinical experience in the medical specialty or area of practice about which he or she is testifying and during the two-year period immediately preceding the occurrence which led to the lawsuit, such person must have been actively engaged in clinical practice in the medical specialty or area of medicine about which he or she is testifying.
4. At least one physician expert witness for the plaintiff and one physician expert for the defendant should be in the same clinical specialty as the defendant physician.

Similar but less detailed guidelines are offered by the AMA (Opinion 9.07—Medical Testimony, Dec 2004).[39]

8.11 CASE REPORTS DEMONSTRATING THE APPLICATIONS OF CAUSATION PRINCIPLES

Treaters and retained experts (physicians, pharmacologists, clinical pharmacists, and toxicologists) are frequently tasked with determining whether or not a drug caused an alleged injury, as well as whether or not the treater (physician, pharmacist, nurse) complied with the applicable standard of care. The following case reports are presented as examples of determinations of causation.

8.11.1 Case Report: Acyclovir Overdose—Pharmacist-Recommended Overdose

George Patient ("Mr. Patient") presented to his physician with complaints of a rash on his trunk on 11/20/15. George was anephric, meaning without kidney function, and had been undergoing hemodialysis three times weekly for a sustained period of time secondary to bilateral nephrectomies. His physician was aware of George's lack of kidney function on 11/20/15 and further aware that George was actively engaged in efforts to obtain renal transplant.

The physician suspected Herpes Zoster (shingles) and prescribed Valtrex (valacyclovir). According to the prescription and medication bottle provided by counsel, George was prescribed 3,000 mg of Valtrex daily (1 gm TID). George took his first dose on 11/20/15 and two doses on 11/21/15. George's wife found him weak and incoherent on the family room floor with broken furniture surrounding him. She called an ambulance, and George was taken to an Emergency Department. He was admitted to the hospital not long after his presentation.

8.11.1.1 Facts of the Case

1. Q full dose of Valtrex 3,000 mg daily (1,000 mg TID) was prescribed; Valtrex is a pro-drug. It is converted to acyclovir in the body.
2. George was admitted to the ED with an altered mental state (AMS).
3. George's medication history was noted to include a recent prescription for Valtrex (1,000 mg TID) and the altered mental and health state of the preceding day and morning were noted.
4. A medical resident physician ordered 850 mg IV acyclovir Q 8 H (2,550 mg/day) at 18:17 (6:17 pm). The order was discontinued at 19:15 (7:15 pm) after a hospital pharmacist's intervention. The order was changed by another physician at 19:14 (7:15 pm) to a single dose of 850 mg IV acyclovir to be given after dialysis and was confirmed/acknowledged by the hospital pharmacist at 19:18 (7:18 pm). This single 850-mg dose, although subsequently a different dose was ordered (–500 mg—see #6), was never discontinued; it was prepared and provided by the hospital pharmacy and was administered at 619 am on 11/23/15, after hemodialysis was complete. The Medication Administration Record documents that this 850-mg IV acyclovir dose was administered at 06:19 am by a nurse on the morning of 11/23/15.
5. At 20:15 (8:15 pm) on 11/22/15, a second medical resident issued a verbal order for acyclovir, which was re-calculated for "renal" dosing—500 mg IV daily on dialysis days after dialysis. This was calculated according to the Renal Monitoring and Dosage Adjustment Policy, by the same hospital pharmacist at 20:25 (8:25 pm) on 11/22/15, and ordered to be given daily q 24 h after dialysis. This 500 mg IV acyclovir dose was administered to the Patient on 11/23/15 at 21:01 (9:01 pm). This order is noted to be discontinued by another physician at 23:50 (11:50 pm) on 11/25/15.
6. On 11/23/15, the patient received 850 mg IV acyclovir at 06:19 am and 500 mg at 21:01, that is, 1,350 mg total acyclovir within 15 hours of his last dialysis.
7. All 1,350 mg of IV acyclovir administered to Mr. Patient on 11/23 was verified and confirmed by the same hospital pharmacist.
8. Valtrex toxicity was considered as the cause of the patient's encephalopathy on 11/23/15. Viral encephalitis was also considered in the differential.
9. Acyclovir IV was continued until the end of November, with the exception of 11/26/15, when the dose was held for one day and then restarted at 250 mg/day.
10. Valtrex encephalopathy was considered frequently as an alternative diagnosis to viral encephalitis until 11/26, at which time the Valtrex encephalopathy was confirmed.
11. George's mental state/encephalopathy improved when the acyclovir dose was discontinued.

8.11.1.2 Opinions

The expert held the following opinions with reasonable pharmacological and pharmaceutical certainty:

1. The appropriate renal dosing of oral Valacyclovir for an individual with no kidney function is 500 mg per day.
2. The appropriate renal dosing of IV acyclovir for an individual with no kidney function is 425 mg per day.
3. No reason existed from a pharmaceutical standpoint to deviate from renal dosing protocols specific to Acyclovir. Moreover, the patient's medical records do not evidence any physician requesting the pharmacy to deviate from renal dosing to orchestrate a deliberate plan of care. The depositions of defendant physicians in the case reflect this as well.
4. The 1,000 mg TID dose of Valtrex was an overdose in this anephric/dialysis patient.
5. The prescription for 1,000 mg Valtrex caused severe neurotoxicity, encephalopathy, confusion, and physical impairments and necessitated his admission to the hospital Emergency Department.
6. The initial Emergency Department assessment of the patient noted the acute alteration of his mental state. His renal status (dialysis), his encephalopathy, and his Valtrex (valacyclovir) 3,000 mg/day dose were noted.
7. The initial order for 850 mg q 8 hours of intravenous acyclovir was a toxic/overdose and ignored the patient's lack of renal function and dependence on dialysis and the need for a significantly reduced dose, recommended in the prescribing information (package insert) and the literature as 500 mg/day. This was changed to a single dose, which still is a toxic overdose, and finally lowered to a 500 mg dose. Even this reduction to 850 mg/day dose calculation is twice the dosing recommendation recommended in the hospital Renal Dosing Protocol (425 mg) as well as in the FDA-approved prescribing information.
8. The 850-mg acyclovir IV single dose was never discontinued by the pharmacist. This being despite his involvement with consulting, verifying, and confirmation of the subsequent 500-mg "renal dose." On its own, the 850-mg dose is an overdose in a patient without kidney function. When combined with the 500-mg dose 15 hours later and with no hemodialysis occurring in the

interim, the overdose is multiplied, and the effects exacerbated.

9. The pharmacist, who provided the renal dosing consult, verified and modified the orders for IV acyclovir and was ultimately responsible for approving the dispensing 1,350-mg of IV acyclovir to be administered the following day to a patient without kidney function, was negligent and departed from the standard of care of a reasonable and prudent hospital pharmacist. The pharmacist's work and decision-making also directly conflicted with the Hospital Renal Monitoring and Dosage Adjustment Policy. This negligence was a direct and proximate cause of the cardiac arrest that George suffered on 11/24/15.
10. The Patient received a second dose of acyclovir (500 mg) on the second hospital day (11/23/15), essentially an overdose of the acyclovir, considering his renal failure. Hemodialysis can remove up to 33–60% of acyclovir. This means that 30–60% of the remaining acyclovir from the 3,000 mg/day treatment of Valtrex remained after the dialysis. Additional acyclovir, with dosages of 850 mg at 06.19 am and 500 mg at 2100 hours, was administered on 11/23, adding to the neurotoxicity of acyclovir.
11. George's encephalopathy improved after the acyclovir was discontinued.
12. George's morbidity and complications that developed after his admission were caused by the initial (physician—Valtrex) and continued excessive and incorrect administration of acyclovir. Had he been administered the correct renal dosing for Valtrex, he would not have become encephalopathic, which precipitated the ED admission. Had the incorrect 850 mg IV acyclovir plus a second dose not been administered on 11/23, George would have avoided the extreme acyclovir toxicity from which he suffered and further avoided the significantly increased risk of cardiac arrest that was ultimately realized.

8.11.1.2.1 Hemodialysis

In anuric (anephric) patients, acyclovir is slowly eliminated with a terminal plasma half-life of approximately 20 hours. The acyclovir total body clearance (29 ml/min/1.73m^2) is only 10% of that seen in patients without renal impairment. Acyclovir is readily hemodialyzed with an extraction coefficient of 0.45. A single hemodialysis (6 h) reduces acyclovir concentrations by up to 33, 45, or 60%.

8.11.1.2.2 Need for Pharmacist Monitoring

The hospital recognized the need for dosage adjustment based upon compromised (or absent) renal function, as described in the Renal Monitoring and Dosage Adjustment Policy. Unfortunately, the pharmacist in question did not discontinue the incorrectly calculated 850-mg acyclovir dose. Since the acyclovir 850-mg IV single dose was not discontinued, it was treated as an active order, prepared by the pharmacy, delivered to the floor, and administered at 06:19 am by a nurse, according to the MAR.

All of the opinions expressed above were stated to a reasonable degree of pharmaceutical certainty and were based on the records received to date. The expert reserved the right to amend or supplement this report if additional information is made available. The case was settled by the hospital (employer of the pharmacist) on the eve of trial.

Case References:

1. *http://www.globalrph.com/anti_herpetic.htm*
2. *Kitching AR, Fagg D, Hay NM, Hatfield PJ, Macdonald A. Neurotoxicity associated with acyclovir in end stage renal failure. N Z Med J. 1997 May 9;110(1043):167–9.*
3. *Haefeli WE, Schoenenberger RA, Weiss P, Ritz RF. Acyclovir-induced neurotoxicity: concentration-side effect relationship in acyclovir overdose. Am J Med. 1993 Feb;94(2):212–5.*
4. *Leikin JB, Shicker L, Orlowski J, Blair AT, McAllister K. Hemodialysis removal of acyclovir. Vet Hum Toxicol. 1995 Jun;37(3):233–4.*
5. *Laskin OL. Clinical Pharmacokinetics of Acyclovir. Clinical Pharmacokinetics of Acyclovir. June 1983, Volume 8, Issue 3, pp 187–201.*

8.11.2 Case Report: Challenging Cause of Death in a Malpractice Matter

8.11.2.1 Facts of the Case

On Thursday, November 29, 2007, Anthony Patient, a 42-year-old, 110-pound, cerebral palsy afflicted, developmentally delayed male resident at a group home, was found unresponsive and shortly thereafter declared dead at the Emergency Department, after unsuccessful resuscitation efforts. An autopsy and toxicology were performed, and a high level of sertraline, 2,000 μg/L (200 μg/L), was noted, with normal and untested (and therefore) no toxic levels for other medications being administered to Anthony (lorazepam, olanzapine). The autopsy (and therefore the toxicology specimens) was performed beginning at 12:10 pm on 12/30/07, ~36 hours after Anthony Patient's death. A forensic pathologist ruled the causes of death as 1) Bronchopneumonia (principle), with 2) sertraline toxicity, and 3) partial bowel obstruction as contributing causes of death. At autopsy, two plastic "stars" were found embedded in the wall of his small intestine at the junction of the jejunum and ileum. The pathologist described necrotic tissue, a small fistula, and partial bowel obstruction caused by these stars.

The patient started having respiratory complaints and signs and symptoms of acute respiratory disease in September 2007 and was seen frequently (11 times) at a local urgent care center for his complaints. He was also treated for his respiratory complaints (albuterol nebulizer/oral albuterol tablets, Z-Pak, prednisone, cephalexin, Mucinex). His last visit was on November 28, 2007, the evening before he was found dead. An X-ray demonstrated excess intestinal gas that was pushing up on his diaphragm. Anthony was last seen at 5:00 am by the home staff, 90 to 120 minutes he was found unresponsive/in cardiac arrest. For several days before his death, the patient was experiencing diarrhea. There are no notations in the records that he was not eating and drinking, and the records indicate that sertraline (maximum dose—200 mg/day) and other medications were being administered.

The Coroner related that he inquired of a forensic toxicologist—Laboratory Director—who performed the post mortem toxicology and the pathologist as to the cause of the excessive sertraline level. He was told that the sertraline tablets must have "accumulated at the site of the bowel obstruction and were released in one acute dose." Further,

> [T]he thought process in terms of why other medications didn't accumulate—I believe that answer falls within the fact the other medications were given on a prn basis. But both the toxicologist and the pathologist stated that they truly could not explain why other medications didn't do that, except for the fact that they were being given on a different dosing schedule.

Later in the inquest, the Coroner related that neither the pathologist nor the toxicologist would speculate on how much Sertraline the toxicology report concentration represented. "Neither physician felt comfortable coming up with a number that would actually be accurate."

8.11.2.2 Opinions

1. Zoloft/sertraline probably did not contribute or cause Anthony's death.
2. The patient was seen clinically the evening before—with no signs of Serotonin Syndrome, which likely would be present if sertraline was accumulating; Anthony was observed two hours before death was discovered. Serotonin Syndrome onset could not be that fast—i.e., 1.5 to 2 hours. Indeed, he may have died in the interim period between 5 am and the time he was discovered unresponsive.
3. The 2,000 μg/L sertraline level is probably inaccurate, an artificial elevation that occurs post-mortem (post-mortem distribution—PMD), as a result of the release of stored sertraline from muscles, liver, and other organs and tissues. While the PMD phenomenon is more pronounced in central (body) blood draws, it does occur in peripheral sampling, due to release from the large muscle masses in the femoral area of the lower extremity.
4. The pathologist and toxicologist both offered an explanation that "the sertraline pills accumulated at the obstruction" and "a toxic dose was released all at once," but neither felt confident in that explanation, as the sertraline was the only toxic level found, and an obstruction would not select one tablet and allow others to pass. Neither was attempting to calculate the amount consumed—it could not be done. Indeed, calculating pre-mortem levels from post-mortem concentrations is fraught with uncertainty.
5. The patient had a partial obstruction. Sertraline would disintegrate in the stomach and dissolution (change from tablet fragments to a liquid mixed with intestinal juices) would occur in the duodenum and jejunum, and substantial portions of sertraline doses administered would most likely be absorbed before the "obstruction." This is a biopharmaceutical fact—this is how drug absorption works—tablets do not accumulate at a partial obstruction several feet into the small bowel. Indeed, it was not a total obstruction—it was a partial obstruction. That means that medicine and foods would be digested in the bowel and pass through the obstruction.
6. The 2,000 μg/L level of sertraline is not predictive for lethality; survival has been reported at much higher levels (~ 2,900 μg/L) in a patient who overdosed with 80 × 100 mg tablets (8,000 mg). Sertraline, and other drugs in its class, are surprisingly well-tolerated and considered much safer than earlier types of antidepressants.
7. A reasonable cause of death was present—bronchopneumonia, along with partial obstruction. Indeed, the intestinal gas inflating the loops of bowel and pressing up on the diaphragm would compromise the patient's breathing, already compromised by his bronchopneumonia.
8. The medication count for Zoloft (sertraline) was accurate—no doses were missing or unaccounted for. Doses are charted as being administered daily for the period before the patient's death.
9. Several authoritative sources supported the expert's opinions, as referenced.

Summary and Conclusion

Not surprisingly, the "lethal level of sertraline" piqued everyone's interest. However, careful and informed analyses of this case caused the expert to conclude that this patient's death was not caused or contributed to by sertraline. The "lethal" sertraline level was most likely an artifact. The clinical condition of the patient does not support sertraline toxicity on the day before his death. The explanation of "all at once absorption" of a toxic dose is incompatible with known pharmaceutical sciences. Further, there was no missing sertraline to explain an accidental overdose of sertraline.

Case References:

1. *Goeringer KE, Raymon L, Christian GD, and Logan BK. Postmortem Forensic Toxicology of Selective Serotonin Reuptake Inhibitors: A review of Pharmacology and Report of 168 Cases. J Forensic Sciences. 2000; 45: (3): 633–648.*
2. *Leiken JB, and Watson WA. Post-mortem Toxicology: What the Dead Can and Cannot Tell Us. J of Toxicology/Clinical Toxicology, Vol 41, No 1. 47–56, 2003.*
3. *Baselt RC.Ed. Disposition of Toxic Drugs and Chemicals in man, Eighth Edition. Biomedical Publications. Foster City, CA. 2009*
4. *Brendel DH, Bodkin JA, and Yang JM. Massive Sertraline Overdose. Annals of Emergency Medicine 36/5. November 2000, 524–526.*
5. *Mackay FR, Dunn NR, Martin RM, Freemantle SN, and Mann RD. Newer antidepressants: A Comparison of tolerability in general practice. British Journal of General Practice, Vol 49, November 1999. 892–896.*
6. *Levine B, Jenkins AJ, and Smialek JE. Distribution of Sertraline in Postmortem Cases. J. Analyt Tox, Vol 18, September 1994. 272–274.*

8.11.3 Case Report: Determination of the Effects of Morphine in a Will Contest

Evaluating, assessing, and determining what effect(s) morphine administration had on the decedent during the period of October 1—October 6, 2020.

8.11.3.1 Facts of the Case

The decedent died on October 6, 2020, two weeks after discharge (9/25/20) to Hospice care at home from a local hospital with a terminal diagnosis (widespread fallopian tube cancer). While hospitalized, she was started on morphine sublingual dosage (2 mg every (q) one hour) for analgesia purposes.

At home, morphine (liquid concentrate 20 mg/ml) was ordered, both as a Scheduled dose, and a "PRN"—as needed:

- 2 mg every 1 hours as needed for pain and accelerating every few days.
- On September 28, 2020, the order was changed to morphine 4 mg q 4 hours Scheduled—PRN morphine 2 mg/hour was also available.
- On September 29, 2020, the order was changed to Morphine 8 mg q 4 hours (PRN dose also available)
- On October 2 or 3, 2020, a dosage increase for morphine (10 mg q 4 hour Scheduled) was ordered and her morphine dose was 2 mg q 1 hours as needed for pain. For certain, the morphine dose was raised to 10 mg q 4 hours the next day, on October 3, 2020.

8.11.3.2 Opinions

The expert's opinions were expressed with reasonable pharmacological certainty.

1. As a result of cognitive impairing and disinhibiting effects of morphine on October 2, 2020, any decisions made by the decedent were subject to the influence of morphine. Her ability to deliberate and consider the consequences of changing her estate plan on her death bed were suspect and fraught with risk.
2. Morphine, a strong opiate narcotic, disinhibits (releases) controls—through a loss of inhibition. Morphine is well-known to impair higher brain functions, deliberation, and memory and cause clouding of the sensorium and judgment. The patient need not "appear" to be impaired. Executive functions, or the effects of impairment or inhibition, were not manifest in physical signs, levels of attention, communication, or responsiveness.
3. Drug-induced cognitive impairment is most commonly linked to opiates and some other Central Nervous System depressants. Opiates are known to cause confusion and a number of other adverse behavioral (cognitive) impairments/effects. Acute and chronic opioid use is associated with neuropsychological dysfunction that impacts attention, executive functions, concentration, visuospatial skills, recall, and psychomotor speed. Higher cortical executive functions are the first brain functions to be impaired; impairment of this level of brain functioning is not apparent to even a trained observer.
4. Cells in the prefrontal cortex are involved in cognitive function. It is posed that each frontal cortical region may be associated with a different aspect of the learning process, evaluation of choices, and subsequent selection of actions. An alternative view suggests that decision-making circuits work in parallel within the frontal lobes to organize different types of decision-making.
5. On October 2, morphine was prescribed at a Scheduled dose of 48–60 mg/day, and a PRN dose of 48 mg/day.

Case References

1. *Gruber SA, Silveri MM, Yurgelun-Todd, DA. Neuropsychological consequences of opiate use. Neuropsychol Rev 2007;17:299–315.*
2. *http://dailymed.nlm.nih.gov/dailymed/lookup.cfm?setid=554baee5-b171-4452-a50a-41a0946f956c#nlm34084-4, access 9/25/13.*
3. *http://www.worstpills.org/includes/page.cfm?op_id=459*
4. *http://dailymed.nlm.nih.gov/dailymed/lookup.cfm?setid=554baee5-b171-4452-a50a-41a0946f956c#nlm34084-4, access 9/25/13.*

5. *Gruber SA, Silveri MM, Yurgelun-Todd, DA. Neuropsychological consequences of opiate use. Neuropsychol Rev 2007;17:299–315.*
6. *J L Giacchino, S J Henriksen Opioid effects on activation of neurons in the medial prefrontal cortex. Prog Neuropsychopharmacol Biol Psychiatry. 1998 Oct;22(7):1157–78.*
7. *Rushworth MF, Kolling N, Sallet J, Mars RB. Valuation and decision-making in frontal cortex: one or many serial or parallel systems? Curr Opin Neurobiol. 2012 Dec;22(6):946–55.*

8.11.4 Case Report: Proof of Drug-Induced Mental Changes in Complainant in Sexual Abuse Case

Ms. Complainant, at age 17, accused Joseph Defendant, her former stepfather, of alleged sexual abuse during the period when she was 5 or 6 until 12 years of age, during part of the period that Ms. Complainant lived in the Defendant's residence while Ms. Complainant's mother was married to the Defendant. The Defendant vehemently denies any abuse, sexual or otherwise, occurred in the home or anywhere else.

Ms. Complainant "told" (led/prompted by) a school guidance/counselor of the alleged abuse in November 2010, which precipitated a notification of child protective services, who notified the police. During the interview, because Ms. Complainant was crying, the guidance counselor claims she could not speak, so the guidance counselor asked her if her father (Defendant) abused her. Ms. Complainant merely nodded in the affirmative. Thus, the guidance counselor put the allegations into the mouth of Ms. Complainant while in an apparent vulnerable state. A police detective subsequently interviewed Ms. Complainant; the police subsequently arranged for recording a telephone conversation between Ms. Complainant and Defendant in which Ms. Complainant repeatedly attempted to solicit discussions about and admissions to the sexual abuse. No admissions were made. Indeed, during the call, once Defendant realized and clarified Ms. Complainant's questions and statements, he was "shocked and numb," in disbelief, that Ms. Complainant would ever make those accusations.

Shortly after the recorded call between Ms. Complainant and Defendant, the police interviewed the Defendant and arrested him.

There have been no persons identified who witnessed any of the alleged abuse, and, indeed, the alleged abuse was disclosed to the school Guidance Counselor in November 2010, more than 5 years after the last alleged abuse. Ms. Complainant did not report any specifics, rather nonverbally (nodding) answered questions from the Guidance Counsellor, suggesting certain behaviors/abuses. It has thus been approximately nine years since the alleged abuse ceased. Ms. Complainant and 2 friends stated/testified that Ms. Complainant instant messaged or texted (indirectly told them) that "something went on with her father"—but no details were provided.

In the police interview, Ms. Complainant was extremely vague about what happened, where it happened, how frequently it happened, ranging from a few times a week to as little as 10 or 12 times total.

In a houseful of up to ten people plus various nannies and babysitters, no one in the family reported, witnessed, or was aware or even suspected any alleged sexual abuse by the. Even complainant's mother stated, "I never noticed anything unusual or suspected him—Defendant of any sexual behavior with my daughter."

The arrest and the indictment are based exclusively upon the allegations of abuse by Ms. Complainant. The concept of CSAAS (Child Sexual Abuse Accommodation Syndrome) was offered. CSAAS provides an explanation for delayed, accommodated, secretive, and/or recantation statements regarding child sexual abuse, when the usual signs and symptoms of child sexual abuse are absent (discussed in detail later in this report). It was introduced by an expert who has correctly identified CSAAS as a *non-diagnostic* report, only describing the phenomenon.

CSAAS is defined by an expert who provides the caveat that "clearly it is not the purpose of this testimony to provide a diagnostic formulation or predictive statement in this matter." CSAAS, as defined, is offered only as an explanation for Ms. Complainant's repressed and delayed recitation of alleged repetitive sexual abuse by her stepfather Defendant. CSAAS is considered controversial and is not accepted by all Courts and Jurisdictions as a basis for expert testimony.

Controversy exists over the reliability and scientific acceptance of CSAAS. Insofar that CSAAS is one explanation, there are others:

> The Complainant was taking Accutane at the time of the accusations. A pharmacologist expert (JTOD) was retained by the defendant to review this matter and, if able, provide expert opinion related to any toxic and psychiatric effects Accutane had on Ms. Complainant, and if, in the expert's opinion, the Accutane adversely affected her memory and psyche, leading to false allegations of sexual abuse by Defendant. The expert discussed the psychiatric toxicity effects on Ms. Complainant during and following the period of her treatment with Accutane (isotretinoin), a drug prescribed for cystic acne.

The expert notes that no mental, psychological, or psychiatric experts have opined that the Complainant was sexually abused. The expert requested permission to interview Ms. Complainant, but she declined the invitation (letter of the Prosecutor).

8.11.4.1 Facts of the Case

1. Accutane is considered a drug with significant and substantial psychiatric toxicities, including depression, psychosis, suicidality, delusions, and nightmares. The US FDA MedWatch analysis for Accutane/Isotretinoin documents the drug's

psychiatric toxicity; so does the published scientific literature, as well as books and published articles by the pharmacologist experts in the field document the Accutane psychiatric toxicity.

2. The Complainant did not begin to experience or be observed to have any behavior changes through her early years until after the Accutane was prescribed and consumed for a period of 6 to 7 months during the third and fourth Quarter of 2008.
3. The Complainant's accusations followed a period of significant Accutane toxicity (dermatology records, investigation of Accutane Class action lawsuit). The Complainant testified that she became depressed and wanted to take her own life.
4. The Complainant and her friends and family have stated/testified that she was not depressed and withdrawn through her early years until she was exposed to Accutane.
5. Even after the accusation of the alleged sexual abuse, the Complainant behaved erratically and ambiguously toward the Defendant. For example, she acted positively toward the Defendant after her separation from his household, went to his house, interacted on the sports fields, hugged him publicly, etc. Even after his arrest, she visited his next-door neighbor several times where she could run into him, including overnight visits and sunning herself on their deck which his kitchen window and deck overlooked (excerpts from the Accutane Psychiatric toxicity chapter from one of the experts' books).
6. No dispute was raised about the known causation relationship of the psychiatric toxicity of Accutane.

8.11.4.2 Opinions

Comments on the individual Riddell criteria for establishing causation in the Accutane case under discussion:

1. Temporal Eligibility: Ms. Complainant had no psychiatric toxicity before the administration of Accutane; Accutane toxicity does not always diminish with the cessation of the drug.
2. Latent Period: Ms. Complainant developed toxicity while taking Accutane and which continued after the Accutane was discontinued.
3. Exclusion: It is important to rule out the effect of concurrent medications or underlying medical conditions as alternative hypotheses. Comment: The Complainant developed psychiatric toxicity after starting Accutane. No other possible causes were known. Accutane was known to cause psychiatric toxicity. The accusations of alleged sexual abuse surfaced in the form of a fresh complaint, whose validity the defense disputes, six months after the Accutane was discontinued, according to a date determined by the court in deciding the admissibility of the fresh complaint. This alleged fresh complaint happened during and after the behaviors associated with the psychological and psychiatric toxicities attributable to Accutane were occurring.
4. De-challenge: The disappearance or improvement of an adverse event after the withdrawal of the treatment is a positive indication of relatedness. Adverse events can however persist after the treatment is withdrawn, which indicates either that there was no relatedness, or that the adverse effect is a persistent injury. Comment: Psychiatric toxicities are often persistent, frequently lasting long after the intoxicating agent is removed.
5. Re-challenge: Re-Introduction of a treatment which is associated with the same or similar adverse event is a good indication of causation. If the adverse event does not reappear, this can be a sign of lack of causation, but it may also indicate the development of tolerance. Of course, since the potential association in the first place may prevent the reintroduction of the suspect treatment (re-administration of penicillin to a person with an allergic history to penicillin), re-challenge is not intentionally done.
6. Singularity of the drug: It is important to determine whether there is something unique about the adverse reaction experience that is not consistent with any other drug taken or any existing disease condition. There is no evidence that the Complainant took any other drugs that could have caused these psychological or psychiatric behaviors. There is overwhelming evidence that Accutane causes psychiatric toxicity, and a close chemical, high-dose Vitamin A, is also known to cause similar brain and psychiatric toxicities.
7. Pattern: It is important to determine whether similar adverse effects have been described in the literature with the treatment in question or another in the same therapeutic class, or it may refer to a morphologic pattern in a target organ that suggests an association with a particular drug or group of drugs.
8. Drug Identification: There is no question of drug identification in this case. Ms. Complainant acknowledges that she took Accutane. The pharmacy records clearly note the dispensing of Accutane. The Complainant inquired into participating in a Class Action lawsuit for injuries caused by Accutane.

The expert pharmacologist testified at the criminal trial of the Defendant. The following opinions were provided to the Court and Jury.

1. The facts and determinants in this matter meet the requirements of a causation determination between Accutane and psychiatric toxicity in Ms. Complainant.

2. Ms. Complainant does *not* present with the usual pattern of a sexually abused child (thus the introduction/suggestion of CSAAS); Behaviors reported in a child that suggests sexual abuse includes a sudden change in eating habits, sudden mood swings—rage, fear, insecurity, or withdrawal, nightmares or other sleep problems without an explanation, language and knowledge, has new words for private body parts, distracted or distant behavior at odd times, plays or dreams of sexual or frightening images, new or unusual fear of certain people or places, talks about a new older friend, suddenly has money, leaves clues that seem likely to provoke a discussion about sexual issues, writes, draws, toys or other gifts without reason, thinks of self or body as repulsive, dirty or bad, exhibits adult-like sexual behaviors, resists removing clothes when appropriate, asks other children to behave sexually or play sexual games, mimics adult-like sexual behaviors with toys or stuffed animals, and wetting and soiling accidents unrelated to toilet training. Indeed, Ms. Complainant's pattern of behavior differs from that of a sexually abused child, e.g., visiting the next-door neighbor, writing a letter stating she wanted to keep seeing him, hugging and kissing him on the sports field after making allegations against him, and continuing to come over to the Defendant's Residence after she, her mother, and brother moved out in July 2008.
3. The Complainant's reports of (and observations of her being) depressed and "dreams and memories" and allegations of sexual abuse are probably (more likely than not) caused by her exposure to Accutane, suffering significant toxicity to Accutane, including psychiatric toxicity, "schizophrenic-like" actions, and psychosis—a "loss of contact with reality." The fact that her mother was separated from and being divorced by Mr. Defendant can exacerbate any psychological or psychiatric toxicity (such as the Accutane toxicity). Additionally, she exhibited moodiness, irritability, crying spells, staring episodes, inconsistent attitudes regarding wanting to socialize and interact with Mr. Defendant and her stepbrothers, and other personality disorders as set forth by the father and a brother.
4. The Complainant's dreams and memories began after she experienced significant toxicity to Accutane. Distortion of dreams and thoughts are manifestations of drug-related dreams; stress (divorce) increases the vulnerability to and likelihood of psychiatric effects, including agitation, delusions, and depression.
5. Ms. Complainant's attribution of guilt to Defendant is probably distorted by her Accutane psychiatric toxicity (see #4).
6. The temporal relationship (exposure before disclosure) of Accutane is more likely the cause of her depression and mental changes than CSAAS behaviors. Accutane is well-known to cause significant psychiatric toxicity.
7. Ms. Complainant does not fit the profile of someone who was sexually abused and, in fact, appears to not have been sexually abused.

This case went to a criminal trial. The author of this causation report (James T. O'Donnell) testified on behalf of the Defendant. The Jury acquitted the Defendant of all charges against him.

Several other chapters in this book contain causation opinions that apply these criteria in the factual settings of the cases.

Case References

1. *Child Sexual Abuse Accommodation Syndrome: Issues of Admissibility in Criminal Trials—Arthur H. Garrison, Institute for Psychological Therapies (IPT), Vol 10, 1998.*
2. *Psychosis occurs when a person loses contact with reality. The person may have false beliefs about what is taking place, or who one is (delusions). They may also see or hear things that are not there (hallucinations).—cited from the US National Library of Medicine: http://www.nlm.nih.gov/medlineplus/ency/article/001553.htm, accessed August 29, 2014.*
3. *Marks MH and Middelkoop T. Psychiatric Toxicities of Accutane. In O'Donnell JT, Ed. Drug Injury: Liability, Analysis, and Prevention, 2nd Ed. L&J Publications, Tucson, 2005.*
4. *O'Donnell JT: Overview of Existing Research and Information Linking Accutane (Isotretinoin), Depression, Psychosis and Suicide". American Journal of Therapeutics, Vol 10, Number 2, March/April 2003, 148–159.*
5. *O'Donnell JT. Testimony—Overview of Existing Research and Information Linking Accutane (Isotretinoin), Depression, Psychosis and Suicide. Hearing Proceedings: Accutane-Is This Acne Drug Treatment Linked to depression and Suicide? Committee on Government Reform, One Hundred Sixth Congress, Second Session, Serial No. 106–248. U.S. Government Printing Office.73 924 DTP, pp. 71–96.*
6. *http://www.stopitnow.org/warning_signs_child_behavior, accessed 09/07/14.*
7. *http://www.healthline.com/health/psychosis#Overview1, accessed 09/07/14.*

8.12 SUMMARY AND CONCLUSIONS

The determination of causation of an adverse effect by a medical treatment is complex. Only by applying a structured, scientific approach consistent with established criteria can an accurate causal assessment be reached.

NOTES

1 Code of Federal Regulations. *Title 21: Food and drugs;* part *310.305(b): New drugs; records and reports; definitions.* Washington, DC: U.S. Government Printing Office, May 16, 2025.
2 Camilleri M. Safety concerns about alosetron. Arch Intern Med. 2002 Jan 14;162(1):100–101.
3 Karch FE and Lasagna L. Towards the operational identification of adverse drug reactions. Clin Pharmacol Ther. 1977 Mar;21(3):247–254.
4 Marks DH. Depression leading to suicide as an adverse effect of metoclopramide. Internet J Gastroenterol [peer-reviewed serial on the Internet]. 2007;5(2). www.ispub.com/ostia/index.php?xmlFilePath=journals/ijge/vol5n2/depression.xml
5 Code of Federal Regulations. *Title 21: Food and drugs; part 310.305(b): New drugs; records and reports; definitions.* Washington, DC: U.S. Government Printing Office.
6 Code of Federal Regulations. *Title 21: Food and drugs; part 310.305(b): New drugs; records and reports; definitions.* Washington, DC: U.S. Government Printing Office.
7 Ma P, Marinovic I and Karaca-Mandic P. Drug manufacturers' delayed disclosure of serious and unexpected adverse events to the US Food and Drug Administration. JAMA Intern Med. Published online July 27, 2015. DOI: 10.1001/jamainternmed.2015.3565.
8 Hutchinson TA and Lane DA. Assessing methods for causality assessment. J Clin Epidemiol. 1989;42:5–16.
9 Robert K. Über den augenblicklichen Stand der bakteriologischen Choleradiagnose (in German). Zeitschrift für Hygiene und Infectionskrankheiten. 1893;14:319–333; Robert K. 2 Die Aetiologie der Tuberkulose. Mitt Kaiser Gesundh. 1884:1–88.
10 Doll R. Sir Austin Bradford Hill and the progress of medical science. BMJ. 1992 Dec 19;305(6868):1521–1526.
11 Morabia A. On the origin of Hill's causal criteria. Epidemiology. 1991 Sep;2(5):367–369.
12 Riddell RH, ed. *Pathology of drug-induced and toxic diseases.* New York: Churchill Livingstone, 1982, pp. 3–9.
13 Horwitz RI, Feinstein AR and Harvey MR. Temporal precedence and other problems of the exposure-disease relationship. Arch Intern Med. 1984 Jun;144(6):1257–1259.
14 Connolly HM, Crary JL, McGoon MD, Hensrud DD, Edwards BS, Edwards WD and Schaff HV. Valvular heart disease associated with fenfluramine–phentermine. N Engl J Med. 1997 Aug 28;337(9):581–588.
15 Jick H and Vessey MP. Case-control studies in the evaluation of drug-induced illness. Am J Epidemiol. 1978 Jan;107(1):1–7.
16 Jones JK. Determining causation from case reports. In BL Strom (ed.), *Pharmacoepidemiology*, 2nd edition. New York: Wiley, 1994.
17 Austin H, Hill HA, Flanders D and Greenberg RS. Limitations in the applications of case-control methodology. Epidemiol Rev. 1994;16(1):65–76.
18 Breslow NE and Day NE. *Statistical methods in cancer research. Volume I: The analysis of case-control studies.* Lyon: International Agency for Research on Cancer, 1980.
19 Schlesselman JJ. *Case-control studies: Design, conduct, analysis.* New York: Oxford University Press, 1982.
20 Kazdin A. *Single-case research designs.* New York: Oxford University Press, 1982.
21 Yun H and Curtis JR. New methods for determining comparative effectiveness in rheumatoid arthritis. Curr Opin Rheumatol. 2013 May;25(3):325–333.
22 Robert K. Über den augenblicklichen Stand der bakteriologischen Choleradiagnose (in German). Zeitschrift für Hygiene und Infectionskrankheiten. 1893;14:319–333; Robert K. *2 Die Aetiologie der Tuberkulose.* Mitt Kaiser Gesundh, 1884, pp. 1–88.
23 Robert K. Über den augenblicklichen Stand der bakteriologischen Choleradiagnose (in German). Zeitschrift für Hygiene und Infectionskrankheiten. 1893;14:319–333; Robert K. *2 Die Aetiologie der Tuberkulose.* Mitt Kaiser Gesundh, 1884, pp. 1–88.
24 Hill AB. The environment and disease: Association or causation. Proc R Soc Med. 1965 May;58(5):295–300.
25 Riddell RH, ed. *Pathology of drug-induced and toxic diseases.* New York: Churchill Livingstone, 1982, pp. 3–9.
26 Hill AB. The environment and disease: Association or causation. Proc R Soc Med. 1965 May;58(5):295–300.
27 Riddell RH, ed. *Pathology of drug-induced and toxic diseases.* New York: Churchill Livingstone, 1982, pp. 3–9.
28 Girard M. Conclusiveness of rechallenge in the interpretation of adverse drug reactions. Br J Clin Pharmacol. 1987 Jan;23(1):73–79.
29 s Stevens M. Deliberate drug rechallenge. Hum Toxicol. 1983 Oct;2(4):573–577.
30 Causality assessment of adverse events following immunization. *Weekly Epidemiology Record.* WHO, March 23, 2001.
31 Marks DH. Neurologic complications of vaccination with outer surface protein A (OspA). Int J Risk Saf Med. 2011 Jan 1;23(2):89–96.
32 Daubert v. Merrell Dow Pharmaceuticals, Inc., 509 U.S. 579, 113 S.Ct. 2786, 125 L.Ed.2d 469 (1993).
33 Daubert v Merrill Dow Pharmaceuticals, Inc., 43 F.3d 1311, 1317 (9th Cir. 1995).

34 *Reference Manual on Scientific Evidence,* 2nd ed. National Research Council, Federal Judicial Center, National Academies Press, Center, 2000
35 Thames LD and Martin L. The Pharmacologist as an Expert Witness. In-House Defense Quarterly Winter, 2009, pp. 28–31. Chicago: Defense Research Institute.
36 www.abcp.net
37 Agee, 2004 WL 5352989 at *2, McClain, 401 F.3d at 1240-44, Tidwell, 626 So. 2d at 1300, Ashman. SK&F Lab Co., 702 F.Supp. at 1405, Crisostomo 857 F.2d at 1153, Hermes 848F.2d at 69, Holley 348 S.E.3d at 776-77).
38 AAFP. Physician expert witness in medical liability suits. http://www.aafp.org/about/policies/all/physician-expert.html
39 AMA Opinion 9.07. Medical Testimony, December 2004.

9 General Principles of Pharmacology

James J. O'Donnell III, James T. O'Donnell, and Vanessa Juettner

SYNOPSIS

DOI: 10.1201/9781003615323-10

9.1 INTRODUCTION

Pharmacology can be defined as the study of drug action on a living organism through chemical processes. It involves the analysis of normal and abnormal interactions between the substance and the living organism. These substances may be administered to achieve either therapeutic or toxic effects on the patient's metabolic processes or hosted parasites, respectively. To achieve an effect, the substance binds, or attaches, to specific targets within the body, which then causes a specific activation or inhibition of chemical processes.

The concept of rational therapeutics (e.g., the administration of the correct dose to achieve the desired effect) was introduced into medicine only about 65 years ago. Only then did it become possible to accurately evaluate therapeutic claims. The effectiveness of therapeutic agents referenced within this chapter is based on experimental evidence and supported by the scientific method.

During the last 50 years, many fundamentally new drug group categories and new members of old groups were introduced. Drugs are derived from a number of sources: chemicals, animals, minerals, proteins, carbohydrates, and fats. All drugs can be toxic; chemicals in botanicals (plants) and natural/organic products can be just as toxic as synthetic chemicals. As stated by Paracelsus, the father of toxicology, "All things are poison, and nothing is without poison; only the dose permits something not to be poisonous." This is more commonly summarized as "The dose makes the poison." The location of the drug in the body can also lead to toxicity; a drug may exert therapeutic effects in one organ system while causing unwanted side effects in another.

The last three decades have seen a rapid growth in information and understanding of the molecular basis for drug action. Studies of the local molecular environment of receptors have shown that receptors, effectors (molecules that interact with receptors), and other proteins do not function in isolation—they are strongly influenced by surrounding regulatory proteins.

9.2 BASIC PRINCIPLES

In the broadest sense, human pharmacology can be considered as the interaction between a drug and the body. At the next level of complexity, the interaction can be broken down into pharmacodynamics and pharmacokinetics (Figure 9.1).

Pharmacodynamics is defined as the drug's effect on the body. In other words, it is the mechanism of action of that specific drug/substance. Pharmacokinetics is defined

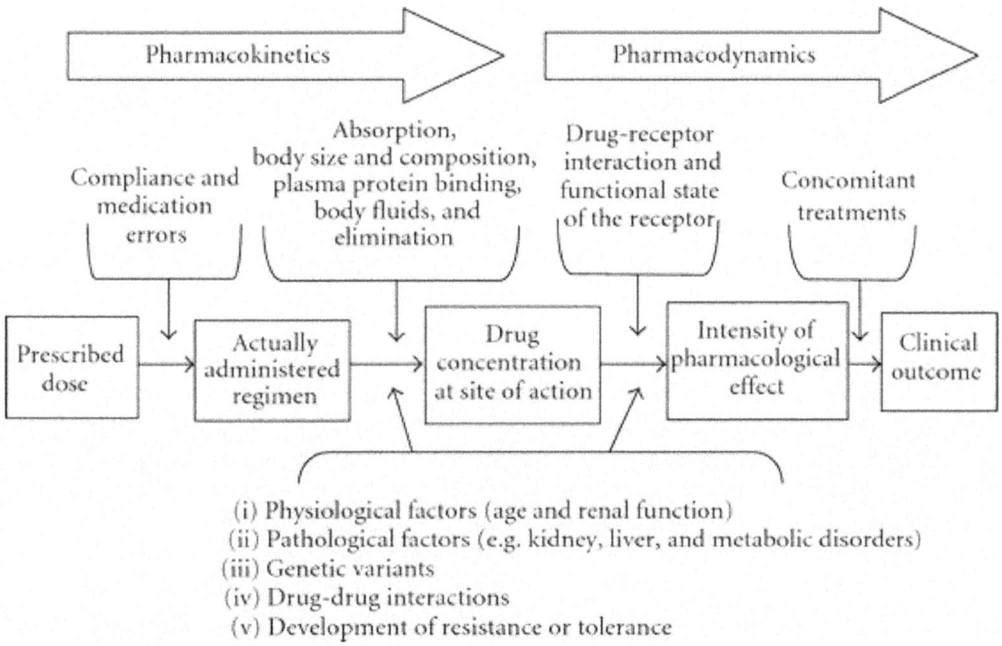

FIGURE 9.1 Pharmacological Pathways.

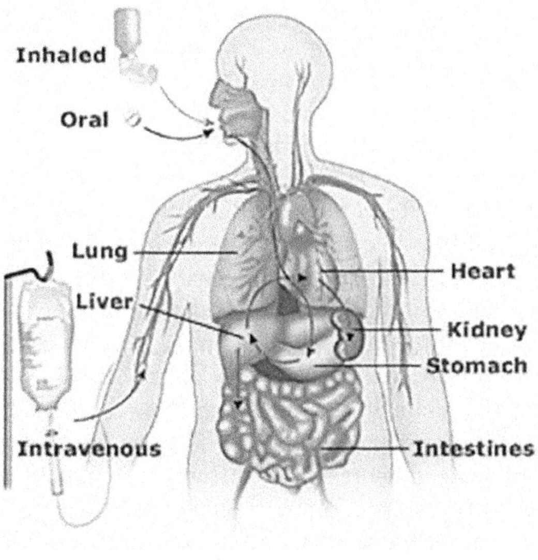

FIGURE 9.2 Drug's Absorption in the Body.

as the effect that the body has on the drug, which includes the processes of absorption, distribution, metabolism, and elimination/excretion (ADME). Both pharmacodynamics and pharmacokinetics are interconnected.

When a drug is administered, it undergoes absorption within the body. Drugs administered orally usually undergo a first pass effect in the liver which alters the drug's bioavailability or the amount of unchanged drug that reaches the circulation blood (systemic circulation). The drug is then distributed to a number of physical sites. While there is some diversity in the mechanism of action, the drug most commonly binds to a specific receptor in lock-and-key fashion on the cell surface in a particular bodily tissue or organ. Binding of a drug to a receptor changes the conformation (shape) of the receptor, and this may activate molecules bound to the receptor on the inside of the cell. Processes induced by this interaction may include the release of secondary messengers as part of a signal transduction cascade, which amplify this signal and lead to a particular cellular response. A secondary messenger is a small biomolecule which relays information from the receptor (e.g., on the cell surface) to effector molecules within the cell. In addition to amplifying the signal, these layers of complexity allow the drug to have different target molecules and thus effects in different cell types and/or organs even though they may bind to the same receptor. For example, opioids cause euphoria through effects on the brain but can also cause constipation through effects on the GI tract, even though they bind to the mu receptor in both cases. This suggests the importance of the distribution of the drug.

Subsequent to drug action, the drug is metabolized, or biotransformed, by key enzymes. This metabolic biotransformation causes the drug to be more easily excreted from the body and often causes it to be inactivated. Naturally, to maintain the desired therapeutic effects, the drug that has been metabolized needs to be replaced by another dose. In order to determine how much and how often this dose should be administered to be safe and effective, one needs to develop a pharmacokinetic model describing the distribution and elimination of the drug.

9.2.1 Absorption

Absorption can be defined as the process by which a drug enters systemic circulation from the site of administration.

Generally, a drug is absorbed orally (mouth), dermally (skin), or by inhalation (Figure 9.2). Following absorption is migration to the site of action in another bodily compartment (e.g., the brain, in the case of an anti-seizure medication). This inter-compartmental navigation requires permeation through various barriers including the stomach/intestine, the blood vessels, and the blood–brain barrier.

9.2.2 Lipid Diffusion

Lipid bilayer diffusion, or passage, is the most important limiting factor for drug permeation. The compartments or organs of the body are separated by cellular membranes, or walls, made up of lipids. These cellular membranes are made up of two layers of lipids called the lipid bilayer. Lipids are a group of naturally occurring molecules which include fats, waxes, and fat-soluble vitamins (A, D, E, and K). Another term for diffusing through lipid bilayers is simple diffusion.

In addition to simple diffusion, there are other ways in which a drug may be moved from once side of a lipid bilayer to the other; drug transport may be mediated by a carrier either by facilitated diffusion or active transport. Both facilitated diffusion and active transport require specific binding to carrier proteins embedded within the lipid bilayer, which then release the drug to the inside of the cell. In facilitated diffusion, like simple diffusion, no energy is required for this process; molecules flow down their concentration gradient. In active transport, however, energy derived from chemical reaction, such as the hydrolysis of ATP, drives the transport of the drug.

9.2.3 Determinants of Absorption

There are several physical characteristics of a drug which determine its ability to absorb across cellular membranes. These determinants can be divided into two categories: mechanical and physiochemical.

Mechanical

- Disintegration—the time for the preparation (e.g., pill) to be reduced to fragments.
- Dissolution—the time for the drug to disperse into a solution, i.e., to dissolve.

Mechanically, both disintegration and dissolution are significant determinants of drug absorption. Disintegration, the reduction of the drug into small fragments, results in increased mobility. The efficacy of a dosage form depends on the time it takes for the tablet or capsule to disintegrate in the patient's gastrointestinal tract. Dissolution is the dispersion of the drug within a solvent or digestive fluid. The rate of the dissolution is the primary variable used to control the onset of action and duration of a drug. Also extended-release tablets have a longer dissolution time and therefore take longer to achieve maximal effect.

Physiochemical

- Molecular size—the larger the molecule, the less likely it is to cross membranes.
- Degree of ionization—the stronger the charge, the less likely it is to cross membranes.
- Polarity—the more polar the molecule, the less likely it is to cross membranes.

Physiochemically, molecular size and degree of ionization are significant determinants of drug absorption. Molecular size or molecular weight (MW), critical for cellular receptor fit and activation, is inversely proportional to a drug's ability to diffuse across cellular membranes.

The MW of drugs varies from very small (lithium-ion MW = 7 kDal) to very large (alteplase protein MW = 59,050 kDal). However, most therapeutic drugs have molecular weights between 100 kDal and 1,000 kDal. Drugs beyond this range (usually proteins) do not diffuse readily between compartments of the body and therefore must often be administered directly into the compartment where they have their effect. For example, alteplase, a clot-dissolving enzyme, is administered directly into the affected blood vessel by intravenous (IV) administration.

In addition to molecular size, drugs which are similar in composition to lipids have more affinity for lipids (lipophilic) and are more likely to be able to pass through lipid bilayers. In a sense, these drugs are able to dissolve into the lipid membrane. What makes a drug similar in composition to a lipid? Drugs that contain no net charge and are nonpolar (the electron density is *not* concentrated on one side of the molecule) tend to be more lipophilic. Concerning net charge, a drug's ability to become ionized or charged is another key physiochemical determinant of absorption. Molecules can hold a positive charge, a negative charge, or no charge at all (neutral). If the molecules within the drug mixture gain a positive or negative charge, they are not capable of diffusing across cellular membranes and less likely to reach a specific compartment within the body. Neutral molecules, on the other hand, more readily diffuse through membranes and can easily reach a number of compartments.

Nonpolar molecules are also more likely to diffuse through a lipid membrane. Halogens such as fluorine (F) or chlorine (Cl) pull electron density through the bonds toward these atoms, which can result in an imbalance of the electron density distribution overall if these atoms are on one side of the molecule; such a polar molecule would be less able to diffuse through lipid membranes. Hydrocarbons (carbon- and hydrogen-containing molecules) are nonpolar and devoid of charge, so the presence of a large hydrocarbon chain would make a drug more lipophilic. For example, steroids are uncharged molecules with only carbon and hydrogen atoms, and, not surprisingly, these drugs can diffuse through lipid membranes easily. All these properties make a drug more likely to be able to pass directly through a lipid membrane.

Most drugs are organic (carbon-containing) compounds and can be categorized as/by:

- Nonelectrolytes, e.g., glucose. These drugs do not ionize, and pH changes do not affect the absorption and distribution of this kind of drug.
- Weak acids or bases. Those drugs that donate protons (positively charged molecules) are weak acids (aspirin, barbiturates). Those drugs that accept protons are weak bases (epinephrine (adrenaline)). Strong acids or bases are not used systemically as medicines. Found in the stomach, hydrochloric acid (HCl) is the body's only strong acid. The most important point to remember is that ionized drugs do not readily pass through membranes.

9.2.3.1 Lipid/Aqueous Partition Coefficient and pH

Because lipid barriers separate aqueous compartments, the lipid/aqueous partition coefficient of a drug determines how readily the molecule can move between aqueous and lipid media. This is important to drug absorption because a drug may be very hydrophobic and pass through lipid membranes easily, but it may not dissolve enough in the aqueous lumen of body compartments in order to interact with the barrier of the compartments and thus pass through it. In the case of weak acids and weak bases, the ability to move from aqueous to lipid media, or vice versa, varies with the pH of the medium, because charged molecules attract the water molecules. The pH is quantified on a scale between 1 and 14. A water-friendly, or aqueous, environment has a more neutral pH (~7). Acidity is inversely proportional to pH (less than 7), while basicity is directly proportional to pH (greater than 7).

The ratio of the lipid-soluble form to water-soluble form for a weak acid or weak base is expressed by the Henderson–Hasselbalch equation. The equation exists in two forms, one for an acidic drug and another for a basic drug.

9.2.3.1.1 Acidic Drug

$$pH = pKa + log\left(\frac{[A^-]}{[HA]}\right) \tag{9.1}$$

Where:

$A^{\bar{n}}$ = the conjugate base of the corresponding acid HA

$pK_a = -\log(K_a)$, where K_a = acid dissociation constant

$[A^{\bar{n}}]$ = molar concentration of $A^{\bar{n}}$.

$[HA]$ = molar concentration of HA.

9.2.3.1.2 Basic Drug

$$pOH = pK_b + log\left(\frac{[BH^+]}{[B]}\right) \tag{9.2}$$

Where:

BH^+ = the conjugate acid of the corresponding base B

$pK_b = -\log(K_b)$, where K_b = base dissociation constant

$[BH^+]$ = molar conc entration of BH^+.

$[B]$ = molar concentration of B.

9.2.3.2 Bioavailability

The amount and means by which one absorbs a drug determine bioavailability or the unchanged drug concentration in the blood. Our first and simplest task is to relate a dose to the concentration of the drug in the body. For the purposes of pharmacokinetic calculations, we will assume the one-compartment model. That is, we will assume that once the drug is absorbed into systemic circulation, it distributes instantaneously and homogenously throughout the vascular space. The first thing we need to find is the amount of the dose that reaches systemic circulation. This is simply the fraction of drug that reaches systemic circulation (bioavailability, *F*) multiplied by the dose.

Bioavailability is determined by how easily the drug is absorbed as well as the amount lost due to first pass metabolism. Maximum absorption occurs when a drug is hydrophobic enough to pass through the lipid bilayer of cell membranes but hydrophilic enough to be soluble. Bioavailability is 100 percent for intravenous (IV) injection. For simplicity's sake, pharmacokinetic (PK) equations are sometimes represented in the form assuming IV injection as this obviates the need to explicitly include the bioavailability. However, a PK equation that contains dose and assumes IV administration can be modified for oral or other routes of administration by simply replacing (dose) by the expression $F \times dose$.

Some reasons for bioavailability are as follows:

1. Tableting—the dosage form must disintegrate and dissolve to be absorbed
2. Stability in the stomach
3. Degradation by bacterial enzymes
4. First pass effect

9.2.3.3 First Pass Effect

Due to its anatomical arrangement, the blood supply from the GI tract goes first to the liver. Drugs taken orally can therefore be metabolized in the GI tract, the liver, or both before absorption to systemic circulation. This phenomenon is variously known as first pass effect or pre-systemic drug elimination. In some cases, the majority of a drug dose can be lost this way, necessitating an increased dosage or different routes of administration (e.g., IV).

Following absorption across the gut, the portal blood delivers the drug to the liver before entering systemic circulation. A drug is metabolized in the gut in addition to the portal blood. Most commonly, the liver is the primary site for metabolism. In addition, the liver is able to excrete the drug into the bile. All of these metabolic precursors may contribute to a reduced rate of drug bioavailability. The effects of first-pass hepatic elimination are expressed as the extraction ratio (ER).

A drug such as morphine is almost completely absorbed, so that loss in the gut is negligible. However, the hepatic extraction ratio for morphine is 0.67, so the ER value is 0.33. The bioavailability of morphine is therefore expected to be about 33 percent, which is close to the observed value.

The clinical value of this phenomenon is that a 10-mg IV dose of morphine is equivalent to a 30-mg oral dose.

9.3 ROUTES OF ADMINISTRATION

Drug administration can be divided into two broad categories—intravascular (within the vein) and extravascular (outside the vein).

Intravascular (e.g., intravenous injection) is the type of administration in which the drug is placed directly into systemic circulation. Because there is no drug lost upon administration, bioavailability is 100 percent.

Extravascular (e.g., oral dosing, intramuscular injections) may be associated with drug loss due to the first pass effect. When a drug is administered extravascularly, the time of onset and intensity of action are determined by the characteristics of absorption from the site of administration.

Bioavailability (*F*) is determined by dividing the amount of a drug which reached systemic circulation after extravascular administration by the amount of a drug which reached systemic circulation after IV administration (same drug, same dose). This is done by taking blood samples at timed intervals, measuring the concentration of the drug and plotting concentration versus time on a graph (Figure 9.3). The resulting area under the curve (AUC) is proportional to the total mass which reached systemic circulation between the first and last sampling intervals. If the oral and IV doses are unequal, one can normalize by dividing the AUC for each administration by the respective dose:
For equal doses:

$$F = \frac{AUC\_Oral}{AUC\_IV} \tag{9.3}$$

For different doses:

$$F = \left(\frac{\left(AUC\_Oral / _{\text{Dose\_Oral}} \right)}{\left(AUC\_IV / _{\text{Dose\_IV}} \right)} \right) \tag{9.4}$$

For direct comparison of two drugs:

$$\text{Relative Bioavailability} = \left(\frac{\left(AUC\_T / _{\text{Dose T}} \right)}{\left(AUC\_Q / _{\text{Dose\_Q}} \right)} \right) \tag{9.5}$$

9.4 EXTRAVASCULAR ADMINISTRATION

9.4.1 Oral Administration

Approximately 80 percent of drugs prescribed in the United States are for oral administration. This route is used largely for convenience, ease of administration, minimal toxicity, and lower expense (Figure 9.4). The first oral absorptive surface is the buccal mucosa (between the inside cheek and gums). Due to the rapid transit time, usually very little absorption takes place here. Special drug formulations are sublingual (SL) or under the tongue. Nitroglycerin is an example of a drug which is formulated to dissolve quickly in the mouth and is rapidly absorbed in approximately one to two minutes. This route will also eliminate the first pass effect.

The next absorptive surface is the stomach/gastric pouch. The minimum absorption time for drugs in the absence of food is about 20 minutes. With food, absorption time becomes quite variable depending upon fat content, viscosity (resistance of a fluid), and volume. The pH of gastric contents is 1–2 (highly acidic). However, the absorbing surface (gastric mucosa) appears to absorb drugs best at pH 3–3.5. Weak acids (aspirin), water, and lipid-soluble nonelectrolytes (ethyl alcohol) are readily absorbed by passive diffusion.

Because some drugs would be adversely affected by acid and digestive enzymes, many are formulated with an enteric coating which resists dissolution in low pH environments. The enteric coating provides a protective effect which, depending on the extent and type, may provide for a delayed or sustained absorption. It at least prevents destruction by gastric acid, thus allowing the dosage form to pass into the small intestine. Enteric coatings, such as those used

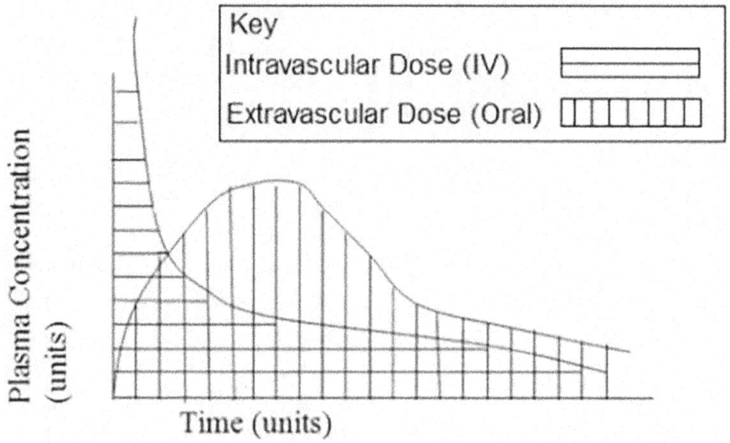

FIGURE 9.3 Difference in Blood Plasma Concentration of an Intravascular versus Extravascular Drug Dose.

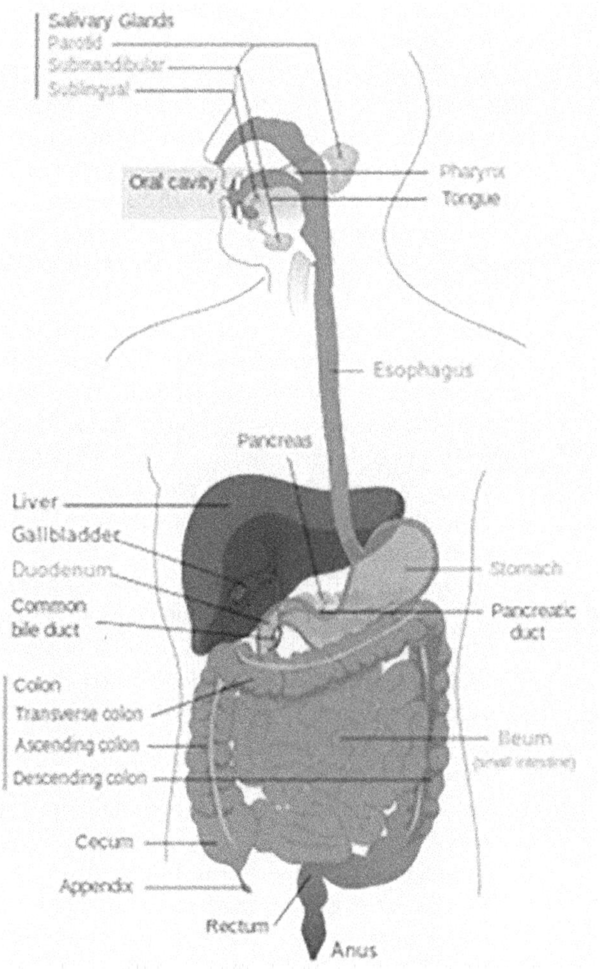

FIGURE 9.4 The Gastrointestinal Tract.

on aspirin, also provide protection of the gastric pouch from irritation leading to possible ulcerations.

Absorption from the small intestine takes 30 to 90 minutes. The rate at which drugs reach the small intestine will depend upon gastric emptying time. Emptying time is decreased by taking a drug with 6–8 oz. of water and increased by the presence of food. These pharmaceutical characteristics will prompt instructions such as "take on empty stomach" or "take with food."

The small intestine, with its large blood circulation, is the primary absorptive surface for most orally administered drugs, largely because its surface, covered with thousands of cellular membrane protrusions, or microvilli has an area of approximately 120 m^2 (≈ 1,000 times that of the stomach).

Malabsorptive function, due to reduced residence time in the small intestine, may be caused by disease, genetics, or a side effect of other (or the same) medication. The pH of the small intestine is more alkaline (pH 6.3–6.5) than the stomach. Therefore, drugs which have a pKa in this range will be better absorbed.

Usually very little drug is absorbed in the large intestine, either because most of the drug has already been absorbed or because of the smaller surface area and blood supply relative to the small intestine. All drugs absorbed in the stomach or small intestine will undergo the first pass (hepatic) effect mentioned before.

9.4.2 Rectal Administration

Rectal administration is useful for drugs which may be inactivated via the oral route and for drugs which are irritating (cause nausea and vomiting). Rectal administration can be used for giving antiemetics to control nausea and vomiting. This route is not used frequently for other types of drugs because absorption is less predictable. It does have the advantage of avoiding the first pass effect intrinsic to the oral route.

9.4.3 Other Routes of Administration

Other routes of administration exist and are presented in Table 9.1.

TABLE 9.1
Other Routes of Administration

Intrathecal	Injection into cerebral spinal fluid (CSF) to obtain effective concentration in the central nervous system (CNS).
Intradermal	Injection into the skin (e.g., local anesthesia with lidocaine).
Intramuscular (IM)	Injection into muscles of the arm or buttocks; used for irritating drugs, drugs not absorbed by the oral route or when a depot of drug is required. The rate of absorption can be altered by formulation (type of suspension and size of crystal) and the application of heat, cold, or exercise. This route of administration was quite popular before the onset of the AIDS/HIV epidemic, and, as a caution against occupational needle sticks, a switch to intravenous administration occurred. Risks of IM include local infections, accidental intravascular administration, and pain experienced by the patient.
Subcutaneous (SQ)	Injection under the skin; absorption is slower than for IV or IM and less predictable. Insulin and heparin are administered subcutaneously.
Topical	Application on the skin; usually for local effect such as rash.
Transdermal	Patches used with drugs like fentanyl, nicotine, nitroglycerin, scopolamine, and hormones are applied topically for sustained absorption into systemic circulation. This is an area of rapid product development.
Inhalation	Gaseous anesthetics are often given by this route for systemic effect. This route is rapid due to the large surface area of the lung. Used with gaseous anesthetics, bronchodilators for asthma, and emergency administration of resuscitative medications.
Eye and Ear Drops	Applied topically for local effects. May lead to systemic toxicity.

9.5 INTRAVASCULAR ADMINISTRATION

Intravenous (IV) and intra-arterial (IA) administration involves introducing a drug directly into the blood vessel and therefore into the systemic circulation. The bolus IV push (hypodermic needle) is the fastest means of getting a drug into the systemic circulation. Circulation throughout the body takes about two minutes. One must take precautions with any bolus injection as the dose cannot be recovered. Other disadvantages include:

a) Transient high blood level concentrations.
b) Only small volumes can be injected.

IV infusion (Figure 9.5) is a useful means to both control the rate of administration and obtain a desired response (even over an extended period of time). This method is used when drugs would be inactivated by gastric enzymes or acid. It is also used for drugs which are poorly absorbed or can cause irritation in tissues if injected intramuscularly. IV infusion is fast and can be used to maintain a desired blood level over a long period of time. IV drip is a special case where the drug is administered dropwise (i.e., drops per unit time). By increasing the time over which the dose is given, one can obtain a lower concentration for a longer period of time.

Due to inherent difficulty and risk, the intra-arterial route is used only for special circumstances (e.g., vasodilator drugs in the treatment of vasospasm and thrombolytic drugs for treatment of embolism).

9.6 DISTRIBUTION

This section will discuss how drugs distribute throughout the body and what factors can affect this distribution. The extent of distribution of a drug away from the blood is indicated by the volume of distribution (V_D). Once the drug has been absorbed, it can be distributed to the rest of the body. This distribution is done in two main ways:

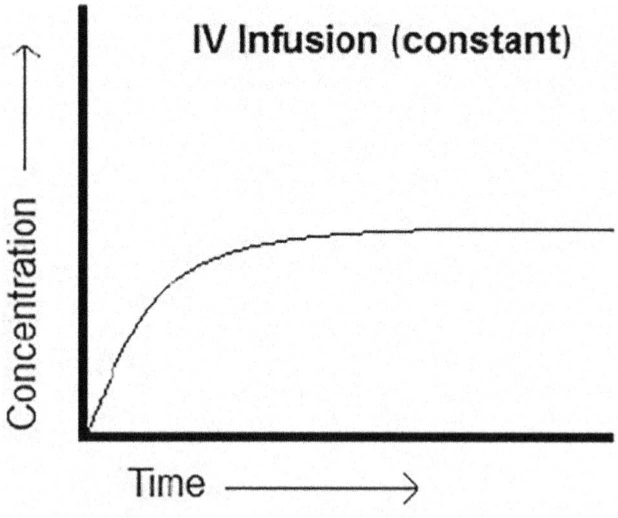

FIGURE 9.5 IV Diffusion is Rapid and Used to Maintain a Target Drug Level in the Blood over Time.

1. *Bulk flow* via the blood. In this phase, the physiochemical (i.e., drug size) properties are not important. However, this phase can result in patterns of distribution. The tissues that are well-perfused will receive more of the drug than the less well-perfused tissues. This is highly relevant in intravascular administration.
2. *Diffusional transfer* determines where and how quickly the drug distributes. This depends upon the drug's ability to cross the cell membranes that separate the various aqueous compartments of the body. In general, there are four ways by which most drug molecules cross cell membranes.
   a. Simple Diffusion: Diffusion through lipid membranes.
   b. Facilitated Diffusion: Carrier-mediated transport of molecules into or out of cells; molecules move down their concentration gradient and therefore require no input of energy.
   c. Active Transport: Carrier-mediated transport across the membrane into or out of cells. This transport may move molecules up their concentration gradient, so it requires the input of energy.
   d. Pinocytosis or phagocytosis: Pinocytosis is the process of engulfing fluid and nutrients by a cell. Phagocytosis is the engulfing of particulates by a cell. Both require cellular energy. Drugs with large MW (>900 kDal) may cross tissue barriers by these processes.

9.6.1 Diffusion

Drugs move across biological barriers by diffusion. The driving force is the concentration gradient. Drugs move down the concentration gradient (from high to low concentration). It is only the concentration of the unbound, unionized drug which contributes to the concentration gradient.

9.6.2 Volume of Distribution

Now that we have determined how much of the dose reaches the systemic circulation, how can we determine the drug concentration? Since concentration is mass/volume, concentration is related to mass (drug dose) through the volume in which it is dissolved (volume of distribution). Since we are assuming the one-compartment model where the drug is homogenously distributed throughout all the space it occupies in the body, the volume of distribution is a theoretical abstraction.

In reality, the drug will only be homogenously distributed within the bloodstream; it will be heterogeneously distributed to the tissues and other spaces of the body depending on the physical composition of the patient and the properties of the drug. Drug concentration, which counts both free molecules and those bound to proteins, can only be measured in the blood compartment. The concentration in other compartments cannot be measured. By necessity, we assume that the drug is just as concentrated (or just as diluted) in the other compartments of the body as it is in the blood compartment; our estimate of volume of distribution is derived from this assumption. As such, the volume of distribution (V_D) is given by the following equation:

$$V_D = \text{total amount of drug in the body} / \text{drug blood plasma concentration} \quad (9.6)$$

An organizing principle for how the volume of distribution changes in various conditions is as follows: Anything that causes the distribution of the drug to shift from the blood compartment to the tissues and other compartments will increase the volume of distribution. This is not due to the patient receiving a blood transfusion—it is merely a mathematical adjustment used to account for the drug's behavior. In the same manner, the actual volume of water in a patient's body may change (dehydration or over-hydration) when factors cause a shift in drug distribution from tissues and other compartments to the bloodstream but is adjusted to more accurately calculate the dosage (Table 9.2).

For example, the more lipophilic a drug, the more affinity it will have for fatty tissues and the more it will be pulled out of the blood, increasing V_D. Similarly, the more obese a patient is, the more drug molecules will be pulled out of the blood and distributed in the fatty tissues, increasing V_D. A drug which has a high degree of protein binding will be pulled into the blood compartment more, decreasing V_D. Affinity or binding of the drug in the blood compartment versus the other compartments of the body causes a shift in distribution in accordance with the basic chemical law of Le Chatelier's principle—" if a chemical system at equilibrium experiences a change in concentration, temperature,

TABLE 9.2
Physical Volumes (in L/kg Body Weight) of Some Body Compartments into Which Drugs or Toxins May Be Distributed.

Compartment and Volume Water	Examples of Drugs or Toxins
Total body water (0.6 L/kg)	Small water-soluble molecules: E.g., ethanol.
Extracellular water (0.2 L/kg)	Larger water-soluble molecules: E.g., gentamicin.
Blood (0.08 L/kg); plasma (0.04 L/kg)	Strongly plasma protein-bound molecules and very large molecules: E.g., heparin.
Fat (0.2–0.35 L/kg)	Highly lipid-soluble molecules: E.g., DDT.
Bone (0.07 L/kg)	Certain ions: E.g., lead, fluoride.

volume, or partial pressure, then the equilibrium shifts to counteract the imposed change and a new equilibrium is established." Once the pharmacokinetic parameter of volume of distribution has been established, concentration can be calculated by dividing the mass of drug (dose in systemic circulation) by the volume of distribution.

Values over 40 L represent a drug which is mostly found somewhere in the body other than the plasma. So the larger the V_D, the more of the drug dose is outside of systemic circulation. In the equation,

$$V_D = \text{total amount of drug in the body} / \text{drug blood plasma concentration} = D / C_0 \quad (9.7)$$

—there are three parameters. Knowing any two of them allows the calculation of the third. In medicine, for descriptive purposes, one can use a standard patient weighing 70 kg. The major compartments of this body are shown in Figure 9.6.

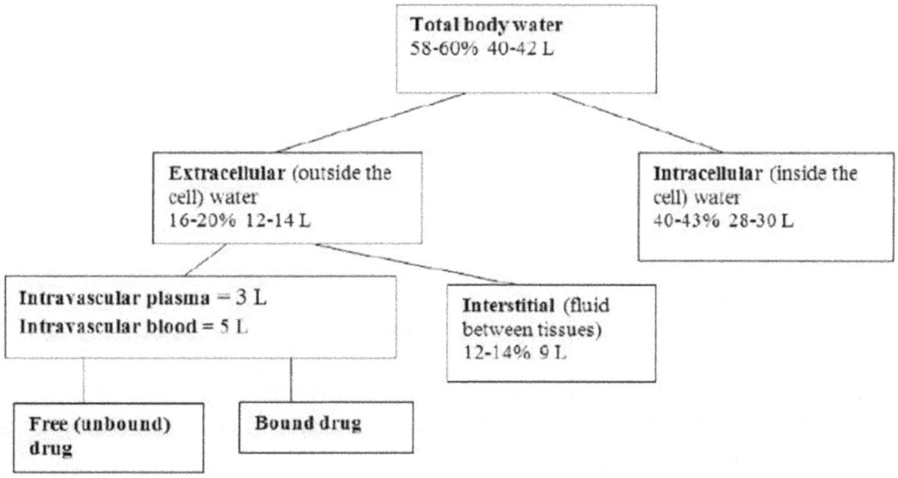

FIGURE 9.6 Bodily Compartments.

Example: If 40 mg of drug is given by IV push to a 70 kg man and the drug distributes into total body water, what was the starting drug concentration in the plasma?

$$V_D \times C_O = D$$

$$Co = D / V_D$$

Where:
V_D = Volume of distribution
D = Dose
Co = Initial concentration

From Figure 9.6, we can determine that the volume of distribution for a 70 kg patient, total body water, is 40 L.

9.6.3 Binding to Plasma Proteins and Cellular Constituents

Plasma, a yellow fluid component of the blood that surrounds the blood cells, contains mostly water but also proteins, glucose, minerals, and hormones. Plasma albumin constitutes about 50 percent of the plasma proteins and is usually responsible for drug binding. Binding to plasma albumin is generally reversible and involves ionic, hydrogen, and Van der Waals forces. There are multiple binding sites with differing polarities so different drugs may bind. Albumin usually binds acidic drugs while alpha-1-acid-glycoprotein binds basic drugs. Equilibrium is established between the free and the bound drug.

9.6.4 Redistribution

Highly lipid-soluble drugs will move into muscles and fat where they have no physiological activity, and this represents a type of sink. This movement will tend to show an increased V_D for the drug, but it will also have an effect upon the duration of the drug's action. For drugs that act in the CNS, sequestration into fat deposits represents a loss of activity. For example, the drugs diazepam and lorazepam (benzodiazepines) are used for epilepsy. They have a long half-life in the blood. But they have only a limited duration of action in epilepsy because they come out of the CNS and are sequestered into the fat where they are physiologically inert. Therefore, the duration of action is not associated with the half-life of the drug but rather with the rate of sequestration into the fat deposits.

9.6.5 Blood–Brain Barrier (BBB)

The blood–brain barrier separates the circulating blood from the brain extracellular fluid. Not all substances present in the bloodstream can gain access to the brain. The endothelial cells lining the inside of the capillary blood vessels perfusing the brain are a particular tight barrier which prevent some drugs and substances from entry into the brain. Inflammation may increase the permeability of the blood–brain barrier, and under these conditions even ionized compounds may penetrate.

Some of the properties which determine drug entry into the brain are:

a) Molecular weight—compounds with MW > 60,000 Dal will not penetrate.
b) Lipid solubility—the greater the lipid solubility, the better the penetration.
c) Fraction of drug unionized at physiological pH—the larger the unionized fraction, the greater the penetration since only unionized drug can cross cell membranes; the larger the concentration gradient of the un-ionized drug there is, the more penetration of the drug across the BBB there will be.
d) Protein binding—only the free fraction contributes to the concentration gradient.

9.6.6 Placental Barrier

The blood supply of the mother is separated from the blood supply of the fetus by several tissue layers known as the "placental barrier." Drugs must diffuse across this barrier to enter fetal circulation.

Passage across the placental barrier is regulated by the same requirements as passage across the blood–brain barrier. However, only very large molecules (e.g., Heparin, proteins, etc.) do not cross the placenta. Small molecules, which represent the overwhelming majority of therapeutic agents, will cross the placenta and represent potential risk to the fetus. In this case, with rare exception, the "barrier" is a myth!

9.6.7 Therapeutic Range

The therapeutic range is the broadness of plasma concentrations within which the plasma drug levels produce the maximum benefit and the least toxicity. Important factors indicated in a drug's therapeutic range are:

- Time to onset of activity: Time from first taking the drug until it starts to work.
- Duration of action: Time during which the dose is effective in the body.

9.6.8 Bioequivalence versus Bioinequivalence

Bioequivalence compares two different manufacturers' products of the same drug (e.g., brand name Drug A versus generic preparation Drug B) or two different drugs. Bioinequivalence may occur even if Drugs A and B have equal bioavailability. Bioequivalence has two requirements:

a) Same maximum bioavailability
b) Same maximum rate of absorption

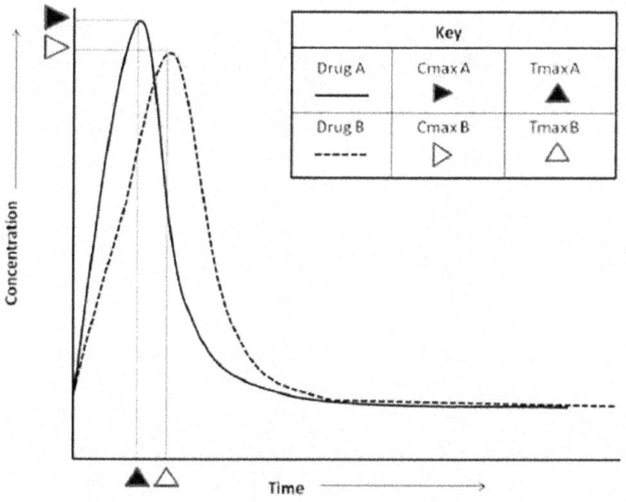

FIGURE 9.7 Bioequivalence of Drugs A and B.

Drug A and Drug B have similar bioavailability according to their AUC's and similar rates of absorption. Drug B, however, is slightly slower. The slower rate of absorption has a lower maximum concentration (*Cmax B*) attained over a longer period of time (*Cmax* and *Tmax*). To quantify the bioequivalence ratio, Drug A's AUC and Drug B's AUC are calculated. The FDA allows for a leeway in the *Cmax* and *Tmax* in approving generic equivalents; equality is not required. To be accepted as bioequivalent, the area ratio would need to fall between 0.8 and 1.25 (see Figure 9.7).

9.7 DRUG METABOLISM (BIOTRANSFORMATION)

Drug metabolism, or biotransformation, is the process by which a drug is converted to another form which is more amenable to excretion, which usually negates the drug's action. Drugs or foreign chemicals are also called xenobiotics. Membrane-associated proteins called cytochrome P450s play an important role in xenobiotic metabolism, especially for lipophilic drugs. The metabolism of these compounds occurs in two phases.

Phase I reactions (Figure 9.8), which usually convert the parent drug to an increasingly polar metabolite by introducing or unmasking a functional group (e.g., –OH, –NH2, –SH),

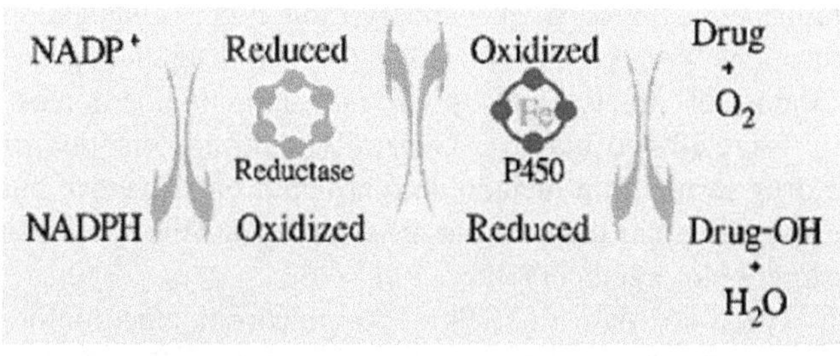

FIGURE 9.8 Phase 1 Drug Oxidation.

are mediated by the cytochrome P450 liver enzymes. Phase I entails a chemical modification in order to add a functional group that can be used to attach a conjugate. The conjugate increases the modified compound to make it more water soluble so it can be excreted in urine. Many P450s tend to add a hydroxyl group (-OH) during a Phase I step of drug metabolism. The hydroxyl then serves as the site for further modifications in Phase 2 drug metabolism—the conjugation.

Endogenous substrates (e.g., glucuronic acid, sulfuric acid, acetic acid, or amino acids) combine with newly incorporated functional groups to form a highly polar conjugate. These conjugations or synthetic reactions are the hallmarks of Phase II metabolism.

The liver is the primary site of drug metabolism, although there is some metabolism in the intestinal wall. Furthermore, there may be some metabolism in the lungs, skin, kidneys, and the brain. Some orally administered drugs (clonazepam, chlorpromazine, and cyclosporine) are more extensively metabolized in the intestines than the liver.

Both intestinal and hepatic metabolism contribute to the first-pass effect. First-pass effects may reduce the bioavailability of orally administered drugs to such a degree that alternative routes of administration must be used to achieve therapeutically effective blood levels.

Mutations in cytochrome P450 genes or deficiencies of the enzymes have been identified and are linked to several human diseases. This is termed a polymorphism. Induction of some endogenous P450s is a risk factor in several cancers since these enzymes can convert procarcinogens to carcinogens.

9.7.1 PHASE I REACTIONS

A larger majority of drug-metabolizing enzymes are located in the lipophilic endoplasmic reticulum membranes of the liver and in other tissue systems. Biotransformation acts upon endogenous (already found within the body) as well as exogenous substrates (also termed xenobiotics).

Biotransformation (drug metabolism) is the process by which a drug is chemically converted in the body to its metabolite. Cytochrome P450s (CYP450s) are the main Phase I endogenous proteins that act as drug-metabolizing enzymes and also have endogenous enzymatic processes that are used to make cholesterol, steroids, and other important lipids such as prostacyclins and thromboxane A2.

P450 enzymes are primarily located in the liver but are also found in the kidneys, lungs, intestines, skin, and eyes. The name cytochrome P450 derives from the fact that these proteins have a heme group and an unusual spectrum. Mammalian cytochrome P450s are membrane bound. They were originally discovered in rat liver microsomes, hence the name microsomal enzymes.

P450s catalyze three main types of chemical reactions: oxidation reduction, and hydrolysis. The reaction that is most important, however, is hydroxylation.

A quick biotransformation rate may be due to the affinity of the drug molecule for the enzyme receptor. Other drugs biotransform slowly, and thus a high molecular burden cannot be tolerated. The CYP enzyme(s) which degrade it will become saturated, and the drug may accumulate in the body. If enzymes cannot metabolize a drug quickly, toxicity can result. Sometimes, a drug may be biotransformed at a decent rate, but the drug has low potency, which means the effective dose must be high. Thus, the molecular burden will be high, which may push the kinetics into a different elimination scheme by order.

Different biotransformation rates may be due to the structure of the drug molecule, as different drugs metabolized by the same CYP isoform (such as, for example, CYP3A4) may have different affinities for the enzyme and therefore different metabolization rates. Alternatively, in some cases, the enzyme itself may have a different structure in different people (polymorphisms of the enzyme). In the latter case, some people may be fast metabolizers, and others may be slow metabolizers. The most prominent CYP enzyme which has different drug metabolism polymorphisms is CYP2D6, which metabolizes most of the neurological drugs and is second only to CYP3A4 in the number of drugs it metabolizes.

9.7.1.1 The Families of Human P450s

The P450 proteins can be classified into family and subfamily categories based on their sequence similarities. Sequences that are greater than 40 percent identical at the amino acid level are categorized into the same family. Sequences that are greater than 55 percent identical are further categorized into the same subfamily. There are more than 2500 cytochrome P450 sequences known.

Biotransformation-utilizing P450 pathways are integral to the biosynthesis of many mammalian compounds such as bile acids and hormones. These enzymes tend to be in families with one or two members, and they have only one substrate. Most of these enzymes use steroids or steroid precursors as their substrates.

9.7.1.2 Induction of P450 Enzymes

Inducers of P450 enzymes accelerate metabolism, and the resultant lowering of the effect of the substrate drug may rob the patient of the beneficial effect. P450 enzymes influence a multitude of gene regulatory mechanisms. Genes can be turned on or induced by a chemical signal thereby driving cellular change. An example is the induction of steroid biosynthetic P450s by ACTH adrenocorticotropic hormone.

Some of the chemically dissimilar P450 substrate drugs, on repeated administration, induce P450 expression by enhancing the rate of its synthesis or reducing the rate of P450 degradation. Induction accelerates substrate metabolism, which usually hinders the pharmacologic action of the inducer and co-administered drugs. However, in the case of drugs metabolically transformed to reactive metabolites, enzyme induction may exacerbate metabolite-mediated toxicity. For example, ethanol induces the CYP2E enzymes.

The CYP3A subfamily is one of the most important drug-metabolizing families and is "the most abundantly expressed P450 in human liver." CYP3A4 is known to metabolize at least 120 known drugs.

Examples of CYP3A4 substrates are:

- Acetaminophen (Tylenol)
- Codeine (opiate analgesic)
- Lidocaine (anesthetic)
- Lovastatin (HMGCoA reductase inhibitor, a cholesterol-lowering drug)
- Taxol (cancer drug)
- Warfarin (anticoagulant)

9.7.1.3 P450 Inhibition

P450 inhibitors slow down metabolism, increase the effect of the substrate drug, and may cause toxicity of the substrate.

There are common drugs given for special purposes, which inhibit P450 enzymes. These include erythromycin (an antibiotic), ketoconazole, and itraconazole (both antifungals that inhibit the fungal CYP51 and unintentionally inhibit CYP3A4). If these drugs are given with other drugs that are normally metabolized by P450 enzymes, the lifetime (half-life) of these other drugs will be prolonged, and plasma levels will be increased, since they will not be cleared as fast.

If these drugs affect heart rhythms or other critical systems, the result can be fatal. For example, the inhibition of CYP3A4 in a patient taking warfarin can cause bleeding (common cause of adverse drug interactions).

An important factor in drug dosage is the interference from food. Grapefruit juice contains a CYP3A4 inhibitor that causes about a twelvefold increase in some drug concentrations. The effect may last several days. It is advisable to discourage your patients from eating grapefruit or drinking grapefruit juice while on medication metabolized by CYP3A4. Pharmacists will automatically place caution labels on prescriptions for such medications (e.g., cholesterol-lowering "statins").

9.7.2 Phase II Reactions

Parent drugs, or their Phase I metabolites that contain certain chemical groups, may undergo coupling or conjugation reactions with another substance to yield drug conjugates. Conjugates are typically polar molecules that are readily excreted and inactive. Generally, biotransformation of a drug results in a metabolite that is not only inactive but also more polar than the parent compound. This facilitates excretion of the metabolite.

There are five main Phase II reactions: glucuronidation, acetylation, glutathione conjugation, sulfation, and methylation.

9.7.2.1 Metabolism of Drugs to Toxic Products

The metabolism of drugs may not always be a safe biochemical event resulting in detoxification and elimination of the compound. Certain compounds are metabolically transformed to reactive intermediates that are toxic to different organ systems. These toxic reactions may not always be present at low levels of parent compound exposure when there are different detoxification mechanisms available. This may include the availability of endogenous detoxifying co-substrates (GSH, glucuronic acid, sulfate); however, when these resources are exhausted, the toxic pathway may prevail and cause organ toxicity.

9.8 FACTORS IMPACTING DRUG METABOLISM

9.8.1 Disease

Diseases such as hepatitis, alcoholic liver disease, fatty liver, and biliary cirrhosis can decrease biotransformation pathways and affect drug metabolism. Decrease in hepatic blood flow as a result of cardiac insufficiency or use of beta blockers may also affect metabolism. Therefore, caution must be exercised when treating hepatic-disease-afflicted patients with drugs which are extensively metabolized in the liver, such as lidocaine, verapamil, or morphine.

9.8.2 Age

Newborns typically have slower rates of Phase 1 biotransformation versus adults. Impairment of bilirubin conjugation (Phase 2), a primary cause of jaundice, is not uncommon in newborns. Older adults demonstrating decreased liver mass and hepatic blood flow have an overall slower rate of biotransformation. Once again, this slow rate of biotransformation may potentiate the effect of drugs extensively metabolized by the liver.

9.8.3 Gender

Androgenic and estrogenic hormones may influence drug metabolism. Clinical reports suggest that sex-dependent differences in drug metabolism exist in humans for ethanol, propranolol, some benzodiazepines, estrogens, and salicylates.

9.8.4 Genetic Factors

Genetic factors that influence enzyme levels also influence drug metabolism. Succinylcholine, for example, is metabolized only half as rapidly in people with genetically determined defects in pseudocholinesterase (see Table 9.3).

9.9 DRUG EXCRETION

Through the concepts of bioavailability and volume of distribution, we have established the relationship between drug dosage and plasma concentration. How can we determine how this drug concentration will change with time? The increase in drug concentration due to drug absorption is countered by the simultaneous elimination of the drug. For our purposes, we assume that the drug absorption is

TABLE 9.3
Examples of Genetic Polymorphisms in Drug Metabolism.

Defect	Enzyme Involved	Drug and Therapeutic Use	Clinical Consequences (Observed or Predictable)
Oxidation	CYP2D6	Bufuralol (-adrenoceptor blocker)	Exacerbation of blockade, nausea
Oxidation	CYP2D6	Codeine (analgesic)	Reduced analgesia
Oxidation	CYP2D6	Debrisoquin (antihypertensive)	Orthostatic hypotension
Oxidation	Aldehyde dehydrogenase	Ethanol (recreational drug)	Facial flushing, hypotension, tachycardia, nausea, vomiting
N-Acetylation	N-acetyl transferase	Hydralazine (antihypertensive)	Lupus erythematosus-like syndrome
N-Acetylation	N-acetyl transferase	Isoniazid (antitubercular)	Peripheral neuropathy
Oxidation	CYP2C19	Mephenytoin (antiepileptic)	Overdose toxicity
S-Methylation	Thiopurine methyltransferase	Mercaptopurines (cancer chemotherapeutic)	Myelotoxicity
Oxidation	CYP2A6	Nicotine (stimulant)	Lesser toxicity
Oxidation	CYP2D6	Nortriptyline (antidepressant)	Toxicity
O-Demethylation	CYP2C19	Omeprazole (proton pump inhibitor)	Increased therapeutic efficacy
Oxidation	CYP2D6	Sparteine	Oxytocic symptoms
Ester hydrolysis	Plasma cholinesterase	Succinylcholine (neuromuscular blocker)	Prolonged apnea
Oxidation	CYP2C9	S-warfarin (anticoagulant)	Bleeding
Oxidation	CYP2C9	Tolbutamide (hypoglycemic)	Cardiotoxicity

instantaneous (though this is only true for IV administration). Elimination of the drug is primarily governed by the metabolism in the liver and excretion from the kidney.

The termination of drug activity in the body occurs when:

- The drug is metabolized.
- The redistribution of the drug into other tissues removes it from its site of action, e.g., redistribution of thiopental into fat.
- The drug is excreted.

As a very general rule, polar compounds are excreted unchanged, and nonpolar compounds are metabolized to more polar compounds. There is a difference between elimination and excretion. In a minority of drug classes, for example, elimination via metabolism without excretion may occur.

In drug excretion, the main routes are via urine and feces, with the kidney (urine producer) being the principal excretion organ. Volatile drugs, such as inhalation anesthetics, are mostly excreted via the lungs, but lungs play only a very small part in elimination for the remainder of drugs.

Excretion via sweat and breast milk has very small contributions to the overall elimination of drugs but can have very important clinical consequences (breast milk excretion with toxicity to the neonate/infant).

With fecal excretion, the passage of drugs and metabolites may occur by passive diffusion or active transport. In passive diffusion, the same physiochemical factors that affect absorption and distribution of the drugs are important (e.g., pH, pKa, and protein binding).

With biliary excretion, the mechanisms by which the body directs some compounds to the bile and others to urine are not clear. Two of the important requirements for biliary excretion are a fairly large MW (>300 kDal) and some polar characteristics.

Some conjugates such as glucuronides (formed by Phase II metabolism) and amino acid conjugates are principally excreted into the bile. From the bile, these compounds pass into the GI tract where they are exposed to bacteria. The bacteria can act on these drugs, sometimes resulting in recovery of the parent drug which can be reabsorbed to again exert its effect. This is known as enterohepatic recycling and is thought to be responsible for the prolongation of action of drugs such as ethinyl, estradiol, and digoxin.

9.9.1 Urinary Excretion

The three processes involved in urinary excretion are glomerular filtration, tubular secretion, and tubular reabsorption.

9.9.1.1 Glomerular Filtration

The overall rate of filtration depends on the plasma concentration and the glomerular filtration rate (GFR) within the kidney. Only the free drug fraction is filtered; therefore, binding of drug to plasma proteins retards excretion, while displacement from proteins enhances filtration. Disease may affect filtration; however, drugs usually do not.

9.9.1.2 Tubular Secretion (Active Secretion)

Proximal tubules in the kidney (nephrons) actively transport a lot of drugs, for example, glucose and amino acids. There are also two nonspecific systems: One for anions (negatively charged, e.g., organic acids) and one for cations (positively charged, e.g., organic bases). Consequently, drugs being eliminated via the same system may compete for the same transport sites. This may be good or bad. There have been no clinically significant drug interactions reported for the basic system, but there are some problems with the acid secretion system, for example, some diuretics compete with the active secretion of uric acid, leading to hyperuricemia.

On the other hand, probenecid, a uricosuric (increases uric acid excretion) agent that prevents the nephrotic reabsorption of uric acid, can also inhibit the anion secretory pathway. This delay in excretion has been used to clinical advantage for dozens of years with a variety of therapeutic agents. It can be used to prevent the secretion of acidic drugs such as penicillin, thereby decreasing their excretion and prolonging their action.

In active secretion, as the free drug is secreted, the plasma level of the drug decreases. This leads to the dissociation of the drug–protein complexes in the plasma, thus increasing the free drug's supply (see Figure 9.9).

9.9.1.3 Tubular Reabsorption

There are specific active transport mechanisms for some drugs (e.g., glucose), but most pass back into the body by passive diffusion in the kidney's distal tubules. By then, urine has been concentrated so that a concentration gradient exists. Only the unionized drug contributes to the gradient. The ionized drug acts as a pool from which more unionized drug may be obtained. Consequently, the pH of urine is very important because of the degree of ionization that will occur. Ionized drugs are not passively reabsorbed.

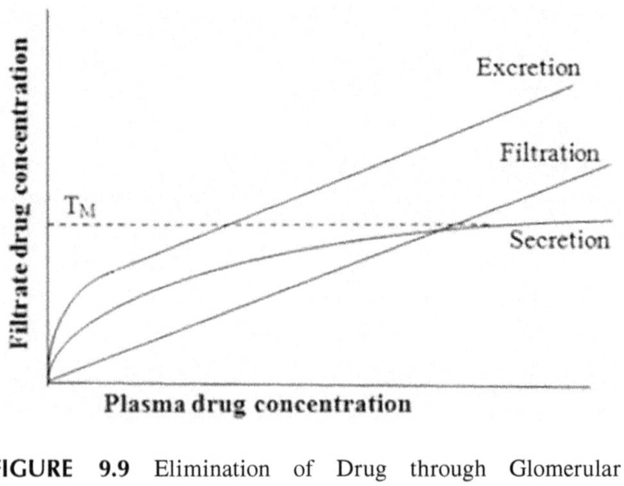

FIGURE 9.9 Elimination of Drug through Glomerular Filtration.

The amount of the drug going out via the urine will then be the net sum of the three processes:

$$Urinary\ excretion = GFR + Active\ secretion - Reabsorption \tag{9.8}$$

Note that reabsorption refers to both active and passive processes.

9.9.1.4 Effects of pH on Urinary Excretion of Ionizable Drugs

Ionization increases renal clearance of drugs:

1. Both ionized and unionized drugs are filtered.
2. Passive reabsorption is only associated with unionized drugs.
3. Ionized portions of a drug are water-soluble and can be filtered but cannot be reabsorbed. They are therefore trapped in the filtrate. This trapping increases the removal of the drug from the body. For example, in acute toxicity from aspirin overdose, alkalinization of the urine will increase the ionization of salicylic acid in the filtrate and thus eliminate it faster by decreasing reabsorption.

9.10 PHARMACOKINETICS

9.10.1 Introduction

Pharmacokinetics (PK) is the study of the how the concentration of a drug changes in the various compartments of the body over time. Pharmacokinetics describes how the body acts upon a drug. In contrast, pharmacodynamics is the relationship between drug concentration at the site of action and the pharmacologic responses (i.e., the intensity and time course of therapeutic and adverse effects). Pharmacodynamics describes what the drug does to the body.

The study of pharmacokinetics is not purely academic. One of the responsibilities of a physician is to prescribe how much (dose) and how often (dosing interval) a drug should be taken by the patient. To determine the proper dose and dosing interval of a drug, one must (1) know what drug concentration this dose would correspond to after absorption and distribution and (2) be able to predict how quickly this concentration will decrease due to elimination. Too much drug or too short a dosing interval could be toxic or fatal. In fact, too much therapy is the most common cause of toxicity. For example, if the dose and thus effects of the anticoagulant warfarin get too high, the patient could have an intracranial bleed. Conversely, if the dose is too small or the dosing interval is too long, the drug will not be effective, and clotting may occur. Other possible consequences of insufficient dosage include an antibiotic not controlling an infection, a blood pressure medication not being able to prevent blood pressure from rising to dangerous levels, or a birth control pill not preventing pregnancy.

The basic assumption in utilizing pharmacokinetics is that drug responses are proportional to blood levels that one can measure. Therefore, PK can be used for predictive purposes to answer the following questions:

- What is the appropriate dose or dosing interval to maintain adequate blood levels, thereby optimizing the therapeutic response?
- How would a disease (such as renal failure) affect the drug concentration in the body?
- Is therapeutic failure due to the use of the wrong drug or inadequate dosing?

Using PK principles, one may predict plasma concentration at any future time, thereby achieving optimal dosing with minimal oversight. For drugs in which the dosage required for therapeutic effect is close to the dosage eliciting toxicity and thus have a small safety margin (i.e., narrow therapeutic index), PK-predicted concentrations may be verified by measuring the drug concentration clinically (therapeutic drug monitoring—TDM).

9.10.2 Therapeutic Window and Therapeutic Index

Indeed, it is vital to operate in a therapeutic window of drug concentration—high enough to be effective but not so high that it is toxic. This is determined by the average responses of the larger population to a drug. The median effective dose, ED50, is the dose at which the drug is effective in 50 percent of individuals. Naturally, toxic and lethal doses are not established by experimenting on human patients! Rather, they are modeled using animal studies. The median lethal dose, LD50, is the dose at which death would result in 50 percent of the population. The median toxic dose, TD50, is the concentration at which 50 percent would experience a specific side effect. Since a drug can have many different side effects, it can have different TD50s—one corresponding to each side effect.

The safety of a drug is expressed as the therapeutic index (TI) or the ratio of TD50/ED50. A high TI indicates that the drug may be safe even if the drug concentration unexpectedly rises somewhat (as could happen due to a drug interaction). If a drug has a low TI, such as is the case for anesthetics, then even a relatively small increase in concentration could lead to toxicity or death. In other words, TI is an indication of the size of the safety margin a drug possesses in terms of its dosage (see Figure 9.10).

Where:
TD = Toxic dose
ED = Effective dose

Narrow therapeutic index drugs are as follows:

- Warfarin
- Phenytoin
- Valproic acid
- Carbamazepine

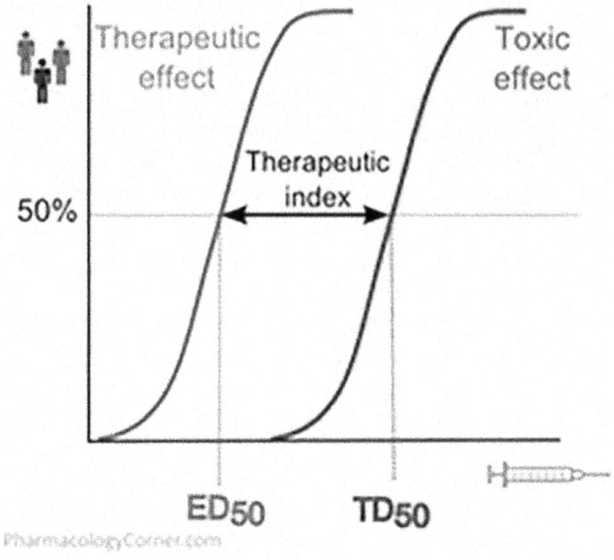

FIGURE 9.10 Therapeutic Index Compares the Amount of Drug that Causes a Therapeutic Effect versus a Toxic Effect in Humans.

- Cyclosporine
- Digoxin

With narrow therapeutic index (NTI) drugs, slight alterations in systemic concentration can lead to significant changes in a patient's pharmacodynamic response. This may result in toxic effects, especially in patients who are receiving a number of medications, are ill, or are of old age. Bioavailability between generic and brand drug products does not equal bioequivalence, especially when referring to NTI drugs. Warfarin is an anticoagulant NTI drug for which substitution is now available and may indeed be substituted without the knowledge of the patient or the practitioner. When the brand name drug is preferred by the practitioner, "no substitution" must be clearly indicated on the prescription to avoid the generic replacement of warfarin and other NTI drugs.

9.10.3 Blood Levels for Narrow Therapeutic Index (NDI) Drugs

When a dose of a drug is given orally, rectally, or intravenously, it ultimately accumulates in the blood (plasma or serum). One may measure drug concentrations by obtaining blood specimens at various times. Of course, the concentration of the drug in blood is constantly changing, so it is important to know when the last dose was given when evaluating serum or plasma drug concentration.

The minimum effective concentration is the concentration below which a drug is known to lack effectiveness. Likewise, the maximum effective concentration indicates the level above which increasing the drug concentration has no additional therapeutic benefit. This latter dose phenomenon is called a maximum effect. The maximum effective concentration is less than or equal to the toxic concentration. The area between the minimum and maximum effective concentrations is termed the therapeutic window.

9.10.4 Kinetic Modeling

Kinetic models attempt to quantify how the body acts upon a drug over time, utilizing mathematical "compartment" models. In compartment modeling, one assumes that the body is equivalent to one or more compartments in which the drug moves. A change in drug concentration in any one body compartment will affect the concentration in any other model compartment. In these models, a change in the concentration within a single compartment results in an immediate re-equilibration of the drug within the compartment (see Figure 9.11).

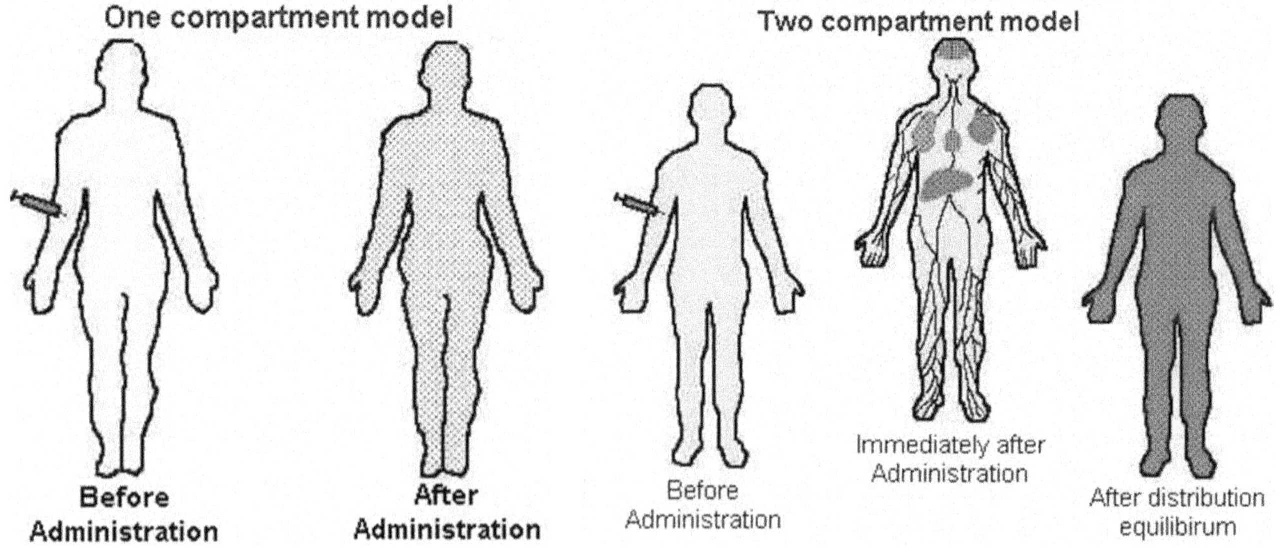

FIGURE 9.11 (A) One-Compartment Model and (B) Two-Compartment Model.

The number of compartments a drug exhibits may be estimated by the examination of the plasma drug concentration versus time curve. Each break in the absorption or elimination curves represents a body compartment.

The concentration decay (kinetics) over time usually proceeds by first-order kinetics (explained below). First-order elimination occurs when the amount of drug eliminated from the body in a specific time is dependent on the amount of drug in the body at that time. For first-order elimination, the fraction of drug eliminated in the body per unit of time remains constant.

9.10.5 Drug Absorption and Elimination

Absorption rate depends on many factors such as dosage form, drug dissolution, and gastric emptying time. The absorption rate constant (ka) is the fraction of the administered dose that leaves the site of administration per unit time. The larger the *ka* the faster the drug is absorbed. The time required for a drug to reach maximal blood concentration is termed T_{max}. The concentration of drug in the blood at this time is termed C_{max}.

9.10.5.1 Absorption Rate

9.10.5.1.1 Zero Order

Absorption rate is constant, independent of amount of drug administered:

$$ko = \text{mg/min or mg/ml/min}$$

Intravenous (IV) infusion demonstrates zero-order absorption kinetics.

9.10.5.1.2 First Order

Absorption rate is proportional to the amount of drug present. *Ka* is the fraction of drug absorbed per unit of time. The larger the *ka*, the faster the drug is absorbed. (see Figure 9.12).

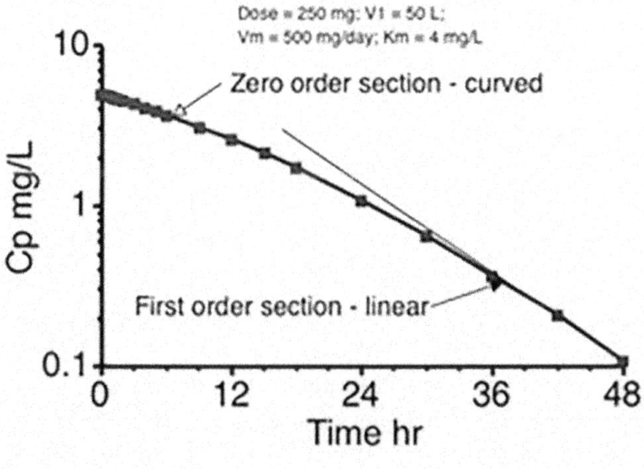

FIGURE 9.12 First- and Zero-Order Elimination.

9.10.5.2 Elimination Rate

Like absorption rate, the rate of elimination for drugs follows either first-order or zero-order kinetics. First order means the rate of elimination is proportional to the amount of drug. The concentration versus time graph will exhibit exponential decay. Zero order means that the rate of elimination is constant. The concentration versus time graph for zero order will be a straight line. Almost all drug elimination is governed by first-order kinetics, although some notable exceptions are alcohol, phenytoin, and some cardiac drugs (at high concentrations); these follow zero-order kinetics. Also, drugs can follow first-order kinetics at one dosage but then transition to zero-order kinetics at higher doses. To understand why a drug would follow first-order or zero-order kinetics, one must examine drug elimination at a molecular level.

As mentioned, most drug metabolism takes place in the liver. A drug molecule is metabolized by binding with a CYP enzyme, where it is cleaved or otherwise modified (elimination). Initially, the more drug molecules that are presented to the liver, the more they bind to CYP enzymes and are degraded. Hence, the rate of the elimination or processing of the drug molecules is proportional to the number of drug molecules. However, the number of CYP enzymes is finite. As the number of drug molecules increases, the CYP enzymes are increasingly occupied until saturation occurs and no more receptor sites are open. Before any more drug molecules can bind to enzymes and be eliminated, the bound drug molecules must be degraded.

At this point, the elimination follows zero-order kinetics. It does not matter how many drug molecules are presented to the liver; the elimination rate is constant as the drug molecules are in essence waiting in line to get processed by the CYP enzymes. In this sense, the elimination of drug molecules by the numerous liver CYP enzymes is analogous to getting into a football stadium through the numerous turnstiles at the gate. Instead of molecules being processed through degradation or chemical modification, people are "processed" from one side of the gate to the inside of the stadium.

Assume there are ten turnstiles at a gate, and it takes a person one second to get through them. If one person shows up to the gate, then that person will be processed in one second, and the rate of processing (elimination) is one person per second. If two people show up to the gate, then the two people go through two separate turnstiles, and the rate of processing is two people per second. Hence, the rate of elimination is proportional to the number of people, so by definition it follows first-order kinetics.

If this is a game between the Bears and the (abysmal) Cleveland Browns, perhaps the number of people showing up to the gate will not exceed ten people per second, and therefore no one has to wait for a turnstile. However, for a Bears-Packers game, a ton of people will show up at the gate to see the game—more than ten people per second. However, the turnstiles will be saturated, and the rate of processing of people from one side of the gate to the other will be constant as the people are slowly funneled through the ten turnstiles. Whether there are 10,000 or 20,000 people that show up, the rate of processing people in the stadium will be constant at 10 people per second. This describes zero-order kinetics. Further, if a few people show up early to beat the lines and the bulk of the people show up later, then the rate of processing would transition from first-order to zero-order kinetics.

9.10.5.2.1 First Order

The rate of drug elimination is proportional to the amount of drug remaining. The rate constant k relates the rate of drug elimination to the amount in the body at any time t:

$$k = \text{rate of elimination/amount of drug in body}$$

By definition, first-order kinetics means that the rate of change in concentration (elimination) is proportional to the concentration. Mathematically, this is represented as follows:

$$\text{Rate of elimination (mg/ min.)} = d[C]/\text{dt} = k_e[C]$$

Where:
k_e = the rate constant (min^{-1})
$[C]$ = concentration
t = time

From the equation, it is clear that the rate constant is the fraction of drug eliminated per unit time. This concept is very useful in developing PK equations, as the rate constant is part of many of them.

A more useful equation for first-order kinetics is represented by the following equation for exponential decay, which will allow one to calculate the concentration of drug remaining after a certain period of time:

$$[C] = C_o e^{-kt} \quad (9.10)$$

Where:
$[C]$ = concentration
C_o = initial concentration
k = the rate constant (also called k_e or rate of elimination)
t = time

A similar equation applies if you are dealing with the amount of drug rather than concentration, though it should be noted that the mass of the drug refers to that which has reached systemic circulation (*F* × *dose*):

$$m_{drug} = m_O e^{-kt} \quad (9.11)$$

Other versions of the first-order equation can be converted from concentration to mass of drug in the same fashion by merely substituting $[C]$ for m_{drug} and the initial concentration for the initial mass. If you are solving for time, the following integrated equation is more useful:

$$-kt = ln([C]/C_o) \quad (9.12)$$

9.10.5.2.2 Zero Order

Zero-order elimination means the mass of drug decreases at a constant rate (e.g., a decline in serum concentration of 5 mg/ml per hour). The units of rate of elimination are mg/hour or mg/ml/hour.

Zero-order kinetics means that the rate of elimination is constant. Therefore, the amount eliminated is just this constant multiplied by the time:

$$\text{Amount of drug eliminated} = (\text{elimination rate}) \times (\text{time}) \quad (9.13)$$

Elimination rate in this case is in units of mg/min. The following expression is an example of how the mass of a zero-order elimination drug would change with time, with the arrows representing a given interval of time:

50 mg => 40 mg => 30 mg => 20 mg => 10 mg => 0 mg

Dividing by volume yields a similar equation for concentration:

$$(\text{Change in drug concentration}) = (\text{elimination rate}) \times (\text{time})$$

Elimination rate is in units of mg/ml/min.

One way to check that your equation is probably correct is to make sure the units cancel to yield the same thing on each side of the equation.

The most useful case of zero-order kinetics is alcohol elimination.

9.10.5.3 Clearance (*CL*)

Clearance is a volume of blood from which the drug is completely removed per unit time. Instead of the drug remaining homogenous throughout the volume of distribution as it becomes more dilute, clearance is modeled as if repeatedly a certain volume of blood has drug completely removed from it. Since the rate constant k_e is the fraction of drug removed per unit time, and the total volume the drug is dissolved in is estimated as the volume of distribution (V_D), then the volume being cleared per unit time is $ke \times V_D$.

$$CL = ke \times V_D \quad (9.14)$$

Units for clearance are volume per unit time (ml/min).

$$\text{Rate of elimination (mg / min)} = CL(\text{ml / min}) \times \text{concentration (mg/ml)} \quad (9.15)$$

Since the total amount eliminated is the dose, the total body clearance can also be calculated from the AUC.

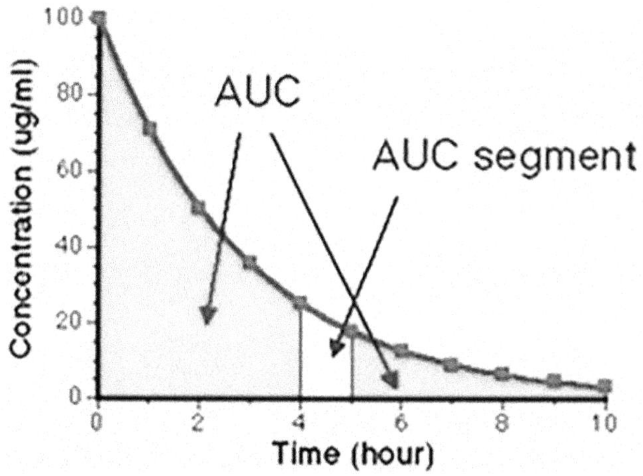

FIGURE 9.13 Area under the Curve (AUC) Graph.

9.10.5.4 Area under the Curve (AUC)

As mentioned previously, the AUC is the area under the plot of plasma concentration of drug versus time after drug administration (see Figure 9.13). The AUC is of particular use in estimating the bioavailability of drugs and in estimating total clearance of drugs (CL). Following single intravenous doses, $AUC = dose / CL$, for single-compartment systems obeying first-order elimination kinetics. For routes other than the intravenous:

$$\text{AUC} = F \times (\text{Dose}) / \text{CL} \tag{9.16}$$

where F is the bioavailability of the drug

$$\text{AUC} = \text{Dose} / \text{CL} = \text{Mg/mL}$$

Where:
F = The bioavailability of the drug
For equal doses:
For different doses:

$$F = \left(\frac{(AUC\_Oral \,/\, \text{Dose Oral})}{(AUC\_IV \,/\, \text{Dose IV})} \right) \tag{9.17}$$

9.10.5.5 Elimination (k)

You have already learned about concepts and processes of hepatic and renal elimination. In this context, elimination is simply defined as follows:

k = rate of drug elimination/amount of drug in the body (i.e., the fractional rate of drug removal per unit time).

Elimination may be broken into two components: Metabolism and excretion.

Metabolism: Chemical biotransformation of the parent drug within the body to one or more products or compounds.

Excretion: Physical removal of parent drug or metabolite from the body.

9.10.5.6 Elimination Half-Life

Elimination half-life ($t^{1/2}$) is the time it takes for 50 percent of the concentration of the drug to be eliminated from the body. It is only constant for first-order kinetics, so it is only used in that context. Elimination half-life is dependent upon volume of distribution (V_D) and clearance (CL) just as k is.

The half-life is inversely proportional to the rate constant:

$$t_{1/2} = ln(2) / k_e = 0.7 \times V_D / CL \tag{9.18}$$

There are two methods to determine half-life: Calculation and graphical. Graphically, half-life is determined by measuring drug concentrations periodically, plotting them as in Figure 9.14, and determining the time it takes for the concentration to be halved. Calculation of half-life is shown next.

The percent of drug lost in a certain number of half-lives is as follows:

$$\text{Percent of drug eliminated} = 1 - (1/2)^n \tag{9.19}$$

$$\text{Percent of steady state achieved} = 100 \times \left[1 - (1/2)^n\right] \tag{9.20}$$

Where:
n = number of half-lives elapsed

9.10.5.7 Steady State

Steady state is a condition of equilibrium in which the rate of drug administration equals the rate of elimination. We may assume that steady state is reached after five half-lives of the drug have elapsed, regardless of the dosing regimen. The figures that follow will serve to discuss these concepts of half-life, steady state, the size of the dose, and the frequency at which it is given to determine the height of the plateau.

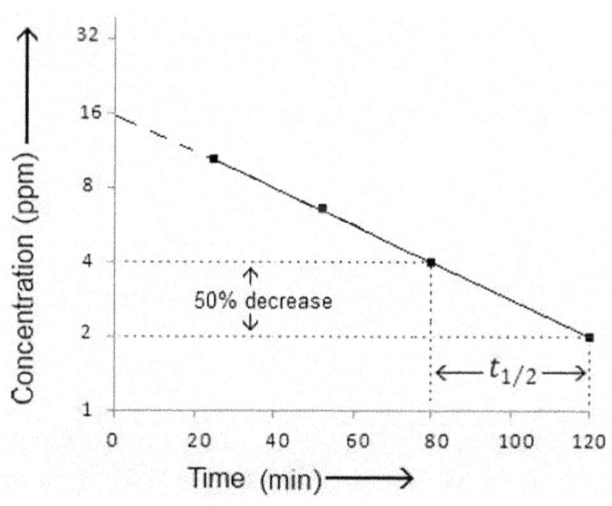

FIGURE 9.14 Drug Elimination Half-Life.

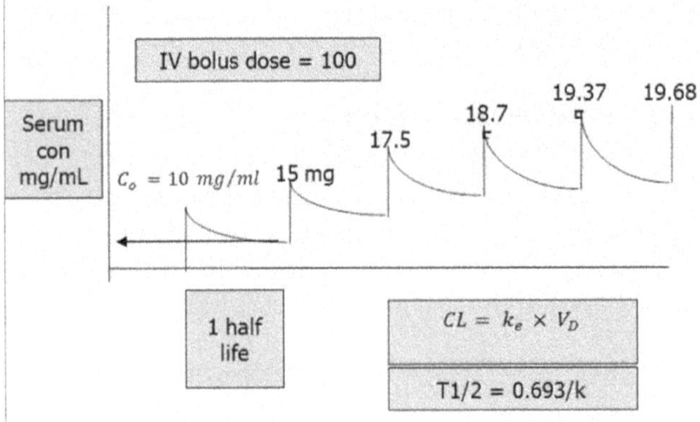

FIGURE 9.15 Steady State.

As successive doses of drug are administered, drug begins to accumulate in the body. The amount of drug added to the system with each administration is the same (Figure 9.15, the concentration increases by 10 mg/mL with every dose). However, the drop in concentration during the elimination phase is greater with each subsequent dose. This is because the concentration at the beginning of the elimination phase (right after the dose) is higher with each subsequent dose, and first-order elimination dictates that the amount of drug eliminated per unit time is proportional to the amount of drug in the body. Therefore, drug in the body will accumulate until the rate of elimination equals the rate of drug entering the body—steady state.

As the rate of drug elimination approaches that of drug administration (i.e., approach steady state), the maximum (peak) and minimum (trough) drug concentrations in the blood increase until equilibrium is reached. At this point, no more drug will accumulate in the body, and the peak and trough drug concentrations will be constant. When peak and trough drug concentrations are roughly the same in two or more successive doses, steady-state (Css) has been reached (Figure 9.16). This occurs after approximately five half-lives.

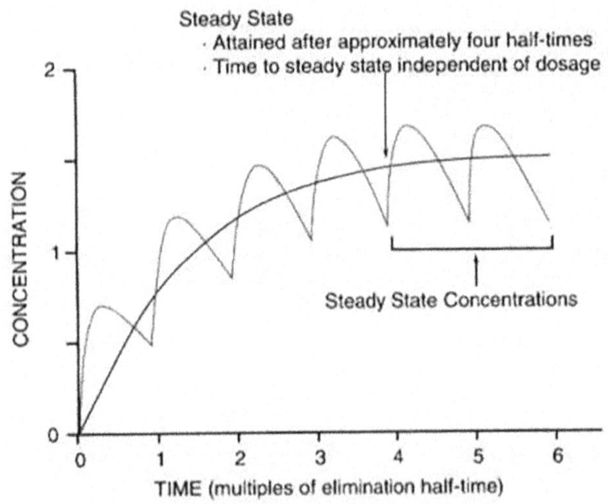

FIGURE 9.16 Steady State Curve.

TABLE 9.4
Number of Half-Lives and Percent Steady State.

Number of Half-Lives	Percent Steady-State
1	50
2	75
3	87.5
4	93.75
5	96.88
6	98.44
7	99.22

Table 9.4 represents graphical data in which the time required to reach steady state is predicted on the basis of a drug's half-life.

Drugs with a higher comparative k_e (shorter half-life) will reach steady state sooner than drugs with a lower k_e (longer half-life). Drugs eliminated quicker reach steady state quicker because the time it takes for the rate of drug elimination to equal the rate of drug absorption is faster compared to drugs eliminated slowly.

9.10.6 Dosing

Now that the important concepts of pharmacokinetics have been established, we can discuss the calculation of dosage. Loading dose is the dose to immediately establish therapeutic levels. Maintenance dose is the amount of drug and dosing interval needed to keep the drug concentration in the therapeutic range.

When a continuous intravenous infusion (IV drip) of a drug is started, it takes approximately five half-lives to reach the steady state. In some cases, an immediate drug response is required that cannot wait five half-lives. If a very large dose is given immediately, followed by smaller doses, the result is that therapeutic concentrations can be immediately achieved. This initial dose is termed a "loading dose." The subsequent smaller doses are termed "maintenance doses" (*MD*).

9.10.6.1 Loading Dose

Loading dose, the amount of drug that needs to be in the systemic circulation to establish a certain desired concentration, can be found using the formula for concentration:

$$(\text{Loading Dose in systemic circulation}) = C \times V_D \quad (9.21)$$

For IV administration, the dose in systemic circulation equals the dose prescribed:

$$\text{Loading Dose} = C \times V_D \quad (9.22)$$

For other routes of administration, the equation must include the bioavailability F.

$$F \times (\text{Loading Dose}) = C \times V_D \quad (9.23)$$

9.10.6.2 Maintenance Doses (*MD*)

For some drugs, the maintenance of a specific blood concentration is imperative to therapeutic success. Therefore, we can administer drugs at specific times on an ongoing basis to maintain adequate blood concentration. The goal of the maintenance dose is to replace the drug lost through elimination. If 10 mg of drug is lost in an hour, then the maintenance dose must be 10 mg every hour (10 mg/hour). Hence, the maintenance dose is calculated by finding the amount of drug eliminated per unit time.

In multiple dosing, the second dose is given before the first dose is completely eliminated; therefore, the maximum concentration after the second dose is higher than the first. Patient compliance is greatest with once-a-day dosing. Ideally, the dose interval should be selected as a factor of 24; so doses can be given at the same time each day.

We have already established that the volume cleared of drug per unit time is the clearance. The total volume cleared is the clearance multiplied by the time. Let the time equal the dosing interval (tau); so the volume cleared is equal to $CL \times tau$. The amount of drug in this cleared volume is the maintenance dose. The amount of drug in any specific volume is given by Mass of drug = Volume cleared × Concentration. Substituting for the volume cleared (volume cleared = $CL \times tau$), the expression becomes:

$$\text{Mass of drug} = \text{concentration} \times CL \times tau \quad (9.24)$$

Taking bioavailability into account, the equation for the maintenance dose (*MD*) is as follows:

$$F \times MD = \text{concentration} \times CL \times tau \quad (9.25)$$

For IV administration, $F = 1$, so the maintenance dose is:

$$MD = \text{concentration} \times CL \times tau \quad (9.26)$$

The clinical difference between the infusion rate and maintenance dose is that the maintenance dose yields a sawtoothing of concentration, while infusion is more tightly controlled. Maintenance doses have more potential for toxicity (right after the dose) or loss of effectiveness (right before the next dose) in comparison to infusion.

Units of the continuous infusion rate have the same units as the zero-order rate constant (e.g., mg/min).

9.10.6.3 Example—Dosage Adjustment in Renal Impairment

Diseases such as renal impairment can reduce clearance, and so the maintenance dose must be adjusted in these cases to compensate for this. The loading dose remains the same as that for healthy patients.

In order to estimate glomerular filtration and, therefore, identify renal impairment, one must look at certain markers within the urine, such as insulin or creatinine. Creatinine is an endogenous compound secreted by the muscle and is usually produced at a constant rate by the body depending on body mass.

Creatinine is filtered out of the blood by the kidneys by glomerular filtration and proximal tubular secretion, and there is minimal reabsorption (entrance back into the blood) from the kidney. If kidney filtration is deficient, then creatinine blood levels increase. Therefore, creatinine levels in the blood or in the urine are a reliable marker to reflect glomerular filtration rates (GFR).

For patients with renal impairment, alteration in dosing regimen is determined from creatinine clearance calculations.

Calculation of kidney function (*KF*) is done on the basis of the following:

- Individualized kidney function assessment
- A comparison of an impaired individual to one with "normal" kidney function
- $KF = \text{Creatinine } CL\,(\text{impaired}) / \text{Creatinine } CL\,(\text{normal})$

Normalize $CrCL$ to a 70-kg individual:

$$\text{CrCL} = [(140 - \text{age}) \times L\text{BW}] / (72 \times S\text{rCr})$$

Normalize to 70 kg:

$$\text{CrCL(mL / min / 70 kg)} = (140 - \text{age}) / S\text{rCr}$$

Assume:

$$CrCL = 120\text{ml/ min/ 70 kg} \text{ in normal renal function}$$

Dosage adjustment for renal impairment determined to compensate for the associated reduction in clearance.

For renal impairment, the magnitude of impact on drug clearance depends on:

- The degree of kidney dysfunction
- The fraction of drug excreted unchanged in kidney (fe)

Changes in drug clearance can be estimated by determining kidney function and the fraction of drug excreted renally:

$$(CL \text{ renally impaired}) = [1 - fe \times (l - KF)] \times (CL \text{ normal}) \quad (9.27)$$

Where:
fe = fraction of drug excreted unchanged in urine

9.10.7 Therapeutic Drug Monitoring (TDM)

The goal of therapeutic drug monitoring (TDM) is to use serum or plasma drug concentrations as an aid to optimize drug therapy and maximize the probability of an appropriate therapeutic effect while minimizing the chance for toxicity.

The therapeutic range (window) is defined as the range of drug concentration in the serum or plasma necessary to achieve a therapeutic response. Although the therapeutic range defines a desirable concentration in the majority of patients, the specific concentration may vary greatly from patient to patient (idiosyncrasy). Moreover, some patients may require dosage in an otherwise toxic or subtherapeutic range.

Some common misconceptions regarding the therapeutic range are as follows:

1. Drug concentrations in the therapeutic range automatically result in the desired therapeutic response.
2. Toxicity is not encountered in the therapeutic range.

In general, the therapeutic range should be considered as a probability, that is, there is high probability of therapeutic success without toxicity. However, therapeutic ranges are derived from population-based studies and are only general guidelines for the general population. Conditions such as age, disease, or drug interaction may alter therapeutic range for a particular patient. The patient's response is always more important than absolute serum or plasma drug concentrations and should be used as a basis for altering dosing patterns.

9.10.8 Pharmacokinetics Summary

Pharmacokinetics is a valuable tool to accurately determine the dosage of a drug to target the therapeutic concentration. It utilizes physiological parameters of the patient and chemical properties of the drug in kinetic models to achieve this end and accounts for the effects of renal impairment on drug elimination kinetics. While pharmacokinetics has a great predictive power, ultimately the patient's response should determine how the dose should be adjusted.

9.11 DRUG RECEPTOR AND PHARMACODYNAMICS

Both the therapeutic and adverse or toxic effects of drugs result from the drug's interactions with molecular tissue systems. Most drugs act by associating with specific macromolecules to induce changes in biochemical or biophysical outcomes. This engagement is embodied in the term receptor. The receptor is the component of a cell or organism that engages with a drug and initiates the chain of events, leading to the clinical effect of the drug.

9.11.1 Agonists and Antagonists

Most drugs exert their effects on the body by interacting with discrete parts of a cell called receptors. Receptors are the central focus of investigation of drug effects and their mechanisms of action (pharmacodynamics) (see Figure 9.17).

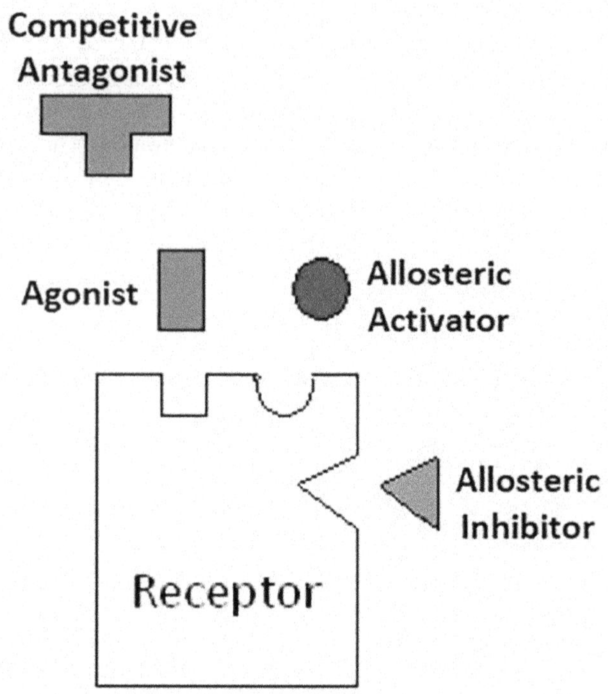

FIGURE 9.17 Receptor and Ligands (Pharmaceutical Modifiers).

Receptors determine the quantitative relationships between dose, or concentration, of the drug and the pharmacological response. They do so by having selectivity for a drug. That is, they recognize distinct drugs or ligands. Affinity for binding a drug determines the concentration of a drug required to form a significant drug–receptor complex (see Figure 9.18).

Mediating the actions of a drug, or ligand, by transducing information from the binding of the drug to a response within the cell produces the physiological effect. Drugs modify only naturally occurring effects and do not generate new effects.

9.11.2 Drug–Receptor Interactions

There are three variables involved in drug–receptor interactions: Dose, effect, and time. Time is eliminated as a variable by considering the effect at maximal response. When quantifying the dose response, the following assumptions are made:

1. The intensity of the response is directly proportional to the number of receptors occupied.
2. One drug molecule binds to one receptor.
3. The amount of drug binding to the receptors is so small compared to the total drug available that practically the amount of uncombined drug equals the total drug present.
4. The binding is reversible and of short duration.
5. The binding of one receptor does not affect another.

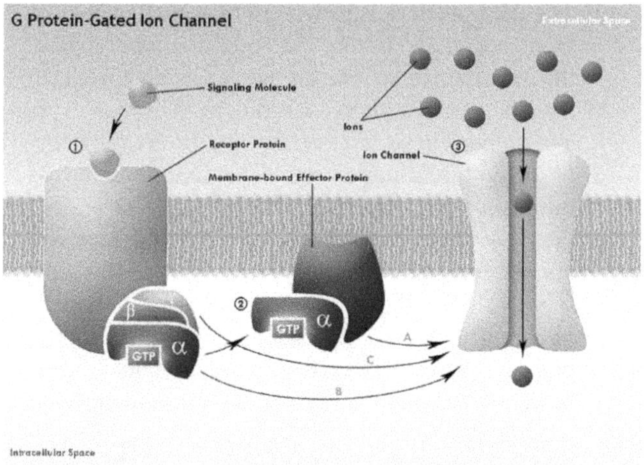

FIGURE 9.18 Drug–Receptor Interactions. Ligand-gated channels are bound by a specific ligand/drug (i.e., acetylcholine), which causes the activation of the channel. In this case, acetylcholine is opening the channel and inducing the influx of Na+ ions. G-protein-activated channels are attached to G proteins within the cell and cause signal transduction or an alteration of intracellular molecules to create a certain response.

Source: Clarson, Craig W. Basic Principles of Pharmacology: Direct Activation of Ion Channel and G-Protein Activation of an Ion Channel. Digital Images. Tulane Pharmwiki, 2009. Web 20 Dec. 2015. http://tmedweb.tulane.edu/pharmwiki/doku.php/drug_receptor_theory. Reproduced by permission from Craig W. Clarkson. @2011 Craig W. Clarkson, Tulane University, New Orleans, LA (with permission).

Mathematically, the drug–receptor interaction can be represented by:

$$D + R \underset{K_2}{\overset{K_1}{\rightleftarrows}} DR = \overset{K_3}{-----\rightarrow} \text{Response} \quad (9.28)$$

Where:
D = Drug
R = Receptor
The preceding equations demonstrate two principles:

1. Affinity is k_1 / k_2 and is a measure of the preference that a drug exhibits for a receptor.
2. Efficacy (intrinsic activity) is k_3 and describes the biological effectiveness of the drug–receptor complex in generating a response.

9.12 DOSE RESPONSES

Dose responses (DRs) are an integral aspect of the drug and effect relationship. DRs are used ubiquitously to determine the therapeutic, toxic, and lethal effects of a particular drug on the body. These tests are done in animals and are an essential step before a drug is tested in humans.

Several statistical concepts are used as a guideline to categorize the safety of a drug. As mentioned before, the therapeutic index plays a significant role in determining drug safety.

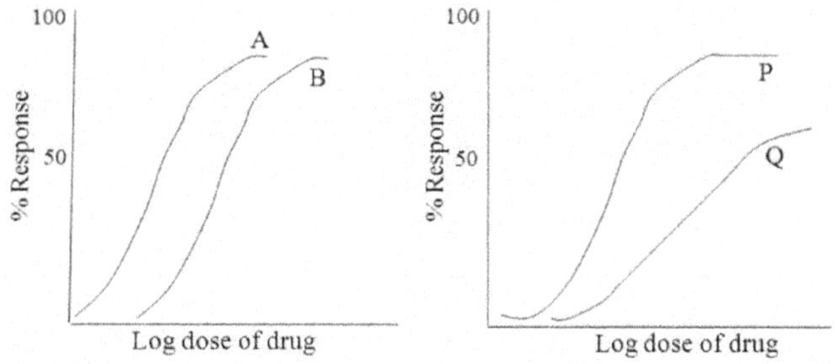

FIGURE 9.19 Log Dose–Response Curves.

There are responses to a drug which can be quantified by a yes/no response, for example, sleep, protection from a seizure, etc. Continuous responses may be changed to quantal responses by setting a goal—for example, a drug (will/will not) decrease blood pressure by 20 mm Hg. The construction of a quantal dose–response curve is associated with the measurement of population responses. Because of individual variations, a single dose of a drug will then exhibit a variance of responses in the population.

The response (given enough individuals) will be the familiar bell-shaped curve found in statistics and can be defined by knowing the median and standard deviation. Note that in a large enough population, a single dose can elicit a response gradient from no effect to toxicity. Log dose response curves (LDRs—see Figure 9.19) can be useful in identifying similarly acting drugs.

Regarding Figure 9.19:

1. If the two drugs have the same pharmacological mechanism in the body, they will produce parallel curves. Therefore, A and B are likely to have the same mechanism, while P and Q do not.
2. Potency can be measured only for drugs binding to the same receptor and producing the same physiological activity. Therefore, the potencies of A and B can be compared. On a graph, affinity is indicated by the position of the LDR on the X axis. The closer to the Y axis, the greater is the potency (i.e., a lower dose is needed for a given response). Therefore, A has a greater potency than does B. Because P and Q have different slopes, they have different mechanisms of action, and therefore their potencies cannot be compared.
3. Efficacy is measured by the maximum response of the LDR. One looks at the size of response and not how it is produced. Therefore, in the graphs in the figure, A and B have the same efficacy, and P has greater efficacy than Q.

9.12.1 POTENCY

Potency is the measure of the amount of drug necessary for a given response. The less drug needed to elicit a response, the more potent the drug. It is important not to equate greater potency with therapeutic superiority since other factors like side effects have to be considered.

Potency of a drug can be dependent on the affinity (1/Kd) of receptors for binding the drug and also on the efficiency with which the drug–receptor interaction responds. Potency refers to the concentration or dose of a drug required to produce 50 percent of that drug's maximal effect (ED50).

9.12.2 Agonism and Antagonism

An agonist is a drug that, when combined with a receptor, leads to a physiologic response, essentially causing a specific action. An antagonist is a drug that, when combined with a receptor, blocks the agonist's (drug or natural agonist) action and leads to no physiologic response.

Pharmacologic antagonists bind to receptors but do not activate the generation of a signal; they interfere with the agonist's capacity to activate the receptor. The effect of a so-called "pure" antagonist depends on its ability to prevent the binding of agonist molecules and subsequent blockade of their biologic actions. Some of the most useful drugs in clinical medicine are pharmacological antagonists.

9.12.2.1 Partial Agonists

Most drugs fall in the range between a full agonist and an antagonist. Those drugs are known as partial agonists, and they exhibit affinity and only moderate efficacy.

Partial agonists exhibit dose-response curves that are similar to those of full agonists, but their maximal response is less.

Many drugs used clinically as antagonists are actually weak partial agonists. For example, buprenorphine, a partial agonist of the mu-opioid receptors, is a generally safer analgesic drug than morphine because it produces less respiratory depression in overdose.

9.12.2.1.1 Duality of Partial Agonists

Regarding Figure 9.20:

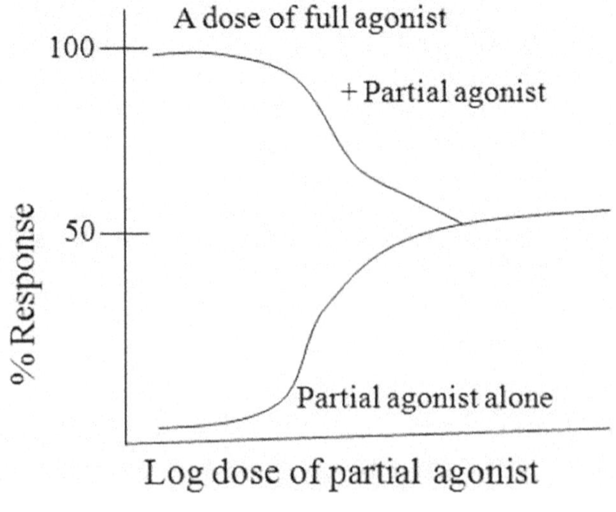

FIGURE 9.20 Partial Agonism.

1. The bottom curve is generated by a partial agonist being added to a tissue. The response maxes out at the maximum response for the partial agonist. The net is a gain in activity or agonism.
2. The upper curve is generated by pretreating the tissue with a full agonist and obtaining the maximum possible response. The full agonist is discontinued and replaced with a partial agonist. As the full agonist is displaced from the receptors by the partial agonist, the response declines. Eventually, all of the full agonist will be displaced, and the response will be completely due to the partial agonist. The net is a loss of activity or antagonism.
3. The partial agonist is the only class of drug that can be used either to stimulate a pharmacological action or block it.

9.13 COMPETITIVE ANTAGONISM

An antagonist alone produces no response. An agonist alone produces its normal LDR curve. The addition of antagonist to tissue before the addition of agonist will result in some receptors being occupied by antagonist. Therefore, more agonist is necessary to displace the antagonist from those receptors. Eventually, given high enough doses of agonist, all of the antagonist will be displaced, and the maximum response will be elicited (curves parallel and of same height).

Changes in agonist concentration–effect (dose–response) curves are produced by a competitive antagonist or by an irreversible antagonist. In the presence of a competitive antagonist, higher concentrations of agonist are required to produce a given effect. Thus, the agonist concentration required for a given effect is shifted to the right, as shown in Figure 9.21 (A and B). High agonist concentrations can overcome inhibition by a competitive antagonist. This is not the case with an irreversible (or noncompetitive) antagonist, which reduces the maximal effect the agonist can achieve, although it may not change its EC50.

9.14 NONCOMPETITIVE ANTAGONISM

Noncompetitive antagonism occurs when the antagonist cannot be displaced from the receptor, and consequently the number of possible receptors available to the agonist decreases. This means that the agonist can never obtain full effect. The resulting curve has a lower slope and height (nonparallel and unequal heights) (see Figure 9.22).

There are three different types of antagonism:

1. Pharmacological antagonism (one receptor)—both the agonist and antagonist compete for the same receptor.
2. Physiological antagonism (two receptors)—two agonists bind to two different receptors. Each

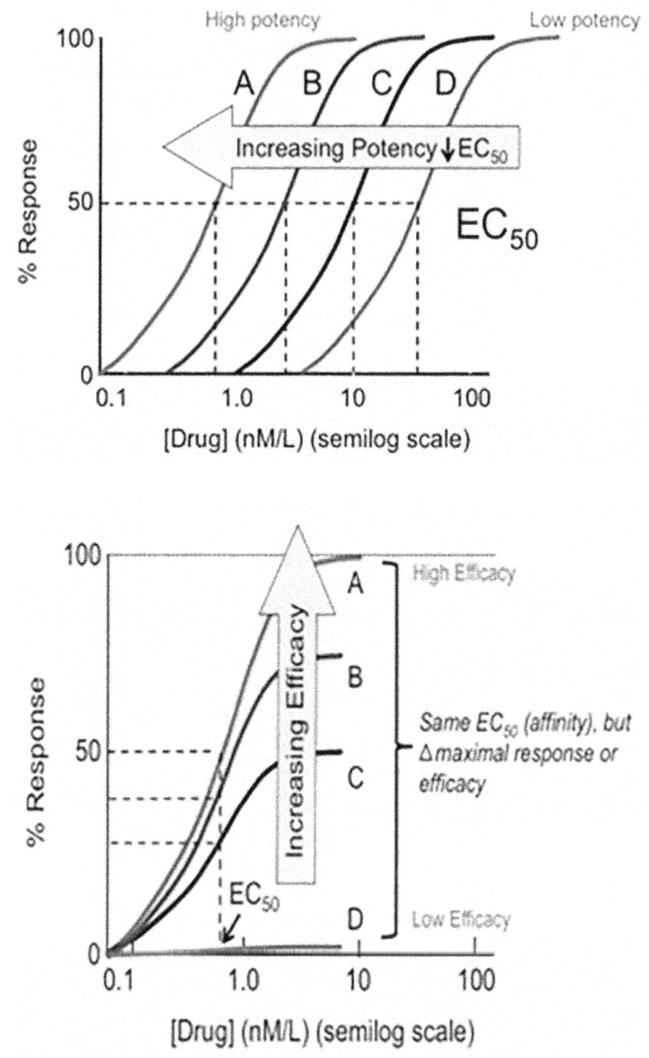

FIGURE 9.21(A AND B) ANTAGONIST INHIBITION.

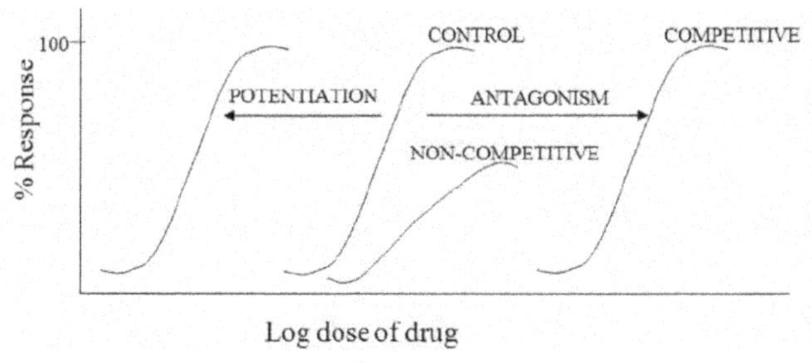

FIGURE 9.22 Effects of Antagonism and Potentiation.

agonist elicits a physiological response. Those responses tend to oppose each other. Although the actions of glucocorticoids and insulin engage distinct receptor–effector systems, insulin is sometimes administered to oppose the hyperglycemic effects of a glucocorticoid hormone.

3. Chemical antagonism (zero receptors)—the antagonist directly interacts with the agonist, for example, antacids neutralizing HCl or chelating agents (e.g., protamine, a positively charged protein that neutralizes negatively charged heparin, thus making the heparin unavailable for interactions with proteins involved in blood clotting).

Classical theories have to be modified to explain things like:

a. Partial agonists
b. Tachyphylaxis—a sudden unresponsiveness to a drug; a phenomenon in which the repeated administration of some drugs results in a rapid and marked decrease in effectiveness.
c. Signaling mechanisms (see Figure 9.23) and drug action:
   1. A lipid-soluble drug crosses the plasma membrane and acts on an intracellular (inside the cell) receptor *R* (which may be an enzyme or a regulator of gene transcription) such as for steroids, Vitamin D, and thyroid hormone.
   2. The drug ligand binds to the extracellular (outside of the cell) domain of a transmembrane receptor, thereby activating an enzymatic activity (AB) of its cytoplasmic domain.
   3. The ligand binds to the extracellular domain of a transmembrane receptor bound to a protein kinase enzyme (*Y*), which it activates.
   4. The ligand binds to and directly regulates the opening of an ion channel such as sodium, calcium, and potassium channels. Many drugs act by mimicking or blocking the actions of endogenous ligands that regulate ion flow through plasma membrane channels. Natural ligands include acetylcholine, serotonin, GABA, and glutamate which are all synaptic transmitters.
   5. The ligand binds to a cell-surface receptor linked to an effector enzyme (E) by a G protein,

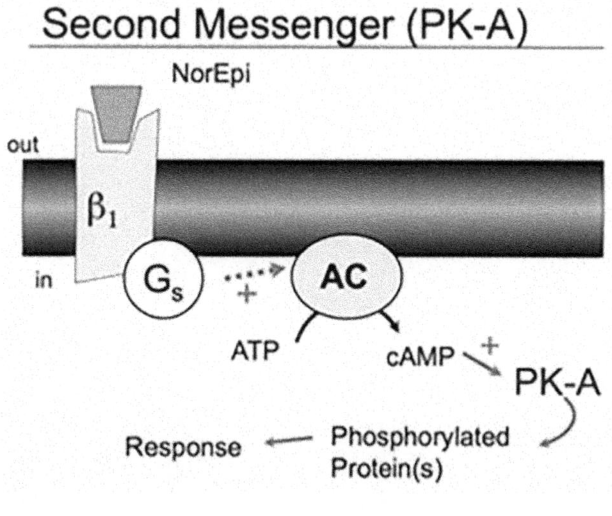

FIGURE 9.23 Signaling Mechanism.

a signal relay protein that is attached to the receptor and acts during receptor activation.

9.15 SUMMARY AND CONCLUSIONS

These general principles (absorption, distribution, metabolism, excretion [ADME], kinetics, and drug receptor site activity) serve as a foundation for all learning and understanding in pharmacology. Separate and apart from the specific action of a particular drug, if there are interferences in ADME, then the drug may have no effect or be toxic. Several examples of alterations or interferences in the ADME are presented throughout the book. A good understanding of these principles will assist the reader in appreciating the example.

Part II

High-Risk Drug Therapies Resulting in Injury and Litigation

10 Allergic Drug Reactions

James T. O'Donnell and James J. O'Donnell III

SYNOPSIS

DOI: 10.1201/9781003615323-12

10.1 ADVERSE DRUG REACTIONS: HOW LARGE IS THE PROBLEM? WHAT DRUGS ARE INVOLVED? WHAT ARE THE INJURIES?

Although there is no doubt that therapeutic agents such as vaccines and antibiotics have changed the course of modern medicine and prolonged the average lifespan of the population, we must still assume that all drugs can potentially be harmful. Pharmacovigilance is a relatively new term that describes efforts to monitor human drug experience. In the United States, the Food and Drug Administration's (FDA) MedWatch system maintains a database of voluntary reports of post-marketing (i.e., after the manufacturer's data has been reported and published in the drug's package insert) adverse drug reactions (ADRS). Pharmacoepidemiology is "the application of epidemiologic knowledge, methods and reasoning to the study of the effects (beneficial and adverse) and uses of drugs in human populations."[1] This task involves the identification, analysis, research, and interventions intended to decrease the incidence and severity of drug-induced injuries. Appendix 10.1 (Terminology Concerning Drug Misadventures) provides the definitions of terms which will be helpful to the reader.

10.1.1 Historical Perspective

The reported incidence and frequency of ADRs vary, depending on the source of the report and on the methods used to describe the event. One reason for these discrepancies is that it is sometimes difficult to determine the causality of the ADR with absolute certainty. Hospital-admission reports have ranged from between less than 1 percent and up to 28 percent. However, most studies report an incidence of between 10 and 20 percent. This disparity reflects differences in the methods used to detect and report ADRs.

The first ADRs probably occurred when humans began to experiment with plants as medications and learned how to brew alcohol and to smoke tobacco. However, the history of ADRs remained relatively sparse until this century. ADRs slowly grew in frequency until the end of the Second World War. Since that time, there has been an explosion of new drugs and a corresponding increase in ADRs.

The increasing prevalence of acute and chronic illnesses attributed to allergies[2,3] and asthma has precipitated[4,5] the widespread use of all kinds of drugs[6]—including drugs that are prescribed, over-the-counter (OTC), or (not infrequently) shared with others similarly afflicted. The cost may indeed represent a socioeconomic "injury." At this point, neither the pharmaceutical industry nor the healthcare practitioners can adequately monitor, control, or prevent possible adverse reactions[7] from the use, misuse, or, at times, the failure to use necessary medications for the respiratory, dermatological, or other systemic manifestations attributable to allergy.[8,9] Nevertheless, the recognition of possible or actual adverse reactions to medication—some common and predictable and others extraordinary and unexpected—continues to be the duty of the providers, as well as of the consumers of pharmaceutical healthcare.[10] Errors, regrettably, are not uncommon. In fact, a recent survey of 36 healthcare facilities detected a 19 percent incidence of incorrect therapy (due to wrong dose in 3 percent of the cases and timing in 8 percent).[11]

10.1.2 Incidence of Adverse Drug Reactions

The human lifespan has increased tremendously over the last several hundred years. Most attribute this life extension to the development of life-saving medications and medical devices, in addition to industrialization. There are currently 4,750 drugs available on the US market in a total of 17,992 drug products.[12] With so many drugs, it is no surprise that the medication-error rate is high in this country, estimated at nearly one in five doses at the typical hospital and skilled nursing facility (different studies report different rates). The percentage of errors rated potentially harmful is 7 percent—more than 40 per day per 300 in-patients, on the average, according to one study. Drug allergies and introductions are an important subset of these errors, representing 5 to 10 percent of all drug injuries that occur, estimates show.

In a review article, the incidence rate of drug-related hospital admissions was reported to vary from 0.2 to 21.7

percent, with the median rate of drug-related hospitalizations at 4.9 percent.[13] The author defined drug-related hospitalizations as adverse events that could cause a side effect,[14] excessive effect, idiosyncratic effect, or hypersensitivity. In another review, the rate of drug-related hospital admissions ranged from 0.3 to 16.8 percent of all hospital admissions, with a median value of 5.6 percent.[15]

A *New England Journal of Medicine* article reviews the topic of emergency hospitalizations for adverse drug events in older Americans.[16] The authors analyzed adverse event data from the National Electronic Injury Surveillance System—Cooperative Adverse Drug Event Surveillance project (2007 through 2009) to estimate the frequency and rates of hospitalization after emergency department visits for ADRs in older adults. The review included nearly 100,000 emergency hospitalizations, half of which were in-patients over 80 years of age. Two-thirds were due to unintentional overdoses. Four medications or medication classes were implicated alone or in combination: Warfarin (33.3 percent), insulins (13.9 percent), oral antiplatelet agents (13.3 percent), and oral hypoglycemic agents (10.7 percent). Frequently, warfarin and anti-platelet medications were combined. Other medications classes reported include opiates (4.8 percent), antibiotics (4.2 percent), digoxin (3.5 percent), renin angiotensin inhibitors (2.9 percent), and sedative hypnotics (2.5 percent). The authors recommend that the improved management of antithrombotic and antidiabetic drugs has the potential to reduce hospitalizations for adverse drug events in older adults. The reader will find extensive discussions of anticoagulant toxicity in *Anticoagulants*, diabetic drug toxicity in *Adverse Effects of Diabetic Drugs,* and of opiate toxicity in *Dangers of Opioids* chapters elsewhere in this book.

Following a 1999 report by the Institute on Medication Safety entitled "To Err is Human," drug-injury prevention has become a major focus of healthcare organizations nationally.[17] This has resulted in many innovative ideas, including the use of bar coding—both at the bedside, as well as on the medication labeling (and sometimes on the administrator of the drug itself), as well as drug-counting/weighing machines and complicated software products. Drug-injury prevention has become a multi-million dollar industry.

A drug-induced disease is an unintended effect of a drug that may result in mortality or morbidity with symptoms sufficient to prompt a patient to seek medical attention and/or require hospitalization. Fortunately, many drug-induced diseases are preventable.

Every healthcare student learns the "Five Basic Rights of Medication Administration" (Table 10.1). These "rights" represent the "right" way to administer medication without errors.

Furthermore, healthcare practitioners should also know the "Four Additional Rights of Medication Administration": (1) Right Documentation, (2) Right Reason, (3) Right to Know (Patient Education), and (4) Right to Refuse.

TABLE 10.1
The Five Basic Rights of Medication Administration.

Right Patient
Right Medication
Right Dosage
Right Time (Frequency)
Right Route of Administration

Unfortunately, this simple system cannot catch every error. In fact, although covered under "right medication," the system offers no way to determine whether that "right medication" might produce a drug allergy in any particular patient at any particular time. Likewise, without being able to predict allergic reactions, it is almost impossible to predict cross-reactions (reactions with similar drugs in the same class).

Hopefully, with today's pharmacy software and checks and balances, the number of interactions will continue to decrease. Pharmacy software flags such interactions, helping medical personnel prevent them before they occur. According to the American Heart Association, total estimated morbidity and mortality cost for drug-related diseases was $76.6 billion in 1995.[18] A follow-up study in 2001, using the same cost-of-illness model, reported annual drug-related morbidity and mortality cost (in 2000 dollars) of $177.4 billion.[19] In comparison, the cost of cardiovascular diseases and stroke was estimated to be $393.5 billion in 2005, and the cost for all cancers in 2004 was about $190 billion.[20]

Due to the limited sample size, clinical trials usually uncover only the more frequent ADRs. For example, a trial with a sample size of 10,000 patients (no adverse reactions) will only yield a 95 percent confidence interval that an ADR with a frequency of 1 in 10,000 will occur. In order to increase the confidence interval for detecting an ADR of the same frequency (1 in 10,000) to 99 percent, a sample size of 46,000 is needed.[21] These numbers lie in stark contrast to a 2005 FDA standard which recommends that the clinical trial of a drug used to treat a non-life-threatening condition expose 1,500 subjects to the investigational product (with 300 to 600 exposed for 6 months and 100 exposed for 1 year).[22]

Delays in sounding an alert are a function of the need for verification and the initiation of any regulatory action. Alerting others usually occurs through published anecdotal reports. Voluntary reporting and other early-warning systems have made a negligible contribution to alerting. The MedWatch system is valuable for generating and forming hypotheses for epidemiological studies. Routine monitoring for drug safety should include patients in various subsets (the elderly, children, and patients with specific disease states, such as kidney or liver disease), where there may be a particular liability to ADRs. The elderly is the group taking the largest amount of drugs and suffering the greatest number of ADRs. Life expectancy—the probability of living a longer life—has increased from around 50 years at the dawn of the twentieth century to an anticipated 75 years at the turn of the twenty-first century. With the greater life expectancy, both the total number of elderly, as well as the number of elderly as a percentage of the population, increases. In actual numbers, this means that the number of people of 75 years of age and over will rise from about 10 million (or 4.4 percent of the population) in 1980 to close to 30 million (9.1 percent of the population) in 2050. For the population over 85 years of age, these values will change from about 3 million in 1980 (1 percent) to about 18 million (5.2 percent) in 2050. This latter group, then, represents the most rapidly growing segment of the population. With the growth in the elderly population, the number of ADRs occurring per year would be expected to grow in the future as well. Remarkably, even though there were more than 650,000 reports submitted to the FDA in 2010, only a small minority of suspected ADRs are reported to the FDA.

10.1.3 Food and Drug Administration Reporting Requirements

Currently, the United States has a voluntary, spontaneous reporting system called MedWatch. Healthcare professionals and drug companies report ADRs to the FDA with the MedWatch Drug Experience Report Form (see Chapter 5, *Important Code of Federal Regulations Applicable to Drug Product Liability Suits*). Since 1962, drug manufacturers have been required to report all ADRs brought to their attention. The drug companies file the majority of the 200,000-plus ADRs reported annually.

The FDA is interested in receiving reports of serious new reactions associated with the use of drugs and biologic products used in the course of medical practice. In addition, there is interest in reactions to new drugs during their first three years of marketing in the United States. The FDA does not collect reports of inappropriate use, prescriber errors, or administration errors. "Serious" reports are generally considered to be those that are life-threatening or those that result in death, hospitalization or prolonged hospitalization, or permanent or severe disability. The determination of seriousness is up to the discretion of the reporter. If there is any doubt, the report should be considered serious and should be submitted to the FDA—a causality assessment is not required.

The ICH (International Conference on Harmonization) Technical Requirements for Registration of Pharmaceuticals for Human Use brings together as equal partners the regulatory authorities of Europe, Japan, and the United States with experts from the pharmaceutical industry in these regions to discuss scientific and technical aspects of product registration. The United States' spontaneous reporting system has many good features. The input is global—covering the entire population of patients treated with drugs. Thus, it includes all drugs and all physicians in "real-life" situations of drug use, unlike the controlled settings of clinical drug trials. It is inexpensive, requires a minimum amount of time, and does not interfere with the practice of the physician. Unfortunately, the overall effectiveness of the Drug Experience Report system has been found to be wanting.[23],[24] Leading a list of its limitations is underreporting—few physicians ever fill out reports. It has been conservatively estimated that 95 percent of ADRs go unreported.[25] Some of the reasons that doctors may neglect to report ADRs are listed in the next section.

The FDA has been under fire from at least two different sides. First, the industry (as well as certain patient groups) argues that the agency takes far too long to approve new drugs. Second, public-interest groups argue that the agency is not thorough enough in its reviews of new drugs. Before drugs can be sold in the United States, the manufacturers must apply to the FDA for the right to test them in humans, submit their test results to the agency, and then apply for the right to sell the drugs. Experts agree that the clinical trials completed before approval cannot detect all side effects that may be caused by the drugs. Because the testing is done in groups of people ranging from a few hundred to a few thousand, it is unlikely that clinical testing will uncover side effects that occur in, say, 1 person in 10,000.

10.1.4 The "Seven Deadly Sins": Why Doctors Fail to Report Adverse Drug Reactions

The following are the main failures of MedWatch, the FDA's voluntary reporting system[26]:

1. **Complacency**—the result of a mistaken belief that only safe drugs are allowed in the market.
2. **Fear of involvement** in litigation or of an investigation of prescribing habits.
3. **Guilty feelings** about the damage physicians may have caused their patients.
4. **Ambition** to collect and publish a personal series of cases.
5. **Ignorance** about what should be reported, the reporting process, and the value of the reporting.
6. **Difference** in reporting mere suspicions.
7. **Indifference** to the responsibility that an individual doctor has to contribute to the general body of knowledge about the effects of drug treatment.

Most drugs are sold to hundreds of thousands (sometimes millions) of people, so rare side effects are often seen only after the drug reaches the market. These side effects are then reported to the FDA by the drug's manufacturers and—to a lesser extent—by healthcare professionals. A General Accounting Office (GAO) study counted as "serious" all those "adverse reactions that could lead to hospitalization, increases in the length of hospitalization, severe or permanent disability, or death."[27] These reactions, whether they are seen in a small or large number of patients, have caused the FDA to withdraw drugs from the market or to add warnings to their labels so that doctors might avoid their use or be more careful in deciding who should use them.

A GAO report suggests that some lives could be saved if the FDA monitored after-market hazards more closely and communicated them more quickly to doctors and the public. Critics of the agency say it can take up to five years from the time a serious side effect is observed to the time that doctors and the public are told. Among the reactions noted by the GAO were a great variety of ailments, including heart failure, shock, respiratory arrest, convulsions, kidney and liver failure, birth defects, and blindness. Some cases have become quite well known, like the birth defects that can be caused by the anti-acne drug Accutane.

The GAO study found that certain classes of drugs, including heart, anti-inflammatory, psychopharmacologic, fertility, dermatologic, and antibiotic drugs, had a much higher percentage of post-approval risks and adverse reactions than other categories of medications.

10.1.5 Attitudes toward Adverse Drug Reactions

Fitzgerald, while researching crisis management and ADRs, said:

> The initial response of those working within an organization, particularly product champions, both technical and commercial, is that of denial. Until this moment, the whole culture within the pharmaceutical company has been positively and energetically to promote the advantage of the drug. Thus, before accepting that the drug is associated with a potentially serious disadvantage, drug champions tend to demand, firstly, proof of causality; secondly, to seek out alternative explanations for the clinical syndrome; and thirdly, to try to implicate other agents in the same drug class, in order to diminish the impact on the specific product.[28]

Replies published by companies concerning published ADRs are not too dissimilar to this pattern, giving a very one-sided viewpoint and certainly not giving the reader a balanced opinion of the problem. These letters usually contain some of the following:

- No admission of a causal relationship.
- No acknowledgment of the validity of any of the comments in the original publication.
- A list of all possible alternatives, however tenuous.
- No mention of the number of cases that the company has received.
- References, some of which seem to have little to do with the original problem.
- Implications that it is a class effect.
- Remarks from a clinician who has been involved with the company as a trialist or adviser, without any acknowledgment of an association with the pharmaceutical company.

In an editorial in *Risk and Safety in Medicine*, Dr. M.N.G. Dukes said there are still "serious instances where risk data have been concealed in the interests of commerce."[29]

10.1.6 Investigator Fraud

Another problem in detecting and reporting ADRs has been the discovery of numerous instances of proven investigator fraud. In the field of ADRs, the investigator's attitude can vary from bewildered ignorance to deliberate dishonesty:

- Some fail to document and report what they should clearly recognize as an ADR.
- Some are so "invested" in the study drug, believing so strongly in its safety, that their enthusiasm overshadows sound scientific and regulatory standards.
- Some choose not to report ADRs—either because it requires too much effort or because they are deliberately attempting to defraud.
- Some are confused over what constitutes an ADR.
- Many ADR reports lack essential information.
- Most are weak in causality assessment (did the drug actually cause the ADR?).

10.2 CLASSIFICATION OF ADVERSE DRUG REACTIONS

In essence, an ADR is any unintended and undesirable response obtained from the appropriate dose of a drug or diagnostic agent. Adverse drug reactions have been conventionally classified as: (1) Overdosage, (2) intolerance, (3) unexpected side effects, (4) secondary effects, (5) idiosyncrasy, and (6) hypersensitivity reactions.

Drug interactions have been categorized into those occurring (1) outside the body, (2) at the site of entry, (3) at storage sites within the body, (4) at the site of action, (5) by the inhibition of metabolizing enzymes, (6) by stimulation of enzymes, and (7) by impacting drug excretion. Drug interactions are also included with other ADRs. Although these classifications have been used both in reviews and textbooks, it is unnecessary and confusing to separate ADRs from drug interactions.

The term "drug–drug interactions" refers to interactions between prescription or nonprescription drugs. The broader term "drug interaction" is often substituted. Many drug interactions cause undesirable effects and account for a significant number of adverse events. They can also limit bioavailability or block desired effects (see Table 10.2).

All serious or unexpected ADRs must be promptly reported. This applies to reports from spontaneous sources and from any type of clinical or epidemiological investigation—independent of design or purpose. It also applies to cases not reported directly to a sponsor or manufacturer (e.g., those found in regulatory authority-generated ADR registries or in publications). The source of a report (investigation, spontaneous, other) should always be identified.

Expedited reporting of reactions that are serious, but expected, will ordinarily be inappropriate. Expedited reporting is also inappropriate for serious events from clinical investigations that are considered unrelated to the study product, regardless of whether the event is expected or not.

There are situations, in addition to single case reports of "serious" adverse events or reactions, that may necessitate rapid communication to regulatory authorities. Appropriate medical and scientific judgment should be applied for each situation. In general, this includes information that might materially influence the risk–benefit assessment of a medicinal product, or that would be sufficient to consider changes in medicinal product administration or overall conduct of a clinical investigation. The following are some examples:

- A clinically important increase in the rate of occurrence for an "expected" serious ADR
- A significant hazard to the patient population—such as lack of efficacy with a medicinal product used in treating life-threatening diseases
- A major safety finding from a newly completed animal study (such as a study on carcinogenicity)

10.2.1 Categories of Adverse Drug Reactions

Traditionally, ADRs have been divided into two types. Type A reactions are dose-related and arise from the normal pharmacological action of a drug. Type B reactions represent an abnormal or novel response to a drug. Adverse drug reactions may broadly be stratified into types A and B. Type A reactions encompass the majority of reactions and can affect anyone. These reactions predictably occur from the known pharmacology of a drug. Type B are less common; however, occurrence in susceptible patients cannot be predicted. Allergic or immunological drug reactions are a group of Type B ADRs. Based on the time of onset, allergic drug reactions can be categorized into immediate and delayed. Based on their underlaying immunological mechanism, they can be further subdivided into four groups: Immediate and mediated by IgE, delayed and caused by anti-body facilitative cell destruction, delayed and caused by immune complex deposition and complement activation, and delayed and T-cell mediated.[30],[31]

10.2.1.1 Type A Reactions: Augmentation of the Pharmacological Response

These reactions are usually the result of an exaggerated, but otherwise normal, pharmacological action of a drug given in the usual therapeutic doses. An example of this type of reaction would be the postural and exercise hypotension (low blood pressure) in a patient taking an adrenergic neuronal blocking agent such as guanethidine (used to treat severe high blood pressure) or drowsiness in those taking phenobarbital (a barbiturate central nervous system depressant used as a sedative hypnotic and also commonly as an anticonvulsant). Type A reactions are largely predictable on the basis of the known pharmacological properties of a drug. They are frequently dose-dependent. Although the incidence of morbidity (side effects) in the population is often high, the mortality rate is usually low.

10.2.1.2 Type B Reactions: Bizarre (Idiosyncratic)

These reactions are unusual effects that would not be expected from known pharmacological actions of a drug when it is given in the accepted therapeutic doses to such a patient whose body handles that drug in a normal manner.[32] Example of this type of reaction includes malignant hyperthermia caused by anesthesia. Many of the immunological (allergic-hypersensitivity) reactions would fall into this category, although these would constitute medication errors if the allergy is known. Anaphylaxis—a classic Type B hypersensitivity reaction—is one of the most serious, potentially life-threatening ADRs.[33] This IgE-mediated reaction generally occurs within 20 minutes of exposure to an antigen. It is most common after an injection, but it can occur with any route of administration. The symptoms of anaphylaxis are produced by a variety of chemical mediators, most notably histamine.[34] While the incidence of anaphylaxis is low, the mortality rate from these reactions is high. These reactions are usually unpredictable and are not observed during conventional toxicological screening programs. Table 10.2 provides a list of immunopathologies of allergic drug reactions.

10.3 TYPES OF DRUG ALLERGY AND HYPERSENSITIVITY

In the United States, patients fill more than 300 million drug prescriptions and purchase millions of over-the-counter medications each month.[35] In many cases, patients are using these medications for the first time. Cutaneous reactions represent one of the most common adverse reactions with drugs. These reactions are associated with penicillins, cephalosporins, sulfonamide antimicrobial agents, allopurinol, and particularly the aromatic amine antiseizure medications, including carbamazepine, phenytoin,

TABLE 10.2
Immunopathology of Allergic Reactions to Drugs.

Type I	Anaphylaxis, urticaria, angioedema, asthma, rhinitis.
Type II	Immune cytopenias. Some organ inflammation.
Type III	Serum sickness, vasculitis.
Type IV	Contact dermatitis. Some exanthems.

Source: Adapted from Kay, A. Concepts of allergy and hypersensitivity. In: Kay, A. Allergy and allergic diseases. Oxford, UK: Blackwell Science, 1997:23.

and lamotrigine. Drug-related rash is reported for nearly all prescription medications, usually at rates exceeding 10 cases per 1,000 new users. These reactions can range from asymptomatic mild eruptions to life-threatening conditions. Cutaneous reactions may be difficult to distinguish from common rashes that are unrelated to medication use, particularly viral exanthems.[36]

Although allergic reactions to antibiotics account for only a small proportion of reported adverse drug reactions, they are associated with substantial morbidity and mortality and increased healthcare costs.[37] Estimates of the prevalence of antibiotic allergy vary widely. Any organ may be affected, but the skin is most common. Data from the Boston Collaborative Drug Surveillance Program indicate a 2.2 percent frequency of cutaneous drug reactions among hospitalized patients, with the antibiotics amoxicillin, trimethoprim–sulfamethoxazole, and ampicillin the most commonly implicated agents. More recently, a six-month prospective analysis in France showed a prevalence of cutaneous drug eruptions of 3.6 per 1,000 hospitalized patients; antibiotics accounted for 55 percent of cases.[38]

10.3.1 The Nature of Drug Allergy

Drug allergies are the body's overreaction to a foreign substance, be it dust, pollen, or a medication. Histamine is released in response to what the body perceives as a threat, and the results can be deadly. Of course, the immune system is designed to protect the body from dangerous invaders, which are usually viruses and bacteria, but they can also be medications on occasion.[39]

Unfortunately, there is no way to predict with 100 percent accuracy who will develop an allergic reaction to a medication. Allergies may develop at any time, even when an agent has been taken in the past. Indeed, multiple exposures actually raise the odds of developing an allergy to a particular substance. Additionally, some allergies do not develop for days or weeks after ingestion of or injection with a medication, which can make the reaction difficult to trace to the substance. Causation assessment can be challenging due to all these variables. Although some other ADRs are dependent upon the amount of the drug administered, this is not the case with a drug allergy. Even a tiny amount of the medication can trigger a life-threatening anaphylactic episode.

Some types of drugs induce allergic reactions more readily than others and result in a spectrum of symptoms that may affect a range of tissues and organs. Medications with larger drug molecules seem to be more likely to cause reactions than those with smaller drug molecules.

Some examples of medications comprising larger drug molecules include:

- Insulin
- Antiserum-containing antibodies
- Recombinant proteins produced by genetic engineering

Many other allergens have molecules too small to set off alarm bells for the immune system. For example, antibiotic molecules cannot induce an immune response themselves—they must combine with a body cell or a carrier protein in the blood. Drug allergies often result from breakdown by-products or metabolites of the drug instead of the drug itself. Sometimes, the same drug (e.g., penicillin) can induce multiple types of allergic reactions. The most common drug sensitivity is to aspirin (ASA). Nearly one million Americans, primarily adults, are sensitive to ASA. However, many medications, including ASA and other nonsteroidal anti-inflammatory drugs (NSAIDs) such as ibuprofen (Advil, Motrin, and others), can trigger an asthma attack in children. It is estimated that up to ten percent of all people develop allergies to penicillin or other antibiotics at some point in their lives. Multi-medication use or frequent courses of antibiotics is associated with a higher risk for developing drug allergies.

Children represent a large segment of the population that is affected by drug allergy. Many times, these allergies manifest as asthma—a common chronic respiratory condition that affects children. An asthma attack can occur when the air passages from the lungs to the nose and mouth are restricted causing difficulty breathing. ASA and ASA-like medications are common triggers for asthma attacks and affect up to 30 percent of asthmatic children.[40]

Children also frequently develop allergies to the following agents:[41]

- Barbiturates
- ASA
- Anticonvulsants
- Sulfa-based drugs
- Dyes that are injected into blood vessels before taking X-rays
- Insulin preparations

Insect stings and the intravenous injection of specific drugs are the most common causes of anaphylaxis—the most severe form of an allergic response. Anaphylactic reactions are often marked by respiratory distress (swelling of the throat, preventing breathing) and death. Skin conditions, including a measles-like rash, hives, and photosensitivity, are the most common drug reactions.

Uncommon—but more serious—symptoms of a drug allergy include the following:[42]

- Fever
- Muscle and joint aches
- Lymph node swelling
- Inflammation of the kidney
- Difficulty breathing and wheezing
- Low blood pressure and fainting
- Rapid or irregular heartbeat
- Swelling of face, tongue, lips, throat, joints, hands, or feet

10.3.2 Dangerous Drug-Allergy Reactions

- Angioedema usually occurs within a few minutes of exposure to a drug, often in conjunction with urticaria. Angioedema often is asymmetrical: For example, only one side of the lip may be affected. This allergic symptom may become life-threatening if the swelling affects the larynx and the air passages become blocked. Emergency symptoms of a drug allergy include the obstruction of the throat from swelling, severe asthma attack, and/or anaphylaxis. Angioedema is the most well-known and serious of the drug-induced throat disorders. Ototoxicity is manifested by hearing loss, tinnitus (continued ringing in the ear), and vertigo. Hyposmia is a diminished ability to detect or recognize a smell, while anosmia is the absolute absence of the sense of smell. All of these may be symptoms of angioedema.
- Anaphylaxis involves a response from the entire body. Although it is rare, hundreds of Americans die each year from anaphylaxis. These deaths are most common in children who are allergic to penicillin and similar antibiotics—drugs that cause 97 percent of all deaths from drug allergies. Anaphylaxis, by definition, requires a prior exposure to the drug acting as the allergen.
- Allergic reactions to drugs are the most common cause of tubulo-interstitial nephritis, which can occur between five days and five weeks after exposure to penicillin, sulfonamides, diuretics, ASA, and other NSAIDs.

10.3.3 Drug Sensitivities Mimic Allergy Symptoms

Sometimes, an allergy is not an allergy—it is actually just a hypersensitivity reaction. However, these types of reactions, especially pulmonary hypersensitivity, can still be dangerous and often mimic the symptoms of an actual drug allergy (such as rashes, urticaria, and angioedema). Anaphylactoid drug reactions present similarly to anaphylactic reactions. In this case, they are caused by drug sensitivity (rather than a drug allergy) and commonly occur after the first drug exposure. Anaphylactoid reactions are associated with the following:

- Opiates
- Radiopaque dyes (radiocontrast media) used in X-ray procedures; 2 to 3 percent of patients have immediate generalized reactions to these dyes
- ASA and other NSAIDs in some people, usually adults
- Pentamidine

Drug-induced diseases have a considerable impact on the American society. They cost billions of dollars annually, cause considerable morbidity, and are often fatal. Some adverse drug effects are not clinically significant; however, many people would contend that any condition that results in hospitalization is significant.

With so many types and manifestations of drug allergies, they can be difficult to detect, and, if missed, the reaction can worsen. The most important factor is awareness. With vigilance (being aware of patient's allergies and cross-allergies), most drug reactions can be caught early or prevented altogether.

10.3.4 Definitions of Allergic/Hypersensitivity Reactions

The definition of an ADR is any response to a medication that was not desired or intended by its prescriber. These reactions occur at doses that would normally—according to package instructions—bestow a positive benefit on the patient, be it therapeutic, diagnostic, or prophylactic. Allergic drug reactions comprise less than 10 percent of ADRs, but they have a substantial negative impact on clinical outcomes and cost of care.[43] These reactions also usually occur within a proximate time of administration of the medication. Studies show that allergic drug reactions account for only 6 to 10 percent of all observed ADRs. Yet, as many as 15 percent of adults believe themselves to be allergic to one or more drugs. The danger? A lifesaving medication may be withheld because of a faulty belief. Although many patients with a history of reacting to a drug could safely receive that drug again, the outcome could be serious if that patient is truly allergic. Hence, a suspicion of drug hypersensitivity must be evaluated carefully. For example, some ADRs that are perceived to be allergy related (but are not) may influence the future use of a particular medication, when, in fact, a drug-induced side effect may be corrected simply by reducing its dose. However, it is important to keep in mind that if the reaction was indeed an allergy, the drug cannot be used or may require other special considerations.[44]

There are two major categories of ADRs used to define and distinguish between the different types. The first is predictable adverse reactions, which are often dose-dependent, appear in otherwise normal patients, and are common enough to fall into this category. The other type is unpredictable reactions, which are usually dose-independent, unrelated to the drug's pharmacological properties, or related to a patient's immunological responsiveness or susceptibility due to genetics. Something else to watch out for are reactions that are unrelated to the drug administered but can be caused by the administration (either events that occur or through the route of administration). For example, sometimes, the parenteral administration of a drug can cause psycho-physiologic reactions (hysteria, vasovagal, hyperventilation, etc.). Some of these reactions may be attributable to the placebo effect (even anaphylactoid symptoms have been observed in placebo-treated patients). And, of course, ADRs may be mistaken for other, coincidental health conditions.

10.3.5 Idiosyncratic Reactions

Idiosyncratic reactions are qualitatively abnormal, unexpected responses to a drug, which are uncharacteristic of its pharmacologic actions and that resemble hypersensitivity. These ADRs do not involve allergy. In contrast, allergic drug reactions are unpredictable and quantitatively abnormal, and they are unrelated to the pharmacologic action of the drug. They involve immune responses to a drug following previous exposure to the same drug or to an immunochemically related substance that had resulted in the formation of specific antibodies, of sensitized T lymphocytes, or of both.[45]

10.3.6 Intolerance

Another type of ADR is intolerance, a characteristic pharmacologic effect of a drug that is quantitatively increased and/or produced by an unusually small dose of a medication. Although similar to intolerance, idiosyncratic and allergic reactions are qualitatively aberrant and often inexplicable in terms of the normal pharmacology of the drug given in usual therapeutic doses.[46]

10.3.7 Toxicity

One type of predictable ADR is related directly to dosage. These ADRs can be expected in almost any patient administered too much or too little of a drug. Additionally, side effects from this type of ADR are usually known to be characteristic of the drug itself. Every drug's overdosage symptoms are different.[47]

Sometimes, a drug overdose is not an acute event. It can be chronic, due in some cases to accumulation resulting from a patient's inability to process and excrete the medication properly. For example, a patient with a liver disorder may render a particular medication (such as morphine) even more toxic than a particular dose would be for another person.

As discussed earlier,[48] drugs with high molecular weight are most likely to cause reactions. Fortunately, most drugs are simple organic chemicals of low molecular weight, usually less than 1.000 Daltons. For such low molecular weight drugs to become immunogenic, the drug or a drug metabolite must be bound to a macromolecular carrier, often by covalent bonds, for an effective antigen processing. Macromolecular drugs, such as heterologous, antisera, and insulin, are complex antigens and can potentially sensitize any patient.

10.3.8 Hypersensitivity Vasculitis

Characterized by inflammation and necrosis of blood vessels, vasculitis is a condition that often involves organs or systems with a rich supply of blood vessels. Thus, the skin is often involved in vasculitic syndromes. According to Ditto:

> *In the systemic necrotizing vasculitis group (polyarteritis nodosa. allergic granulomatosis of Churg-Strauss) and granulomatous vasculitides (Wegener granulomatosis, lymphomatoid granulomatosis, giant cell arteritides), cutaneous involvement is not as common a presenting feature as seen in the hypersensitivity vasculitides (HSV).*[49]

Drugs do appear to be causative or associated with HSV—especially in patients over 50, who are more frequently prescribed medications that have been associated with this syndrome (e.g., diuretics or cardiac drugs). Other frequently implicated agents include penicillin, sulfonamides, thiouracils, hydantoins, iodides, and allopurinol, the author contends. Signs and symptoms to watch out for include fever, malaise, rash, hepatocellular injury, renal failure, leukocytosis, and eosinophilia. That said, the most common clinical feature of HSV is palpable purpura, making the skin the most likely place where vasculitis is recognized. The lesions are usually distributed in a symmetric pattern on the lower extremities and sacral area.[50]

10.3.9 Predominantly Organ-Specific Reactions

10.3.9.1 Dermatologic Manifestations

Studies show that skin lesions are among the most common ADRs, occurring in between 2 and 3 percent of hospitalized in-patients.[51] The most common culprits include:

- Anticonvulsants and central-nervous system depressants
- Sulfonamides (especially TMP-SMX)
- NSAIDs
- Beta-lactam antibiotics (especially ampicillin and amoxicillin)

With cutaneous reactions, eruptions are usually exanthematous or morbilliform in nature. Outside of Stevens–Johnson syndrome and toxic epidermal necrolysis (TEN), most are of mild or moderate severity, abate within a few days, and pose no threat to life or subsequent health. Most rashes due to medications are self-limited and only mildly symptomatic. The majority of skin events attributed to drugs are either exanthematous (maculopapular or morbilliform) eruptions (>80 percent) or urticaria (5 to 10 percent), but these percentages vary among medications and among patient groups.[52] Among patients who are not immunologically compromised, severe cutaneous reactions to medications are rare (with an incidence of <1 case per 1,000 new users), even with high-risk medications.[53]

10.3.10 Urticaria

Urticaria is the second most frequent drug-induced eruption. It may occur alone or may be part of an acute reaction such as anaphylaxis or serum sickness. An allergic IgE-mediated mechanism is often suspected, but it may be the result of other mechanisms.[54]

10.3.11 Fixed Drug Eruptions

Fixed drug eruptions are lesions that continue to appear in the same places each time a medication is administered and are indications of drug hypersensitivity. Men and children appear to be more frequently affected than women. The lesions are usually well-defined and rounded, varying in size, and usually presenting as a purple, raised spot.[55]

10.3.11.1 Assessing the Likelihood of a Severe Reaction

"Lesions are most common on the lips and genitals but may occur anywhere on the skin or mucous membranes," Ditto writes.

> *Usually, a solitary lesion is present, but the lesions may be more numerous, and additional ones may develop with subsequent administration of the drug. The length of time from exposure to the drug to the onset of symptoms is 30 minutes to 8 hours (mean, 2.1 hours). The lesions usually resolve within 2 to 3 weeks after drug withdrawal, leaving transient desquamation and residual hyper pigmentation.*[56]

Because it is so difficult to absolutely prove the presence or the absence of a drug allergy, it remains the physician's responsibility to collect whatever evidence he can and evaluate it thoroughly. Only the skillful and practiced physician will notice the subtle signs of any cutaneous hypersensitivity reaction. To make sure you know how to recognize cutaneous drug hypersensitivity reactions, review the clinical criteria and manifestations. Most of these cases are very treatable, especially when recognized early.

With Stevens–Johnson syndrome, some studies show effective early management with high-dose corticosteroids (160- to 240-mg methylprednisolone a day, initially). This is a bit controversial, however. Proponents say that corticosteroids hasten recovery, produce few major side effects, and can result in almost a 100 percent survival and full recovery. This strategy should never be used for the management of TEN drug challenges to establish whether a patient can tolerate a drug following a reaction.

10.3.12 Photosensitivity Reactions

Almost regardless of the route of administration (topical, oral, parenteral), photosensitivity reactions are always a possibility. These reactions occur when a drug present in the skin interacts with the light energy from direct sunlight or filtered or artificial light with sufficient UV light. Individuals with lighter skin seem most susceptible to these reactions, which are most likely to occur on the face, the neck, the forearms, and the backs of the hands. Usually, photosensitivity is a phototoxic, non-immunologic reaction caused by oxidative energy being transferred to tissues, resulting in damage to tissues. Every drug has its own specific light-absorption spectrum. These types of reactions look a lot like bad sunburns—occasionally with vesiculation. A photosensitivity reaction should be expected if the patient has been taking tetracycline or amiodarone.[57]

When a photosensitive reaction is the result of a photoallergic immunologic reaction, the picture is slightly altered. In this scenario, the radiant light energy alters the drug in the skin to form reactive metabolites that combine with cutaneous proteins to form a complete antigen, provoking an immunologic response. These reactions may be difficult to trace because they can occur or recur days to months after light exposure (even without continuing the drug). Unlike non-immunologic reactions, window glass cannot protect against a reaction. A patch test can confirm the presence of such a reaction. The most likely culprits are sulfonamides (antibacterials, hypoglycemics, diuretics), phenothiazines, NSAIDs, and griseofulvin.

10.3.13 Generalized Exfoliative Dermatitis

A potentially life-threatening skin disease, exfoliative dermatitis presents as excessive scaling of the skin, resulting in peeling over virtually the entire body, including hair and nails. Symptoms can include fever, chills, and malaise, as well as large extra-renal fluid loss. Fatalities occur most frequently from this type of reaction in elderly or debilitated patients. Pre-existing skin disorders (psoriasis, seborrheic dermatitis, etc.) may be at the root of this reaction, but it is often difficult to track down. The reaction does not immediately cease upon stopping the drug. It may continue for months after withdrawal of the culprit. Most frequent causes are sulfonamides, penicillins, barbiturates, carbamazepine, phenytoin, phenylbutazone, allopurinol, and gold salts.[58]

10.3.14 Thrombocytopenia

A well-recognized complication of drug therapy, thrombocytopenia is not usually fatal. Clinical manifestations include petechiae and ecchymoses and, upon occasion, gastrointestinal bleeding, hematuria, and/or vaginal bleeding. This complication can be identified through an examination of bone marrow, which will show normal or increased numbers of normal appearing megakaryocytes. Prompt recovery (within two weeks) is expected upon the withdrawal of the drug.[59]

10.3.15 Hemolytic Anemia

There are three mechanisms for the provocation of drug-induced immune hemolytic anemia. The first is an immune complex type, the second is a hapten or drug adsorption type, and the final is an autoimmune reaction. In general, however, the immune complex mechanism is the most frequent mechanism for the development of this reaction.[60]

10.3.16 Agranulocytosis

Usually occurring six to 10 days after initial drug therapy, patients suffering from agranulocytosis may experience high fever, chills, arthralgias, and severe prostration. The granulocytes disappear within a matter of hours or persist five to ten days after withdrawal. This drug-induced neutropenia is mediated by immunologic mechanisms.[61]

10.3.17 Treatment: Withdrawal of the Suspected Drug

If an allergic drug reaction is suspected, a detailed history of all drugs taken within the past month or two should be examined. Upon reasonable suspicion, treatment should be discontinued. If the reaction resolves, the answer is clear.[62]

10.3.18 Symptomatic Treatment

Some drug-induced allergy or hypersensitivity reactions do not require any treatment at all. Other types may be uncomfortable or dangerous enough so that they will require treatment aimed at alleviating the symptoms until the reaction subsides. The best examples are probably urticaria, which can be treated with corticosteroids, and drug-induced serum sickness, which can be treated with antihistamines and NSAIDs. More severe manifestations require treatment with prednisone 40 to 60 mg daily to start, with tapering over 7 to 10 days. The most prominent types of reactions—those that may lead to anaphylaxis or anaphylactoid reactions—require the most aggressive treatment or in many cases withdrawal from the suspect drug(s).[63]

10.3.19 Prevention of Allergic Drug Reactions

The best way to prevent drug allergy is to limit exposure to medications, prescribing only those that are clinically essential. Also, prescribing as few medications as possible simplifies the identification of a potential allergen. Studies show that the number of ADRs is proportional to the number of drugs prescribed. It is also possible to administer antihistamines and/or corticosteroids (alone or in combination with adrenergic agonists) in advance; this has been found to reduce the number and severity of anaphylactoid reactions.[64]

Alternatively, desensitization is employed to help the patient better tolerate the drug. This is only for patients with a history of an IgE-mediated immediate generalized reaction to a drug, confirmed by skin testing. The desensitization produces a temporary, nonresponsive state lasting as long as therapy continues. Anaphylactic sensitivity may return within 48 hours of withdrawing the drug. Caution and continuation of an agent, such as insulin, are therefore advised. Drugs that are not clearly indicated should also be stopped. If a drug is necessary but possibly cross-reactive, it may be prudent to search for a non-cross-reactive drug in the same class.

With allergies, this means the mechanism should be based on the identification of specific antibodies and/or sensitized lymphocytes. Although many drugs will evoke an immune response, only a small number of patients will actually experience a clinical hypersensitivity reaction. Penicillin alone has been associated with many of these reactions.

Anaphylaxis and urticaria following penicillin administration are examples of type I reactions, and associated with high-dose penicillin therapy is a type II reaction. A serum sickness-like reaction, now most commonly associated with penicillin treatment, is a type III reaction. Finally, the contact dermatitis that occurred when penicillin was used topically in the past is an example of a type IV reaction.

Anaphylaxis occurs most commonly after parenteral administration, but it has also followed oral, percutaneous, and respiratory exposure. Symptoms usually appear within 30 minutes of exposure. Although these symptoms can be ameliorated with treatment, they may last 24 hours or longer or recur several hours after apparent resolution. Without treatment, death can occur within minutes of initial presentation.

Preclinical testing is a potential tool for limiting exposure to medications which might induce an allergic response. Immune-mediated hypersensitivity reactions include exaggerated humoral or cell-mediated responses to specific antigens and may culminate in adverse, potentially life-threatening effects. The host immune status and accompanying presence of infections can influence the response of immune-mediated side effects. Variability in the immune status may impact the type of idiosyncratic reaction(s) that manifest. The issues commonly encountered in drug development include contact hypersensitivity, systemic hypersensitivity, respiratory sensitivity, photoallergy, and pseudoallergy. There are no accepted preclinical models to measure and predict all types of hypersensitivity reactions that may occur when a drug is tested in humans. Development of preclinical models would be of great interest to predict all types of hypersensitivity reactions in humans. Preclinical testing for topical and inhalational drugs is recommended prior to human studies.[65]

10.3.20 Pseudoallergy

Some reactions mimic an allergy but are not associated with antibody production or sensitized T-lymphocytes. This is difficult, if not impossible, to observe clinically or distinguish from hypersensitivity. Pseudoallergy is an inflammatory reaction originating from mast cells, basophils, or other body tissues.[66] A few examples:

- Skin flushing
- Local red skin rashes
- Bronchospasm
- Angioedema
- Hypotension

Pseudoallergy is also called drug intolerance or anaphylactoid reactions (e.g., bronchospasm, angioedema, urticaria, hypotension), although the anaphylactoid reactions are non-IgE mediated.

10.3.21 Angioedema

Angioedema is a reaction causing swelling in the tissue just below the surface of the skin, most often around the lips and eyes. It generally results from an allergic reaction to either a food or medication, wherein histamine causes blood vessels to swell. Sometimes, the condition is unilateral, impacting only one side of the body and not the other. The condition is mild in most cases, but severe angioedema can cause bronchoconstriction or swelling of the tongue, both of which can block the airway and cause death.[67]

According to the University of Maryland Medical Center,

> The characteristic lesion is well delineated and round or oval; it varies in size from a few millimeters to 25 to 30 cm. Edema appears initially, followed by erythema, which then darkens to become a deeply colored, reddish purple, dense raised lesion. . . . Lesions are most common on the lips and genitals but may occur anywhere on the skin or mucous membranes.[68]

Angioedema usually presents as a solitary lesion. Sometimes, however, the lesions may be more numerous, and additional ones may develop with re-exposure to the drug. Angioedema usually develops between 30 minutes and 8 hours after the administration of the offending substance. The average is about two hours.

Common symptoms of angioedema include:[69]

- Sudden appearance of red welts, especially near the eyes and lips, but also on the hands, feet, and the inside of the throat.
- Burning, painful, swollen areas; sometimes itchy.
- Hoarseness, tight or swollen throat, breathing trouble.
- Discolored patches or rash on the hands, feet, face, or genitals.
- Vomiting, abdominal pain, diarrhea, and reduced appetite.
- In a form called angioedema-eosinophilia syndrome, hives, itching, fever, muscle pain, decreased urine, weight gain, and high white blood cell count occur (UNM).

Studies show that more than 50 percent of patients presenting to the ED with angioedema were taking ACE inhibitors. In patients with idiopathic anaphylaxis, ACE inhibitors are contraindicated at least on a relative basis until it has been ruled out as a cause of the reaction.[70]

10.3.22 Hypersensitivity Reactions

Allergies and drug reactions that elicit immune responses are not completely understood, perhaps because of the lack of a validated animal model for hypersensitivity. It is also difficult to isolate the antigenic components and metabolites of potential drug allergens. Although much is unknown about the mechanisms of hypersensitivity reactions, it is known that a drug can cause a number of different hypersensitivity reactions (via different mechanisms, even). On the basis of current evidence and existing models of hapten-mediated allergy, a number of complex stages appear to be involved in the generation of an immune response to a drug.[71] These stages are:

1. Formation of a complete antigen.
2. Processing of the complete antigen by antigen-presenting cells.
3. Recognition of the antigenic determinant by the T lymphocytes.
4. Generation of a drug-specific antibody or sensitized T-cells.
5. Elicitation of a clinical immune response.

Sylvia writes:

> *To be recognized by the immune system, a drug must bind, usually covalently, to a high molecular weight carrier protein, thereby forming a complete antigen. The hapten hypothesis, first described in 1966, offers an understanding of this stage of immune processing. The parent drug rarely has the ability to bind to tissue or cellular proteins and serve as a hapten. For most low molecular weight drug allergens, the hapten is a reactive metabolite of the parent drug, formed via metabolism in the liver, skin keratinocytes, or white blood cells. 1M-55 As an example, sulfamethoxazole is well recognized as a highly allergenic compound; however, a reactive metabolite, the nitroso-sulfamethoxazole derivative, not the parent compound, serves as the primary hapten.*[72]

10.4 RISK FACTORS, DRUGS, AND PATIENTS

10.4.1 Hypersensitivity Risk Factors

Drug hypersensitivity usually involves contributory or predisposing factors—usually drug or patient (host) related. Although numerous studies and ample controversy continue to highlight the influence of these factors on the risk of hypersensitivity, causes still remain largely unknown.[73]

Besides molecular weight over 4,000 Da, other factors may include chemical composition consisting of protein or peptides and the ability of the drug to form a covalent bond with a carrier protein. The presence of proteins of nonhuman origin or the inclusion of antigenic excipients (peanuts, for example) also increases the risk of drug reactivity. As mentioned earlier in this course, another possible hypersensitive provocateur may include the route of drug administration, as well as the dose and/or frequency of administration.

For example, parenteral routes of administration—perhaps because they provide a higher rate of drug delivery than oral or other routes of administration—seem to provoke more severe reactions (after an initial sensitization). Dosage also plays a role in provoking hypersensitivity. In general, the amount given is usually proportional to the immune response mounted by the patient's body.

Certain allergic reactions are reported more frequently among specific age groups. For example, anaphylaxis with penicillin has been reported more commonly in patients between the ages of 20 and 49 years compared with children. It is thought, however, that this fact is related more to the possibility of more exposures to the drug throughout an adult individual's lifetime, creating a higher risk of sensitivity.

Overprescription of antibiotics can also cause hypersensitivity, particularly in those who receive frequent courses of antibiotics (e.g., children with chronic otitis media or bronchitis). So, the frequency and number of exposures are more likely to increase risk compared with age.

Gender may be a risk factor for drug allergy. Bigby et al. reported a 35 percent higher incidence of drug-induced allergic cutaneous reactions in women than in men.[74] More recently, in a study of penicillin allergy, Macy et al. also found that women were more likely to present with hypersensitivity reactions.[75]

10.4.2 Identification of a Drug Allergy

Drug allergies can sometimes be difficult to identify because so many factors may be involved and contributing to the patient's reaction. Additionally, some symptoms of drug allergy mimic other conditions such as hypersensitivity reactions.

The key distinguishing factor with allergies, however, is an exaggerated immune response. The physiopathology of these diseases is not well understood. For this reason, physicians must immediately identify risk factors—before an allergic response ever happens. Although clinical and biologic tests are helpful diagnostic tools, they cannot predict who will develop an allergic reaction. For this reason, we must turn to the epidemiological characteristics of the demographic that develops a reported drug allergy reaction.

The factors most associated with drug allergies are:[76]

- Female gender
- Concomitant infections (HIV, herpes)
- Concurrent illnesses (systemic lupus erythematosus)
- Genetic predisposition (certain ethnic groups have been found to have similar allergies and sensitivities among individuals. For example, some ethnic groups seem to be prone to certain types of ADRs. A study by Easterbrook[77] found that being a member of the Caucasian race raised the incidence of hypersensitivity to abacavir. African Americans were found to be more susceptible to developing ACE-related angioedema than other ethnic groups)[78]
- Use of anticonvulsants
- Insulin-dependent diabetics
- Use of local injectable anesthetics
- Use of topical anesthetics
- Host-related factors can predispose to drug allergy especially by acting on the way the drug is processed
- Frequent exposure to a drug (such as an anti-retroviral drug used to treat a patient with HIV)

Certain drugs also seem to be more prone to causing reactions than others. The drugs that seem to cause the most problems include:[79]

- Penicillin
- Sulfa drugs
- Anticonvulsants
- Insulin preparations (particularly animal sources of insulin)
- Iodinated X-ray contrast dyes (these iodine-containing dyes can cause allergy-like anaphylactoid reactions)

10.4.3 Allergy to Antibiotics

Antibiotics are the most common cause of life-threatening immune-mediated drug reactions considered off-target. These include anaphylaxis and organ-specific and severe cutaneous adverse reactions. These ADRs and hypersensitivity reactions (HSRs) result through a variety of mechanisms. Antibiotic allergies are frequently documented in the electronic health record, which results in changes to the care of future infectious diseases. A common caution in the allergy literature states that inaccurately determined allergies might result in the use of unnecessarily broad-spectrum or inferior antibiotics, posing a threat to patient safety and public health. Despite these threats, the histories associated with documented allergies are rarely reconciled, or acted on, by the healthcare team.[80]

Penicillins, cephalosporins, and sulfa drugs are the antibiotics most frequently associated with allergic reactions.

10.4.3.1 Penicillins and Cephalosporins

It is estimated that 10 percent of the population is allergic to penicillin. Healthcare students are always taught to specifically ask about an allergy when penicillin is considered. This risk is exacerbated by the fact that more than a dozen other "penicillins" are marketed, but their names do not specifically include "penicillin." A patient allergic to one type of penicillin is at risk for an allergic reaction to another. To further complicate the issue, there is a group of drugs that share the beta lactam ring—the cephalosporins. As a result of this common chemical structure, there is a risk of "cross-allergenicity" when cephalosporins are given to penicillin-allergic patients and vice versa.[81]

Since Beta-lactam antibiotics share common structures, there is a risk of cross-reactivity. Patients with a history of penicillin allergy are at a higher risk for adverse reaction to any additional antibiotics (including cephalosporins and sulfa). An explanation for not having higher cross-reactivity is that the alpha rings between the different classes vary, allowing for different antigenic determinants to be created when the agents bind to carrier proteins in the systemic circulation (haptenization). Penicillins contain a thiazolidine ring, whereas cephalosporins have a dihydrothiazine ring, and carbapenems contain a modified thiazolidine ring. Monobactams do not contain an alpha ring. Common side chains also contribute to cross-reactivity. The degree of cross-reactivity appears to be greater among the same class of antibiotics than between classes. The greatest risk of cross-reactivity is among penicillins. The penicillins and monobactams have an R1 side chain, while the cephalosporins and carbapenems have both an R1 and R2 side chain. For the majority of cephalosporins, the R1 side chain is more clinically relevant for cross-reactivity than the R2 side chain as the R2 side chain acts as a leaving group during carrier protein conjugation, and therefore it cannot contribute to the epitope for IgE binding. The similarity of R1 side chains between agents is considered the major predictor of cross-reactivity between the beta-lactam antibiotics.[82]

Available data, although based on small numbers, suggest an increased risk of cephalosporin reactions among patients with positive results on penicillin skin tests. In a review combining data from 11 studies of cephalosporin administration in patients with a history of penicillin allergy,[83] cephalosporin reactions were found to have occurred in 6 of 135 patients with positive skin-test results for penicillin allergy (4.4 percent), as compared with only 2 of 351 with negative skin tests (0.6 percent). Indiscriminate administration cannot be recommended, especially for patients who have had life-threatening reactions. Among 12 cases of fatal anaphylaxis caused by antibiotics in the United Kingdom from 1992 to 1997, 6 cases occurred after the first dose of a cephalosporin, and 3 of the 6 patients were known to have penicillin allergy.[84]

In addition to being the most common cause of drug allergy in general, Beta-lactam antibiotics are also considered to be the most common non-serum causes of serum sickness-like reactions. Other drugs occasionally incriminated include ciprofloxacin, metronidazole, streptomycin, sulfonamides, allopurinol, carbamazepine, hydantoins, methimazole, phenylbutazone, propranolol, and thiouracil.

10.4.3.2 Sulfonamide Allergic Reactions and Cross-Sensitivity

For patients who have a history of allergy to sulfonamide antibiotics, concern has been raised about the use of other sulfonamide-containing drugs (diuretics, sulfonylureas, and celecoxib). However, sulfonamide antimicrobial agents (sulfamethoxazole, sulfadiazine, sulfisoxazole, and sulfacetamide) differ from other sulfonamide-containing medications by having an aromatic amine group at the N4 position and a substituted ring at the N1 position; these groups are not found in nonantibiotic sulfonamide-containing drugs. Thus, despite product-labeling warnings, cross-reactivity between these two groups of sulfonamides is believed to be unlikely.[85,86]

10.4.4 Case Report: Cross-Allergenicity

A case in Montana demonstrates the serious nature of allergic reactions and cross-allergenicity of drugs (*Re: Estate of Frank Hamilton v. F. John Allaire, M.D.*, Montana Eighth Judicial District Court, Cascade County CDV-91-303). In this case, a 51-year-old patient suffered anaphylaxis and death in the Montana Deaconess Medical Center following one intramuscular (IM) dose of Ancef (cefazolin). He had a history of penicillin allergy, which he had noted on consent forms to receive drugs and treatments. His physician was aware of the allergy, and the pharmacist also called the physician's attention to the allergic caution. According to Mr. Randy Dix, the attorney representing the family, the hospital pharmacist stated that it was not his job to "second guess" the doctor and filled the Ancef as ordered. The order read "penicillin sensitive, give one-gram Ancef IM." The pharmacist filled the order, and the nurse administered the injection. Shortly thereafter, the patient suffered a cardiopulmonary arrest and died.

In his defense, the physician stated that the patient said that he had suffered a mild rash reaction to previous penicillin. Mild reactions (delayed hypersensitivities) are not a contraindication to cephalosporin. However, when the attending nurse was deposed, she specifically remembered the patient always anxious and asking to be sure that he was not receiving penicillin, because he had a serious reaction to penicillin in the past. The nurse testified that she was not aware of the penicillin-cephalosporin cross-reactivity and obvious contraindication in her patient.

Before the initiation of cephalosporin therapy, careful inquiry should be made concerning previous hypersensitivity reactions to cephalosporins, penicillins, and other drugs. Cephalosporins should be avoided in patients who have had an immediate-type (anaphylactic) hypersensitivity reaction to penicillins and should be administered with caution to patients who have had a delayed-type (e.g., rash, fever, eosinophilia) reaction to penicillin.

Experts in the case, including a physician (infectious-disease specialist) and a former hospital pharmacist, stated that other non-cross-reactive drugs were available to treat the patient's suspected pneumonia.

The case was presented to the Montana Medical Legal Panel, who found substantial evidence that such acts or omissions constituted a departure from the accepted standards of healthcare and that there was a reasonable probability that the claimant was injured by such a departure. The hospital settled the lawsuit early in the case. The physician settled the case after experts for the plaintiff gave their reports and depositions.

Unfortunately, it seems that there exists an almost cavalier attitude about this well-described risk of cross-reactivity. Pharmacists should realize that it is their responsibility to monitor for allergic cross-reactivity. Perhaps if the pharmacist in this case had advised the physician of the danger, had called the nurse, or had interviewed the patient, he would have discovered the history of this serious reaction, and this death could have been avoided.

10.5 ERYTHEMA MULTIFORME, STEVENS–JOHNSON SYNDROME, AND TOXIC EPIDERMAL NECROLYSIS

10.5.1 Fixed Drug Eruptions

In contrast to most other drug-induced dermatoses, fixed drug eruptions (lesions that continue to recur in the same locations on the body every time a specific allergen is encountered) are considered to be a certain indicator of drug hypersensitivity. Men and children seem to be affected by this reaction more frequently than women. Drugs that have frequently been found to be associated include:

- Phenolphthalein
- Sulfonamides
- Tetracycline
- Barbiturates
- Lamotrigine (Lamictal)
- NSAIDs

10.5.2 Erythema Multiforme-Like Eruptions

Erythema multiforme (EM minor) is often a benign cutaneous illness with or without minimal mucous membrane involvement. A more severe cutaneous reaction that does affect mucous membranes (at least two mucosal surfaces) and constitutional symptoms is called *erythema multiforme major* (EM major).

In the past decade, advances have been made for the diagnosis of severe cutaneous adverse reactions (SCARs) to drugs, management, identification of their pathogenetic mechanisms, and populations at risk. The early detection of SCARs is critical in the identification of culprit drugs. SCARs are potentially life threatening and associated with various clinical patterns and morbidity during the acute state of Stevens–Johns syndrome (SJS) and TEN, drug reactions with eosinophilia and systemic symptoms, and acute generalized exanthematous pustulosis.[87]

Most instances of drug-induced erythema multiforme can be classified as EM major or SJS. This form of EM produces bulbous-erosive lesions and is usually accompanied by high fever, headache, and malaise. It also affects mucosal surfaces. There is often more pronounced truncal involvement. Painful oral and pharyngeal mucous membrane lesions may stop patients from eating. The border of the lips all but disappears and develops serosanguinous crusts. Eighty-five percent of patients develop hyperemia and/or extensive pseudomembrane formation.

Both SJS and TEN are most commonly caused from drugs, especially the following:[88]

- Sulfonamides
- Cephalosporins
- Penicillins
- Fluoroquinolones
- Anticonvulsants (phenytoin, phenobarbital, and carbamazepine)
- Allopurinol
- Lamotrigine (Lamictal)
- NSAIDs

TEN (Lyell syndrome) is a sudden, potentially lethal condition presented by widespread blistering of the skin, extensive epidermal necrosis, and exfoliation. Some research suggests that TEN may represent the extreme manifestation of EM major. Other studies challenge this position. Further, some write that TEN is a worsening of SJS. All agree that extensive skin involvement with SJS and TEN is best treated in a burn unit.

10.5.2.1 Case Report: Lamictal Induced Stevens–Johnson Syndrome

10.5.2.1.1 Opinions

1. Lamictal was the cause of this patient's SJS reaction, in particular, following a rapid dosage acceleration. The bases for this opinion are as follows:
   a. Lamictal, as an anticonvulsant, is listed with drugs with the highest risk and frequency of SJS. Simply noting (MedWatch) 1,276 SJS reports for Lamictal, 34 for Adderall, and 490 for Cipro demonstrates the overwhelming greater risk of Lamictal than Adderall or Cipro.
   b. The risk of SJS is increased with rapid dosage acceleration. (Manufacturer's official package insert; published literature, including *New England Journal of Medicine*, *Journal of Clinical Neurology,* and *Drug Safety Journal*). This is linked to an accumulation of a toxic intermediary metabolite, or an inability to completely metabolize, due to an overload of the glucuronidation (Phase II) pathway, leading to an increase in toxic metabolites.
   c. The risk of Lamictal for SJS and serious skin reactions is increased in adolescents and children (manufacturer's official package insert and literature; supported by MedWatch analyses). Lamictal is not an approved FDA indication for bipolar disorder in adolescents.
   d. Clinical diagnosis of SJS secondary to Lamictal is replete in the clinical records for the patient.
   e. The initial dosage, the interval between dosage accelerations, and the increased dose acceleration all exceeded the manufacturer's dosage acceleration instructions and resulted in a 400 percent dose escalation (*Strong Temporal Relationship*). The increased dosage and the rapid accelerations all increase the risk of SJS/TEN and are proximate causes of the patient's SJS/TEN.
   f. The risks listed here for Lamictal were not disclosed to the patient or her mother; the

Lamictal was a proximate cause of the SJS/TEN.

2. Cipro is not the cause or contributor to the patient's SJS.
   a. Cipro was started after the second dose acceleration of Lamictal and, after the prodrome (beginning signs of toxicity), manifest as a number of complaints, including urinary. The patient was clinically diagnosed as having a urinary tract infection, for which Cipro was prescribed.
   b. Even ignoring the lack of a temporal relationship for Cipro, MedWatch report analysis demonstrates the following: SJS/TEN is reported 1.9-fold more frequently for Lamictal than for Cipro ($p < 0.0001$).
      Lamictal: 1,276 SJS/TEN reports in 32,578 total MedWatch reports (3.92 percent).
      Cipro: 490 SJS/TEN reports out of 23,481 total MedWatch reports (2.07 percent).
3. Adderall is not the cause or contributing cause of the patient's SJS.
   a. She was taking Adderall for a prolonged time before and after the SJS illness. Adderall is therefore unlikely to be even a contributing cause.
   b. MedWatch report analysis demonstrates that SJS/TEN is reported 6.3-fold more frequently for Lamictal than Adderall ($p < 0.0001$)
   c. 34 SJS/TEN reports out of a total 5,453 MedWatch reports.
4. Lamictal's SJS/TEN reporting incidence is twice in children under 18 (8.49%/3.72% = 2.28%) compared to adult patients (> 18 years old).
5. The Causation analysis criteria of biological plausibility, strong temporal relationship, literature precedent, challenge, and de-challenge are met. The final criteria of re-challenge are (hopefully) never fulfilled! Indeed, in this case, the patient's medical records are flagged with "Lamictal Allergy" to avoid a re-challenge.

10.5.3 Fluoroquinolones

Effective against both negative and gram-positive organisms, fluoroquinolones are antimicrobial agents with a broad range of activity. Adverse reactions may include skin rash and pruritis, phototoxicity, and/or Achilles's tendon inflammation and rupture.

10.5.4 ASA and NSAIDs

Second to the Beta-lactam antibiotics, ASA and NSAIDs are the most likely drugs to cause allergic drug reactions. Reactions may include exacerbated urticaria (in 21 to 30 percent of patients who suffer from idiopathic urticaria or angioedema), bronchoconstriction in patients with nasal polyps, persistent erythema, and anaphylaxis. Sometimes, in perfectly healthy patients, there have been reports of urticaria and anaphylactoid reactions within minutes after taking ASA or a nonselective NSAID. Respiratory reactions occur in about 10 to 20 percent of asthmatic patients older than 10 years. That said, those with known sensitivities present with reactions in 66 to 97 percent of cases.[89] There is less risk of reaction in asthmatic children under the age of 10, but the risks appear to increase in the teenage years, equaling the number of asthmatic adults who suffer an ADR. Usually, the patients who suffer from respiratory reactions already had established respiratory problems for months or years before a clear, causative reaction from ASA or NSAIDs. Reactions usually occur within two hours of drug ingestion. These reactions may be quite severe, even fatal. They consist of severe nasal congestion, rhinorrhea, and eye problems.

10.5.5 NSAID Cross Reactivity Case Report

The following is a preliminary report prepared in a case in which an aspirin-allergic patient suffered a serious allergic reaction when prescribed Naproxen, an NSAID. Pharmacists' duties and responsibilities are discussed in the report.

10.5.5.1 Facts of the Case

Mr. S, a 64-year-old, complained of back and leg pain which prompted him to seek care at the Emergency Department (ED). He was evaluated and prescribed Lortab (hydrocodone and acetaminophen) and Naprosyn (naproxen), 500 mg twice a day. He filled the prescriptions at a local pharmacy (Naprosyn 500 mg, #30). At home, he took one capsule/tablet of naproxen and reported that within five minutes, he had difficulty breathing and returned to the ED. At the ED, he required mechanical ventilation for several days and was discharged home again. A few days later, he again had severe respiratory complaints, which prompted his return to the ED, where he entered a long and complicated treatment for airway complications following his intubation.

An examination of the Neighborhood Healthcare records indicates an aspirin/ASA allergy, as well as prior treatment for an allergic reaction to Advil (ibuprofen—an NSAID). NSAIDs were also listed in his allergy history following an allergic reaction to Advil.

After the litigation began, the ED resident physician who prescribed Naproxen was deposed. He testified that he was unaware of the cross-allergenicity between aspirin and naproxen, and if the pharmacist had called, he would have discontinued the naproxen and avoided NSAIDs in this aspirin-allergic patient.

10.5.5.2 Opinions

1. Naprosyn/naproxen, an NSAID, is contraindicated in a patient with a history of aspirin allergies. Contraindication means—DO NOT USE!

The cross-reactivity of aspirin and NSAIDs is well known and promulgated.
2. The initial allergic/anaphylactic reaction with angioedema was caused by the allergic reaction to Naprosyn.
3. Mr. S's history of aspirin allergy (anaphylaxis) was known to Walgreens. Salicylate is listed in the allergy window. Aspirin is listed in another pharmacy profile location. Entry of Naprosyn (naproxen) in the pharmacy system therefore should have precipitated a serious warning to the technician and/or pharmacist. Such a warning should have prompted the pharmacist to inquire further with Mr. S regarding his allergy history, which would have verified the aspirin allergy, thus contraindicating the dispensation (SHOULD NOT FILL). The pharmacist(s) who over-rode the computer alert and verified and checked/verified/dispensed the Naprosyn prescription for this patient violated the standard of care of pharmacists. This violation is a proximate cause of his allergic reaction. This violation put Mr. S in danger of a fatal anaphylactic reaction to Naprosyn, which we know occurred.

10.5.5.3 Case Conclusion

Had the pharmacist(s) exercised their duty and complied with the standard of care for screening allergies with all prescriptions and responding to the allergy warning, Mr. S would not have suffered his acute life-threatening allergic reaction and the subsequent morbidity.

10.5.6 Radiographic Contrast Media

Nonfatal, immediate generalized reactions to non-iodinated, gadolinium-based contrast agents for magnetic resonance imaging (MRI) occur in about 1 to 2 percent of cases. Severe anaphylactoid reactions are rare (1:350,000 infections). This is another instance in which risk factors are the best predictors of a possible reaction. The following groups are most likely to suffer an ADR after receiving an injected radiographic contrast media (RCM):[90]

- History of a previous reaction to these agents
- Severe coronary artery disease
- Unstable angina
- Advanced age
- Female gender
- Exposure to large volumes of contrast media
- Atopic individuals
- Asthmatics

The following patients are just slightly more likely to suffer an ADR after RCM administration:

- Patients who react to iodides
- Patients with allergies to shellfish

The most common side effects are nausea and vomiting. More generalized reactions include:

- Pruritus
- Urticaria
- Angioedema
- Bronchospasm
- Hypotension
- Syncope
- Contrast Media Neurotoxicity

10.5.7 Local Anesthetics

Patients who experience any ADR following the administration of a local anesthetic are often told that they are allergic to the entire range of agents in this classification. This is untrue and dangerous, considering that such patients may not be able to receive routine dental care or outpatient surgical procedures.

The most common reactions to local anesthetics include:

- Vasovagal reactions
- Toxic reactions
- Hysterical reactions
- Epinephrine side effects
- Contact dermatitis

To manage these patients, a different local anesthetic agent should be used. For example, an amide should be substituted for an ester. Amides are not known to cross react with other amides.

As a side note, latex-containing products—such as gloves and rubber dams—are often used in dental and surgical practices. If a patient is allergic to latex, this factor should be considered while testing for adverse reactions that might otherwise be attributed to the local anesthetic. Among other analgesics, morphine and codeine are most likely to activate mast cells and cause flushing or acute urticaria. Meperidine, tramadol, and fentanyl are much less likely to cause mast-cell activity. Sometimes, the side effect of opioid painkillers may mimic hypersensitivity. However, if a patient has a history of codeine- or morphine-induced urticaria, alternative agents are recommended when narcotics are required.

10.5.8 Anticonvulsants (AED)

Adverse cutaneous reactions caused by mostly aromatic anti-epileptic drugs (AEDs) affect 50,000 people a year in the United Kingdom with an incidence of 75.7 per 100,000. Optical optimal management of these cases is often difficult, as a patient may report symptoms to a general practitioner and attend the emergency department or Informa specialist over the telephone or via email. When clinical assessment is limited, it is thought safest to withdraw the offending medication after informing the patient of a new drug allergy. This may unjustifiably restrict further treatment choices and increased cost. Most frequent offenders are aromatic AEDs: Carbamazepine, oxcarbazepine, eslicarbazepine, phenytoin, lamotrigine, phenobarbital, primidone, and the sulfa derivative zonisamide.[91]

Phenytoin hypersensitivity syndrome is rare. It usually begins a couple of months after the initiation of the drug. Reactions may include fever, marked erythematous papules that may blister, necrosis from vasculitis, liver enlargement, and mouth ulcers. These symptoms may actually be an indicator of SJS. Lab tests may reveal atypical lymphocytes, elevation of serum creatinine, eosinophilia (sometimes pulmonary), leucopenia, and hepatic abnormalities.

Carbamazepine can cause similar reactions and is contraindicated in patients who are hypersensitive to phenytoin, because of their shared structures and metabolism.

According to Ditto:

> The mechanism may relate to inadequate detoxification by epoxide hydrolase of hepatic microsome-generated metabolites of phenytoin and carbamazepine. The relatives of affected patients who are themselves non-epileptic and not exposed to phenytoin may have findings of delayed metabolism. The metabolites are thought to cause neoantigen formation with the clinical hypersensitivity syndrome.[92]

Additional information on erythema multiforme, SJS, and TEN can be found in the following references:[93,94,95,96,97,98,99,100,101,102,103].

10.6 SUMMARY AND CONCLUSIONS

Allergic reactions to drugs may be deadly. Initial dose reactions cannot be avoided. For drugs with high risk for severe allergic reactions, close monitoring, and even pretreatment with an antihistamine and corticosteroid is common (contrast media), or observation of the patient (injections of penicillin). Once an allergic reaction is experienced, the patient should be advised to write down the reaction; tell it to all physicians, pharmacists, and other health providers; and wear a medic alert bracelet. Providers should inquire of allergies, without relying on the patient to volunteer. Allergies should be prominently posted on the patient chart, over the patient's bed, on all drug order and medication administration sheets.

Serious allergic reactions to drugs for which the patient had a known or knowable history is an avoidable adverse reaction—it should not happen. Finally, patients allergic to one drug in a class (penicillin, aspirin) are at risk for an allergic reaction to another drug in the same class (ampicillin, ibuprofen). This is known as a cross-allergenicity. History of hypersensitivity to a member of the class should be considered as a contraindication—do not do it.

APPENDIX 10.1

Terminology Concerning Drug Misadventures

Adverse Event (or Adverse Experience): Any untoward medical occurrence in a patient or clinical-investigation subject administered a pharmaceutical product. It is not necessary for the event to have a causal relationship with this treatment.

Adverse Drug Reaction (ADR): In the preapproval clinical experience with a new medicinal product or its new usages, particularly as the therapeutic doses may not be established, "all noxious and unintended responses to a medicinal product related to any dose should be considered adverse drug reactions."

Unexpected Adverse Drug Reaction: An adverse reaction, the nature or severity of which is not consistent with the applicable product information (e.g., an investigator's brochure for an unapproved investigational medicinal product).

Serious Adverse Event: A serious adverse event, experience, or reaction is any untoward medical occurrence that at any dose may: (1) Result in death, (2) be life-threatening, (3) require in-patient hospitalization or prolongation of existing hospitalization, (4) result in persistent or significant disability or incapacity, and (5) results in a congenital anomaly or birth defect. (Note: The term "life-threatening" refers to an event in which the patient was at risk of death at the time of the event; it does not refer to an event which hypothetically might have caused death if it were more severe.)

NOTES

1 Trontel, A. CDER/CBER PDUFA3 risk management working group, April 9, 2003.
2 Litaker, John R., and James P. Wilson. "Epidemiology and public health impact of drug-induced diseases." In *Drug-Induced Diseases: Prevention, Detection, and Management*, edited by James E. Tisdale and Douglas A. Miller. Bethesda, MD: American Society of Health-System Pharmacists, 2005:3. Print.
3 Hallas, J. "Drug related hospital admissions in subspecialities of internal medicine." Dan Med Bull. 1996;43:141–155.
4 Einarson, T. R. "Drug-related hospital admissions." Ann Pharmacother. 1993;27:832–840.
5 Johnson, Jefferey A., and Lyle Bootman. "Drug-related morbidity and mortality: A cost-of-illness model." J Manag Care Pharm. 1996;2(1):39–47. Print.
6 Budnitz, Daniel S., Maribeth C. Lovegrove, Nadine Shehab, and Chesley L. Richards. "Emergency hospitalizations for adverse drug events in older Americans." N Engl J Med. 2011;365(21):2002–2012. Print.
7 Stelfox, H. T., S. Palmisani, C. Scurlock, E. J. Orav, and D. W. Bates. "The 'to err is human': Report and patient safety literature." Qual Saf Health Care. 2006;15(3):174–178.
8 "Drug-related morbidity and mortality: A cost-of-illness model, 9 October 1995." Johnson and Bootman. 1949;155(18).

9 Ernst, F. R., and A. J. Grizzle. "Drug-related morbidity and mortality: Updating the cost-of-illness model." J Am Pharm Assoc (Wash). 2001 Mar–Apr;41(2):192–199. doi:10.1016/s1086-5802(16)31229-3. PMID: 11297331.
10 Jacobsen, Thomas M., and Albert I. Wertheimer. *Modern Pharmaceutical Industry: A Primer*. Sudbury, MA: Jones and Bartlett, 2010. Print.
11 O'Donnell, J. T. "Adverse drug reaction: Focus on drug allergy." In *Drug Injury: Liability, Analysis, and Prevention*, 3rd edition. Tucson: Lawyers & Judges Publishers Inc., 2012.
12 Litaker, John R., and James P. Wilson. "Epidemiology and public health impact of drug-induced diseases." In *Drug-Induced Diseases: Prevention, Detection, and Management*, edited by James E. Tisdale and Douglas A. Miller. Bethesda, MD: American Society of Health-System Pharmacists, 2005:3. Print.
13 Hallas, J. "Drug related hospital admissions in subspecialities of internal medicine." Dan Med Bull. 1996;43:141–155.
14 Einarson, T. R. "Drug-related hospital admissions." Ann Pharmacother. 1993;27:832–840.
15 Johnson, Jefferey A., and Lyle Bootman. "Drug-related morbidity and mortality: A cost-of-illness model." J Manag Care Pharm. 1996;2(1):39–47. Print.
16 Budnitz, Daniel S., Maribeth C. Lovegrove, Nadine Shehab, and Chesley L. Richards. "Emergency hospitalizations for adverse drug events in older Americans." N Engl J Med. 2011;365(21):2002–2012. Print.
17 Stelfox, H. T., S. Palmisani, C. Scurlock, E. J. Orav, and D. W. Bates. "The 'to err is human': Report and patient safety literature." Qual Saf Health Care 2006 June;15(3):174–178.
18 "Drug-related morbidity and mortality: A cost-of-illness model, 9 October 1995." Johnson and Bootman. 1949;155(18).
19 Go, A. S., et al. "Heart disease and stroke statistics-2014 update: A report from the American Heart Association." Circulation. 2014 Jan 21;129(3).
20 Go, A. S., et al. "Heart disease and stroke statistics-2014 update: A report from the American Heart Association." Circulation. 2014 Jan 21;129(3).
21 Jacobsen, Thomas M., and Albert I. Wertheimer. *Modern Pharmaceutical Industry: A Primer*. Sudbury, MA: Jones and Bartlett, 2010. Print.
22 *Guidance for Industry Premarketing Risk Assessment*. Rockville, MD: U.S. Department of Health and Human Services, Food and Drug Administration, Center for Drug Evaluation and Research, 2005. Print.
23 Paul, H. "Risks vs. benefits: How a drug firm deals with disputes over its medicines." NEJM. 1979;300:1046.
24 Wardell, P., et al. "Postmarketing surveillance of new drugs II: Case study." J Clin Pharm. June 1, 1984:1.
25 Wardell, P. "Can post marketing surveillance permit earlier approval?" Drug Ther. February 1992:143.
26 Schiff, G. "Monitoring and reporting adverse drug reaction." Infusion. 1985;9(6).
27 Seligman, P. *Risk Management: The FDA Role*. Office of Pharmacoepidemiology and Statistical Science, Center for Drug Evaluation and Research. GAO, January 17, 2002.
28 Fitzgerald, G. (former FDA officer in the Center for Drug Evaluation and Research). Personal communication, 1992.
29 Dukes, M. N. G., ed. *Side Effects of Drugs Annual 8: A Worldwide Yearly Survey of New Data and Trends*. New York: Elsevier, 1984.
30 Ditto, Marie Anne. "Drug allergy." In *Patterson's Allergic Diseases*, edited by Roy Patterson, Leslie Carroll Grammer, and Paul A. Greenberger, 7th edition. Baltimore, MD: Wolters Kluwer Health/Lippincott Williams & Wilkins, 2009:238–270.
31 Likic, R., and D. B. Glibo. "Pathophysiology of allergic drug reactions." Psychatr Danub. 2019 Mar;31(Suppl 1):66–69.
32 Bohm, R., E. Proksch, T. Schwarz, and I. Cascorbi. "Drug hypersensitivity: Diagnosis, theetics, and prevention." Dtsch Arztebl Int. 2018;115:501–512.
33 Sylvia, Lynne M. "Drug allergy and pseudoallergy." In *Drug-Induced Diseases: Prevention, Detection, and Management*, edited by James E. Tisdale and Douglas A. Miller. Bethesda, MD: American Society of Health-System Pharmacists, 2005:27–50. Print.
34 Savitsky, M. E. "Recognizing hospital adverse drug reactions." J Pharm Pract. 1989;2(4):203–208.
35 Stern, R. S. "Clinical practice: Exanthematous drug eruptions." N Engl J Med. 2012 Jun 28;366(26): 2492–2501.
36 Stern, R. S. "Clinical practice: Exanthematous drug eruptions." N Engl J Med. 2012 Jun 28;366(26): 2492–2501.
37 Gruchalla, R. S., and M. Pirmohamed. "Clinical practice: Antibiotic allergy." N Engl J Med. 2006 Feb 9;354(6):601–609.
38 Gruchalla, R. S., and M. Pirmohamed. "Clinical practice: Antibiotic allergy." N Engl J Med. 2006 Feb 9;354(6):601–609.
39 Alic, Margaret. "Drug allergies/sensitivities: Information from Answers.com." Answers.com: Wiki Q&A Combined with Free Online Dictionary, Thesaurus, and Encyclopedias. Answers Corporation. Web. 13 Jan 2009. www.answers.com/topic/drug-allergies-sensitivities.
40 Alic, Margaret. "Drug allergies/sensitivities: Information from Answers.com." Answers.com: Wiki Q&A Combined with Free Online Dictionary, Thesaurus, and Encyclopedias. Answers Corporation. Web. 13 Jan 2009. www.answers.com/topic/drug-allergies-sensitivities.
41 Alic, Margaret. "Drug allergies/sensitivities: Information from Answers.com." Answers.com: Wiki Q&A Combined with Free Online Dictionary,

Thesaurus, and Encyclopedias. Answers Corporation. Web. 13 Jan 2009. www.answers.com/topic/drug-allergies-sensitivities.
42 Keim, Samuel M. "Drug allergy causes, symptoms, treatment: Drug allergy symptoms on EMedicineHealth." In *EMedicineHealth*, edited by Melissa C. Stoppler. WebMD, Inc. Web. 8 Dec 2011. www.emedicinehealth.com/drug_allergy/page3_em.htm.
43 Saff, Rebecca R., Yu Li, Nikita Santhanakrishnan, Carlos A. Camargo Jr, Kimberly G. Blumenthal, Li Zhou, and Aleena Banerji. "Identification of inpatient allergic drugs reactions using ICD-9-CM codes." J Allergy Clin Immunol Pract. 2019 Jan;7(1):259–264.
44 Ditto, Marie Anne. "Drug allergy." In *Patterson's Allergic Diseases*, edited by Roy Patterson, Leslie Carroll Grammer, and Paul A. Greenberger, 7th edition. Baltimore, MD: Wolters Kluwer Health/Lippincott Williams & Wilkins, 2009:238–270.
45 Ditto, Marie Anne. "Drug allergy." In *Patterson's Allergic Diseases*, edited by Patterson Roy, Leslie Carroll Grammer, and Paul A. Greenberger, 7th edition. Baltimore, MD: Wolters Kluwer Health/Lippincott Williams & Wilkins, 2009:238–270.
46 Ditto, Marie Anne. "Drug allergy." In *Patterson's Allergic Diseases*, edited by Roy Patterson, Leslie Carroll Grammer, and Paul A. Greenberger, 7th edition. Baltimore, MD: Wolters Kluwer Health/Lippincott Williams & Wilkins, 2009:238–270.
47 Ditto, Marie Anne. "Drug allergy." In *Patterson's Allergic Diseases*, edited by Roy Patterson, Leslie Carroll Grammer, and Paul A. Greenberger, 7th edition. Baltimore, MD: Wolters Kluwer Health/Lippincott Williams & Wilkins, 2009:238–270.
48 Ditto, Marie Anne. "Drug allergy." In *Patterson's Allergic Diseases*, edited by Roy Patterson, Leslie Carroll Grammer, and Paul A. Greenberger, 7th edition. Baltimore, MD: Wolters Kluwer Health/Lippincott Williams & Wilkins, 2009:238–270.
49 Ditto, Marie Anne. "Drug allergy." In *Patterson's Allergic Diseases*, edited by Roy Patterson, Leslie Carroll Grammer, and Paul A. Greenberger, 7th edition. Baltimore, MD: Wolters Kluwer Health/Lippincott Williams & Wilkins, 2009:238–270.
50 Ditto, Marie Anne. "Drug allergy." In *Patterson's Allergic Diseases*, edited by Roy Patterson, Leslie Carroll Grammer, and Paul A. Greenberger, 7th edition. Baltimore, MD: Wolters Kluwer Health/Lippincott Williams & Wilkins, 2009:238–270.
51 Ditto, Marie Anne. "Drug allergy." In *Patterson's Allergic Diseases*, edited by Roy Patterson, Leslie Carroll Grammer, and Paul A. Greenberger, 7th edition. Baltimore, MD: Wolters Kluwer Health/Lippincott Williams & Wilkins, 2009:238–270.
52 Stern, R. S. "Clinical practice: Exanthematous drug eruptions." N Engl J Med. 2012 Jun 28;366(26):2492–2501.
53 Stern, R. S. "Clinical practice: Exanthematous drug eruptions." N Engl J Med. 2012 Jun 28;366(26):2492–2501.
54 Ditto, Marie Anne. "Drug allergy." In *Patterson's Allergic Diseases*, edited by Roy Patterson, Leslie Carroll Grammer, and Paul A. Greenberger, 7th edition. Baltimore, MD: Wolters Kluwer Health/Lippincott Williams & Wilkins, 2009:238–270.
55 Ditto, Marie Anne. "Drug allergy." In *Patterson's Allergic Diseases*, edited by Roy Patterson, Leslie Carroll Grammer, and Paul A. Greenberger, 7th edition. Baltimore, MD: Wolters Kluwer Health/Lippincott Williams & Wilkins, 2009:238–270.
56 Ditto, Marie Anne. "Drug allergy." In *Patterson's Allergic Diseases*, edited by Roy Patterson, Leslie Carroll Grammer, and Paul A. Greenberger, 7th edition. Baltimore, MD: Wolters Kluwer Health/Lippincott Williams & Wilkins, 2009:238–270.
57 Ditto, Marie Anne. "Drug allergy." In *Patterson's Allergic Diseases*, edited by Roy Patterson, Leslie Carroll Grammer, and Paul A. Greenberger, 7th edition. Baltimore, MD: Wolters Kluwer Health/Lippincott Williams & Wilkins, 2009:238–270.
58 Ditto, Marie Anne. "Drug allergy." In *Patterson's Allergic Diseases*, edited by Roy Patterson, Leslie Carroll Grammer, and Paul A. Greenberger, 7th edition. Baltimore, MD: Wolters Kluwer Health/Lippincott Williams & Wilkins, 2009:238–270.
59 Ditto, Marie Anne. "Drug allergy." In *Patterson's Allergic Diseases*, edited by Roy Patterson, Leslie Carroll Grammer, and Paul A. Greenberger, 7th edition. Baltimore, MD: Wolters Kluwer Health/Lippincott Williams & Wilkins, 2009:238–270.
60 Ditto, Marie Anne. "Drug allergy." In *Patterson's Allergic Diseases*, edited by Roy Patterson, Leslie Carroll Grammer, and Paul A. Greenberger, 7th edition. Baltimore, MD: Wolters Kluwer Health/Lippincott Williams & Wilkins, 2009:238–270.
61 Ditto, Marie Anne. "Drug allergy." In *Patterson's Allergic Diseases*, edited by Roy Patterson, Leslie Carroll Grammer, and Paul A. Greenberger, 7th edition. Baltimore, MD: Wolters Kluwer Health/Lippincott Williams & Wilkins, 2009:238–270.
62 Ditto, Marie Anne. "Drug allergy." In *Patterson's Allergic Diseases*, edited by Roy Patterson, Leslie Carroll Grammer, and Paul A. Greenberger, 7th edition. Baltimore, MD: Wolters Kluwer Health/Lippincott Williams & Wilkins, 2009:238–270.
63 Ditto, Marie Anne. "Drug allergy." In *Patterson's Allergic Diseases*, edited by Roy Patterson, Leslie Carroll Grammer, and Paul A. Greenberger, 7th edition. Baltimore, MD: Wolters Kluwer Health/Lippincott Williams & Wilkins, 2009:238–270.
64 Ditto, Marie Anne. "Drug allergy." In *Patterson's Allergic Diseases*, edited by Roy Patterson, Leslie Carroll Grammer, and Paul A. Greenberger, 7th

edition. Baltimore, MD: Wolters Kluwer Health/Lippincott Williams & Wilkins, 2009:238–270.
65 Bala, S., J. Weaver, and K. L. Hastings. "Clinical relevance of preclinical testing for allergic side effects." Toxicology. 2005 Apr 15;209(2):195–200.
66 Ditto, Marie Anne. "Drug allergy." In *Patterson's Allergic Diseases*, edited by Roy Patterson, Leslie Carroll Grammer, and Paul A. Greenberger, 7th edition. Baltimore, MD: Wolters Kluwer Health/Lippincott Williams & Wilkins, 2009:238–270.
67 Blankenship, Crystal S. "Auditory nose and throat disorders." In *Drug-Induced Diseases: Prevention, Detection, and Management*, edited by James E. Tisdale and Douglas A. Miller. Bethesda, MD: American Society of Health-System Pharmacists, 2005:752. Print.
68 Ehrlich, Steven D. *Angioedema*. University of Maryland Medical Center, University of Maryland Medical System. Web. 23 Jan 2009. www.umm.edu/altmed/articles/angioedema-000011.htm.
69 Blankenship, Crystal S. "Auditory nose and throat disorders." In *Drug-Induced Diseases: Prevention, Detection, and Management*, edited by James E. Tisdale and Douglas A. Miller. Bethesda, MD: American Society of Health-System Pharmacists, 2005:752. Print.
70 Gibbs, Lip and Beevers. "Angioedema due to ACE inhibitors: Increased risk in patients of African origin." Br J Clin Pharmacol. 1999;48:861–865.
71 Sylvia, Lynne M. "Drug allergy and pseudoallergy." In *Drug-Induced Diseases: Prevention, Detection, and Management*, edited by James E. Tisdale and Douglas A. Miller. Bethesda, MD: American Society of Health-System Pharmacists, 2005:27–50. Print.
72 Sylvia, Lynne M. "Drug allergy and pseudoallergy." In *Drug-Induced Diseases: Prevention, Detection, and Management*, edited by James E. Tisdale and Douglas A. Miller. Bethesda, MD: American Society of Health-System Pharmacists, 2005:27–50. Print.
73 Sylvia, Lynne M. "Drug allergy and pseudoallergy." In *Drug-Induced Diseases: Prevention, Detection, and Management*, edited by James E. Tisdale and Douglas A. Miller. Bethesda, MD: American Society of Health-System Pharmacists, 2005:27–50. Print.
74 Bigby, M., S. Jick, H. Jick, and K. Arndt. "Drug-induced cutaneous reactions; a report from the Boston Collaborative Drug Surveillance Program on 152,438 consecutive in-patients, 1975 to 1982." JAMA. 1986;256:3358–3363.
75 Macy, Eric, Ripdeep Mangat, and Raoul J. Burchette. "Penicillin skin testing in advance of need: Multiyear follow-up in 568 test result-negative subjects exposed to oral penicillins." J Allergy Clin Immunol. 2003;111(5):1111–1115. Print.
76 Joint Task Force on Practice Parameters. "Disease management of drug hypersensitivity: A practice parameter." Ann Allergy Asthma Immunol. 1999;83:665–700.
77 Easterbrook, P. J., A. Waters, S. Murad, N. Ives, C. Taylor, D. King, A. Vyakarnam, and D. Thorburn. "Epidemiological risk factors for hypersensitivity reactions to abacavir." HIV Med. 2003;4:321–324.
78 Gibbs, Lip and Beevers. "Angioedema due to ACE inhibitors: Increased risk in patients of African origin." Br J Clin Pharmacol. 1999;48:861–865.
79 "Drug allergies." University of Pennsylvania Health System|Penn Medicine. Web. 9 Dec 2011. www.pennmedicine.org/encyclopedia/em_PrintArticle.aspx?gcid=000819.
80 Blumenthal, K. G., J. G. Peter, J. A. Trubiano, and E. J. Phillips. "Antibiotic allergy." Lancet. 2019 Jan 12;393(10167):183–198.
81 "Penicillin allergy—Amoxicillin allergy—Cephalosporin allergy." Allergies ó Allergy. 1 Nov 2010. Web. 9 Dec 2011. http://allergies.about.com/od/medicationallergy/a/penicillin.htm.
82 Joint Task Force on Practice Parameters; American Academy of Allergy, Asthma and Immunology; American College of Allergy, Asthma and Immunology; Joint Council of Allergy, Asthma and Immunology. "Drug allergy: An updated practice parameter." Ann Allergy Asthma Immunol. 2010 Oct;105(4):259–273.
83 Gruchalla, R. S., and M. Pirmohamed. "Clinical practice: Antibiotic allergy." N Engl J Med. 2006 Feb 9;354(6):601–609.
84 Gruchalla, R. S., and M. Pirmohamed. "Clinical practice: Antibiotic allergy." N Engl J Med. 2006 Feb 9;354(6):601–609.
85 Brackett, C. C., H. Singh, and J. H. Block. "Likelihood and mechanisms of cross-allergenicity between sulfonamide antibiotics and other drugs containing a sulfonamide functional group." Pharmacotherapy. 2004;24:856–870.
86 Knowles, S., L. Shapiro, and N. H. Shear. "Should celecoxib be contraindicated in patients who are allergic to sulfonamides? Revisiting the meaning of 'sulfa' allergy." Drug Saf. 2001;24:239–247.
87 Fuon, T. A., L. Valeryie-Allanore, P. Wolkenstein, and O. Chosidow. "Severe cutaneous adverse reactions to drugs." Lancet. 2017;390(10106):1996–2011.
88 Sylvia, Lynne M. "Drug allergy and pseudoallergy." In *Drug-Induced Diseases: Prevention, Detection, and Management*, edited by James E. Tisdale and Douglas A. Miller. Bethesda, MD: American Society of Health-System Pharmacists, 2005:27–50. Print.
89 Ditto, Marie Anne. "Drug allergy." In *Patterson's Allergic Diseases*, edited by Roy Patterson, Leslie Carroll Grammer, and Paul A. Greenberger, 7th edition. Baltimore, MD: Wolters Kluwer Health/Lippincott Williams & Wilkins, 2009:238–270.

90 https://www.acr.org/-/media/ACR/files/clinical-resources/contrast_media.pdf (2022). Accessed June 30, 2022.
91 Fowler, T., A. S. Bansal, and D. Lozadi. "Risks and management of antiepileptic drug induced skin reactions in an adult out-patient setting." Seizure Eur J Epilepsy. 2019;72:61–70.
92 Ditto, Marie Anne. "Drug allergy." In *Patterson's Allergic Diseases*, edited by Roy Patterson, Leslie Carroll Grammer, and Paul A. Greenberger, 7th edition. Baltimore, MD: Wolters Kluwer Health/Lippincott Williams & Wilkins, 2009:238–270.
93 Tripathi, A., N. T. Peters, and R. Patterson. "Chapter 16: Erythema multiforme, Stevens-Johnson syndrome, and toxic epidermal necrolysis." In *Patterson's Allergic Diseases*, edited by L. C. Grammer and P. A. Greenberger. Philadelphia: Lippincott Williams & Wilkins, 2002.
94 Margolis, Randall J., Marcia G. Tonnesen, Terence J. Harrist, Atul K. Bhan, Bruce U. Wintroub, Martin C. Mihm Jr, and Nicholas A. Soter. "Lymphocyte subsets and langerhans cells/indeterminate cells in erythema multiforme." J Invest Dermatol. 1983;81:403–406.
95 Patterson, Roy, Mark S. Dykewicz, Armand Gonzalzles, Leslie C. Grammer, David Green, Paul A. Greenberger, Kris G. McGrath, and Cheryl L. Walker. "Erythema multiforme and Stevens-Johnson syndrome, descriptive and therapeutic controversy." Chest. 1990;98:331–336.
96 Shiohara, Tetsuo, Machiko Chiba, Yukiko Tanaka, and Masaji Nagashima. "Drug-induced, photosensitive, erythema multiforme-like eruption: Possible role for cell adhesions molecules in a flare induced by Rhus dermatitis." J Am Acad Dermatol. 1990;22:647–650.
97 Levenson, D. E., K. A. Arndt, and R. S. Stern. "Cutaneous manifestations of adverse drug reactions." J Allergy Clin N Am. 1991;II(3):493–507.
98 Patterson, R., et al. "Stevens-Johnson Syndrome (SJS): Effectiveness of corticosteroids in management and recurrent SJS." Allergy Proc. 1992;13(2):89–95.
99 Patterson, R., M. Miller, and M. Kaplan. "Effectiveness of early therapy with corticosteroids in Stevens-Johnson syndrome: Experience with 41 cases and a hypothesis regarding pathogenesis." Ann Allergy. Jul 1994;73:27–34.
100 Cheriyan, Sarah, Roy Patterson, Paul A. Greenberger, Leslie C. Grammer, and John Latall. "The outcome of Stevens-Johnson syndrome treated with corticosteroids." Allergy Proc. 1995;16(4):151–155.
101 Schlienger, R. G., S. R. Knowles, and N. H. Shear. "Lamotrigine-associated anticonvulsant hypersensitivity syndrome." Neurology. 1998;51:1172–1175.
102 Tripathi, A., A. M. Ditto, and L. C. Grammer. "Corticosteroid therapy in an additional 13 cases of Stevens-Johnson syndrome: A total series of 67 cases." Allergy Asthma Proc. 2000;21:101–105.
103 Pichler, W. J. "Delayed drug hypersensitivity reactions." Ann Intern Med. 2003;139:683–693.

11 Drug-Induced Falls

James J. O'Donnell III and James T. O'Donnell

SYNOPSIS

11.1 INTRODUCTION

Falls pose a major health risk in the elderly as well as those individuals impaired by drug and alcohol. Every 15 seconds, an older adult is treated in an Emergency Department for a fall-related injury, and every 29 minutes, an older adult dies from a fall. Maintaining one's balance while walking or standing requires a complex, coordinated effort from numerous cognitive and motor functions. Both age and drug/alcohol use (or both) can impair these functions, leading to falls. As a result, falls can be a major source of liability. This chapter will discuss the various ways in which age and specific drugs lead to falls. Also, tools to assess fall risk and proper preventative strategies will be discussed.

11.2 THE DEFINITION OF FALL

The most widely accepted definition of a fall is that of the Kellogg International Working group. It defines a fall as "unintentionally coming to the ground or some lower level other than as a consequence of sustaining a violent blow, loss of consciousness, sudden onset of paralysis as in stroke or an epileptic seizure" [1]. Many researchers have used this or a broader definition of falls depending on

DOI: 10.1201/9781003615323-13

the focus of study. The broader definition of fall addresses cardiovascular events such as postural hypotension and transient ischemic attacks. There are differences in the definition and methods of recording falls. Falls resulting from environmental factors sometimes are included and excluded in the studies. Some studies count falls that lead to body contact with the floor, while others include contact with a wall.

11.3 EPIDEMIOLOGY

Falls are a serious problem for the elderly. They can result in hospitalization and often adversely continue to affect the quality of life. It is estimated that 30% of people fall at least once in a year [2, 3] and account for 85% of all injury-related admissions to hospitals [4]. The Center for Disease Control and Prevention (CDC) estimated that one out of three adults [5] and 40% of people [6] with age ≥ 65 years living at home will fall at least once each year. Falls are a common cause of debilitating injuries and loss of independence and often lead to death. The rate of falls and related complications rises with the increase in age.

11.4 CAUSES AND RISK FACTORS

There are many different causes of falls with accidents being one of the most significant causes. Impaired cognitive and motor functions are predictive of falls. These functional deficits may be due to advanced age, recreational or prescription drugs, or both. In fact, the elderly may be expected to be taking more prescription medication in comparison to younger people, making age a causative factor even in falls resulting from medication. Health Canada has published and widely disseminates a flow diagram on medications and fall risk (Figure 11.1) and a table of medications most likely associated with fall risk (Figure 11.2).

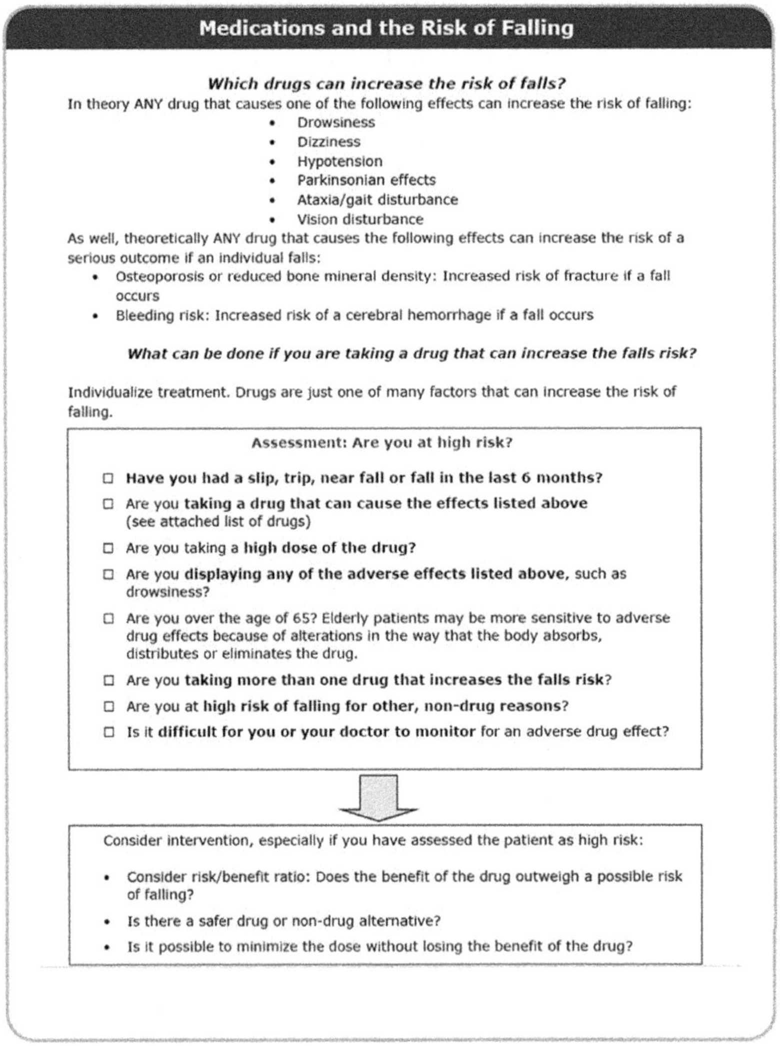

FIGURE 11.1 Flow Diagram on Medications and Fall Risk.

Medications and the Risk of Falling

Examples of drugs that can increase the risk of falling, or of a serious outcome if a fall occurs (and possible mechanisms)

ACE Inhibitors (3)
Benazepril
Captopril
Cilazapril
Enalapril/enalaprilat
Fosinopril
Lisinopril
Perindopril
Quinapril
Ramipril
Trandolapril

Alcohol (1,5)

Alpha Receptor Blockers (2,3, especially initial doses)
Alfuzosin
Doxazosin
Prazosin
Tamsulosin
Terazosin

Anticoagulants (8)
Dalteparin
Danaparoid
Enoxaparin
Heparin
Nadroparin
Nicoumalone
Tinzaparin
Warfarin

Anticonvulsants (1,2,5,6,7)
Carbamazepine (1,2,6)
Ethosuximide (1,2,5)
Fosphenytoin (1,2,5,7)
Gabapentin (1,2,5,6)
Lamotrigine (1,2,6)
Levetiracetam (1,2,5)
Methsuximide (1,2,5)
Oxcarbazepine (1,2,5,6)
Phenobarbital (1,2)
Phenytoin (1,2,5,7)
Primidone (1,2)
Topiramate (1,2)
Valproic acid (1,2,5)
Vigabatrin (1,2)

Antidepressants (1,2,3,6)
Amitriptyine
Bupropion
Citalopram
Clomipramine
Desipramine
Doxepin
Escitalopram
Fluoxetine
Fluvoxamine
Imipramine
Maprotiline
Mirtazapine
Moclobemide
Nortriptyline
Paroxetine
Phenelzine 1,2,3
Sertraline
Tranylcypromine 2,3
Trazodone
Trimipramine
Venlafaxine

Antihistamines, sedating (1)
Cold Medications that contain sedating antihistamines (1)
Azatadine
Brompheniramine
Cetirizine
Chlorpheniramine
Clemastine
Cyproheptadine
Diphenhydramine
Hydroxyzine
Meclizine
Promethazine
Trimeprazine

Antipsychotics (1,3,4)
Chlorpromazine
Clozapine
Flupenthixol
Fluphenazine
Haloperidol
Loxapine
Methotrimeprazine
Olanzapine
Paliperidone
Perphenazine
Pimozide
Pipotiazine
Prochlorperazine
Quetiapine
Risperidone
Thioproperazine
Thiothixene
Trifluoperazine
Zuclopenthixol

Corticosteroids, oral (7)
Corticosteroids, inhaled, high-dose (7)
Beclomethasone
Betamethasone
Budesonide
Cortisone
Dexamethasone
Fludrocortisone
Fluticasone
Hydrocortisone
Methylprednisolone
Prednisolone
Prednisone
Triamcinolone

Digoxin (mechanism unknown)

Eye drops (6)

Herbal and Natural health products
Natural sleep aids
Natural products for sexual enhancement (possible adulteration with undeclared drugs)

Metoclopramide (1,2,4)

Muscle Relaxants (1,2)
Baclofen
Carisoprodol
Chlorzoxazone
Cyclobenzaprine
Dantrolene
Methocarbamol
Orphenadrine
Tizanidine

Nitrates (2,3)
Isosorbide dinitrate
Isosorbide mononitrate
Nitroglycerin

NSAIDs
ASA/acetylsalicylic acid (8)

Opiates/narcotics (1,2,3)
Alfentanil
Butorphanol
Codeine
Fentanyl
Hydromorphone
Meperidine
Methadone
Morphine
Oxycodone
Oxymorphone
Nalbuphine
Pentazocine
Propoxyphene
Sufentanil

Proton Pump Inhibitors (9)
Esomeprazole
Lansoprazole
Omeprazole
Pantoprazole
Rabeprazole

Sedative/hypnotics
Benzodiazepines
Barbiturates (1,2,5)
Alprazolam
Bromazepam
Chloral hydrate
Clorazepate
Diazepam
Diphenhydramine
Doxylamine
Flurazepam
Lorazepam
Midazolam
Nitrazepam
Oxazepam
Pentobarbital
Phenobarbital
Temazepam
Triazolam
Zopiclone

Thiazolidinediones (7)
Pioglitazone
Rosiglit

Possible mechanisms (often unclear): (1) Drowsiness; (2) Dizziness; (3) Hypotension; (4) Parkinsonian effects; (5) Ataxia/gait disturbance; (6) Vision disturbance; (7) Osteoporosis or reduced bone mineral density increases the fracture risk if a fall occurs; (8) Risk of serious bleeding if a fall occurs. Drugs are listed by generic (chemical) name under each drug group. For Brand (manufacturer's) names, check in the CPS to find the generic name. This list includes only those drugs for which there is evidence of increased risk of falls or their consequences. There may be other drugs that increase this risk in certain patients.

Barbara Cadario and BC Falls and Injury Prevention Coalition. Drugs and the Risk of Falling: Guidance Document. Revised August 2011.

FIGURE 11.2 Medications Associated with Fall Risk.

11.4.1 Physiological Risk Factors for Falls in the Elderly

Increased reaction time and decreased peripheral vision significantly contribute to accident-related falls. Gait and balance problems are the next common precipitating cause of falls in the elderly. A number of studies have identified changes in gait patterns that differentiate between elderly fallers and non-fallers. These gait patterns are predictive of falling in older people. Elderly people are less likely to be able to walk fast enough to safely cross a busy intersection [7]. A number of studies have identified variability in cadence and step length in elderly patients. According to studies by Hausdorff et al., decreased ankle plantar flexor torque and increased hip flexion, hip adduction, knee extension, and knee varum ankle dorsiflexion are commonly reported in fallers [8, 9]. Impaired sensor motor function and reduced step length are associated with reduced head stability which can increase the risk of falling [10]. Tripping and slipping are the most common gait-related mechanism of falls in older people [11–14]. Ten percent of fatal falls are reported in elderly people during walking on stairs [15]. Further research is needed to determine the exact gait patterns related to postural instability and risk of fall. Dizziness is also reported as one of the major cause of falls; this symptom is commonly seen with problems like cardiovascular disorders, hyperventilation, orthostasis, drug side effect, anxiety, or depression.

Age-related decline in sensorimotor functions is also commonly seen in elderly people; it is associated with instability and contributing to falls [16]. Impairment in physiological systems such as vestibular sense, peripheral sensation, vision, and reaction time is a common predictor of falls in elderly people. Some studies have found a significant association [17–19] between visual field loss and falls but the other did not (21).

Some studies have shown an association of reduced peripheral sensation with falls. Reduced proprioceptive acuity at the knee [20], sensory abnormalities [21], and peripheral neuropathy [22] are associated with the risk of falls. Vestibular system is important in maintaining posture through the vestibulo-ocular and vestibulo-spinal pathways [23]. Vestibular asymmetry was associated with falls in two case control studies [24, 25]. It has been found that muscle strength declines with age in both sexes [26]. Few studies [25, 27] have shown that lower limb muscle weakness is a major risk factor for falling in older people. These studies demonstrated that ankle muscle weakness was a significant contributor to falls in the elderly [28]. Increased reaction time is also associated with the risk of falls in the older community [29]. Elderly people who report slow reaction time are more susceptible to falls. Thus, these studies suggest that the impairment in physiological systems contributes to falls in the elderly. Though less common in younger people, these physiological deficiencies, if present in younger people, would be also expected to contribute to falls. In particular, prescription and recreational drugs, including alcohol, would be expected to reproduce many of the physiological impairments which are present in the elderly. As such, studies of the relationship of reaction time, balance, cognitive slowness, and other deficiencies and falls in the elderly are also highly suggestive of relevance in younger people impaired by drugs.

11.4.2 Psychological Risk Factors

Attentional limitations, fear of falling, cognitive impairment, and depression are associated with impaired stability. It is evident that multi-tasking requires greater attention with a reduction in performance in primary or secondary task. Dual-tasking ability has been identified as risk factors for falls in elderly [30].

Postural and cognitive tests are important predictors of falls. In elderly people, if the primary task of maintaining postural stability is impaired, it can lead to increased risk of falls. Elderly people require more attention resources for postural control which leads to an inability to perform a cognitive (secondary) task. Performance of a cognitive task requires diversion from the postural task which may contribute to postural instability. Fear of falling causes a restriction of daily activities and contributes to prospective falls [31, 32]. Fear of falling is more common in older people, but it is not an independent risk factor for falls. It also contributes to poor health status, functional decline, and frailty.

11.4.3 Medical Conditions

Medical conditions have been reported to be associated with the risk of falls. Cerebrovascular disease such as stroke is associated with an increased risk of falls [11, 33]. People who have had a stroke are more predisposed to tripping due to lack of coordination between lower limb muscles. Parkinson's disease, dementia, and depression have all been shown to be associated with increased risk of falls. Many people with Parkinson's disease suffer from falls due to their rigid posture and abnormal gait [34]. Dementia increases the risk of falling due to cognitive impairment; it is strongly associated with falls leading to hip fractures in the elderly [35]. Studies have shown that severe depression increases the risk of multiple falls [36]. People with depression are not involved in physical activity and thus suffer from falls due to improper coordination and balance. They also exhibit higher risk of hip fracture [37]. Osteoarthritis causes reduced knee extension which increases the risk of falls in older population [36]. Studies have shown that peripheral vascular disease [38], foot problems [14] and urinary incontinence are also associated with falls [39].

11.5 MEDICATION-RELATED FALLS

Falls are one of the major problems in long-term care facilities. A large number of people suffer from injuries and fractures related to falls. A total of 10,300 fatal fall injuries and an estimated 2.6 million non-fatal fall injuries occurred in

2000 in the United Sates which incurred an estimated cost of US$179 million and US$19 billion, respectively [40]. There are a large number of studies that have focused on prescription medication like benzodiazepines, antipsychotics, antidepressants, antidepressants, and cardiovascular medications. There are several over-the-counter medications for pain, cold, and insomnia which also increase the risk of falls. These over-the-counter products contain alcohol or anticholinergics which can adversely affect the psychomotor function or can interact with other medications to increase the risk of falls.

There is an absence of good randomized controlled trial data which could provide concrete evidence to support medication-associated falls. Numerous studies [2, 11, 13, 41–60] have looked at the relationship between falls, medication, and diagnoses. These studies focused on medication use and risk of falls or fall-related fractures. The majority of the studies were observational which include 4 cross-sectional [43, 54, 55, 57], 8 case control [11, 13, 44, 46–48, 51, 52], and 15 [12, 42, 45, 49, 50, 53, 56, 58–65] cohort studies.

In the cross-sectional studies, data on falls was retrospective, and information on the current drug use was obtained from the participants. These studies were conducted in community-based settings and required the subjects to recall a fall event in the previous 12 months. Retrospective studies are subject to criticism because of the concern that one-third of older people forget about experiencing a fall one year later [66]. Researchers and clinicians should consider alternative methods to count the number of falls considering the inability of the subjects to recall past events.

Retrospective case control type studies [11, 13, 44, 46, 47, 51, 54] included hospital admissions due to injurious falls and data from medication use extracted from the prescription databases. Two of the case control studies were prospective and involved medication use in hip fracture.

Twelve of the 15 cohort studies were prospective. Participants were contacted every few months in the five community-based prospective cohort studies, and data were collected by fall calendars [58, 62, 64] and questionnaires or phone calls [42, 59]. Six of the prospective cohort studies were performed in institutional settings, and data on falls were registered by the staff of the institutional care facility [12, 45, 60, 61, 63, 65]. The several limitations observed in these studies include small sample size, questionable reliability, and confounding by indication. It is difficult to identify whether relation between falls and medication is due to the drug or the disease.

There is a concern about the reliability of the prescription records in the studies. One study [67] reported higher number of patients using benzodiazepines after serum analysis than documented in their records. The serum was tested positive in 41% of 82 community-dwelling patients; however, prescription records detected benzodiazepines usage in only 18% patients. Therefore, prescription records may not be reliable in some cases. It is also important to keep track of the individual medication on a daily basis. In one cohort study that included 2,510 nursing home residents, aged 65 years or greater [68], a high rate of misclassification was reported. Nursing home incident reports and medical records were used in identifying falls. A lot of patients had stopped some medications, or some had started new medications. There is a need for more studies to confirm the association of medication and falls.

Two meta-analyses [69] were published in 1999 by Leipzig et al. These meta-analyses showed a strong association of psychotropic drugs with falls but little or no correlation with cardiac or analgesic drugs. It was also found that multiple medications increase the risk of recurrent falls. These studies indicated that some drug classes are associated with an increase in risk of falls in older people.

11.6 TYPES OF MEDICATIONS THAT INCREASE THE RISK OF FALL

Medications which cause some effects like confusion, depression, sedation, arrhythmia, hypovolemia, orthostatic hypotension, impairment in gait and balance, and delayed reaction time increase the risk of falls. Fall-risk increasing drugs (FRIDs) include drugs for cardiovascular diseases (such as digoxin, type 1a anti-arrhythmics, and diuretics), benzodiazepines, antidepressants, antiepileptic, antipsychotics, antiparkinsonian drugs, opioids, and urological spasmolytics. Psychotropic and benzodiazepine drug use is most consistently associated with falls [70].

11.6.1 Centrally Active Medications

Psychotropic drugs include antipsychotics, anxiolytics, hypnotics, and antidepressants. They are indicated for depression, anxiety, psychosis, and sleep disorders. During the last decade, the utilization of antipsychotics and antidepressants has increased among elderly [71, 72]. Several studies have identified an increased risk of falling [73, 74] and hip fracture [75] when using psychotropic medications. The meta-analysis published by Leipzig et al. [76] also showed an association of psychotropic drugs with falls. The aim of this meta-analysis was to evaluate the association of psychotropic drugs in relation to falls in the elderly. It included 40 studies of non-randomized controlled trial. The odds ratio was calculated which showed an association between the psychotropic drugs usage and falls.

These studies have shown that psychoactive medications are associated with falls, but little work has been done to explain the physiological mechanism linked with the association of these drugs. A one-year prospective study was undertaken to identify possible mediating physiological mechanisms for the association between psychoactive medication use and falls in 414 women aged 65 to 99 years who were randomly selected from the community [77]. This study showed impaired sensori-motor measures in subjects taking psychoactive medications in comparison to control subjects. There was a relationship between factors such as tactile sensitivity, lower limb muscle strength, reaction time, and postural stability with the risk of falls. The path analysis model used in this study showed that reduced physiological functioning is involved in the fall after adjusting for the confounding factors such as increased age and inactivity.

11.6.2 Benzodiazepines

Several studies have shown an association of benzodiazepines with an increased risk of falls [12, 13, 42, 45, 50, 54–56, 58, 61–63] and hip fractures [46–48, 50–52] (see Section 11.9 for more discussion of this topic). These medications are commonly prescribed for anxiety in nursing home settings. They are commonly used for patients more than 65 years of age. In a patient cohort of patients 85 years of age or older, a study showed prescription of benzodiazepines carried a ten-fold higher risk of falls [78].

For nursing home patients, short-acting benzodiazepines are often preferred to avoid the risk of falls. A cohort study of 2,510 residents of nursing homes was conducted to determine the relationship of falls and the elimination half-life of benzodiazepines used [79]. There was a 44% increase in the risk of falls in benzodiazepines users in comparison to non-users. Risk of falls was associated with the drug elimination half-life. Overall, long-acting benzodiazepines showed higher risk compared to short-acting drugs.

However, short-acting benzodiazepines are not devoid of risk of falls. For example, short-acting benzodiazepines were associated with increased risk of nocturnal falls [79]. Some studies have shown a higher association of short-acting benzodiazepines with falls in comparison to long-acting benzodiazepines [73]. Temazepam, alprazolam, diazepam, and lorazepam, but not triazolam, chlordiazepoxide, or clorazepate were significantly associated with falls. There was 2.7 times likelihood of usage of psychotropics in fallers as identified in this study. There were no significant differences between short- and long-acting benzodiazepines users in a multicenter cohort study including community dwelling women [80].

11.6.3 Antipsychotics

Antipsychotics are commonly prescribed psychotropic medications for schizophrenia, delusional disorder, psychotic symptoms in mood disorders, and for a number of organic psychoses. A study conducted in Australia which included nursing home patients found an increased risk for falls in patients taking antipsychotic medication (odds ratio 4.4, 95% confidence interval 1.2–16.5) [44]. Confounding factors like age, sex, health status, depression, dementia, incontinence, ambulatory status, gait and balance problems, length of stay, and use of other medications were adjusted. The data includes medication used within 24 hours from the fall event. A case control study evaluating the risk of injurious falls requiring hospitalization also found significant association of antipsychotics with falls [91, 92]. Meta-analysis from Leipzig et al. also found the association of antipsychotics and falls [69]. It is always difficult to determine whether the underlying disease or the medication is involved in the increased risk of fall. A prospective six-month study in the rehabilitation setting found that antipsychotic drugs decrease the risk of falling [93].

Recently, research has focused on the association of atypical antipsychotics and falls. These drugs are widely prescribed in older people with dementia. Atypical antipsychotics are preferred over typical antipsychotics due to less risk of extrapyramidal and anticholinergic effects. Several randomized trials have shown that olanzapine and risperidone are useful for people suffering from dementia [94]. A prospective cohort study was conducted in Australia to determine whether the use of atypical antipsychotics is associated with lower risk of falls than the use of typical antipsychotics [95]. The confounding factors such as dementia and Parkinson's disease were adjusted because these conditions make one more susceptible for falls. This study did not find any difference in risk of falls associated with the use of atypical antipsychotics compared to conventional antipsychotics. Typical antipsychotics are known to cause side effects like postural hypotension and sedation. Therefore, typical and atypical antipsychotics may reasonably increase the risk of falls. The advantage of this study is the baseline evaluation of risk factors associated with fall and the short follow-up period. The participants were taking the medications at the time of evaluation. Olanzapine users were found to be more likely to fall than risperidone users. However, a major limitation of this study was the confounding by indication. Subjects with higher risk of falling were prescribed atypical antipsychotics with the belief that they cause less extrapyramidal side effects. A large epidemiological study compared the risk of fall among olanzapine and risperidone users. The percentage of people who fell was higher in the olanzapine group as compared to the risperidone group.

The risks of fall with the use of antipsychotics are more commonly seen in the long-term care facilities. However, studies conducted in the community have not found strong association of falls with antipsychotic drugs [96]. The possible reason suggested was that the number of antipsychotics were not sufficient to detect a significant relationship.

11.6.4 Antihypertensives

Antihypertensive drugs are implicated as a potential cause of falls in the elderly. There are fewer studies investigating the effects of cardiovascular medications on falls in the elderly compared to the psychotropic drugs. Diuretics were found to be weakly associated with falls in a meta-analysis published in 1999. This study included community dwelling and long-term care patients. The confounding factors were not adjusted in this study [69]. In another study published in 2004, no association was found between diuretics use and falls [97]. In contrast to these two studies, one study conducted in the UK found an association of diuretics with the risk of falls [98]. This study found an increased risk of falling from the use of diuretics within three weeks after the prescription. No risk was associated with use of calcium channel blockers, ACE inhibitors, and ARBs.

A study conducted in Japan found an increased risk of falls associated with the initial use of antihypertensives over a three-day period [99]. This study collected the data from the prescription rather than the actual usage of the medication.

A study involving 376,061 hypertensive elderly (aged ≥65 years) undergoing single-use antihypertensive drug therapy showed an association of fractures with different kind of antihypertensive [100]. The fracture rate was higher among the patients using loop diuretics (49.0 per 1000 person-years, 95% CI 46.1–52.1) in comparison to those using thiazide diuretics (28.5 per 1000 person-years, 95% CI 25.4–31.9). The subjects were identified from the Medicare administrative database and followed for more than a year. This study showed an increased association of ARBs and thiazide diuretics with the risk of fractures. Recently, HYVET trial examined the use of indapamide-sustained release dosage form with or without perindopril 2–4 mg on fractures involving hypertensive elderly aged ≥80 years [101]. A total of 3,845 participants were studied, and total of 104 fractures were reported. The results showed that a thiazide diuretic and an ACE inhibitor may decrease fracture rate. The major drawback of the study was that the data was collected after six months, and it could be possible that some of the fractures were missed. The data on the association of antihypertensive and risk of falls is conflicting, and more research needs to be done.

11.6.4.1 Orthostatic Hypotension and the Risk of Fall

Orthostatic hypotension is also known as postural hypotension. It is most commonly defined as a reduction in systolic blood pressure of at least 20 mmHg or in diastolic pressure of at least 10 mmHg occurring in response to a change from a supine to an upright position. The symptoms of orthostatic hypotension include dizziness, light headedness, or faintness during a drop in blood pressure. The prevalence of orthostatic hypotension is highly variable in the elderly because of the techniques of the blood pressure measurement. The prevalence of orthostatic hypotension varies with age and has been found to be 5–34% in community dwelling elderly people [102, 103]. A major limitation of this study that they have taken into account the drugs known to cause orthostatic hypotension. After adjusting for the confounding variables, the prevalence of orthostatic hypotension was reduced to 6% [104]. The decrease in the prevalence suggests that orthostatic hypotension might be associated with the disease or the antihypertensive medications. A study involving 3,775 women aged 60–80 years has found that the prevalence of orthostatic hypotension was 28%. This study found the association between beta blockers after adjusting for the confounding factors. Multiple comorbidities, uncontrolled hypertension, and use of multiple antihypertensives were risk factors for orthostatic hypotension [105].

Antihypertensiveness causes a variety of adverse effects like dizziness, fatigue, weakness, falls, anorexia, and orthostasis. Orthostatic hypotension is associated with patients presenting with syncope in the emergency department [106]. Antihypertensives are associated with an increased risk of orthostatic hypotension, but ACE inhibitors, angiotensin-receptor antagonists, and beta-adrenoceptor antagonists with intrinsic sympathomimetic activity are less likely to cause orthostatic hypotension [107].

Major types of antihypertensives are involved with the risk of falls. A study was conducted in 9,682 people aged more than 60 years to determine the association of antihypertensive with the risk of fall [98]. The main prescription medications included were thiazide-type diuretics, calcium channel blockers, angiotensin-converting enzyme (ACE) inhibitors, angiotensin-II receptor antagonists, and beta blockers. This large case control study showed that the risk of fall was 25% higher in people who were prescribed diuretics in comparison to nonusers. The risk of falls was higher during the first week of prescription. ACE inhibitors also increased the risk of fall, but the majority of people in this group had underlying disease that also the increased risk of fall. Beta blockers were not found to increase the risk of falls. The major advantage of this study is that data was collected prospectively and did not involve patient recall. This study found the association of diuretics with the falls during the first three weeks of exposure. The mechanism of fall was not clear.

Earlier studies found a hypotensive response during the first few weeks of diuretic use, followed by the decrease in the plasma volume and cardiac output. The blood pressure returns to the normal level after a few weeks due to the hemodynamic reaction to the volume-depleted state in one study [108]. The other possible reasons might be that the medication may have been taken off after the patients reported the problem. This study found a weak association of diuretics with the falls but, due to the high incidence of prescription, could lead to a significant effect on the population. A study involving nursing home residents who had a previous fall found that there is double risk of fall in patients who had orthostatic hypotension [109]. There was no association between the risk of falls and orthostatic hypotension in subjects who had no previous falls. The timing of orthostatic hypotension does not produce a significant impact on the fall. It might be possible that orthostatic hypotension may not be the sole factor leading to falls. The presence of other disabilities may increase risk of fall such as, for example, cerebrovascular disease leading to a decrease in the perfusion to the brain. This study found an increased risk of recurrent fall in nursing home residents who had previous fall(s) and episodes of orthostatic hypotension.

It is also believed that the treatment of hypertension by antihypertensive drugs could worsen orthostatic hypotension in elderly people, which increases risk of falls. The prevalence of orthostatic hypotension is lower in people with controlled hypertension [61]. The data are conflicting for association between falls and orthostatic hypotension. Some studies have defined orthostatic hypotension as a decrease in 20 mmHg or more in systolic BP (SBP) or a decrease of 10 mmHg or more in diastolic BP (DBP) after standing for three minutes (after rising from a supine position). Some of these studies found an association of orthostatic hypotension with fall [61, 110]. Other studies did not find any association between fall and orthostatic hypotension using this definition [111, 112]. These studies found that there was no association between falls and orthostatic hypotension in patients with controlled hypertension. These studies suggest that the treatment with antihypertensive medications may lead to orthostatic hypotension and increase the risk of falls in elderly.

More studies are required to validate the association of falls and orthostatic hypotension. Regardless, it may be wise to identify patients who are at risk of orthostatic hypotension and take preventive measures. It is necessary to provide adequate hydration and avoid using antihypertensive medications along with psychoactive medications.

11.6.5 Opioids

Opiates were associated with falls in a prospective cohort study. CNS medications are known to increase the risk of falls and fractures, but many of the relevant studies did not control for potential confounding factors. The data collected from administrative databases did not take into account the confounding variables that may modify the association of medications and fall risk like cognition, depressive symptoms, physical function, and bone mineral density [88, 113, 114]. One study has taken into account the confounding factor where the indications for use may play a role in the increased risk of falls [115]. CNS depression itself may increase the risk of falls rather than the medications itself.

A cohort study was conducted in 8,127 elderly women to examine the effects of 4 classes of medications including benzodiazepines, antidepressants, anticonvulsants, and narcotics on risk of fractures [116]. The participants were followed prospectively for incident non-spine fractures, including hip fractures. This study found an increased risk of fractures associated with narcotics. This study found slower gait speed as the mechanism for an increased risk of falls, but it should be noted that narcotic use was independently associated with the risk of any non-spine fracture despite adjustment for several potential confounders, including age, health status, estrogen use, comorbid medical conditions, physical activity, functional impairment, dizziness, fall history, depressive symptoms, weight change, neuromuscular performance, and hip bone density. Kaiko et al reported that narcotics can increase the risk of falls through CNS effects like sedation and dizziness [117]. Two other studies looked at risk of fractures with use of opioids. A study evaluated the risk of fractures with the use of opioid prescription drugs like propoxyphene and codeine [118]. The relative risk (95% CI) of hip fracture in current users of codeine or propoxyphene was 1.6 as compared to non-users. However, there was no difference between relative risks of fracture among the current users of codeine and propoxyphene. The second study found 80% association of increased risk of hip fractures with the use of opioid analgesics like propoxyphene [119]. Use of narcotics is accompanied by several side effects like low bone density, poor health status, weight loss, and impairments in neuromuscular function which may modify the association of fractures with the use of opioid analgesics. A population-based study found an increase in fracture risk at very low dose of opioids. It might be possible that the increase in fracture risk is due to the fall because the time interval was not long enough to cause any change in bone structure [120].

Opioids are used for various indications, and these drugs can increase the overall risk of fracture. Morphine and tramadol were associated with an increased risk of fracture compared to dextropropoxyphene. Despite the higher half-life of dextropropoxyphene compared to tramadol, the risk of fracture is higher with tramadol, indicating that half-life is not driving this difference. The increase in fracture might be possible due to the change in postural balance.

11.7 MARIJUANA

Marijuana is mainly obtained from hemp plant, Cannabis sativa, and contains the active cannabinoid compound tetrahydrocannabinol (THC). It has a major effect on cardiovascular system, increasing heart rate and supine blood pressure and causing postural hypotension. Marijuana can cause peripheral vasodilation, orthostatic hypotension, and tachycardia. Marijuana may exacerbate cardiovascular diseases because marijuana increases cardiac work, catecholamine levels, carboxyhemoglobin, and postural hypotension [121]. For in-depth discussions of marijuana pharmacology and intoxication, see Chapters 49 and 50 in *O'Donnell's Drug Injury*, Fourth Edition (2016), and Chapter 35 (Marijuana) in this book.

11.8 ALCOHOL

There have been 21 studies published from 1950 to 1985 on the subject of alcohol consumption and falls [122]. Type 1 studies examined the association of alcohol exposure and fall cases. It was found that 21 to 77% of fatal falls and 17–53% of non-fatal falls were related to alcohol exposure. Type II studies found that the ratio of observed to expected deaths ranged from 2.9 to 16, assessing fatal falls among alcohol users. A type IV study found the relative risk of 1, 3, and 60 at blood alcohol levels of 50–100 mg/dl, 100–150 mg/dl, and greater than 160 mg/dl, respectively. This study examined blood alcohol levels of fall subjects with respect to controls. These four types of studies have provided evidence that alcohol consumption may increase the risk for falls; however, more case control studies are needed.

A study from Brenner in 1967 reported that alcohol-dependent persons are 16 times more likely to die from a fall [123]. Alcohol was the reason behind 42% of injury fatalities and 18% of those who died of illness [124]. Epidemiological studies identifying the risk of falls from alcohol are not well-designed. The majority of these studies reported higher percentage of falls due to alcohol, but detectable blood alcohol concentrations were found in few subjects. Many studies were inconsistent in their findings regarding the association of alcohol and falls. Some of the studies did not find any association between falls and alcohol consumption in the elderly [13, 125]. In contrast, another study showed that older adults are susceptible to fall for postural imbalance due to alcohol ingestion [126].

A study was conducted to determine the cross-sectional and longitudinal associations between alcohol consumption and risk of falls in older adults. The cross-sectional analysis did not show the association between risk of falls and alcohol consumption, but longitudinal analysis indicated a 25% higher risk of fall in people who consumed more than 14 or more drinks per week (95% CI 3—52%). Several reasons have been postulated for the lack of association between risk of falls and alcohol in cohort study. It is possible that elderly people who consider themselves to be at high risk for falls may stop heavy alcohol consumption. Also, heavy drinkers do not get enrolled in cohort studies. Thus, the population of heavy drinkers is depleted due to the drinkers who had cut back on their use. This study enrolled elderly people who are healthy; disparities in health may also account for the discrepancy between cross-sectional and longitudinal analyses. Heavy drinkers with health complications might be underrepresented in cohort studies. Future long-term prospective studies are needed to confirm these findings.

Some studies examined the mechanism of falls related to alcohol. Alcohol consumption was found to be associated with postural hypotension [127], which was shown to lead to falls in the Cardiovascular Health Study [104]. Blood alcohol concentration was related to the loss of balance, leading to head and limb injury [128]. It is very important to maintain stable upright balance, and this requires coordination, feedback, and feed forward control and adaptation. The risk of falling can be predicted by the ability of the person to maintain the upright standing position [129]. Segmental body movement coordination is important for maintaining balance [130]. A study found that a blood alcohol concentration of 0.10% affected the body movement coordination pattern and adaptation. There is a correlation between the subjective feeling of drunkenness and changed upper body movements but not with the increased knee movements. It might be possible that the inability to relate the feeling of drunkenness with change in knee movements may lead to an increased risk of falls. Increased consumption of ethanol can impair the conduction of nerve impulse at the synapse [131]. This could lead to the delay in the balance responses, making balance control difficult [132]. Studies have also tried to find the severity of injury sustained during falls in alcohol-consuming patients in comparison to people who abstain from drinking. There is higher incidence of craniofacial injury in people who fall due to alcohol consumption [128]. The intoxicated patients are not able to outstretch their hands to prevent the fall, leading to more head injuries.

11.9 HIP FRACTURES

Hip fractures are one of the serious consequences of falls [133] with a lifetime incidence of 11 to 23% for women and 3 to 11% for men [134]. Hip fractures are common in elderly people more than 70 years of age. It is found that 90% of hip fractures are related to falls; another study estimated this number as 97% [137]. It is estimated that 5% of falls lead to fractures in older people [135]. Hip fractures constitute 1% of all fall incidents [136]. Hip fractures are more commonly seen in women than men [82]; the age-adjusted incidence is equal for both men and women in the institutional setting, [138] but the rate is higher for women than men in community dwellers (164). After adjusting for age and gender, the incidence is higher in institution dwellers than home dwellers (164).

Hip fractures are associated with significant morbidity and mortality. Many people die as a result of hip fracture within six months. People who survive still experience a decrease in the quality of life. It is estimated that 50% of the survivors are taken to nursing home, and half of them stay in nursing home for more than a year (92). It is one of the most common fall-related injuries that can lead to increases in the length of hospitalization, permanent disability, and death [83]. Fall-related injuries cost $19 billion in 2000 [84], and more than $8.7 billion/year was spent on hip fractures by the U.S. health care system [85]. These costs may increase in the future, as the incidence of hip fractures is estimated to increase to 2.6 and 4.5 million for the years 2025 and 2050, respectively [139].

Psychotropic drugs are known to increase the risk of hip fractures. Benzodiazepines were found to increase the risk of hip fractures in elderly by 50%, and this drug class accounts for 10% of hip fractures among community dwellers [81]. These drugs are more commonly given to the elderly and have attracted more attention in the past. Benzodiazepines are associated with many adverse events including cognitive deficits, ataxia, dysarthria, diplopia, and vertigo; as these conditions increase the risk of a fall, it is no surprise that benzodiazepines also increase the risk of falls and hip fractures. There is still controversy regarding the characteristics of benzodiazepines which increase the risk of hip fractures. Some studies in the past investigated the effect of short- and long-acting benzodiazepines on the risk of hip fracture with conflicting results. While all studies showed that both short- and long-acting benzodiazepines increased the risk of falls [86–89, 90], one large study showed that long-acting benzodiazepines carried greater increased hip fracture risk than short-acting ones [86], while other studies demonstrated that short-acting benzodiazepines carried more risk [87–89]. It was found that there is higher risk with increase in dose of benzodiazepines [88]. The risk was higher in the people who were not chronic users of the medications, and risk increases with the increase in the dose [140]. There are few studies conducted to find the association between antipsychotic use and hip fractures. A study from Ray et al. found two-fold increased risk for hip fracture with the use of conventional antipsychotics [75]. The risk was higher with prolactin-increasing antipsychotics [141].

In addition to the fall itself, a decrease in bone mineral density can make a hip fracture more likely. Alcohol consumption can affect both these factors. The association of alcohol and fractures has been inconsistent in the past. Some studies have shown higher [142, 143], lower [144, 145], or no [146, 147] association between alcohol consumption and risk for fall. These studies are limited due to the lack of number of cases. A significant U-shaped relation was found between risks of hip fracture and alcohol intake in the Cardiovascular Health Study. Alcohol intake was positively associated with bone mineral density. There was no decrease in the risk of fractures; however, it might be possible that the increased risk of fracture observed with alcohol use might be due to the effect of alcohol on cerebellar or peripheral nerve function [148, 149].

11.10 POLYPHARMACY

Polypharmacy is usually defined as the use of more than three or four medications [150]. Several studies have shown multiple medications as a risk factor for falls [44, 60, 61, 66, 96, 151–156, 180–187]. Ziere et al. conducted a study to evaluate the associations between the use of commonly taken medications and groups of medications and the risk of falls in elderly people living in the community [150]. The relative risk of a fall with the use of one, two, and three medications was 1.4, 2.2, and 2.4, respectively. Diazepam [odds ratio (OR): 3.7, 95% confidence interval (CI): 1.5–9.3], diltiazem (OR: 1.8, 95% CI: 0.8–4.1), diuretics (OR: 1.8, 95% CI: 1.2–2.8), and laxatives (OR: 2.1, 95% CI: 1.0–4.5) were associated with an increased risk of multiple falls. A study from Lawlor et al. found that risk of falls increased with the increase in the number of drugs and chronic diseases; however, a stronger association was found with multiple diseases in comparison to multiple prescriptions of drugs [157]. This study showed that polypharmacy is not an independent risk factor of falls, and the prevention of chronic diseases may be a better approach toward the prevention of falls. Sedatives/hypnotics and antidepressants were associated with increased risk of falling. The major limitation of this study was that the respondents were younger than nonrespondents and thus less likely to have a medical record of diabetes and stroke. Fall risk increases with chronic diseases, and these chronic diseases may have been underestimated due to the lack of record of the disease pathology.

It is found that polypharmacy with at least one high-risk medication is associated with an increased risk of falling [150]. Falls were more common in women than men. The risk also increased with several factors including increasing disability, staying indoors because of health, joint complaints, dizziness, gait or postural disturbance, orthostatic hypotension, history of diabetes mellitus, hypertension, Parkinson's disease, stroke, depressive episodes, and the presence of memory complaints. The odds ratio increased from 1.4 (95% CI 1.0, 2.0) to 1.6 (95% CI 1.1, 2.1) by increasing the number of drugs from 3 to 4 or more medications (p-value for trend = 0.008). Diuretics cause dizziness as a result of orthostatic hypotension, leading to a fall. Benzodiazepines affect the central nervous system and can result in a fall. The adjustment was made for comorbid conditions and disability, but polypharmacy (i.e., the number of drugs) remained a significant risk factor for falling.

The rate of adverse drug reactions is related to the number of medications. The adverse drug events may include falls, fractures, cognitive dysfunction, postural hypotension, electrolyte disorders, and cardiac failure and are responsible for up to 23% of hospital admissions in the elderly [158]. Adverse drug reactions are more common in the elderly population and result in more hospital admissions compared to other age groups [159, 160]. Elderly people use a higher number of prescription medications and are thus more likely to be affected by adverse drug reactions. Some classes of medications such as benzodiazepines, antipsychotics, and antidepressants are likely to predispose older people to falls. These drugs are an independent risk factor of falls despite adjusting for underlying disease.

11.11 FALL RISK ASSESSMENT

The incidence of falls is three times higher among older people in residential aged care settings in comparison to community settings [161]. Intrinsic and extrinsic factors can cause an increase in the risk of falls. Cognitive impairment/psychological status, acute/chronic illness and mobility, sensory deficits, and fall history are identified as some of the important intrinsic risk factors in 21 studies reviewed by Rawsky [162]. According to Robbins et al., predicted 1-year risk of falling increased from 12% in long-term care residents with no risk factors to 100% in residents who had all three risk factors (hip weakness, poor balance, and number of prescribed medications) [21]. Factors for post hospitalization such as decline in mobility, use of assistive device, cognitive impairment, and self-report of confusion are identified upon discharge from the hospital [163]. Extrinsic factors such as environmental hazards (e.g., walking on slippery/rough surfaces, obstacles, inadequate light, or loose carpets) affect most community dwelling elderly people [164]. History of a previous fall is an important predictor of falling; people with a previous fall are three times more likely to fall than people without such a history [165].

11.12 TYPES OF ASSESSMENTS

Fall risk assessment is performed to identify persons at higher risk of falls. The three most common types of assessment relevant to fall and mobility are performed on the basis of patient setting (outpatient, nursing homes, and hospitals). The first type of assessment is performed by geriatricians or nurse practitioners in the outpatient or nursing home setting to evaluate and treat patients at risk for falls or who have recently fallen. It identifies risk factors including gait and balance disorders, weakness, dizziness, environmental hazards, confusion, visual impairment, postural hypotension as well as others, leg weakness, gait and balance instability, poor vision, cognitive and functional impairment, and sedating and psychoactive medications that predispose the patients to falls, but do not provide the fall risk index [161].

The second type of assessment is completed in hospital and nursing home settings. It employs several instruments or forms to identify who is likely to fall on the basis of intrinsic or medical characteristics of the patient such as psychological status, mobility dysfunction, fall history, elimination frequency/dependence, acute/chronic illnesses, and sensory deficits. The instruments include Morse Fall Scale, STRATIFY, Resident Assessment Instrument, Fall Risk Assessment Tool, Hendrich Fall Risk Model, High Risk for Falls Assessment Form, or Royal Melbourne Hospital Risk Assessment Tool [166–169]. Nurses employ these instruments or forms after patient admission to the hospitals or long-term care facility and update them regularly.

The third type of assessment is performed by physical therapists for outpatient, community-dwelling patients regardless of medical diagnosis. These instruments include Tinetti Performance Oriented Mobility Assessment [36], Berg Balance Test [170], Functional Reach [171], or Dynamic Gait Index [172]. They measure intrinsic factors like gait and balance and require patients to walk, get up from a chair, and/or perform other functional activities.

According to a review article, the following criteria are important for choosing the most appropriate assessment tool for a specific setting: High sensitivity, specificity, and interrater reliability; similarity of patient population to ones in which the instrument was developed or studied; written procedures explicitly outlining appropriate use of the form; reasonable time required to administer the scale; and established thresholds identifying when to initiate interventions [173]. The acute care setting requires an assessment that is easy and quick to complete due to the repeated assessment required during an inpatient stay. Nursing assessment tools were found to be most appropriate in these settings. This review found 2 out of 14 assessment tools which have high sensitivity and specificity [166, 174]. The STRATIFY tool is one of the widely used tools in the hospital setting. In outpatient settings, the severity of illness and medications do not vary over a short time. Mobility and balance are quite predictive of falls, and thus functional assessment tools are more predictive of falls. Elderly Fall Screening Test [175] and the Timed Up & Go [176] have both sensitivity and specificity. In long-term care settings, a higher number of patients are at risk of falls, and hence they require precautionary measures on a large scale. Nursing assessment tools like Morse fall scale and the functional assessment instruments like Timed Up & Go are suitable in these settings. In outpatient settings, functional assessment tools are the most important because they focus on mobility and balance.

Further research is needed to determine the most important assessment tools that match the severity and changing medical condition of the patient. Often different institutions develop their own fall risk assessment scale, but they lack reliability or validity determination.

11.13 STRATEGIES FOR FALL PREVENTION IN INSTITUTIONALIZED SETTINGS

Multifaceted intervention programs are important to reduce rate of falls after fall risk screening tools identify high-risk patients. Two randomized control trials conducted in hospitals [177, 178] and three conducted in nursing homes [179–181] have found that prevention programs are essential in reducing the rate of falls.

The strategies of fall risk prevention have been incorporated into best practice guidelines by Australian Council for Safety and Quality in Health Care.

11.13.1 Screening

Elderly people who had previous falls should be questioned about falls on a periodic basis. It is important to know the complete history of the patient to determine the mechanism of falling. Fall risk screening helps in classifying people to low- and high-risk group. Elderly people admitted to the hospital should be screened for their risk of fall as soon as they are admitted. The appropriate fall risk assessment tools should be identified for the screening. The outcomes of the screen should be documented. Risk factors increase the likelihood of falls [182]; therefore, it is important to identify the risk factors.

11.13.2 Addressing Risk Factors

Interventions may be successful in preventing falls. In the case of balance and mobility limitations, walking aids are helpful. Exercise is important to prevent deterioration in motor function [177]. Cognitive impairment increases the risk factor for falls; regular checking for delirium is essential. Impaired cognition is commonly seen in people residing in residential care facilities. Vitamin D supplementation plays an important role in preventing both hospital and residential care settings. A meta-analysis examined the effectiveness of Vitamin D supplementation in preventing falls in elderly people [183]. Injury minimization by using hip protectors or vitamin D and calcium supplementation could be instituted. Physical training programs are important to improve gait, balance, mobility, and flexibility [184]. Urinary incontinence has been identified as the risk factor of falls [174] and should be treated. Walker, canes, and shoes are helpful for patient with gait and balance disturbances.

Footwear is identified as a risk factor for falls [185]. Foot and footwear should be assessed for safety during admission to hospitals. Psychoactive medications should be withdrawn gradually to reduce risk of falls and should be used cautiously with the lowest effective dose prescribed for the specific symptoms. Regular exercise reduced the risk of falls in long-term residential care facilities [186]; however, it is unclear whether the provision of exercise as a single intervention affects falls in hospital patients. Risk factors such as confusion, agitation, comorbidity, psychoactive medication use, adverse drug reactions, reduced muscle strength, poor balance, and poor vision should be addressed and treated.

11.13.2.1 Monitoring Patients

It is important to identify patient falls. Improved surveillance may reduce the risk of falls. A staff member should stay with the patient who is at an increased risk of fall. These high-risk patients should be checked regularly. The risk of falling should be flagged without interfering with the privacy of the patient.

11.13.2.2 Environmental Interventions

Environmental hazards should be minimized. Patients with limited mobility should have their personal belongings and equipment closer to them to make it easy and safe for them to access. Chairs should be height adjustable to make it easy for the person to stand up. People should have easy access to personal effects to minimize the risk of fall in an attempt to reach for them in an unsafe manner. Long handled reachers should be provided to those who can carry out their daily tasks independently. These strategies may prevent people from falling but also restrict walking, leading to reduced mobility. Hence, exercise programs should be carried out to improve mobility. It is important to ensure that the flooring pattern does not create an illusion of slope or steps for patients with impaired eyesight or cognitive impairment.

11.13.2.3 Educational Programs

It is important to provide awareness about the patient's risk factors to the hospital staff and caregivers. Hospital staff should discuss with patient caregivers about the need for close monitoring. They should not be allowed to perform the activities which increase the risk of falls.

11.13.2.4 Reducing Fall Injury

Patients' need for hip protectors should be assessed considering the patient's recent fall history, age, mobility and steadiness of gait, disability status, and whether they have osteoporosis or a low body mass index. Hospitals should be training the staff regarding the correct application of hip protectors. It is important to wear hip protectors at bedtime due to the increased risk of falling at night.

11.13.3 Discharge Planning

Interventions to reduce the risk of falls should be considered in discharge planning for patients who have an increased risk of falls during hospital admission. There are high risks of falls in patients who are functionally dependent and need professional help after discharge [163]. It should be completely assured that a person can safely manage household tasks without assistance before getting discharged from hospital. There is evidence that risk assessment and fall prevention programs are effective in reducing the risk of falls; however, benefits from interventions are generally seen after six months of implementation. More studies are needed to validate the effectiveness of fall prevention programs in elderly people with cognitive decline living in residential care facilities.

11.13.4 Disseminating Evidence: Awareness and Intervention Work!

Tinetti et al. studied fall risks and changes in rates of falls and injuries before and after the study [187]. The interventions encouraged clinicians and staff involved in outpatient rehabilitation, home care, and senior centers to implement effective risk assessments and strategies for the prevention of falls (e.g., medication reduction, balance, and gait training). The outcomes assessed included rates of serious fall-related injuries and fall-related use of medical services. Initially (prior to interventions), the adjusted rates of serious fall-related injuries were 31.2 per 1,000 person-years in the usual-care region and 31.9 in the intervention region. With the interventions and during the evaluation period, the adjusted rates were 31.4 and 28.6, respectively. Between the pre-intervention period and the evaluation period, the rate of fall-related use of medical services increased from 68.1 to 83.3 in the usual care region and from 70.7 to 74.2 in the intervention region. The total percentages of clinicians who received the interventional visits ranged from 62% to 100%. The authors concluded that the dissemination of evidence about fall prevention, in tandem with interventions to change clinical practice, may reduce fall-related injuries in the elderly.

11.14 CONCLUSIONS

The definition of a fall should be simple in order for a lay person to understand and document it. There is need for daily recording of falls, surveillance of documentation, and ascertainment of details of falls. Further research is needed to identify the mechanisms by which drug use leads to falls. Most of the studies which have examined medication use and risk of fall are observational studies. There is a need of more randomized controlled trials for assessing the reliability and validity of the association between the use of medications and falls. There is a need to include falls as an adverse effect in clinical trials of medicines intended for elderly people to examine the relationship between medications and risk of falls. There is strong evidence of an association between the use of psychotropic medications and increased risk of falls. Benzodiazepines and antipsychotics are associated with falls despite adjusting for the underlying disease. There is also evidence about the physiological mechanisms which mediate these causal connections between medications and falls. Impairment of sensorimotor systems, postural hypotension, neuromuscular incoordination, and impaired balance are physiological mechanisms that lead to medication use and falls.

Polypharmacy is considered as an important risk factor for falling. It increases the risk of the sedation, confusion, balance disorders, and complications caused by pharmacological interactions. Increased risk of falls is more likely with the polypharmacy regimen having at least one established fall-risk-increasing drug. It is important to establish a definition of polypharmacy which could be linked as a risk factor associated for fall.

Accurate assessment of risk is also important to prevent falls in people. There are a few identifiable and potentially reversible risk factors identified in multiple studies. These risk assessment tools lack validation, and the heterogeneity of settings reduces their effectiveness. It is important to develop a strategy to identify and reverse the common risk factors of falls. There is a need to consider environmental risk factors during risk assessment. Post-fall assessment, combined with the identification of modifiable risk factors, is a better strategy of reducing the risk of falls. Fall risk programs have been found to decrease rate of falls in elderly. A number of these programs have been evaluated in randomized controlled trials. Interventions are required six months in advance for better results. More studies are required to prove the usefulness of fall interventions in older people with cognitive impairment living in residential care. The individual strategies for the prevention of falls need to be tested for their cost effectiveness.

Additional readings

National Council on Aging (NCOA) Toolkit is available https://www.ncoa.org/page/falls-prevention-awareness-week-toolkit/

O'Donnell's Drug Injury, Fourth Edition, is available from L&J Publications (Tucson, Arizona) at https://www.lawyersandjudges.com/products/odonnells-drug-injury-fourth-edition?variant=25630934022

REFERENCES

1. The Prevention of Falls in Later Life. A report of the Kellogg International Work Group on the prevention of falls by the elderly. *Dan Med Bull* 1987; 34 Suppl 4: 1–24.
2. Tinetti ME, Speechley M, and Ginter SF. Risk factors for falls among elderly persons living in the community. *N Engl J Med* 1988; 319: 1701–1707.
3. O'Loughlin JLRY, Boivin JF, and Suissa S. Incidence of risk factors for falls and injurious falls among the community dwelling elderly. *Am J Epidemiol* 1993; 137: 342–354.
4. Weir E and Culmer L. Fall prevention in the elderly population. *CMAJ* 2004; 171: 724.
5. Hornbrook MC, Stevens VJ, Wingfield DJ, Hollis JF, Greenlick MR, and Ory MG. Preventing falls among community-dwelling older persons: Results from a randomized trial. *Gerontologist* 1994; 34: 16–23.
6. Rubenstein LZ. Falls in older people: Epidemiology, risk factors and strategies for prevention. *Age Ageing* 2006; 35 Suppl 2: ii37–ii41.
7. Hoxie RE and Rubenstein LZ. Are older pedestrians allowed enough time to cross intersections safely? *J Am Geriatr Soc* 1994; 42: 241–244.
8. Hausdorff JM, Edelberg HK, Mitchell SL, Goldberger AL, and Wei JY. Increased gait unsteadiness in community-dwelling elderly fallers. *Arch Phys Med Rehabil* 1997; 78: 278–283.
9. Hausdorff JM, Rios DA, and Edelberg HK. Gait variability and fall risk in community-living older adults: A 1-year prospective study. *Arch Phys Med Rehabil* 2001; 82: 1050–1056.
10. Menz HB, Lord SR, and Fitzpatrick RC. A structural equation model relating impaired sensorimotor function, fear of falling and gait patterns in older people. *Gait & Posture* 2007; 25: 243–249.
11. Prudham D and Evans JG. Factors associated with falls in the elderly: A community study. *Age Ageing* 1981; 10: 141–146.
12. Campbell AJ, Reinken J, Allan BC, and Martinez GS. Falls in old age: A study of frequency and related clinical factors. *Age Ageing* 1981; 10: 264–270.
13. Lord SR, Ward JA, Williams P, and Anstey KJ. An epidemiological study of falls in older community-dwelling women: The Randwick falls and fractures study. *Aust J Public Health* 1993; 17: 240–245.
14. Gabell A, Simons MA, and Nayak US. Falls in the healthy elderly: Predisposing causes. *Ergonomics* 1985; 28: 965–975.
15. Startzell JK, Owens DA, Mulfinger LM, and Cavanagh PR. Stair negotiation in older people: A review. *J Am Geriatr Soc* 2000; 48: 567–580.
16. Lord SR, Rogers MW, Howland A, and Fitzpatrick R. Lateral stability, sensorimotor function and falls in older people. *J Am Geriatr Soc* 1999; 47: 1077–1081.
17. Klein BE, Moss SE, Klein R, Lee KE, and Cruickshanks KJ. Associations of visual function with physical outcomes and limitations 5 years later in an older population: The Beaver Dam eye study. *Ophthalmology* 2003; 110: 644–650.
18. Felson DT, Anderson JJ, Hannan MT, Milton RC, Wilson PW, and Kiel DP. Impaired vision and hip fracture: The Framingham study. *J Am Geriatr Soc* 1989; 37: 495–500.
19. Dargent-Molina P, Favier F, Grandjean H, Baudoin C, Schott AM, Hausherr E, Meunier PJ, and Breart G. Fall-related factors and risk of hip fracture: The EPIDOS prospective study. *Lancet* 1996; 348: 145–149.
20. Hurley MV, Rees J, and Newham DJ. Quadriceps function, proprioceptive acuity and functional performance in healthy young, middle-aged and elderly subjects. *Age and Ageing* 1998; 27: 55–62.
21. Robbins AS, Rubenstein LZ, Josephson KR, Schulman BL, Osterweil D, and Fine G. Predictors of falls among elderly people: Results of two population-based studies. *Arch Intern Med* 1989; 149: 1628–1633.

22. Buchner DM and Larson EB. Falls and fractures in patients with Alzheimer-type dementia. *JAMA* 1987; 257: 1492–1495.
23. Stelmach GE and Worringham CJ. Sensorimotor deficits related to postural stability. Implications for falling in the elderly. *Clin Geriatr Med* 1985; 1: 679–694.
24. Kristinsdottir EK, Jarnlo GB, and Magnusson M. Asymmetric vestibular function in the elderly might be a significant contributor to hip fractures. *Scand J Rehabil Med* 2000; 32: 56–60.
25. Kristinsdottir EK, Nordell E, Jarnlo GB, Tjader A, Thorngren KG, and Magnusson M. Observation of vestibular asymmetry in a majority of patients over 50 years with fall-related wrist fractures. *Acta Otolaryngol* 2001; 121: 481–485.
26. MacLennan WJ, Hall MR, Timothy JI, and Robinson M. Is weakness in old age due to muscle wasting? *Age Ageing* 1980; 9: 188–192.
27. Whipple RH, Wolfson LI, and Amerman PM. The relationship of knee and ankle weakness to falls in nursing home residents: An isokinetic study. *J Am Geriatr Soc* 1987; 35: 13–20.
28. Studenski S, Duncan PW, and Chandler J. Postural responses and effector factors in persons with unexplained falls: Results and methodologic issues. *J Am Geriatr Soc* 1991; 39: 229–234.
29. Lord SR, McLean D, and Stathers G. Physiological factors associated with injurious falls in older people living in the community. *Gerontology* 1992; 38: 338–346.
30. Shumway-Cook A and Woollacott M. Attentional demands and postural control: The effect of sensory context. *J Gerontol A Biol Sci Med Sci* 2000; 55: M10–M16.
31. Murphy SL, Dubin JA, and Gill TM. The development of fear of falling among community-living older women: Predisposing factors and subsequent fall events. *J Gerontol A Biol Sci Med Sci* 2003; 58: M943–M947.
32. Lachman ME, Howland J, Tennstedt S, Jette A, Assmann S, and Peterson EW. Fear of falling and activity restriction: The survey of activities and fear of falling in the elderly (SAFE). *J Gerontol B Psychol Sci Soc Sci* 1998; 53: P43–P50.
33. Jorgensen L, Engstad T, and Jacobsen BK. Higher incidence of falls in long-term stroke survivors than in population controls: Depressive symptoms predict falls after stroke. *Stroke* 2002; 33: 542–547.
34. Paulson GW, Schafer K, and Hallum B. Avoiding mental changes and falls in older Parkinson's patients. *Geriatrics* 1986; 41: 59–62, 67.
35. Brody EM, Kleban MH, Moss MS, and Kleban F. Predictors of falls among institutionalized women with Alzheimer's disease. *J Am Geriatr Soc* 1984; 32: 877–882.
36. Tinetti ME, Williams TF, and Mayewski R. Fall risk index for elderly patients based on number of chronic disabilities. *Am J Med* 1986; 80: 429–434.
37. Whooley MA, Kip KE, Cauley JA, Ensrud KE, Nevitt MC, and Browner WS. Depression, falls, and risk of fracture in older women: Study of osteoporotic fractures research group. *Arch Intern Med* 1999; 159: 484–490.
38. Gardner AW and Montgomery PS. Impaired balance and higher prevalence of falls in subjects with intermittent claudication. *J Gerontol A Biol Sci Med Sci* 2001; 56: M454–M458.
39. Brown JS, Vittinghoff E, Wyman JF, Stone KL, Nevitt MC, Ensrud KE, and Grady D. Urinary incontinence: Does it increase risk for falls and fractures? Study of Osteoporotic Fractures Research Group. *J Am Geriatr Soc* 2000; 48: 721–725.
40. Cashin RP and Yang M. Medications prescribed and occurrence of falls in general medicine inpatients. *Can J Hosp Pharm* 2011; 64: 321–326.
41. Lee JS, Kwok T, Leung PC, and Woo J. Medical illnesses are more important than medications as risk factors of falls in older community dwellers? A cross-sectional study. *Age Ageing* 2006; 35: 246–251.
42. Fernie GR, Gryfe CI, Holliday PJ, and Llewellyn A. The relationship of postural sway in standing to the incidence of falls in geriatric subjects. *Age and Ageing* 1982; 11: 11–16.
43. Dyer CA, Taylor GJ, Reed M, Robertson DR, and Harrington R. Falls prevention in residential care homes: A randomised controlled trial. *Age and Ageing* 2004; 33: 596–602.
44. Yip YB and Cumming RG. The association between medications and falls in Australian nursing-home residents. *Med J Aust* 1994; 160: 14–18.
45. Nurmi I, Sihvonen M, Kataja M, and Luthje P. Falls among institutionalized elderly: A prospective study in four institutions in Finland. *Scand J Caring Sci* 1996; 10: 212–220.
46. Luukinen H, Koski K, Laippala P, and Kivela SL. Risk factors for recurrent falls in the elderly in long-term institutional care. *Public Health* 1995; 109: 57–65.
47. Thapa PB, Gideon P, Fought RL, and Ray WA. Psychotropic drugs and risk of recurrent falls in ambulatory nursing home residents. *Am J Epidemiol* 1995; 142: 202–211.
48. Rubenstein LZ, Josephson KR, and Robbins AS. Falls in the nursing home. *Ann Intern Med* 1994; 121: 442–451.
49. Aizen E, Shugaev I, and Lenger R. Risk factors and characteristics of falls during inpatient rehabilitation of elderly patients. *Arch Gerontol Geriatr* 2007; 44: 1–12.
50. Dromerick A and Reding M. Medical and neurological complications during inpatient stroke rehabilitation. *Stroke* 1994; 25: 358–361.
51. Teasell R, McRae M, Foley N, and Bhardwaj A. The incidence and consequences of falls in stroke patients during inpatient rehabilitation: Factors associated

with high risk. *Arch Phys Med Rehabil* 2002; 83: 329–333.
52. Nyberg L and Gustafson Y. Patient falls in stroke rehabilitation: A challenge to rehabilitation strategies. *Stroke* 1995; 26: 838–842.
53. American Geriatrics Society, British Geriatrics Society, and American Academy of Orthopaedic Surgeons Panel on Falls Prevention. Guideline for the prevention of falls in older persons. *J Am Geriatr Soc* 2001; 49: 664–672.
54. Ganz DA, Bao Y, Shekelle PG, and Rubenstein LZ. Will my patient fall? *JAMA* 2007; 297: 77–86.
55. Luukinen H, Koski K, and Jokelainen J. Temporal changes in the frequency of falling accidents among the elderly during the 1990s: A population-based study. *Public Health* 2006; 120: 418–420.
56. Kannus P, Parkkari J, Koskinen S, Niemi S, Palvanen M, Jarvinen M, and Vuori I. Fall-induced injuries and deaths among older adults. *JAMA* 1999; 281: 1895–1899.
57. Luukinen H, Koski K, Laippala P, and Kivela SL. Predictors for recurrent falls among the home-dwelling elderly. *Scand J Prim Health Care* 1995; 13: 294–299.
58. Aoyagi K, Ross PD, Davis JW, Wasnich RD, Hayashi T, and Takemoto T. Falls among community-dwelling elderly in Japan. *J Bone Miner Res* 1998; 13: 1468–1474.
59. Kallin K, Jensen J, Olsson LL, Nyberg L, and Gustafson Y. Why the elderly fall in residential care facilities, and suggested remedies. *J Fam Pract* 2004; 53: 41–52.
60. Lipsitz LA, Jonsson PV, Kelley MM, and Koestner JS. Causes and correlates of recurrent falls in ambulatory frail elderly. *J Gerontol* 1991; 46: M114–M122.
61. Campbell AJ, Borrie MJ, and Spears GF. Risk factors for falls in a community-based prospective study of people 70 years and older. *J Gerontol* 1989; 44: M112–M117.
62. Salgado RI, Lord SR, Ehrlich F, Janji N, and Rahman A. Predictors of falling in elderly hospital patients. *Arch Gerontol Geriatr* 2004; 38: 213–219.
63. Blake AJ, Morgan K, Bendall MJ, Dallosso H, Ebrahim SB, Arie TH, Fentem PH, and Bassey EJ. Falls by elderly people at home: Prevalence and associated factors. *Age Ageing* 1988; 17: 365–372.
64. Luukinen H, Koski K, Honkanen R, and Kivela SL. Incidence of injury-causing falls among older adults by place of residence: A population-based study. *J Am Geriatr Soc* 1995; 43: 871–876.
65. Downton JH and Andrews K. Prevalence, characteristics and factors associated with falls among the elderly living at home. *Aging (Milano)* 1991; 3: 219–228.
66. Cummings SR, Nevitt MC, and Kidd S. Forgetting falls: The limited accuracy of recall of falls in the elderly. *J Am Geriatr Soc* 1988; 36: 613–616.
67. Schwab M, Roder F, Aleker T, Ammon S, Thon KP, Eichelbaum M, and Klotz U. Psychotropic drug use, falls and hip fracture in the elderly. *Aging (Milano)* 2000; 12: 234–239.
68. Ray WA, Thapa PB, and Gideon P. Misclassification of current benzodiazepine exposure by use of a single baseline measurement and its effects upon studies of injuries. *Pharmacoepidemiol Drug Saf* 2002; 11: 663–669.
69. Leipzig RM, Cumming RG, and Tinetti ME. Drugs and falls in older people: A systematic review and meta-analysis: II. Cardiac and analgesic drugs. *J Am Geriatr Soc* 1999; 47: 40–50.
70. Huang AR, Mallet L, Rochefort CM, Eguale T, Buckeridge DL, and Tamblyn R. Medication-related falls in the elderly: Causative factors and preventive strategies. *Drugs Aging* 2012; 29: 359–376.
71. Trifiro G, Sini G, Sturkenboom MC, Vanacore N, Mazzaglia G, Caputi AP, Cricelli C, Brignoli O, Aguglia E, Biggio G, and Samani F. Prescribing pattern of antipsychotic drugs in the Italian general population 2000–2005: A focus on elderly with dementia. *Int Clin Psychopharmacol* 2010; 25: 22–28.
72. Rosholm JU, Gram LF, Isacsson G, Hallas J, and Bergman U. Changes in the pattern of antidepressant use upon the introduction of the new antidepressants: A prescription database study. *Eur J Clin Pharmacol* 1997; 52: 205–209.
73. Mendelson WB. The use of sedative/hypnotic medication and its correlation with falling down in the hospital. *Sleep* 1996; 19: 698–701.
74. Gales BJ and Menard SM. Relationship between the administration of selected medications and falls in hospitalized elderly patients. *Ann Pharmacother* 1995; 29: 354–358.
75. Ray WA, Griffin MR, Schaffner W, Baugh DK, and Melton LJ 3rd. Psychotropic drug use and the risk of hip fracture. *N Engl J Med* 1987; 316: 363–369.
76. Leipzig RM, Cumming RG, and Tinetti ME. Drugs and falls in older people: A systematic review and meta-analysis: I. Psychotropic drugs. *J Am Geriatr Soc* 1999; 47: 30–39.
77. Sheahan SL, Coons SJ, Robbins CA, Martin SS, Hendricks J, and Latimer M. Psychoactive medication, alcohol use, and falls among older adults. *J Behav Med* 1995; 18: 127–140.
78. Caramel VM, Remarque EJ, Knook DL, Lagaay AM, and Van den Brande KJ. Benzodiazepine users aged 85 and older fall more often. *J Am Geriatr Soc* 1998; 46: 1178–1179.
79. Ray WA, Thapa PB, and Gideon P. Benzodiazepines and the risk of falls in nursing home residents. *J Am Geriatr Soc* 2000; 48: 682–685.
80. Ensrud KE, Blackwell TL, Mangione CM, Bowman PJ, Whooley MA, Bauer DC, Schwartz AV, Hanlon JT, and Nevitt MC. Central nervous system-active medications and risk for falls in older women. *J Am Geriatr Soc* 2002; 50: 1629–1637.

81. Cumming RG and Le Couteur DG. Benzodiazepines and risk of hip fractures in older people: A review of the evidence. *CNS Drugs* 2003; 17: 825–837.
82. Melton LJ 3rd. Who has osteoporosis? A conflict between clinical and public health perspectives. *J Bone Miner Res* 2000; 15: 2309–2314.
83. Mahoney JE. Immobility and falls. *Clin Geriatr Med* 1998; 14: 699–726.
84. Stevens JA, Corso PS, Finkelstein EA, and Miller TR. The costs of fatal and non-fatal falls among older adults. *Inj Prev* 2006; 12: 290–295.
85. Ray NF, Chan JK, Thamer M, and Melton LJ 3rd. Medical expenditures for the treatment of osteoporotic fractures in the United States in 1995: Report from the National Osteoporosis Foundation. *J Bone Miner Res* 1997; 12: 24–35.
86. Ray WA, Griffin MR, and Downey W. Benzodiazepines of long and short elimination half-life and the risk of hip fracture. *JAMA* 1989; 262: 3303–3307.
87. Cumming RG and Klineberg RJ. Psychotropics, thiazide diuretics and hip fractures in the elderly. *Med J Aust* 1993; 158: 414–417.
88. Herings RM, Stricker BH, de Boer A, Bakker A, and Sturmans F. Benzodiazepines and the risk of falling leading to femur fractures: Dosage more important than elimination half-life. *Arch Intern Med* 1995; 155: 1801–1807.
89. Wang PS, Bohn RL, Glynn RJ, Mogun H, and Avorn J. Hazardous benzodiazepine regimens in the elderly: Effects of half-life, dosage, and duration on risk of hip fracture. *Am J Psychiatry* 2001; 158: 892–898.
90. Wagner AK, Zhang F, Soumerai SB, Walker AM, Gurwitz JH, Glynn RJ, and Ross-Degnan D. Benzodiazepine use and hip fractures in the elderly: Who is at greatest risk? *Arch Intern Med* 2004; 164: 1567–1572.
91. Mustard CA and Mayer T. Case-control study of exposure to medication and the risk of injurious falls requiring hospitalization among nursing home residents. *Am J Epidemiol* 1997; 145: 738–745.
92. Cumming RG. Epidemiology of medication-related falls and fractures in the elderly. *Drugs Aging* 1998; 12: 43–53.
93. Mion LC, Gregor S, Buettner M, Chwirchak D, Lee O, and Paras W. Falls in the rehabilitation setting: Incidence and characteristics. *Rehabil Nurs* 1989; 14: 17–22.
94. De Deyn PP, Rabheru K, Rasmussen A, Bocksberger JP, Dautzenberg PL, Eriksson S, and Lawlor BA. A randomized trial of risperidone, placebo, and haloperidol for behavioral symptoms of dementia. *Neurology* 1999; 53: 946–955.
95. Le Hien TT, Cumming RG, Cameron ID, Chen JS, Lord SR, March LM, Schwarz J, Le Couteur DG, and Sambrook PN. Atypical antipsychotic medications and risk of falls in residents of aged care facilities. *J Am Geriatr Soc* 2005; 53: 1290–1295.
96. Cumming RG, Miller JP, Kelsey JL, Davis P, Arfken CL, Birge SJ, and Peck WA. Medications and multiple falls in elderly people: The St Louis OASIS study. *Age Ageing* 1991; 20: 455–461.
97. Woolcott JC, Richardson KJ, Wiens MO, Patel B, Marin J, Khan KM, and Marra CA. Meta-analysis of the impact of 9 medication classes on falls in elderly persons. *Arch Intern Med* 2009; 169: 1952–1960.
98. Gribbin J, Hubbard R, Gladman JR, Smith C, and Lewis S. Risk of falls associated with antihypertensive medication: Population-based case-control study. *Age Ageing* 2010; 39: 592–597.
99. Shuto H, Imakyure O, Matsumoto J, Egawa T, Jiang Y, Hirakawa M, Kataoka Y, and Yanagawa T. Medication use as a risk factor for inpatient falls in an acute care hospital: A case-crossover study. *Br J Clin Pharmacol* 2010; 69: 535–542.
100. Solomon DH, Mogun H, Garneau K, and Fischer MA. Risk of fractures in older adults using antihypertensive medications. *J Bone Miner Res* 2011; 26: 1561–1567.
101. Peters R, Beckett N, Burch L, de Vernejoul MC, Liu L, Duggan J, Swift C, Gil-Extremera B, Fletcher A, and Bulpitt C. The effect of treatment based on a diuretic (indapamide) +/– ACE inhibitor (perindopril) on fractures in the Hypertension in the Very Elderly Trial (HYVET). *Age Ageing* 2010; 39: 609–616.
102. Masaki KH, Schatz IJ, Burchfiel CM, Sharp DS, Chiu D, Foley D, and Curb JD. Orthostatic hypotension predicts mortality in elderly men: The Honolulu Heart Program. *Circulation* 1998; 98: 2290–2295.
103. Schoenberger JA. Drug-induced orthostatic hypotension. *Drug Saf* 1991; 6: 402–407.
104. Rutan GH, Hermanson B, Bild DE, Kittner SJ, LaBaw F, and Tell GS. Orthostatic hypotension in older adults. The Cardiovascular Health Study. CHS Collaborative Research Group. *Hypertension* 1992; 19: 508–519.
105. Kamaruzzaman S, Watt H, Carson C, and Ebrahim S. The association between orthostatic hypotension and medication use in the British Women's Heart and Health Study. *Age Ageing* 2010; 39: 51–56.
106. Sarasin FP, Louis-Simonet M, Carballo D, Slama S, Junod AF, and Unger PF. Prevalence of orthostatic hypotension among patients presenting with syncope in the ED. *Am J Emerg Med* 2002; 20: 497–501.
107. Hajjar I. Postural blood pressure changes and orthostatic hypotension in the elderly patient: Impact of antihypertensive medications. *Drugs Aging* 2005; 22: 55–68.
108. Roos JC, Boer P, Koomans HA, Geyskes GG, and Dorhout Mees EJ. Haemodynamic and hormonal changes during acute and chronic diuretic treatment in essential hypertension. *Eur J Clin Pharmacol* 1981; 19: 107–112.
109. Harris T, Lipsitz LA, Kleinman JC, and Cornoni-Huntley J. Postural change in blood pressure associated

with age and systolic blood pressure. The National Health and Nutrition Examination Survey II. *J Gerontol* 1991; 46: M159–M163.
110. Graafmans WC, Ooms ME, Hofstee HM, Bezemer PD, Bouter LM, and Lips P. Falls in the elderly: A prospective study of risk factors and risk profiles. *Am J Epidemiol* 1996; 143: 1129–1136.
111. Chu LW, Chi I, and Chiu AY. Incidence and predictors of falls in the Chinese elderly. *Ann Acad Med Singapore* 2005; 34: 60–72.
112. Luukinen H, Koski K, Kivela SL, and Laippala P. Social status, life changes, housing conditions, health, functional abilities and life-style as risk factors for recurrent falls among the home-dwelling elderly. *Public Health* 1996; 110: 115–118.
113. Ray WA, Griffin MR, and Malcolm E. Cyclic antidepressants and the risk of hip fracture. *Arch Intern Med* 1991; 151: 754–756.
114. Liu B, Anderson G, Mittmann N, To T, Axcell T, and Shear N. Use of selective serotonin-reuptake inhibitors or tricyclic antidepressants and risk of hip fractures in elderly people. *Lancet* 1998; 351: 1303–1307.
115. Cumming RG, Nevitt MC, and Cummings SR. Epidemiology of hip fractures. *Epidemiol Rev* 1997; 19: 244–257.
116. Ensrud KE, Blackwell T, Mangione CM, Bowman PJ, Bauer DC, Schwartz A, Hanlon JT, Nevitt MC, and Whooley MA. Central nervous system active medications and risk for fractures in older women. *Arch Intern Med* 2003; 163: 949–957.
117. Kaiko RF, Wallenstein SL, Rogers AG, Grabinski PY, and Houde RW. Narcotics in the elderly. *Med Clin North Am* 1982; 66: 1079–1089.
118. Shorr RI, Griffin MR, Daugherty JR, and Ray WA. Opioid analgesics and the risk of hip fracture in the elderly: Codeine and propoxyphene. *J Gerontol* 1992; 47: M111–M115.
119. Guo Z, Wills P, Viitanen M, Fastbom J, and Winblad B. Cognitive impairment, drug use, and the risk of hip fracture in persons over 75 years old: A community-based prospective study. *Am J Epidemiol* 1998; 148: 887–892.
120. Vestergaard P, Rejnmark L, and Mosekilde L. Fracture risk associated with the use of morphine and opiates. *J Intern Med* 2006; 260: 76–87.
121. Jones RT. Cardiovascular system effects of marijuana. *J Clin Pharmacol* 2002; 42: 58S–63S.
122. Hingson R and Howland J. Alcohol as a risk factor for injury or death resulting from accidental falls: A review of the literature. *J Stud Alcohol* 1987; 48: 212–219.
123. Waller JA. Nonhighway injury fatalities. I. The roles of alcohol and problem drinking, drugs and medical impairment. *J Chronic Dis* 1972; 25: 33–45.
124. Lord SR, Anstey KJ, Williams P, and Ward JA. Psychoactive medication use, sensori-motor function and falls in older women. *Br J Clin Pharmacol* 1995; 39: 227–234.
125. Nelson DE, Sattin RW, Langlois JA, DeVito CA, and Stevens JA. Alcohol as a risk factor for fall injury events among elderly persons living in the community. *J Am Geriatr Soc* 1992; 40: 658–661.
126. Vogel-Sprott M and Barrett P. Age, drinking habits and the effects of alcohol. *J Stud Alcohol* 1984; 45: 517–521.
127. Burke V, Beilin LJ, German R, Grosskopf S, Ritchie J, Puddey IB, and Rogers P. Postural fall in blood pressure in the elderly in relation to drug treatment and other lifestyle factors. *Q J Med* 1992; 84: 583–591.
128. Johnston JJ and McGovern SJ. Alcohol related falls: An interesting pattern of injuries. *Emerg Med J* 2004; 21: 185–188.
129. Granata KP and Lockhart TE. Dynamic stability differences in fall-prone and healthy adults. *J Electromyogr Kinesiol* 2008; 18: 172–178.
130. Patel M, Modig F, Magnusson M, and Fransson PA. Alcohol intoxication at 0.06 and 0.10% blood alcohol concentration changes segmental body movement coordination. *Exp Brain Res* 2010; 202: 431–443.
131. Treistman SN, Bayley H, Lemos JR, Wang XM, Nordmann JJ, and Grant AJ. Effects of ethanol on calcium channels, potassium channels, and vasopressin release. *Ann N Y Acad Sci* 1991; 625: 249–263.
132. Woollacott MH. Effects of ethanol on postural adjustments in humans. *Exp Neurol* 1983; 80: 55–68.
133. Marks R, Allegrante JP, Ronald MacKenzie C, and Lane JM. Hip fractures among the elderly: Causes, consequences and control. *Ageing Res Rev* 2003; 2: 57–93.
134. Johnell O and Kanis J. Epidemiology of osteoporotic fractures. *Osteoporos Int* 2005; 16(Suppl 2): S3–S7.
135. Salva A, Bolibar I, Pera G, and Arias C. Incidence and consequences of falls among elderly people living in the community. *Med Clin (Barc)* 2004; 122: 172–176.
136. Sattin RW. Falls among older persons: A public health perspective. *Annu Rev Public Health* 1992; 13: 489–508.
137. Tamblyn R, Reid T, Mayo N, McLeod P, and Churchill-Smith M. Using medical services claims to assess injuries in the elderly: Sensitivity of diagnostic and procedure codes for injury ascertainment. *J Clin Epidemiol* 2000; 53: 183–194.
138. Lofthus CM, Osnes EK, Falch JA, Kaastad TS, Kristiansen IS, Nordsletten L, Stensvold I, and Meyer HE. Epidemiology of hip fractures in Oslo, Norway. *Bone* 2001; 29: 413–418.
139. Gullberg B, Johnell O, and Kanis JA. World-wide projections for hip fracture. *Osteoporos Int* 1997; 7: 407–413.
140. Schneeweiss S and Wang PS. Claims data studies of sedative-hypnotics and hip fractures in older people: Exploring residual confounding using survey information. *J Am Geriatr Soc* 2005; 53: 948–954.

141. Liperoti R, Onder G, Lapane KL, Mor V, Friedman JH, Bernabei R, and Gambassi G. Conventional or atypical antipsychotics and the risk of femur fracture among elderly patients: Results of a case-control study. *J Clin Psychiatry* 2007; 68: 929–934.
142. Hernandez-Avila M, Colditz GA, Stampfer MJ, Rosner B, Speizer FE, and Willett WC. Caffeine, moderate alcohol intake, and risk of fractures of the hip and forearm in middle-aged women. *Am J Clin Nutr* 1991; 54: 157–163.
143. Felson DT, Kiel DP, Anderson JJ, and Kannel WB. Alcohol consumption and hip fractures: The Framingham Study. *Am J Epidemiol* 1988; 128: 1102–1110.
144. Cummings SR, Nevitt MC, Browner WS, Stone K, Fox KM, Ensrud KE, Cauley J, Black D, and Vogt TM. Risk factors for hip fracture in white women. Study of Osteoporotic Fractures Research Group. *N Engl J Med* 1995; 332: 767–773.
145. Johnell O, Gullberg B, Kanis JA, Allander E, Elffors L, Dequeker J, Dilsen G, Gennari C, Lopes Vaz A, Lyritis G, and Mazzuoli G. Risk factors for hip fracture in European women: The MEDOS Study. Mediterranean Osteoporosis Study. *J Bone Miner Res* 1995; 10: 1802–1815.
146. Turner LW, Wang MQ, and Fu Q. Risk factors for hip fracture among southern older women. *South Med J* 1998; 91: 533–540.
147. Cumming RG and Klineberg RJ. Case-control study of risk factors for hip fractures in the elderly. *Am J Epidemiol* 1994; 139: 493–503.
148. Mukamal KJ. Alcohol consumption and abnormalities of brain structure and vasculature. *Am J Geriatr Cardiol* 2004; 13: 22–28.
149. Kucera P, Balaz M, Varsik P, and Kurca E. Pathogenesis of alcoholic neuropathy. *Bratisl Lek Listy* 2002; 103: 26–29.
150. Ziere G, Dieleman JP, Hofman A, Pols HA, van der Cammen TJ, and Stricker BH. Polypharmacy and falls in the middle age and elderly population. *Br J Clin Pharmacol* 2006; 61: 218–223.
151. Kerman M and Mulvihill M. The role of medication in falls among the elderly in a long-term care facility. *Mt Sinai J Med* 1990; 57: 343–347.
152. Neutel CI, Perry S, and Maxwell C. Medication use and risk of falls. *Pharmacoepidemiol Drug Saf* 2002; 11: 97–104.
153. Ebly EM, Hogan DB, and Fung TS. Potential adverse outcomes of psychotropic and narcotic drug use in Canadian seniors. *J Clin Epidemiol* 1997; 50: 857–863.
154. Wells BG, Middleton B, Lawrence G, Lillard D, and Safarik J. Factors associated with the elderly falling in intermediate care facilities. *Drug Intell Clin Pharm* 1985; 19: 142–145.
155. Close JC, Hooper R, Glucksman E, Jackson SH, and Swift CG. Predictors of falls in a high risk population: Results from the prevention of falls in the elderly trial (PROFET). *Emerg Med J* 2003; 20: 421–425.
156. Lim KD, Ng KC, Ng SK, and Ng LL. Falls amongst institutionalised psycho-geriatric patients. *Singapore Med J* 2001; 42: 466–472.
157. Lawlor DA, Patel R, and Ebrahim S. Association between falls in elderly women and chronic diseases and drug use: Cross sectional study. *BMJ* 2003; 327: 712–717.
158. Grymonpre RE, Mitenko PA, Sitar DS, Aoki FY, and Montgomery PR. Drug-associated hospital admissions in older medical patients. *J Am Geriatr Soc* 1988; 36: 1092–1098.
159. Chutka DS, Evans JM, Fleming KC, and Mikkelson KG. Symposium on geriatrics: Part I: Drug prescribing for elderly patients. *Mayo Clin Proc* 1995; 70: 685–693.
160. Pouyanne P, Haramburu F, Imbs JL, and Begaud B. Admissions to hospital caused by adverse drug reactions: Cross sectional incidence study. French Pharmacovigilance Centres. *BMJ* 2000; 320: 1036.
161. Rubenstein LZ, Josephson KR, and Osterweil D. Falls and fall prevention in the nursing home. *Clin Geriatr Med* 1996; 12: 881–902.
162. Rawsky E. Review of the literature on falls among the elderly. *Image J Nurs Sch* 1998; 30: 47–52.
163. Mahoney J, Sager M, Dunham NC, and Johnson J. Risk of falls after hospital discharge. *J Am Geriatr Soc* 1994; 42: 269–274.
164. Connell BR. Role of the environment in falls prevention. *Clin Geriatr Med* 1996; 12: 859–880.
165. Kiely DK, Kiel DP, Burrows AB, and Lipsitz LA. Identifying nursing home residents at risk for falling. *J Am Geriatr Soc* 1998; 46: 551–555.
166. Oliver D, Britton M, Seed P, Martin FC, and Hopper AH. Development and evaluation of evidence based risk assessment tool (STRATIFY) to predict which elderly inpatients will fall: Case-control and cohort studies. *BMJ* 1997; 315: 1049–1053.
167. Morris JN, Nonemaker S, Murphy K, Hawes C, Fries BE, Mor V, and Phillips C. A commitment to change: Revision of HCFA's RAI. *J Am Geriatr Soc* 1997; 45: 1011–1016.
168. Hendrich A, Nyhuis A, Kippenbrock T, and Soja ME. Hospital falls: Development of a predictive model for clinical practice. *Appl Nurs Res* 1995; 8: 129–139.
169. Fife DD, Solomon P, and Stanton M. A risk/falls program: Code orange for success. *Nurs Manage* 1984; 15: 50–53.
170. Berg K. Balance and its measure in the elderly: A review. *Physiother Can* 1989; 41: 240–246.
171. Duncan PW, Weiner DK, Chandler J, and Studenski S. Functional reach: A new clinical measure of balance. *J Gerontol* 1990; 45: M192–M197.
172. Whitney SL, Hudak MT, and Marchetti GF. The dynamic gait index relates to self-reported fall history in individuals with vestibular dysfunction. *J Vestib Res* 2000; 10: 99–105.
173. Perell KL, Nelson A, Goldman RL, Luther SL, Prieto-Lewis N, and Rubenstein LZ. Fall risk assessment

measures: An analytic review. *J Gerontol A Biol Sci Med Sci* 2001; 56: M761–M766.
174. Schmid NA. 1989 Federal Nursing Service Award Winner. Reducing patient falls: A research-based comprehensive fall prevention program. *Mil Med* 1990; 155: 202–207.
175. Cwikel JG, Fried AV, Biderman A, and Galinsky D. Validation of a fall-risk screening test, the Elderly Fall Screening Test (EFST), for community-dwelling elderly. *Disabil Rehabil* 1998; 20: 161–167.
176. Shumway-Cook A, Brauer S, and Woollacott M. Predicting the probability for falls in community-dwelling older adults using the Timed Up & Go Test. *Phys Ther* 2000; 80: 896–903.
177. Haines TP, Bennell KL, Osborne RH, and Hill KD. Effectiveness of targeted falls prevention program in subacute hospital setting: Randomised controlled trial. *BMJ* 2004; 328: 676.
178. Healey F, Monro A, Cockram A, Adams V, and Heseltine D. Using targeted risk factor reduction to prevent falls in older in-patients: A randomised controlled trial. *Age Ageing* 2004; 33: 390–395.
179. Jensen J, Lundin-Olsson L, Nyberg L, and Gustafson Y. Fall and injury prevention in older people living in residential care facilities: A cluster randomized trial. *Ann Intern Med* 2002; 136: 733–741.
180. Becker C, Kron M, Lindemann U, Sturm E, Eichner B, Walter-Jung B, and Nikolaus T. Effectiveness of a multifaceted intervention on falls in nursing home residents. *J Am Geriatr Soc* 2003; 51: 306–313.
181. Ray WA, Taylor JA, Meador KG, Thapa PB, Brown AK, Kajihara HK, Davis C, Gideon P, and Griffin MR. A randomized trial of a consultation service to reduce falls in nursing homes. *JAMA* 1997; 278: 557–562.
182. Tinetti ME, Doucette J, Claus E, and Marottoli R. Risk factors for serious injury during falls by older persons in the community. *J Am Geriatr Soc* 1995; 43: 1214–1221.
183. Bischoff-Ferrari HA, Dawson-Hughes B, Willett WC, Staehelin HB, Bazemore MG, Zee RY, and Wong JB. Effect of Vitamin D on falls: A meta-analysis. *JAMA* 2004; 291: 1999–2006.
184. Shaw FE. Prevention of falls in older people with dementia. *J Neural Transm* 2007; 114: 1259–1264.
185. Berg WP, Alessio HM, Mills EM, and Tong C. Circumstances and consequences of falls in independent community-dwelling older adults. *Age and Ageing* 1997; 26: 261–268.
186. Schnelle JF, Kapur K, Alessi C, Osterweil D, Beck JG, Al-Samarrai NR, and Ouslander JG. Does an exercise and incontinence intervention save healthcare costs in a nursing home population? *J Am Geriatr Soc* 2003; 51: 161–168.
187. Tinetti ME, Baker DI, King M, Gottschalk M, Murphy TE, Acampora D, Carlin BP, Leo-Summers L, and Allore HG. Effect of dissemination of evidence in reducing injuries from falls. *N Engl J Med* July 17, 2008; 359: 252–261.

12 Drug-Induced Movement Disorders[1]

Jadwiga Najib and Meagan Bailey

SYNOPSIS

[1] Special thanks to Deborah A. Hall (M.D., Ph.D.) for clinical review and case reports included in this chapter.

DOI: 10.1201/9781003615323-14

12.1 INTRODUCTION

Drug-induced movement disorders (DIMDs) represent a variety of iatrogenic and clinically distinct movement disorders and are a major problem in clinical neuropsychiatry and medicine. DIMDs refer to a variety of treatment-emergent, involuntary motor symptoms including dystonia, dyskinesia, akathisia, parkinsonism, tremor, asterixis, chorea, and serotonin syndrome. DIMDs were first described in the 1950s, shortly following the introduction of antipsychotic agents, and more recently have been described with other psychotropic agents and central nervous system medications. Metoclopramide, used for gastrointestinal motor dysfunction and as an antiemetic, is now a recognized major cause of DIMDs. Although most of the offending agents are primarily characterized as dopamine receptor-blocking agents (DRBAs), which primarily block D2 receptors, various other agents including central nervous system stimulants, anticonvulsants, antidepressants, H2-receptor antagonists, antiemetics, hormones, antiarrhythmics, and calcium channel blockers can affect motor behavior and cause movement disorders. Various drugs may either cause a new movement disorder or potentially activate a subclinical degenerative process or underlying brain disorder.

To highlight that neuroleptics are one of the most important causes of DIMDs, *Diagnostic and Statistical Manual of Mental Disorders*, fifth edition, text-revised (DSM-V-TR) published by the American Psychiatric Association (APA), contains a separate section involving medication-induced movement disorders, including neuroleptic-induced parkinsonism, neuroleptic malignant syndrome, neuroleptic-induced acute dystonia, medication-induced acute akathisia, tardive dyskinesia, tardive dystonia, tardive akathisia, medication-induced postural tremor, antidepressant discontinuation syndrome, and other medication-induced movement disorders, and adverse effects of medication.[1] How best to manage DIMDs remains controversial including using the lowest effective dosage of the agent, treating the reactions with medications, and changing the neuroleptic to one with a lower potential for inducing DIMDs.

12.2 PRESENTATION

DIMDs are divided into three main categories reflecting time periods: 1) Acute and intermediate, which occur shortly following exposure to the offending agent, usually within two to five days, and quickly reach maximal severity and intensity; 2) chronic, which are non-acute syndromes that appear after variable exposure to the offending agent and last as long as the agent is administered; and 3) tardive, which appear following a long-term exposure (several months to the offending agent and continue even after the causative agent is discontinued.)[2]

The symptomatology of DIMDs is often indistinguishable from that of idiopathic movement disorders; hence the diagnosis of DIMDs requires a careful observation and description of symptoms, a thorough medication history, as well as a neurologic and general physical examination.[3,4] Recognition of the abnormal movement, as well as the identification of the temporal relationship of the initiation of therapy with a causative agent (acute onset) or exposure to such an agent within the previous several months (tardive) and the onset of the abnormal movement is important in diagnosing DIMDs.

A 2014 Centers for Disease Control (CDC) report that evaluated antipsychotics and adult emergency room visits noted that 19 percent of such visits resulted in hospitalization and 49 percent involved patients aged 19 to 44 years. When the estimated numbers of outpatient prescription visits were taken into account, antipsychotics were implicated at a three-fold higher rate than sedatives and anxiolytics, a four-fold higher rate than stimulants, and almost five-fold higher rate than antidepressants. Typical antipsychotics were implicated at almost a 3-fold higher rate than atypical antipsychotics. Movement disorders, including dystonia and trismus, were the most common adverse effects among antipsychotic-related emergency room visits.[5]

12.3 AGENTS ASSOCIATED WITH DRUG-INDUCED MOVEMENT DISORDERS

Since various medications may induce movement disorders, the estimated rates of DIMDs have been inconsistent and difficult to quantify. However, DRBAs account for most cases of DIMDs, with neuroleptics (also referred to as antipsychotics) accounting for the majority of the reported cases of DIMDs. Neuroleptics are utilized in clinical practice not only for the treatment of schizophrenia, or psychosis, but also for conditions such as various anxiety and mood disorders, including bipolar and depressive disorders. Some reports note that approximately 60 to 75 percent of patients who receive acute treatment with neuroleptic agents develop clinically significant DIMDs in one form or another, with some patients developing more than one form at the same time.[5,7] One study noted a range of 2–60 percent with typical neuroleptics and 2–3 percent with atypical neuroleptics.[8] Another study noted that nearly two-thirds (62 percent) of institutionalized chronic schizophrenic patients were known to suffer neuroleptic-induced movement disorders from conventional neuroleptics: Approximately one-quarter had parkinsonism, one-third had tardive dyskinesia, and another one-third reported akathisia.[9]

Antipsychotics work primarily by blocking dopamine neurotransmission in the brain, specifically in the mesolimbic tract. However, when dopamine blockade occurs in other dopaminergic tracts, notably in the nigrostriatal pathway, the degree of blockade is associated with the incidence of extrapyramidal syndromes (EPS). The typical antipsychotics, also referred to as conventional or first-generation antipsychotics (FGAs), have traditionally been utilized for the treatment of schizophrenia and have a narrow range between the therapeutic dose and toxicity. Typical antipsychotics exhibit a higher degree of D_2 receptor blockade than the atypical antipsychotics, and patients treated with conventional antipsychotics have been known to exhibit a higher incidence of EPS. Such variations are associated with each drug's unique pharmacology, as noted by their different degree of blockade of specific receptors, leading to differences in their potential for DIMDs. The milligram potency is highly correlated with the type of adverse effects noted with conventional antipsychotics. Low-milligram, high potency antipsychotics such as haloperidol and trifluoperazine produce more EPS but fewer anticholinergic adverse effects due to their strong activity at dopamine receptors. Whereas high-milligram, low-potency agents such as chlorpromazine and thioridazine, which have weak activity at dopamine receptors and strong activity at anticholinergic sites, produce fewer extrapyramidal side effects (EPS) but more anticholinergic adverse effects such as sedation and hypotension.[10]

Atypical antipsychotics also referred to as second-generation antipsychotics (SGAs) generally have a broader range between the dose that controls symptoms and the one that produces EPS. They have Food and Drug Administration (FDA)-approved indications for the treatment of schizophrenia, schizoaffective disorder, mood disorders including bipolar and depressive disorders, irritability in patients with autistic disorder, as well as treatment of Tourette syndrome. Additionally, many antipsychotics are being prescribed for off-label uses and in patient populations that may be particularly vulnerable to their adverse events, especially the very young and very old. The atypical antipsychotics not only are antagonists at the D_2 receptors but are also antagonists at serotonin (5-HT) receptors, particularly the 5-HT_{2A} receptors. Their effect on the 5-HT receptors has been implicated in their role for managing mood disorders, either as adjuncts to antidepressants for major depression or as monotherapy and/or adjuncts to moods stabilizers in bipolar disorders. Additionally, the degree and duration of their blockade on D_2 receptors are lessened compared to the FGAs. It is thought that this combined effect of lower degree and decreased duration of D_2 receptor blockade and their 5-HT receptor antagonism accounts for their lower risk of developing EPS as well as their antipsychotic effect. The degree to which these receptors are affected differs among the antipsychotics, and the amount of receptor blockade can also be influenced by dose. For example, increasing the dose of risperidone, a high-potency atypical antipsychotic, above 6 mg/day increases risk for EPS due to greater degree of D_2 receptor blockade.[11] Likewise, the level of EPS observed with risperidone at 16 mg/day was shown to be comparable to that observed with haloperidol at 10 mg/day.[12] High-potency typical and atypical antipsychotics are associated with a higher potential for inducing EPS, while having lower anticholinergic activity. Low-potency typical and atypical antipsychotics are noted to have more anticholinergic effects, more weight gain, dizziness, and orthostatic symptoms compared to high-potency typical and atypical antipsychotics. Both clozapine and quetiapine, two low-potency atypical antipsychotics, exhibit a broad degree of separation between efficacy and induction of EPS and hence are associated with a low risk of EPS across their entire clinical dosage range; whereas the incidence of movement disorders for risperidone, paliperidone, olanzapine, and ziprasidone appears to be dose-related as they have a narrower separation between antipsychotic effect and EPS. Thus, EPS effects may be masked at low doses and be more pronounced at the higher dosage range with some antipscyhotics.[13]

Antipsychotic-induced movement disorders are estimated to occur in 19 percent and 42 percent of patients receiving atypical and typical antipsychotic drugs, respectively.[14] Generally, the SGAs or atypical antipsychotics are associated with a lower risk for DIMDs than the conventional or typical high-potency neuroleptics (e.g., haloperidol).[15] The reduced risk of DIMDs associated with the atypical antipsychotics, when compared with the low-potency neuroleptics (e.g., chlorpromazine), appears to be less robust, with the exception of clozapine (Clozaril®) and quetiapine (Seroquel®).[16] Although as a class, atypical neuroleptics [i.e., risperidone (Risperdal®), olanzapine (Zyprexa®), ziprasidone (Geodon®), aripiprazole (Abilify®), paliperidone (Invega®), iloperidone (Fanapt®)], lumateperone (Caplyta®), Asenapine (Saphris®), lurasidone (Latuda®), cariprazine (Vraylar®), and brexpiprazole (Rexulti®) are associated with a lower risk of treatment-emergent EPS, data shows that the consistency with which atypicals cause this may be varied.[16,17] A meta-analysis noted that the relative risk for EPS among the SGAs compared to haloperidol was as follows (from least risk to highest risk): Clozapine, sertindole, olanzapine, quetiapine, aripiprazole, ziprasidone, amisulpride, zotepine, and risperidone.[17] (Sertindole, amisulpride, and zotepine are not commercially available in the United States, and the analysis did not include some of the more recently approved SGAs.) In another meta-analysis, risperidone was associated with more use of anti-parkinsonian medication than clozapine, olanzapine, quetiapine, and ziprasidone. Ziprasidone was associated with more use of anti-parkinsonian medications than olanzapine and quetiapine. Quetiapine was associated with significantly less use of anti-parkinsonian medications than olanzapine, risperidone, or ziprasidone.[18] Data on the newest agents, namely asenapine, brexpiprazole, iloperidone, lurasidone, paliperidone, lumateperone, and cariprazine, is limited. Since paliperidone is the active metabolite of risperidone, its EPS profile is similar to that of risperidone.[19,20]

Data from the Clinical Antipsychotic Trials of Intervention Effectiveness (CATIE) in schizophrenia showed that patients treated with perphenazine, a conventional typical high-potency agent, had the highest rate of drug discontinuation due to EPS (8.4 percent) than those receiving any of the atypical antipsychotics.[21] However, a secondary analysis noted no significant differences in incidence or change in rating scales for akathisia, dystonia, parkinsonism, or tardive dyskinesia when comparing the atypical antipsychotics with perphenazine or comparing between atypical antipsychotics. Thus, these findings show that atypical antipsychotics appear less advantageous in schizophrenia then they initially did, especially when compared to a typical antipsychotic (perphenazine) that is less potent than haloperidol.[22] Additionally, the advantages initially implied with atypical antipsychotics in reducing the risk of EPS may be lessened when compared with modest doses of lower potency typical antipsychotics, and that both typical and atypical antipsychotics may need to be looked as a single drug class with a potential for causing DIMDs that are dependent upon receptor-binding affinities as well as specific patient susceptibility.[23] A meta-analysis noted that the atypical antipsychotics do not necessarily have greater efficacy than their typical counterparts, with haloperidol being the predominant comparator, and that improvements in efficacy are selective at best, with all atypicals inducing EPS.[17] Some investigators have found the SGAs to be superior to the FGAs regarding quality of life issues.[24,25] However, some clinicians have noted that atypical neuroleptics did not improve the quality of life in schizophrenia more so than the typical neuroleptics.[26]

Some atypical antipsychotics have been FDA approved for indications other than psychosis. Aripiprazole, quetiapine, olanzapine and brexpiprazole have been approved for adjunctive therapy in major depressive disorder; risperidone, and aripiprazole have been approved for use in autism spectrum disorders; quetiapine, aripiprazole, lurasidone, cariprazine, as well as olanzapine in combination with fluoxetine have been approved for use in bipolar disorder. Despite FDA approval for limited diagnoses, atypical antipsychotics are also being prescribed for anxiety, insomnia, eating disorders, attention deficit hyperactivity disorder, agitation and psychosis in dementia, obsessive compulsive disorder, post-traumatic stress disorder, and substance abuse. Many of these uses have limited evidence for their effectiveness but continue to be widely prescribed. With the use of these medications increasing in these populations, DIMDs are being seen in many other patient populations.[27]

Clozapine, an atypical neuroleptic utilized at doses of 150 to 900 mg/day, produces low levels of EPS; however, it is associated with an increased incidence of anticholinergic adverse effects, weight gain and metabolic effects, seizures, sedation, orthostatic hypotension, drooling, myocarditis, and other cardiovascular and respiratory effects. Agranulocytosis, a life-threatening blood disorder, is a major treatment problem, and hence stringent blood monitoring is warranted. Clozapine, like quetiapine, can be used to effectively treat drug-induced psychosis in patients with Parkinson's disease without potentially worsening their symptoms. Clozapine appears to be the least likely to produce tardive dyskinesia and has been shown to reduce dyskinetic movements in patients with tardive dyskinesia. Thus, in some instances, it has been invoked in patients with tardive movement syndromes from exposure to other antipsychotics but who still require treatment with an antipsychotic.[28]

Most antipsychotics and antidepressants lower the seizure threshold and may cause seizures. The risk is greater with clozapine than with most other atypical antipsychotics and greater with the tricyclic antidepressants (TCAs) than with the selective serotonin reuptake inhibitors (SSRIs).[15] A retrospective cohort study of cases involving acute toxic ingestion of FGAs and SGAs noted that the odds of a major adverse outcome or death were significantly greater for the SGAs than the FGAs. The odds of respiratory depression, coma, and hypotension were higher in patients who ingested the SGAs, whereas the odds of dystonia and rigidity were higher in patients who ingested the FGAs, suggesting that the SGAs appear no safer than FGAs in case of acute overdose.[29]

A variety of other drugs have been associated with hyperkinetic movement disorders. DRBAs such as metoclopramide and prochlorperazine, commonly prescribed for nausea and vertigo, have been associated with various DIMDs. It is estimated that 1 in 500 people who take metoclopramide will likely develop EPS. The length of exposure and total cumulative exposure to metoclopramide also increase the risk of developing EPS or tardive dyskinesia.[30]

The antiepileptic drug phenytoin has been associated with chorea, dystonia, tremors, and myoclonus. Other antiepileptic drugs such as carbamazepine, oxcarbazepine, and eslicarbazepine have been associated with dystonias and myoclonus, while dyskinesias and tics have only occurred in association with carbamazepine.[31] Adrenergics, stimulants, lithium, lamotrigine, theophylline, and TCAs may cause postural tremor, a rhythmic alteration in movement. The prevalence of lithium-induced tremor is about 40 percent and may take the form of twitching in the arms and legs. TCAs and SSRIs have been reported to cause myoclonus. Oral buccal lingual dyskinesias have also been reported with oral contraceptives, fentanyl, digoxin, cimetidine, diazoxide, lithium, TCAs, and methadone.[32–34] Amiodarone, an antiarrhythmic agent, is associated with various neurological adverse effects including tremor, ataxia, and peripheral neuropathy, with the incidence of neurotoxicity reportedly varying from 3.2 to 74 percent.[35]

Anticholinergic toxicity can occur from therapeutic or toxic doses of various medications with anticholinergic properties, including antihistamines (e.g., diphenhydramine), atropine, benztropine (commonly used with neuroleptics to prevent/manage DIMDs and in patients with Parkinson's disease), oxybutynin (medication used for overactive bladder), low potency antipsychotics, TCAs, quinidine, and disopyramide. Additionally, anticholinergic toxicity may occur when diphenhydramine, benztropine, phenylpropanolamine, and salicylate or lysergic acid (LSD) are added to illegal drugs. Toxicity from anticholinergic drugs causes both central (confusion, tremor, myoclonus, agitation, seizures, coma) and peripheral effects (dry mouth, blurry vision, urinary retention, increased heart rate). Hyperthermia associated with anticholinergic toxicity may occur due to muscular rigidity secondary to agitation and seizures.[36] Midazolam, a short-acting benzodiazepine used for induction and maintenance of general anesthesia and as an adjunct to regional anesthesia, has been noted to induce muscle tremor, athetoid movements, and tonic clonic movements.[37]

DRBAs, dopamine-depleting drugs (e.g., reserpine, tetrabenazine), may be associated with drug-induced parkinsonism. SPECT imaging of the dopamine transporter may aid in determining whether the neuroleptic-induced parkinsonism is entirely drug-induced or an exacerbation of subclinical Parkinson's disease.[38]

Bupropion, an antidepressant structurally related to amphetamines and also utilized for seasonal affective disorder and smoking cessation, has been implicated in various movement disorders. A recent systematic review on this antidepressant assessed reports from 16 countries and noted its association with dyskinesia, dystonia, parkinsonism, myoclonus, tics, stuttering, rapid eye movement sleep disorders, ballism, and bruxism.[39] The same authors also reviewed pregabalin, a drug originally approved for focal-onset seizures but currently utilized for fibromyalgia, neuropathic pain associated with diabetic peripheral neuropathy, neuropathic pain associated with spinal cord injury, postherpetic neuralgia, and as an adjunctive therapy for treatment of partial seizures and noted over 300 cases from 17 countries with ataxia, tremors, myoclonus, parkinsonism, dystonia, dyskinesia, and akathisia being attributed to this medication.[40]

Although SSRI-induced movement disorders are less common, they may occur, and with the continued increasing use of SSRIs, the clinician should be aware of this complication. EPS induced by antidepressants and neuroleptics are identical in manifestation and response to treatment. In fact, the only difference between the two is that antidepressant-induced extrapyramidal symptoms (such as akathisia, bruxism, parkinsonism, or dystonia) are relatively rare and thus often underdiagnosed/misdiagnosed. It has been estimated that the risk of EPS with antidepressant use is less than 1 in 1000, and a study using a large health claims database in the United States from 2006 to 2015 noted a harmful association between the incidence of EPS and use of antidepressants, with rate ratios with respect to EPS as follows: Duloxetine (5.68), mirtazapine (3.78), citalopram (3.47), escitalopram (3.23), paroxetine (3.07), sertraline (2.57), venlafaxine (2.37), bupropion (2.31), and fluoxetine (2.03).[R] A review utilizing VigiBase®, the World Health Organization (WHO) international database of suspected adverse drug reactions to identify DIMDs, noted that citalopram, paroxetine, duloxetine, and mirtazapine were associated most frequently with DIMDs, while mirtazapine, vortioxetine, amoxapine, phenelzine, tryptophan, and fluvoxamine were associated with the highest level of movement disorders.[41] Risk factors associated with antidepressant-induced EPS appear to be similar to those risk factors associated with neuroleptic-induced EPS, which include advanced age, women, patients with Parkinson's disease, patients concurrently treated with certain psychotropics, and patients with a history of affective disorders.[42]

Abrupt discontinuation of neuroleptic medication can cause a motor withdrawal syndrome. Dyskinesia has been reported with abrupt discontinuation of clozapine, haloperidol, quetiapine, risperidone, and aripiprazole. Akathisia has also been reported after discontinuing olanzapine. Frequently, there is a resolution of these movements after a period of several weeks; however, most of this data comes from individual case reports or case series.[43,44]

12.4 RISK FACTORS

Although not all DRBAs carry the same risk for DIMDs, various populations have been determined to be at an increased risk for developing DIMDs.[45] Patients with bipolar depression are at an increased risk of acute antipsychotic-induced movement disorders. Male sex, use of FGA, and exposure to lithium have been associated with DIMDs in patients with depressive disorders.[46] Generally, the elderly have a decreased functional reserve and may be susceptible to or have neuronal loss that may render them vulnerable to the effects of the DRBAs. Additionally, advanced age may reduce the capacity for metabolizing medications, increasing the risk for EPS by increasing the levels of exposure to the offending agents. Many DRBAs can produce hyperprolactinemia, which may lead to decreased estrogen and amenorrhea, potentially increasing the risk for DIMDs in women. Patients with phenylketonuria have increased phenylalanine levels, which may predispose them to DIMDs. Diabetic patients, independent of their use of DRBAs, are at a high risk for developing DIMDs, although the risk increases with the use of these agents due to impaired glucose metabolism. Also, chronic exposure to a DRBA for more than three months puts patients at an increased risk for DIMDs. Children and adolescents, compared to adults, are more sensitive to the development of DIMDs when treated with typical antipsychotics.[47] Generally, young males are more susceptible to dystonic reactions, older patients are more likely to develop drug-induced parkinsonian symptoms, and older women are more susceptible to develop tardive dyskinesia. The duration of medication exposure and total cumulative dose of the psychotropic agents utilized seem to increase the risk of emergence of tardive dyskinesia.[48] Smoking may also increase the risk for tardive dyskinesia.[49]

12.5 SEQUELAE OF DRUG-INDUCED MOVEMENT DISORDERS

Symptoms of DIMDs involve abnormalities in the coordination and integration of body movements and can be both painful and disfiguring. Both drug-induced dystonia and dyskinesia can be very noticeable and cause patients social stigma, adding to the stigma of psychiatric illness. Patients with DIMDs may experience difficulty with social functioning, interpersonal communication, performance of motor tasks, and activities of daily living. The DIMDs can cause patient distress, impair quality of life, and in severe cases lead to secondary morbidity and even death. For example, severe drug-induced parkinsonism may impair dexterity and impinge on occupational and social activities. Higher rates of mortality and increased rates of respiratory tract infection are observed in patients with tardive dyskinesia. Akinesia is known to produce depression, fatigue, and psychomotor retardation, while akathisia has been associated with inducing anxiety, psychomotor agitation, aggression, and insomnia.[50] Anecdotal reports have linked drug-induced akathisia to violence and suicide attempts, although it is not possible to categorically prove either association.[51] Patients with DIMDs may also be less likely to adhere to a medication regimen, increasing the risk of relapse and rehospitalization. Additionally, neuroleptic-induced movement disorders are an important cause of psychiatric malpractice lawsuits.[52,53]

12.6 THEORIES OF CAUSATION

The extrapyramidal system contains multisynaptic neurons which are involved in controlling and integrating motor and cognitive function; contributing to the unconscious stability of movement and balance; and providing coordination of gait, posture, and voluntary movement. The pathophysiology of DIMDs is complex and multifactorial and not clearly understood. It is likely related to a combination of genetic predisposition, dopaminergic system hypersensitivity, overactivation of the cholinergic system, and decreased function reserve. Various other hypotheses have been proposed including a dysfunction in gamma-aminobutyric acid (GABA) neurons and oxidative stress resulting in neurotoxicity. Since the use of DRBAs increases the turnover of neurotransmitters, the overproduction of free radicals created as a byproduct of catecholamine metabolism may participate in the genesis of tardive dyskinesia.[6]

The diversity in EPS potential noted with various antipsychotics is thought to be due to differences in D_2 receptor antagonism, speed of dissociation from the D_2 receptor, selectivity for limbic versus nigrostriatal D_2 receptors, and activity at other receptors, including serotonergic and or muscarinic receptors. Antipsychotics block dopamine in the mesocortical, tuberoinfundibular, nigrostriatal, and mesolimbic pathways, with the latter blockade exerting the medication's therapeutic antipsychotic effects. Traditionally, it has been postulated that greater than 75–80 percent blockade of nigrostriatal D_2 receptors is required for EPS to occur. The risk for drug-induced parkinsonism with antipsychotics appears to directly correlate to occupancy at nigrostriatal dopamine receptors, potentiating an imbalance between dopamine and acetylcholine which may result in DIMDs. Compared to the conventional antipsychotics, the atypical antipsychotics possess lower affinities for nigrostriatal dopaminergic receptors and more rapidly dissociate from the D_2 receptors. However, the risk of EPS from antipsychotics is dose-dependent and varies among drugs in the typical and atypical classes.[54]

Dopamine blockade in the mesocortical dopamine pathway and the involvement of adrenergic neurotransmitters systems, with relative excess of serotonergic activity, have been hypothesized as the underlying cause of akathisia. Support for this model is noted as akathisia is observed with the use of central acting DRBAs and serotonergic agents, such as the selective serotonin reuptake inhibitors (SSRIs). Some primary dystonias appear to be caused by specific genetic mutations, impacting dopamine D3 allele, and further research involving the genetic basis of primary dystonias will assist in understanding the pathophysiology of dystonic movement related to antipsychotics and potentially aid in suggesting effective means for treatment.[55,56]

Pharmacogenomics, the effect of genetic polymorphisms of drug-metabolizing enzymes, drug transporter, and drug target receptor genes on medication pharmacokinetics and pharmacodynamics in DIMDs, is ongoing and of interest. In single studies, genetic polymorphisms in the alpha-1A adrenergic receptor (*ADRA1A*), G-protein signaling regulator (*RGS9*), solute family carrier 19 (*SLC18A2*), cannabinoid receptor (*CNR1*), and beta-arrestin (*ARRB2*) have been associated with tardive dyskinesia (TD). Additionally, with dopamine receptor 2 (*DRD2*), an increased risk for TD was noted for carriers of the A2 allele of the TaqlA polymorphism in two meta-analyses. Additionally, the TaqlA1 allele is associated with higher prolactin levels and hyperprolactinemia-associated adverse events in patients receiving risperidone. Gene polymorphisms associated with a decreased risk of TD include manganese-dependent superoxide dismutase-2 (*MnSOD*), nitric oxide synthase 3 (*NOS3*), *CYP3A5*, serotonin receptor 2A (*5-HT2A*), and dopamine receptor 4 (*DRD4*). Likewise, variants of the ATP-Binding Cassette, subfamily B, member 1 (*ABCB1*) gene also hold promise as biomarkers for dosing considerations.[57,58] Genome-wide screening has noted that the genes associated with the gamma-aminobutyric acid (GABA) receptor signaling pathway are involved in drug-induced TD secondary to antipsychotics in patients with schizophrenia, suggesting that genetic factors may predispose to both drug-induced parkinsonism and TD.[59]

The cytochrome P450 2D6 enzyme (CYP2D6) is responsible for the metabolism of various antidepressants and neuroleptics, and many medications that are substrates for CYP2D6 (i.e., are metabolized by the enzyme) are themselves strong inhibitors of the enzyme. Medications which inhibit CYP2D6, or individuals with poor metabolizer status, may have increased serum concentrations of medications which require the enzyme for proper metabolism, and make them more susceptible to EPS. CYP2D6 is responsible for the metabolism of 1-methyl-4-phenyl-1,2,3,6-tetrahydropyridine (MPTP), a dopamine neurotoxin, which, together with its metabolite MPP+, has the ability to produce symptoms of parkinsonism and is now used on a research basis to create lab models of Parkinson's disease. Inhibition of CYP2D6 by psychotropic agents may cause the accumulation of these neurotoxins and increase the possibility of DIMDs. All SSRIs to some extent are inhibitors of CYP2D6; however, paroxetine, fluoxetine, and, its active metabolite, norfluoxetine, are potent inhibitors of this isoenzyme. Citalopram and sertraline also inhibit this enzyme but to a lesser extent. Bupropion and duloxetine, two different antidepressants, are noted to be moderate inhibitors of CYP2D6. Medications whose major metabolic pathway involves metabolism with CYP2D6 include beta-blockers, antidepressants, antipsychotics (especially risperidone), opioids, dextromethorphan (a common antitussive agent), and Class I antiarrhythmics. Additionally, aripiprazole, haloperidol, iloperidone, paliperidone, perphenazine, risperidone, and thioridazine are antipsychotics with noted elevated serum levels in CYP2D6 poor metabolizers. Concomitant use of these substrates with medications which are potent CYP2D6 inhibitors may result in increased levels of the substrates, exposing the patient to an increased risk of adverse effects.[60–62] Interestingly, most of the non-psychotropic agents that are CYP2D6 isoenzyme inhibitors induce EPS: Quinidine induces psychosis and hallucinations, quinine induces ataxia and restlessness, quinolone antibiotics may cause restlessness, captopril may induce hallucinations, lidocaine may cause psychosis and tremors, cimetidine may cause EPS and hallucinations, and dextromethorphan may induce hallucinations.[63] Ethnicity is a factor in the phenotypical variability of CYP2D6, and the prevalence of CYP2D6-poor metabolizers is approximately 7 to 10 percent in Caucasians, 3 to 8 percent in African Americans, 6 to 10 percent in Asians, and less than 0.5 percent in Japanese and Koreans. However, the occurrence of CYP2D6 ultra-rapid metabolizers appears to be greater among the individuals of North African and Middle Eastern descent. Although CYP2D6 is the main cytochrome enzyme responsible for the metabolism of many typical and atypical antipsychotics, CYP1A2 is the primary metabolizer for olanzapine and clozapine. Thioridazine and perphenazine also are metabolized by CYP1A2, in addition to CYP2D6. Smoking has been associated with accelerating the metabolism of drugs that are metabolized by CYP 1A2. Quetiapine is metabolized primarily by CYP3A4, while haloperidol and loxapine are metabolized by both CYP2D6 and CYP3A4.[60]

12.7 DRUG-INDUCED MOVEMENT DISORDERS IN CHILDREN AND ADOLESCENTS

In recent years, there has been a remarkable increase in prescription rates of psychoactive medications used in children and adolescents by both general practitioners and child psychiatrists. Stimulants, antidepressants, antipsychotics, mood-stabilizing medications including anticonvulsants, and benzodiazepines are the most commonly prescribed psychoactive medications in this patient population. Although most antipsychotics are used to treat psychotic symptoms and schizophrenia spectrum disorders, their use extends to various nonpsychotic disorders, including treatment for a variety of neuropsychiatric disorders, as well as behavioral issues in individuals with intellectual and developmental disabilities.[64]

Since safety and tolerability profiles of psychoactive medications have not been thoroughly assessed in the younger patient population, much of the current data on the prevalence of movement disorders in children and adolescents treated with neuroleptics is unsatisfying, with evidence gaps for some drugs and outcomes, especially with regards to safety outcomes.[65] One European study examined the prevalence of DIMDs, namely akathisia, parkinsonism, and tardive dyskinesia, in an adolescent population with schizophrenia and in relationship to predominantly atypical antipsychotic treatment. The number of patients treated with atypical, typical, or a combination of atypical/typical antipsychotics was 76, 10, and 7, respectively. Movement disorder symptoms were noted in 37 out of the 93 patients (40 percent), fulfilling strict/subthreshold criteria for akathisia (8 percent), parkinsonism (8 percent), or tardive dyskinesia (42 percent).[66] These prevalence rates are similar with results from other studies, noting that symptoms of movement disorders are less prevalent and less pronounced under treatment with atypical antipsychotics than with typical antipsychotics. However, some former studies have reported higher prevalence rates, namely for tardive dyskinesia, most likely because of treatment with predominately typical antipsychotics, different assessment methods, and heterogeneous patient populations which included patients suffering from intellectual disability or autism. Given the scarcity of data in managing pediatric DIMDs, recent treatment recommendations have been published in managing EPS associated with atypical antipsychotics.[67]

Another concern in children exposed to the long-term use of antipsychotics, specifically the atypicals, is the risk of the development of metabolic and endocrine dysfunction. Weight gain, hyperglycemia, and dyslipidemia (including hypercholesterolemia and hypertriglyceridemia) are associated with the use of atypical antipsychotics as well as with schizophrenic disorders.[68–70] Chronic exposure to these agents may pose a higher risk of cardiovascular morbidity and mortality in adult life. Elevated prolactin levels, often seen with typical antipsychotics and risperidone, and their possible long-term repercussions on reduced bone mineral density, hypogonadism, and sexual dysfunction remain uncertain.[65,71,72] A retrospective cohort study of over 43,000 patients between ages of 6 and 24 years who were prescribed an antipsychotic had a three-fold increased risk for type 2 diabetes within the first year of use, and there was a dose-response relationship that remained elevated for up to one year after the medications were discontinued.[73]

EPS are very rare in neonates but have been reported in babies born to mothers who received antipsychotic drugs for extended periods during pregnancy. Although metoclopramide administered to mothers in labor usually has no significant effects on newborns, a case of dystonia in a newborn due to placental transfer of metoclopramide following a single standard dose has been reported.[74]

Since DIMDs may be a result of individual vulnerability, some patients may be more susceptible to symptoms of movement disorders, just as some patients may be more susceptible to body weight gain from atypical neuroleptics. In view of the fact that the long-term safety of the application of psychoactive medications on the developing brain needs to be clarified, the risks and benefits of the treatment need to be assessed in each patient. It may be best to avoid using these agents to treat conditions in the pediatric patient population that can be adequately treated with medications presenting less risk of serious adverse effects.

A 2015 CDC report on pediatric emergency room visits due to adverse events from antipsychotics noted that atypical and typical antipsychotics were implicated in 98 percent and 83 percent, respectively. Haloperidol caused nearly 4 times more emergency room visits for adverse drug events than antipsychotics as a group, and haloperidol caused more than 5 and 13 times more DIMDs than other typical and atypical antipsychotics, respectively, relative to the number of outpatient visits at which the drugs were prescribed. Overall, emergency room visits by children and adolescents due to adverse events from antipsychotics were noted to be at a 3.8-fold higher rate than stimulants. In adolescents, antipsychotics were implicated at a rate 2.7-fold higher than antidepressants. Dystonia, EPS, and muscle spasticity were the most common events occurring in 48 percent of child and adolescent antipsychotic-related emergency room visits.[75] A study in Canada assessed the risk of movement disorders in children who received either risperidone or quetiapine, the two most frequently utilized antipsychotics prescribed to children in Canada, and noted a lower risk of EPS with the latter antipsychotic. The unadjusted and adjusted hazard ratios (95% confidence interval (CI)) for quetiapine compared to risperidone were 0.83 (0.56–1.25) and 0.53 (0.34–0.83), respectively.[76]

12.8 DRUG-INDUCED MOVEMENT DISORDERS IN THE ELDERLY

The elderly tend to have more co-morbidities and consume more drugs, including medications bought over-the-counter, than any other age group. They may have compromised renal and/or hepatic function resulting in a change in how a particular medication is metabolized (by the liver) or eliminated (by the kidney). Additionally, patients with compromised mental capacity may not adhere to their medication regimen and can require aids to improve their compliance. All these factors may make the elderly patient more prone to adverse side effects and drug interactions.

Sedation from medications, in combination with unsteadiness, may make elderly patients more prone to falls and other aspects of motor incoordination. Medications with strong anticholinergic properties can lead to confusion in the geriatric patient population and complicate delirium or dementia. Patients with Parkinson's disease may have worsening of their disease state with the use of DRBAs which may exacerbate the symptoms of parkinsonism. Debilitated patients may be at an increased risk for neuroleptic malignant syndrome.[77] DIMDs, especially tardive dyskinesia, are more persistent in the elderly than in younger patients. A report from the Agency for Healthcare Research and Quality in 2011 noted that olanzapine was associated with the greatest risk of causing EPS in elderly patients, where 1 of every 10 patients who received olanzapine experienced EPS, compared to risperidone with 1 case for every 20 patients treated.[78]

The association of higher mortality risk in dementia patients was initially noted with the typical antipsychotics and later with the atypical antipsychotics, which led the FDA to issue warnings of their use in elderly patients with dementia.[79] Antipsychotics are not approved for the treatment of dementia-related psychosis; yet, many elderly patients receive typical and atypical antipsychotics to ameliorate behavioral and psychological symptoms of dementia. Recently, pimavanserin (Nuplazid®), an atypical antipsychotic whose effects are mediated on serotonin receptors and not on dopamine receptors, was approved for the management of hallucinations associated with Parkinson's disease psychosis.[80] Compared to the typical antipsychotics, the atypical antipsychotics appear to have a lesser propensity to cause EPS when combined with the acetylcholinesterase inhibitors in managing symptoms of Alzheimer disease.[81] Their off-label use in elderly patients with dementia has led to deaths from heart-related events, such as heart failure, or infections, chiefly pneumonia, and will require drug manufacturers to label the drugs with a black box warning against such off-label use.[82,83]

A Government Accountability Office (GAO) report published in 2015 noted that approximately one-third of older adults with dementia who spent more than 100 days in a nursing home in 2012 were receiving an antipsychotic, and 14 percent of Medicare Part D enrollees with dementia who resided outside of a nursing home were prescribed an antipsychotic.[84] Antipsychotics with a high binding affinity for alpha-2-adrenergic and M1-muscarinic receptors (e.g., risperidone) have been associated with a greater risk for stroke in older patients with and without dementia. Additionally, the association appears to be dose-related and noted only in the first 28 days of antipsychotic use.[85] Data from nearly 91,000 older U.S. veterans with dementia noted that the use of haloperidol, risperidone, olanzapine, and quetiapine was associated with an increase mortality risk of 3.8 percent, 3.7 percent, 2.5 percent, and 2.0 percent, respectively. Haloperidol had the highest risk, with the number needed to harm (i.e., the number of people who had to be taking the drug in order for one of them to die within six months) being 26. Risperidone, olanzapine, and quetiapine had numbers needed to harm of 27, 40, and 50, respectively.

The concomitant use of antipsychotics with acetylcholinesterase inhibitors may enhance the neurotoxic effect of the antipsychotics.[86] A population-based cohort study of nearly 200,000 older adults noted that those prescribed an atypical antipsychotic were more likely 90 days later to have a 52 percent increased risk for a serious fall and a 50 percent increased risk for non-vertebral osteoporotic fractures. The use of antipsychotics and other drugs that may cause hypotension, orthostasis, sedation, and gait abnormalities is a concern in the elderly who are already at an increased risk for falls.[87]

12.9 ACUTE/INTERMEDIATE DRUG-INDUCED MOVEMENT DISORDERS

These DIMDs usually occur shortly after an exposure to the drug and are of such rapid evolution reaching maximal severity that patients may present to the emergency room necessitating hospitalization. Failure to accurately diagnose them and treat them appropriately may result in unnecessary pain and distress, increased morbidity, and, in severe cases, even death.[2]

12.9.1 Dystonia

12.9.1.1 Presentation

Acute dystonic reactions are manifested by an abrupt onset of sustained, often painful muscular spasms producing twisting movements and abnormal postures of the muscles of the eyes, face, neck, throat, or extremities. The symptoms are often distressing and frightening for the patient and may interfere with ambulation, respiration, vision, speaking, and swallowing. Dystonic movements may interfere with motor performance by superimposing an unwanted posture, which causes discomfort and anxiety in the affected patients. The involuntary movements could include rigid contractions and arching of the back muscles called opisthotonos; a spasm in which the eye(s) turns upward called oculogyric crisis; a spasm of the neck in which the head is turned backward or sideways, called retrocollis or torticollis, respectively; forced opening of the mouth or jaw clenching (trismus); and tongue protrusion, which may cause slurred speech due to hypertonic tongue called dysarthria and macroglossia.[6,88] Laryngospasm with compromise of the airway, which is the most severe acute dystonic reaction, may lead to stridor, dyspnea, and choking and may create a medical emergency.[79] Sustained muscle contractions may lead to aching pain and even rhabdomyolysis. These acute dystonic reactions are terrifying to the patient who has no prior experience with these problems or knowledge of this adverse effect. When a dystonic reaction does occur in a psychotic patient, the fragile trust developed between psychiatrist and patient may be irrevocably harmed, leading to a deteriorating compliance with the neuroleptic agents and further diminishing the patient's willingness to take the medications.[89] Malpractice suits are usually based on dystonic reactions that persist.

The signs or symptoms of acute dystonic reactions develop within seven days of initiating therapy or rapidly raising the dose of a neuroleptic agent or reducing a medication being used to treat or prevent acute EPS, that is, an anticholinergic agent. Over 50 percent of acute dystonic reactions occur within 48 hours, and 90 percent within five days, following the exposure to DRBAs.[90] The risk of an acute dystonic reaction dramatically decreases with the duration of therapy and is minimal beyond one month after initial therapy or dose increase. Acute dystonic reactions may also develop in the third to seventh day, following each depot neuroleptic injection.

Acute dystonic reactions last anywhere from a few seconds to several hours and may present with a diurnal variation with the symptoms being markedly worse in the afternoon and evening. Acute dystonic reactions differ from tardive dystonias in that the former are sudden in onset, cause acute discomfort and stress to the patient, and are rapidly resolved following the administration of anticholinergic agents. Dystonic movements may occur anywhere in the body and may fluctuate and spread over time to involve other parts of the body. Dystonias generally intensify during voluntary movements, excitement, nervousness, and psychological stress; they decrease during periods of relaxation and disappear during sleep. They can also occur as bursts with return to normal function between attacks, hence "paroxysmal dystonias."

Drug-induced Pisa syndrome is a rare form of dystonia characterized by sustained truncal lateroflexion and has been associated with prolonged treatment with typical and atypical antipsychotics. However, it has also been reported in patients who received cholinesterase inhibitors and antiemetics. It may occur following the addition of another neuroleptic to an established regimen of neuroleptics, or it may subtly occur in neuroleptic-treated patients. It may be acute or tardive and develops predominately in women and older patients with neurodegenerative disease.[91,92]

12.9.1.2 Implicated Agents

The reported prevalence of acute dystonic reactions in patients exposed to neuroleptics has varied with estimates ranging from a low 2.3 percent to a high 94 percent.[90] The discrepancies are most likely due to differences in the examined patient population including age and gender, concurrent treatment with other medications, the design of the study, and the type of neuroleptic drug and dosage utilized. Generally, the increased incidence of acute dystonic reactions is attributed to the more frequent use of high-potency antipsychotics and the use of higher doses. The atypical antipsychotic agents, clozapine, risperidone, olanzapine, quetiapine, aripiprazole, ziprasidone, paliperidone, and most recently iloperidone, are less likely to induce acute dystonic reactions than their typical antipsychotic counterparts at clinically effective dosages.[7] The risk of dystonias and other extrapyramidal adverse effects associated with risperidone therapy appear to be dose-related and generally observed with doses above six mg/day.[12] A Cochrane review and meta-analysis noted that dystonia was recorded for all SGA reviewed, with the exception of clozapine, for which no data was available. The review noted that the prevalence estimates of dystonia were 1.4 percent, 1.6 percent, 2.2 percent, 2.4 percent, 2.8 percent, 5.0 percent, and 5.5 percent, for quetiapine, olanzapine, ziprasidone, paliperidone, asenapine, risperidone, and aripiprazole, respectively. However, for the FGA, the prevalence percentages for chlorpromazine and haloperidol were 10.9 percent and 16.5 percent, respectively.[16]

The relationship between dose and risk of a dystonic reaction is less clear, however, as lower dosages appear to produce fewer extrapyramidal side effects than moderate dosages, and moderate dosages appear to produce more extrapyramidal adverse effects than very high doses. An inverted U-shaped curve function between the prevalence of dystonia and neuroleptic dose appears to exist. Thus, most dystonia occurs with moderate-to-high doses of neuroleptics, while the very low doses and the very high doses of neuroleptics (approximately over 2,000 mg/day of chlorpromazine equivalence) produce the least dystonia.[92] Dystonic reactions usually begin reversing after a few hours and tend to disappear 24 to 48 hours after the antipsychotic agent is withdrawn.[90]

Levodopa and dopamine-stimulating agents such as amphetamines and cocaine may induce acute dystonic reactions. Paroxysmal dystonias have also been reported following the ingestion of amphetamines and related compounds. A wide range of abnormal movements including choreiform movements, multifocal tics, dystonias, akathisia, and opsoclonus-myoclonus have been reported in patients abusing cocaine and other central nervous stimulants and depressants.[93] Since amphetamines and other non-amphetamine stimulants, like methylphenidate, may increase the risk of dystonia, the combination of antipsychotics with these stimulants may also increase the risk for this drug-induced reaction during treatment and upon withdrawal. As the concomitant use of stimulants and atypical antipsychotics has increased in treating attention deficit hyperactivity disorders, this is a concern especially in children and adolescents. Not only is the risk increased with the concurrent use of these two classes of medications, but also there have been at least five case reports of dystonic reactions occurring following the discontinuation of the stimulant in patients receiving antipsychotics.[94]

Antiemetic compounds, with dopamine receptor-blocking activity, such as metoclopramide, prochlorperazine, promethazine, trimethobenzamide, and thiethylperazine, are well-recognized for their dystonia-producing capacity. A profound acute dystonic reaction may occur after only one or two doses of a dopamine-blocking antiemetic.[95] This is particularly common in children, young adults, and adolescents. Patients with AIDS on metoclopramide may be at an increased risk for developing EPS than others receiving the same therapies.[96] Droperidol, also a dopamine receptor antagonist, is used as a preanesthetic anxiolytic agent and precipitates acute dystonic reactions.[97] There are a handful of reports implicating type-2 histamine antagonists (H2 antagonists) as causative agents of dystonias and other EPS. Cimetidine, one such agent, utilized widely for peptic ulcer disease as well as acid reflux, has been noted to induce dystonic reactions. Predisposing factors for such reactions included advanced age, renal and hepatic impairment, higher doses, preexisting psychiatric illness, and the concurrent use of psychotropic medications.[98]

Serotonergic antidepressants have also been implicated in causing dystonic reactions since initial reports in 1958, and case reports associating them with EPS, including dystonias, continue to be published in literature, with the majority (over 80 percent) involving SSRIs, followed by SNRIs.[99] A review of published reports of SSRI-induced dystonic reactions noted that the time to onset of symptoms was 1.5 days to 8 months following the initiation of SSRI therapy, with a mean of 70 days. Steps for managing the reactions included dosage reduction; discontinuing the SSRI; or the coadministration of a benzodiazepine, anticholinergic agent, or botulinum toxin with partial-to-complete resolution observed within one day to six months.[100] The long half-life of fluoxetine and its active metabolite, norfluoxetine, may be implicated in delaying the appearance of extrapyramidal adverse effects associated with the antidepressant. As serum levels slowly rise to the steady state, there may be a delay in acute dystonic reactions, and the movements may represent a delayed acute reaction rather than tardive dyskinesia, an important distinction since the latter effect implies irreversibility.[101] Amoxapine, an antidepressant with dopamine receptor-blocking properties, may cause acute dystonias, other extrapyramidal adverse effects, and tardive dyskinesias. Although tricyclic antidepressants (TCAs) are not reported to affect dopamine metabolism, they have been noted to produce dystonic reactions in patients.[102]

Other agents that have been implicated in producing acute dystonic reactions include buspirone, bupropion, disulfiram, carbamazepine, erythromycin, flecanide, bethanechol, reserpine, ergotamine, and monoamine oxidase inhibitors.[98,103,104] Dystonia, secondary to carbamazepine therapy, has been associated with abnormal movements restricted to the tongue.[105] Duloxetine, a serotonin and norepinephrine reuptake inhibitor utilized for depression, anxiety disorders, peripheral neuropathy, fibromyalgia as well as chronic musculoskeletal pain, has been reported to cause acute dystonia following a single 30 mg dose in a 19 year-old patient. The clinical presentation was noted as dystonia with an Abnormal Involuntary Movement Scale score of 22, necessitating parenteral 5-mg biperiden administration to resolve the dystonia.[106] Likewise, a 60-year old woman developed neck dystonia and dyskinesias of face, neck, and jaw after an increase in the dose of duloxetine to 60 mg, following a dose of 30 mg for three weeks.[107]

12.9.1.3 Risks

Risk factors for developing acute dystonic reactions include men, young age, a primary psychotic disorder, history of electroconvulsive therapy, intellectual disability, use of potent DRBAs without concomitant anticholinergic prophylaxis, and a past history of dystonias.[89,108] The frequency of acute dystonic reactions is more commonly associated with the high-potency neuroleptics in the butyrophenone class (e.g., haloperidol), as compared with the lower potency neuroleptics in the phenothiazine class (chlorpromazine, thioridazine). Electrolyte or metabolic disorders such as hypocalcemia, hyperthyroidism, and hyperparathyroidism have been reported as risk factors in several cases.[3] Concurrent use of cocaine or ecstasy with a DRBA appears to predispose patients to acute dystonic reactions and can also cause dystonia when used alone.[109] If acute dystonia is encountered as a recurring problem with stable neuroleptic treatment, then one should have a high index of suspicion and search for alternate explanations. Perhaps the patient has ingested a larger neuroleptic dose than prescribed, has combined the neuroleptic with other central nervous system depressants or alcohol, or has suddenly discontinued anticholinergic or antihistaminic medications. Alcohol ingestion may trigger dystonia in patients receiving neuroleptics who have not previously experienced dystonic episodes.[110] Children and adolescents are at risk for acute dystonic reactions not only from prescribed DRBAs but also from various scenarios leading to inadvertent ingestion of agents which may cause these DIMDs.[5] For example, acute dystonic reactions have been reported following the ingestion of "street Xanax" tablets that actually contained haloperidol.[111]

12.9.1.4 Management

Patients initiating therapy with antipsychotics should be warned about the possible occurrence of acute dystonic reactions and should receive instructions on how to deal with these adverse events. Management of acute dystonias includes the administration of intravenous or intramuscular antimuscarinic drugs with anticholinergic (e.g., benztropine) or antihistaminic (e.g., diphenhydramine) properties. These agents are very effective and rapid in managing the dystonic reaction, and a prompt therapeutic response to either parenteral agent is virtually diagnostic of acute dystonic reactions. Other agents which may be utilized in managing a dystonic reaction include a benzodiazepine (e.g., lorazepam, diazepam, clonazepam), a dopaminergic agent (amantadine), or a beta-blocker (e.g., propranolol, metoprolol). If anticholinergics are ineffective or not tolerable, then benzodiazepines may be administered intravenously. Since antipsychotic agents have long half-lives and duration of action, and all anticholinergic drugs given parenterally will wear off after several hours, additional oral anticholinergic drugs (e.g., diphenhydramine, benztropine, biperiden, procyclidine, or trihexyphenidyl) should be continued for prophylaxis at least two to four weeks after the dystonic reaction has resolved, especially if a long-acting DRBA was used or if therapy with a DRBA will need to be continued.[92,111] Alternative strategies include lowering the psychotropic dosage or switching to a psychotropic from a different class with a lower potential for dystonic reactions. There is an inverse relationship between the incidence of drug-induced acute dsytonias and age, and also the efficacy of anticholinergic agents for prophylaxis appears to be inversely related to the patient's age.[89] Thus, the use of prophylactic anticholinergic agents in older patients for primary prevention of acute dystonias is not favored and should be utilized in patients at high risk for developing dystonia.[33]

The American Psychiatric Association (APA) guidelines suggest that the use of prophylactic anticholinergics may be considered especially for those patients receiving high-potency agents with a prior history of experiencing acute EPS, patients who prefer preventive treatment to avoid discomfort or distress, or patients for whom the occurrence of adverse effects would lead to poor compliance and adversely affect their disease state.[89] A consensus statement updated in 2012 by the World Health Organization recommends against routine prophylactic use of anticholinergic for preventing EPS, and short-term use of anticholinergics may be considered only in patients with significant EPS when dose reduction and switching strategies have not proven effective or when the side effects are acute or severe. Additionally, they recommend against the use of anticholinergics in pregnant women except for acute short-term use.[110]

In all patients, the benefit of using prophylactic antimuscarinic agents should be weighed against the potential for adverse effects. As a class, antimuscarinic agents are associated with tachycardia, urinary retention, constipation, and mydriasis and should be used with caution in patients with heart disease, prostatic disease, ileus, and glaucoma. They may also impair cognitive function in elderly patients, worsen the severity of tardive dyskinesia, and exacerbate existing psychosis. Additionally, anticholinergics may mask some EPS, an indicator for the future development of tardive dyskinesia in some susceptible patients.[89,112]

12.9.2 Ataxia

Ataxia refers to unsteady gait and lack of coordination usually associated with cerebellar dysfunction and is marked by clumsy movement. Ataxia may affect any part of the body, and the movements are jerky and uncoordinated, without the smooth flow of normal motion. Symptoms are quite variable and may include swaying while standing, a wide-based gait sometimes likened to a "drunken reeling," and an uneven gait with steps of various uneven lengths and lateral deviations. Additionally, patients may present with dysarthric speech and nystagmus. Medications that may cause ataxia include aminoglycosides, benzodiazepines, sedatives, and anticonvulsants (e.g., phenytoin, carbamazepine). A systematic literature search of drug-induced cerebellar ataxia identified the most common groups of medications as anti-epileptics, benzodiazepines, and antineoplastics. Although ataxia was commonly reversible after discontinuing the offending agent, persistent symptoms were associated with lithium, phenytoin, and cytarabine.[113]

12.9.3 Bruxism

Bruxism is the involuntary grinding or gnashing of teeth and clenching of the jaw that can occur during daytime or at night. Medications reported to cause bruxism include SSRIs, selective norepinephrine reuptake inhibitors (SNRIs) (e.g., venlafaxine, duloxetine), amphetamines, flecanide, flunarizine, haloperidol, levodopa/carbidopa, bupropion, and vortioxetine.[39,41] Of all these medications, the most frequently cited cause is the use of SSRIs, SNRIs, bupropion, or vortioxetine, with the DIMD detected as early as 1 day to as late as 11 months following the start of therapy. Most reports of drug-induced bruxism have resolved with either the dose adjustment of the offending medication or the use of buspirone or gabapentin. A case report of a seven-year follow-up of a patient with venlafaxine-induced diurnal bruxism treated with an occlusal splint was reported.[114] Bruxism may also occur due to drug interactions, and two reports in literature cite bruxism in children within hours following concomitant valproic acid for seizure disorder and methylphenidate for attention-deficit hyperactivity disorder.[115,116]

12.9.4 Neuroleptic Malignant Syndrome

Neuroleptic malignant syndrome (NMS) is a rare idiosyncratic adverse drug reaction which may occur from the use of medications that involve the dopaminergic system. Neuroleptic agents are by far the biggest culprits in NMS, although the disorder may also occur with other dopamine-depleting agents such as metoclopramide or after the withdrawal from levodopa therapy.[88] Antidepressants, including TCAs, SSRIs, and lithium, either alone or in combination, have been implicated in causing a syndrome resembling NMS.[117,118] Likewise, a similar syndrome has been reported in patients using cocaine. The incidence of this adverse effect is low, with a reported prevalence ranging from 0.07 percent to 2.2 percent of patients receiving neuroleptics. Likewise, the mortality associated with this reaction is lower in patients receiving atypical antipsychotics compared to patients receiving typical antipsychotics (3 percent versus 16 percent).[119,120]

The disorder may occur hours to months after the initial dose, and the syndrome usually lasts five to ten days after the oral antipsychotic is discontinued and two to three times longer upon withdrawal of depot medications.[119] NMS develops acutely, and the essential feature is hyperpyrexia which occurs in conjunction with or shortly after the onset of muscular rigidity. Temperatures of 101°F (38.3°C) to 103°F (39.4°C) typically occur and, in some cases, may rise above 107°F (41.6°C).[5] The muscular hypertonicity is usually described as a "lead pipe" rigidity and may be associated with dyskinetic or choreiform movements. The symptomatology may also consist of diaphoresis, dysphagia, tremor, incontinence, and mental status changes that may range from confusion to coma, mutism, tachycardia, elevated or labile blood pressure, leukocytosis, and elevated creatine phosphokinase (CPK).[120] CPK levels increase as a result of muscular activity and myonecrosis from intense and sustained muscle contractions. Myoglobinuria may occur secondary to severe myonecrosis, and this can lead to acute renal failure. Metabolic acidosis may occur, and liver function tests may be elevated suggesting acute fatty acid changes in the liver secondary to hyperthermia.[119–121] Other sequelae include respiratory complications such as pneumonia and pulmonary embolism and cardiovascular complications such as cardiac arrest and arrhythmias.[120] Even among patients who recover from NMS, persistent symptoms, such as residual catatonia, may occur in a small percentage of patients.[121]

Certain antipsychotics have been implicated more than others in this disorder, which may reflect their frequency of usage or potency. Haloperidol, a high-potency neuroleptic, either as monotherapy or with other agents, has been cited as a causative agent in 49 percent to 65 percent of NMS cases. This high incidence may reflect its use in rapid neuroleptization (rapid escalation of the dose of the drug in order to see a quick response) and its relatively high dopamine blockade.[119] The atypical neuroleptics including aripiprazole, clozapine, olanzapine, quetiapine, risperidone, and ziprasidone also have been implicated as causative agents in NMS. A systematic review noted that NMS from atypical antipsychotics is characterized by lower incidence, lower clinical severity, and less frequent lethal outcome compared to NMS from typical antipsychotics. Additionally, NMS associated with clozapine and aripiprazole may present with atypical features from other atypical antipsychotics, notably less intense EPS with clozapine and less severe fever and autonomic symptoms with aripiprazole.[122]

Potential risk factors include the male gender, dehydration, severe agitation, mood disorder, high drug dosage, and intramuscular administration of the drug. Patients with preexisting Parkinson's disease may even be at an increased risk of this disorder since further depletion of dopamine occurs secondary to the neuroleptic. Intellectually disabled patients and those with preexisting brain disease also appear to be at a greater risk for NMS.[121] Catatonia may also be a risk factor for the development of NMS.[123]

Treatment of NMS depends on the recognition and immediate withdrawal of the offending neuroleptic agent. General medical supportive measures should be initiated including hydration, fever reduction, and treatment of any concomitant infection. Pharmacologic agents such as bromocriptine will reduce parkinsonian symptoms, and benzodiazepines may facilitate muscle relaxation. Symptoms of muscular rigidity may be decreased using dantrolene, which is also effective in reducing the fever.[121]

Once an episode of NMS is treated, at least two weeks should pass before restarting neuroleptics in patients who absolutely require such agents. Guidelines for restarting neuroleptics have been proposed by clinicians. A higher occurrence rate of NMS is observed in patients restarted on a high potency agent than in those administered lower potency agents. Upon restarting a neuroleptic, the occurrence of NMS may be as high as 83 percent in patients who receive a neuroleptic of the same potency as the initial offending drug. The rate may be as low as 10 percent when lower-potency neuroleptics are used in such patients.[123] The low potency or atypical neuroleptics should be utilized while avoiding the long-acting depot agents. Therapy should be initiated with the lowest possible dose, and patients should be monitored for any signs of the disorder upon re-challenge with neuroleptics.[117]

12.9.5 Serotonin Syndrome

Drugs that block serotonin reuptake or have serotonin-like activity may induce a rare, but potentially lethal, serotonin syndrome. This syndrome is characterized by cognitive and behavioral changes (e.g., confusion, elevated mood, agitation, insomnia, coma), autonomic symptoms (e.g., increased heart rate, fever, labile blood pressure), and neurological symptoms (e.g., myoclonus, rigidity, hyperreflexia, tremor, ataxia, akathisia).[123]

Symptoms of serotonin syndrome usually appear very rapidly, and in a review of published cases, approximately 60 percent of patients presented with symptoms within six hours of the causative medication initiation, change in dose, or overdose.[124] Serotonin syndrome may occur with a single serotonergic drug but is more severe when two or more drugs with serotonergic properties are co-prescribed. It has also been reported to occur following the administration of a single dose of a serotonergic drug.[125,126] Drugs that increase serotonin transmission include antidepressants [monoamine oxidase inhibitors (MAOIs), selective serotonin/norepinephrine reuptake inhibitors (SNRIs), selective serotonin reuptake inhibitors (SSRIs), tricyclic antidepressants (TCAs)]; buspirone and migraine medications (e.g., triptans and ergotamines); drugs of abuse (e.g., cocaine, LSD, MDMA, or "ecstasy"); and dietary supplements (St. John's wort, ginseng) when taken in combination with SSRIs or triptans.[124,127] Other medications include tramadol, tryptophan, meperidine, lithium, amphetamines, linezolid, selegiline, sibutramine, methylene blue, metoclopramide, and dextromethorphan (a cough suppressant found in many over-the-counter cough preparations). The atypical antipsychotics have been shown to cause serotonin syndrome when prescribed in combination with SSRIs.[89,126,128–130]

The management of serotonin syndrome includes discontinuing the causative drug(s). Depending on the severity of symptoms, patients may require supportive care. Complications include renal failure from muscle breakdown. Benzodiazepines may help control the agitation and limit the excessive muscle activity.[15] Patients may also be managed with cyproheptadine, propranolol, chlorpromazine, diphenhydramine, and methysergide.[89,128]

12.10 CHRONIC DRUG-INDUCED MOVEMENT DISORDERS

Chronic DIMDs are non-acute syndromes that persist only while the offending agent is being administered and remit when the offending agent is discontinued. Various medications may produce single movement disorders such as tremor, myoclonus, or chorea and are considered simple side effects. Drug-induced akathisia and parkinsonism are of intermediate-onset, usually occurring within the first three months of initiation of therapy with the causative agent, and represent more complex syndromes.

12.10.1 Akathisia

12.10.1.1 Presentation

The most poorly understood of all extrapyramidal side effects and the most challenging to manage is akathisia. It is reported to occur in 8 to 76 percent of patients treated with neuroleptics with 20 to 30 percent being a conservative estimate.[89,131] The disorder is classified into acute, chronic, tardive, and withdrawal subtypes based on the epidemiology and presentation of the movements. The disorder is characterized by a subjective inner feeling of anxiety, restlessness, and an irresistible urge to be in motion to satisfy the urge to move. Objective signs of motor overactivity are manifested as pacing, fidgety movements or swinging of the legs, crossing and uncrossing one's legs, "walking on the spot" while standing, hand wringing, rocking back and forth, and other purposeless repetitive motions where patients have an inner urge to move various parts of their bodies. Although akathisia literally means inability to remain seated, most patients describe that the condition worsens when they are standing still.[89,132]

The onset of acute akathisia is associated within days to weeks of drug initiation, with most symptoms occurring within six weeks of initiating neuroleptic medication. However, it may occur within the first few hours of increase of dose of neuroleptic medication or reduction of medication used to treat (or prevent) acute EPS. Tardive akathisia starts during long-term neuroleptic treatment and is not related to a change in the medication or dose. Withdrawal akathisia refers to akathisia that begins after the neuroleptic agent is reduced in dose or discontinued. Regardless of the onset—whether acute, tardive, or withdrawal—akathisia may persist. No major differences in the motor phenomena of acute and chronic akathisia are observed; however, patients with chronic akathisia may have a less intense subjective sense of restlessness.[15]

A common problem with assessing patients with akathisia is distinguishing it from psychomotor agitation associated with the psychoses. This poses a clinical challenge since mistaking akathisia for psychotic agitation may worsen akathisia, if the dose of the neuroleptic is increased. As drug-induced akathisia may be difficult to clinically distinguish from medical conditions associated with restlessness (e.g., restless leg syndrome), it should be suspected if symptoms occur soon after the implicated drug is initiated in the absence of such other conditions. Although it has been reported that mild akathisia may be difficult to differentiate from generalized anxiety, it has been noted that complaints concerning the legs discriminate most effectively between mild akathisia and restlessness due to an underlying psychiatric disorder.[6]

Symptoms of akathisia can cause severe distress for affected patients and, if left untreated, may lead to serious complications including aggression, medication nonadherence, dysphoria, and worsening of psychosis. A patient may experience significant mental distress if asked not to move or if restrained from moving. If the akathisia occurs early in treatment or after increases in doses, it may be more troublesome and distressing for the patient.[132] Akathisia has also been associated with depressive mood, suicidal or assaultive ideation, depersonalization, and severe agitation.[133] Given the implications of untreated akathisia, it is important to recognize early signs as one of the gravest consequences of this movement disorder is its reported association with suicide. Several reports have looked at the relationship between suicidal ideation and akathisia, and it is thought that sudden suicidal ideation emerges as a response to the intolerable feelings of restlessness.[132,133]

12.10.1.2 Case Study: Trazodone-Induced Akathisia

A 58-year-old male with bipolar disorder was hospitalized for a recurrent depressive episode. At the time of admission, the patient described depressed mood, feelings of hopelessness, guilt, and insomnia. It was noted that the patient's past depressive episodes were characterized by profound anergia and psychomotor retardation; however, at the present time, his primary complaints were of restlessness and dysphoria. The restlessness was associated with a marked inability to sit still for more than a few moments and the inability to find a comfortable position to fall asleep; hence, insomnia. His medical history was noncontributory. For at least one year prior to this episode, the patient was maintained on lithium carbonate with a plasma level of 0.8 mEq/L and trazodone 200 mg/day. However, just prior to the onset of his decompensation, the patient's daily dose of trazodone was increased to 300 mg. The antidepressant was tapered and subsequently discontinued, while the lithium was maintained. Within a few days, the patient's symptoms improved regarding his motor restlessness and anxiety and completely remitted by the tenth day after the discontinuation of trazodone.

12.10.1.3 Implicated Agents

Medications commonly associated with acute akathisia include typical and atypical neuroleptics, and phenothiazine antiemetics, with the majority of tardive akathisia cases involving the neuroleptic agents.[134] Additionally, many medications used in the palliative care setting, including antiemetics (metoclopramide, prochlorperazine) and antidepressants (tricyclic, SSRIs, venlafaxine), may cause significant akathsia.[117]

Although atypical antipsychotics may induce akathisia, they do so at a much lower rate compared with the conventional antipsychotics. A pooled analysis of 4, 6-week studies reported akathisia in 2.4 percent of patients treated with olanzapine (dose range from 5 to 20 mg/day) compared with 10 percent in patients treated with chlorpromazine (dose range from 200 to 800 mg/day).[135] Another study noted the point prevalences of akathisia associated with conventional neuroleptics, risperidone, and clozapine to be 24 percent, 13 percent, and 7 percent, respectively.[136] The CATIE study showed that akathisia is still a problem and occurred at a frequency of 5 percent in patients treated with olanzapine or quetiapine, 7 percent for patients who received risperidone or perphenazine (a typical antipsychotic), and 9 percent for patients treated with ziprasidone. Akathisia is the main extrapyramidal syndrome reported in patients with schizophrenia and mania who are taking aripiprazole. Lurasidone, a more recently approved atypical antipsychotic, has been associated with akathisia in 11 percent of patients.[19] Compared to older atypical antipsychotics, a recent meta-analysis noted that the relative risk of akathisia was highest with lurasidone, asenapine, and aripiprazole having individual relative risks reported at 2.7, 2.22, and 1.52, respectively.[137]

As clozapine is not used as a first-line agent in managing psychosis but rather when treatment with other agents fails, a caveat in relation to clozapine studies is that patients have previously received other antipsychotic medications and some may have persistent akathisia as a result of exposure to the earlier agents.[138] A rare case of acute nocturnal akathisia induced by clozapine has been reported in a 43-year-old man with schizophrenia that was successfully treated with propranolol 40 mg/day, while the patient continued on clozapine at a dose of 350 mg/day.[139]

The discontinuation of SGAs may be associated with sudden EPS, and sudden emergence of akathisia has been reported in four women with bipolar disorder following sudden ziprasidone dose reduction.[140] The newer SGA, iloperidone, when compared to zipasidone, was shown to be associated with lower incidence of EPS, particularly akathisia.[141] Four randomized placebo-controlled double-blind trials evaluated the prevalence of EPS and akathisia in quetiapine-treated bipolar manic patients and concluded that quetiapine treatment was similar to placebo in terms of occurrence of akathisia in such patients.[142,143] Additionally, another study noted significant reduction in parkinsonism and akathisia when patients with schizophrenia and preexisting EPS were switched from previous antipsychotics to quetiapine.[143] A review of various antipsychotics noted the prevalence percentage for drug-induced akathisia as follows: Paliperidone (3.3 percent), quetiapine (5.2 percent), ziprasidone (8.3 percent), aripiprazole (8.5 percent), olanzapine (8.7 percent), risperidone (14.2 percent), chlorpromazine (15.9 percent), and haloperidol (24.8 percent).[16] Another recent systematic review evaluating the newer SGA noted that the estimated weighted mean incidence rate of akathisia was 3.9 percent for iloperidone, 6.8 percent for asenapine, 10.0 percent for brexpiprazole, 12.7 percent for lurasidone, and 17.2 percent for cariprazine. Most cases of drug-induced akathisia with cariprazine were reported in patients with bipolar mania compared to schizophrenia, and most occurred during the first two to six weeks of treatment initiation. Overall, less than 1 percent of patients with schizophrenia and less than 5 percent of patients with bipolar disorder discontinued cariprazine due to akathisia, suggesting that akathisia is manageable for most patients. The report also noted that evening administration of lurasidone may be associated with lower rates of akathisia, and the incidence of this movement disorder seem to be dose-related: 6 percent for lurasidone 20 mg/day; 11–12 percent for lurasidone 40–80 mg/day; and 22 percent for lurasidone 120 mg/day.[144] Lumateperone, a newer SGA that simultaneously modulates serotonin, dopamine, and glutamate neurotransmission, was noted to have a low incidence of EPS, with akathisia reported at 0.3 percent.[145] A tolerability profile of several atypical antipsychotics noted the incidence of akathisia statistically higher in patients with affective disorders for quetiapine and ziprasidone; however, differences compared to patients with schizophrenia were not significant.[146] Reports also note that severe akathisia has been associated after the initiation of a low-dose quetiapine regimen for the management of insomnia.[147]

Aripiprazole, which is approved by the FDA as an adjunct for the treatment of major depressive disorder in patients taking antidepressants, has been associated with treatment-related akathisia. One study noted that akathisia occurred in 4.5 percent of patients who received an antidepressant and adjunct placebo, compared with 23 percent of those who took an antidepressant and adjunct aripiprazole.[148] Similarly, another study using aripiprazole in refractory bipolar depression noted that 42 percent of patients had treatment-related akathisia, suggesting that SGAs in combination with other psychotropic medications may increase the risk of developing akathisia.[149,150]

The SSRIs are also implicated in acute akathisia, but rarely in tardive akathisia with fluoxetine and paroxetine reported most commonly as the offending agent.[99] As more and more non-psychiatrists prescribe SSRIs for various psychiatric conditions, there is the potential for akathisia to be misdiagnosed, further complicating the patient's condition. This is illustrated in a case involving a 21-year-old man prescribed sertraline for depression who developed akathisia, which was misdiagnosed as an anxiety disorder. The prescriber doubled the patient's dose, but the symptoms got worse, and then his sertraline was changed to paroxetine with no improvement in symptoms. After being referred to a psychiatrist who diagnosed the patient as having drug-induced akathisia, the patient's akathisia resolved following the discontinuation of paroxetine.[151]

SSRI-induced akathisia appears to occur in at least 4.5 percent of exposed patients. More reports of SSRI-induced movement disorders have been cited in women than men; however, this may be due to sex bias since epidemiologic studies indicate a two-fold greater incidence of depression in women than men, causing more women to be likely to be prescribed an SSRI. There is interpatient variability regarding the development of akathisia in response to exposure time. The onset of akathisia has been reported from half a day to three months after initiating therapy with the SSRI, with a mean of two weeks, and in some cases, symptoms were noted after a dose increase. Most cases resolve within two weeks of discontinuing therapy or decreasing the dose of the SSRI, adding a benzodiazepine (e.g., lorazepam) or beta-blocker (e.g., propranolol).[100,152]

Since many treatment emergent adverse effects associated with SSRIs include agitation, anxiety, and restlessness, it is possible that a subset of these patients may be experiencing akathisia. Several patient case reports have noted suicide attempts, which may be a means to end the restlessness that akathisia provokes. For example, a patient on sertraline for three weeks developed akathisia and attempted suicide "to escape from the profound discomfort and restlessness."[153] An 83-year-old male with SSRI-induced akathisia described it as a "restless nightmare" that if it would not stop, he would "rather be dead."[154] Another case report noted a woman as having a good mood but being afraid that "she would kill herself because of these restless and out-of-control feelings."[155] Following a dose increase of fluoxetine, a 22-year old female experienced akathisia and had an "elaborate suicidal ideation revolving around her own violent death."[156] It has been hypothesized that the suicidal ideation at times observed in patients treated with an SSRI may, at least in part, be attributable to akathisia.[157–159]

Metoclopramide is a DRBA that is not used as an antipsychotic but is an antiemetic and gastroprokinetic agent associated with numerous reports of drug-induced akathisia.[160,161] Its uses include the management of severe nausea, diabetic gastroparesis, esophageal reflux, dyspepsia, neurogenic bladder, orthostatic hypotension, hiccups, and nonprolactinemic amenorrhea among others. Following a single dose of intravenous metoclopramide as pulmonary aspiration prophylaxis prior to endoscopic sinus surgery, akathisia, accompanied by motor restlessness, flushing, and diaphoresis, was noted to occur in a male patient who experienced occasional gastro-esophageal reflux.[162] Likewise, in 25 percent of healthy volunteers, a 10-mg intravenous bolus dose of metoclopramide produced complaints of akathisia, usually within 15 to 30 minutes, and the effect lasted for three to four hours.[163]

12.10.1.4 Other Drugs

Although akathisia is generally not considered to be an adverse effect of heterocyclic antidepressants, a few case reports have cited this effect.[164,165] Amoxapine, a dibenzoxapine antidepressant with intrinsic neuroleptic activity used in managing patients with psychotic depression, has been associated with producing akathisia.[166] Mirtazapine, a tetracyclic antidepressant, has been cited as a cause of akathisia four hours after the first dose is administered.[167] However, two small studies with small numbers of patients noted the efficacy of mirtazapine for the management of antipsychotic-induced acute akathisia, with one in four patients showing a partial response and one in five patients showing a complete remission.[168] Droperidol, a dopamine antagonist with some histamine and serotonin antagonist activity used for post-operative nausea and vomiting, has been noted to produce acute akathisia within 90 minutes following oral administration.[169] Several case reports have also cited serotonin antagonists such as cyproheptadine, methysergide, and buspirone in inducing akathisia in patients treated with such agents.[170–173] Additionally, calcium channel blockers (cinnarizine, flunarizine, diltiazem [the former two are not available in the United States]), carbamazepine, ethosuximide, and methysergide may occasionally be associated with akathisia.[128,174] Akathisia associated with atomoxetine, a non-stimulant medication used in managing attention-deficit hyperactivity disorders (ADHD), may be misinterpreted as an increase in the severity of ADHD symptoms and thus may complicate the management of ADHD in these patients.[175]

12.10.1.5 Risks

Risk factors for drug-induced akathisia include drug dosage, rate of dosage increment, and drug potency.[135] Other risk factors not well-delineated include advanced age, women, cognitive impairment, iron deficiency, intellectual disability, and history of affective disorder.[33,176] Also, use of multiple akathisia-inducing drugs may increase the risk of drug-induced akathisia. Patients with cancer or those with terminal illness receiving palliative care and taking antipsychotics for managing delirium may also be at a higher risk for the development of akathisia.[177] Simultaneous use of an SSRI has been shown to increase the number of cases of akathisia in patients who receive FGAs either as oral or as depot injections.[178] Patients with bipolar mood disorders, especially bipolar depression, are at an increased risk of developing akathisia with both FGAs and SGAs.[179] This is relevant to practice since several atypical antipsychotics are currently used in managing bipolar disorders. Akathisia can potentially be mistaken for agitated psychosis which may lead to the dose escalation of the antipsychotic drug and the potential for worsening of the restlessness. Some clinicians have suggested that drugs with greater anticholinergic properties may reduce the risk for developing akathisia, as anticholinergics may be used in managing akathisia.[180] The worsening of akathisia has been associated with atypical neuroleptics other than clozapine, thus atypicals, especially risperidone at doses greater than 6 mg/day, continue to carry notable risks for akathisia, and unfortunately this DIMD may be overlooked as an adverse effect of second-generation antipsychotics.[181]

12.10.1.6 Management

The optimal pharmacologic management for neuroleptic-induced akathisia is yet to be determined, and the most effective treatment for acute akathisia is to discontinue the offending drug. Alternatively, a clinician may lower the dosage of the offending agent or, if a neuroleptic is the causative agent, change it to a lower potency agent with higher anticholinergic properties. Although the treatment of choice is to lower the antipsychotic dose or switch to a different antipsychotic, this may lead to worsening psychosis or relapse, and various adjunctive medications to treat akathisia may be the best treatment option for some patients. When switching to another antipsychotic, the one with a lower potential for akathisia is recommended (e.g., SGA such as quetiapine or clozapine or an FGA such as chlorpromazine).[145]

Looking at predisposing factors, examining symptoms, and using the Barnes Akathisia Rating Scale can aid in recognizing akathisia.[182] Various agents including benzodiazepines, lipophilic beta-blockers, anticholinergic agents, cyproheptadine, and clonidine have been utilized in the management of neuroleptic-induced akathisia. Some clinicians hypothesize that beta-blockers act peripherally to relieve the somatic manifestations of akathisia via their action on beta-adrenergic receptors located in the muscle, while the subjective signs of akathisia are ameliorated with either beta-blockers or benzodiazepines.[183] Benzodiazepines, most commonly lorazepam at a dose of 1.5–3.0 mg/day in divided doses or clonazepam 0.5 mg once daily, are also used; however, most benzodiazepines may be beneficial in managing this disorder. Centrally acting (lipophilic) beta-blockers are regarded by some as the most effective treatment for akathisia, and propranolol is the most common agent administered at a dose of 30 to 120 mg/day titrated to produce clinical response while monitoring blood pressure and pulse rate.[89] Generally, benzodiazepines or beta-blockers are preferred for patients who do not have symptoms of Parkinson's disease, and anticholinergics may be used in patients with Parkinson's disease. Amantadine can also be tried, although there is some evidence that the akathisia becomes refractory after several weeks of treatment, and in patients with cognitive impairment it may worsen confusions.[152] A Cochrane review concluded that there was insufficient data based on good-quality research to support the use of anticholinergics in neuroleptic-induced akathisia, and current guidelines note that akathisia tends not to respond to anticholinergics.[89] A concern, however, with anticholinergics is the potential for significant adverse effects such as cognitive impairment, constipation, blurry vision, and urinary retention.[145] Alternative agents that have been equivocally shown to be effective include amantadine, opiates, and buspirone.[152] Amelioration of akathisia has been associated with current clozapine therapy.[179] The role of mitrazapine in the treatment of antipsychotic-induced akathisia has been evaluated, and it may be useful for patients with contraindications or intolerability to beta-blockers and for those patients with comorbid depression or negative symptoms associated with schizophrenia.[184]

12.10.2 Parkinsonism

12.10.2.1 Presentation

Drug-induced parkinsonism (DIP) presents very similar to the symptom complex associated with idiopathic Parkinson's disease (PD). The constellation of tremor, bradykinesia, rigidity, and postural instability constitutes parkinsonism. Bradykinesia is defined as slowness of movement, which may manifest in impaired movement initiation. This global slowing and slowness in initiating movements are the most common presenting symptoms. Rigidity is defined as an increased resistance to passive stretch and manifests in decreased arm swinging, decreased eye blinking, a mask-like face, and drooling. Parkinsonian muscular rigidity involves excessive firmness and tensing of resting muscles. It may affect all skeletal muscles or only discrete muscular areas. Two kinds of rigidity may occur: Continuous or "lead-pipe" rigidity in which the limb or joint resists movement and feels locked in place and cogwheel rigidity which involves the muscle stretched around a joint to cause a rhythmic resistance that interrupts the usual smooth motion of the joint. Parkinsonian tremor consists of low-frequency oscillations occurring mainly at rest and may look as if the patient is rolling a pill between their fingers and thumb. The incidence of this rest tremor has been reported to be as high as 50 percent in DIP, while the incidence is much higher in PD. Although resting tremor may be less prominent, it can be as vigorous as in PD. Additionally, in PD, an asymmetrical presentation is more common, while drug- or toxin-induced tremors tend to be bilateral as they represent an exacerbation of physiologic tremor. A highly characteristic although not pathognomonic sign of DIP is a low-frequency perioral high-amplitude tremor known as the rabbit syndrome.[2,4,185]

In the majority of cases, symptoms of DIP often appear in the first month after the offending agent has been started, and most symptoms will resolve within one to two months after the implicated agent has been discontinued. However, some patients may require up to one year for complete resolution of symptoms. Although tremor is the most visible feature of DIP, it is generally the least disabling. Bradykinesia is associated with much of the difficulty observed in carrying out activities of daily living. Even mild symptoms of DIP may cause impaired dexterity which may impinge on occupational and social tasks. Functional impairment can lead to increased caregiver burden and significant reductions in quality of life.[15] In the institutionalized elderly population, DIP was reported at a prevalence rate of 0.5 percent to 3 percent, with essential tremor being the most common movement disorder observed in that population.[186–188]

12.10.2.2 Case Study: Neuroleptic-Induced Parkinsonism

A 67-year-old woman with a 40-year history of bipolar disorder presented with problems with walking and balance. Her bipolar disorder was well-controlled with lithium for many years. One year prior to her clinic presentation, she developed colitis and stopped her lithium. She became suicidal and required prolonged psychiatric hospitalization, which resulted in electroconvulsive therapy. She was started on olanzapine, and it controlled her psychosis, allowing her to be discharged home. Over the next six months, she noticed that her walking was much slower and her posture more stooped. Her balance was also significantly affected, and she required a walker when leaving the house because of frequent falls. On examination, she exhibited bilateral bradykinesia, rigidity, stooped posture with small steps, and fell back on the pull test. The patient was diagnosed with drug-induced parkinsonism, and the olanzapine was tapered off by her psychiatrist and replaced with clozapine. Three months later, her gait and posture had improved, and she was no longer using a walker; however, she still had some rigidity on examination.

12.10.2.3 Implicated Agents

DIP may be due to drugs that deplete dopamine from intraneuronal storage sites (e.g., reserpine), drugs that act as dopamine "false neurotransmitters" (e.g., alpha-methyldopa), or drugs that block striatal dopamine receptors (e.g., neuroleptics and metoclopramide) resulting in an imbalance of dopamine and acetylcholine in the nigrostriatum.

The prevalence of DIP associated with typical and atypical antipsychotics ranges from 20 percent to 35 percent, with higher rates in elderly patients.[4,189] A retrospective cohort study of adults 66 years and older noted that the risk of development of DIP was similar among those patients who received a high-dose atypical antipsychotic and those patients who received a higher-potency typical antipsychotic. Thus, when potency and dose of antipsychotics are considered, atypical antipsychotics are not necessarily safer than typical antipsychotics in relation to DIP.[190] DIP typically presents earlier in antipsychotic treatment, with 50 to 75 percent of cases occurring within the first month, and 90 percent of cases within the first three months.[4] A Cochrane review and meta-analysis of various antipsychotics noted the prevalence percentage for drug-induced parkinsonism as follows: Aripiprazole (7.2 percent), olanzapine (8.1 percent), quetiapine (8.8 percent), ziprasidone (10.0 percent), risperidone (12.1 percent), chlorpromazine (21.1 percent), and haloperidol (22.6 percent).[16] Although aripiprazole's partial agonist activity has been postulated to induce less EPS, more case reports and case series outlining aripiprazole's role in movement disorders are published.[191]

The atypical neuroleptics, olanzapine, and risperidone may cause DIP and have been shown to worsen the primary motor manifestations of the disease, especially at high doses. Generally, clozapine has a low incidence of EPS, including parkinsonism. Clozapine produces sialorrhea, due to an increase in salivary flow, which is independent of EPS, and this is in contrast to conventional antipsychotics which typically cause dry mouth due to bradykinesia of the swallowing muscles.[192] Quetiapine and ziprasidone appear to be associated with a low incidence of DIP. Quetiapine has not been shown to significantly cause or exacerbate parkinsonism, even at relatively higher doses, and, like clozapine, has been shown to effectively reduce psychotic symptoms in PD patients without worsening the primary motor manifestations of the disease.[193]

A review of SSRI-induced parkinsonism suggests that SSRIs may have the potential to worsen symptoms in patients with PD; however, establishing a definitive role is difficult. Since the disease is slow and subtle, any worsening of symptoms thought to be drug-related may be attributed directly to the progression of the disease. A review of published reports of SSRI-induced movement disorders noted that patients experienced cogwheel rigidity, resting tremor, bradykinesia, akinesia, or gait disturbances. The time of onset of symptoms was found to be from three days to four months after initiating therapy with the SSRI. DIP was reported most commonly in patients receiving treatment with sertraline, citalopram, or escitalopram, and 37 percent of cases occurred within seven days of treatment initiation or dose increase.[99] One patient developed irreversible DIP within two months of initiating treatment with sertraline. Even with the discontinuation of the SSRI, the patient steadily over the next three years progressed with symptoms of gait disturbance, tremor, rigidity, and cognitive deficits.[194] Other antidepressants, such as SNRIs (e.g., duloxetine), and trazodone, a compound chemically unrelated to tricyclic or tetracyclic antidepressants often used as a sedative, have also been reported to induce DIP, with the latter antidepressant potentially inhibiting midbrain dopaminergic neurotransmission, leading to DIP.[195,196]

Chronic treatment with valproate, an antiepileptic agent utilized for seizures and mood disorders, has been associated with parkinsonism.[197,198] Dopamine-blocking antiemetic agents, including prochloperazine and metoclopramide, may induce reversible parkinsonism when these agents are used at therapeutic doses for nausea.[199] Toxins are also implicated in DIP and are often associated with irreversible structural damage to the basal ganglia and include MPTP, organophosphate pesticides, methanol, manganese, carbon monoxide, and carbon disulphide.[200–202]

12.10.2.4 Other Drugs

Calcium channel blockers, such as diltiazem, verapamil, flunarizine and cinnarizine, have also been implicated in DIP; however, the latter two agents are relatively potent dopamine blockers that are not marketed in the United States but are prescribed in Europe and Latin America for various disorders, including vertigo, migraine, and tinnitus.[199]

DIP has been reported in four patients with schizophrenia exposed to high doses of diazepam (> 100 mg/day).[203] Cisapride, a parasympathomimetic and gastroprokinetic agent no longer marketed in the United States (voluntarily removed from the U.S. market in 2000 due to concerns of QT prolongation), has also been associated with DIP. Other medications known to cause or worsen parkinsonism include amphotericin B, amiodarone, bethanechol, captopril, lovastatin, meperidine, methyldopa, phenelzine, phenytoin, and procaine. Lithium, a mood stabilizer, commonly produces a postural tremor; however, it is not firmly established if it can induce parkinsonism.[204]

12.10.2.5 Risks

Factors that increase the risk of DIP include patients with advanced age, dementia, preexisting parkinsonism, exposure to DRBAs, exposure to higher doses of neuroleptics, and female gender (twice as common in women than men).[204] Patients with basal ganglia dysfunction may also be at risk, and some individuals may be more susceptible to DIP due to a preexisting deficiency of nigrostriatal dopamine.[152] DIP has a significantly higher incidence in patients with AIDS psychosis who are receiving DRBA, and one study noted that the likelihood of developing EPS was 2.4 times higher in psychotic patients with AIDS compared to psychotic patients without AIDS.[205] Other proposed risk factors include trauma, infection, premorbid personality, and emotional stress. An inverse association between cigarette smoking and Parkinson's disease has been noted to be present in the majority of case-control studies.[206,207]

12.10.2.6 Management

The most effective management of DIP involves the discontinuation of the offending agent, and symptoms will usually resolve within one to two months. Rarely, however, some patients may require up to one year for complete resolution of symptoms. Some patients may never recover, and this raises the question as to whether they had subclinical PD that was uncovered by the use of DRBA. Autopsy findings of typical histologic features of PD in patients with a past history of DIP support this concept, and, thus, concomitant PD should be kept in mind if parkinsonism persists after the implicated agents are discontinued.[208]

If discontinuing the agent is not feasible, or if discontinuing the agent does not improve symptoms, then the management of symptoms of DIP involves lowering the dosage of the offending agent to the lowest effective dosage or adding an antiparkinsonian medication. Switching to a neuroleptic that is a low-potency agent with anticholinergic properties, or an atypical antipsychotic such as quetiapine or clozapine, may also be helpful. The most common drug treatment modalities for neuroleptic-induced parkinsonism are anticholinergics and the indirect dopamine agonist amantadine. Pimavanserin, approved for the management of hallucinations and delusions associated with Parkinson's disease psychosis, is an atypical antipsychotic whose effects are mediated on serotonin receptors as opposed to dopamine, making it an effective alternative treatment for managing psychosis in patients with PD.[80,209]

Anticholinergic agents currently available for managing DIP are all effective but differ somewhat in adverse effects and duration of action. These include diphenhydramine, benztropine, trihexphenidyl, biperiden, and procyclidine. Diphenhydramine is the most sedating, while trihexphenidyl is the least. All of the anticholinergics need to be administered two to four times a day except benztropine which may be administered once daily due to its long duration of action. Amantadine may be used as an alternative to anticholinergics due to its indirect dopaminergic properties. Advantages of amantadine over anticholinergics are that it may be better tolerated, it does not adversely affect memory, and it may be an alternative in patients for whom anticholinergics are contraindicated, such as in patients with narrow angle glaucoma or benign prostatic hypertrophy. Amantadine is administered in doses of 100 to 400 mg daily in divided doses with dosage adjustments required in renal dysfunction. Although the incidence of adverse effects is low, some patients may experience dizziness, nervousness, insomnia, anxiety, and impaired concentration during treatment. Livedo reticularis, a skin discoloration which is reversible upon the discontinuation of amantadine, has also been noted in some patients especially those in colder climates. Rarely, hallucinations and abnormal dreams may also occur in patients treated with amantadine. Levodopa, which is generally utilized in managing idiopathic PD, is generally not utilized for neuroleptic-induced parkinsonism due to insufficient efficacy and increased risk of exacerbating an underlying psychiatric disorder.[89,210,211]

The use of clozapine in the management of drug-induced psychosis in patients with Parkinson's disease has become increasingly popular.[212] Numerous open trials have demonstrated an improvement in psychosis in more than 80 percent of patients with Parkinson's disease who received clozapine. Clozapine will not worsen Parkinson's disease, and a surprising effect has been an improvement of motor features, notably tremor in such patients. It appears to improve tremors in a majority of patients with Parkinson's disease and completely ameliorates Parkinson's disease tremor in some cases.[213] Additionally, the use of clozapine in treating psychosis in patients with Parkinson's disease has been associated with dramatic improvements in facial and truncal dystonias.[212]

12.10.3 Myoclonus, Tremor, Tics, Asterixis

Other continuous DIMDs, including tremor, chorea, and myoclonus, may be associated with various medications, and a dose reduction or discontinuation of the offending medication will typically relieve the symptoms.

Myoclonus is defined as sudden, brief, shock-like, or lightning-like involuntary movements caused by muscular contractions. Although various disorders—including neurodegenerative, systemic metabolic disorders—and infections may cause myoclonus, this involuntary movement may also be drug-induced. Evidence is available to indicate that levodopa, bismuth salts, and cyclic antidepressants alone or in combination with lithium may induce reversible myoclonus. SSRIs can also induce myoclonus, although this DIMD is most frequently associated with serotonin syndrome. Other drugs that have been reported to induce myoclonus include typical and atypical antipsychotics, MAOIs, metoclopramide, anticonvulsants (valproic acid, carbamazepine, phenytoin, gabapentin, lamotrigine), opiates (morphine, fentanyl, methadone, hydrocodone), general anesthetics (propofol, enflurane, etomidate), antineoplastics (chlorambucil, prednimustine, ifosfamide), cardiovascular drugs (propafenone, flecainide, diltiazem, nifedipine), and anti-infectives (penicillins, cephalosporins, imipenem, quinolones, isoniazid, and acyclovir). Anxiolytics, such as buspirone, carisoprodol, and benzodiazepines, have also been implicated in myoclonus. High doses of morphine and meperidine and opioids have been implicated as causative agents of myoclonus; however, these studies usually cite concomitant factors such as malignancies, renal failure treated with hemodialysis, and exposure to neuroleptics.[214,215] Withdrawal from benzodiazepine treatment may also induce drug-induced myoclonus. Withdrawal of the offending drug usually leads to gradual resolution of the drug-induced myoclonus, although some cases may require treatment with serotonin antagonists such as methysergide and cyproheptadine.[216]

Tremor is rhythmic and usually monomorphic, and, unlike myoclonus, it does not unpredictably and chaotically change in direction. Tremor is a recognized complication of antidepressant therapy, and it is estimated that up to 10 percent of patients on a tricyclic antidepressant, such as imipramine, may experience it.[217] The mechanism may be the enhancement of physiologic tremor as propranolol ameliorates the tremor. However, generalized choreoathetoid movements may be a manifestation of tricyclic antidepressant poisoning.[218] The recognition of the serotonin syndrome has been associated with the use of serotonin reuptake inhibitors, tricyclic antidepressants, monoamine oxidase inhibitors, and other agents known to increase the biologic activity of serotonin. Symptoms associated with serotonin syndrome may be confused with neuroleptic malignant syndrome and include myoclonus, ataxia, agitation, altered mental status, shivering, and hyperreflexia. Symptoms may be minor or life-threatening in severity and noted to occur in about 15 percent of patients overdosing on SSRIs.[219] A Cochrane review and meta-analysis of various antipsychotics noted the prevalence percentage for drug-induced tremors to be: Paliperidone (2.7 percent), quetiapine (6.0 percent), aripiprazole (6.1 percent), ziprasidone (6.5 percent), olanzapine (7.9 percent), risperidone (8.2 percent), chlorpromazine (18.4 percent), and haloperidol (22 percent).[16]

Occasional episodes of tremors have been reported with phenytoin and carbamazepine. Psychostimulants such as cocaine, amphetamine, methamphetamine, methylphenidate, and MDMA have also been associated with tremors.[220] Amiodarone, a cardiac antiarrhythmic agent, may produce a tremor, typically of the postural type, and may also cause ataxia. Cyclosporine-A, an immunosuppressive agent utilized in organ transplantation, may produce a tremor of low amplitude and high frequency. Alcohol use or withdrawal may be associated with tremors, ataxia, myoclonus, parkinsonism, and orolingual dyskinesias. Drugs used in the management of asthma can often produce tremors as an adverse effect. Agents known to cause this effect include isoproterenol, aminophylline, theophylline, terbutaline, and other beta agonists utilized in the management of asthma. Lithium, utilized for the prophylaxis and management of manic depressive disorders, is known to produce enhancement of physiological tremor. The incidence is from 33 to 65 percent, and the occurrence increases with increasing lithium levels and is seen in 100 percent of lithium toxicity cases. Valproic acid is the most common tremor-inducing agent among the antiepileptic drugs. Approximately 25 percent of patients receiving chronic valproic acid therapy will experience tremor, which is generally postural.[217] Alcohol ingestion may lead to an improvement in some primary movement disorders, including essential tremor and myoclonic dystonia.[221] Tranquilizers, including benzodiazepines, are often utilized in the management of tremor; however, tremors may occur during benzodiazepine withdrawal. Additionally, many medications that are renally eliminated may produce disturbances in the central nervous system when utilized in individuals with some degree of renal impairment.

SSRIs such as fluoxetine, paroxetine, sertraline, and escitalopram have been associated with the appearance of tics.[222] Abnormal involuntary choreiform movements have been reported in an elderly male on chronic maintenance hemodialysis who received valacyclovir and famciclovir.[221] Stimulants such as cocaine, even in small doses, can exacerbate or cause the recurrence of motor tics in patients with different movement disorders, including Tourette's syndrome and tardive dyskinesia. Some clinicians have concluded that cocaine addiction is a predisposing factor for the development of tics and dystonias upon exposure to neuroleptics. As over 30 million Americans have used cocaine and over 5 million use it regularly, it may be regarded as an important cause or trigger of hyperkinetic movement disorders, especially if there is a sudden onset or an acute exacerbation.[223,224] Amphetamines may also lead to movement disorders commonly described as stereotypies.[224]

Asterixis is a movement disorder that presents as loss of muscle tone, resulting in a coarse "flapping tremor." It appears as an involuntary jerk superimposed on a postural or intentional movement and is also referred to as "negative myoclonus." The symptoms are most obvious when the patient stands still with outstretched arms and dorsiflexed wrists, and the extremities are usually asynchronously affected. Although metabolic disorders and hepatic encephalopathy are the most common causes for asterixis, some anticonvulsants, medications, and mood stabilizers such as carbamazepine, gabapentin, and lithium have been associated with this disorder.[225–227] In most patients, a cessation or reduction of the medication has led to cessation of asterixis.[98]

12.11 PERSISTENT/TARDIVE DRUG-INDUCED MOVEMENT DISORDERS

DIMDs may be persistent and tardive, appearing during long-term exposure to the offending agent, hence the term "tardive" meaning "late-onset." These DIMDs are patterned and periodic and persist beyond the discontinuation of the causative agent. The term tardive syndrome encompasses tardive stereotypies, which present as involuntary, repetitive, rhythmic, purposeless movements, which may appear purposeful or ritualistic. Tardive dyskinesia (TD) is the most common type, followed by tardive dystonia, akathisia, tremor, chorea, and myoclonus.[228,229]

12.11.1 Tardive Dyskinesia

12.11.1.1 Presentation

TD is a syndrome characterized by repetitive muscle movements that are purposeless in nature and can impair the patient's ability to function socially and, rarely, physiologically. Most movements are rapid unsustained movements variously described as choreic, with the former referring to movements that are unpredictable and rapid and flow from one body region to another, while the latter are rhythmic, reproducible, and regular, remaining generally restricted in their anatomic distribution. Athetoid movements may also occur, and these are slow, sinuous, and continual. Any area of the body may be affected, but the orofacial area is commonly involved, affecting more than 75 percent of patients with TD. Symptoms include lip-smacking and puckering, tongue protrusion, chewing, sucking, grimacing, blinking, puffing of cheeks, and frowning. Other abnormal movements involve the extremities and trunk and are observed in 50 percent and 25 percent of patients, respectively. Symptoms manifested include shoulder shrugging, rocking, incessant flexion-extension movements, wrist flexion or torsion, ankle flexion or rotation, or ballistic movements. In the elderly patient population, orofacial dyskinesias are more common whereas limb or truncal dyskinesias without orofacial involvement are more commonly observed in younger patients.

Over the past 20 years, the prevalence of TD has increased dramatically. This may be because more patients are receiving DRBAs, patients may be starting medication at an earlier age and taking them longer, the doses are higher, and drug holidays are more likely.[196] To fit the definition of TD, patients must have a history of at least three months of total cumulative exposure to at least one DRBA with exposure being continuous or intermittent. In patients over the age of 60, the history of neuroleptic use should be for at least one month. The signs or symptoms of TD develop during exposure to neuroleptic or within four weeks of withdrawal from an oral neuroleptic agent. In the case of depot preparation, the time of withdrawal is extended to eight weeks.[230]

The symptoms of TD tend to be worsened by stimulants and may be transiently worsened by emotional arousal, stress, and distraction during voluntary movements in unaffected parts of the body. The abnormal body movements are transiently reduced by relaxation and are generally absent during sleep. Symptoms of TD may appear during neuroleptic treatment, after dosage reduction, or after discontinuation of the neuroleptic agent. Upon neuroleptic withdrawal, the symptoms of this disorder may appear to be aggravated; however, with time, their severity usually subsides. TD may be irreversible, and improvement of TD after drug withdrawal is variable in reported studies, with remission rates reported lower in the elderly. One study noted that only 2 percent of patients who withdrew from neuroleptics had a significant recovery, and another 20 percent reported some level of improvement within one year.[231]

In severe cases, TD may be associated with medical problems such as ulcers in cheeks and tongue, ill-fitting dentures, loss of teeth, macroglossia, difficulty in walking, swallowing, or breathing, weight loss, depression, and suicidal ideation. Although most cases of TD are of minor functional significance, the disorder is cosmetically and socially disfiguring, and by the very nature of these constant odd movements, patients may be hindered from fully participating and functioning successfully within the community setting.[232,233]

Spontaneous dyskinesias may resemble TD and have been observed in patients with schizophrenia long before the discovery of antipsychotics. Their reported rate has been as high as 53 percent. However, the development of dyskinesias has also been associated with normal aging, with 4 to 8 percent of healthy elderly men experiencing them.[234–237]

12.11.1.2 Case Study: Neuroleptic-Induced Oral Buccal Dyskinesia and Akathisia

A 67-year-old woman with longstanding history of bipolar disorder, well-controlled on mood stabilizers such as valproic acid or lamotrigine, with various selective serotonin reuptake inhibitors, presented to clinic with abnormal movements. At the age of 65, her symptoms became uncontrolled with the lamotrigine and sertraline, so lurasidone was started. The medication was very helpful in treating her bipolar disorder, but she began to feel that she could not sit still and she had to continuously move her legs at all times or she developed an uncomfortable sensation. This began to interrupt her sleep. Three months after the initial restlessness began, she started having uncontrolled movements of her lips and tongue. On examination, she had opening and closing of her mouth and lip pursing, as well as writhing movements of her tongue that were viewed with her mouth open. Her psychiatrist diagnosed akathisia as well as tardive orobuccal dyskinesia, and she began a slow taper off of the lurasidone. However, both the akathisia and the orobuccal dyskinesia persisted. Several other medical treatments were tried for both the akathisia and the dyskinesia, such as clonazepam and amantadine, but none were successful in providing significant improvement in her movement.

12.11.1.3 Implicated Agents

Neuroleptics are by far the biggest culprits in causing the symptoms of TD. Increased risk of TD has been associated with the cumulative amount of neuroleptic agent, the number of interruptions in neuroleptic treatment as well as the cumulative amount of anticholinergic agents. Generally, if the treatment with neuroleptics is required, then treatment should not be given intermittently, as the risk of TD is three times as great for patients with more than two interruptions as for patients with two or less interruptions in treatment.[238] The incidence of persistent TD was noted to increase with longer duration of treatment in a study of antipsychotic-naïve patients with first-episode schizophrenia. The cumulative incidence of TD after one year, two years, and four years was reported at 4.8 percent, 7.2 percent, and 15.6 percent, respectively.[239] A review noted that the annualized TD incidence was 3.9 percent for atypical antipsychotics and 5.5 percent for typical antipsychotics. Stratified by age, annual TD incidence rates were 0.35 percent with atypical antipsychotics in children, 3 percent with atypical antipsychotics versus 7.7 percent with typical antipsychotics in adults, and 5.2 percent with typical antipsychotics in the elderly. TD in four adult studies noted TD prevalence rates were 13.1 percent for atypical antipsychotics, 15.6 percent for antipsychotic-free patients, and 32.4 percent for typical antipsychotics.[240]

The expectation that the atypicals would reduce the threat of TD has received considerable support in reviews and several clinical trials, although some of the latter have been industry sponsored. Reports of TD associated with the use of atypical antipsychotics are increasing, as more patients are exposed to these agents for longer time periods. For example, risperidone demonstrated a lower incidence of acute EPS during initial clinical trials; however, postmarketing data indicates that EPS liability is dose-dependent. In the absence of longer-term data, the limited evidence available indicates that the atypical antipsychotics have a decreased liability of TD, approximately 1 percent compared with 5 percent for typical antipsychotics annually.[239] The apparent incidence of TD with risperidone is between 0.03 and 2.4 percent; the risk of EPS increases when risperidone is dosed above 6 mg/day.[240–243] Cases have been reported demonstrating a relationship between this atypical neuroleptic and TD, and in one trial, a jury awarded a 45-year-old woman $6.7 million who was on risperidone and developed TD over a 15-month period.[244] In a two-year prospective study with risperidone or olanzapine in antipsychotic-naïve patients aged more than 55 years, the cumulative TD rate was 5 percent and 7 percent after one year and two years, respectively, with risperidone, while the rate was 7 percent and 11 percent after one and two years, respectively, with olanzapine.[241] Although quetiapine has been associated with a lower risk of inducing EPS, it has been reported to precipitate TD in patients never exposed to typical neuroleptics.[245] The incidence of TD with olanzapine is 0.5 to 1 percent compared with 4.5 to 7.5 percent for haloperidol, and some reports cite that the rate of TD with quetiapine is similar to olanzapine and significantly less than that associated with haloperidol in all age groups.[241] Ziprasidone has been reported to induce TD in a patient with a long history of treatment with traditional antipsychotics.[246] Aripiprazole has been implicated in causing TD in a patient following 18 months of treatment for refractory depression and in a patient following 9 months of treatment for schizophrenia.[247,248] In another care series, aripiprazole was implicated in causing akathisia, chorea, orobuccolingual dyskinesia, and acute dystonia.[249] However, aripiprazole has also been noted to improve symptoms of TD in a patient who developed TD while on quetiapine and later on ziprasidone.[248] Clozapine, although less likely to cause EPS, may also induce TD in rare cases.[250]

The relationship between initiating therapy with either a typical or atypical antipsychotic agent and subsequent new diagnosis of a DIMD other than parkinsonism in older patients with dementia was evaluated. In the one-year follow-up period, it was noted that the risk of developing TD or another DIMD other than parkinsonism, while being treated with an atypical agent, was not statistically different from that with a typical antipsychotic.[45] More recently, a records-based case control study did not find a significant difference in the risk of TD between atypical and typical antipsychotic medication users in adult patients at the Veterans Administration Puget Sound Health Care System after adjusting for age, race, gender, schizophrenia, schizoaffective disorder, depression, and anti-parkinsonian drugs.[251] Thus, the relative risk for TD may be smaller with the atypicals; however, they cannot be said to have an absolute advantage over the typical antipsychotics.

Reports also show that low doses of clozapine are effective in the management of neuroleptic-induced EPS (TD, DIP, and chronic akathisia) in neuroleptic-resistant chronic schizophrenic patients.[252] A few case reports note the onset of TD following clozapine treatment; however, in all those cases, patients had exposure to other antipsychotic drugs, and the dyskinesia can be considered an idiosyncratic reaction to clozapine.[253,254] Since clozapine is utilized in patients who have previously been exposed to neuroleptics as this is not a first-line agent but one reserved for patients who are treatment resistant or cannot tolerate any of the other neuroleptics, such patients may already have been sensitized to develop TD as a result of their exposure to various other neuroleptics.

Metoclopramide, a dopaminergic receptor blocker, is also implicated in causing TD. It is used in the treatment of diabetic gastroparesis and esophageal reflux and as an antiemetic. It may cause or exacerbate TD, and the course of the disorder is similar to that observed with neuroleptic usage. Symptoms of the movement disorder may disappear following drug withdrawal, or they may be irreversible. The majority of the cases reported with metoclopramide as a causative factor in TD are in elderly women.[255–258] One study noted a higher incidence of TD in diabetic patients treated with metoclopramide than in nondiabetics treated with the agent.[98] Although metoclopramide has been available for over 30 years, the manufacturers did not adequately study the long-term safety of this drug and grossly underestimated the risk of TD and other related movement disorders associated with its use. Analyses published recently have cited metoclopramide as the most common cause of DIMDs, and exposure greater than 12 weeks was evident in a majority of those reports.[259] The FDA now requires manufacturers of metoclopramide to add a boxed warning to the drug's labeling advising of the risk of TD associated with long-term, high-dose use and to implement a risk evaluation and mitigation strategy so patients are provided a guide to address the risk.[260]

12.11.1.4 Case Study: Metoclopramide-Induced Oral Buccal Lingual Dyskinesia

An 83-year-old woman was placed on metoclopramide for symptoms of nausea for seven months. Her dentist noticed that her jaw was moving around during a routine dental examination, but she was not bothered by this. She discontinued the medication as she no longer had nausea. One year later, she was hospitalized for an ileostomy, and metoclopramide was restarted. She had complications from the surgery and was in the hospital for several weeks. After she was discharged, the metoclopramide was stopped again, but she had developed more severe jaw movements, bruxism, and tongue thrusting. She began to have severe jaw pain, as well as difficulty eating because of food being pushed out of her mouth by her tongue. On examination, she had prominent jaw opening and tongue thrusting. Botulinum toxin was used for her jaw movements, which alleviated pain, but the movements remained several years later. Tongue movement was targeted with botulinum toxin as well, but the patient developed dysphagia, so this was not repeated.

Oral facial dyskinesias, described as persistent involuntary movements of the face and mouth, have been linked to extended use of antihistaminic decongestants.[261] Amiodarone, an antiarrhythmic agent, is associated with various neurologic adverse effects including severe cases of dyskinesia.[35] Choreoathetotic movements as well as facial dyskinesia have been reported with gabapentin, an anticonvulsant utilized for seizure disorders and pain management and as a mood stabilizer.[262]

SSRI-induced movement disorders have been reported as involuntary movements of the face, limbs, or trunk, as well as facial grimacing. Dyskinesias were noted to occur within one day to two months of initiating therapy with the offending SSRIs, while the latent dyskinesias (i.e., TD) were noted to occur within six months to four years of initiating the antidepressant. A majority of the patients were receiving a neuroleptic concurrently or had done so in the past.[100] Most of the cases involved fluoxetine, used alone and in conjunction with neuroleptics, and several dozen spontaneous reports of TD have been recorded by the manufacturer.[263] TD has been associated with most classes of antidepressant agents, and, in contrast to neuroleptics, dyskinesia associated with antidepressant treatment appears to be typically rapid in onset and disappears rapidly after the withdrawal of the offending antidepressant.[264–266]

12.11.1.5 Risks

Advanced age has always been cited as a major risk factor for TD, and elderly patients have a greater likelihood that the TD may be more severe or more generalized with continued neuroleptic usage compared to younger patients. Other risk factors for TD have cited women, duration and cumulative amount of antipsychotic medication, organic brain damage (neurodegenerative disease), alcohol abuse, recent drug-free intervals, a diagnosis of affective disorder and subsequent adjunctive neuroleptic use for such disorders other than their use in schizophrenia or schizoaffective disorders, and early development of EPS, particularly DIP. Diabetic patients have been noted to have an increased risk of spontaneous dyskinetic movements and TD compared to non-diabetics.[267]

Genetic factors responsible for differences in inter-individual vulnerability have also been implicated, with a higher risk in African Americans.[268] Alcohol and/or drug abuse has been found to increase the risk of TD by threefold, particularly the orofacial subtype involving the head and upper extremities in patients with a long history of alcohol abuse or dependence.[269] An association has been noted between the level of cigarette consumption and the current severity of TD and requires further exploration considering the high prevalence of smoking in psychiatric patients.[270] Since smoking induces hepatic enzymes and accelerates the metabolism of antipsychotics, patients may require higher doses of prescribed neuroleptics which may contribute to the increased prevalence of TD in smokers.

The perception has existed that patients treated with conventional neuroleptic medications may be at an increased risk of developing a diagnosis for TD compared to patients treated with atypical neuroleptics.[192] The purported TD-suppressing and TD-preventive effects of atypical neuroleptics cannot be endorsed, as recent data has shown that compared to typical neuroleptics, atypical neuroleptics do not have a reduced risk of causing TD nor do they have an ability to suppress the preexisting TD.[181] Additionally, among patients with a diagnosis of TD, the same incidence of use of atypical neuroleptics as typical neuroleptics was noted, even after adjustments were made for age, sex, race, diagnosis, and anti-parkinsonian drugs. Thus, there was no significant difference in risk of TD between patients who received atypical and typical neuroleptics.[271] According to a multivariate analysis, the only variable for the long-term evolution of tardive dyskinesia was dependent on illness duration, independent of age.[237]

12.11.1.6 Management

Recently, newer agents have been studied and approved for managing the symptoms of TD. Valbenazine (Ingrezza ®) and deutetrabenazine (Austedo ®) were both approved by the FDA as treatment for TD in April 2017 and August 2017, respectively. Both are reversible specific inhibitors of vesicular monoamine transporter 2 (VMAT2), a protein in the brain that transports monoamine neurotransmitters (i.e., dopamine, serotonin, norepinephrine, histamine) into vesicles for release into the synapse. Both drugs are related to tetrabenazine, an FDA-approved drug for the treatment of Huntington's chorea. The inhibitory effects of these VMAT2 inhibitors may lower monoamine neurotransmitter concentrations in the synaptic cleft, reducing the availability of dopamine to hypersensitive postsynaptic receptors and thus decreasing the occurrence of dyskinetic movements.[272]

Valbenazine does not require genotyping and enables once-daily dosing, with recommendations starting at 40 mg daily with or without food and increasing the dose after one week to 80 mg once daily. Concomitant use with MAOI should be avoided, and use with strong CYP3A4 inhibitors or strong CYP2D inhibitors requires a dose of 40 mg once daily. Concomitant use of strong CYP3A4 inducers is not recommended. There were no differences reported in low incidences of depression or suicidality between valbenazine and placebo, and compared to placebo, the most common adverse reaction was noted to be somnolence (11 percent versus 4 percent, respectively). Deutetrabenazine is related to tetrabenazine with improvements in tolerability aided by slower drug metabolism, and low incidences of depression and suicidal ideation were noted. Deutetrabenazine also does not require genotyping, and the dose is determined individually for patients based on reduction of TD symptoms and tolerability, with the recommended starting dose at 6 mg twice daily, administered with food. The dose may be increased at weekly intervals in increments of 6 mg/day to a maximum daily dose of 48 mg. A maximum daily dose of 36 mg (18 mg twice daily) is recommended with the concomitant use of strong CYP2D6 inhibitors. Alcohol and other sedatives may cause additive sedation and somnolence. The most common adverse reactions with deutetrabenazine compared to placebo were nasopharyngitis (4 percent versus 2 percent) and insomnia (4 percent versus 1 percent). Deutetrabeanzine is contraindicated in suicidal patients or those untreated/inadequately treated for depression with Huntington's disease. Both valbenazine and deutetrabenazine treatment may potentially prolong QT interval, and patients should be monitored for a fast, slow, or irregular heartbeat; shortness of breath; dizziness; or fainting.[273–275]

In years past, various agents have been utilized for managing symptoms of TD, and the treatment of TD was an unmet clinical need prior to 2017 as few options demonstrating efficacy and safety in managing this condition were available. In 2013, American Academy of Neurology evidence-based guidelines for managing TD noted that interventions with some evidence to support their use in managing symptoms of TD included clonazepam, Gingko biloba, amantadine, and tetrabenazine.[274] Later in 2018, they updated their guidelines to include deutetrabenazine and valbenazine as established effective treatments for TD, and the use of pallidal deep brain stimulation as a consideration for intractable TD.[276]

Ginkgo biloba, an herbal product, has free radical scavenging action and has been studied in managing tardive syndromes at doses 80 to 240 mg/day. Although sold over the counter as an herb, caution is advised with ginkgo biloba due to its antiplatelet effect which may lead to increased bleeding, including cerebral bleeding and hemorrhagic complications.[277] Other agents that have been associated with a reduction in the magnitude of symptoms include baclofen, valproic acid, vitamin E, vitamin B6, melatonin, branch-chain amino acids, and essential fatty acids. However, there is no convincing evidence that any of these pharmacologic interventions or dietary supplements are successful treatment options, as their success rate is low.[15,278] It is also recommended that anticholinergics be discontinued since these agents may at times worsen TD. Case reports cite possible improvement in neuroleptic-induced TD after changing to the atypical antipsychotic aripiprazole.[279,280] Clozapine has been shown to be the most effective antipsychotic in managing tardive syndrome and noted not to be associated with worsening of any tardive syndrome.[281]

The continued need for chronic neuroleptic treatment needs to be regularly assessed, and their use should be discontinued when their efficacy is uncertain or when alternative agents can be used instead.[230,282,283] Treatment of TD primarily consists of discontinuing the causative agent, although an abrupt cessation of a neuroleptic should be avoided as acute withdrawal may induce transient worsening of symptoms.

It is important to minimize exposure to DRBAs in an attempt to prevent the occurrence of this movement disorder. Clinicians should follow best practice guidance for use of antipsychotics, limit prescription to specific indications, use effective doses, and minimize the duration of therapy.[284] Periodic evaluations of patients on long-term neuroleptics should be undertaken, and patients should be examined regularly, at least every three to six months, for dyskinesia as well as other types of neurological disorders. The nature and severity of the movement disorder should be noted to serve as a baseline for ongoing evaluations. The Abnormal Involuntary Movement Scale (AIMS) is the most widely recommended and utilized tool for evaluating TD in clinical practice.[89,285] The AIMS consists of 12 items, with the first 1 to 7 items assessing the severity of abnormal movements in different body areas (e.g., face, jaw, tongue, lips, trunk and upper and lower extremities) and are scored on a 5-point scale (0 = none and 4 = severe). The latter 8 to 12 items include three clinician-based questions assessing global severity, patient incapacitation, and patient awareness, and two questions addressing dental status. As items 8 to 12 are subjective with no conventional scoring, they are not included in the total score of items 1 through 7. In recent years, malpractice suits have resulted in substantial judgments for the plaintiffs over the development of TD in psychiatric patients. Plaintiffs are successful in approximately 50 percent of all TD-related malpractice cases, compared with only about 10 to 20 percent of all medical malpractice suits. The lawsuits have cited improper administration of neuroleptic agents, including the misdiagnosis of a medical condition that did not warrant therapy with a DRBA. Physicians have been known to either fail to monitor patients or poorly monitor patients' body movements while being under treatment.[286] It is essential that periodic assessment of abnormal movements be undertaken for the early detection of TD. Additionally, proper documentation of the indication of drug therapy and obtaining an informed consent are equally important in avoiding liability. Hospital policies and state law mandate that patients be informed of the potential benefits and risks of psychotropic agents, and it has been recommended that informed consent be obtained every six months due to the fluctuating mental competence of patients with schizophrenia and other chronic mental illnesses.[287–291] Patients receiving antipsychotics should be monitored utilizing the AIMS and need to be treated promptly if TD is present. About 10 percent of patients with TD remain severely disabled even with pharmacologic treatment, and data shows that deep brain stimulation of the globus pallidus internus may be considered in patients whose TD symptoms are not responsive to pharmacotherapy.[284]

12.11.2 Tardive Akathisia

Chronic, tardive, and withdrawal akathisia commonly are reported with long-term use of neuroleptic agents. Reported rates for tardive akathisia are approximately 30 percent, similar to the 20 to 30 percent reported for acute akathisia.[291] The incidence with atypical antipsychotics appears to be lower compared to the typical antipsychotics; however, no systematic data are currently available, and studies are limited.[89,276]

Although the temporal criteria for tardive akathisia are debatable, symptoms of tardive akathisia may occur after three months on a stable medication regimen or several months after drug withdrawal or dose reduction. The term chronic akathisia refers to the duration of akathisia, irrespective of whether the type of onset is acute, tardive, or withdrawal. Withdrawal akathisia, however, is restricted to akathisia which may develop when the dose of a neuroleptic is withdrawn or reduced. Risk factors for the development of chronic and tardive akathisia are poorly understood, but female sex, old age, iron deficiency, negative symptoms, cognitive dysfunction, and affective disorder may increase the risk of tardive or chronic akathisia.[132,292,293]

Management strategies for tardive akathisia are very similar to those used for acute akathisia and include beta-blockers, antimuscarinic agents, and benzodiazepines, although improvement may be equivocal.[33,89] A case of aripiprazole-induced tardive akathisia responding to the dopamine agonist ropinirole has been reported.[294] Chronic akathisia due to risperidone has been cited as a reason for a patient to become extremely irritable, easily agitated, and at times violent.[132]

12.11.3 Tardive Dystonia

Tardive dystonia occurs after chronic exposure, usually months to years, of treatment with DRBA or within three months of treatment discontinuation. Symptoms are generally more insidious, and severity may vary. Tardive dystonia may occur as a result of chronic neuroleptic exposure with preferential involvement of axial muscles and characteristic rocking movements of the trunk and pelvis. Facial dystonia can present as blepharospasm or facial grimacing, while involvement of the mandible may present in tonic deviation, protrusion, bruxism, or sustained opening or closing of the jaw. Tardive dystonia appears to be most prominent in younger adults and in men. This DIMD frequently persists even after the discontinuation of the causative agent, and patients are often refractory to medical management. It is important to exclude neurological causes of dystonia (e.g., Wilson disease) while making the diagnosis. Most reports of tardive dystonias have been associated with typical neuroleptics; however, cases have been reported with atypical agents including olanzapine, risperidone, and aripiprazole.[15] Many tardive dystonias involve the craniocervical region, which constitutes the most common and most severely affected region. Anticholinergics such as trihexyphenidyl may be utilized for managing tardive dystonia; however, their use may worsen dyskinesia. Botulism toxin injection may be beneficial for certain forms of focal movements impacting the tongue, jaw muscles, or cervical musculature. Clozapine has been shown in several uncontrolled observations to benefit about 40 percent of patients with TD, particularly those with tardive dystonia.[295]

12.11.3.1 Case Report: Neuroleptic-Induced Cervical Dystonia

A 39-year-old African American man with schizophrenia presented to clinic for neck spasms that started seven years prior when the patient was on haloperidol 50 mg daily. He was on this medication for three years, and he began to notice that his head would preferentially turn to the right. He began to have pain with this, and it was progressively more difficult for him to turn his head to the left. Before haloperidol, he had been on olanzapine, ziprasidone, clozapine, and risperidone without efficacy nor adverse effects. He was switched to aripiprazole, and his neck turning improved but did not resolve. He used a soft collar to help alleviate some of the pain associated with the neck turning. Physical examination revealed head turn to the right with some decrease in range of motion with the patient attempting to turn his head to the left, and he was diagnosed with tardive cervical dystonia. The patient responded well to botulinum toxin injections but was unable to wean off aripiprazole because of the poor control of schizophrenia without this medication.

12.11.4 Other Tardive Variants

Other tardive variants less commonly reported in literature include tardive myoclonus, tardive tics, tardive Tourette syndrome, tardive parkinsonism, and tardive tremors.[2,293] Tardive gait has also been reported and may be part of the TD spectrum. Patients with tardive gait present with different gait abnormalities, including "unsteadiness," "pelvic thrust," stiffness," "dancing gait," and a "duck-like" gait. This type of heterogeneous neurological disorder has been noted to occur in patients who had taken DRBAs such as prochloperazine, metoclopramide, as well as antipsychotics for a number of years.[296,297] Benzodiazepines may be beneficial in managing some symptoms, particularly when used for tardive myoclonus. Deep brain stimulation may be beneficial in severe and refractory cases of some tardive syndromes including tardive dyskinesia, tardive dystonia, and tardive tourettism.[277] Clozapine may be a treatment option in patients with tardive syndromes who may require continued treatment with an antipsychotic, as its beneficial effects in such syndromes are greater than its role in causing or worsening tardive syndromes.[281]

12.12 DRUGS USED FOR MOVEMENT DISORDERS

Restless leg syndrome (RLS) is characterized by an irresistible urge to move, usually the legs, to stop an uncontrollable sensation. If affects women twice as often as men. RLS may be primary, where the pathophysiology is not established, although impaired iron metabolism and abnormal dopaminerigic neurotransmission have been proposed. Secondary causes of RLS include iron deficiency anemia, folate deficiency, chronic kidney disease, diabetes mellitus, pregnancy, peripheral neuropathy, and drug-induced causes. Medications which have been reported as causative agents in drug-induced RLS include analgesics (NSAIDS), anti-epileptic agents (phenytoin, topiramate, zonisamide), antidepressants (SSRIs, TCAs, trazodone, mirtazapine, venlafaxine), atypical antipsychotics (clozapine, olanzapine, quetiapine, risperidone), donepezil, lithium, metoclopramide, interferon-alfa, anesthetics, nicotine, caffeine, and thyroid hormones and tramadol.[298–300] Generally, antidepressants are the drugs most commonly implicated in secondary RLS, and symptoms occur shortly, usually within one week, after drug initiation or dose increase.

A review of literature of RLS induced by quetiapine noted that in almost all cases, the DIMD occurred when the antipsychotic was added to the existing antidepressant therapy in patients with affective disorders, appearing to increase the risk for RLS in this patient population.[301] With regard to other drug-induced RLS, the onset of symptoms varies widely. Symptoms have been shown to occur one to five days following drug initiation or dose increase with antipsychotics, while symptoms following supplementation with thyroid hormones may take two months to appear.[302]

Long-term treatment with levodopa for PD may lead to levodopa-induced abnormal movements in patients with PD. Monophasic dyskinesia occurs at the time of maximal clinical improvement and is usually of the choreic type commonly referred to as "peak-dose" dyskinesia, whereas diphasic dyskinesia is of the dystonic or ballistic type and is referred to as the "onset" or "end-dose" dyskinesia. Adjusting the dosing of dopaminergic medications, such as lowering the dose, may be beneficial. Discontinuing selegiline (deprenyl) may reduce dyskinesias, and reducing the dose of or discontinuing treatment with a dopamine agonist may also be beneficial.[303] Amantadine is commonly used in levodopa-induced dyskinesia and can be effective for some patients.[304] Newer agents that are reversible vesicular monoamine transporter type 2 inhibitors such as valbenazine and deutetrabenazine have recently been approved by the FDA for the treatment of tardive dyskinesia in adults.[16]

12.13 MONITORING

Patients receiving DRBAs should be examined regularly for DIMDs as a component of a regular evaluation of extrapyramidal symptoms (EPS). Hence, the documentation of informed consent is critical in reducing liability, and consent forms have been developed to aid in providing appropriate documentation of the risk of TD and the benefits of antipsychotic medications.[305] The Mount Sinai guidelines on the pharmacotherapy of schizophrenia represent a minimal level of monitoring and recommend that patients be evaluated for EPS and tardive dyskinesia prior to starting on new medications, every three to six months for patients who receive typical antipsychotics, and every

12 months for patients who receive an atypical antipsychotic agent. Additionally, the guidelines call for more frequent monitoring for patients who are at a higher risk for EPS.[306] Recently updated guidelines from the American Psychiatric Association stress regular assessments of patients for tardive dyskinesia and other movement disorders.[89] Examination of EPS can be performed easily by clinicians trained to recognize the various manifestations and movements associated with DIMDs.[307] These DIMDs are assessed formally in clinical trials using several different standardized rating scales such as the Barnes Akathisia Scale, Simpson Angus Scale, Extrapyramidal Symptom Rating Scale and the Abnormal Involuntary Movement Scale, and the Rush Dyskinesia Rating Scale, which detect and quantify these movement disorders.[308–312]

Clinicians frequently overlook many DIMDs, hence it is important to consider this complication among other secondary and tertiary conditions, as most DIMDs are potentially reversible with discontinuation of the offending agent. Listing all potential medications if a DIMD is suspected is necessary as is grading the implicated medications according to their potential to cause the identified DIMD. The offending agent should be discontinued, and, if not possible, then a reduction in dose should be made, or a substitution of the offending agent to an alternative agent with a better adverse effect profile.[6]

12.14 CLINICAL AND LEGAL ISSUES IN PSYCHIATRY

Unfortunately, DIMDs may be undiagnosed, misdiagnosed, and untreated even among psychiatrists and neurologists.[313] In one study of 25 representative schizophrenic patients who underwent a standardized neurological examination to detect EPS, two-thirds were prescribed an atypical neuroleptic, and 18 of the 25 had EPS. Upon a review of the clinician's notes for the past 12 months, it was noted that only half of the patients had documented evidence of a management plan addressing the EPS. However, only 1 patient of the 25 during that time period had a documented physical examination recording the presence or absence of EPS.[314] Likewise, a review of medical records of 204 hospitalized patients showed a high rate of failure to document the assessment and course of EPS.[315] These findings suggest that clinicians do not recognize the importance of documentation of these significant adverse effects, and it highlights the fact that although screening for EPS is recommended by the American Psychiatric Association, it may not be routine. Possible reasons for this may be that clinicians may lack the knowledge and skills to accurately diagnose and appropriately manage EPS, they may underestimate the distress the DIMDs may produce, or they may simply lack the time to address this aspect of patient care. Additionally, lack of understanding of DIMDs, complacency among prescribers of DRBAs, the increased use of DRBAs in populations that had never previously been exposed to such agents (e.g., children, adolescents, elderly), and wider use in the adult population may increase the number of cases of DIMDs.[316]

From a legal standpoint, the greater the risk of any treatment, the greater is the duty to warn, monitor, or look for other alternatives.[317] However, there is evidence that the fear of litigation may influence treatment methods to a greater degree than sound medical evidence and best practice guidelines. A report in 2005 noted that up to 93 percent of physicians in high-liability specialties report practicing defensive medicine.[318] To avoid this counterproductive trend, physicians should be concerned first with safety and efficacy and should manage the risk of malpractice liability by following the traditional golden standards of medicine of informed consent, use of evidence-based medicine, integration of specialized medicine, and thorough patient follow-up care.[319]

Prevention and early recognition of the symptoms are the best methods of managing DIMDs. First, patients and, if appropriate, their family members need to be informed of the risks of DIMDs and benefits of treatment before starting therapy with a DRBA. Second, the use of the DRBAs should be restricted to only those patients for whom no alternative treatment is available. Third, the exposure should be limited by keeping the dose of the DRBA to the lowest possible effective level. Fourth, the patient should be assessed every three months, and the patient's need for continued treatment with a DRBA should be reassessed. Fifth, whenever possible, the patient's medication should be switched to one that has limited antagonism of dopamine receptors (e.g., use an antiemetic such as ondansetron instead of metoclopramide or compazine). And last, but not least, every patient who is taking a DRBA should be examined every three months for symptoms of DIMDs.

The plaintiff in a medical malpractice suit must prove by a preponderance of the evidence that the physician was negligent. What is sometimes referred to as " the four D's" must be established: The physician had a duty to care for the patient, the physician breached that duty, the injuries caused were the direct and proximate result of the physician's breach, and the injuries suffered by the plaintiff are compensable damages resulting from the physician's malpractice.[320–323] The prescription of psychotropics exposes the clinician to significant professional liability claims, and the psychiatrist's prescription liability pertains largely to two areas: negligence and informed consent.[324–326] A patient may claim malpractice liability based on the intentional tort of battery or on grounds of negligence for unwarranted use of medications without the patient's meaningful consent to the treatment course. Prescribing psychiatrists risk negligence liability in various areas such as failure to obtain an adequate medical and psychiatric history; failure to obtain an adequate physical examination; failure to obtain adequate laboratory tests; lack of indication for a prescribed medication; contraindication to a prescription; prescription of an improper dosage; prescription for an improper duration; failure to recognize, monitor, and treat medication side effects; failure to abate drug reactions and interactions; and failure to consult with other physicians.[327] Negligence may also be claimed if the prescriber misdiagnosed the patient's condition or if the patient was subjected to an excessive dosage or duration of treatment. Prescribers who misdiagnose patients and treat them with psychotropics may be held liable for negligent malpractice when a patient develops a DIMD. A forensic non-treating expert may express an opinion that a different diagnosis would have been more accurate than the one provided by the treating prescriber, and the correct diagnosis would not have required treatment with the psychotropic in question. A patient may also bring suit against the drug manufacturer on product liability grounds associated with defective design, testing, or warning information relating to the medication that may have caused the DIMD. In many states, products liability law holds every person who transmits a defectively made drug product from manufacture to the injured patient liable without fault for administering the drug. Patients who are committed to a state or federal governmental agency (e.g., the Department of Veterans Affairs, a state mental hospital, or a state detention center) may also claim that their civil rights under the Eighth and Fourteenth Amendments to the Constitution were violated by the physician treating them if the patient is under some type of legal restraint at the time of treatment such as confinement to prison, a pretrial detention center, a mental institution, or a psychiatric ward in any hospital. The allegation is that the treating physician under the Civil Rights Act (42 USC 1983) violated the patient's civil rights as the patient was under the control of the state. A patient treated in prison or in a state mental institution who develops a DIMD may also claim that the prescriber was "deliberately indifferent" to the patient's condition, a separate "Constitutional Tort" that permits the recovery of damages for pain, suffering, impairment of functioning, and loss of earnings. State-created medical malpractice claims based on negligence may be joined to a Federal Civil Rights Act suit.

With the advent of managed care and the dramatic changes in health care produced by it, more and more managed care organizations are increasingly named as defendants in malpractice suits. Such malpractice suits against managed care organizations have focused mainly on the negligent selection of unqualified panel clinicians, inappropriate medication usage evaluations seen as substandard medical care, and negligent provision of care usually for staff model health maintenance organizations in which the physicians are "supervised" employees.[328,329] As medical records are legal as well as clinical documents, record keeping is as much a part of providing health care as the underlying care activity itself. In addition to an initial evaluation and examination before diagnosing a patient, clinical consultations may be necessary and appropriate before and/or during treatment. The clinician requesting the consultation should document any discussion, especially if the consultant is not likely to keep notes. Permission should be obtained from the consultant to record his name, and if a formal consultation is requested, the consultant should write a note in the chart or treatment record, especially if the consultant has seen the patient or is seeking reimbursement for his intervention.[330]

Physicians, since the beginning of the twentieth century, have been required to obtain the consent of their patients before undertaking a proposed procedure or treatment. However, for the past several decades, physicians have also been legally required to provide information to patients about the proposed intervention prior to proceeding. Together, consent and disclosure of information help promote increased autonomy regarding the variety of medical treatment options available. Additionally, adequate informed consent can aid to maximize patient compliance with treatment and improve the psychiatrist–patient relationship.[331–333]

Elements of informed consent in medical care are threefold: Information, competency, and voluntariness of decision-making. According to the legal doctrine of informed consent, sufficient information is needed to make an adequate consent, as accepting a consent based on insufficient information may constitute malpractice.[334] This applies to diagnostic evaluation procedures as well as treatment. The question for physicians is how much and what information are needed for a patient to make an informed choice.[335] It appears that the most common answer is what a "reasonable person" would want to know to accept or reject treatment such as: The nature or diagnosis of the patient's condition; the nature of the proposed intervention; the purpose of the proposed intervention; the benefits of the proposed intervention; the risks of the proposed intervention, including incidence, severity, and significance; the possible alternatives to the proposed intervention, including no treatment; the benefits of the alternative interventions; and the risks of the alternative interventions, including incidence, severity, and significance.[336] With regard to information about the risks of treatment, disclosure is warranted when the risks are frequent, significant, severe, or life-threatening. Since package inserts for antipsychotics clearly state that TD is a possible side effect, the issue of informed consent is crucial. Obtaining informed consent for antipsychotics, however, poses difficulty to psychiatrists due to their potential for severe adverse effects and the impaired judgment and potential incompetence of acutely psychotic patients for whom those agents are usually prescribed.[288,337]

Voluntariness, the second component of informed consent, requires the patient to give consent freely, without coercion. The last component, competency, is a legal concept not yet defined in a consistent or clinically instructive manner. It generally refers to the ability to understand and manipulate relevant information in a rational way regarding the informed consent provided. Four components in considering competency include understanding the information, appreciating its relevance for the person's particular situation, expressing a consistent choice, and rationally manipulating the relevant information in the final decision-making process. Competency is dependent on time and context and varies with the patient's changing status.[338,339] Once a patient is said to be incompetent, a substitute decision-maker is appointed to make any treatment choices. This decision-maker may be the physician, a guardian, a neutral third party, or the judge.[340] Generally, an involuntarily committed patient is presumed competent unless legally adjudicated otherwise. Additionally, both voluntary and involuntary patients have the right to accept or reject proposed treatment with medications.[341] The courts recognize four exceptional situations in which the usual requirements of informed consent do not apply: Medical emergencies, waivers, therapeutic privileges, and incompetence.[342]

The difference between battery and negligent failure to disclose is outlined in *Lackey v. Bressler*,[343] a combined negligent medical malpractice, assault and battery, and breach of contract for the use of antipsychotics which caused the patient to develop TD. The court provided the following explanation of the difference between negligent failure, negligent failure to warn, and intentional battery:

> Where a medical procedure is completely unauthorized, it constitutes an assault and battery, i.e., trespass to the person. . . . If, however, the procedure is authorized, but the patient claims a failure to disclose the risks involved, the cause of action is bottomed on negligence.

Numerous suits have been brought against nonpsychiatric physicians, psychiatrists, hospitals, and manufacturers regarding cases of DIMDs. Pharmaceutical reference guides, package inserts, and regulations of the U.S. Food and Drug Administration are valuable sources in malpractice litigations.[317] As only legal cases constituting those that have been tried and then appealed by the losing party are published in the legal literature, many that are settled out of court are sealed from disclosure by the settlement agreement. As TD is neither too infrequent nor too insignificant a risk of treatment to avoid disclosure, informative discussions regarding movement disorders should occur as soon as clinically feasible. Failure to detect early signs of TD and to intervene early once it occurs and is diagnosed have been a significant area of malpractice litigation.[289,326] The doctrine of *res ipsa loquitur* ("the thing speaks for itself") does not apply to cases with TD in establishing fault, since TD may occur in the absence of negligence.[317] The following cases demonstrate patient–plaintiff allegations of psychiatrist's failures to properly prescribe and monitor treatment outcomes with neuroleptic agents and make a timely diagnosis of a DIMD.

In *Collins v. Cushner*, a 56-year-old housewife sought treatment for anxiety from a family practitioner. She was diagnosed by the physician with "spastic colon" and prescribed low doses of trifluoperazine for a period of six years. For almost 2.5 years, the patient received phone renewals on her antipsychotic without being seen by the defendant physician. She subsequently developed abnormal movements in her arms and hands, and the defendant discontinued the antipsychotic for two months but reinstated it and doubled the dose. Six months later, the defendant prescribed benztropine to treat the patient's involuntary movements of the face. In the lawsuit, the plaintiff stated that the defendant continued to prescribe the antipsychotic despite product information warnings stating its use in anxiety and potential for TD in long-term treatment of women in the patient's age group. This case combines the elements of negligence, failure to warn of side effects, and failure to monitor. The plaintiff also stated that the anticholinergic, benztropine, further aggravated her condition and the litigation was settled for $125,000.[344]

In another case, *Clites v. Iowa*, the parents of an intellectually disabled man at a state residential facility sued the state for negligence and for treatment without adequate informed consent. The patient was institutionalized since age 11, and from the age of 18 to 23, the patient was treated with various neuroleptics for "aggressive behavior" under the auspices of several physicians. The patient received medications for five years before TD was diagnosed of the face and extremities. The trial court noted that the severe aggression and self-destructive behavior justifying the use of antipsychotics argued by the defendant were lacking and that the medications were used inappropriately for the staff's convenience and not for the patient's treatment. In addition, the court cited that the patient was improperly monitored because he was not "regularly visited" by a physician, and for a period of three years, no physical examinations were conducted. It further cited that staff at the facility "ignored the known risks of uninterrupted use of major tranquilizers," and the medical staff failed to react to the patient's symptoms of TD and change the drug management program accordingly. Also, the court stated that polypharmacy was not warranted in this case nor the use of the particular agents involved. Furthermore, the attending physician, who was not familiar with TD, failed to obtain appropriate consultation. The trial court also noted that the patient's parents, his legal guardians, "were never informed of the potential side effects of the use, and prolonged use, of major tranquilizers, nor was consent to their use obtained" and thus violated the "standard that requires some form of informed consent prior to the administration of major tranquilizers." The trial court ruled for the plaintiff and awarded $385,165 for future medical expenses and $375,000 for past and future pain and suffering.[345] Two years later, the district court's ruling was subsequently upheld in the Iowa Court of Appeals.[346] The judge in the case commented that

> Although the evidence may have justified a higher award, such is not controlling. The determinative question posed is whether on the record, giving the jury its right to accept or reject whatever portions of the conflicting evidence it chose, the verdict effects substantial justice between the parties.

In *Hedin v. United States*, another case involving TD, the plaintiff was treated with thioridazine and later chlorpromazine as an outpatient following a two-month psychiatric hospitalization for alcohol abuse. He continued to take 600 mg of chlorpromazine daily for almost four years before his physicians noted his movement disorder and subsequently discontinued his drug therapy. The movements involved the face, mouth, trunk, and extremities, and the patient stated he had been aware of these movements, but that he was not aware that they were due to the medication. The defendant, the U.S. Veterans Administration, admitted that it was negligent in prescribing the neuroleptics in excessive amounts for prolonged periods without proper supervision. The plaintiff who had become functionally disabled due to the TD was awarded damages of nearly $2.2 million.[347]

In *Barclay v. Campbell*,[348] the defendant psychiatrist admitted to not disclosing the risks of TD to a young schizophrenic patient. The court sided with the psychiatrist, and the decision was upheld on appeal, on the basis that he was justified in not disclosing this risk because it was not "medically feasible" to do so and that the patient was not a "reasonable person." This was reversed on appeal to the Texas Supreme Court in 1986 on the grounds that the psychiatrist could not use the therapeutic-privilege exception to the informed-consent disclosure requirement. It was also cited that although the patient's young age posed a small risk for TD, it did not negate the psychiatrist's duty to disclose this movement disorder. At trial, the jury found the defendant had not informed the patient of the risk of TD; however, the patient would have consented to the treatment anyway. Subsequently, the case was settled out of court.[349]

In the case *Ronald Bloom v. Will Creed, M.D.*, Dr. Bloom allegedly called in a prescription for an antipsychotic medication while covering for a colleague.[350] Dr. Bloom had never met nor treated Mr. Creed, and Mr. Creed did not know Dr. Bloom. The patient contended that the physician failed to warn him of side effects or to monitor his condition while using antipsychotic medication. The Supreme Court of Mississippi ruled 7–2 in favor of Dr. Bloom. Since many physicians provide coverage for one another frequently without access to full medical records, this case suggests a duty to provide an informed consent when a prescription is filled for a patient treated by a colleague prescriber.

Psychiatrists and the members of the mental health treatment team have many means and opportunities to provide information about neuroleptic agents and TD to patients. Medication counseling can be provided by pharmacists as well as psychiatrists as a matter of sound clinical practice.[341] Additionally, pharmacists may provide a warning label regarding involuntary movements on prescription bottles as well as instructions to the patient on how to recognize movement disorders and report such to the psychiatrist.[342]

The Task Force Report of the American Psychiatric Association on TD makes the following recommendations for the prevention and management of TD:

1. review the reasons why neuroleptics are chosen and consider alternative treatments if available; to educate patients and family members regarding the benefits and risks and obtain informed consent for long-term treatment, with documentation provided in the medical record;
2. establish objective evidence of the benefit of antipsychotic medications and review it periodically, at least every three to six months, in order to assess ongoing need and benefit;
3. administer the lowest effective dosage for chronic management; to exercise particular caution with children, elderly patients, and those with affective disorders;
4. examine patients regularly for early signs of dyskinesia and note such in the medical record;
5. consider alternative neurologic diagnosis if dyskinesia does occur;
6. reevaluate the indications for continued neuroleptic treatment and obtain informed consent from patients regarding continuing or discontinuing antipsychotic therapy if presumptive TD is present;
7. attempt to decrease the dosage if a neuroleptic is continued; to consider discontinuing the neuroleptic, or switching to an atypical neuroleptic if dyskinesia worsens;
8. utilize more benign agents first such as benzodiazepines, or vitamin E, if treatment for TD is indicated and to keep abreast of new treatment developments;
9. consider obtaining a second opinion if movement disorder is severe or disabling.[230]

As many as 60 percent of atypical antipsychotics and 64 percent of typical antipsychotics are prescribed off-label and hence used for indications not approved by the FDA.[3] To address this issue, the American Psychiatric Association released a list of specific uses of antipsychotic medications that are common, but potentially unnecessary and sometimes harmful, as part of the *Choosing Wisely* initiative, established by the American Board of Internal Medicine, to advance medical professionalism and to improve health care. This list identifies five evidence-based recommendations that should prompt conversations between patients and their health care providers about the appropriate use of antipsychotics. The five questions inform providers when *not* to prescribe antipsychotics: (1) For any indication without appropriate initial evaluation and appropriate ongoing monitoring; (2) if two or more antipsychotic medications are used concurrently; (3) as first choice to treat behavioral and psychological symptoms of dementia; (4) routinely as a first-line intervention for insomnia in adults; and (5) as a first-line intervention for children and adolescents for any diagnosis.[351] The legal aspects of psychiatric practice continue to evolve dramatically with changes observed in the health-care system and vary from state to state. Obtaining informed consent, disclosing adverse effects, and proper management of such adverse effects along with documentation are all activities the clinician needs to undertake while treating patients with antipsychotic agents.

12.15 CONCLUSION

Movement disorders occur as a heterogeneous group of conditions in which abnormalities in the form and speed of movements of the body predominate. DIMDs have gradually emerged as a major problem in clinical psychiatry and medicine. A number of various types of movement disorders have been identified and associated with different dopamine receptor blockers, namely DRBAs. The clinical spectrum of these movement disorders ranges from slight embarrassment or discomfort to life-threatening conditions such as neuroleptic malignant syndrome and other potentially detrimental disorders. DIMDs are among the most common iatrogenic disorders to result in malpractice suits and continue to remain among the most distressing of all drug-induced disorders. The potential for medications to induce movement disorders has to be balanced against their benefits. Simple measures, such as ensuring that the lowest effective dose of medication is used, that dosages are titrated gradually, that the potential for drug interactions is considered, and that unnecessary polypharmacy is avoided, may reduce the risk of DIMDs. It is imperative for clinicians to continuously monitor for the emergence of DIMDs and to treat them, so that patients are not distressed or uncomfortable and to facilitate medication adherence with proper therapy management.

Since antipsychotics are being prescribed increasingly as monotherapy, and off-label for a multitude of problems, the risk of DIMDs is observed with both typical and atypical neuroleptics. Some of the initial superiority of atypical neuroleptics compared with conventional neuroleptics may be biased by the use of inappropriately high doses of the latter agents. Now as the doses of atypical antipsychotics used in clinical practice are increasing, the EPS advantage of these agents narrows with the continuous frequent use of these higher doses. Movement disorders associated with new-generation antipsychotics and antidepressants are not rare, and better monitoring is required to assess their potential on patients' quality of life and to prevent under-ascertainment. DIMDs remain a significant concern for patients, and a preventive approach is preferable as the treatment of some DIMDs may be challenging.

REFERENCES

1. *Diagnostic and Statistical Manual of Mental Disorders*, 5th edition (DSM-V). Washington, DC: American Psychiatric Association; 2013.
2. Rodnitzky RL. Drug-induced movement disorders. Clin Neuropharmacol. 2002;25:142–152.
3. Sachdev PS. Neuroleptic-induced movement disorders: An overview. Psychiatr Clin North Am. 2005;28: 255–274.
4. Ward KM, Citrome L. Antipsychotic-related movement disorders: Drug-induced parkinsonism vs. tardive dyskinesia-key differences in pathophysiology and clinical management. Neurol Ther. 2018;7(2):233–248.
5. Hampton LM, Daubresse M, Chang HY, Alexander GC, Budnitz DS. Emergency department visits by adults for psychiatric medication adverse events. JAMA Psychiatry. 2014 Sep;71(9):1006–1014.
6. Zádori D, Veres G, Szalárdy L, Klivényi P, Vécsei L. Drug-induced movement disorders. Expert Opin Drug Saf. 2015 Jun;14(6):877–890.
7. Divac N, Prostran M, Jakovcevski I, Cerovac N. Second-generation antipsychotics and extrapyramidal adverse effects. Biomed Res Int. 2014;2014:Article ID 656370.
8. Burkhard PR. Acute and subacute drug-induced movement disorders. Parkinsonism Relat Disord. 2014;20:S108–S112.
9. Janno S, Holi M, Tuisku K, Wahlbeck K. Prevalence of neuroleptic-induced movement disorders in chronic schizophrenia inpatients. Am J Psychiatry. 2004;161:160–163.
10. Rybakowski JK, Vansteelandt K, Remlinger-Molenda A, Fleischhacker WW, Kahn RS, Peuskens J; EUFEST Study Group. Extrapyramidal symptoms during treatment of first schizophrenia episode: Results from EUFEST. Eur Neuropsychopharmacol. 2014 Sep;24(9):1500–1505.
11. Li C, Xia J, Wang J. Risperidone dose for schizophrenia. Cochrane Database Syst Rev. 2009 Oct 7;4:CD007474.
12. Conley RR. Risperidone side effects. J Clin Psychiatry. 2000;61(supplement 8):20–23.
13. Gerlach J. The continuing problem of extrapyramidal symptoms: Strategies for avoidance and effective treatment. J Clin Psychiatry. 1999;60(supplement 23):20–24.
14. De Leon J. The effect of atypical versus typical antipsychotics on tardive dyskinesia: A naturalistic study. Eur Arch Psychiatry Clin Neurosci. 2007;257: 169–172.
15. Haddad PM, Dursun SM. Neurological complications of psychiatric drugs: Clinical features and management. Hum Psychopharmacol. 2008;23:15–26.
16. Martino D, Karnik V, Osland S, Barnes TRE, Pringsheim TM. Movement disorders associated with antipsychotic medication in people with schizophrenia: An overview of Cochrane reviews and meta-analysis. Can J Psychiatry. 2018 Jan 1;63(11):706743718777392. doi: 10.1177/0706743718777392. Epub ahead of print. PMID: 29758999; PMCID: PMC6299187.
17. Leucht S, Corves C, Arbter D, Engel RR, Li C, Davis JM. Second-generation versus first-generation antipsychotic drugs for schizophrenia: A meta-analysis. Lancet. 2009;373:31–41.
18. Rummel-Kluge C, Komossa K, Schwarz S, Hunger H, Schmid F, Kissling W, Davis JM, Leucht S. Second-generation antipsychotic drugs and extrapyramidal side effects: A systematic review and meta-analysis of head-to-head comparisons. Schizophr Bull. 2012 Jan;38(1):167–177.
19. Werner FM, Coveñas R. Safety of antipsychotic drugs: Focus on therapeutic and adverse effects. Expert Opin Drug Saf. 2014 Aug;13(8):1031–1042.
20. Suzuki H, Gen K, Otomo M, Inoue Y, Hibino H, Mikami A, Matsumoto H, Mikami K. Relationship between the plasma concentration of paliperidone and the clinical and drug-induced extrapyramidal symptoms in elderly patients with schizophrenia. Hum Psychopharmacol. 2014 May;29(3):244–250.

21. Lieberman JA, Stroup TS, McEvoy JP, Swartz MS, Rosenheck RA, Perkins DO, Keefe RS, Davis SM, Davis CE, Lebowitz BD, Severe J. Effectiveness of antipsychotic drugs in patients with chronic schizophrenia. N Engl J Med. 2005;353:1209–1223.
22. Miller DD, Caroff SN, Davis SM, Rosenheck RA, McEvoy JP, Saltz BL, Riggio S, Chakos MH, Swartz MS, Keefe RS; Clinical Antipsychotic Trials of Intervention Effectiveness (CATIE) Investigators. Extrapyramidal side effects of antipsychotics in a randomized trial. Br J Psychiatry. 2008;193:279–288.
23. Caroff SN, Hurford I, Lybrand J, Campbell EC. Movement disorders induced by antipsychotic drugs: Implications of the CATIE schizophrenia trial. Neurol Clin. 2011 Feb;29(1):127–148.
24. Ritsner M, Gibel A, Perelroyzen G, Kurs R, Jabarin M, Ratner Y. Quality of life outcomes of resperidone, olanzapine, and typical antipsychotics among schizophrenia patients treated in routine clinical practice. J Clin Psychopharmacol. 2004;24:582–591.
25. Mortimer AM, Al-Abib AOA. Quality of life in schizophrenia on conventional versus atypical antipsychotic medication: A comparative cross-sectional study. Int J Soc Psychiatry. 2007;53:99–107.
26. Kilian R, Dietrich S, Toumi M, Angermeyer MC. Quality of life in persons with schizophrenia in outpatient treatment with first-of second-generation antipsychotics. Acta Psychiatr Scand. 2004;110:108–118.
27. Maher AR, Theodore G. Summary of the comparative effectiveness review on off-label use of atypical antipsychotics. J Manag Care Pharm. 2012;18(5 Suppl B):S1–S20.
28. Lee D, Baek JH, Bae M, Choi Y, Hong KS. Long-term response to clozapine and its clinical correlates in the treatment of tardive movement syndromes: A naturalistic observational study in patients with psychotic disorders. J Clin Psychopharmacol. 2019 Nov/Dec;39(6):591–596.
29. Ciranni MA, Kearney TE, Olson KR. Comparing acute toxicity of first-and second-generation antipsychotic drugs: A 10-year, retrospective cohort study. J Clin Psychiatry. 2009;70:122–129.
30. Kennedy C, Hunter C, Davidson A. Metoclopramide, an increasingly recognized cause of tardive dyskinesia. J Clin Pharamcol. 2008;48:379–384.
31. Rissardo JP, Caprara ALF. Carbamazepine-, oxcarbazepine-, eslicarbazepine-associated movement disorder: A literature review. Clin Neuropharmacol. 2020 May/Jun;43(3):66–80.
32. Tarsy D. Chapter 17: Miscellaneous drug induced movement disorders. In: *Drug Induced Movement Disorders*, Edited by Factor, Lang and Weiner, 2nd edition. Blackwell Future Publishing; 2005:430–441.
33. Claxton KL, Chen JJ, Swope DM. Drug-induced movement disorders. J Pharm Pract. 2007;20:415–429.
34. Detweiler MB, Kalafat N, Kim KY. Drug-induced movement disorders in older adults: An overview for clinical practioners. Consult Pharm. 2007;22:149–165.
35. Charness ME, Morady F, Scheinman MM. Frequent neurologic toxicity associated with amiodarone therapy. Neurology. 1994;34:669–671.
36. Stotter Cuddy ML. The effects of drugs on thermoregulation. AACN Clin Issues Adv Pract Acute Crit Care. 2004;15:238–253.
37. Vorsanger GJ, Roberts JT. Midazolam-induced athetoid movements of the lower extremities during epidural anesthesia reversed by physostigmine. J Clin Anesth. 1993;5:494–496.
38. Lorberboym M, Treves TA, Melamed E, Lampl Y, Hellmann M, Djaldetti R. [123I]-FP/CIT SPECT imaging for distinguishing drug-induced parkinsonism from Parkinson's disease. Mov Disord. 2006;21:510–514.
39. Rissardo JP, Caprara ALF. Bupropion-associated movement disorders: A systematic review. Ann Mov Disord. 2020;3:86–98.
40. Rissardo JP, Caprara ALF. Pregabalin-associated movement disorders: A literature review. Brain Circ. 2020;6(2):96–106.
41. Revet A, Montastruc F, Roussin A, Raynaud JP, Lapeyre-Mestre M, Nguyen TTH. Antidepressants and movement disorders: A postmarketing study in the world pharmacovigilance database. BMC Psychiatry. 2020 Jun 16;20(1):308.
42. Guo MY, Etminan M, Procyshyn RM, Kim DD, Samii A, Kezouh A, Carleton BC. Association of antidepressant use with drug-related extrapyramidal symptoms: A pharmacoepidemiological study. J Clin Psychopharmacol. 2018 Aug;38(4):349–356.
43. Ahmed S, Chengappa KNR, Naidu VR, Baker RW, Parepally H, Schooler NR. Clozapine withdrawal-emergent dystonias and dyskinesias: A case series. J Clin Psychiatry. 1998;59:472–477.
44. Salomon C, Hamilton B. Antipsychotic discontinuation syndromes: A narrative review of the evidence and its integration into Australian mental health nursing textbooks. Int J Ment Health Nurs. 2014;23(1):69–78.
45. Lee PE, Sykora K, Gill SS, Mamdani M, Marras C, Anderson G, Shulman KI, Stukel T, Normand SL, Rochon PA. Antipsychotic medications and drug-induced movement disorders other than parkinsonism: A population-based cohort study in older adults. J Am Geriatr Soc. 2005;53:1374–1379.
46. Rey MV, Molina L, Recinos B, Paz B, Rovelo M, Rodriguez Elias FE, Calderón J, Arellano A, Perez-Lloret S; CA-APD Study Team. Movement disorders after exposure to antipsychotic drugs in patients with depressive disorders. Clin Neuropharmacol. 2018 Sep/Oct;41(5):177–180.
47. McConville BJ, Sorter MT. Treatment challenges and safety considerations for antipsychotic use in children and adolescents with psychoses. J Clin Psychiatry. 2004;65(Suppl 6):20–29.

48. Najib, J. Tardive dyskinesia: A review and current treatment options. Am J Ther. 1999;6:51–60.
49. Diehl A, Reinhard I, Schmitt A, Mann K. Does the degree of smoking effect the severity of tardive dyskinesia? A longitudinal clinical trial. Eur Psychiatr. 2009;24:33–40.
50. Chouinard G, Chouinard V. Atypical antipsychotics: CATIE study, drug-induced movement disorder and resulting iatrogenic psychiatric-like symptoms, supersensitivity rebound psychosis and withdrawal discontinuation syndromes. Psychother Psychosom. 2008;77:69–77.
51. Hansen L. A critical review of akathisia, and its possible association with suicidal behaviour. Hum Psychopharmacol. 2001;15:139–141.
52. Shriqui CL, Bradwejn J, Jones BD. Tardive dyskinesia: Legal and preventive aspects. Can J Psychiatry. 1990;35:576–580.
53. Slovenko R. Update on legal issues associated with tardive dyskinesia. J Clin Psychiatry. 2000;61:45–57.
54. Briles JJ, Rosenberg DR, Brooks BA, Roberts MW, Diwadkar VA. Review of the safety of second-generation antipsychotics: Are they really "atypically" safe for youth and adults? Prim Care Companion CNS Disord. 2012;14(3).
55. Casey D. Pathophysiology of antipsychotic drug-induced movement disorders. J Clin Psychiatry. 2004;65(suppl 9):25–28.
56. Fiorentini C, Savoia P, Bono F, Tallarico P, Missale C. The D3 dopamine receptor: From structural interactions to function. Eur Neuropsychopharmacol. 2015 Sep;25(9):1462–1469.
57. Chang FC, Fung VS. Clinical significance of pharmacogenomic studies in tardive dyskinesia associated with patients with psychiatric disorders. Pharmgenomics Pers Med. 2014 Oct 13;7:317–328.
58. Ezquerra M, Compta Y, Marti MJ. Identifying the genetic components underlying the pathophysiology of movement disorders. Appl Clin Genet. 2011 Jun 23;4:81–92.
59. Shin HW, Chung SJ. Drug-induced parkinsonism. J Clin Neurol. 2012 Mar;8(1):15–21.
60. Jose de Leon MD, Susce MT, Pan RM, Fairchild M, Koch WH, Wedlund PJ. The CYP2D6 poor metabolizer phenotype may be associated with risperidone adverse drug reactions and discontinuation. J Clin Psychiatry. 2005;66:15–27.
61. Brennan MD. Pharmacogenetics of second-generation antipsychotics. Pharmacogenomics. 2014 Apr;15(6):869–884.
62. Brandl EJ, Kennedy JL, Müller DJ. Pharmacogenetics of antipsychotics. Can J Psychiatry. 2014 Feb;59(2):76–88.
63. Vandel P, Bonin B, Vandel S, Sechter D, Bizouard P. CYP 2D6 phenotype hypothesis of antidepressant extrapyramidal side-effects. Med Hypotheses. 1996;47:439–442.
64. Olfson M, Blanco C, Liu L, Moreno C, Laje G. National trends in the outpatient treatment of children and adolescents with antipsychotic drugs. Arch Gen Psychiatry. 2006;63:679–685.
65. Krause M, Zhu Y, Huhn M, Schneider-Thoma J, Bighelli I, Chaimani A, Leucht S. Efficacy, acceptability, and tolerability of antipsychotics in children and adolescents with schizophrenia: A network meta-analysis. Eur Neuropsychopharmacol. 2018 Jun;28(6):659–674.
66. Gebhardt S, Härtling F, Hanke M, Mittendorf M, Theisen FM, Wolf-Ostermann K, Grant P, Martin M, Fleischhaker C, Schulz E, Remschmidt H. Prevalence of movement disorders in adolescent patients with schizophrenia and in relationship to predominantly atypical antipsychotic treatment. Eur Child Adolesc Psychiatry. 2006;15:371–382.
67. Pringsheim T, Doja A, Belanger S, Patten S; Canadian Alliance for Monitoring Effectiveness and Safety of Antipsychotics in Children (CAMESA) Guideline Group. Treatment recommendations for extrapyramidal side effects associated with second-generation antipsychotic use in children and youth. Paediatr Child Health. 2011 Nov;16(9):590–598.
68. Newcomer JW. Second-generation (atypical) antipsychotics and metabolic effects: A comprehensive literature review. CNS Drugs. 2005;19(Suppl 1):1–93.
69. Fedorowicz VJ. Metabolic side effects of atypical antipsychotics in children: A literature review. J Psychopharmacol. 2005;19:533–550.
70. Patel JK, Buckley PF, Woolson S, Hamer RM, McEvoy JP, Perkins DO, Lieberman JA; Cafe Investigators. Metabolic profiles of second-generation antipsychotics in early psychosis: Findings from the CAFE study. Schizophr Res. 2009;111:9–16.
71. Pappagallo M, Silva R. The effect of atypical antipsychotic agents on prolactin levels in children and adolescents. J Child Adolesc Psychopharmacol. 2004;14:359–371.
72. Laita P, Cifuentes A, Doll A, Llorente C, Cortés I, Parellada M, Moreno D, Ruiz-Sancho A, Graell M, Arango C. Antipsychotic-related abnormal involuntary movements and metabolic and endocrine side effects in children and adolescents. J Child Adolesc Psychopharmacol. 2007;17:487–501.
73. Bobo WV, Cooper WO, Stein CM, Olfson M, Graham D, Daugherty J, Fuchs DC, Ray WA. Antipsychotics and the risk of type 2 diabetes mellitus in children and youth. JAMA Psychiatry. 2013;70(10):1067–1075.
74. Gokhale SG, Panchakshari MB. Maternal medication causing drug dystonia in a newborn: Placental transfer of drugs. J Matern-Fetal Neo Med. 2004;16:215–217.
75. Hampton LM, Daubresse M, Chang H, Alexander G, Budnitz DS. Emergency department visits by children and adolescents for antipsychotic drug adverse events. JAMA Psychiatry. 2015;72(3):292–294.
76. Biscontri RG, Jha S, Collins DM, Bugden S, Katz LY, Alessi-Severini S. Movement disorders in children

and adolescents receiving antipsychotic pharmacotherapy: A population-based study. J Child Adolesc Psychopharmacol. 2017 Dec;27(10):892–896.
77. Cancelli I, Beltrame M, Gigli GL, Valente M. Drugs with anticholinergic properties: Cognitive and neuropsychiatric-side effects in elderly patients. Neurol Sci. 2009;30:87–92.
78. Maglione M, Maher AR, Hu J, Wang Z, Shanman R, Shekelle PG, Roth B, Hilton L, Suttorp MJ, Ewing BA, Motala A. *Off-Label Use of Atypical Antipsychotics: An Update* [Internet]. Rockville, MD: Agency for Healthcare Research and Quality (US); 2011 Sep. Report No.: 11-EHC087-EF. PMID: 22132426.
79. Yan J. FDA extends black-box warning to all antipsychotics. *Psychiatry News*, July 18, 2008;43:1. http://psychnews.psychiatryonline.org.
80. Zhang H, Wang L, Fan Y, Yang L, Wen X, Liu Y, Liu Z. Atypical antipsychotics for Parkinson's disease psychosis: A systematic review and meta-analysis. Neuropsychiatr Dis Treat. 2019;15:2137–2149.
81. Shimizu S, Mizuguchi Y, Sobue A, Fujiwara M, Morimoto T, Ohno Y. Interaction between anti-Alzheimer and antipsychotic drugs in modulating extrapyramidal motor disorders in mice. J Pharmacol Sci. 2015 Apr;127(4):439–445.
82. Gill SS, Bronskill SE, Normand SL, Anderson GM, Sykora K, Lam K, Bell CM, Lee PE, Fischer HD, Herrmann N, Gurwitz JH. Antipsychotic drug use and mortality in older adults with dementia. Ann Intern Med. 2007;146:775–786.
83. Schneeweiss S, Setoguchi S, Brookhart A, Dormuth C, Wang PS. Risk of death associated with the use of conventional versus atypical antipsychotic drugs among elderly patients. CMAJ. 2007;176:627–632.
84. United States Government Accountability Office. *Antipsychotic Drugs and Older Adults. Antipsychotic Drug Use: HHS Has Initiatives to Reduce Use Among Older Adults in Nursing Homes, But Should Expand Efforts to Other Settings*. GAO 15–1211. http://www.gao.gov/assets/670/668221.pdf.
85. Wu CS, Wang SC, Gau SS, Tsai HJ, Cheng YC. Association of stroke with the receptor-binding profiles of antipsychotics-a case-crossover study. Biol Psychiatry. 2013 Mar 1;73(5):414–421.
86. Maust DT, Kim HM, Seyfried LS, Chiang C, Kavanagh J, Schneider LS, Kales HC. Antipsychotics, other psychotropics, and the risk of death in patients with dementia: Number needed to harm. JAMA Psychiatry. 2015 May;72(5):438–445.
87. Fraser LA, Liu K, Naylor KL, Hwang YJ, Dixon SN, Shariff SZ, Garg AX. Falls and fractures with atypical antipsychotic medication use: A population-based cohort study. JAMA Intern Med. 2015 Mar;175(3):450–452.
88. Clark GT. Medical management of oral motor disorders: Dystonia, dyskinesia and ndrug-induced dystonic extrapyramidal reactions. J Calif Dent Assoc. 2006 Aug;34(8):657–667.
89. Keepers GA, Fochtmann LJ, Anzia JM, Benjamin S, Lyness JM, Mojtabai R, Servis M, Walaszek A, Buckley P, Lenzenweger MF, Young AS, Degenhardt A, Hong SH; Systematic Review. The American Psychiatric Association practice guideline for the treatment of patients with schizophrenia. Am J Psychiatry. 2020 Sep 1;177(9):868–872.
90. Grebb JA. Medication-induced movement disorders. In: *Comprehensive Textbook of Psychiatry*, Edited by Kaplan HI, Sadock BJ, 6th edition. Baltimore: Williams & Wilkins; 1995:1909–1915.
91. Suzuki T, Matsuzuka H. Drug-induced Pisa syndrome (pleurothotonus): Epidemiology and management. CNS Drugs. 2002;16:165–174.
92. Nishimura, K, Mikami Y, Tsuchibuchi S, Horikawa N. Pisa syndrome resolved after switching to olanzapine. J Neuropsychiatry Clin Neurosci. 2007;19:202–203.
93. Weiner WJ, Rabinstein A, Levin B, Weiner C, Shulman LML. Cocaine-induced persistent dyskinesias. Neurology. 2001;56:964–965.
94. Guler G, Yildirim V, Kutuk MO, Toros F. Dystonia in an adolescent on risperidone following the discontinuation of methylphenidate: A case report. Clin Psychopharmacol Neurosci. 2015 Apr 30;13(1): 115–117.
95. Incecik F, Önlen Y, Özer C, Özcan K. Metoclopramide induced acute dystonic reaction: Two case reports. Marmara Med J. 2008;21:159–161.
96. van Der Kleij FG, de Vries PM, Stassen PM, Sprenger HG, Gans RO. Acute dystonia due to metoclopramide: Increased risk in AIDS (letter). Arch Intern Med. 2002;162:358–359.
97. Park CK, Choi HY, Oh IY, Kim MS. Acute dystonia by droperidol during intravenous patient-controlled analgesia in young patients. J Korean Med Sci. 2002;17(5):715.
98. Zesiewicz TA, Sullivan KL. Drug-induced hyperkinetic movement disorders by nonneuroleptic agents. Handb Clin Neurol. 2011;100:347–363.
99. Hawthorne JM, Caley CF. Extrapyramidal reactions associated with serotonergic antidepressants. Ann Pharmacother. 2015 Oct;49(10):1136–1152.
100. Gerber PE, Lynd LD. Selective serotonin-reuptake inhibitor-induced movement disorders. Ann Pharmacother. 1998;32:692–698.
101. Coulter DM, Pillans PI. Fluoxetine and extrapyramidal side effects. Am J Psychiatry. 1995;152:122–125.
102. Garcia de Yebenes J, Sanchez Pernaute R, Tabernero C. Symptomatic dystonias. In: *Movement Disorders-Neurologic Principles and Practice*, Edited by Watts RL, Koller WC. New York: McGraw Hill; 1997:455–475.
103. Ganzini L, Casey D, Hoffman W, McCall A. Prevalence of metoclopramide-induced tardive dyskinesia and acute extrapyramidal movement disorders. Arch Intern Med. 1993;153:1469–1475.

104. Dhikav V, Anand KS. Acute dystonic reaction with rivastigmine. Int Psychogeriatr. 2013 Aug;25(8): 1385–1386.
105. Scully C, Bagan JV. Adverse drug reactions in the orofacial region. Crit Rev Oral Biol Med. 2004;15: 221–239.
106. Karakaş Uğurlu G, Onen S, Bayındırlı D, Cayköylü A. Acute dystonia after using single dose duloxetine: Case report. Psychiatry Investig. 2013;10(1):95–97.
107. Siddiqui SH, Memon NA, Shanker R. Drug-induced movement disorder and confusion associated with duloxetine. BMJ Case Rep. 2018 Mar 28;2018:bcr2016216746.
108. Derinoz O, Caglar AA. Drug-induced movement disorders in children at pediatric emergency department: 'dystonia'. Emerg Med J. 2013 Feb;30(2):130–133.
109. Hegarty AM, Lipton RB, Merriam AE, Freeman K. Cocaine as a risk factor for acute dystonic reactions. Neurology. 1991;41:1670.
110. Freed E. Alcohol-triggered neuroleptic induced tremor, rigidity and dystonia. Med J Aust. 1981;2: 44–45.
111. Hendrickson RG, Morocco AP, Greenberg MI. Acute dystonic reactions to "street Xanax". N Engl J Med. 2002;346:1753.
112. World Health Organization. Role of anticholinergic medications in patients requiring long-term antipsychotic treatment for psychotic disorders. Updated June 2012. http://www.who.int/mental_health/mhgap/evidence/resource/psychosis_q6.pdf.
113. Van Gaalen J, Kerstens FG, Maas RP, Härmark L, van de Warrenburg BP. Drug-induced cerebellar ataxia: A systematic review. CNS Drugs. 2014 Dec;28(12):1139–1153.
114. Chen JM, Yan Y. Long-term follow-up of a patient with venlafaxine-induced diurnal bruxism treated with an occlusal splint: A case report. World J Clin Cases. 2019 Feb 26;7(4):516–524.
115. Pearson NL. A grinding issue: Drug-induced bruxism. CPJ/RPC. 2008;141:300–301.
116. Ranjan S, Chandra PS, Prabhu S. Antidepressant-induced bruxism: Need for buspirone? Int J Neuropsychopharmacol. 2006;9:485–487.
117. Jackson N, Doherty J, Coulter S. Neuropsychiatric complications of commonly used palliative care drugs. Postgrad Med J. 2008;84:121–126.
118. Burkhard PR. Acute and subacute drug-induced movement disorders. Parkinsonism Relat Disord. 2014 Jan;20(Suppl 1):S108–S112.
119. Dickey W. The neuroleptic malignant syndrome. Prog Nuerobiol. 1991;36:425–436.
120. Modi S, Dharaiya D, Schultz L, Varelas P. Neuroleptic malignant syndrome: Complications, outcomes, and mortality. Neurocrit Care. 2015 Jul 30;24: 97–103.
121. Najib, J. Neuroleptic malignant syndrome: A case report and review of treatment. Hosp Pharm. 1997; 32:512–518.
122. Belvederi Murri M, Guaglianone A, Bugliani M, Calcagno P, Respino M, Serafini G, Innamorati M, Pompili M, Amore M. Second-generation antipsychotics and neuroleptic malignant syndrome: Systematic review and case report analysis. Drugs RD. 2015 Mar;15(1):45–62.
123. White DAC, Robins AH. Catatonia: Harbinger of the neuroleptic malignant syndrome. Brit J Psychiatr. 1991;158:419–421.
124. Evans CE, Sebastian J. Serotonin syndrome. Emerg Med J. 2007;24:e20; Mason PJ, Morris VA, Balcezak TJ. Serotonin syndrome: Presentation of 2 cases and review of the literature. Med (Baltimore). 2000;79:201–209.
125. Phan H, Casavant MJ, Crockett S, Lee A, Hall MW, Nahata MC. Serotonin syndrome following a single 50 mg dose of sertraline in a child. Clin Toxicol. 2008;46:845–849.
126. Isenberg D, Wong SC, Curtis JA. Serotonin syndrome triggered by a single dose of suboxone. Am J Emerg Med. 2008;26:840.
127. Borrelli F, Izzo AA. Herb–drug interactions with St John's wort (Hypericum perforatum): An update on clinical observations. AAPS J. 2009;11(4):710–727.
128. Boyer EW, Shannon M. The serotonin syndrome. N Engl J Med. 2005;352:112–1120.
129. Bartlett D. Drug-induced serotonin syndrome. Crit Care Nurse. 2017 Feb;37(1):49–54.
130. Wang RZ, Vashistha V, Kaur S, Houchens NW. Serotonin syndrome: Preventing, recognizing, and treating it. Cleve Clin J Med. 2016 Nov;83(11):810–817.
131. Sachdev P. The epidemiology of drug-induced akathisia: Part 1. Acute akathisia. Schizophrenia Bull. 1995;21(3):431–449.
132. Bratti IM, Kane JM, Marder SR. Chronic restlessness with antipsychotics. Am J Psychiatry. 2007; 164:1648–1654.
133. Atbasoglu EC, Schultz SK, Andreasen NC. The relationship of akathisia with suicidality and depersonalization among patients with schizophrenia. J Neuropsychiatry Clin Neurosci. 2001;13:336–341.
134. Kane JM, Fleischhacker WW, Hansen L, Perlis R, Pikalov III A, Assunção-Talbott S. Akathisia: An updated review focusing on second-generation antipsychotics. J Clin Psychiatry. 2009;70:627–643.
135. Dossenbach M, Treuer T, Kryzhanovskaya L, Saylan M, Dominguez S, Huang X. Olanzapine versus chlorpromazine in the treatment of schizophrenia: A pooled analysis of four 6-week, randomized, open-label studies in the Middle East and North Africa. J Clin Psychopharmacol. 2007;27:329–337.
136. Miller CH, Mohr F, Umbricht D, Woerner M, Fleischhacker WW, Lieberman JA. The prevalence of acute extrapyramidal signs and symptoms in patients

treated with clozapine, risperidone, and conventional antipsychotics. J Clin Psychiatry. 1998;59:69–75.
137. Thomas JE, Caballero J, Harrington CA. The incidence of Akathisia in the treatment of schizophrenia with aripiprazole, asenapine and lurasidone: A meta-analysis. Curr Neuropharmacol. 2015;13(5):681–691.
138. Kumar R, Sachdev PS. Akathisia and second-generation antipsychotic drugs. Curr Opin Psychiatry. 2009;22:293–299.
139. Sahoo S, Ameen S. Acute nocturnal akathisia induced by clozapine. J Clin Psychopharmacol. 2007;27:205.
140. Oral ET, Altinbas K, Demirkiran S. Sudden akathisia after a ziprasidone dose reduction. Am J Psychiatry. 2006;163:546.
141. Cutler AJ, Kalali AH, Weiden PJ, Hamilton J, Wolfgang CD. Four-week, double-blind, placebo- and ziprasidone-controlled trial of iloperidone in patients with acute exacerbations of schizophrenia. J Clin Psychopharmacol. 2008;28:S20–S28.
142. Nasrallah HA, Brecher M, Paulsson B. Placebo-level incidence of extrapyramidal symptoms (EPS) with quetiapine in controlled studies of patients with bipolar mania. Bipolar Disord. 2006;8:467–474.
143. Cortese L, Caligiuri MP, Williams R, Schieldrop P, Manchanda R, Malla A, Harricharan R. Reduction in neuroleptic-induced movement disorders after a switch to quetiapine in patients with schizophrenia. J Clin Psychopharmacol. 2008;28:69–73.
144. Demyttenaere K, Detraux J, Racagni G, Vansteelandt K. Medication-induced akathisia with newly approved antipsychotics in patients with a severe mental illness: A systematic review and meta-analysis. CNS Drugs. 2019 Jun;33(6):549–566.
145. Correll CU, Vanover KE, Davis RE, Chen R, Satlin A, Mates S. Safety and tolerability of lumateperone 42 mg: An open-label antipsychotic switch study in outpatients with stable schizophrenia. Schizophr Res. 2021 Feb;228:198–205.
146. Moteshafi H, Stip E. Comparing tolerability profile of quetiapine, risperidone, aripiprazole and ziprasidone in schizophrenia and affective disorders: A meta-analysis. Expert Opin Drug Saf. 2012 Sep;11(5):713–732.
147. Catalano G, Grace JW, Catalano MC, Morales MJ, Cruse LM. Acute akathisia associated with quetiapine use. Psychosomatics. 2005;46:291–301.
148. Lenze EJ, Mulsant BH, Blumberger DM, Karp JF, Newcomer JW, Anderson SJ, Dew MA, Butters MA, Stack JA, Begley AE, Reynolds CF. Efficacy, safety, and tolerability of augmentation pharmacotherapy with aripiprazole for treatment-resistant depression in late life: A randomised, double-blind, placebo-controlled trial. The Lancet. 2015;386(10011):2404–2412.
149. Berman RM, Marcus RN, Swanink R, McQuade RD, Carson WH, Corey-Lisle PK, Khan A. The efficacy and safety of aripiprazole as adjunctive therapy in major depressive disorder: A multicenter, randomized, double-blind, placebo-controlled study. J Clin Psychiatry. 2007;68:843–853.
150. Kemp DE, Gilmer WS, Fleck J, Straus JL, Dago PL, Karaffa M. Aripiprazole augmentation in treatment resistant bipolar depression: Early response and development of akathisia. Prog Neuropsychopharmacol Biol Psychiatry. 2007;31:574–577.
151. Walker L. Sertraline-induced akathisia and dystonia misinterpreted as a panic attack. Psychiatr Serv. 2002;53:1477–1478.
152. Salem H, Nagpal C, Pigott T, Teixeira AL. Revisiting antipsychotic-induced akathisia: Current issues and prospective challenges. Curr Neuropharmacol. 2017;15(5):789–798.
153. Settle EC. Akathisia and sertraline. J Clin Psychiatry. 1993;54:321.
154. Hansen L, Wilkinson DG. Drug induced akathisia, suicidal ideation and its treatment in the elderly. Int J Geriatr Psychiatry. 2001;16:231–232.
155. Hamilton MS, Opler LA. Akathisia, suicidality, and fluoxetine. J Clin Psychiatry. 1992;53:401–406.
156. Hansen L. Fluoxetine dose-increment related akathisia in depression: Implications for clinical care, recognition and management of selective serotonin reuptake inhibitor-induced akathisia. J Psychopharmacol. 2003;17:451–452.
157. Opler LA. Akathisia and suicide. Am J Psychiatry. 1991;148:1259.
158. Wirshing WC, Van Putten T, Rosenberg J, Marder S, Ames D, Hicks-Gray T. Fluoxetine, akathisia, and suicidality: Is there a causal connection? Arch Gen Psychiatry. 1992;49:580–581.
159. Koliscak LP, Makela EH. Selective serotonin reuptake inhibitor-induced akathisia. J Am Pharm Assoc. 2009;49:e28–e38.
160. Allen JC, Gralla R, Reilly L, Kellick M, Young C. Metoclopramide: Dose related toxicity and preliminary antiemetic studies in children receiving cancer chemotherapy. J Clin Oncol. 1985;3:1136.
161. Miller LG, Jankovic J. Metoclopramide induced movement disorders: Clinical findings with a review of the literature. Arch Intern Med. 1989;149:2486–2492.
162. Moos DD, Hansen DJ. Metoclopramide and extrapyramdial symptoms: A case report. J Peri Anesthesia Nurs. 2008;23:292–299.
163. Jungmann E, Schoffling K. Akathisia and metoclopramide. Lancet. 1982;2:221.
164. Zubenko GS, Cohen BM, Lipinski JF Jr. Antidepressant-related akathisia. J Clin Psychopharmacol. 1987;7:254–257.
165. Pohl R, Yeragani VK, Balon R, Lycaki H. The jitteriness syndrome in panic disorder patients with antidepressants. J Clin Psychiatry. 1988;49:100–104.
166. Ross DR, Walker JL, Patterson J. Akathisia induced by amoxapine. Am J Psychiatry. 1983;140:115–116.
167. Gulsun M, Doruk A. Mirtazapine-induced akathisia. J Clin Psychopharmacol. 2008;28:467.

168. Praharaj SK, Kongasseri S, Behere RV, Sharma PS. Mirtazapine for antipsychotic-induced acute akathisia: A systematic review and meta-analysis of randomized placebo-controlled trials. Ther Adv Psychopharmacol. 2015 Oct;5(5):307–313.
169. Barnes TRE, Braude WM, Hill DJ. Acute akathisia after oral droperidol and metoclopramide preoperative medication. Lancet. 1982;2:48–49.
170. Bernick C. Methysergide-induced akathisia. Clin Neuropharmacol. 1988;11:87–89.
171. Calmels JP, Sorbette F, Montastruc JL. Iatrogenic hyperkinetic syndrome caused by an antihistaminic (letter). Nouvelle Presse Medicale. 1982;11(30):2296–2297.
172. Patterson, JF. Akathisia associated with buspirone. J Clin Psychopharmacol. 1988;8:296–297.
173. Ritchie EC, Bridenbaugh RH, Jabbari B. Acute generalized myoclonus following buspirone administration. J Clin Psychiatry. 1988;49:242–243.
174. Blaisdell GD. Akathisia a comprehensive review and treatment summary. Pharmacopsychiatry. 1994;27: 139–146.
175. Yazici KU, Percinel I. Atomoxetine-associated akathisia: A case report. J Clin Psychopharmacol. 2014 Dec;34(6):770–772.
176. Kane JM, Fleischhacker WW, Hansen L, Perlis R, Pikalov A 3rd, Assunção-Talbott S. Akathisia: An updated review focusing on second-generation antipsychotics. J Clin Psychiatry. 2009 Apr 21;70(5): 627–643.
177. Espi Forcen F, Matsoukas K, Alici Y. Antipsychotic-induced akathisia in delirium: A systematic review. Palliat Support Care. 2015 Jun 19;14:77–84.
178. Markkula J, Helenius H, Lauerma H. On the relationship of atypical and low-dose conventional antipsychotics with akathisia in a clinical patient population. Nord J Psychiatry. 2007;61:152–157.
179. Gao K, Kemp DE, Ganocy SJ, Gajwani P, Xia G, Calabrese JR. Antipsychotic-induced extrapyramidal side effects in bipolar disorder and schizophrenia: A systematic review. J Clin Psychopharmacol. 2008; 28:203–209.
180. Rathbone J, Soares-Weiser K. Anticholinergics for neuroleptic-induced acute akathisia. Cochrane Database Syst Rev. 2006:CD003727. doi:10.1002/14651858. CD003727.pub3.
181. Modestin J, Wehrli MV, Stephan PL, Agarwalla P. Evolution of neuroleptic-induced extrapyramidal syndromes under long-term neurolpetic treatment. Schizophr Res. 2008;100:97–107.
182. Koliscak LP, Makela EH. Selective serotonin reuptake inhibitor-induced akathisia. J Am Pharm Assoc 2009 Mar–Apr;49(2):e28–e36;quiz e37–e38.
183. Ratey JJ, Sorgi P, Polakoff S. Nadolol as a treatment for akathisia. Am J Psychiatry. 1985;142:640–642.
184. Hieber R, Dellenbaugh T, Nelson LA. Role of mirtazapine in the treatment of antipsychotic-induced akathisia. Ann Pharmacother. 2008;42:841–846.
185. Brigo F, Erro R, Marangi A, Bhatia K, Tinazzi M. Differentiating drug-induced parkinsonism from Parkinson's disease: An update on non-motor symptoms and investigations. Parkinsonism Relat Disord. 2014 Aug;20(8):808–814.
186. Morley JF, Pawlowski SM, Kesari A, Maina I, Pantelyat A, Duda JE. Motor and non-motor features of Parkinson's disease that predict persistent drug-induced Parkinsonism. Parkinsonism Relat Disord. 2014 Jul;20(7):738–742.
187. Moghal S, Rajput AH, Meleth R, D'Arcy C, Rajput R. Prevalence of movement disorders in institutionalized elderly. Neuroepidemiology. 1995;14: 297–300.
188. Tse W, Libow LS, Neufeld R, Lesser G, Frank J, Dolan S, Tarshish C, Gracies JM, Olanow CW, Koller WC, Hälbig TD. Prevalence of movement disorders in an elderly nursing home population. Arch Gerontol Geriat. 2008;46:359–366.
189. Halliday J, Farrington S, MacDonald S, MacEwan T, Sharkey V, McCreadie R. Nithsdale schizophrenia surveys 23: Movement disorders: 20-year review. Br J Psychiatry. 2002;181:422–427.
190. Rochon PA, Stukel TA, Sykora K, Gill S, Garfinkel S, Anderson GM, Normand SL, Mamdani M, Lee PE, Li P, Bronskill SE. Atypical antipsychotics and Parkinsonism. Arch Intern Med. 2005;165: 1882–1888.
191. Selfani K, Soland VL, Chouinard S, Huot P. Movement disorders induced by the "atypical" antipsychotic aripiprazole. Neurologist. 2017 Jan;22(1):24–28.
192. Pierre JM. Extrapyramidal symptoms with atypical antipsychotics: Incidence, prevention and management. Drug Saf. 2005;28:191–208.
193. Targum SD, Abbot JL. Efficacy of quetiapine in Parkinson's patients with psychosis. J Clin Psychopharmacol. 2000;20:54–60.
194. Gregory RJ, White JF. Can sertraline induce parkinson's disease? Psychosomatics. 2001;42:163–164.
195. Bayrak A, Cetin B, Meteris H, Kesebir S. Parkinsonism secondary to duloxetine use: A case report. North Clin Istanb. 2015;2(3):243–246.
196. Sarwar AI. Trazodone and parkinsonism: The link strengthens. Clin Neuropharmacol. 2018 May/Jun; 41(3):106–108.
197. Masmoudi K, Gras-Champel V, Douadi Y, Masson H, Andrejak M. Parkinsonism and/or cognitive impairment with valproic acid therapy: A report of ten cases. Pharmacopsychiatry. 2006;39:9–12.
198. Jamora D, Lim SH, Pan A, Tan L, Tan EK. Valproate-induced Parkinsonism in epilepsy patients. Mov Disord. 2007;22:130–133.
199. Mena MA, de Yebenes JG: Drug-induced parkinsonism. Expert Opin Drug Saf. 2006;5:759–771.
200. Wyckoff J, McBride M. Manganese exposure from welding: An emerging liability risk. Environmental Claim J. 2004;16:117–134.

201. Triano AR, Micheli FE, Alarcon F, Teive H. Movement disorders in Latin America. Parkinsonism Relat Disord. 2006;12:125–138.
202. Montgomery EB Jr. Heavy metals and the etiology of Parkinson's disease and other movement disorders. Toxicology. 1995;97:3.
203. Suranyi-Cadotte BE, Nestoros JN, Nair NP, Lal S, Gauthier S. Parkinsonism induced by high doses of diazepam. Biol Psychiatry. 1985;20:451–460.
204. López-Sendón J, Mena MA, de Yébenes JG. Drug-induced parkinsonism. Expert Opin Drug Saf. 2013 Jul;12(4):487–496.
205. Hriso E, Kuhn T, Masdeu JC, Grundman M. Extrapyramidal symptoms due to dopamine-blocking agents in patients with AIDS encephalopathy. Am J Psychiatry. 1991;148:1558–1561.
206. Baron JA. Cigarette smoking and Parkinson's disease. Neurology. 1986;36:1490–1496.
207. Koller W, Vetere-Overfield B, Gray C, Alexander C, Chin T, Dolezal J, Hassanein R, Tanner C. Environmental risk factors in Parkinson's disease. Neurology. 1990;40:1218–1221.
208. Rajput AH, Rozdilsky B, Hornykiewicz O, Shannak K, Lee T, Seeman P. Reversible drug-induced parkinsonism, clinicopathologic study of two cases. Neurology. 1982;39:644–646.
209. Duma SR, Fung VS. Drug-induced movement disorders. Aust Prescr. 2019 Apr;42(2):56–61.
210. López-Sendón JL, Mena MA, de Yébenes JG. Drug-induced parkinsonism in the elderly: Incidence, management and prevention. Drugs Aging. 2012 Feb 1;29(2):105–118.
211. Al Dakheel A, Beaulieu-Boire I, Fox SH. Emerging drugs for levodopa-induced dyskinesia. Expert Opin Emerg Drugs. 2014 Sep;19(3):415–429.
212. Factor SA, Brown D. Clozapine prevents recurrence of psychosis in Parkinson's disease. Mov Disord. 1992;7:125–131.
213. Factor SA, Friedman JH. The emerging role of clozapine in the treatment of movement disorders. Mov Disord. 1997;12(4):483–496.
214. Cardoso F, Jankovic J: Movement disorders. Neurol Clin. 1993;11:625–638.
215. Mercadante S. Pathophysiology and treatment of opioid-related myoclonus in cancer patients. Pain. 1998;74:5–9.
216. Jimenez-Jimenez FJ, Puertas I, de Toledo-Heras M. Drug-induced myoclonus: Frequency, mechanisms and management. CNS Drugs. 2004;18:93–104.
217. Morgan JC, Sethi KD. Drug-induced tremors. Lancet Neurol. 2005;4(12):866–876.
218. Kronfol Z, Greden JF, Zis AP. Imipramine-induced tremor: Effect of a beta-adrenergic blocking agent. J Clin Psychiatry. 1983;44:225–226.
219. Friedman JH. Movement disorders induced by psychiatric drugs that do not block dopamine receptors. Parkinsonism Relat Disord. 2020 Aug 26;79:60–64.
220. Asser A, Taba P. Psychostimulants and movement disorders. Front Neurol. 2015 Apr 20;6:75.
221. Lou JS, Jankovic J. Essential tremor: Clinical correlates in 350 patients. Neurology. 1991;41:234–238.
222. Altindag A, Yanik M, Asoglu M. The emergence of tics during escitalopram and sertraline treatment. Int Clin Psychopharmacol. 2005 May;20(3):177–178.
223. Cardoso FEC, Jankovic J. Cocaine related movement disorders. Mov Disord. 1993;8:175–178.
224. Lopez W, Jeste DV. Movement disorders and substance abuse. Psychiatr Serv. 1997;48:634–637.
225. Rittmannsberger H, Leblhuber F. Asterixis induced by carbamazepine therapy. Biol Psychiatry. 1992;32: 364–368.
226. Sechi G, Murgia B, Sau G, Peddone L, Tirotto A, Barrocu M, Rosati G. Asterixis and toxic encephalopathy induced by gabapentin. Prog Neuro-Psychopharmacol Biol Psychiatry. 2004;28:195–199.
227. Stubblefield BM, Herklotz M, Hand M. Asterixis related to gabapentin as a cause of falls. Am J Phys Med Rehabil. 2005;84:136–140.
228. Stacy M, Cardoso F, Jankovic J. Tardive stereotypy and other movement disorders in tardive dyskinesias. Neurology. 1993;43:937–941.
229. Bhidayasiri R, Fahn S, Weiner WJ, Gronseth GS, Sullivan KL, Zesiewicz TA; American Academy of Neurology. Evidence-based guideline: Treatment of tardive syndromes: Report of the Guideline Development Subcommittee of the American Academy of Neurology. Neurology. 2013 Jul 30;81(5):463–469. Erratum in: Neurology. 2013 Nov 26;81(22):1968.
230. Kane JM, Jeste DV, Barnes TR, Casey DE, Cole JO, Davis JM, Gualtieri CT, Schooler NR, Sprague RL, Wettstein RM (eds). *American Psychiatric Association Task Force Report on Tardive Dyskinesia*. Washington, DC: American Psychiatric Press; 1992.
231. Glazer WM, Morgenstern H, Schooler N, Berkman CS, Moore DC. Predictors of improvement in tardive dyskinesia following discontinuation of neuroleptic medication. Br J Psychiatry. 1990;157:585–595.
232. Fetner DE, Hertzman M. Progress in the treatment of tardive dyskinesia; theory and practice. Hosp Community Psychiatry. 1993;1:25–34.
233. Kane JM, Jeste DV, Barnes TR, Casey DE, Cole JO, Davis JM, Gualtieri CT, Schooler NR, Sprague RL, Wettstein RM (eds). *American Psychiatric Association Task Force Report on Tardive Dyskinesia*. Washington, DC: American Psychiatric Press; 1992.
234. Kane JM, Weinhold P, Kinon B, Wegner J, Leader M. Prevalence of abnormal involuntary movements ("spontaneous dyskinesias") in the normal elderly. Psychopharmacology. 1982;77:105–108.
235. Klawans HL, Barr A. Prevalence of spontaneous lingual-facial-buccal dyskinesias in the elderly. Neurology. 1982;32:558–559.
236. Waln O, Jankovic J. An update on tardive dyskinesia: From phenomenology to treatment. In: *Tremor and*

Other Hyperkinetic Movements. Edited by Louis ED; 2013;3:tre-03-161-4138-1.
237. Merrill RM, Lyon JL, Matiaco PM. Tardive and spontaneous dyskinesia incidence in the general population. BMC Psychiatry. 2013 May 28;13:152.
238. Van Harten PN, Hoek HW, Matroos GE, Koeter M, Kahn RS. Intermittent neuroleptic treatment and risk for tardive dyskinesia: Curacao extrapyramidal syndromes study III. Am J Psychiatry. 1998;155:565–567.
239. Chakos MH, Alvir JM, Woerner MG, Koreen A, Geisler S, Mayerhoff D, Sobel S, Kane JM, Borenstein M, Lieberman JA. Incidence and correlates of tardive dyskinesia in first episode of schizophrenia. Arch Gen Psychiatry. 1996;53:313–319.
240. Correll CU, Schenk EM. Tardive dyskinesia and new antipsychotics. Curr Opin Psychiatry. 2008;21: 151–156.
241. Woerner MG, Correll CU, Alvir JM, Greenwald B, Delman H, Kane JM. Incidence of tardive dyskinesia with risperidone or olanzapine in the elderly: Results from a 2-year, prospective study in antipsychotic-naive patients. Neuropsychopharmacology. 2011;36(8):1738–1746.
242. Buzan R. Risperidone-induced tardive dyskinesia. Am J Psychiatry. 1996;153:734–735.
243. Jeste DV, Lacro JP, Bailey A, Rockwell E, Harris MJ, Caligiuri MP: Lower incidence of tardive dyskinesia with risperidone compared with haloperidol in older patients. J Am Geriatr Soc. 1999;47:716–719.
244. White A. *Woman Whose Face is Disfigured by Drugs Awarded $6.7 Million*. Philadelphia, PA: The Legal Intelligencer; 2000;222:104.
245. Glazer WM, Morgenstern H, Pultz JA, Yeung PP, Rak IW. Incidence of tardive dyskinesia is lower with quetiapine treatment than with typical antipsychotics in patients with schizophrenia and schizoaffective disorder. Schizophr Resour. 2000;41:206–207.
246. Rosenquist KJ, Walker SS, Gjhaemi SN. Tardive dyskinesia and ziprasidone (letter). Am J Psychiatry. 2002;159:1436.
247. Maytal G, Ostacher M, Stern TA. Aripiprazole-related tardive dyskinesia. CNS Spect. 2006;6:435–439.
248. Abbasian C, Power P. A case of aripirpazole and tardive dyskinesia. J Psychopharmacol. 2009;23: 214–215.
249. Hall DA, Agarwal P, Griffith A, Segro V, Seeberger LC. Movement disorders associated with aripiprazole use: A case series. Int J Neurosci. 2009;119(12): 2274–2279.
250. Hazari N, Kate N, Grover S. Clozapine and tardive movement disorders: A review. Asian J Psychiatry. 2013;6(6):439–451.
251. Marshall DL, Hazlet TK, Gardner JS. Neuroleptic drug exposure and incidence of tardive dyskinesia: A records-based case-control study. J Man Care Pharm. 2002;8:259–265.
252. Spivak B, Mester R, Abesgaus J, Wittenberg N, Adlersberg S, Gonen N, Weizman A. Clozapine treatment for neuroleptic-induced tardive dyskinesia, parkinsonism, and chronic akathisia in schizophrenic patients. J Clin Psychiatry. 1997;58:318–322.
253. Uzun O, Doruk A. Tardive oculogyric crisis during treatment with clozapine: Report of three cases. Clin Drug Investig. 2007;27:861–864.
254. Kumet R, Freeman MP. Clozapine and tardive dyskinesia (letter). J Clin Psychiatry. 2002;63:167–168.
255. Beauclair L, Fontaine R. Tardive dyskinesia associated with metoclopramide. Can Med Assoc J. 1986;134:613–614.
256. Modrego PP, Perez TJM. Acute dyskinesia after metoclopramide withdrawal. J Am Geriatric Soc. 1997;45(4):536.
257. Wiholm BE, Mortimer O, Boethius G, Häggström JE. Tardive dyskinesia associated with metoclopramide. Br Med J. 1984;288:545–547.
258. Kenney C, Hunter C, Davidson A, Jankovic J. Metoclopramide, an increasingly recognized cause of tardive dyskinesia. J Clin Pharmacol. 2008;48:379–384.
259. Pasricha PJ, Pehlivanov N, Sugumar A, Jankovic J. Drug insight: From disturbed motility to disordered movement—A review of the clinical benefits and medicolegal risks of metoclopramide. Nat Clin Pract Gastroenterol Hepatol. 2006 Mar;3(3):138–148.
260. United States Food and Drug Administration. FDA requires boxed warning and risk mitigation strategy for metoclopramide-containing drugs. https://www.fda.gov/media/74425/download. Accessed June 11, 2021.
261. Thach BT, Chase TN, Bosma JF. Oral facial dyskinesia associated with prolonged use of antihistaminic decongestants. N Engl J Med. 1975;293:486–487.
262. Buetefisch CM, Gutierrez A, Gutmann L. Choreathetotic movements: A possible side effect of gabapentin (Letter). Neurology. 1996;46:851.
263. Sandler NH. Tardive dyskinesia associated with fluoxetine. J Clin Psychiatry. 1996;57:91.
264. Albayrak Y, Ekinci O. Duloxetine-associated tardive dyskinesia resolved with fluvoxamine: A case report. J Clin Psychopharmacol. 2012 Oct;32(5):723–724.
265. Arya DK. Extrapyramidal symptoms with selective serotonin re-uptake inhibitors. Br J Psychiatry. 1994;165:728–733.
266. Yassa R, Camille Y, Belzile L. Tardive dyskinesia in the course of antidepressant therapy: A prevalence study and review of the literature. J Clin Psychopharmacol. 1987;7:243–246.
267. Ganzini L, Heintz RT, Hoffman WF, Casey DE. The prevalence of tardive dyskinesia in neuroleptic-treated diabetics. Arch Gen Psychiatry. 1991;48:259–263.
268. Rosengarten H, Schweitzer JW, Friedhoff AJ. Possible genetic factors underlying the pathophysiology of tardive dyskinesia. Pharmacol Biochem Behav. 1994;49:663–667.
269. Lucey JL, Dinan TG. Orofacial dyskinesia and the alcohol dependence syndrome. Psychol Med. 1992;22:79–83.

270. Diehl A, Reinhard I, Schmitt A, Mann K, Gattaz WF. Does the degree of smoking effect the severity of tardive dyskinesia? A longitudinal clinical trial. Eur Psychiatry. 2009 Jan;24(1):33–40.
271. Marshall, DL, Hazlet TK, Gardner JS, Blough DK. Neuroleptic drug exposure and incidence of tardive dyskinesia: A records-based case-control study. J Man Care Pharm. 2002;4(8):259–265.
272. Citrome LL. Medication options and clinical strategies for treating Tardive Dyskinesia. J Clin Psychiatry. 2020 Jan 28;81(2):TV18059BR2C.
273. Factor SA, Remington G, Comella CL, Correll CU, Burke J, Jimenez R, Liang GS, O'Brien CF. The effects of valbenazine in participants with tardive dyskinesia: Results of the 1-year KINECT 3 extension study. J Clin Psychiatry. 2017 Nov/Dec;78(9): 1344–1350.
274. Citrome L, Saklad SR. Revisiting tardive dyskinesia: Focusing on the basics of identification and treatment. J Clin Psychiatry. 2020 Feb 18;81(2):TV18059AH3C.
275. Correll CU, Kane JM, Citrome LL. Epidemiology, prevention, and assessment of tardive dyskinesia and advances in treatment. J Clin Psychiatry. 2017 Sep/Oct;78(8):1136–1147. doi:10.4088/JCP.tv17016ah4c. PMID:29022654.
276. Bhidayasiri R, Jitkritsadakul O, Friedman JH, Fahn S. Updating the recommendations for treatment of tardive syndromes: A systematic review of new evidence and practical treatment algorithm. J Neurol Sci. 2018 Jun 15;389:67–75.
277. Aquino CC, Lang AE. Tardive dyskinesia syndromes: Current concepts. Parkinsonism Relat Disord. 2014 Jan;20 Suppl 1:S113–S117.
278. Margolese HC, Chouinard G, Kolivakis TT, Beauclair L, Miller R, Annable L. Tardive dyskinesia in the era of typical and atypical antipsychotics. Part 2: Incidence and management strategies in patients with schizophrenia. Can J Psychiatry. 2005;50:703–713.
279. Grant MJ, Baldessarini RJ. Possible improvement of neuroleptic-associated tardive dyskinesia during treatment with aripiprazole. Ann Pharmacother. 2005;39:1953.
280. Caykoylu A, Ekinci O, Yilmaz E. Resolution of risperidone-induced tardive dyskinesia with a switch to aripiprazole monotherapy. Prog Neuro-Psychopharmacol Biol Psychiatry. 2009;33:571–572.
281. Hazari N, Kate N, Grover S. Clozapine and tardive movement disorders: A review. Asian J Psychiatr. 2013 Dec;6(6):439–451.
282. Bhidayasiri R, Boonyawairoj S. Spectrum of tardive syndromes: Clinical recognition and management. Postgrad Med J. 2011 Feb;87(1024):132–141.
283. Cloud LJ, Zutshi D, Factor SA. Tardive dyskinesia: Therapeutic options for an increasingly common disorder. Neurotherapeutics. 2014 Jan;11(1):166–176.
284. Ricciardi L, Pringsheim T, Barnes TR, Martino D, Gardner D, Remington G, Addington D, Morgante F, Poole N, Carson A, Edwards M. Treatment recommendations for tardive dyskinesia. *Can J Psychiatry.* 2019;64(6):388–399.
285. Munetz MR, Benjamin S. Who should perform the AIMS examination. Hosp Community Psychiatry. 1990;41:912–915.
286. Kaye NS, Reed TJ. Tardive dyskinesia: Tremors in law and medicine. J Am Acad Psychiatry Law. 1999;27: 315–333.
287. Heaton H. Plaintiffs win half of suits involving tardive dyskinesia. Clin Psychiatry News. 1990;18:12–17.
288. Mills MJ, Eth S: Legal liability with psychotropic drug use: Extrapyramidal syndromes and tardive dyskinesia. J Clin Psychiatry. 1987;48(Suppl 9):28–33.
289. Mills MJ, Norquist GS, Shelton RC, Gelenberg AJ, Van Putten T. Consent and liability with neuroleptics: The problem of tardive dyskiensia. Int J Law Psychiatry. 1986;8:243–252.
290. Rinck C, Guidry J, Calkins CF. Review of states' practices on the use of psychotropic medication. Am J Ment Retard. 1989;93:657–668.
291. Schwartz HI. Legal and ethical issues in neuroleptic noncompliance. Psychiatr Ann. 1986;16:588–595.
292. Sachdev P. The epidemiology of drug-induced akathisia: II: Chronic, tardive, withdrawal akathisias. Schizophr Bull. 1995;21:451–461.
293. Sachdev P. The epidemiology of drug-induced akathisia: Part II. Chronic, tardive, and withdrawal akathisias. *Schizophr Bull.* 1995;21(3):451–461.
294. Hettema JM, Ross DE. A case of aripiprazole-related tardive akathisia and its treatment with ropinirole. J Clin Psychiatry. 2007;68:1814–1815.
295. Mehta SH, Morgan JC, Sethi KD. Drug-induced movement disorders. Neurol Clin. 2015 Feb;33(1):153–174.
296. Jankovic J. Tardive syndromes and other drug-induced movement disorders. Clin Neuropharmacol. 1995;18:197–214.
297. Kuo SH, Jankovic J. Tardive gait. Clin Neurol Neurosurg. 2008;110:198–201.
298. Giudice M. Drug-induced restless leg syndrome. CPJ/RPC. 2009;142:41–42.
299. Hoque R, Chesson AL Jr. Pharmacologically induced/exacerbated restless legs syndrome, periodic limb movements of sleep, and REM behavior disorder/REM sleep without atonia: Literature review, qualitative scoring, and comparative analysis. J Clin Sleep Med. 2010 Feb 15;6(1):79–83.
300. Rissardo JP, Caprara ALF. Mirtazapine-associated movement disorders: A literature review. Tzu Chi Med J. 2020 Jul 13;32(4):318–330.
301. Rittmannsberger H, Werl R. Restless legs syndrome induced by quetiapine: Report of seven cases and review of the literature. Int J Neuropsychopharmacol. 2013 Jul;16(6):1427–1431.
302. Harris MK, Shneyder N, Borazanci A, Korniychuk E, Kelley RE, Minagar A. Movement disorders. Med Clin N Am. 2009;93:371–388.

303. Durif F. Treating and preventing levodopa-induced dyskinesias. Drugs Aging. 1999;14:337–345.
304. Sawada H, Oeda T, Kuno S, Nomoto M, Yamamoto K, Yamamoto M, Hisanaga K, Kawamura T; Amantadine Study Group. Amantadine for dyskinesias in Parkinson's disease: A randomized controlled trial. PLoS One. 2010;5(12):e15298.
305. Gupta S, Frank B, Madhusoodanan S. Tardive dyskinesia: Legal issues and consent. Psychiatr Ann. 2002;32:245–248.
306. Marder SR, Essock SM, Miller AL, Buchanan RW, Davis JM, Kane JM, Lieberman J, Schooler NR. The Mount Siani conference on the pharmacotherapy of schizophrenia. Schizophr Bull. 2002;28:5–16.
307. Loonen AJM, van Praag HM. Measuring movement disorders in antipsychotic drug trials: The need to define a new standard. J Clin Psychopharmacol. 2007;27:423–430.
308. Barnes TR. A rating scale for drug-induced akathisia. Br J Psychiatry. 1989;154:672–676.
309. Simpson GM, Angus JW. A rating scale for extrapyramidal side effects. Acta Psychiatr Scand. 1970(suppl);212:11–19.
310. Chouinard G, Cosci F, Chouinard VA, Alphs L. Extrapyramidal symptom rating scale [abstract]. Can J Neurol Sci. 1980;7:233.
311. Chouinard G, Margolese HC. Manual for the extrapyramidal symptom rating scale (ESRS). Schizophr Res. 2005;76:247–265.
312. Lane RD, Glazer WM, Hansen TE, Berman WH, Kramer SI. Assessment of tardive dyskinesia using the Abnormal Involuntary Movement Scale. J Nerv Ment Dis. 1985;173:353–357.
313. Dixon L, Weiden P, Frances AJ, Rapkin B. Management of neuroleptic-induced movement disorders: Effects of physician training. Am J Psychiatry. 1989;146:104106.
314. Mitra S, Haddad PM. Documentation of extrapyramidal symptoms. Psychiatr Bull. 2007;31:76–77.
315. Cortese L, Jog M, McAuley TJ, Kotteda V, Costa G. Assessing and monitoring antipsychotic-induced movment disorders in hospitalized patients: A cautionary study. Can J Psychiatry. 2004;49:31–36.
316. Day JC, Kinderman P, Bentall R. A comparison of patients' and prescribers' beliefs about neuroleptic side-effects: Prevalence, distress and causation. Acta Psychiatr Scand. 1998;97:93–97.
317. Slovenko R. Update on legal issues associated with tardive dyskinesia. J Clin Psychiatry. 2006;61(suppl 4):45–57.
318. Studdert DM, Mello MM, Sage WM, DesRoches CM, Peugh J, Zapert K, Brennan TA. Defensive medicine among high-risk specialist physicians in a volatile malpractice environment. JAMA. 2005;293:2609–2617.
319. Bailey RK, Adams JB, Unger DM. Atypical antipsychotics: A case study in new era risk management. J Psychiatr Pract. 2006;12:253–258.
320. Bonnie R. Professional liability and the quality of mental health care. Law Med Health Care. 1988;16:229–240.
321. Klein JI, Glover SI. Psychiatric malpractice. Int J Law Psychiatry. 1983;6:131–157.
322. Simon RI, Sadoff RL. *Psychiatric Malpractice: Causes and Comments for Clinicians*. Washington, DC: American Psychiatric Press; 1992.
323. Meyer DJ. Psychiatry malpractice and administrative inquiries of alleged physician misconduct. Psychiatr Clin N Am. 2006;29:615–628.
324. Brackins LW. The liability of physicians, pharmacists, and hospitals for adverse drug reactions. Defense Law J. 1985;34:273–344.
325. Dukes MNG, Swartz B. *Responsibility for Drug-Induced Injury*. Amsterdam: Elsevier; 1988.
326. Wettstein RM. Legal aspects of neuroleptic-induced movement disorders. In: *Legal Medicine*. Edited by Wecht CH. New York: Praeger; 1985:117–179.
327. Wettstein RM. Tardive dyskinesia and malpractice. Behav Sci Law. 1983;1:85–107.
328. Applebaum PS. Legal liability and managed care. Am Psychol. 1993;48:251–257.
329. Applebaum PS. Managed care and the next generation of mental health law. Psychiatr Serv. 1996;47:27–28.
330. Garrick TR, Weinstock R. Liability of psychiatric consultants. Psychosomatics. 1994;35:474–484.
331. Applebaum PS, Lidz CW, Meisel A. *Informed Consent: Legal Theory and Clinical Practice*. New York: Oxford University Press; 1987.
332. Faden RF, Beauchamp TL. *A History and Theory of Informed Consent*. New York: Oxford University Press; 1986.
333. Tietz GF. Informed consent in the prescription drug context: The special case. Washington Law Rev. 1986;61:367–417.
334. Munetz MR, Roth LH. Informing patients about tardive dyskinesia. Arch Gen Psychiatry. 1985;42: 866–871.
335. Laugharne J, Davies A, Arcelus J, Bouman WP. Informing patients about tardive dyskinesia: A survey of clinicians' attitudes in three countries. Int J Law Psychiatry. 2004;27:101–108.
336. Rozovsky F. *Consent to Treatment: A Practical Guide*, 2nd edition. Boston, MA: Little Brown; 1990.
337. Applebaum PS, Schaffner K, Meisel A. Responsibility and compensation for tardive dyskinesia. Am J Psychiatry. 1985;142:806–810.
338. Applebaum PS, Grisso T. Assessing patients' capacities to consent to treatment. N Engl J Med. 1988;319:1635–1638.
339. Grisso T, Applebaum PS. Comparison of standards for assessing patient's capacities to make treatment decisions. Am J Psychiatry. 1995;152:1033–1037.
340. Gutheil TG, Bursztajn HJ. Clinician's guidelines for assessing and presenting subtle forms of patient incompetence in legal settings. Am J Psychiatry. 1986;143:1020–1023.

341. Applebaum PS. The right to refuse treatment with antipsychotic medication: Retrospect and prospect. Am J Psychiatry. 1988;145:413–419.
342. Applebaum PS, Gutheil TG. *Clinical Handbook of Psychiatry and the Law*, 2nd edition. Baltimore: Williams & Wilkins; 1991.
343. *Lackey v. Bressler*, 358 S.E. 2d 560 (Court of Appeals of North Carolina 1987).
344. *Collins v. Cushner Montgomery County Maryland*, Circuit Court, Number 48751 (October 20, 1980).
345. *Clites v. Iowa*, Law #46274 Iowa District Court, Pottawattamie County (August 7, 1980).
346. *Clites v. State of Iowa*, 322 N.W. 2d 917 (Court of Appeals of Iowa 1982).
347. *Hedin v. U.S.*, Number 5–83 CIV 3 (D. Minn.) (1985).
348. *Barlay v. Campbell*, 683 SW2d 498, Texas (1984).
349. *Barclay v. Campbell*, 704 S.W. 2d 8 (Supreme Court of Texas 1986).
350. *Ronald Bloom v. Will Creed, M.D.*, 724 So. 2d 357 (Supreme Court of Mississippi 1998).
351. American Psychiatric Association. Choosing Wisely: Five things physicians and patients should question. http://www.choosingwisely.org/wp-content/uploads/2015/02/APA-Choosing-Wisely-List.pdf. Accessed June 14, 2021.

13 Acute Adverse Drug Events in Critical Care, ED, and ICU

Gourang P. Patel

SYNOPSIS

13.1 BACKGROUND

13.1.1 EPIDEMIOLOGY

The critical-care area of medical practice is fast-paced and presents challenges when applying the treatment recommendations at the bedside. Adverse drug events (ADEs) have a significant impact on morbidity and mortality. In the United States, ADEs account for approximately $150 billion in costs annually.[1] The Institute of Medicine's (IOM) 1999 report "To Err is Human" reported approximately 100,000 deaths each year as a result of medical errors. This number is steadily increasing.[1] Generally, there are five categories of ADE: (1) Adverse drug reactions, (2) medication errors, (3) therapeutic failures, (4) adverse drug withdrawal events, and (5) overdoses.[2] A medication error is defined as a preventable event that occurs as a result of inappropriate use by a healthcare professional. The advent of hundreds of new medications in the market each year has resulted in an increase in the occurrence of untoward outcomes attributable to these errors.

The IOM describes the need to further improve safety within the healthcare system.[1] Since the reduction of medication errors is a priority for patient safety, the IOM published another report specifically addressing this topic.[1] It indicated that a hospitalized patient is subjected to at least one medication error per day. In the intensive care unit, the median error rate is approximately 106 per 1,000 patient days (range = 1.2 to 947 per 1,000 patient days).[3] Due to the large number of medications prescribed for patients in the emergency department (ED) and intensive care unit (ICU)—as well as the acuity and severity of the patient population—it is necessary to focus resources in areas where there is a high risk and high potential benefit from prevention efforts. The Joint Commission (formerly the Joint

DOI: 10.1201/9781003615323-15

Commission on Accreditation of Healthcare Organizations or JCAHO) has focused its efforts on providing standards for healthcare institutions. One of its areas of specialization is the utilization of medications in the emergency department (ED) and ICU. The Joint Commission provides oversight to medical institutions through the process of accreditation. That process includes the establishment of numerous patient-safety goals developed to ensure consistent evaluations among evaluators. Several patient safety goals focus on medication utilization. In addition, the Joint Commission provides the rationale, strategies, and recommendations for the implementation of these patient-safety goals.[4]

The Joint Commission has several goals addressing components of medication safety. The National Patient Safety Goals, which are updated annually, focus on areas of improved care (e.g., patient identification, safety of medication use, medication reconciliation, and reducing patient fall risk). These goals are a constructive and consistent way to evaluate a patient's condition. They also include components of clinician education.[4]

13.1.2 Environment

One tool developed for such a task is provided by the Institute for Safe Medication Practices (ISMP). ISMP is currently organized to aid healthcare institutions around the world in establishing safe medication practices. It has developed a list of "high-alert" medications to serve as a reference and starting point for ICU and ED clinicians.[2,5] The medications on this list include the following medication classes: Vasoactive agents, intravenous sedation and analgesia, anticoagulants, insulin, total parenteral nutrition, intravenous electrolytes, epidurals, and chemotherapeutic agents. The purpose of intense surveillance over these medication classes is because of their potential to cause significant morbidity and mortality when they are prescribed, prepared/dispensed, administered, and/or monitored incorrectly.

Medication errors can occur during any stage of the process—prescription, distribution/operations, administration, or monitoring. The first stage, prescribing, describes how the original order for a medication was obtained. Many institutions have not yet developed a process for computerized prescription order entry (CPOE). Often, the process of medication ordering and transcription is still a manual one. As a result, the probability of error increases. Administration errors occur the most frequently compared to other stages of the medication-use process. The utilization of automation—including bar-coding and advanced infusion pumps—reduces the occurrence of these errors and, therefore, improves patient safety.[5]

The final stage in which medication errors occur is within the monitoring process.[3] For example, clinicians need to be aware that when patients are receiving anticoagulation with unfractionated heparin (UFH) infusion, Activated Partial Thromboplastin Time (APTT) or Heparin antiXa levels need to be monitored to avoid supra or subtherapeutic levels of the anticoagulant. Monitoring errors are reported to occur the least frequently compared to other stages. Rather than an indication of positive performance, however, this statistic most likely points to a deficient error detection mechanism. A single center study of 134 patients identified 178 ADEs with an incidence rate of 52%. The study identified several triggers that identified potential medication-related events. Triggers for ADRs include the following: Extravasation, hypoxia, hypotension, protamine, decrease in hemoglobin or hematocrit, and hypoglycemia.[6]

13.2 HIGH-RISK MEDICATION-RELATED EVENTS

The ISMP has provided a guide to direct our attention to a group of medications that—if prescribed, distributed, administered, and/or monitored inappropriately—can result in temporary or permanent harm.[2] In fact, in some cases, these events and reactions can result in fatality.

13.2.1 Hypersensitivity Reactions

Hypersensitivity reactions can encompass a variety of clinical presentations. In this section, there will be particular focus on the following types of life-threatening hypersensitivity reactions: Anaphylaxis, angioedema, and dermatologic manifestations (i.e., Steven–Johnsons Syndrome [SJS] and Toxic Epidermal Necrolysis [TEN]). (See the "Allergic Drug Reactions" Chapter 10 for more information on dermatologic manifestations from medications.) In summary, the dermatologic reactions of SJS and TEN often involve an immune reaction in the body in response to a drug. Often, the drugs implicated in SJS and TEN are similar and can include any of the following: Sulfonamides, phenytoin, penicillin (and its associated derivatives), barbiturates, phenothiazines, thiazides, and NSAIDs. Both SJS and TEN can have devastating outcomes for a patient; however, the distinguishing factor between TEN and SJS is the percentage of skin detachment.[7,8] The treatment for SJS and TEN is to identify and remove the offending agent and provide supportive care in a specialized unit that is prepared to treat severely burned patients, as the physiology and infection risk are similar between these two patient groups.

Anaphylaxis is a rare reaction to a drug but carries devastating consequences if unrecognized. (See Chapter 10 for further details.) In summary, anaphylaxis is a severe allergic reaction to a food or drug. The reaction can turn fatal once the respiratory and/or circulatory systems are affected. The reaction has an onset of minutes. The main cellular mediator of this reaction is histamine. Histamine affects changes in blood-vessel permeability. Histamine acts very quickly in the body and generally described as defining a reaction within a couple of minutes. Additional cellular mediators are activated as well. The result of changes in vessel permeability can manifest either in edema of the airway—leading to respiratory compromise—and/or vasodilation of blood vessels (which manifests as a clinical presentation of hypotension, low blood pressure).[9,10] The treatment of anaphylactic reactions involves the administration of intravenous, intramuscular, or oral antihistamine (i.e., diphenhydramine) and/or epinephrine via a subcutaneous or intramuscular route, depending on the severity of the reaction. Drugs/therapies that have been more widely documented to cause this type of reaction are antibiotics, sulfa drugs, opioids, chemotherapy, and immune therapies used in rheumatoid arthritis or gastrointestinal disorders (e.g., infliximab).

Angioedema is a reaction that involves respiratory complications as a result of stimulation of upper airway-edema (i.e., tongue and larynx) that can result in impaired carbon dioxide and oxygen exchange. This can potentially be fatal. The classification of the types of hypersensitivity reactions are categorized in either Type I (IgE-mediated) and Type II (T-cell-mediated hypersensitivity) reactions which are named on the basis of the etiology of the reaction. For example, the IgE-mediated reactions generally trigger a physiologic response after 30 minutes of exposure and rarely are reported beyond 120 minutes. Angioedema typically occurs with the administration of an anti-hypertension drug class called angiotensin inhibitors or angiotensin receptor blockers. The angioedema reaction can be life-threatening and cause closure of the patient's airway. Oftentimes, the reaction can be managed with supportive care but, occasionally, requires a surgical intervention to restore airway patency. There are many drugs in this class, although the reaction is more likely to occur in African-Americans. It does not have a time-onset, although the majority of these reactions are thought to occur within the first few weeks of therapy.[11] The treatment for these types of reactions can include an antihistamine, epinephrine, and/or an H2 antagonist.[9,10] As with the other types of hypersensitivity reactions, it is imperative that such a hypersensitivity be documented in patients' hospital medical records under the class of allergies. The patient's retail out-patient pharmacy should also be notified in order to avoid an unwanted encounter in the future. In the same respect, it is very important for clinicians to evaluate for drug allergies prior to the prescription, dispensing, and administration of medications, as the consequences of any of these reactions can be fatal. The treatment of these reactions does vary; however, with anaphylaxis and angioedema, the use of an antihistamine (i.e., diphenhydramine), H2 receptor antagonist (i.e., ranitidine or famotidine), and epinephrine 0.3 mg (pediatric) or 0.5 mg (adults) are given either subcutaneously or via intramuscular route. Intravenous administration of epinephrine is not advised as the systemic adverse reactions (i.e., ventricular arrhythmias) are more likely to occur. Another hypersensitivity type that has been reported are those associated with vasculitis. The vasculitis reactions are generally delayed and present weeks after the initial exposure. The medications reported to have triggered vasculitis reactions are the following: Allopurinol, beta-lactams antibiotics, sulfonamides, thiazide diuretics, and phenytoin.[10]

13.2.2 Cardiovascular Reactions

Cardiovascular reactions can have a variety of presentations as either a change in blood pressure (BP), heart rate (HR), and/or heart rhythm. The cardiovascular changes can be classified as minor, moderate, or severe. The degree of the cardiovascular compromise dictates the relative changes in BP and HR or heart rhythm.

13.2.2.1 Blood Pressure (BP)

Blood pressure is primarily regulated via the selective constriction or dilation of arteries and veins. Therefore, drugs that can affect the degree of artery resistance or venous capacitance greatly affect the degree of blood-pressure control. The reactions that affect BP are generally accidental or iatrogenic (i.e., caused by healthcare provider). An iatrogenic reaction with antihypertensive medications often occurs when multiple providers are prescribing drugs to lower a patient's blood pressure. Often, one prescriber is unaware that another is prescribing a similar medication. The blood pressure has a vital role in determining the amount of oxygen carried by the red blood cells to vital organs such as the brain and heart. The two categories of blood pressure that are concerning are those readings that are very high (i.e., SBP >180 mmHg or DBP >110 mmHg) or those that are very low (i.e., a decrease of 40 mmHg from baseline BP or SBP <90 mmHg). The blood pressure readings reported as high are secondary to patient-related factors (i.e., nonadherence to medication) and generally present in the ED or post-operatively. These situations are best handled via intravenous or oral medication administration, depending on the degree of end-organ damage. End-organ damage is defined as clinical evidence of damage to the brain (e.g., stroke), heart (e.g., heart attack), eyes (e.g., evidence of edema), or kidney (e.g., evidence or kidney failure). The necessary response to the evidence of end-organ damage is the administration of intravenous medication to lower blood pressure.[12] On the other hand, low blood pressure can also induce accidental or iatrogenic adverse events. When patients are admitted to the hospital or examined in the ED, they may be prescribed additional antihypertensive therapy if the prescriber is unaware of the patient's current medications. Another scenario involves the too rapid upward titration of medication which may result in overmedication, hypotension, or harm.

13.2.2.2 Heart Rate (HR)

Heart rate is a component of cardiovascular function and determines the ability of the body to maintain optimal blood pressure and appropriate blood flow. Heart rates that are often high (i.e., greater than 100) or low (i.e., less than 60) are often benign unless associated with a particular disease state or symptoms. High heart rates are often experienced by many who exercise or have stress. High heart rates can be problematic in conjunction with patients with a cardiac history and/or prior stroke. Clinically relevant low heart rate is defined as HR less than 40 beats per minute (BPM). However, if a patient has subjective complaints (i.e., syncope or shortness of breath) with a heart rate of less than 60 BPM, investigation is warranted. The vast majority of these reactions are (again) mediated by antihypertensive or anti-angina medications. If a high or low heart rate goes untreated, it may lead to cardiac arrest.

13.2.2.3 Arrhythmias

The American Heart Association (AHA) describes heart rhythms that have been identified as being incompatible with life. The heart rhythms of ventricular tachycardia (VT), pulseless electrical activity (PEA), and asystole carry a high rate of mortality. They require prompt medical attention or may cause fatality. The treatment of VT, PEA, or asystole requires the use of an Advanced Cardiac Life Support (ACLS) in order to increase the chance of reversal of the acute situation.[13] The initiation of ACLS is key, as minutes are critical to a patient's neurological and physical outcomes. The incidence of VT is highest for people outside a medical facility, which is why there are often automated external defibrillators (AEDs) placed in public facilities such as shopping malls, airports, schools, and universities, as well as in medical facilities that serve patients in remote areas of a hospital campus.

13.2.3 Nephrotoxicity

Kidney damage, or nephrotoxicity, has a variety of definitions. The implications are that some types are permanent (requiring life-long dialysis) and other types are reversible over a short time period. The following section will address two anti-infective drug classes: Aminoglycosides and amphotericin B.

13.2.3.1 Aminoglycosides

The aminoglycosides are a class of antibiotics that are utilized for a variety of gram-negative and gram-positive bacterial infections. Although drugs in this class are effective in killing bacteria, they carry the risk of ototoxicity (hearing loss) and nephrotoxicity (decreased kidney function). The nephrotoxicity of the amino glycosides has been described in the order of greatest to least: Neomycin > tobramycin > gentamicin > amikacin.[14] The functionality of a patient's renal system is monitored by measuring urine output (GFR—glomerular filtration rate) and serum creatinine throughout the course of treatment. The onset of kidney damage is variable, with elderly individuals (age >65 years) exhibiting a higher susceptibility. Prompt recognition is often accomplished not only by a routine monitoring of the renal function, but also the drug levels (i.e., trough) of the amino glycoside are utilized in this regard. Successful reduction of nephrotoxic incidents, and improved patient care, are therefore accomplished through the collaboration of the dedicated pharmacist and the prescribing clinician. For A more thorough review of drug induced nephrotoxicity, see Chapter 14 – Nephrotoxic Drugs.

13.2.3.2 Amphotericin B

Polyenes or amphotericin B (ampho B) are a class of anti-infectives used to treat fungal infections most often associated with patients who are immuno-compromised (i.e., suffering from HIV and cancer or using steroids). Ampho B has several different formulations, including deoxycholate, colloidal dispersion, lipid complex, and liposomal. All the formulations can cause nephrotoxicity (deoxycholate > colloidal dispersion > lipid complex > liposomal); however, the liposomal formulation carries the lowest risk. Ampho B also requires frequent renal function monitoring (i.e., urine output and serum creatinine) in order to detect nephrotoxicity from drug therapy. Inadequate monitoring of ampho B therapy can result in a life-long dialysis as a result of irreversible injury to the kidney tubules. In addition to nephrotoxicity, infusion-related reactions, countered by antihistamine and acetaminophen, pose a risk for patients who are prescribed drugs in this class. For the prevention of nephrotoxicity, an intravenous hydration infusion of normal saline (osmolarity = 0.9%) or sodium bicarbonate ($NaHCO_3$–) infusion is administered prior to and post administration of amphotericin B.[15]

13.2.3.3 Intravenous Contrast

Intravenous (IV) contrast is associated with three main types of reactions: Anaphylaxis, tissue extravasations (skin injury), and nephrotoxicity (kidney damage). IV contrast is useful in several diagnostic procedures for the detection of blood clots in the lung (pulmonary embolism) and for cardiac procedures (percutaneous coronary intervention in cath-lab). The use of IV contrast is widespread; therefore, monitoring for one of the three types of reactions during this diagnostic therapy is warranted.

The anaphylaxis presentation is similar to what has already been described in this chapter. The presentation is within minutes of the infused contrast and results in shortness of breath and tongue swelling. The treatment includes prompt administration of an antihistamine and epinephrine as described before.

Tissue injury (extravasations) resulting from IV contrast administration depends on the osmolarity of the solution (available in forms ranging from hyper-osmolar to iso-osmolar) and the site of infusion (the type of line access the patient has for the infusion). Management of tissue extravasation includes supportive care and consultation with a plastic surgeon to determine if surgery is necessary.

The other type of event to monitor with IV contrast is the occurrence of nephrotoxicity. The occurrence of kidney injury can be prevented by the administration of normal saline (osmolarity = 0.9%), sodium bicarbonate infusion, or N-acetylcysteine therapy prior to the patient receiving IV contrast. Kidney injury is more likely to occur in the elderly and in patients who are already receiving nephrotoxic drugs (aminoglycosides or amphotericin B). Management includes hydration and the monitoring of urine output. In the worst cases, temporary dialysis is required until the kidney recovers physiologic function (Chapters 10 and 21 discuss contrast media toxicity).

13.2.4 Hypoglycemic Events

The utilization of insulin and/or oral medication to effectively control a patient's blood sugar while they are admitted to a hospital is increasing. The one untoward consequence of using either an insulin preparation or oral hypoglycemic agent (glyburide, glimepiride, etc.) is hypoglycemia. The blood sugar used to define hypoglycemia is variable, as patients may experience signs and/or symptoms (such as perspiration, fast heart rate, tremor, and so on) of hypoglycemia without having a blood sugar that may be low. Low blood sugar can be defined as blood sugar less than 60 mg/dL or, alternatively, what is commonly used in clinical trials within the medical literature which is a blood sugar level less than 40 mg/dL. The reader is also referred to Chapter 18, which describes adverse events with diabetic therapy. The emphasis for the management of hypoglycemia revolves around the premise of prevention and appropriate monitoring of a patient while on therapy. For example, the prevention of hypoglycemia requires an analytical review of blood-sugar protocols for drug therapy and developing criteria for selecting an insulin regimen based on organ function (i.e., kidney and liver). In addition, the development of appropriate criteria for monitoring patients receiving insulin or oral diabetic therapy is critical for safe and effective blood sugar management.

The utilization of insulin infusions to maintain goal blood glucose levels has been a focus as a supportive care measure for critically ill patients. The clinical literature originally had supported an aggressive goal of blood glucose levels of 110–140 mg/dL. However, after additional research had been completed in more acutely ill patients, it was clear that the goal was leading to more harm than benefit.[17] Recent literature reviewing 11 studies demonstrated that a more aggressive blood sugar management strategy by the clinicians in the ICU ultimately led to more hypoglycemic events. In fact, the study revealed a five-fold increase in hypoglycemia/severe hypoglycemia when this approach was implemented.[17] The current recommendation by the Society of Critical Care Medicine (SCCM) is an approach utilizing a protocol which would be activated after two consecutive blood glucose levels are more than 180 mg/dL. The protocol should target an upper blood glucose level ≤180 mg/dL rather than an upper target blood glucose level ≤110 mg/dL. The available methods for achieving these goals can be attained with either a paper (manual calculation) or computer algorithm method. Due to the complexity of the calculations and the environment in the ICU, it would be recommended to utilize a computer algorithm module when possible. After the initiation of the protocol, the blood glucose values should be monitored every one to two hours until glucose values and insulin infusion rates are stable and then every four hours thereafter. The clinician should be cautious in the interpretation of blood glucose measurements obtained with point-of-care testing as such measurements may not accurately reflect the arterial blood or plasma glucose values.[18] Additional concerns that have been raised include the preparation of insulin infusions for administration in the ICU. The preparation is dependent on a hospital's resources, distribution channel to the ICU, availability of pre-mix insulin, and technician training, which are all variables to consider in an event when there is an error with insulin intravenous infusions.

13.2.5 Infusion-Related Reactions

13.2.5.1 Extravasations

Risk factors for extravasations include the following: pH (acid pH<5/Base pH>9), cytotoxicity, vasoconstrictive (ex. catecholamines), and those medications which have extreme osmolarity. Various formulations of medications possess properties described before; therefore, it is critical that this is reviewed in any reported extravasation event to triage management appropriately and efficiently to prevent any delays in care. In addition, many intensive care units will have policies and procedures which can outline the appropriate infusion site (peripheral versus central line) to ensure that the appropriate mechanism for drug delivery is utilized as well.[19] Intravenous infusions of catecholamine may be required to increase a patient's blood pressure in order to maintain perfusion to the brain and heart. The vasoactive infusions (i.e., dopamine, norepinephrine, epinephrine, and so on) are utilized to attain this goal. The intravenous infusions described have the capability to migrate outside the vein, termed extravasation, and consequently cause tissue necrosis. The extravasations more often occur when a peripheral line (as opposed to a central line access) is utilized for drug administration. The management of extravasations secondary to catecholamine infusions is done by the use of phentolamine intravenously and/or subcutaneous injections around the site of injury. Phentolamine provides a reversal effect (i.e., alpha antagonist activity) of the catecholamines, so that the vein can stay patent and there is a minimal progression of tissue necrosis. The prevention of extravasations requires appropriate monitoring by the nursing staff each time there is an infusion started in order to detect subtle changes in the patient's physical exam and line site.[20] Extravasation can also occur secondary to the chemical itself (doxycycline) or a diluent in the intravenous drug, such as diazepam or lorazepam, which contains propylene glycol. Several extravasations secondary to drugs require supportive care, which may include raising the affected limb or applying compression to increase the process of drug diffusion from the affected tissue site.

13.2.5.2 Propofol-Related Infusion Syndrome (PRIS)

Propofol infusion syndrome (PRIS) is described as a cascade of events leading to cardiovascular collapse and death. The triad of events which center around PRIS include metabolic acidosis, hypotension, bradycardia, and hyper-triglyceridemia. PRIS is more likely to be prominent in patients receiving higher dosing of propofol (i.e., 4 mg/kg/hr) for more than 48 hours.[21,22] The supportive evidence of the events related to propofol infusion center around the pharmacology that propofol is composed of a commercial preparation which is 10 percent lipid emulsion which can predispose to hypertriglyceridemia. Propofol can also inhibit beta-receptors on the heart, and calcium receptors on the blood vessels, which can lead to bradycardia and hypotension, respectively. The progression to metabolic acidosis is secondary to the ability of propofol to inhibit mitochondrial activity and increase anaerobic metabolism, consequently leading to the formation of lactic acid.[21–23] Since propofol can impact the mitochondrial chain transport system, the metabolism within the body transitions from aerobic to anaerobic metabolism, triggering a number of clinical consequences which ultimately lead to cardiovascular collapse. PRIS can be prevented with appropriate monitoring by clinicians to ensure that the dose and duration of drug infusion are tailored to patient requirements. Some strategies used to assist in facilitating this goal are the utilization of multiple sedative strategies to ensure that the propofol infusion dose stays at a minimum amount required to maintain the sedation goals. Another strategy is utilizing a sedation holiday (when clinically safe to do so) in patients on the continuous infusion to limit the overall exposure to the drug.[22] In the event that PRIS does occur, there is not a specific treatment for this reaction. The management of PRIS is supportive care by keeping the organ systems from failing to a catastrophic, fatal level.

13.2.5.3 Intravenous N-Acetylcysteine (NAC)

Intravenous NAC can be used for the prevention of contrast-induced nephropathy and the treatment of acetaminophen toxicity and drug-induced liver injury. Currently, there are two preparations of NAC, one that has an FDA-approved indication for intravenous administration (i.e., Acetadote®) and another preparation—NAC solution—which can be administered orally. NAC assists to convert the toxic metabolite of acetaminophen (APAP) which is NAPQI via glutathione donation. Once the glutathione storage becomes depleted in the liver, the elimination becomes prolonged, leading to a buildup of the toxic APAP metabolite NAPQI. The utilization of NAC for the management of APAP overdose integrates the Rumack–Matthew nomogram when the time of ingestion is clearly identified and the ingestion is non-sustained released preparation and occurs all at one time. Prior to the NAC solution, Acetadote was also given via intravenous infusion via an infusion filter.[24,25] The occurrence of infusion reactions is minimal; however, the reactions most commonly reported include anaphylaxis (as described earlier), itching, and flushing. The patient can be pretreated for the non-anaphylaxis type of reactions; however, clinicians need to be aware that these reactions are more likely to occur when given via the intravenous route and used in the treatment of acetaminophen toxicity or drug-induced liver injury in which the dosing (mg/kg) and frequency (number of doses) required are significantly higher.[24,25] In 2015, there was the introduction of a FDA-approved IV formulation of NAC which was supposed to help reduce the expense for the product as well as limit any concerns regarding an infusion-related reaction during administration.

13.2.6 Reversal Agents

The management of patients in an emergency department or a critical-care area often requires the administration of anticoagulants for the management of a blood clot, opioids for the management of pain, or benzodiazepines for the management of anxiety. All of these conditions require a careful approach, as excessive dosing and/or frequency can have untoward effects leading to patient harm and even death.

13.2.6.1 Protamine

Protamine is by nature a basic compound used to neutralize the effects of a parenteral anticoagulant unfractionated heparin (UFH) or low-molecular weight heparin (LMWH), which are both acidic compounds. Either UFH or LMWH can be used to treat patients with suspected or documented blood clots in the lower extremity or lung (i.e., venous thromboembolism) or acute coronary syndrome (heart attack).[26,27] Protamine intravenous infusion requires prompt administration and must be monitored for infusion-related reactions as well. The infusion of protamine can cause decreased blood pressure, decreased heart rate, and flushing.[26,27] Therefore, the decision to prescribe and administer protamine requires careful consideration in relation to the time of the administration of UFH or LMWH to ensure that the medication will continue to be safe and effective after administration.

13.2.6.2 Vitamin K

A form of anticoagulation which patients may be administered at home or in the hospital for blood clots (pulmonary or deep venous thromboembolism) is a vitamin K antagonist, such as warfarin. Warfarin is used as an anticoagulant for a variety of blood coagulation disorders. Generally, the medication may be started in the hospital, and then patients are followed up on an out-patient basis to ensure that the drug is effective (in the appropriate INR range) and safe (without the evidence of over-anticoagulation or bleeding). Warfarin is an oral vitamin K antagonist that shows an anticoagulant activity via the inhibition of vitamin K clotting factors (Factors II, VII, IX, and X) through the inhibition of the carboxylation of glutamic residues. The drug is monitored by an INR blood test. Over-anticoagulation can occur when patients are at home, and they may present to the ED. The other instance is when a patient receives over-anticoagulation in the hospital and presents to the ICU. Either scenario may require the administration of vitamin K. Vitamin K is an adjunct therapy, which means that, often, the patient is also receiving blood products for a high INR or active bleeding. Vitamin K is available as an oral tablet that can be given to patients with no evidence of active bleeding with an INR greater than 9.[26,28] Vitamin K is also a parenteral product that can be administered either subcutaneously or via intravenous infusion. The subcutaneous route is not recommended for patients with or without active bleeding as the drug absorption, activity, and effectiveness are questionable, at best. The preferred route of administration of vitamin K in a patient with an elevated INR with active bleeding is intravenous infusion. The intravenous push route is no longer recommended, secondary to infusion hypersensitivity reactions and cardiovascular manifestations; therefore, the infusion is not the selected route. In patients requiring vitamin K for INR reversal, the routes of administration would be either oral tablet (slow onset) or intravenous infusion (fast onset) in combination with adjunct therapy (blood-product administration).[26,28] The dosing for vitamin K is dependent on the INR and the clinical scenario of the patient presentation.

13.2.6.3 Naloxone

Naloxone is an opioid antagonist, generally used for opioid reversal. Naloxone is given via intravenous push administration at a dose of 0.4 mg for opioid naive patients. Naloxone has a short half-life and can be given repeated times. In some cases, a continuous infusion may be required for patients having difficulty eliminating opioid metabolites and drug interactions, or who have long-acting opioid preparations. In documented opioid overdose cases, the metabolism shifts in the body from first order to zero order. The enzymes in the liver responsible for the metabolism and breakdown of the drug to have it eliminated from the body become saturated. Once saturated, the enzymes have limited activity, thus prolonging the effects of the opioid implicated in the overdose. Many emergency support staff (EMS) and now law enforcement around the country have requirements of having the nasal narcan available and ready to administer by the first responder when they arrive on the scene to attempt to reverse the effects of the opioid.[29] The effects of opioids are primarily seen on the mu receptor. The opioids act on the mu1 receptor to provide relief for analgesia and pain relief. The effect of the opioids on the mu2 receptor is responsible for the adverse effects that are observed with respiratory depression and gastrointestinal complications of therapy.[30,31] Naloxone is also not to be confused with naltrexone, which is the oral preparation of the medication. Longer courses also have been described in the management of patients with liver toxicity, which may or may not be secondary to a medication. Generally, the infusion of NAC would continue until the liver enzymes (AST/ALT) are less than 1,000.

13.2.6.4 Flumazenil

Flumazenil is a GABA-antagonist used to reverse the side effects of sedation and disorientation from GABA-agonist activity or benzodiazepines. Flumazenil is generally dosed at 0.2 mg intravenous push. The main monitoring effect from flumazenil administration is seizures. The science behind why seizures may develop is that often when GABA activity is reversed too quickly, it lowers the seizure threshold. The concept is similar to the scenario when patients with a significant alcohol history abruptly stop drinking. The consequence is the development of seizure activity; therefore, the decision to administer flumazenil should be carefully reviewed in order to prevent this side effect.[30,31] In addition, a recent meta-analysis was performed, reviewing the utilization of flumazenil therapy in the emergency department in patients with suspected or confirmed benzodiazepine overdose. The authors reported that based on the review of all the literature, there was an increased risk of an adverse event secondary to the administration of flumazenil and that the therapy did not outweigh the safety/risk to the patient.[32] Flumazenil does not have an established role for the reversal of benzodiazepine overdose, and caution should be advised if administering it during the course of an emergency for this intention. In an event flumazenil is administered, depending on the benzodiazepine targeted for reversal, there may be re-sedation effects that need to be monitored for as the drug has a shorter half-life, and many benzodiazepines have longer half-lives. Flumazenil's effects are evident within 1–2 minutes and peak within 10 minutes after administration.[29]

13.3 SUMMARY

The use of medications in the emergency department (ED) and critical care (ICU) areas can often improve patient care. However, clinicians should maintain careful vigilance and monitoring to ensure patient safety and to avoid unnecessary harm or risk. Clinicians in the ED and ICU need to be aware of clinical data that helps make the selection of a therapy more effective. However, a balance must be maintained to provide a safe medication therapy. In addition, the consideration of all aspects of the medication process—prescribing, distribution, administration, and monitoring—is recommended in order to achieve and maintain this balance.

REFERENCES

1. L.T. Kohn, J.M. Corrigan, M.S. Donaldson. To Err is Human: Building a Safer Health-System. Washington, DC: Institute of Medicine, National Academy of Press, 1999.
2. Institute of Safe Medication Practices (ISMP). High Alert Medications. www.ismp.org/Tools/highAlertMedications.asp. Accessed 4 February 2012.
3. S. Kane-Gill, R.J. Weber. Principles and Practices of Medication Safety in the ICU. Crit. Care Clin. 2006; 22:273–290.
4. Joint Commission. www.jointcommission.org. Accessed 4 February 2012.
5. G.P. Patel, S. Kane-Gill. Medication Error Analysis: A Systematic Approach. Curr. Drug Saf. 2010;5:2–5.
6. F.J. Molina, P.T. Rivera, A. Cardona, D.C. Restrepo, O. Monroy, D. Rodas, J.G. Barrientos. Adverse Events in Critical Care: Search and Active Detection Through the Trigger Tool. World J. Crit. Care. 2018;7:9–15.
7. M. Mockenhaupt. Severe Drug-Induced Skin Reactions: Clinical Pattern, Diagnostics and Therapy. J. Detsch Dermatol. Ges. 2009;7:142–162.
8. L. French. Toxic Epidermal Necrolysis and Steven-Johnson Syndrome: Our Current Understanding. Allergol. Int. 2006;55:9–16.
9. B. Schnyder. Approach to a Patient with Drug Allergy. Immunol. Allergy Clin. N. Am. 2009;29:405–418.
10. S. Kanji, C. Chant. Allergic and Hypersensitivity Reactions in the Intensive Care Unit. Crit. Care Med. 2010;38:s162–s168.

11. B.G. Katzung. Basic and Clinical Pharmacology, 11th edition, McGraw-Hill Medical, New York. 2009.
12. J. Varon. The Diagnosis and Treatment of Hypertensive Crises. Postgrad. Med. 2009;121:5–13.
13. P.J. Kiel, M. Lo, D. Stockwell, G.P. Patel. An Evaluation of Amikacin Nephrotoxicity in the Hematology/Oncology Population. Am. J. Ther. 2008;15(2):131–136. doi: 10.1097/MJT.0b013e31815adfde
14. P.K. Kiel, M. Lo, D. Stockwell, G.P. Patel. An Evaluation of Amikacin Nephrotoxicity in the Hematology/Oncology Population. Am. J. Ther. 2008;15:131–136.
15. A. Lemke, A.F. Kiderlen, O. Kayser. Amphotericin B. Appl. Microbiol. Biotechnol. 2005;68:151–162.
16. R.W. Katzberg, R. Lamba. Contrast-Induced Nephropathy After Intravenous Administration: Fact or Fiction? Radiol. Clin. N. Am. 2009;47:789–800.
17. T. Yamada, N. Shojima, H. Noma, T. Yamauchi, T. Kadowaki. Glycemic Control, Mortality, and Hypoglycemia in Critically Ill Patients. Intens. Care Med. 2017;43:1–15.
18. P.R. Dellinger, M.W. Levy, A. Rhodes, D. Annane, H. Gerlach et al. Surviving Sepsis Guidelines for Severe Sepsis and Septic Shock 2012. Crit. Care Med. 2013;41:580–637.
19. D. Doellman, L. Hadaway, L.A. Bowe-Geddes, M. Franklin, J. LeDonne, L. Papke-O'Donnell, J. Pettit, L. Schulmeister, M. Stranz. Infiltration and Extravasation. J. Nurs. Infusion. 2009;32:203–211.
20. R.A. Phillips, P. Andrades, J.H. Grant, P.D. Ray. Deep Dopamine Extravasation Injury: A Case Report. J. Plast. Reconstr. Aesthet. Surg. 2009;62:222–224.
21. J. Orsini, A. Nadkarnia, J. Chen, N. Cohen. Propofol Infusion Syndrome: Case Report and Literature Review. Am. J. Health. Syst. Pharm. 2009;66:908–915.
22. A. Fudickar, B. Bein. Propofol Infusion Syndrome: Update of Clinical Manifestations and Pathophysiology. Minerva Anestesiol. 2009;75:339–344.
23. A.E. Mirrakhimov, P. Voore, O. Halytskyy, M. Khan, A.M. Ali. Propofol Infusion Syndrome in Adults: A Clinical Update. Crit. Care Res. Pract. 2015;2015: 1–10.
24. A.J. Whyte, T. Kehrl, D.E. Brooke, K.D. Katz, D. Sokolowski. Safety and Effectiveness of Acetadote for Acetaminophen Toxicity. J. Emerg. Med. 2008 Nov 18. E-pub ahead of print.
25. M. Kanter. Comparison of Oral and i.v. Acetylcysteine in the Treatment of Acetaminophen Poisoning. Am. J. Health. Syst. Pharm. 2006;63:1821–1827.
26. American College of Chest Physicians (ACCP). Guidelines on Antithrombotic Therapy. Chest. August, 2008. Supplement:1–793.
27. M. Levi. Emergency Reversal of Antithrombotic Treatment. Intern Emerg. Med. 2009;4:137–145.
28. A. Lubetsky, H. Yonath, D. Olchovsky, R. Loebstein, H. Halkin, D. Ezra. Comparison of Oral vs. Intravenous Phytonadione (vitamin K1) in Patients with Excessive Anticoagulation. Arch. Intern. Med. 2003;163: 2469–2473.
29. S. Patel. Toxicologic Emergencies in the Intensive Care Unit. Crit. Care Nurs. Q. 2013;36:335–344.
30. L. Brunton, J. Lazo, K. Parker. Goodman and Gilman's The Pharmacological Basis of Therapeutics, 11th edition, 2006. McGraw Hill.
31. American Hospital Formulary Service (AHFS). 2010. American Society of Health-System Pharmacists. Bethesda.
32. E. Penninga, N. Graudal, M.B. Ladekarl, G. Jürgens. Adverse events associated with flumazenil treatment for the management of suspected benzodiazepine intoxication: A systematic review with meta-analyses of randomised trials. Basic Clin. Pharmacol. Toxicol. 2016; 118(1):37–44.

14 Nephrotoxic Drugs

Jason M. Kidd, Domenic A. Sica, and Todd W. B. Gehr

SYNOPSIS

14.1 INTRODUCTION

Nephrotoxicity is an expansive term that implies some form of kidney damage. The expression nephrotoxicity does not in any way stipulate the mode of renal damage; thus, in a strict sense, this term has come to be used to describe any of a number of forms of renal injury. When nephrotoxicity occurs it can be expected to involve both kidneys. A nephrotoxic reaction can proceed at a casual pace and be present for months to years. This pattern oftentimes goes undetected even by the most astute clinician. Alternatively, nephrotoxicity can emerge suddenly and progress rapidly within a matter of weeks to months. This latter pattern is one which requires prompt attention.

Nephrotoxicity can be idiosyncratic as occurs when an antibiotic—such as a sulfa drug—damages the kidneys. In other cases, it can have a direct cause and effect relationship with an excess of drug as might be the case with a compound such as the antibiotic gentamicin. Nephrotoxicity can occur in isolation without any organ systems other than the kidney being involved, or it can be part of a generalized disturbance involving heart, liver, and skin among other organ systems. Such a generalized disturbance is what can be occasionally seen with the drug allopurinol, which is used in the treatment of gout.

It is important to appreciate that the chronic kidney disease (CKD) patient receives many medications in the hopes of slowing the progression of CKD. On the one hand, these medications can be viewed as important cogs in the treatment regimen for CKD. On the other hand, the use of these same medications—angiotensin-converting enzyme (ACE)

DOI: 10.1201/9781003615323-16

inhibitors or angiotensin-receptor blockers—is not without some risk.

The major such risk with these medications is the development of a life-threatening increase in serum potassium values—otherwise termed hyperkalemia. It remains to be determined as to whether the failure to use these medications in the CKD patient with progressive disease represents a departure from the standard of care.

14.2 FRAMEWORK OF THE PROBLEM

To appreciate the scope of the term nephrotoxicity (Table 14.1), a systematic approach to renal disease and accompanying drug therapy is necessary. The elements of such an analysis include a description of why the kidney is a location prone to adverse drug effects and what patient type is most susceptible to renal damage. Since the preexisting renal disease sets the stage for additional side effects in organs other than the kidney, it is important to recognize the numbers of patients in the United States with CKD. This includes those being treated with either hemodialysis or peritoneal dialysis and individuals having undergone a renal transplant. An additional important consideration is how damage is assessed both once it has occurred and as it progresses. Finally, the list of drugs which are known nephrotoxins is encyclopedic, so appropriate examples of drugs and their accompanying pattern of damage will be provided. The discussion of drug nephrotoxicity patterns will include a description of where errors are most commonly made either in the assessment or treatment of patients so afflicted.

TABLE 14.1
Scenarios of Nephrotoxicity and Adverse Effects Linked to the Kidney.

Scenario	Example
Direct damage to the kidney arising from excessive exposure to a known nephrotoxin	Gentamicin
Secondary damage to the kidney as the result of medication-related muscle cell damage	Cerivastatin (Baycol ®)
Direct but idiosyncratic damage to the kidney as in the case of an allergic reaction	Sulfa drugs
Reversible damage to the kidney	Nonsteroidal anti-inflammatory drugs
Damage to organ systems other than the kidney when drug doses have not been appropriately adjusted for the level of renal function in the patient with chronic kidney disease	Antiarrhythmics
Inadequate treatment of hypertension or chronic kidney disease	Failure to identify the scope of the problem and/or to select appropriate therapies
Inadequate treatment of side effects from medications used in the treatment of renal disease	Inadequate treatment of ACE-inhibitor-related angioedema

14.3 BASIS FOR THE KIDNEY BEING SUSCEPTIBLE TO DAMAGE

While the kidneys make up only 0.4% of body weight, they receive approximately 25% of the cardiac output. Otherwise stated, the kidneys receive a hefty blood flow on a minute-by-minute basis. This large blood flow increases the kidney's exposure and therein susceptibility to a variety of circulating drugs and toxins. The kidneys are routinely exposed to more blood-borne toxins than any organ other than the lungs. The kidney functions to both filter blood-borne substances and to then process this filtrate in a manner, which conserves important substances—such as sodium—and disposes of waste products—such as creatinine and urea nitrogen. Filtration within the kidney occurs via individual units called glomeruli of which there are several millions in both kidneys.

Glomeruli can be damaged by direct exposure to environmental toxins or drugs. The effect of environmental toxins on the kidney can be quite insidious and is an area that is poorly appreciated by many clinicians. The sieving potential of glomeruli is large, and, on average, 125-cc of filtrate is produced each minute. This value of 125-cc is conventionally termed the glomerular filtration rate (GFR). In addition, the kidney is responsible for a number of specialized physiologic functions, which are easily perturbed by medications. These characteristics lend themselves to both immunological and non-immunologically mediated injury such as alterations in renal blood flow, intrarenal drug metabolism, and tubular transport processes.

14.4 PATIENT GROUPS MOST SUSCEPTIBLE TO NEPHROTOXICITY

Irrespective of the cause, a reduction in renal function increases the risk of developing future nephrotoxicity. CKD can potentially predispose to nephrotoxicity for three reasons: First, CKD limits the clearance from the body of a number of medications, which can result in drug accumulation and the potential for drug concentration-dependent renal side effects (unless the medication dose is adjusted according to the level of renal function); second, the kidney in CKD has already been damaged and is in many instances unable to cope with further metabolic and toxic change as may be imposed on it with drug exposure; third, CKD is a condition that often co-exists with other disease states including diabetes, coronary artery disease, and congestive heart failure, and, with such a clustering of diseases, it is inevitable that a requirement for "polypharmacy" arises. Whenever multiple medications are being given—whether it is in the setting of CKD disease or not—the risk of drug–drug toxic interactions rise. The kidney can then become a target for such interactions. Finally, the elderly are a patient group predisposed to drug-related nephrotoxicity. In this regard, this greater risk of nephrotoxicity relates to the sluggish disposal of drugs by both the aging liver and kidney, which, in turn, allows blood levels for many medications to rise albeit somewhat unpredictably.

TABLE 14.2
Stages of Chronic Kidney Disease.

Stage	Description	GFR
1	Chronic kidney damage with normal or increased GFR	>90
2	Mild	60–89
3	Moderate	30–59
4	Severe	15–29
5	Kidney failure	<15 or dialysis

14.5 DEMOGRAPHICS OF CHRONIC KIDNEY DISEASE

CKD is a worldwide public health problem and has recently been recognized as an increasingly common problem in the United States. In the United States, the incidence and prevalence of kidney failure have doubled in the past 10 years, and the condition is associated with poor outcomes and high costs, especially in the elderly. CKD is defined by either kidney damage as manifested by the presence of an abnormal urinalysis, specifically protein or blood in the urine, or a glomerular filtration rate of less than 60 ml per minute per 1.73 m^2 for three months or more. The Third National Health and Nutritional Examination Survey (NHANES III) reported that approximately 6.2 million people are estimated to have a serum creatinine of more than 1.5 mg/dL (see Section 14.6).[1] This same study estimated that 800,000 Americans have a serum creatinine of more than 2.0 mg/dL and that the end-stage renal disease (ESRD) population numbered 326,000. This latter population, which comprises mostly of hemodialysis patients, is increasing at a rate of approximately 10% annually. The primary causes of CKD are diabetes (40%), hypertension (27%), glomerulonephritis (11%), interstitial nephritis (4%), and other urologic diseases (18%) (USRDS Data System, 2003). In an effort to better define this large group of patients, the National Kidney Foundation has developed a new classification system for CKD (Table 14.2). This system assigns patients a stage based on their GFR, which can be estimated from the serum creatinine (see discussion later in the chapter).[2]

14.6 METHODS TO ASSESS RENAL FUNCTION AND/OR DAMAGE

The available tests to detect nephrotoxicity are fairly insensitive; thus it can go unnoticed for some time. Serum creatinine measurements remain one of the most widely used tests for gauging renal function as elevated levels, when indexed for muscle mass, are indicative of kidney disease.

Creatinine is a product of creatine metabolism in muscles, and its daily production correlates closely with muscle mass. Thus, the greater the muscle mass, the higher the "normal serum creatinine." For example, in a heavily muscled male, a serum creatinine value of 1.4 mg/dL might be considered normal, though such a value may be considered grossly abnormal in an individual with less muscles. Furthermore, as the GFR declines, the influence of muscle mass on serum creatinine concentrations becomes even more complex with the result that serum creatinine changes, as measures of progressive renal failure, poorly correlate with GFR changes.[3]

Normal serum creatinine concentrations for a typical population range from 0.5–1.3 mg/dL (40–110 micromole/L) in males to 0.5–1.1 mg/dL (40–100 micromole/L) in females. Although a serum creatinine may fall within these established ranges, it does not automatically follow that renal function is normal, as a specific serum creatinine value can be associated with a wide range of GFR rate values. For example, a small muscle mass individual, such as an elderly female, with normal renal function might be expected to have a serum creatinine value close to 0.5 mg/dL. If this individual presents with a serum creatinine of 1.0 mg/dL, although this value is in the normal "population "range, it represents a significant deviation from the norm for this individual. As creatinine clearance is reciprocally related to serum creatinine concentrations, in this patient, the doubling of serum creatinine would represent an approximate halving of renal function.

Because of the aforementioned limitations of utilizing serum creatinine to estimate kidney function, more reliance on utilizing the estimated GFR has become a standard medical practice. Most laboratories now report an estimated GFR for African Americans and non-African Americans based on the serum creatinine and the demographics of the patient. Most estimations of GFR utilize combinations of the serum creatinine, age, race, sex, and body size. One of these equations, the MDRD (Modification of Diet in Renal Disease) Study equation, has become the most widely used of these equations, and most laboratories use this equation to estimate GFR when a serum creatinine is ordered for a particular patient. Because this equation was developed in a patient population with CKD, the accuracy of the equation is a major limitation, especially at GFR values of over 60 ml/min. Because of these limitations, the estimated GFR is not reported precisely for individuals with GFR values over 60 ml/min. A newly devised equation, the CKD-EPI equation, has been developed to overcome the limitations of the MDRD equation and appears to be more accurate at higher GFR values. This equation or its variation will likely replace the MDRD equation for the estimation of GFR values for individual patients although there will continue to be a distinction made between African Americans and non-African Americans. Suffice it to say, the GFR value has replaced the serum creatinine for the determination of CKD in individual patients. Failure to recognize this would now be considered a breach in the standard of care.

Thus, one of the most common errors on the part of a health care provider is the failure to recognize the limited sensitivity of a serum creatinine value to detect acute functional change as well as its inability to monitor progressive disease. In the setting of progressive kidney disease, it is not uncommon for considerable loss of kidney function to have occurred before referral to a kidney specialist. The exact timing of such referral remains a matter of substantial debate. Alternatively, if an acute process is at play—be it nephrotoxic or otherwise—referral should occur within a matter of days-to-weeks. Failure to refer in a timely fashion can be viewed as a deviation from the standard of care.

14.7 LEVEL OF RENAL FUNCTION AT WHICH DRUG ACCUMULATION OCCURS

The total body clearance (TBC) of a compound is the summed value of individual organ clearances including the liver and kidney among other organs such as skin, intestine, and muscle. Renal clearance is an important contributor to the TBC of several compounds including ACE inhibitors; certain beta-blockers; most diuretics; and a number of antibiotics, antiarrhythmics, and pain medications. To be clinically relevant, the renal clearance of a compound need not be that high in absolute terms as long as the percentage contribution to the TBC from renal elimination is substantial (typically >50%).

Renally cleared compounds begin to accumulate at GFR values less than 60-mL/min (60% of normal), though the precise level of renal function at which clinically relevant changes in drug clearance occur is very compound-specific. A significant decline in drug clearance for a renally cleared drug can be expected by the time filtration falls below 30 mL/min (30% of normal). It is at GFR values below 30 mL/min (30% of normal) that the issue of drug accumulation surfaces though as stated significant accumulation can occur even at higher levels of function.[4]

Drug accumulation is pertinent in a number of ways for CVR compounds. First, if the compound administered has a narrow therapeutic window, its accumulation can quickly exceed the boundaries of the sought-after pharmacologic effect with sometimes hazardous consequences. For instance, accumulation of an antihypertensive compound can lead to an exaggerated fall in blood pressure (BP). If the GFR falls as the result of such a BP drop, the renal clearance of a compound can be incrementally reduced, and, with further accumulation, a vicious cycle of events can ensue. Second, if an administered compound has well-established concentration-related side effects, they will occur more often and with greater severity when a drug accumulates. This is the case with renally cleared beta-blockers and the side effect of sedation. Finally, drug accumulation increases the risk of drug–drug interactions and thereby manufactures a risk from concurrent therapy that otherwise would be absent.

14.8 NEPHROTOXIC DRUGS

The clinician should have a working knowledge of the elimination profile of various medications and any interactions that may arise from drug accumulation.

14.8.1 What Constitutes Prompt Clinical Action in the Face of Nephrotoxicity?

Prompt clinical action in the face of nephrotoxicity means identifying the offending medication and withdrawing it. Discontinuation of the medication alone is not the only step that needs to be taken. In addition, the rate of progression of the underlying disease needs to be established. This typically requires serial assessment of renal function (e.g., serum creatinine measurements), implementation of any of the several recognized therapies, and in most cases appropriate discussion between the primary care physician and the specialist evaluating the patient. As previously mentioned, nephrotoxicity can be sudden, or it can be slowly-to-moderately progressive. It is the former that can prove life-threatening, and/or, if not quickly identified, result in permanent renal demise, if not death, can ensue. It is the latter that can present the greatest challenge to the clinician and where errors of complacency occur.

14.9 NEPHROTOXICITY SCENARIOS

Several medications have nephrotoxic potential. Such tendencies for medications to cause renal damage are for the most part dormant; however, the presence of CKD can trigger and/or increase the risk of injury.

14.9.1 Lithium Toxicity

A 48-year-old Caucasian male with a bipolar disorder has received lithium for over 15 years. His lithium levels have been sporadically checked, in part, because of poor appointment compliance on the part of the patient. His lithium levels have been in high normal to high range when measured. Recently, his lithium dose was reduced because of symptoms of lithium toxicity. A review of his laboratory studies show that he has had a slowly rising serum creatinine value reflecting the progression of kidney disease. Five years back, he had 80% of expected renal function. A more recent measurement now shows him to have 50% of expected normal kidney function. The patient was never informed of his having renal failure and files suit.

14.9.1.1 Discussion

Renal failure is a not an uncommon complication of long-term lithium therapy, which can only be identified by periodic monitoring of renal function.[5] Once renal failure is diagnosed in a lithium-treated patient (oftentimes, it is a diagnosis of exclusion for a lithium-related etiology), a treatment plan should be established. Any such treatment plan should involve the patient in a decision on the advisability of continuing therapy, particularly if the renal failure is at an advanced stage. Failure to do so can be construed to represent a departure from the standard of care. As lithium is being used in a setting where a patient's recall can be called into question, it is prudent to have such discussions on long-term treatment witnessed. Moderately advanced lithium-related renal failure may go undetected if the parties treating such patients are unfamiliar with the relevance of small changes in serum creatinine as a marker of progressive renal failure. This may be the case for psychiatrists who assume primary care for a patient without adequate internal medicine support.

14.9.2 Gentamicin Toxicity

A 70-year-old, 60-kg female is admitted to the hospital with a severe infection for which she is prescribed nafcillin and gentamicin. Nafcillin is prescribed at a dose of 1 gram IV q 4 hours, and gentamicin is prescribed at a dose of 5 mg/kg (300 mg) IV q day. Routine admission labs reveal normal electrolytes and a serum creatinine concentration of 1.4 mg/dL. One week later, she is doing better, and her serum creatinine is now 1.5 mg/dL. Antibiotics are continued without dosage modification for another week. At the end of the second week in the hospital, the patient complains of dizziness and was unable to walk without assistance. Laboratory evaluation reveals a serum creatinine of 5.8 mg/dL, and a consultation is obtained for acute kidney failure.

14.9.2.1 Discussion

Antibiotics often cause acute renal failure. In this case, either nafcillin (causing allergic interstitial nephritis) or the aminoglycoside antibiotic gentamicin (causing acute tubular necrosis) were possibilities although gentamicin toxicity is the most likely. Aminoglycoside antibiotics are intravenous antibiotics, widely prescribed for serious infections. These types of antibiotics are extensively eliminated by the kidneys; therefore, dosage adjustment is necessary in patients with CKD. This patient had a serum creatinine of 1.4 mg/dL, which, although being in the upper range of population normal values, in this case reflected her having only 35% of normal renal function. Her gentamicin dosage should have early on reflected this reduction in GFR and reduced.

The monitoring of plasma gentamicin concentrations is of paramount importance in the accurate dosing of this medication in a patient such as this with preexisting renal disease.[6] In this case, therapeutic drug-level monitoring for gentamicin should have been performed in parallel with the drug's dosing. Aminoglycoside antibiotics cause both acute kidney failure and vestibular toxicity (dizziness and imbalance), side effects which are dependent on dose, duration, age, and the presence of kidney disease.[7] This patient experienced both side effects, which were avoidable. This scenario represented a breach in the standard of care. Although gentamicin toxicity in certain situations may be unavoidable owing to the nature of the infection and sometimes need for a lengthy duration of therapy, its risk can be minimized by a careful monitoring of gentamicin blood levels. When a lengthy course of treatment with gentamicin is anticipated, it is clearly the responsibility of the physician to warn the patient of the possible occurrence of these disabling and potentially life-threatening toxicities. Moreover, the patient should be routinely questioned as to early signs of vestibular toxicity as its early identification affords the opportunity to immediately discontinue gentamicin and thereby improve the chances of vestibular function being recovered.

The treatment modalities used in the management of ESRD can themselves carry risk. An adverse outcome within a dialysis facility can have multiple potential causes as well as a considerable diffusion of blame.

14.9.3 Dialysis-Related Issues

A 40-year-old hemodialysis patient is peacefully sleeping during a routine dialysis procedure. He is covered in a blanket, and all his vital signs were normal at the initiation of dialysis. He has been on hemodialysis for five years, has controlled hypertension, and works in a local bank. Three hours into his dialysis session, a pressure alarm signals from his dialysis machine. The technician caring for him does not disturb him and simply resets the alarm. Ten minutes later, a BP alarm signals that a low BP is present. The technician attempts to arouse the patient but is unsuccessful. An attempt is made to resuscitate the patient, but the patient succumbs. During the resuscitation effort, a large puddle of blood is noted under and behind the patient's chair.

14.9.3.1 Discussion

With such a technical procedure being performed on average three times a week, it is surprising that more such technical mistakes do not occur. This patient had a partially dislodged venous dialysis needle which resulted in his exsanguination.[8] A multitude of avoidable mishaps can and do occur in the dialysis unit, some of which are listed in Table 14.3.[9] These calamities can be the responsibility of the technician/nurse tending to the patient or, on occasion, can be the result of physician error. Physicians are not routinely in attendance for the entirety of a dialysis session and therefore must rely on the hemodialysis staff for the timely and accurate reporting of patient problems. Judgmental errors on the part of the treating physician can occur if the "sense" of a patient's clinical condition is miscommunicated.

TABLE 14.3
Mishaps Related to Hemodialysis.

Dialysate problems
Endotoxin exposure
Chloramine exposure
Fluoride exposure
Dialyzer reactions
First-use syndromes
Reuse-related problems, infection transmission
Anaphylactoid reactions to ACE inhibitors
Process-related problems
Hypotension/hypertension
Blood loss
Access infections
Air embolus

Failure to appreciate the need to avoid certain drugs and/or to adjust medication doses in CKD can prove fatal. In most cases, this represents a failure to appreciate the importance of drug dose adjustment in renal disease. The ultimate responsibility for an appropriate drug therapy in CKD rests in the hands of the primary treating physician.

14.9.4 Drug Clearance in Relationship with Renal Failure

14.9.4.1 Case 1

A young dialysis patient is a victim of a severe automobile accident and admitted to the hospital with multiple fractures. As he had just been dialyzed that day, the dialysis service was not notified of his admission presuming that it would be a couple of days before he would next need to be dialyzed. Because of severe pain, he is begun on meperidine (Demerol ®) 75 mg IM every 4 hours. Two days after he has begun meperidine, he begins to experience twitching and tremors. This is reported to the treating surgeon who instructs the staff to observe the patient. One day later, the patient experiences a series of seizures, aspirates, and dies shortly thereafter.

14.9.4.1 Discussion

Renally cleared drugs and/or their metabolites systemically accumulate in patients with CKD unless the medication dose is adjusted. In many instances, such accumulation is of marginal significance. In other cases when small changes in drug levels carry significant risk (narrow therapeutic index), life-threatening complications may arise.[10] This case is one such instance. Meperidine is metabolized to an active metabolite, normeperidine, that accumulates in dialysis patients.[11] Normeperidine is known to lower the threshold for seizures. However, the breach in the standard of care in this patient went beyond failure to dose adjust this medication. The breach in this case arose from having prescribed this compound without first understanding the risks inherent to its use in advanced renal failure. Moreover, physicians familiar with drug-dosing in renal failure were not consulted in a timely fashion. If such a thing had occurred, this medication would likely have been discontinued and an adverse outcome avoided.

14.9.4.2 Case 2

A 70-year-old patient has an acute myocardial infarction complicated by a life-threatening rhythm disturbance—ventricular tachycardia. An antiarrhythmic procainamide is begun intravenously, and his ventricular tachycardia is controlled. His serum creatinine at the time of admission is 4.5 mg/dL, which reflects his having approximately 25% of normal renal function. He is placed on a conventional maintenance dose of oral procainamide in an amount not adjusted for his level of renal failure. Two days later in the early afternoon, he sustains a fatal arrhythmia. Serum procainamide concentrations obtained the morning of the event were twice the upper limit of normal range, and the serum concentrations of the active metabolite of procainamide N-acetylprocainamide were three times the upper limit of normal.

14.9.4.3 Discussion

In patients with renal failure, lower doses (with the same interval between doses) or longer intervals between doses (without an adjustment of the actual dose amount) are means by which blood levels of medications can be safely controlled. Procainamide and its active metabolite N-acetylprocainamide possess antiarrhythmic properties useful in the treatment of ventricular tachycardia; however, both substances are cleared from the body by the renal route and will accumulate in the renal failure patient unless the standard dose is reduced.[12] The breach in the standard of care in this instance was glaring and involved an inadequate understanding of the dosing of this narrow therapeutic index compound in a patient with advanced renal failure. Moreover, there was a lapse in reporting the blood levels of procainamide and its metabolite to the treating physician. Such critical information being absent, the physician of record was unable to take the necessary steps to avert this catastrophe.

Therapies in common use in renal failure can be etiologic for some very unique side effects. Physicians should be familiar with the manner of presentation for such side effects as well as what represents optimal treatment.

14.9.5 Angioedema with an ACE Inhibitor

A 45-year-old African American male is seen in evaluation for hypertension and CKD. His BP is observed to be 150/105 during a routine office visit. In light of his having CKD, he is started on the ACE inhibitor lisinopril and scheduled for follow-up in two weeks. Two days after beginning lisinopril, he develops swelling of his lower lip, which subsides over several hours without treatment. The next day, he experiences the same symptom, but, this time, his tongue is also noted to be swollen. He goes to an Emergency Room and is treated with an antihistamine, epinephrine, and intravenous steroids. His symptoms abate over the next 12 hours, and he is discharged to follow-up with his treating physician. He is given no instructions at the time of discharge from the Emergency Room (as the discharging physician differed from the admitting physician). The next day, he takes another dose of his lisinopril and, shortly thereafter, experiences profound swelling of his lips and tongue. By the time the Rescue Squad arrives, he is in full arrest and cannot be resuscitated.

14.9.5.1 Discussion

ACE inhibitor-related angioedema (life-threatening lip and tongue swelling) is two to three times more common in African Americans than in Caucasians. Once it has occurred, the risk of a subsequent episode (oftentimes more severe) rises. Although the Emergency Room management was reasonable, there was a breach in the standard of care at discharge. Failure to advise the patient to stop his ACE inhibitor was a significant oversight. Once ACE inhibitor angioedema has occurred, subsequent use of any ACE inhibitor is absolutely contraindicated, and the patient should be so informed. Management errors can also become the basis for filing suits in the case of ACE inhibitor angioedema. Errors are typically made in the floor monitoring of newly admitted patients as well as in the transition of responsibility for care from the Emergency Room physician to the admitting physician. Adverse outcomes in an angioedema patient are usually seen in the several-hour time span, shortly after admission. It is often difficult to identify where the line of responsibility falls at the time of an adverse outcome in an angioedema patient.[13]

Hyperkalemia is becoming a much more common occurrence in renal failure patients with the expanding use of reno- and cardioprotective therapies that also give rise to clinically relevant changes in serum potassium.

14.9.6 Fatal Hyperkalemia with Medications

A 65-year-old male with a history of heart failure is being treated with standard therapy consisting of the ACE inhibitor enalapril, the beta-blocker metoprolol, digoxin, furosemide, and potassium chloride. His serum creatinine is 1.4 mg/dL (approximately 60% of normal renal function), and he weighs 65 kg. He does well until he presents to the Emergency room with an acute myocardial infarction and, after a short hospitalization, stabilizes and is discharged on his pre-admission medications, except for the addition of the potassium-sparing diuretic spironolactone. His serum creatinine at discharge was 2.0 mg/dL (approximately 40% of normal renal function), and his serum potassium was 4.8 mEq/L (normal range—3.5 to 5.0 mEq/L). Once discharged, he develops diarrhea and increasing weakness, which persist for several days. A call to his family physician is made on a Friday, and he is instructed to come into the office on Monday if his symptoms do not improve. Shortly thereafter, he presents to a local Emergency Room with profound weakness and is found to have a serum potassium value of 7.5 mEq/L and a serum creatinine concentration of 4.5 mg/dL (approximately 15% of normal renal function). His BP is 70/40 mm Hg, and an ECG reveals what looks like a "sine wave" pattern (classic pattern for cardiotoxicity with hyperkalemia). Before specific therapy can be started for the hyperkalemia, the patient experiences a cardiopulmonary arrest. Although successfully resuscitated, he suffers permanent anoxic brain injury and thereafter requires permanent nursing home care.

14.9.6.1 Discussion

Patients with complex cardiac disorders often require multiple medical therapies; therefore, the medications used in this patient represented standard therapy. However, as the patient's clinical condition deteriorated, his prescription regimen required adjustment. In particular, when a patient receives multiple therapies known to increase serum potassium values, extra care must be directed to situations where serum potassium values would be expected to rise further. Failure to do so can result in serious elevations in serum potassium going undetected with potentially disastrous consequences. At the time of call-in with complaints of an intercurrent illness, steps were not taken to immediately see this patient. The breach in the standard of care herein was reflected in a failure to appreciate the risk of serious hyperkalemia in this patient. The risk of a life-threatening elevation in serum potassium should have been anticipated for three reasons: First, at the time of discharge following his myocardial infarction, he already had a high normal serum potassium value; second, discharge medications included supplemental potassium, as well as two compounds with known potassium-conserving properties—enalapril and spironolactone; and third, an intercurrent illness which leads to dehydration is one of the lead reasons that severe hyperkalemia develops in a patient multiply-medicated in this fashion. More careful attention to patient instructions was needed (such as advising the patient if significant dehydration develops for any reason [as gauged by weight loss] to contact his physician immediately). An earlier physician visit would have reduced the chances of this patient experiencing a cardiopulmonary arrest.[14]

Certain drugs can cause acute renal failure arising from muscle cell damage. An understanding of the mode of presentation for this form of renal damage should be common knowledge for those medications commonly used—such as statins.

14.9.7 Statin Therapy and the Development of Myopathy

A 70-year-old male with diabetes and hypertension develops hypercholesterolemia and hypertriglyceridemia, and therapy is begun with a statin. At first, he tolerates the medication, and the statin dose is gradually increased. With dose escalation, he develops mild muscle weakness and pain, which he believes to have been a viral syndrome. These symptoms gradually subside and are mentioned to his treating physician at the next office visit. The physician charts the symptoms, and, in further management of the lipid abnormality, gemfibrozil is added to his statin therapy. Two weeks later, he develops muscle pain which gradually increases over several days to marked weakness and is brought to the Emergency Room where he is diagnosed as having muscle damage (rhabdomyolysis) and related acute renal failure. He requires hemodialysis, and four weeks after his episode of rhabdomyolysis, he still requires maintenance dialysis.

14.9.7.1 Discussion

Statins (3-hydroxy-3-methylglutaryl coenzyme A reductase inhibitors) are associated with skeletal muscle complaints, including clinically important myositis and rhabdomyolysis, myalgia, muscle weakness, mild serum creatine kinase (CK) elevations, muscle cramps, and persistent myalgia and CK elevations even after statin withdrawal. The risk of rhabdomyolysis and other adverse effects can be exacerbated by several factors such as concomitant medications. Medications such as the fibrate gemfibrozil alter statin metabolism and increase statin plasma concentration and noticeably increase the risk of rhabdomyolysis. There is no predictable method to determine those at risk for myopathy, nor is there a reliable screening test. Patients should be informed and told to look for generalized muscle pain or weakness. If these symptoms occur, the patient should stop medications and report to a medical professional immediately. The breach in the standard of care was in the failure to recognize that the prior symptoms in this patient were likely to be secondary to statin-linked muscle toxicity. In such patients, subsequent statin–fibrate combination therapy must be undertaken cautiously and only after a careful risk–benefit analysis. Patient counseling on the risks and warning signs of myopathy is critical and did not occur. Left to his own devices, this patient believed that this second wave of symptoms would abate as had previously been the case. Earlier detection, discontinuation of the culprit medications, and directed treatment would likely have changed the outcome in this case.[15]

14.9.8 Nephrotoxicity Related to Checkpoint Inhibitor Use

A 54-year-old female with a history of melanoma is placed on nivolumab and ipilimumab. She has tolerated her initial infusions well without significant side effects, and recent scans have shown an improvement in her disease. One week after her most recent infusion, she develops a low-grade fever and rash on her lower extremities along with swelling. She is directed to the Emergency Room for further evaluation. In the Emergency Room, she is noted to be hypertensive with a blood pressure of 160 mmHg/100 mmHg. She is also noted to have lower extremity edema. Blood work is performed and is notable for a serum creatinine of 2.0 mg/dL without history of antecedent renal failure. She is also noted to have a low serum albumin of 1.8 g/dL. A urinalysis shows significant proteinuria. She is aggressively hydrated and advised to return to her oncologist. A few days later, she sees her oncologist for follow-up. Her symptoms persist. Infusions are stopped, and she is referred to see a nephrologist. Prior to this visit, she develops the acute onset of shortness of breath and suffers a cardiac arrest. She is able to be resuscitated, and during her work up, she is discovered to have a large pulmonary embolism. As a result of her cardiac arrest, she requires a prolonged hospitalization with multiple setbacks, and she is unable to receive further treatment of her melanoma.

14.9.8.1 Discussion

Over the last several years, the treatment of cancer has changed to include highly targeted therapy and immunotherapy. As with other types of chemotherapy, adverse drug effects may occur. Prompt recognition of these effects is imperative in order to decrease the risk of severe side effects. Proteins called checkpoints are made by our immune systems that strike a balance between activating T-cells to destroy foreign cells and suppressing our own T-cells from attacking our normal cells. When these checkpoints are blocked, our own immune systems can be harnessed to kill cancer cells. Immune checkpoint inhibitors (ICIs) have subsequently been developed and have proven to be highly efficacious in the treatment of many cancers. Due to the increased activation of immune system by these drugs, there are significant risks of immune-related adverse events such as rash, diarrhea (colitis), cardiac inflammation (pericarditis), and adrenal insufficiency. These immune-related adverse events can also lead to kidney failure. Furthermore, these drugs have been described to have caused the nephrotic syndrome which leads to heavy protein loss in the urine and places patients at high risk of blood clots.[16]

TABLE 14.4
Common Renal Toxicities Related to Cancer Treatment.

Drug/Class	Adverse Event
Checkpoint Inhibitors/Immunotherapies • Ipilimumab • Pembrolizumab • Nivolumab	Kidney failure, protein in the urine, hypertension
Platinum-based chemotherapy • Carboplatin • Cisplatin	Kidney failure, electrolyte disorders (low magnesium, potassium)
Alkylating agents • Cyclophosphamide • Ifosphamide	Low sodium (hyponatremia), bladder hemorrhage
VEGF inhibitors • Avastin • Bevacizumab	Protein in the urine, high blood pressure, anemia, low platelets
Antimetabolites • Gemcitabine	Kidney failure, high blood pressure, low platelets, anemia

Immune checkpoint inhibitors and other forms of immunotherapy can lead to kidney damage. An understanding of the possible side effects is critical for these drugs as well as the potential nephrotoxic side effects of other chemotherapies (Table 14.4).

14.10 CONCLUSIONS

CKD is steadily growing in its prevalence in the United States. As the patient numbers with this illness increase, the opportunity for adverse medication-related and/or device outcomes is following suit. Not unexpectedly, the management (or the lack of the same) of the CKD patient bears legal ramifications. The management of CKD is in a state of flux with standards of care evolving at a fairly constant pace. Physicians must be aware of the recommended strategies to slow the progress of CKD as well the important role the kidney plays in drug elimination. Moreover, the kidney is a target organ vulnerable to damage by a wide range of chemicals, medications, and environmental toxins. In most cases, evolving kidney disease is asymptomatic; thus, the evaluation of progressive medication-related renal disease necessitates keen interpretive skills of renal function determinants.

NOTES

1. Coresh J, Astor BC, Greene T, et al. Prevalence of chronic kidney disease and decreased kidney function in the adult US population: Third National Health and Nutrition Examination Survey. Am J Kidney Dis 2003; 41: 1–12.
2. National Kidney Foundation. K/DOQI clinical practice guidelines for chronic kidney disease: Evaluation, classification, and stratification. Am J Kidney Dis 2002; 39(2 Suppl 1): S1–S266.
3. Sica DA. Complications of hypertension: Kidney. In: Crawford MH, DiMarco JP, eds. Cardiology (2nd edition). Mosby, London, England, 2004: 501–510.
4. Sica DA. Drug dosing in renal disease. In: Bakris G, ed. The Kidney and Hypertension (1st edition). Martin Dunitz, London. England, 2003: 127–138.
5. Gitlin M. Lithium and the kidney: An updated review. Drug Saf 1999; 20: 231–243.
6. Bartal C, Danon A, Schlaeffer F, et al. Pharmacokinetic dosing of aminoglycosides: A controlled trial. Am J Med 2003; 114: 194–198.
7. Lu CM, James SH, Lien YH. Acute massive gentamicin intoxication in a patient with end-stage renal disease. Am J Kidney Dis 1996; 28: 767–771.
8. Roy T. Patients' safety and haemodialysis devices. Nephrol Dial Transplant 2001; 16: 2138–2142.
9. Bosch X. Medical devices firm offers answer to unexplained haemodialysis deaths. Lancet 2001; 358: 1622.
10. Sica DA, Gehr TWB, Yancy C. Hyperkalemia, congestive heart failure, and aldosterone receptor antagonism. Cong Heart Fail 2003; 9: 224–229.
11. Hagmeyer KO, Mauro LS, Mauro VF. Meperidine-related seizures associated with patient-controlled analgesia pumps. Ann Pharmacother 1993; 27: 29–32.
12. Reiffel JA, Appel G. Importance of QT interval determination and renal function assessment during antiarrhythmic drug therapy. J Cardiovasc Pharmacol Ther 2001; 6: 111–119.
13. Sica DA, Black HR. Current concepts of pharmacotherapy in hypertension: ACE inhibitor-related angioedema: Can angiotensin-receptor blockers be safely used? J Clin Hypertens (Greenwich) 2002; 4: 375–380.
14. Sica DA, Gehr TWB, Yancy C. Hyperkalemia, congestive heart failure, and aldosterone receptor antagonism. Cong Heart Fail 2003; 9: 224–229.
15. Sica DA, Gehr TWB. HMG-CoA reductase inhibitors and rhabdomyolysis: Considerations in the renal failure patient. Curr Opin Nephrol Hypertens 2002; 11: 123–133.
16. Perazella MA, Shirali AC. Immune checkpoint inhibitor nephrotoxicity: What do we know and what should we do? Kidney Int 2020; 97: 62–74.

15 Drug-Induced Liver Disease

James T. O'Donnell, James J. O'Donnell III, Donald H. Marks, and Paul N. Danese

SYNOPSIS

DOI: 10.1201/9781003615323-17

15.1 INTRODUCTION: THE PROBLEM OF DRUG-INDUCED LIVER DISEASE

Drug-induced liver disease is an uncommon but challenging clinical problem with respect to both diagnosis and management. Its incidence is estimated to be 14 to 19 cases per 100,000 persons, with jaundice companying 30% of cases. Drug-induced liver injury is responsible for 3 to 5% of hospital admissions for jaundice, and it is the most frequent cause of acute liver failure in most Western countries, accounting for more than half of the cases.[1] The liver is the primary organ where drug metabolism occurs. Consequently, regardless of the site-of-action for therapeutic effect, most drugs will also interact with the tissues of the liver and thus have potential for liver toxicity. Therefore, it is not surprising that drug-induced liver dysfunction/disease (DILD) is a primary cause of drug-induced death and one of the main reasons for the removal of drugs from the pharmaceutical market. An investigation into drug products withdrawn from the EU market between 2002 and 2011 cites hepatic disorders as the second most common safety reason for withdrawing a drugs. The study report provides safety reasons and the evidence used to support the decision-making.[2]

Liver adverse reactions are linked to approximately 1,100 drugs.[3] These adverse reactions amount to 2–3% of all hospitalizations and 3% of all jaundiced patients.[4] As clinical events of DILD are often nonspecific and have variable latency, accurate diagnosis of DILD requires careful monitoring of the patient.[5]

For an accurate detection of drug hepatotoxicity, an extensive drug history, a low threshold of suspicion, and the elimination of other liver disease causes are integral. An excellent resource for the current status of drug-induced liver toxicity is the *LiverTox*, which is described as a living document and is continuously expanded, revised, and updated by the National Institute of Diabetes and Digestive and Kidney Diseases[6] Given the complexity and importance of the liver's drug-metabolizing systems, the fact that drugs and chemicals can poison the liver is or should be of utmost concern to pharmacists and physicians. An exposition of the metabolic processes promotes an understanding of how certain drug interactions occur and what to do about those interactions.

DILD can mimic many forms of liver disease and can be distinguished by its major pathological pattern of injury: (1) Hepatitis, also known as hepatocellular or cytotoxic, (2) cholestatic, (3) vascular, and (4) neoplastic. Any of these DILD types can be the result of acute or chronic exposure to a particular drug agent.[7]

All the cells present within the liver can be affected by a drug. The type of liver injury is dependent upon the clinical pathologies that arise which are connected to a specific mechanism of hepatic toxicity. The specific drug, the details of treatment (dosing, duration), and patient susceptibility also play a large role. This can rationalize how DILD can result in a wide array of liver diseases which, at first glance, look like natural liver deterioration.[8,9,10,11,12] Given its rarity, drug-related hepatotoxicity may not occur during clinical trials, which are usually limited to a few thousand participants. However, after the approval of a drug for use and subsequent marketing, large numbers of patients are exposed, and rare toxic effects may emerge.[13]

The diversity in the clinical pathology of the DILD contributes to the diagnostic difficulties that arise in discovering the role a specific drug plays in a clinical manifestation. Aside from the plethora of classic drug agents that result in hepatotoxicity,[14] there are many other agents that need to be taken into account. Even the excipients within a formulation are considered, especially with herbal medicines which are being consumed with increased frequency, many of which are undocumented.[15,16,17] Illicit drugs such as cocaine and amphetamines (ecstasy) can also cause DILD.[18] Due to the variety of agents which can precipitate DILD, drug hepatotoxicity remains a significant challenge for the scientific community, namely, physicians, health authorities, and pharmaceutical firms.

15.2 HISTORY OF ADVERSE DRUG REACTIONS

The presence of adverse drug reactions (ADRs) in the liver is a significant challenge to overcome within drug development. DILD can result in a wide variety of liver diseases with the most common syndrome being acute hepatitis. DILD is also one of the most frequent causes of fulminant (end-stage) hepatitis. The majority of liver ADRs are present in only a small percentage of patients which makes it challenging to spot during drug development. Liver dysfunction is mostly recognized due to random reports within the first two years of the newly marketed drug. The presence of DILD is weakly documented by only a few studies. However, even in these cases diagnoses are not absolute.[19]

Both genetic and environmental factors also play into one's susceptibility to DILD, and there are many important avenues to take concerning DILD. These future ventures should include studies of the prevalence of liver ADRs, seeking specific markers and determining the role of the genetic and environmental factors that contribute to patient susceptibility.[20]

A discussion of toxic mechanisms and specific drug-related hepatotoxicity is also important. As contrasted to prescribing physicians, there may be little that the pharmacist can do to prevent that toxicity, other than to recognize patients at risk; understand the meanings and values of certain liver tests and interpretations; recommend to patients when and why liver-function testing is important; and inform the patient what drugs to avoid, why alcohol may make other drugs toxic, and so forth. Just as genetic susceptibility can influence the occurrence of DILD, genetic testing can be applied in drug development to identify the potential for DILDs.[21]

In general, there is no effective treatment against DILD except for stopping the drug and providing general supportive care. The efficient use of *N*-acetylcysteine subsequent to acetaminophen overdose and intravenous carnitine for valproate-induced mitochondrial injury are the exceptions. When a common drug is found to cause even rare hepatotoxicity, it may be removed from clinical use. Although such a drug poses a great danger to only a few patients, its removal leads to the loss of drug availability to many.[22]

For practicing physicians, drug-related hepatotoxicity is a liability risk; for the pharmaceutical industry, it leads to financial losses; and from a regulatory perspective, it is the most common reason for regulatory actions on the part of the Food and Drug Administration (FDA).[23] The US FDA and other regulatory agencies continue to report market withdrawals due to drug-induced liver injury.[24,25,26] The Swiss Pharmacovigilance Agency reported thatrisk of hepatotoxicity associated with Ulipristal.[27]

In a consensus report involving the criteria for detecting drug-induced liver disorders, the term "liver injury" was defined as the increase of greater than or equal to two times the upper limit of normal (ULN) alanine amino transferase (ALT) or conjugate bilirubin (CB). This is also the case for a combined increase in aspartate amino transferase (AST), alkaline phosphatase (ALP), or total bilirubin (TB).[28]

Levels of ALT that are greater than twice the ULN should be taken seriously, and therefore alternate drugs should be used. If there are no alternates, the physician may choose to challenge the patient diagnostically. Clinically, the approach to adverse hepatic reactions is to classify them as either dose-dependent (type I) or dose-independent (type II) (see Table 15.1). Type I usually involves patients who have ingested a sufficient amount of drugs, and Type II is a rare manifestation of therapeutic drug doses.[29]

Liver damage by nonnarcotic analgesics usually manifests into acute hepatitis with a degree of cholestasis. This is often indistinguishable from viral hepatitis and sometimes chronic active hepatitis. Acetaminophen (Tylenol) in overdose may cause acute hepatic necrosis which has the potential to progress to fulminant hepatic failure. Aside from the case of acetaminophen, the mechanisms behind nonnarcotic analgesic liver damage remain to be elucidated.[30]

TABLE 15.1
Examples of Drugs that in Typical Cases Lead to Hepatocellular, Mixed, Cholestatic, or Fatty Injury (See Text for Definition) in a Dose-Dependent (Type I) or Dose-Independent (Type II Manner).

Hepatocellular	Mixed	Cholestatic	Fatty
Type I			Amiadorone
Acetaminophen	Cyclosporine	Tetracycline	Corticosteroids
Methotrexate		Anabolic steroids	Tetracycline
Tetracycline			Valproic acid
Type II			
Allopurinol	Amitriptyline	Ajmaline	
Disulfiram	Captopril	Chlorpromazine	
Halothane	Carbamazepine	Erythromycin	
Enflurane/	Ibuprofen		
Isoniazid	Indomethacin		
Methyldopa	Nitrofurantoin		
Phenytoin	Oxyphenbutazone		
Pirprofen	Phenylbutazone		
Propylthiouracil	Ranitidine		
Salicylates	Sulfonamide		

15.3 OVERVIEW OF DILD, EPIDEMIOLOGY RISK FACTORS, HISTOPATHOLOGY, AND DIAGNOSES

The ability of a wide range of medications to cause DILD is well known to the medical community. Familiar examples include acetaminophen, methotrexate, and statins. The liver is the principal site of drug metabolism and detoxification in the body. Many medications pass through the liver and remain concentrated there, leading to local higher concentrations of potentially hepatotoxic medications. People are genetically diverse, which affects the way each of us metabolizes drugs and other chemicals. Liver toxicity of medication should be taken in the context of the increasing number of different medications available, the rising number of medications individual patients are concurrently taking, the complexity of drug–drug interactions, and the toxicity of drug metabolites.

DILD is a relatively uncommon, but severe, cause of idiosyncratic liver damage that requires special consideration as a safety problem. There are approximately 2,000 cases of acute liver failure each year in the United States, with medications accounting for perhaps 25–50% of these. Thirty-nine percent are due to acetaminophen, and 13% are idiosyncratic reactions due to other medications. DILD accounts for 2–5% of cases of patients hospitalized with jaundice, approximately 10% of all cases of acute hepatitis, and up to a quarter of all cases of chronic hepatitis. DILD has become the leading cause of acute liver failure among patients presenting for evaluation at liver-transplant centers in the United States, and the leading single cause for having to remove approved drugs from the market. In the United States, drug-related hepatotoxicity is now the leading cause of acute liver failure among liver transplants because of a drug overdose. Acetaminophen (paracetamol) is the most common drug in these cases, and the patients often have no prior history of liver disease.

15.3.1 Epidemiology of Drug Hepatotoxicity

There are over 1,100 medicinal agents, herbal remedies, illicit substances, and environmental agents that have been proven to cause DILD. About 10% of mild-to-moderate liver biochemistry alteration cases are caused by medicinal agents.[31] In patients who are older than 50 years of age, this number is increased to 40%. In patients with drug-induced hepatitis including jaundice, the risk for fulminant hepatic injury is 20%, while the risk for patients with acute viral hepatitis and jaundice is 1%. Also, a risk of sub-fulminant hepatic injury is 70% for patients with drug-induced hepatitis with encephalopathy.[32] Approximately 10–15% of patients with end-stage liver failure drug-related. Additionally, reporting systems indicate the relative severity of drug hepatotoxicity. Epidemiological studies show that hepatotoxic reactions are between 1 in 600 and 1 in 3,500, which is 2–3% of all hospital admissions due to adverse drug reactions.[33]

15.3.2 Risk Factors

15.3.2.1 Acquired Factors

- Chronic alcohol intake increases the severity of acetaminophen hepatotoxicity. This is caused by mechanisms involving the induction of Phase I liver enzymes such as CYP2E which generates the toxic metabolite N-acetyl-p-quinone imine (NAPQI) from acetaminophen. Glutathione acts as an antioxidant or electrophilic scavenger. Due to glutathione depletion, the liver has a lower resistance to the toxic metabolites. Alcoholism also potentiates the methotrexate toxicity. Alcohol favors CYP2E1 metabolism, which increases the production of NAPQI, a toxic metabolite responsible for hepatocyte death. Chronic alcoholism, through malnourishment, may decrease the amount of glutathione (GSH), which inactivates NAPQI, and spares liver cells. When the substrate is diminished, hepatocyte death increases. A thorough alcohol use history should always be taken when evaluating possible DILD, and consideration should be given to the wisdom of treating some causes of liver disease (e.g. Hepatitis B or C) if alcohol use/abuse is ongoing.
- Drug–drug interactions can play a role in hepatotoxicity. Enzyme increases can lead to the formation of toxic metabolites from one of the two drugs taken together. For example, the rifampin–isoniazid combination results in the facilitation of isoniazid biotransformation into toxic molecules. Similarly, enzyme induction by a drug such as phenobarbital can cause liver toxicity to antidepressant drugs. Enzyme inhibition by drugs can also impact hepatotoxicity. For example, in the case of troleandomycin–estrogen drug–drug interaction, estrogen metabolism is inhibited by the blockade of CYP3A4 causing an accumulation of estrogen and resultant cholestatic effects (troleandomycin is no longer sold in the United States; it is only sold in Turkey).[34]
- Extrahepatic disease also plays a role in drug-induced liver toxicity. For example, hyperthyroidism causes halothane hepatitis, and HIV (human immunodeficiency virus) increases the risk of adverse reactions such as co-trimoxazole hepatotoxicity. Other liver diseases might influence the hepatotoxicity of drugs such as antiretrovirals and methotrexate. Antiretrovirals also can worsen dormant chronic hepatitis B and C by destabilizing or adversely modifying the immune system.[35] Coinfection of HIV with Hepatitis B or C can leave patients at an increased risk for hepatotoxic effects when treated with antiretroviral therapy. However, data on whether HAART (highly active antiretroviral therapy) can prevent or cause lung injury in HIV-Hepatitis C coinfected patients is conflicting.[36] Patients with cirrhosis have a poor tolerance for hepatotoxic drugs. Patients with HIV can experience drug-related hepatotoxicity from HAART treatment. Up to 90% of HIV patients receive a drug which is hepatotoxic. Additionally, one of the newer and most effective individual treatments which have been incorporated into the HAART cocktail are protease inhibitors, and there is emerging evidence that these carry significant hepatotoxicity.[37,38,39] Direct HAART-related hepatotoxicity events include hypersensitivity reactions and lactic acidosis.[40] In addition to direct drug toxicity, mechanisms can include HIV viral hepatitis, coinfection with Hepatitis B or C, and insulin resistance from HAART medications contributing to the development of steatohepatitis.[41] Additionally, alcohol abuse afflicts a quarter of recently diagnosed HIV patients, and the combination of alcohol and HAART may further injure the liver in comparison to HAART alone.[42] The hepatitis C infection treatments Viekira Pak (AbbVie) and Technivie (AbbVie) increased the risk for serious liver injury, particularly in those with underlying advanced liver disease. As a result of the extensive liver injury associated with both these therapies, both drugs were discontinued in 2018.[43]

15.3.3 Histopathology

DILD does not usually present with a characteristic histopathologic picture, regardless of the causative medication. Although there are a number of distinctive pathologic categories of DILD,[44] rarely it is possible to diagnose DILD from the histopathologic pattern, although causes sometimes can be ruled out. DILD can present with one of several pathologic categories:

1) Impaired liver function
2) Acute hepatocyte necrosis
3) Fatty liver
4) Granulomatous change

5) Acute cholestasis
6) Cholestatic type
7) Chronic parenchymal injury
8) Vascular change
9) Liver tumor

In the presence of suspected DILD, the pathologic picture may help confirm the diagnosis. Knowing the distinctive pathologic category may or may not help in identifying a cause of liver disease, in that one drug can present with different pathologic states, and no pathologic picture seems to be pathognomic for a particular drug or toxin.

It is clear that cirrhosis can follow a number of insults produced by drug intake. The drugs involved are those that lead to types of liver disease that in other circumstances also may progress to cirrhosis. Cirrhosis may be the end result of the prolonged administration of drugs that presumably act as direct toxins, such as methotrexate and isoniazid, or those that may be mediated by hypersensitivity, such as oxyphenisatin and methyldopa.[45] As a result of the liver toxicity risk, oxyphenisatin was ordered to be removed from all over-the-counter laxatives (https://www.ecfr.gov/current/title-21/chapter-I/subchapter-D/part-330/subpart-B/section-330.12). Cirrhosis is most commonly caused by chronic, excessive alcohol use/abuse.

15.3.4 Diagnosis

Drug-induced liver dysfunction is diagnosed by the detection of anomalies in the liver enzymes or by the emergence of hepatitis-like symptoms. End-stage liver failure is usually the first appearance of acute liver injury. Patients might display symptoms such as pruritus, coagulopathy, or malabsorption of vitamins A, D, E, and K. Malnutrition also may contribute to liver dysfunction.[46]

Absolute diagnosis of DILD is usually determined by the deduction of possible causes, onset of action, the state of the symptoms after stopping the drug, and comparison with other reported cases. Liver biopsy can be helpful; however, even this mechanism of diagnosis can fail in determining specifically drug-induced liver dysfunction.[47]

To assess the causality of DILD, there are a number of methods one can employ using factors such as:

- The timeline of drug administration including the time between the beginning treatment and end treatment; onset of drug action
- The effects of stopping or continuing a drug and the role of drug and disease in the etiology when this happened
- Patient response to the drug readministration/rechallenge
- Lab test results
- Background knowledge of drug toxicity

The main purpose of determining causality is to use quantitative lab results to determine the likelihood of liver toxicity.[48] It is also important to know what happens when a drug is stopped or taken in combination with other drugs. It is the responsibility of the physician and pharmacist to keep up to date with new additions to the known hepatotoxic drug list.[49] Determining the cause of drug-induced hepatic injury becomes closely definitive once the aforementioned parameters are investigated and applied to specific patients' cases. In rare circumstances, the cause of liver injury may only be *probable* or *highly probable*.[50] For example, this is true in cases of drug overdose with acetaminophen, relapse after accidental carbamazepine readministration, and drug hepatitis in relation to iproniazid.[51]

More commonly, diagnoses of the cause of liver injury are considered *possible*. In these cases, the liver injury has no distinct features, the timeline hints at the problem, and some general causes of liver injury have been excluded. Far too often, the diagnosis of the cause of liver injury is *doubtful* or *unlikely*. This means that there are no specific features of hepatic injury, and significant pieces of evidence involving timeline are not present. The degree of end-stage hepatic injury needs to be quantified to assess hepatic recovery following either liver transplantation or drug cessation due to poor outcome.[52]

An *excluded* diagnosis is evident when another cause has been established such as a viral infection or when the timeline of hepatic injury does not match up with drug administration. This is the case when the symptoms are present before the drug administration or if there is a delay of symptoms greater than 15 days after the end of treatment. Some exceptions to this include hepatitis caused by halothane, of which reactions can take place several weeks after the first exposure.[53]

Being able to recognize the development of hepatic injury is integral to the prevention of chronic perpetuation of cholestasis or other liver dysfunction. Efficient recognition and withdrawal of the drug will also prevent unnecessary damage-control measures. There are some drugs that do not show the true effects until much later, however. In the case of amoxacillin-clavulante acid, the onset of liver disease may emerge weeks after the interval of therapeutic administration. Also, recovery after drug withdrawal may take months (three or more) and, in certain circumstances, may never come, for example, with progression of vanishing bile duct syndrome (VBDS).[35]

One novel method under development for diagnosis of DILD is evaluating the profile of non-coding RNAs called micro-RNAs (miRNAs).[54,55,56] MiRNAs may be released from injured cells into the blood in vacuoles in which they are relatively stable, and thus they may be used as biomarkers. Elevation or downregulation of these biomarkers may indicate DILD; assays to measure these biomarkers are noninvasive, unlike current biopsy methods.

15.4 HEPATIC DRUG METABOLISM

Human metabolism must deal with a variety of substances that, in excess, can cause diseases. Most of the liver's detoxification is performed on substances that are fat soluble, including drugs, certain vitamins, carcinogens, pesticides, and other environmental pollutants. Many endogenous chemicals, such as fatty acids, prostaglandins, and sex hormones, are also fat soluble and are metabolized by the liver. The duration of the physiological or toxicological action of these lipophilic substances depends on how long they reside intact in the liver. Other substances that are not fat soluble are also metabolized by the liver after a conversion reaction that renders the chemicals into a fat-soluble state on which the liver can act. The cytochrome P450 (CYP450) system of enzymes is the primary enzyme system for the metabolism of drugs. Hepatic microsomal P450s are the mixed function oxidases (MFOs) that activate oxygen for incorporation into lipophilic substrates. Oxidized substrates are then either eliminated from the body or are metabolized further by allied hepatic enzyme system.

This is the collective term for the family of hemoproteins that is found in the hepatic endoplasmic reticulum. Each individual P450 exhibits a characteristic range of turnover numbers with specific substrates.[57] Several hundred isoenzymes of CYP450 have been identified, and this is a very active area of research with significant relevance to drug metabolism.

The drugs that are currently known to cause serious DILD generally are widely prescribed and have a high margin of safety. They include agents such as NSAIDs, antibiotics, anticonvulsants, newer antihypertensive drugs, H_2 Receptor blockers, and psychotropic agents. For these types of drugs, the absolute incidence is in the order of one adverse hepatic drug reaction per 100,000 person years of exposure. Because of the very large number of prescriptions filled for these medications, they are among the most common causes of DILD. Acetaminophen continues to be a drug with widespread prescription and OTC use; however, acetaminophen presents its own set of challenges to the toxicological community. Dose-related toxicity can lead to fatal hepatic failure, and the drug continues to be widely used in suicide attempts. Even when given at normal doses, acetaminophen can still cause hepatotoxicity.

15.5 FDA AND DILD

FDA approval does not ensure that a drug is not hepatotoxic, or that DILD will not occur. Registration trials for pharmaceuticals focus on efficacy. Safety is a secondary endpoint. Study sample sizes are typically small, and if the incidence of DILD is low, then it may not become apparent until post-licensure, which is often collected by spontaneously reported post-marketing data. Some drugs in current or recent use, including many familiar examples, but certainly not all drugs capable of causing DILD, have been discussed in this review. The FDA has taken a number of well-publicized actions concerning hepatotoxic medications in recent years, including the strengthening of warnings, restrictions on use, and the removal from marketing. Examples include glimepiride, interferon beta 1a, trimethoprim sulfamethoxazone, pemoline, bromfenac, duloxetine, felbamate, kava kava, troglitazone, tolcapone, trovafloxacin, and zileuton. Additionally, Rezulin was removed from marketing due to hepatotoxicity.

15.6 TYPES OF LIVER INJURY

15.6.1 Hepatitis

The entire spectrum of liver injury seen in conjunction with viral hepatitis, both morphological and clinical, can also result from drug administration. Hepatic reactions are unpredictable with few exceptions. In contrast to drug-induced cholestasis, which is relatively common and benign, hepatitic (inflammatory) reactions are uncommon and have significant mortality.[58,59]

15.6.2 Massive Hepatic Necrosis (Fulminant Hepatitis)

Massive hepatic necrosis is a rare complication of viral hepatitis that involves the destruction of the entire liver lobule. This form of injury can be accurately mimicked by drugs such as halothane, iproniazid, and isoniazid. When exposed to these agents, hepatocytes within entire hepatic lobules appear to progress through coagulative necrosis. The lesion may begin in the central zones of the lobule and progress to include the entire lobule.[60]

Both the clinical and morphological sides of liver disease can be generated by a number of drugs, many of which can produce massive hepatic necrosis. Some of these drugs include halothane, isoniazid, phenytoin, phenelzine, sertraline, naproxen, diclofenac, kava kava, or ecstasy, and iproniazid. The presence of eosinophilia may be indicative of drug-induced hepatitis; however, this only occurs in less than half the patients. Upon drug cessation, patients generally recover; however, a second exposure might manifest massive liver necrosis.[61]

15.6.3 Drug-Induced Vanishing Bile Duct Syndrome

15.6.3.1 Case Report

A 37-year-old black woman (Ms. W) presented with difficult-to-control diabetes (DM), hypertension, chronic skin abscesses, and morbid obesity. She received trimethoprim/sulfamethoxazole (TMP-SMZ) for the control of her skin abscesses at admission and continued for 30 days post-discharge. She then presented to the hospital for a urinary tract infection and was prescribed antibiotics. Metformin and glimepiride were also added at the time of her hospital discharge, as parenteral insulin was poorly controlling her DM. Soon after, Ms. W developed a cholestatic drug reaction which then progressed to end-stage liver disease (ESLD) that contained the histologic features of vanishing bile duct syndrome (VBDS).

Ms. W's clinical course was characteristic for medication-induced cholestatic liver disease. In general, a slow

TABLE 15.2
Drugs in Current Use that have been Reported in Association with the VBDS[66]

Amoxicillin-clavulanic acid	Estradiol, Norandrostenolone
Ampicillin	Flucloxacillin, Dicloxacillin
Amitryptiline	Imipramine Glycyrrhizin
Azathiopurine	Haloperidol
Barbiturates	Ibuprofen
Carbamezipine	Phenytoin D-penicillamine
Chlorthiazide	Prochlorperazine
Co-trimoxazole	Tetracycline
Clindamycin	Terbinafine
Chlorpromazine	Thiabendazole
Cimetidine	Tiopronin
Cyproheptadine	Tolbutamide
Erythromycin esters	Methyl testosterone

resolution should occur following the discontinuation of the drug. She unfortunately did not recover as expected; the presence of VBDS was identified, leading to a liver transplant.[62] The patient's workup seemed to indicate a hepatocellular mechanism for liver jaundice, as the cause was attributed to be drug-induced. Before the clinical manifestation of the symptoms, she was started on both TMP-SMZ and glimepiride around the same time. Both drugs have been associated with cholestatic jaundice. VBDS is a considered a rare disorder, impacting the intra-hepatic bile ducts. Most patients are asymptomatic, and those who do show symptoms rarely present with jaundice. The alkaline phosphatase level is typically elevated along with GGT (may exceed 600 IU/L). Upon physical examination, pathological features like frontal bossing, triangular facies, butterfly vertebrae, and posterior embryotoxon of the eye may be noted, but none of these findings were observed in this patient. VBDS has been reported in association with the use of chlorpromazine, flucloxacillin, amitriptyline, and TMP-SMZ (Table 15.2). Both TMP-SMZ and glimepiride were temporally associated with the timing of onset for Ms. W's cholestatic jaundice. TMP-SMZ, but not glimepiride, has been reported to be causally related to VBDS. The development of cholestatic jaundice and subsequent VBDS following TMP-SMZ was determined to be probably causative.[63]

Ms. W presented with medication-induced cholestatic jaundice which progressed to VBDS. Although the initial workup and biochemical markers pointed to an obstructive etiology, the cholestatis was drug-induced (TMP-SMZ). Prescribing physicians should always consider the potential for medication-induced liver disease when liver enzymes become abnormal, and immediate withdrawal is necessary for any potentially offending agents if possible.[64]

The clinical and biochemical characteristics of VBDS are similar to that of PBC (primary biliary cirrhosis); however, anti-mitochondrial antibodies that are present in PBC are not detectable in VBDS. The pathological progression of this condition is not known. Potential mechanisms include immune-mediated bile duct damage indicated by the presence of white blood cells and Stevens–Johnson syndrome in some circumstances. Another mechanism includes the presence of toxicity from secondary bile acid retention.[65]

15.7 SPECIFIC DILD PRODUCT AREAS AND CASE DISCUSSIONS

Case reports have appeared of hepatotoxicity by acetaminophen, NSAID use and hepatotoxicity, isoniazid-induced hepatotoxicity, and methotrexate-induced hepatotoxicity.

Several mechanisms of drug-induced toxicity have been discussed, most of which demonstrate different toxic mechanisms, involve special age groups, and may have resulted in removal or threats of removal of drugs from the market. This is certainly demonstrative of the serious nature of drug-induced liver toxicity. Many case series of DILD have involved litigation following some serious injury or fatality related to a drug exposure.

15.7.1 Nonsteroidal Anti-Inflammatory Drugs (NSAIDs) Use and Hepatoxicity

The class termed nonsteroidal anti-inflammatory drugs (NSAIDs) includes anthranilic and arylalkanoic acid derivatives. Serious forms of hepatotoxicity are not currently a common problem with this group of drugs, but drugs such as ibufenac and benoxaprofen had to be withdrawn for this reason. Literature reports of the extent of use and patterns of clinical, biochemical, and pathological anomalies have shown that analgesics of this class seem to have a greater chance of hepatotoxicity; however, liver damage is not a dominant feature of acute NSAID overdosage.[67] NSAIDs have been associated with rare adverse reactions in the liver, including fulminant hepatitis and cholestasis.[68] These reactions are idiosyncratic, mostly independent of the dose administered, and are host dependent. Among the NSAIDs (which excludes acetaminophen), a rank order of relative risk cannot be established, and the incidence in relation to use is not known.[69]

NSAIDs have anti-inflammatory effects along with the inhibition of cyclooxygenase and therefore prostaglandin formation. These drugs are heterogenous when it comes to adverse effects on the liver. A few NSAIDs are thought to cause drug-induced hepatitis, and nearly all NSAIDs are implicated in case-reported liver disease. The risk for NSAID users who also are in contact with other potential hepatotoxic drugs has been shown to be much greater than from additively combining the risks for NSAID and other drug exposure individually, suggesting a synergistic toxicity of combining NSAIDs with other hepatotoxic drugs.[70]

Idiosyncratic hepatotoxic injury is a major clinical concern because a prediction cannot be made based upon preclinical safety studies and because the reactions are host-dependent. Even though the incidence of such injury is low, the resulting injury can be quite significant, sometimes resulting in fulminant liver failure.[71] An emphasis is placed on using minimal analgesic, rather than anti-inflammatory, doses of short-acting NSAIDs and, where possible, avoiding their use in high-risk patients.[72]

15.7.1.1 Diclofenac

The nature of diclofenac-related liver injury is idiosyncratic based on the varying onset of injury after long periods of drug administration. Delayed recurrence of injury after readministration of the drug indicates that metabolic abnormalities may be at play. This postulation is supported by the lack of fever, rash, or eosinophilia in most reported cases. Of the marketed NSAIDs, diclofenac has been identified to have a greater potential for hepatotoxicity.

15.7.1.2 Naproxen

Naproxen has been the culprit in a few cases of liver injury. Hepatocellular jaundice, fulminant hepatic failure, cholestatic jaundice, and indeterminate jaundice have been associated with naproxen.[73]

15.7.1.3 Other NSAIDs

15.7.1.3.1 Sulindac

Sulindac was selected for a study because several hundred cases of hepatic injury which had been reported to the FDA's Adverse Reaction Voluntary Reporting System between 1978 and 1986 had a large number associated with sulindac.[74] The resulting report contained analysis of clinical, biochemical, and histological characteristics of hepatic injury and postulates mechanisms of liver injury.[75]

From 338 reports that were submitted to the FDA, 247 were inadequate or ambiguous for sulindac toxicity. A total of 91 cases of drug reaction were analyzed, and 15 have histological data available. The results of this study indicated four deaths—three with severe hypersensitivity and one with fulminant hepatic failure. Two-thirds had hypersensitivity reactions. Female-to-male ratio was 3.5 to 1; 69% of the patients were over 50 years of age. A total of 67% of patients had jaundice, 43% had cholestasis, and 25% had hepatocellular injury. Eosinophilia was more frequent in patients with cholestatic injury (40%) than in those with cholestasis.

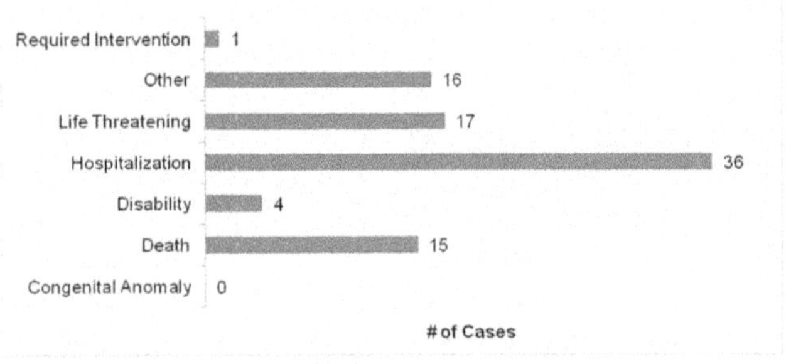

FIGURE 15.1 Sulindac Adverse Event Outcomes.

Source: Distribution of reported patient outcomes within the FDA Adverse Event Reporting System where liver injury is co-reported with sulindac as a suspect medication.

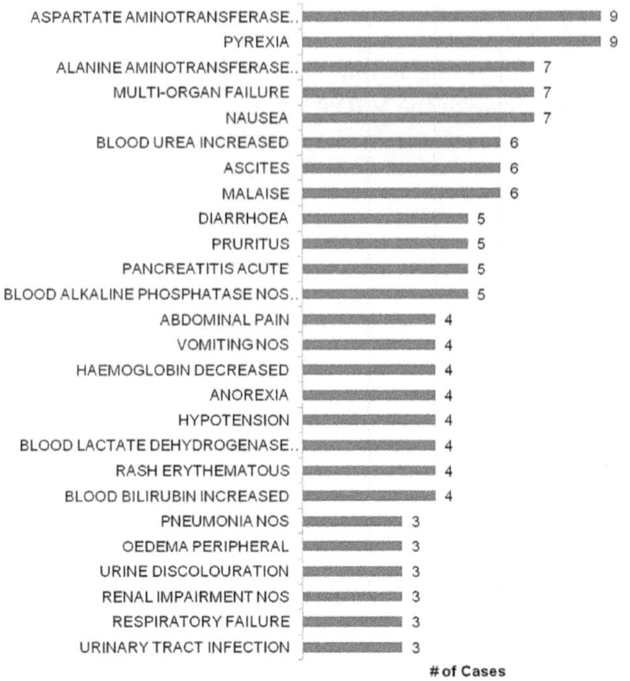

FIGURE 15.2 Top 25 adverse reactions co-reported with liver injury when sulindac is a suspect medication.

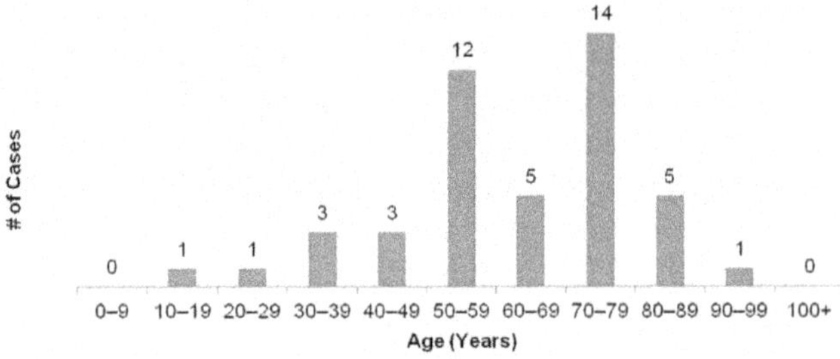

FIGURE 15.3 Age distribution of patients within the FDA AERS where liver injury is co-reported with sulindac as a suspect medication.

15.7.2 Isoniazid-Induced Hepatotoxicity

INH (isoniazid—isonicotinic acid hydrazide) is an important hepatotoxin, especially with the resurgence of tuberculosis. and the public health clinics' protocols for prophylactic use in exposed persons. Close monitoring of patients for liver enzyme elevations and signs of fatigue and jaundice can detect liver toxicities and save the patient from developing an end-stage liver disease.

When isoniazid was introduced in 1952, it represented a major advance in the treatment of tuberculosis. It has remained the mainstay of anti-tuberculous chemotherapy. Isoniazid is potent, bactericidal, and has good clinical efficacy. In addition, it is inexpensive and can be administered orally. Initially, isoniazid was thought to have a low incidence of side effects. This apparent safety, together with the high level of patient acceptability, led to isoniazid becoming extremely popular during the 1960s. This included its use as a chemo-prophylactic agent for tuberculin-reactive individuals, such as household contacts of patients with recently diagnosed tuberculosis, who were thought to be at heightened risk of active tuberculosis.

Studies from the USPHS and others showed that between 10% and 36% of patients have asymptomatic elevations of ALT levels during isoniazid therapy. In most patients, these abnormalities occur within ten weeks, are relatively minor, and resolve spontaneously. They are often associated with trivial histological changes in the liver. The frequency of clinically significant hepatotoxicity is about 1% of all patients exposed. There is, however, a striking age dependence, with isoniazid hepatitis being rare in childhood and occurring in more than 2% of adults over the age of 50. Several observations indicate that the longer the period of isoniazid treatment prior to the recognition of hepatotoxicity, the more severe the liver injury at the time of diagnosis. Isoniazid hepatitis appears to be more severe in African American women, in alcoholics, and in those treated with combined therapy with rifampicin.

Deaths still occur from isoniazid-induced liver injury. Most, if not all, deaths due to isoniazid-induced liver injury could be prevented by the immediate interruption of isoniazid treatment at the onset of the first symptoms of hepatotoxicity. The role of monitoring liver enzymes during the first three months of isoniazid therapy is less clear, although it may indirectly serve a useful function by keeping the specter of dangerous hepatotoxicity in the minds of prescribers and recipients of isoniazid. A 2020 article notes the continuing problem of increased risk of hepatotoxicity and temporary drug withdrawal during treatment of active tuberculosis in pregnant women.[76]

Isoniazid-induced hepatotoxicity is an idiosyncratic form of drug-induced liver injury. It is independent of the total or incremental dose of isoniazid, and several studies have shown no relationship with isoniazid blood levels. Drug allergy is unlikely to be involved. Thus, the onset of the reaction tends to be later than the usual interval for drug-induced allergic reactions (fever, rash, arthralgia, and eosinophilia are uncommon), and drug-induced antibodies or autoantibodies have not been found.[77]

An examination of the FDA's Adverse Event Reporting System suggests that liver injury is strongly associated with isoniazid-related adverse reactions. Specifically, 35% of the 1,925 adverse event cases where isoniazid is reported as a suspect medication report some form of hepatic injury (677 cases). Figure 15.4 shows that both males and females are roughly equally affected by isoniazid-related liver injury. In contrast to gender, patient age appears to play a role in the seriousness of isoniazid-related liver injury, as serious patient outcomes, such as death, are skewed toward more elderly patients (Figure 15.5). As noted before, isoniazid cases that report hepatitis as an adverse reaction are somewhat rare in children, with only 2.4% of isoniazid-hepatitis cases coming from patients aged ten years or less. Also, as

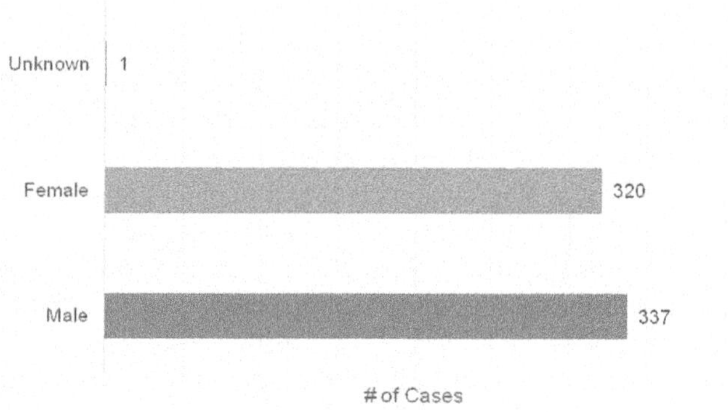

FIGURE 15.4 Distribution of patient gender within the FDA Adverse Event Reporting System where liver injury is co-reported with isoniazid as a suspect medication.

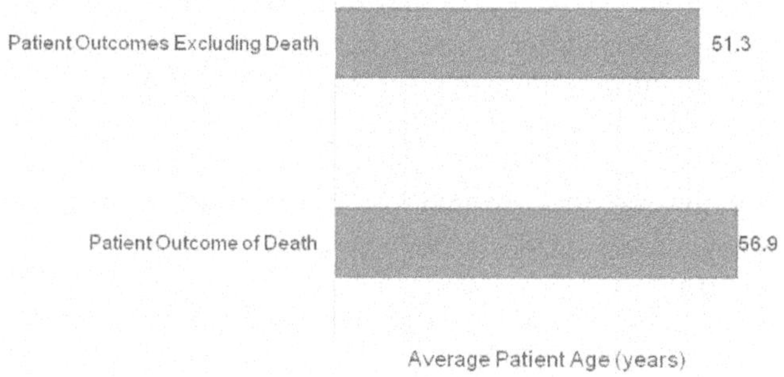

FIGURE 15.5 Comparison of the average age of patients in isoniazid-related liver-injury adverse event cases as a function of whether death is reported as a patient outcome.

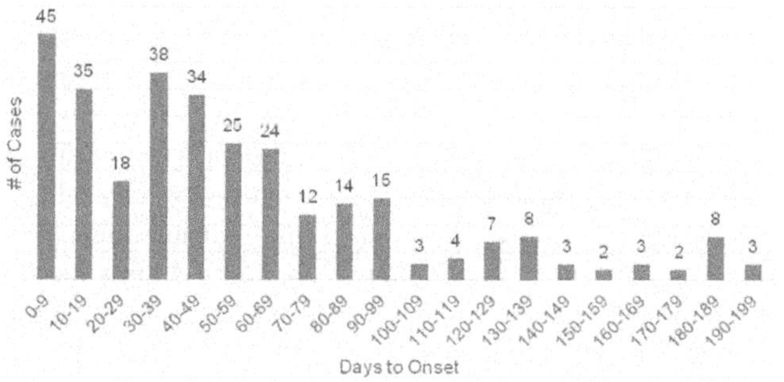

FIGURE 15.6 Distribution of number of days to the onset of liver-injury-related adverse reactions after the commencement of isoniazid therapy.

noted earlier, the time to onset of isoniazid-related adverse reactions can occur months after initial treatment with isoniazid (Figure 15.6). A recent (2021) review documents the continued evaluation of isoniazid as a necessary drug with hepatotoxicity.[78]

15.7.3 Acetaminophen

Acetaminophen, also called paracetamol, is one of the most common pain-relieving over-the-counter drug used and offered in workplaces, schools, and other institutions.

Acetaminophen may not be considered a "real drug" by patients, and a patient may not include it in their drug history reported to hospitals and doctor's offices. Acetaminophen is a well-accepted dose-related hepatotoxic drug and can also possibly cause liver injury even at therapeutic doses.[79] Importantly, acetaminophen is the most common cause of DILD in the United States and United Kingdom.[80]

Acetaminophen differs from NSAIDs in that it is not anti-inflammatory. Although considered relatively non-toxic and taken by as many as 100 million Americans each year, a number of acetaminophen-related liver injuries and deaths are reported every year to poison control centers. These include cases of accidental overdose.

A person's nutritional state can exert a major influence on his or her capacity to metabolize and eliminate drugs and foreign compounds. Chronic alcohol abuse or malnutrition and starvation may lead to a deficiency of glutathione, a substrate necessary for inactivating hepatic toxic substances. In addition to reducing hepatic glutathione, fasting can enhance the activity of P450 2E1 (CYP2E1), which means acetaminophen is converted to its toxic metabolite at a faster rate. The extent to which each of these factors contributes to the increased risk of acetaminophen-induced hepatotoxicity among alcoholics remains unclear.

An important patient variable that influences potential acetaminophen toxicity is the nutritional state—whether a patient has been eating a normal diet or fasting. Several reports have implicated fasting as a factor that enhances the prospect of hepatotoxicity associated with therapeutic doses of acetaminophen. Yet, it is reasonable to expect that an individual who takes acetaminophen for symptoms of a cold, for example, or for other minor illness may not be hungry. That person's decreased food and fluid intake could therefore potentially exacerbate acetaminophen toxicity.

Consider also that nausea is one of the early symptoms of acetaminophen-induced toxicity. Patients who feel nauseated typically stop eating and drinking—further enhancing the very reason that made them stop eating and drinking: Acetaminophen toxicity. This would further exacerbate the acetaminophen toxicity.

Acetaminophen is mostly converted in the liver to inactive compounds by conjugation with sulfate and glucuronide, with a small portion being metabolized via the cytochrome P450 enzyme system. The cytochrome P450 system oxidizes acetaminophen to produce a highly reactive intermediary metabolite, N-acetyl-p-benzo-quinone imine (NAPQI). Under normal conditions, NAPQI is detoxified in the liver by conjugation with glutathione.[81] This mechanism continues to be recognized as the cause of acetaminophen liver toxicity.[82]

There has been a prevalence of increased susceptibility to acetaminophen-induced liver injury in patients who are taking drugs that increase CYP450 hepatic enzymes or are ingesting large quantities of alcohol. In this scenario, even common therapeutic levels of acetaminophen can cause hepatotoxicity.[83]

15.7.3.1 Acetaminophen Toxicity Assessment Nomograms

The Rumack Matthew Nomogram is commonly used to access risk of liver injury from acetaminophen toxicity and is based on time passed since ingestion of the acetaminophen and the plasma level of acetaminophen. As described in the literature, the clinical course after a toxic ingestion follows four stages.

- Stage 1 occurs 12–24 hours post ingestion. Symptoms present include nausea, vomiting, diaphoresis, and anorexia. Children frequently have episodes of vomiting even without toxic levels. Those patients with plasma levels in the toxic range have a mean onset of symptoms by six hours, with 100% showing symptoms by 14 hours. Laboratory studies (liver enzymes as a measure of liver inflammation, clotting time as a measure of hepatic synthetic capacity) are typically normal during this time.
- Stage 2 occurs 24–48 hours post ingestion. By that time, symptoms have decreased, but laboratory abnormalities begin to appear with a rise of liver enzymes (AST and ALT), bilirubin, and prothrombin time.
- Stage 3 occurs between 48 and 96 hours post-ingestion when the peak abnormalities are seen. AST levels as high as 30,000 may be seen, with the definition of hepatotoxicity related to acetaminophen being accepted as AST levels in excess of 1,000. Well under 1% of patients in Stage 3 will develop fulminant hepatotoxicity.
- Stage 4 occurs during the first week after ingestion with hepatic abnormalities returning to near normal by seven or eight days.

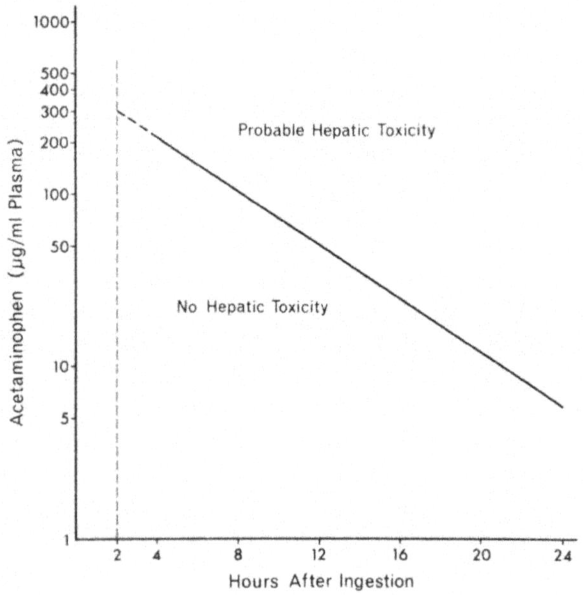

FIGURE 15.7 Acetaminophen Hepatic Toxicity Nomogram.

Early therapeutic intervention is crucial. A number of unfortunate persons with acetaminophen toxicity do not have their symptoms immediately recognized and do not receive appropriate therapy for a number of days.

The warnings present on products containing acetaminophen may include:

> "Alcohol—If you consume 3 or more alcoholic drinks every day, ask your doctor if you should take acetaminophen or other pain reliever/fever reducers."

15.7.3.2 FDA Report—Acetaminophen-Induced Liver Disease

A 2017 FDA guidance acknowledged that acetaminophen is one of the most commonly used medications for treating pain and fever. It states that it is also combined with over-the-counter medicines (often for cold and flu), as well as with the most prescribed drug, such as hydrocodone/acetaminophen. It then identified acetaminophen as the largest cause of acute liver failure in the United States. The report states that in 2005, there were more than 28 billion doses of acetaminophen-containing products purchased by U.S. consumers, who tend to view it as a benign, *safe medication—one that does not cause the gastrointestinal symptoms associated with nonsteroidal anti-inflammatories, such as ibuprofen.*

15.7.3.3 Move of FDA toward Revised Labeling

In the interests of safe and reliable use, FDA published the following notices and recommendations regarding acetaminophen in 2017:[84]

- All manufacturers of prescription combination drug products with more than 325 mg of acetaminophen to discontinue marketing
- FDA drug safety communication: Prescription acetaminophen products to be limited to 325 mg per dosage unit; boxed warning will highlight the potential for severe liver failure
- Federal register notice: Prescription drug products containing acetaminophen; actions to reduce liver injury from unintentional overdose

15.7.3.4 Assessment of Safety After Labeling Changes

The FDA-recommended organ-specific (liver) warnings on acetaminophen labels to heighten public caution in usage of this drug appear to have increased the safety of the public's acetaminophen usage. One study showed that these organ-specific labels enhanced acetaminophen risk perception, though morbidity/mortality was not documented.[85] As acetaminophen is present in many different drugs, another source of danger results from the patient not appreciating the danger of overdose due to combining different acetaminophen-containing drugs. This was attributed to inadequate and variable acetaminophen labeling.[86]

15.7.3.5 Acetaminophen FDA MedWatch Reports

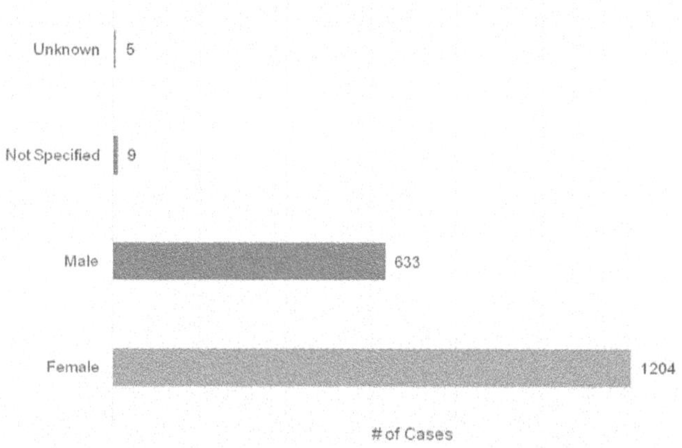

FIGURE 15.8 Distribution of patient gender within the FDA Adverse Event Reporting System Cases where liver injury is co-reported with isoniazid as a suspect medication.

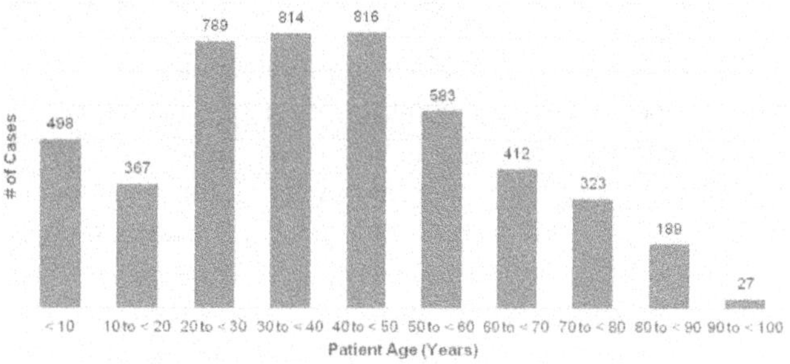

FIGURE 15.9 Distribution of patient ages in adverse event cases where liver injury is co-reported with acetaminophen, and acetaminophen is considered a suspect medication.

Source: Data obtained from the US Food & Drug Administration's Adverse Event Reporting System.

15.7.4 Macrolide Hepatotoxicity

Macrolide-induced hepatotoxicity is characterized by cholestatic hepatitis. The best example of this is erythromycin estolate. The onset of this form of DILD is 2 to 25 days after macrolide exposure. The clinical symptoms include anorexia, nausea, vomiting, and significant right upper quadrant pain. Jaundice also occurs in 50% of patients. Liver biopsies demonstrate that cholestasis with plethora of white blood cells in the portal inflammatory infiltrate. Newer macrolide antibiotics have caused cholestatic jaundice. Examples include roxithromycin, charithromycin, and azithromycin.[87]

15.7.4.1 Biaxin (Clarithromycin)-Induced Fulminant Hepatic Failure and Death

Clarithromycin, along with many other macrolide antibiotics, has the capacity to cause liver cholestasis; however, more uncommonly is hepatocellular injury. In less than 1% of patients, there is an elevation of AST, ALT, bilirubin, and alkaline phosphatase. Animal studies have indicated that large doses of clarithromycin can cause reversible liver dysfunction; however, in humans, there has been no dose relation with hepatotoxicity. Hepatic necrosis is even more rare when associated with macrolide erythromycin.[88]

A published article by Wallace et al.[89] and publications that followed warned about high-dose risk in the elderly and suggested caution. A December 1995 FDA Advisory Committee recommendation for a 1,500-mg/day dosage of Biaxin for the treatment of H. pylori would predictably increase the use of Biaxin.

An FDA Anti-Infective Drug and Gastrointestinal Drugs Advisory committee recommendation was as follows:

> [A] combination therapy of the anti-secretory medication Prilosec and the antibiotic Biaxin be approved for the treatment of Helicobacter pylori (H. pylori) infected patients with active duodenal ulcer to eradicate H. pylori, the bacteria now believed to cause approximately 89% of peptic ulcers. . . . The recommended dosage of eradicating H. pylori is Prilosec 40 mg once daily and Biaxin 500 mg three times daily for the first 14 days.

This FDA Advisory Committee recommendation would predictably increase the use and the dosage of clarithromycin.

The authors recommend "reductions in doses may be required in patients with reduced renal function and/or reduced body mass to prevent hepatic or gastrointestinal toxicity." The elderly fall in both of these categories as a result of their elevated age (normal aging process reduces lean body mass and deceases renal function as a function of age).

Central zonal necrosis is an imminent liver toxic sign, usually associated with a few drugs acting like liver toxins (i.e., acetaminophen). Clarithromycin was the only drug being taken by the patient discussed in this case at the time of his fatal liver toxicity that had central zonal necrosis associated with its use.

Conventional knowledge describes macrolide toxicities, including clarithromycin, to be associated with occasional abnormalities in liver tests and occasional cholestatic jaundice, considered idiosyncratic, and therefore not dose related. Most are described as mild and transient. Shaheen and Grimm[90] described a 25-year-old man who developed fulminant hepatic failure following clarithromycin use; he subsequently required liver transplantation. The authors wrote, "the potential for severe liver injury associated with clarithromycin is of growing concern in the light of recent reports to the FDA. We believe that this case, although not proof of causation, supports a true association."

The Food and Drug Administration's AERS database includes 878 reported cases of liver toxicity where clarithromycin is considered a suspect, including 20 cases where pancreatitis is also reported. Figure 15.10 shows the age distribution of patients reporting clarithromycin-related liver injury cases, with an average patient age of 54.5 years.

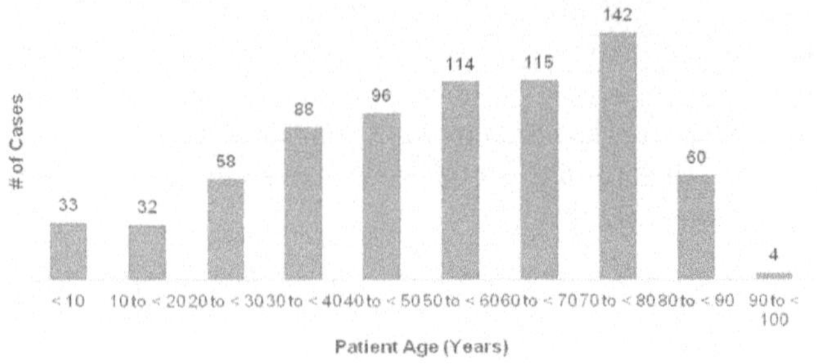

FIGURE 15.10 Distribution of patient ages in adverse event cases where liver injury is co-reported, and clarithromycin is considered a suspect medication.

15.7.5 Methotrexate (MTX) Hepatotoxicity

Methotrexate hepatotoxicity in psoriatic patients is well established; however, there are differences in the incidences and risks for hepatotoxicity.[91] A study on 104 patients in Nova Scotia was performed to look deeper at the connections between MTX hepatotoxicity and risks such as obesity, diabetes, and alcohol consumption.[92]

MTX is commonly used for severe psoriasis and psoriatic arthritis and has an established efficacy and significant degree of patient compliance. Side effects associated with MTX have been shown to greatly decrease by using low, intermittent doses. However, even in this case, if used long term, there is a potential for hepatic fibrosis and cirrhosis. The incidence of cirrhosis in this case can be as much as 25.6%.[93]

With the increasing usage of methotrexate (MTX), a well-defined toxicology profile has been developed, with hepatotoxicity being the most significant adverse reaction that can occur with long-term therapy. Hepatic fibrosis became evident in children and adults with leukemia who were given daily doses of MTX. In the late 1960s, case reports included psoriasis patients who developed cirrhosis that were also treated with MTX. Taken together, this information suggests that MTX had the means to cause hepatotoxicity in patients with nonmalignant conditions that were treated with low doses of methotrexate.[94]

Methotrexate (MTX) is a folic acid antagonist that was approved for use in the treatment of rheumatoid arthritis in 1988. Methotrexate (MTX) is a highly significant and ubiquitous drug treatment for rheumatoid arthritis. Patients with RA usually respond very favorably to low-dose methotrexate therapy, and the probability of patients continuing their treatment beyond five years is greater than for other slow-acting antirheumatic drugs. Thus, given its sustained clinical utility and relatively predictable toxicity profile, low-dose methotrexate is a useful addition to the therapy of RA.[95]

Patients who are about to begin methotrexate treatment have a requirement to abstain from alcohol consumption; however, exceptions include special occasions. Regular alcohol consumption is strictly discouraged due to the lack of data on what is a safe amount of alcohol when taking methotrexate. Patients need to be counseled and guided regarding the risks especially involving alcohol consumption, dose, and age. They should be educated on the reasons and logic behind routine blood monitoring (this four to eight weeks), the need for liver biopsy, and also potential complications; this conversation should be indicated in the patient's records.[96]

Examination of the FDA's Adverse Event Reporting System shows that, of the 2,512 cases reporting methotrexate as a suspect medication with liver injury, there is a bimodal distribution of patient ages, with a minor mode highlighting patients aged less than 20 years (Figure 15.10). The gender distribution of those suffering liver injury is heavily skewed toward females (62% for females versus 38% for males), which likely mirrors the gender composition of patients who are most likely to be prescribed methotrexate. As noted before, declining renal function is commonly associated with methotrexate and liver injury, with 15% of these cases reporting some form of renal function disorder.

15.7.6 Estrogens and Oral Contraceptive Steroids

Estrogen-induced cholestatic liver damage is another prominent condition. In this case, ethnicity plays a role. Ethnic diversity involving these conditions suggests that there are genetic factors that govern one's sensitivity to estrogen-induced cholestasis. This condition is high in Chile and Scandinavia where 1 in 4,000 women are affected. In other countries, the frequency is 1 in 10,000. Additionally, 50% of women who have had pregnancy-derived benign cholestasis develop cholestasis with oral contraceptives.

The estrogen-induced liver dysfunction usually terminates within days or weeks of estrogen cessation, but there have been reported cases of chronic cholestatic progression. Other agents which have produced a similar response include 17-alkylated anabolic steroids, which may also cause chronic cholestasis and tamoxifen.

Estrogens at physiological doses are pertinent in therapies such as hormone replacement therapy (HRT) for menopause and do not cause cholestasis and can be used effectively in patients with chronic cholestasis. This is particularly important because these patients are at risk for osteoporosis.[97]

15.7.7 Statins

Statins are 3-hydroxy-3-methyl glutaryl-coenzyme A reductase inhibitors which commonly cause a rise in angiotensin. The liver disorders that are connected with statin use include mild hepatic injury to end state or fulminant, hepatic failure. However, fulminant hepatic failure is uncommon. Cholestasis is one side effect of this condition and is associated with the statins lovastatin, atorvastatin, and pravastatin. Liver histology indicates acute cholestatic hepatitis, and liver blood test alterations approach normal levels after statin discontinuation.[98]

15.7.8 Ticlopidine

Ticlopidine is a platelet inhibitor that is used for the treatment of vascular-related conditions. In early clinical trials, the liver blood tests indicated anomalies in 4.4% of the patients, and greater than 30 ticlopidine-induced cholestasis patients have been discovered. These individuals were mostly were of ages 55 and above, possibly in connection with atherosclerotic vascular disease. Symptoms begin 2–12 weeks after ticlopidine administration and include pruritis, jaundice, abdominal discomfort, and fever. AP levels increase to three times the normal amount with a moderate rise in AT. Liver blood tests indicate normalization of these levels within three to six months after drug cessation, but full recovery may take greater than one year.[99]

15.7.9 ACE Inhibitors and AT II Receptor Antagonists

Angiotensin-converting enzyme (ACE) inhibitors are also involved in cholestasis and include captopril. The onset of cholestatic symptoms takes about eight weeks after the drug is taken, and symptoms include acute cholangitis with abdominal pain, fever, and jaundice. Angiotensin II receptor antagonists, such as irbesartan, is a new class of antihypertensive, that has also been known to cause cholestatic hepatitis.[100]

15.7.10 Fluoroquinolones

Fluoroquinolones are used ubiquitously, and with this in mind, hepatic dysfunction is lower than expected. Fourteen cases have been discovered with eight of them being cholestasis. Drug examples include ciprofloxacin, norfloxacin, ofloxacin, and enoxacin, with clinical symptom onset between 3 and 12 days after drug administration. The hepatic threat was resolved in all of the patients who presented with cholestasis.[101,102]

15.7.11 Terbinafine

Terbinafine is an antifungal which is used in the treatment of onychomycosis, which is a fungal infection of the nails. Ten percent of treated patients have had elevated AT and bilirubin levels, and four cases of cholestasis have been reported. The onset of hepatic threat occurs between 20 and 40 days after therapy commencement. After drug cessation, liver tests normalize between three and six months. Histological analysis indicated hepatocellular and canalicular cholestasis with different stages of portal vein inflammation. Three cases have shown cholangitis, and one case has shown ductopenia. Other drugs that fit this category include ketoconazole and fluconazole.[103]

Analysis of the FDA Adverse Event Reporting System identifies 953 cases where liver injury is reported with terbinafine as a suspect medication with the majority of these cases reporting some form of abnormal liver enzyme test

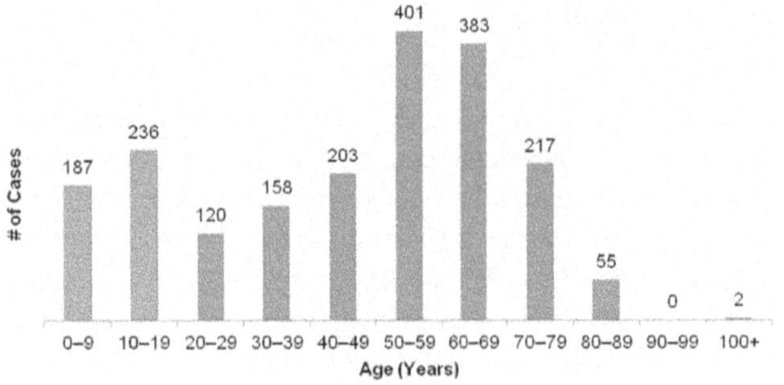

FIGURE 15.11 Distribution of patient ages in adverse event cases within the FDA Adverse Event Reporting System where liver injury is co-reported with methotrexate as a suspect medication.

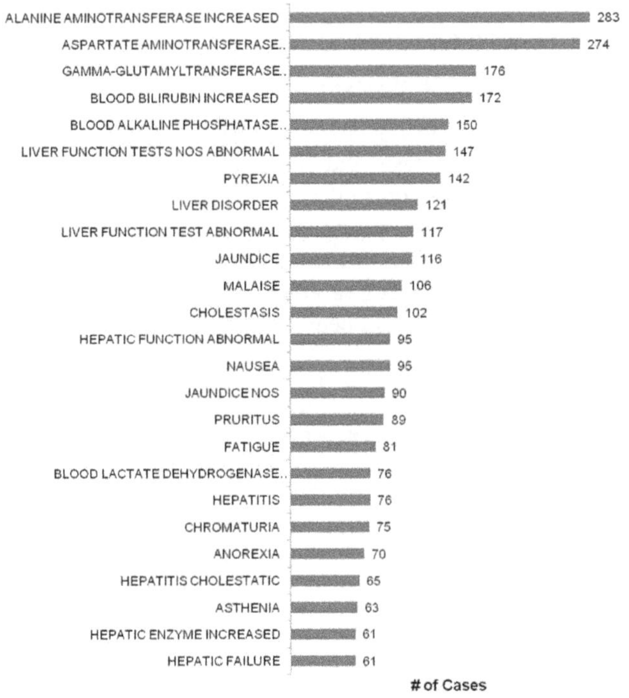

FIGURE 15.12 Top 25 adverse reactions co-reported with liver injury when terbinafine is a suspect medication.

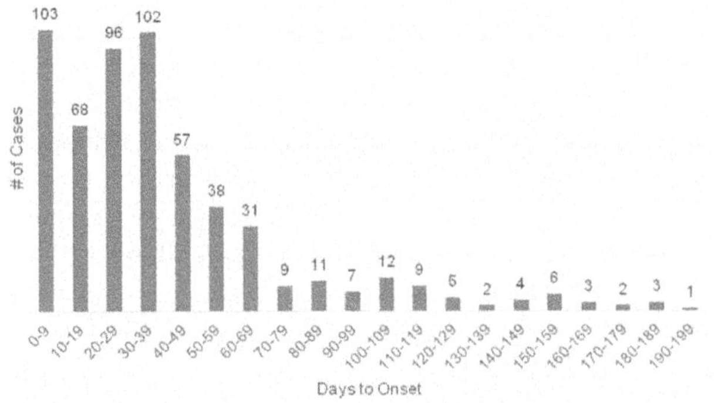

FIGURE 15.13 Distribution of number of days to the onset of liver-injury-related adverse reaction after the commencement of terbinafine therapy.

result (Figure 15.11). The AERS database indicates that terbinafine-related liver injury reactions primarily occur within approximately 40 days from the beginning of terbinafine therapy (Figure 15.12).

15.7.12 Ketoconazole

On July 26, 2013, the United States Food and Drug Administration (FDA) issued a Drug Safety Communication limiting the use of Nizoral (ketoconazole) oral tablets.[104] Until that time, ketoconazole had been an available systemic treatment for a broad range of fungal infections. The FDA's warning highlighted, among other dangers, the risk of potentially fatal drug-induced liver injury (DILI) associated with ketoconazole. The statement concluded that "Nizoral oral tablets should not be a first-line treatment for any fungal infection, [and] Nizoral should be used . . . only when alternative antifungal therapies are not available or tolerated." On the same day, the European Medicines Agency's Committee on Medicinal Products for Human Use (EMA-CHMP) issued a similar directive, stating that the risks of oral ketoconazole outweigh the benefits and that "doctors should not prescribe oral ketoconazole."[105]

The FDA Communication1 goes on to state the following:

> Serious hepatic injury was identified as the major toxicity for Nizoral tablets and was noted to be unrelated to dose, duration, or indication for treatment. In conducting the benefit-risk assessment, spontaneous adverse event reports of ketoconazole-induced liver injury, including fatalities and liver transplantations, retrieved from the FDA Adverse Event Reporting System (AERS) were assessed independently by a hepatology expert in FDA. The overall risk for ketoconazole-induced serious liver injury appeared higher than that associated with other azole antifungal drugs as assessed from pharmacoepidemiologic studies.

This indicates that the information from the AERS was a component of the basis for the agency action. The ARES data is not easily available to the scientific community, and to our knowledge, an analysis of the data has not been published in the biomedical literature.[106]

15.7.13 Selective Serotonin Reuptake Inhibitors—Serzone Liver Toxicity

Cohen and James discuss this issue in Chapter 20, elsewhere in this edition:

> Serzone is a second-generation, non-TCA that has been associated with severe liver disease (hepatotoxicity). The incidence of hepatic injury associated with Serzone is twenty-nine cases per 100,000 patient-years. In 2002, the FDA required a "black box warning" concerning the hepatotoxicity risk for patients taking Serzone. The manufacturer (Bristol-Myers Squibb) also sent out "Dear Doctor" letters that described several instances of liver failure—some of which were fatal or required a liver transplant—with a reported rate in the United States of one case per 250,000 to 300,000 patient–years. The Canadian Adverse Drug Reaction Monitoring Program database

identified thirty-two cases of liver injury due to Serzone, of which 81% were classified as severe. Out of those thirty-two cases, eleven patients were taking only Serzone and liver injury developed in 88% of the cases within the first six months of therapy. Interestingly, 70% of the thirty-two cases of liver injury were women, which is consistent with the greater incidence of depression among women.

Current recommendations suggest caution in prescribing Serzone to any patient taking other drugs metabolized by the hepatic cytochrome P450-3A4 isoenzyme system. This precaution is to avoid drug interaction with Serzone, which is a substrate and an inhibitor of that metabolic pathway. A warning is also issued *not* to prescribe Serzone to any patient with preexisting liver disease. In addition, it is recommended that liver enzyme tests be monitored periodically (the time to liver injury generally ranges from two weeks to six months). Patients should also be advised about the signs and symptoms of liver injury (such as nausea, vomiting, abdominal pain, and yellow discoloration of the skin), so that the drug can be stopped if they occur, and patients can be evaluated. Serzone should be stopped in patients who experience liver enzyme elevations of more than three times the upper limit of normal.

15.7.14 Herbal and Other Dietary Supplements and Hepatotoxicity

The 4th Edition of *Drug Injury* reported on hepatotoxicity caused by Chapparal, Kava, and Oxy-Elite Pro.[107] The problem continues, as noted by the following review:

> Herbal and dietary supplements (HDS) are used increasingly both in the United States and worldwide and HDS induced liver injury in the U.S. has increased proportionally. Current challenges in the diagnosis and management of HDS-induced liver injury were the focus of a 2-day research symposium sponsored by the American Association for the Study of Liver Disease and the National Institutes of Health. HDS-induced liver injury now accounts for 20% of cases of hepatotoxicity in the United States based on research data. The major implicated agents include anabolic steroids, green tea extract, and multi-ingredient nutritional supplements (MINS). Anabolic steroids marketed as bodybuilding supplements typically induce a prolonged cholestatic, but ultimately self-limiting liver injury that has a distinctive serum biochemical as well as histological phenotype. Green tea extract and many other products, in contrast, tend to cause an acute-hepatitis like injury. Currently, however, the majority of cases of HDS-associated liver injury are due to MINS, and the component responsible for the toxicity is usually unknown or can only be suspected. HDS-induced liver injury presents many clinical and research challenges, in diagnosis, identification of the responsible constituents, treatment and prevention. Also important are improvements in regulatory oversight of non-prescription products to guarantee their constituents and insure purity and safety. The confident identification of injurious ingredients within HDS will require strategic alignments among clinicians, chemists, and toxicologists. The ultimate goal should be to prohibit or more closely regulate potentially injurious ingredients and thus promote public safety.

The U.S. Department of Justice reported that five individuals and two companies plead guilty to felony charges in a multimillion-dollar scheme to fraudulently sell popular dietary supplements (including Chapparal) (March 19, 2019). All of the defendants played roles in developing, manufacturing, or marketing the popular workout and weight loss supplements known as Jack 3D and oxy elite pro which were distributed by Dallas-based dietary supplement company USP Labs. The misbranding charges all relate in part to oxy elite pro, which was recalled in 2013 in the wake of an investigation by the FDA into whether the supplement caused liver injuries in consumers.[108]

A report from Australia gives the fact that complementary and alternative medicine use is prevalent in over 60% of the Australian population. Patient education, raising awareness of the potentiality of severe consequences of these often-benign supplements, is critical in reducing the incidence of morbidity and mortality. The relative rarity of these presentations and the lack of definitive diagnostic tests often lead to a prolonged and costly work-up and delay in identifying the underlying etiology of liver injury. Two patient cases are reported. Two patients were admitted to the hospital, following two weeks of generalized cramping abdominal pain, nausea and vomiting, jaundice, and pruritis. Neither patient had reported fevers or any recent risk factors for the acquisition of viral hepatitis. One patient volunteered a history of excess alcohol consumption with abstinence since the onset of icteric illness. On average, the patient consumed three grams of acetaminophen per week, with the last dose of one gram administered three days before the presentation. Patient B had a seizure disorder, secondary to a traumatic brain injury that was controlled by levetiracetam with prior normal liver function tests (LFTs). Both patients noted the use of oral supplements purchased over the Internet. One was taking corydalis for over 18 months for its purported analgesic properties. The second patient used multi-herbal supplement that contained, among other components, Tongkat ali root (Eurycoma longifolia), horny goat week, and saw palmetto fruit extract, for the presumed anabolic effect on skeletal muscle. Both patients while hospitalized and abstaining from their supplements experienced rapid resolution of pruritus and abdominal pain early in their admission and were asymptomatic on discharge. They were advised not to rechallenge with the implicated supplements, given the severity of the presentation.[109]

15.8 SUMMARY AND CONCLUSIONS

Make no mistake. Hepatotoxicity is rare statistically. However, even a rare risk, when a large percentage of the population uses a drug, can become a significant population risk. This comment certainly applies to any analysis of NSAID-induced idiosyncratic adverse reactions indicating that a number of acidic NSAIDs are connected to hepatocellular and cholestatic (rare) liver injury. The risk of unpredictable liver injuries due to NSAIDs at therapeutic levels is minimal. Current NSAID usage has been associated with a twofold increase in the risk of liver injury and an additional risk of 5 per 100,000 person years. Fulminant hepatitis can progress in susceptible patients, and an intriguing task for the future is to pinpoint some of the risks that can be important in producing toxicity. For example, there is evidence that NSAID-induced liver injury is more prevalent in elderly patients compared to other age groups. It is unclear whether this is due to increased usage in elderly patients or a decrease in kidney function which could enhance susceptibility through drug accumulation or increased serum levels of drug glucuronides which would lead to higher levels of a drug irreversibly binding to plasma proteins.[110]

Nonnarcotic analgesics (acetaminophen-Tylenol) can result in a plethora of hepatic lesions; however, clinically significant liver damage is uncommon with normal doses. Hepatotoxicity that is caused by salicylates, NSAIDs, acetaminophen, and pyrazolones varies, but some of these drugs cause generalized liver reactions. The risks of liver injury may vary depending on factors such as age, sex, dosage, and treatment duration. Hepatoxicity from salicylates and most NSAIDs have been frequently associated with females who have collagen diseases. Acetaminophen-induced liver dysfunction almost always is due to overdosage, usually unbeknownst to the patient.

The liver is a vital organ for life and is vital for metabolism of drugs and other substances consumed by patients. When the drugs consumed for a variety of therapeutic purposes cause injury to the patient, it creates a quandary for the therapist. Special monitoring and evaluation of continued benefit over risk may lead to the selection of an alternative but less-toxic agent. Sometimes, the FDA and the manufacturer must make the difficult choice to not bring the product to market, restrict its use after release, or eventually withdraw the product from the market.

A mere 25% of all patients with acute idiosyncratic end-stage liver failure survive a few weeks with no liver transplant. The cause of death includes multi-organ failure, sepsis, cardiac arrest, cerebral edema, and respiratory failure. In the case of mild-to-moderate liver dysfunction, mortality is less common than severe morbidity. As expected, the patient prognosis becomes worse the longer the hepatotoxin is taken.[111]

It is well accepted to monitor patients who are at a special risk, such as patients with alcoholic liver disease. Cost–benefit analysis does not absolve the continuous monitoring of serum transaminases in otherwise healthy individuals. The best method of severe hepatotoxicity prevention is to educate and alert clinicians to be mindful of the DILD diagnosis when a patient develops clinical signs of liver disease.[112]

NOTES

1. Hoofnagle JH, Bjornsson ES. Drug-induced liver injury: Types and phenotypes. N Engl J Med. 2019 Jul 18;381(3):264–273.
2. Larrey D. Epidemiology and individual susceptibility to adverse drug reactions affecting the liver. Semin Liver Dis. 2002;22:145–155.
3. Pirmohamed M, Park KB. Adverse drug reactions: Back to the future. Br J Clin Pharmacol. 2003 May;55(5):486–492.
4. Fattinger K, Roos M, Vergères P, Holenstein C, Kind B, Masche U, Stocker DN, Braunschweig S, Kullak-Ublick GA, Galeazzi RL, Follath F, Gasser T, Meier PJ. Epidemiology of drug exposure and adverse drug reactions in two swiss departments of internal medicine. Br J Clin Pharmacol. 2000;49(2):158–167. PMC.
5. Lee WM, Senior JR. Recognizing drug-induced liver injury: Current problems, possible solutions. Toxicol Pathol. 2005;33(1):155–164.
6. LiverTox. *Clinical and Research Information on Drug-Induced Liver Injury*. Bethesda, MD: National Institute of Diabetes and Digestive and Kidney Diseases; 2012. Updated 2020 Feb 12. https://www.ncbi.nlm.nih.gov/books/NBK548388/
7. MacLaren R. Hepatic and cholestatic diseases. In: Tisdale JE, MillerDA, editors. *Drug-Induced Diseases: Prevention, Detection, and Management*. Bethesda, MD: American Society of Health System Pharmacists; 2005:515–535.
8. Stricker BHCH. *Drug-Induced Hepatic Injury*. 2nd ed. Amsterdam: Elsevier; 1992.
9. Farrell GC. Drug-induced acute hepatitis. In: Farrell GC, editor. *Drug-Induced Liver Disease*. Edinburgh: Churchill Livingstone; 1994:247–299.
10. Pessayre O, Larrey D, Biour M. Drug-induced liver injury. In: Bircher J, Benhamou JP, McIntyre N, Rizzetto M, Rodés J, editors. *Oxford Textbook of Clinical Hepatology*. 2nd ed. Oxford: Oxford University Press; 1999:1261–1315.
11. Zimmerman HJ. Drug-induced liver disease. In: Zimmerman HJ, editor. *Hepatotoxicity: The Adverse Effects of Drugs and Other Chemicals on the Liver*. 2nd ed. Philadelphia: Lippincott Williams & Wilkins; 1999:427–456.
12. Larrey D. Drug-induced liver diseases. J Hepatol. 2000;32:77–88.
13. Navarro VJ, Senior JR. Drug-related hepatotoxicity. N Engl J Med. 2006;354:731–739.
14. Biour M, Poupon R, Grange JD, Chazouilleres O. Hépatotoxicité des medicaments. Gastroenterol Clin Biol. 2000;11:1052–1091.
15. Larrey D. Hepatotoxicity of herbal medicines. J Hepatol. 1997;26:47–51.
16. Schuppan D, Jia JD, Brinkhaus B, Hahn EG. Herbal products for liver diseases: A therapeutic challenge for the new millennium. Hepatology. 1999;30:1099–1104.
17. Seeff LB, Lindsay KL, Bacon BR, Kresina TF, Hoofnagle JH. Complementary and alternative medicine in chronic liver disease. Hepatology. 2001;34:595–603.
18. Larrey D. Drug-induced liver diseases. J Hepatol. 2000;32:77–88.

19 Larrey D. Epidemiology and individual susceptibility to adverse drug reactions affecting the liver. Semin Liver Dis. 2002;22:145–155.
20 Larrey D. Epidemiology and individual susceptibility to adverse drug reactions affecting the liver. Semin Liver Dis. 2002;22:145–155.
21 Wing K, Douglas I, Bhaskaran K, Klungel OH, Reynolds RF, Pirmohamed M, Smeeth L, van Staa TP. Development of predictive genetic tests for improving the safety of new medicines: The utilization of routinely collected electronic health records. Drug Discov Today. 2014 Apr;19(4):361–366.
22 Navarro VJ, Senior JR. Drug-related hepatotoxicity. N Engl J Med. 2006;354:731–739.
23 Navarro VJ, Senior JR. Drug-related hepatotoxicity. N Engl J Med. 2006;354:731–739.
24 Devarbhavi H. An update on drug-induced liver injury. J Clin Exp Hepatol. 2012 Sep;2(3):247–259.
25 Watkins P. Drug safety sciences and the bottleneck in drug development. Clin Pharmacol Ther. 2011;89:788–790.
26 Babai S, Auclert L, Le-Louët H. Safety data and withdrawal of hepatotoxic drugs. Therapie. 2021 Nov–Dec;76(6):715–723.
27 Abo Loha C, Livio F. Pharmacovigilance [Pharmacovigilance update]. Rev Med Suisse. 2019 Jan 9;15(632–633):92–95. French. PMID: 30629378.
28 Standardization of definitions and criteria of causality assessment of adverse drug reactions. Drug-induced liver disorders: Report of an international consensus meeting. Int J Clin Pharmacol Ther Toxicol. 1990;28:317–322.
29 LiverTox. *Clinical and Research Information on Drug-Induced Liver Injury*. Bethesda, MD: National Institute of Diabetes and Digestive and Kidney Diseases; 2012. Updated 2020 Feb 12. https://www.ncbi.nlm.nih.gov/books/NBK548388/
30 Prescott LF. Liver damage with non-narcotic analgesics. Med Toxicol. 1986;1:44–56.
31 Larrey D. Epidemiology and individual susceptibility to adverse drug reactions affecting the liver. Semin Liver Dis. 2002;22:145–155.
32 Bernuau J, Benhamou JP. Fulminant and subfulminant liver failure. In: Bircher J, Benhamou JR, McIntyre N, Rizzetto M, Rodés J, editors. *Oxford Textbook of Clinical Hepatology*. 2nd ed. Oxford: Oxford University Press; 1999:1341–1372.
33 LiverTox. *Clinical and Research Information on Drug-Induced Liver Injury*. Bethesda, MD: National Institute of Diabetes and Digestive and Kidney Diseases; 2012. Updated 2020 Feb 12. https://www.ncbi.nlm.nih.gov/books/NBK548388/
34 Larrey D. Epidemiology and individual susceptibility to adverse drug reactions affecting the liver. Semin Liver Dis. 2002;22:145–155.
35 Krähenbühl S. Mitochondria: Important target for drug toxicity? J Hepatol. 2001;34:334–336.
36 Jones M, Núñez M. HIV and hepatitis C co-infection: The role of HAART in HIV/hepatitis C virus management. Curr Opin HIV AIDS. 2011 Nov;6(6):546–552.
37 Wu X, Li Y, Peng K, Zhou H. HIV protease inhibitors in gut barrier dysfunction and liver injury. Curr Opin Pharmacol. 2014 Dec;19:61–66.
38 Navarro VJ, Senior, JR. Drug-related hepatotoxicity. N Engl J Med. 2006;354:731–739.
39 Kontorinis N, Dieterich D. Hepatotoxicity of antiretroviral therapy. AIDS Rev. 2003 Jan–Mar;5(1):36–43.
40 Núñez M. Clinical syndromes and consequences of antiretroviral-related hepatotoxicity. Hepatology. 2010 Sep;52(3):1143–1155.
41 Heil EL, Townsend ML, Shipp K, Clarke A, Johnson MD. Incidence of severe hepatotoxicity related to antiretroviral therapy in HIV/HCV coinfected patients. AIDS Res Treat. 2010:Article ID 856542.
42 Barve S, Kapoor R, Moghe A, Ramirez JA, Eaton JW, Gobejishvili L, Joshi-Barve S, McClain CJ. Focus on the liver: Alcohol use, highly active antiretroviral therapy, and liver disease in HIV-infected patients. Alcohol Res Health. 2010;33(3):229–236.
43 Da Hee Han. Two hepatitis C virus infection treatments to be discontinued. https://www.empr.com/home/news/two-hepatitis-c-virus-infection-treatments-to-be-discontinued/
44 Kanel GC, Korula J. *Liver Biopsy Evaluation: Histologic Diagnosis and Clinical Correlations*. W.B. Saunders; 2000.
45 Black M, Mitchell JR, Zimmerman HJ, Ishak KG, Epler GR. Isoniazid-associated hepatitis in 114 patients. Gastroenterology. 1975;69:289–302.
46 MacLaren R. Hepatic and cholestatic diseases. In: Tisdale JE, MillerDA, editors. *Drug-Induced Diseases: Prevention, Detection, and Management*. Bethesda, MD: American Society of Health System Pharmacists; 2005:515–535.
47 Lewis JH. Drug-induced liver disease. Med Clin North Am. 2000;84:1275–1311.
48 Standardization of definitions and criteria of causality assessment of adverse drug reactions. Drug-induced liver disorders: Report of an international consensus meeting. Int J Clin Pharmacol Ther Toxicol. 1990;28:317–322.
49 Chitturi S, Farrell GC. Drug-induced cholestasis. Semin Gastrointest Dis. 2001;12:113–124.
50 Marks DH. Evaluation of medical causation. In: O'Donnell JT, O'Donnell JJ, editors. *O'Donnell's Drug Injury*. 4th ed. Tucson: L&J Publishing.
51 Larrey D. Epidemiology and individual susceptibility to adverse drug reactions affecting the liver. Semin Liver Dis. 2002;22:145–155.
52 Larrey D. Epidemiology and individual susceptibility to adverse drug reactions affecting the liver. Semin Liver Dis. 2002;22:145–155.

53 Larrey D. Epidemiology and individual susceptibility to adverse drug reactions affecting the liver. Semin Liver Dis. 2002;22:145–155.
54 Wang K, Zhang S, Marzolf B, Troisch P, Brightman A, Hu Z, Hood LE, Galas DJ. Circulating microRNAs, potential biomarkers for drug-induced liver injury. Proc Natl Acad Sci USA. 2009 Mar 17;106(11):4402–4407.
55 Laterza OF, Lim L, Garrett-Engele PW, Vlasakova K, Muniappa N, Tanaka WK, Johnson JM, Sina JF, Fare TL, Sistare FD, Glaab WE. Plasma MicroRNAs as sensitive and specific biomarkers of tissue injury. Clin Chem. 2009;55(11):1977–1983.
56 Wang Y, Chen T, Tong W. miRNAs and their application in drug-induced liver injury. Biomark Med. 2014;8(2):161–172.
57 Angulo P. Nonalcoholic fatty liver disease. N Engl J Med. 2002;346:1221–1231.
58 Rubin E. Iatrogenic hepatic injury. Hum Pathol. 1980;11:312–331.
59 Rubin E. Iatrogenic hepatic injury. Hum Pathol. 1980;11:312–331.
60 Rubin E. Iatrogenic hepatic injury. Hum Pathol. 1980;11:312–331.
61 Rubin E. Iatrogenic hepatic injury. Hum Pathol. 1980;11:312–331.
62 Marks DH. Case report: Drug toxicity leading to vanishing bile duct syndrome and cholestatic jaundice. Internet J Gastroenterol. 2009;8:6.
63 Marks DH. Evaluation of medical causation. In: O'Donnell JT, O'Donnell JJ, editors. *O'Donnell's Drug Injury*. 4th ed. Tucson: L&J Publishing.
64 Marks DH. Case report: Drug toxicity leading to vanishing bile duct syndrome and cholestatic jaundice. Internet J Gastroenterol. 2009;8:6.
65 Núñez M, Clinical syndromes and consequences of antiretroviral-related hepatotoxicity. Hepatology. 2010 Sep;52(3):1143–1155.
66 LiverTox. *Clinical and Research Information on Drug-Induced Liver Injury*. Bethesda, MD: National Institute of Diabetes and Digestive and Kidney Diseases; 2012. https://www.ncbi.nlm.nih.gov/books/NBK547852/
67 Prescott LF. Liver damage with non-narcotic analgesics. Med Toxicol. 1986;1:44–56.
68 Boelsterli UA, Zimmerman HJ, Kretz-Rommel A. Idiosyncratic liver toxicity of nonsteroidal antiinflammatory drugs: Molecular mechanisms and pathology. Crit Rev Toxicol. 1995;25:207–235.
69 Prescott LF. Liver damage with non-narcotic analgesics. Med Toxicol. 1986;1:44–56.
70 Boelsterli UA, Zimmerman, HJ, Kretz-Rommel A. Idiosyncratic liver toxicity of nonsteroidal antiinflammatory drugs: Molecular mechanisms of pathology. Crit Rev Toxicol. 1995;25(3):207–235.
71 Boelsterli UA, Zimmerman HJ, Kretz-Rommel A. Idiosyncratic liver toxicity of nonsteroidal antiinflammatory drugs: Molecular mechanisms and pathology. Crit Rev Toxicol. 1995;25:207–235.
72 Nuki G. Pain control and the use of nonsteroidal analgesic antiinflammatory drugs. Br Med Bull. 1990;46:262–278.
73 Rapha Group Software, Inc. 1996.
74 O'Donnell JT, Marks DH, Danese P, O'Donnell JJ. Drug-induced liver disease: Primer for the primary care physician. Dis Month. 2014;60(2):49–104.
75 Remien CH, Sussman NL, Adler FR. Mathematical modelling of chronic acetaminophen metabolism and liver injury. Math Med Biol. 2014;31(3):302–317.
76 Beck-Friis J, Studahl M, Yilmaz A, Andersson R, Lönnermark E. Increased risk of hepatotoxicity and temporary drug withdrawal during treatment of active tuberculosis in pregnant women. Int J Infect Dis. 2020 Sep;98:138–143. doi:10.1016/j.ijid.2020.06.069. Epub 2020 Jun 24. PMID: 32592906.
77 Farrell GC. Drug-induced acute hepatitis. In: Farrell GC, editor. *Drug-Induced Liver Disease*. Edinburgh: Churchill Livingstone; 1994:247–299.
78 Anne M Larson. Amy L Graziani, isoniazid hepatotoxicity. https://www.uptodate.com/contents/isoniazid-hepatotoxicity
79 LiverTox. *Clinical and Research Information on Drug-Induced Liver Injury*. Bethesda, MD: National Institute of Diabetes and Digestive and Kidney Diseases; 2012. Updated 2020 Feb 12. https://www.ncbi.nlm.nih.gov/books/NBK548388/
80 Remien CH, Sussman NL, Adler FR. Mathematical modelling of chronic acetaminophen metabolism and liver injury. Math Med Biol. 2014;31(3):302–317.
81 Prescott LF, Critchley JA, Balali-Mood M, Pentland B. Effects of microsomal enzyme induction on paracetamol metabolism in man. Br J Clin Pharmacol. 1981;12:149–153.
82 Yoon E, Babar A, Choudhary M, Kutner M, Pyrsopoulos N. Acetaminophen-induced hepatotoxicity: A comprehensive update. J Clin Transl Hepatol. 2016;4(2):131–142. doi:10.14218/JCTH.2015.00052.
83 Minton NA, Henry JA, Frankel RJ. Fatal paracetamol poisoning in an epileptic. Hum Toxicol. 1988;7:33–34.
84 https://www.fda.gov/drugs/information-drug-class/acetaminophen
85 Goyal RK, Rajan SS, Essien EJ, Sansgiry SS. Effectiveness of FDA's new over-the-counter acetaminophen warning label in improving consumer risk perception of liver damage. J Clin Pharm Ther. 2012 Dec;37(6):681–685.
86 King JP, McCarthy DM, Serper M, Jacobson KL, Mullen RJ, Parker RM, Wolf MS. Variability in acetaminophen labeling practices: A missed opportunity to enhance patient safety. J Med Toxicol. 2015 Feb 20;11:410–414.
87 Chitturi S, Farrell GC. Drug-induced cholestasis. Semin Gastrointest Dis. 2001;12:113–124.

88 Shaheen N, Grimm IS. Fulminant hepatic failure associated with clarithromycin. Am J Gastroenterol. 1996;91:394–395.

89 Wallace RJ Jr, Brown BA, Griffith DE. Drug intolerance to highdose clarithromycin among elderly patients. Diagn Microbiol Infect Dis. 1993;16:215–221.

90 Shaheen N, Grimm IS. Fulminant hepatic failure associated with clarithromycin. Am J Gastroenterol. 1996;91:394–395.

91 VanDooren-Greebe RJ, Kuijpers AL, Buijs WC, Kniest PH, Corstens FH, Nagengasts F, De Boo T, Willems JL, Duller P, Van De Kerkhof PC. The value of dynamic hepatic scintigraphy and serum aminoterminal propeptide of type III procollagen for early detection of methotrexate-induced hepatic damage in psoriasis patients. Br J Dermatol. 1996;134:481–487.

92 Malatjalian DA, Ross JB, Williams CN, Colwell SJ, Eastwood BJ. Methotrexate hepatotoxicity in psoriatics: Report of 104 patients from Nova Scotia, with analysis of risks from obesity, diabetes and alcohol consumption during long term follow-up. Can J Gastroenterol. 1996;10:369–375.

93 Malatjalian DA, Ross JB, Williams CN, Colwell SJ, Eastwood BJ. Methotrexate hepatotoxicity in psoriatics: Report of 104 patients from Nova Scotia, with analysis of risks from obesity, diabetes and alcohol consumption during long term follow-up. Can J Gastroenterol. 1996;10:369–375.

94 West SG. Methotrexate hepatotoxicity. Rheum Dis Clin North Am. 1997;23:883–915.

95 Tett SE, Triggs EJ. Use of methotrexate in older patients: A risk-benefit assessment. Drugs Aging. 1996;9:458–471.

96 Kremer JM, Alarcón GS, Lightfoot RW Jr, Willkens RF, Furst DE, Williams HJ, Dent PB, Weinblatt ME. Methotrexate for rheumatoid arthritis: Suggested guidelines for monitoring liver toxicity. American College of Rheumatology. Arthritis Rheum. 1994;37:316–328.

97 Chitturi S, Farrell GC. Drug-induced cholestasis. Semin Gastrointest Dis. 2001;12:113–124.

98 Chitturi S, Farrell GC. Drug-induced cholestasis. Semin Gastrointest Dis. 2001;12:113–124.

99 Chitturi S, Farrell GC. Drug-induced cholestasis. Semin Gastrointest Dis. 2001;12:113–124.

100 Chitturi S, Farrell GC. Drug-induced cholestasis. Semin Gastrointest Dis. 2001;12:113–124.

101 Fuchs S, Simon Z, Brezis M. Fatal hepatic failure associated with ciprofloxacin. Lancet. 1994;343:738–739.

102 Grassmick BK, Lehr VT, Sundareson AS. Fulminant hepatic failure possibly related to ciprofloxacin. Ann Pharmacother. 1992;26:636–639.

103 Samarasinghe DA, Farrell GC. Drug-induced liver disease. In: Gitnick G, editor. *Current Hepatology.* 1994;14:117–167.

104 FDA Drug Safety Communication. FDA limits usage of Nizoral (ketoconazole) oral tablets due to potentially fatal liver injury and risk of drug interactions and adrenal gland problems. UCM. 2013 Jul 26;36(44).

105 European Medicines Agency recommends suspension of marketing authorizations for oral ketoconazole. Benefit of oral ketoconazole does not outweigh risk of liver injury in fungal infections. EMA/458028/2013, Jul 26, 2013.

106 Greenblatt HK, Greenblatt DJ. Liver injury associated with ketoconazole: Review of the published evidence. J Clin Pharmacol. 2014;54(12):1321–1329.

107 Navarro VJ, Khan IA, Björnsson E, Seeff LB, Serrano J, Hoofnagle JH. Liver injury from herbal and dietary supplements. Hepatology. 2016. doi:10.1002/hep.28813.

108 https://www.fda.gov/inspections-compliance-enforcement-and-criminal-investigations/press-releases/march-13-2019-five-individuals-and-two-companies-plead-guilty-felony-charges-multi-million-dollar

109 Peri V, Yu C, Vaz K, Asadi K, Grace J. Herb-induced liver injury: A report on two Australian cases. Cureus. 2022 May 3;15(4):e24886.

110 Boelsterli UA, Zimmerman HJ, Kretz-Rommel A. Idiosyncratic liver toxicity of nonsteroidal antiinflammatory drugs: Molecular mechanisms and pathology. Crit Rev Toxicol. 1995;25:207–235.

111 MacLaren R. Hepatic and cholestatic diseases. In: Tisdale JE, Miller DA, editors. *Drug-Induced Diseases: Prevention, Detection, and Management.* Bethesda, MD: American Society of Health System Pharmacists; 2005:515–535.

112 LiverTox. *Clinical and Research Information on Drug-Induced Liver Injury*. Bethesda, MD: National Institute of Diabetes and Digestive and Kidney Diseases; 2012. Updated 2020 Feb 12. https://www.ncbi.nlm.nih.gov/books/NBK548388/

16 Antineoplastic Therapy

Kathryn Schultz and Eris Tollkuci

SYNOPSIS

16.1 BACKGROUND

Cancer care is a complex course that can include multiple therapies, routes of administration, and different frequencies of treatment. This complexity, in addition to medications that tend to be toxic and have narrow therapeutic indexes, creates a recipe for high risk of drug toxicity and injury. Estimates of incidence of antineoplastic errors range from 1 to 4 per 1,000 orders and impact both adult and pediatric patients.[1] A major cancer center in the United States sought to better define the rate of adverse events (AEs) and the number with the potential to cause patient harm. They determined that 32% of the AEs identified were probably or definitely preventable. Six percent of all AEs and 4% of the preventable AEs were judged to result in permanent harm, require life-sustaining intervention, or result in death.[2]

Specific groups of high-risk antineoplastics include intrathecal and oral chemotherapy. In fact, of the 16 ISMP Best Practices for Hospitals for 2020–21, 2 pertain to antineoplastic medications—vincristine and oral methotrexate.[3] The administration of drugs inadvertently into the cerebrospinal fluid is infrequent but is well-documented and usually fatal. Despite being part of Institute of Safe Medication Practices Alerts since 1997 and Best Practice recommendations since 2014, sporadic near misses are still of concern. One case of vincristine being administered intrathecally in 2001 resulted in the death of the 18-year-old patient with leukemia.[4] The supervising physician was sentenced for manslaughter. Of note, the supervising physician and physician in training stated that neither had received training in administering cytotoxic drugs.

Oral antineoplastic therapy presents an additional set of errors that can be related to patient self-administration, including taking extra doses or missing doses or misunderstanding directions and duration of treatment. In addition to these administration concerns, there can also be concerns about the safety of oral medications. Thalidomide presents a unique historic case as the drug was initially indicated to treat insomnia and relieve morning sickness for pregnant women. The application to the FDA for thalidomide to be approved in the United States came in 1960, years after it had been approved in Canada, Europe, and South America.[5,6] Upon review by Frances Kelsey of the FDA, she noted that the clinical reports were testimonials instead of well-designed and executed studies, and they were lacking long-term evaluation for toxicity. Shortly thereafter, European physicians noted increasing numbers of deformities in newly born babies and miscarriages. The link between thalidomide and deformities was then uncovered, and the drug was removed from the market in numerous countries. Kelsey's efforts triggered improved regulations on new drug development, and thalidomide eventually resurfaced for the treatment of multiple myeloma, with the addition of a risk evaluation and mitigation strategy

DOI: 10.1201/9781003615323-18

(REMS) program to prevent the medication from causing toxicity to pregnant patients as it had done previously.

16.2 CHEMOTHERAPY—*ANTIMETABOLITES*

Antimetabolites are structurally similar to natural compounds in the body such as amino acids, DNA, and RNA, which inhibit cell growth and proliferation.

Folic acid analogs such as methotrexate (MTX) are utilized in a wide variety of disease states such as acute lymphoblastic leukemia, osteosarcoma, psoriasis, and rheumatoid arthritis (RA).[7] High-dose methotrexate (HD MTX), defined as a dose greater than or equal to 500 mg/m^2, must be followed by leucovorin (folinic acid) rescue in order to decrease toxicity.[8] Leucovorin is periodically subjected to national shortages, secondary to the supply of raw materials, manufacturing, and temporary closure of production lines. The interruptions in supply have triggered clinicians to reevaluate dosing strategies as a rescue therapy to conserve drug and could also be potentially leading to medication errors. Osteosarcoma dosing can be as high as 12 g/m^2, and dosing for psoriasis and RA is significantly lower at 10 to 15 mg once weekly.[9] Concomitant weekly folic acid is recommended to reduce hematologic, gastrointestinal (GI), and hepatic adverse events. MTX is associated with toxicities such as myelosuppression, mucositis, nephrotoxicity, hepatotoxicity, and neurotoxicity.[10] In addition, numerous errors have been reported nationally in regard to low-dose methotrexate prescriptions prescribed for rheumatoid arthritis and other autoimmune conditions. Errors range from drug interactions to dispensing errors both in the in-patient and out-patient settings. Pemetrexed and pralatrexate, two other folic acid analogs, require supplementation with folic acid and vitamin B12 in order to decrease the risk of hematologic toxicities.[11,12]

6-Mercaptopurine (6-MP) is an oral purine analog antimetabolite which can cause adverse events such as myelosuppression, hepatotoxicity, mucositis, and rash.[13] Deficiency of thiopurine S-methyltransferase (TPMT) can increase the risk of adverse events.[14] Dose adjustments must be implemented if concomitant therapy with allopurinol, a xanthine oxidase inhibitor, cannot be avoided in order to decrease the risk of serious adverse events.[15]

5-Fluorouracil (5-FU) and cytarabine are pyrimidine analog antimetabolites. Dihydropyrimidine dehydrogenase (DPD) gene mutations that result in complete or near complete absence of DPD activity increase the risk for acute early-onset toxicity and fatal reactions. 5-FU is administered through a bolus and continuous intravenous (IV) infusion. The bolus infusion is associated with an increased risk of myelosuppression, oral mucositis, diarrhea, and GI toxicity in which the continuous IV infusion is associated with an increased risk of hand-foot syndrome (HFS) and cardiotoxicity. Leucovorin is coadministered with 5-FU in order to increase the efficacy of the medication. HFS or palmar-plantar erythema is a dose-limiting toxicity (DLT) of 5-FU, occurring in one-half to two-thirds of patients and is characterized by redness, pain, blisters, and peeling of the hands and soles of feet.[16] Uridine triacitate is an antidote available in cases of 5-FU overdose.[17,18] Institutions and providers should be aware of this antidote and its utilization for 5-FU overdose.[19] Cytarabine or cytosine arabinoside (ara-C) is associated with myelosuppression. High-dose cytarabine (HiDAC) is defined as a dose of greater than 1,000 mg/m^2. HiDAC is associated with an increased risk of cerebellar toxicity and conjunctivitis.[20]

16.3 CHEMOTHERAPY—ANTIMICROTUBULES

Vinca alkaloids are naturally occurring or semisynthetic nitrogenous bases extracted from the pink periwinkle plant *Catharanthus roseus*. They inhibit the formation of mitotic spindles and prevent cells from completing metaphase. Vinca alkaloids should never be administered intrathecally, and central access is recommended for IV infusion due to their vesicant properties.[21,22,23] Adverse events include peripheral neurotoxicity which is dose-dependent and cumulative, central neurotoxicity (seizures or coma), and myelosuppression which is a DLT of vinblastine and vinorelbine.[24] These agents are cytochrome P450 (CYPs) 3A4 substrates; therefore, caution should be utilized in order to prevent serious drug–drug interactions with strong CYP 3A4 inhibitors such as azole antifungals.[25] Ensure that patients are having regular bowel movements while receiving vinca alkaloids in order to prevent constipation and/or paralytic ileus.[26]

Taxanes are extracted from the bark of the Pacific yew and stabilize microtubules and prevent disassembly. They are poorly water-soluble and require formulation with Cremophor EL (CrEL). CrEL is known to leach plasticizers from polyvinyl chloride (PVC) bags/tubing; therefore, these agents should be prepared with PVC-free material in order to prevent severe hepatotoxicity.[27] Anaphylaxis and severe hypersensitivity reactions have occurred in 2% to 4% of patients receiving paclitaxel in clinical trials. All patients should be premedicated with corticosteroids, diphenhydramine, and histamine-2 antagonists.[28]

16.4 CHEMOTHERAPY—*ALKYLATORS*

Alkylators exert cytotoxic effect by covalently binding to reactive chemical groups in the cells and causing inter- and intrastrand crosslinks. Class adverse events include myelosuppression, GI toxicities, alopecia, infertility, and secondary malignancies.

Nitrogen mustards such as cyclophosphamide and ifosfamide can also cause hemorrhagic cystitis (HC) due to the accumulation of the toxic acrolein metabolite in the bladder. The incidence of HC is higher with ifosfamide.[29,30] HC prevention should include vigorous hydration (2–3 L/m^2/day), maintaining a urine output greater than 100–200 mL/hr and mesna, which binds acrolein to form a stable and nontoxic product. Mesna must always be administered with ifosfamide and should be considered for cyclophosphamide doses greater than or equal to 1,500 mg/m^2.[31] Cyclophosphamide can cause the syndrome of inappropriate antidiuretic hormone (SIADH), and high-dose therapy can increase the risk of cardiotoxicity.[32]

Temozolomide (TMZ) is a highly lipid-soluble oral methylating agent utilized in central nervous system (CNS) malignancies such as glioblastoma. TMZ can cause dose-related myelosuppression, and inadvertent overdoses can be fatal.[33] Letarte et al. evaluated dosing errors related to TMZ from November 1997 to May 2012. MedWatch identified 45 medication errors. Patient errors were most common, followed by dispensing errors and prescribing errors.[34] Caution should be utilized when prescribing TMZ to ensure that the dose/frequency matches the appropriate indication. Patient education requires a special focus to ensure appropriate and safe administration as well as timely identification of adverse events.

Platinum analogues such as carboplatin and cisplatin are utilized in a variety of solid tumor malignancies (e.g., lung cancer, testicular cancer, ovarian cancer) and lymphomas. Cisplatin can cause nephrotoxicity which in certain cases can be irreversible, severe acute and delayed nausea and vomiting as well as neurotoxicity.[35] The neurotoxicity generally presents as a bilateral, high-frequency hearing loss. A number of strategies have been implemented to monitor and manage the side effect. Patients undergo periodic evaluation by an audiologist as well as testing to monitor the progressive nature of the toxicity. Cisplatin-induced nephrotoxicity occurs due to the accumulation of the toxic metabolite, thiol, which results in a reduction in renal blood flow, tubular function, and glomerular filtration rate (GFR). The incidence is about 40% and with an onset of 10 to 20 days post therapy. Renal damage is cumulative and potentially irreversible. Hypersensitivity reactions (HSRs) have been reported with carboplatin, and the risk is increased in patients previously exposed to platinum therapy.[36] Carboplatin desensitizations have been successfully utilized in patients experiencing HSRs.[37]

16.5 CHEMOTHERAPY—TOPOISOMERASE I INHIBITORS

Irinotecan is a camptothecin which causes single-strand DNA breaks and is commonly utilized in colorectal cancer.[38] Diarrhea is a DLT which requires prompt treatment. Early-onset diarrhea occurs due to the direct inhibition of acetylcholinesterase which leads to a cholinergic surge and is managed with atropine. Late-onset diarrhea occurs as a result of the action of active metabolite, 7-ethyl-10-hydroxycamptothecin (SN-38), which accumulates and causes damage to the intestinal mucosa. Late-onset diarrhea can be life threatening, and first-line treatment includes antidiarrheals such as loperamide.[39]

16.6 CHEMOTHERAPY—TOPOISOMERASE II INHIBITORS

Topoisomerase II inhibitors include podophyllotoxins, anthracyclines, and anthracycline analogs. They cause double-strand breaks in the DNA. Podophyllotoxins such as etoposide (VP-16) are utilized in several solid tumor malignancies as well as leukemias and lymphomas. The IV formulation of etoposide can cause anaphylactic-like reactions with an incidence up to 2%. Contributing factors include higher drug concentration, rate of infusion as well as polysorbate 80 and benzyl alcohol in the IV formulation. Hypotension may occur during a rapid administration of etoposide, and secondary acute leukemias have been reported with therapy. Myelosuppression is a common DLT.[40]

Anthracyclines and anthracycline analogs can increase the risk of myocardial damage, including acute left ventricular failure. This class of chemotherapy agents requires a comprehensive assessment prior to administration including a history and physical examination, screening for cardiovascular disease risk, and baseline cardiac function evaluation through an echocardiogram.[41] The risk of cardiomyopathy is proportional to the drug cumulative exposure and is further increased with concomitant cardiotoxic therapy (e.g., trastuzumab).[42]

16.7 CHEMOTHERAPY—ANTITUMOR ANTIBIOTICS

Dactinomycin binds to DNA and intercalates between base pairs, ultimately inhibiting DNA, RNA, and protein synthesis. It is utilized for the treatment of Ewing sarcoma and gestational trophoblastic neoplasms.[43] Dactinomycin may be prescribed in micrograms, although many regimens list the dose in milligrams (e.g., mg/kg). Special caution should be utilized when prescribing this chemotherapy agent in order to prevent dosing errors.

16.8 CHEMOTHERAPY—*MISCELLANEOUS*

There are several clinical scenarios in oncology which warrant emergent initiation of therapy. Patient-specific factors should always be taken into consideration when evaluating emergent cytotoxic chemotherapy. Hydroxyurea is more commonly utilized for the management of sickle cell disease; however, it has an off-label use for cytoreduction in the setting of acute myeloid leukemia (AML).[44] Timely cytoreduction is crucial in preventing the effects of leukostasis in leukemia patients.[45] All-trans-retinoic acid (ATRA, tretinoin) is an oral retinoic acid derivative utilized for the treatment of acute promyelocytic leukemia (APL). Induction treatment of APL with ATRA should be initiated early, and therapy should be discontinued if pending cytogenetic analysis does not confirm t(15;17) translocation or the presence of PMl/RARα fusion protein.[46]

There are two asparagine products currently FDA-approved for the treatment of acute lymphoblastic leukemia (ALL). Dosing and frequency of administration are notably different between these two products and require special attention in order to prevent inadvertent dosing errors. Pegaspargase is an enzyme formulated from a modified version of L-asparaginase, which ultimately leads to the depletion of asparagine in leukemic cells. FDA-approved dosing is 2,000–2,500 units/m^2, administered no more frequently than every 14 days.[47] The asparaginase (*Erwinia*) product is FDA-approved for ALL and can be substituted for pegaspargase at a dose of 25,000 units/m^2 three times weekly (Monday, Wednesday, Friday) for six doses for each planned pegaspargase dose.[48] Both asparagine products require close monitoring for serious hypersensitivity reactions, pancreatitis, and coagulopathies.

16.9 TARGETED THERAPY

16.9.1 Infusion-Related Reactions (IRRs)

Many cancer therapies have infusion-related reactions, ranging from hypersensitivity reactions to cytokine-release syndrome. Monoclonal antibodies specifically can have varying incidence of hypersensitivity reactions depending on the proportion of source protein from mouse versus human. Mild and moderate reactions typically exhibit chills, rash, flushing, fever, and shortness of breath. Severe reactions are less common but can present as anaphylaxis, hypotension, and bronchospasm and have the potential to result in death.[49,50,51]

16.9.2 Immunotherapy (Immune Checkpoint Inhibitors)

Immune checkpoint inhibitors (ICIs) include programmed death-1 (PD-1) inhibitors such as pembrolizumab, nivolumab, and cemiplimab; programmed death-ligand 1 (PD-L1) inhibitors such as atezolizumab, avelumab, and durvalumab; and the CTLA-4 inhibitor (cytotoxic T-lymphocyte-associated protein 4) ipilimumab. Checkpoint inhibitor-based immunotherapy toxicities can be divided into three categories: Infusion reactions, immune-related adverse reactions (irAEs), and adverse events of special interest (AEoSI). The skin, colon, endocrine organs, liver, and lungs are the organs most frequently affected by irAEs.[52]

16.9.2.1 Infusion-Related Reactions

Most infusion-related reactions are mild and are typically associated with low-grade fever, chills, headaches, or nausea. Severe reactions are reported in less than 1% of patients. Infusion-related reactions have most commonly been reported with avelumab with any-grade reactions occurring in 25% of patients. The National Comprehensive Cancer Network (NCCN) guidelines recommend that clinicians reference each product's prescribing information for premedication recommendations.[53] Mild reactions are generally transient and do not require therapy interruption or any other interventions. Moderate reactions are generally managed by holding the infusion or slowing down the rate of infusion per institutional guidelines. Treatment with antihistamines, acetaminophen, nonsteroidal anti-inflammatory drugs (NSAIDs), narcotics, or intravenous (IV) fluids may be utilized but typically are not required for longer than a 24-hour period. Severe reactions require urgent management and permanent discontinuation of the ICI.

16.9.2.2 Immune-Related Adverse Events (irAEs)

Successful management of irAEs begins with toxicity recognition and grading. Clinicians are encouraged to reference national or institution-specific clinical guidelines in order to determine when holding immunotherapy may be an appropriate management option for irAEs.[54,55] Early recognition of symptoms is crucial for prompt intervention and treatment; hence, patient counseling in regard to symptom recognition is important prior to ICI therapy initiation. Immunosuppression with corticosteroids is the mainstay of therapy with the exception of select endocrine irAEs which may be managed with hormonal supplementation.[56] Dosing for systemic steroids such as prednisone or methylprednisolone depends on the toxicity grade/severity and can range between 0.5 to 2 mg/kg/day. Myocarditis is a rare but potentially severe ICI adverse event. Its symptoms are nonspecific, and its management requires pulse-dose methylprednisolone administration at 1,000-mg IV daily for 3–5 days. Additional immunosuppression may be required for severe irAEs not responding to initial corticosteroid therapy within 48 to 72 hours. Consultation with any appropriate and relevant medical specialist is recommended at this point. Tumor necrosis factor (TNF) inhibitors such as infliximab can be utilized in steroid-refractory cases by means of targeting and inhibiting pro-inflammatory cytokines (IL-1 and IL-6).[57] These agents are particularly effective for immune-mediated colitis and inflammatory arthritis. The duration of therapy is not well defined in the setting of irAEs but is typically one single dose. Vedolizumab is a monoclonal antibody which binds and inhibits the interaction of $\alpha 4\beta 7$ integrin with MAdCAM-1 (mucosal addressin cell adhesion molecule-1). Mycophenolic acid and mycophenolate mofetil (MMF) are immunosuppressive agents which decrease the proliferation of B- and T-cells, induce T-cell apoptosis, and suppress dendritic cells and IL-1. These agents have been utilized in steroid-refractory irAEs involving the liver, kidney, pancreas, and eyes.[58] Intravenous immunoglobulin (IVIG), with its immunomodulatory mechanism, can be utilized to manage neurologic inflammatory or autoimmune conditions.[59] Plasmapheresis or IVIG may be considered for severe or steroid-refractory neurological irAEs.[60,61,62] Additional therapies cited in the NCCN guidelines include rituximab, tacrolimus, tocilizumab, cyclosporine, cyclophosphamide, methotrexate, and antirheumatic agents.[63,64,65]

16.10 TUMOR LYSIS SYNDROME

Tumor lysis syndrome (TLS) is considered an oncologic emergency and is the most common disease-related emergency faced by providers caring for adults and children with hematologic cancers.[66] TLS can have laboratory and/or clinical manifestations, but the key is typically preventing TLS rather than treating it, especially preventing clinical manifestations. These clinical manifestations can include renal insufficiency, cardiac arrhythmias, and seizures and can even lead to death if multiorgan failure occurs. The risk of TLS is also impacted by the size of the cancer mass as well as specific cancers that have a high potential for TLS, typically due to rapid proliferation of the cancer. High-grade lymphomas and acute leukemias tend to have a higher risk for TLS. Highly effective treatment therapies can also increase the risk for TLS. This is why some medications noted to have higher risk of TLS in specific disease states include recommendations for dose escalation and monitoring to mediate and monitor those at higher risk.[67]

There are cases of litigation related to clinical TLS, specifically when TLS led to death.[68] Therefore, the monitoring and management of laboratory TLS to mitigate the risk of developing clinical TLS are paramount. Intravascular expansion with fluids and the oral agent allopurinol are key components to prophylaxis. Other options for the management of laboratory TLS are available for the specific electrolytes (potassium, phosphorus, and calcium) affected by TLS. These include medications or procedures to treat hyperkalemia, such as oral sodium polystyrene sulfonate and hemodialysis, respectively. Hypocalcemia can lead to cardiac arrhythmias, and the management of phosphorus levels can aid in preventing hypocalcemia as well as supplementation with calcium replacement. Additionally, in 2009, a medication called rasburicase was approved by the FDA as a form of "treatment" for the hyperuricemia component associated with TLS.[69] Rasburicase is a recombinant form of the enzyme urate oxidase, and it works by breaking down circulating uric acid into the more soluble by-product, allantoin, so that it can be easily excreted by the kidneys.

Many institutions have developed protocols for the prevention and management of TLS as it can occur during the diagnosis of some cancers as well. This risk mitigation strategy is helpful as these types of patients may be seen by generalists prior to referral to oncologists. Specifically, it helps provide guidance for specific labs to monitor, the frequency of monitoring, and risk factors that can lead to an increased risk of TLS. It also can provide supportive care strategies that can help decrease the risk of TLS prior to patients starting anticancer therapy.

16.11 HEPATOTOXICITY

Chemotherapy-induced hepatotoxicity occurs frequently, and the clinical presentation can greatly vary from asymptomatic increase of liver chemistries, cholestatic hepatitis, fibrosis and cirrhosis, sinusoidal obstruction syndrome (SOS), to fulminant hepatic failure.[70] SOS, formerly known as veno-occlusive disease (VOD), is a serious and potentially life-threatening complication and results from damage to the sinusoidal endothelium. The following signs and symptoms should be closely monitored in order to identify SOS promptly: Rapid weight gain, ascites, hepatomegaly, and bilirubin/transaminase elevations.[71] SOS treatment should be conducted according to the guidelines from the British Committee for Standards in Hematology (BCHS) and the British Society for Blood and Marrow Transplantation (BSCMT) as well as the European Society for Blood and Marrow Transplantation (EBMT) recommendations.[72,73] SOS treatment must be initiated as soon as possible, with fluid and sodium balance and careful diuretic utilization, and patients should be evaluated for defibrotide therapy.

Busulfan is an alkylating agent, and high area under the curve (AUC) concentrations versus time curve values are associated with an increased risk of SOS. This toxicity is often encountered in the hematopoietic stem cell transplant (HSCT) setting. Oral busulfan doses above 16 mg/kg and concurrent use with alkylating agents may increase the risk of SOS. Transplant centers routinely utilize busulfan pharmacokinetic-based dosing in order to decrease the risk of SOS.[74] Notable drug interactions which can alter busulfan concentrations include but are not limited to the following: Azole antifungals, phenytoin, acetaminophen, and metronidazole.[75]

Gemtuzumab ozogamicin (GO) is an anti-CD33 antibody drug conjugate utilized for the treatment of CD33-positive AML. GO has US boxed warning alerts for hepatotoxicity, including severe or fatal SOS, especially after HSCT.[76] GO originally received an accelerated approval in 2000; however, due to safety concerns, it was voluntarily pulled front the US market in 2011. GO has subsequently come back on the market at a lower dose. Monitor frequently for signs and symptoms of SOS and other serious adverse events which include myelosuppression, infusion-related reaction, and TLS.

Inotuzumab ozogamicin (InO) is an anti-CD22 antibody drug conjugate utilized for the treatment of B-cell acute lymphoblastic leukemia (B-cell ALL).[77,78] InO has US boxed warning alerts for SOS, myelosuppression, infusion-related reactions, infections, and QT prolongation. An expert panel concluded that patients receiving InO who proceed to HCT are at a high risk of developing VOD, up to approximately 20%.[79]

16.12 CONCLUSIONS

In general, many medications have inherent risks for adverse events. Some adverse events are potentially preventable (partially or fully), and some are not. We hope this chapter helps to outline some of the key areas where adverse events may be potentially mitigated. While many of the earlier comments are related specifically to drug administration or the mechanism of action of the medication, there are technology-related tools that can also aid with providing process prompts to help mitigate some of these risk factors. Order sets and panels are a great tool for including labs, monitoring parameters, and even medications with defaulted doses to help for various work-ups and diagnostics. For example, a common error with neutropenic fever management is the selection of the initial antibiotic, even more so when the patient has documentation of an allergy to an antibiotic. An order set specific for neutropenic fever can provide guidance on a multitude of areas to help select the most appropriate therapy. Some such ideas include a hyperlink to the institutional and/or national guidelines for treatment, recommendations for clarification of the allergy or how to contact pharmacy to help with drug selection with a specific allergy, and then panels of medications to select depending on the signs and symptoms the patient is presenting to determine if monotherapy or multidrug therapy is most appropriate empirically.

NOTES

1 Weingart SN, Zhang L, Sweeney M, Hassett M. Drug safety in oncology: Chemotherapy medication errors. Lancet Oncol. 2018;19:e191–e199.
2 Lipitz-Snyderman A, Pfister D, Classen D, Atoria CL, Killen A, Epstein AS, Anderson C, Fortier E, Weingart SN. Preventable and mitigable adverse events in cancer care: Measuring risk and harm across the Continuum. Cancer. 2017;123:4728–4736.
3 Institute for Safe Medication Practices (ISMP). *ISMP Targeted Medication Safety Best Practices for Hospitals*; 2020. https://www.ismp.org/guidelines/best-practices-hospitals.
4 Dyer C. Doctor sentenced for manslaughter of leukaemia patient. BMJ. 2003;327:123.
5 Bren L. Frances Oldham Kelsey. FDA medical reviewer leaves her mark on history. FDA Consum. 2001;35(2):24–29.
6 Kuehn BM. Frances Kelsey honored for FDA legacy. JAMA. 2010;304(19):2109–2112.
7 Methotrexate. *Lexi-Drugs Online* [database on the Internet]. Hudson, OH: Lexicomp, Inc.; 2016. Updated 25 Dec 2020; cited 28 Dec 2020. http://online.lexi.com. Subscription required to view.
8 Howard SC, McCormick J, Pui CH, Buddington RK, Harvey RD. Preventing and managing toxicities of high-dose methotrexate. Oncologist. 2016;21(12):1471–1482.
9 Methotrexate. *Lexi-Drugs Online* [database on the Internet]. Hudson, OH: Lexicomp, Inc.; 2016. Updated 25 Dec 2020; cited 28 Dec 2020. http://online.lexi.com. Subscription required to view.
10 Methotrexate. *Lexi-Drugs Online* [database on the Internet]. Hudson, OH: Lexicomp, Inc.; 2016. Updated 25 Dec 2020; cited 28 Dec 2020. http://online.lexi.com. Subscription required to view.
11 *Folotyn (Pralatrexate)* [Prescribing Information]. East Windsor, NJ: Acrotech Biopharma LLC; September 2020.
12 *Alimta (Pemetrexed)* [Prescribing Information]. Indianapolis, IN: Eli Lilly and Company; January 2019.
13 *Mercaptopurine Tablets* [Prescribing Information]. Spring Valley, NY: Par Pharmaceuticals; May 2012.
14 Relling MV, Schwab M, Whirl-Carrillo M, Suarez-Kurtz G, Pui CH, Stein CM, Moyer AM, Evans WE, Klein TE, Antillon-Klussmann FG, Caudle KE. Clinical Pharmacogenetics Implementation Consortium guideline for thiopurine dosing based on TPMT and NUDT15 genotypes: 2018 update. Clin Pharmacol Ther. 2019;105(5):1095–1105.
15 *Mercaptopurine Tablets* [Prescribing Information]. Spring Valley, NY: Par Pharmaceuticals; May 2012.
16 *Adrucil (Fluorouracil Injection)* [Prescribing Information]. North Wales, PA: Teva Pharmaceuticals Inc; October 2017.
17 Bamat MK, Tremmel R, von Borstel R, Helton J. Clinical experience with uridine triacetate for 5-FU overexposure: An update [abstract e20592 from 2013 ASCO Annual Meeting]. J Clin Oncol. 2013;31(18s):e20592.
18 von Borstel R, O'Neil J, Bamat M. Vistonuridine: An orally administered, life-saving antidote for 5-fluorouracil (5FU) overdose. J Clin Oncol. 2009;27(15S):9616 [abstract 9616 from 2009 ASCO Annual Meeting].
19 ISMP Canada. *Fluorouracil Incident Root Cause Analysis*; April 30, 2007.
20 *Cytarabine* [Prescribing Information]. Lake Forest, IL: Hospira; June 2018.Grissinger M. Severe harm and death associated with errors and drug interactions involving low-dose methotrexate. PT. 2018;43:191–192. PMID: 29622936.
21 Institute for Safe Medication Practices (ISMP). *FDA Removes Syringe Administration From Vincristine Labeling*. ISMP Medication Safety Alert!Acute Care Edition; 2020:25(12). https://www.ismp.org/acute-care/medication-safety-alert-june-18-2020.
22 Institute for Safe Medication Practices (ISMP). *ISMP Calls on FDA: No More Syringes for Vinca Alkaloids*. ISMP Medication Safety Alert!Acute Care Edition; 2019:24(5). https://www.ismp.org/acute-care/medication-safety-alert-march-14-2019.
23 Jacobson JO, Polovich M, McNiff KK, LeFebvre KB, Cummings C, Galioto M, Bonelli KR, McCorkle MR. American Society of Clinical Oncology/Oncology nursing society chemotherapy administration safety standards. J Clin Oncol. 2009;27(32):5469–5475.
24 *Vincristine Sulfate* [Prescribing Information]. Lake Forest, IL: Hospira Inc; May 2020.
25 Moriyama B, Henning SA, Leung J, Falade-Nwulia O, Jarosinski P, Penzak SR, Walsh TJ. Adverse interactions between antifungal azoles and vincristine: Review and analysis of cases. Mycoses. 2012 Jul;55(4):290–297.
26 Galiana GE, García HB, Ferrándiz CL, Cervera Grau JM. Paralytic ileus due to vinorelbine. Clin Transl Oncol. 2005 May;7(4):169–170.
27 Gelderblom H, Verweij J, Nooter K, Sparreboom A. Cremophor EL. The drawbacks and advantages of vehicle selection for drug formulation. Eur J Cancer. 2001 Sep;37(13):1590–1598.
28 *Taxol (Paclitaxel)* [Prescribing Information]. Princeton, NJ: Bristol-Myers Squibb Company; April 2011.
29 *Cyclophosphamide Injection, Multi-Dose Vial* [Prescribing Information]. Orlando, FL: Ingenus Pharmaceuticals; July 2020.

30 *Ifosfamide* [Prescribing Information]. North Wales, PA: Teva Pharmaceuticals USA, Inc; December 2015.
31 *Mesnex (Mesna)* [Prescribing Information]. Deerfield, IL: Baxter Healthcare Corporation; December 2018.
32 *Cyclophosphamide Injection, Multi-Dose Vial* [Prescribing Information]. Orlando, FL: Ingenus Pharmaceuticals; July 2020.
33 *Temodar (Temozolomide)* [Prescribing Information]. Whitehouse Station, NJ: Merck & Co Inc; November 2019.
34 Letarte N, Gabay MP, Bressler LR, Long KE, Stachnik JM, Villano JL. Analyzing temozolomide medication errors: Potentially fatal. J Neurooncol. 2014;120(1):111–115. doi:10.1007/s11060-014-1523-1.
35 *Cisplatin Solution for Injection* [Prescribing Information]. Schaumburg, IL: Athenex; June 2017.
36 *Carboplatin* [Prescribing Information]. Orlando, FL: Ingenus Pharmaceuticals; August 2017.
37 Tollkuci E, Chalmers A, Schultz K, Basu S, Dewdney S, Usha L. Clinical outcomes using carboplatin desensitizations in patients with gynecologic cancer. J Hematol Oncol Pharm. 2020;10(2):65–72.
38 *Camptosar (Irinotecan)* [Prescribing Information]. New York, NY: Pharmacia & Upjohn Co; January 2020.
39 Stein A, Voigt W, Jordan K. Chemotherapy-induced diarrhea: Pathophysiology, frequency and guideline-based management. Ther Adv Med Oncol. 2010;2(1):51–63.
40 *Etoposide Injection* [Prescribing Information]. Eatontown, NJ: Hikma Pharmaceuticals USA Inc, August 2019.
41 Armenian S, Bhatia S. *Predicting and Preventing Anthracycline-Related Cardiotoxicity.* American Society of Clinical Oncology Educational Book; 2018 May 23;38:3–12.
42 *Doxorubicin* [Prescribing Information]. New York, NY: Pfizer Labs; March 2020.
43 *Cosmegen (Dactinomycin)* [Prescribing Information]. Lebanon, NJ: Recordati Rare Diseases Inc; August 2018.
44 Döhner H, Estey EH, Amadori S, Appelbaum FR, Büchner T, Burnett AK, Dombret H, Fenaux P, Grimwade D, Larson RA, Lo-Coco F. Diagnosis and management of acute myeloid leukemia in adults: Recommendations from an international expert panel, on behalf of the European LeukemiaNet. Blood. 2010;115(3):453–474.
45 Grund FM, Armitage JO, Burns P. Hydroxyurea in the prevention of the effects of leukostasis in acute leukemia. Arch Intern Med. 1977;137(9):1246–1247.
46 *Tretinoin* [Prescribing Information]. North Wales, PA: Teva Pharmaceuticals USA Inc; October 2015.
47 *Oncaspar (Pegaspargase)* [Prescribing Information]. Boston, MA: Servier Pharmaceuticals LLC; June 2020.
48 *Erwinaze (Asparaginase)* [Prescribing Information]. Palo Alto, CA: Jazz Pharmaceuticals; December 2019.
49 CTCAE 4.3.
50 Roumbouts MD, Swart EL, Van Den Eertwegh AJM, Crul M. Systematic review on infusion reactions to and infusion rate of monoclonal antibodies used in cancer treatment. Anticancer Res. 2020;40:1201–1218.
51 Chung CH. Managing premedications and the risk for reactions to infusional monoclonal antibody therapy. Oncologist. 2008;13:725–732.
52 Haanen JB, Carbonnel F, Robert C, Kerr KM, Peters S, Larkin J, Jordan K, ESMO Guidelines Committee. Management of toxicities from immunotherapy: ESMO Clinical Practice Guidelines for diagnosis, treatment and follow-up [published correction appears in Ann Oncol. 2018 Oct 1;29(Suppl 4):iv264–iv266]. Ann Oncol. 2017;28(suppl 4):iv119–iv142.
53 National Comprehensive Cancer Network. Management of immunotherapy-related toxicities (version 1.2020). https://www.nccn.org/professionals/physician_gls/pdf/immunotherapy.pdf (Accessed January 12, 2021).
54 National Comprehensive Cancer Network. Management of immunotherapy-related toxicities (version 1.2020). https://www.nccn.org/professionals/physician_gls/pdf/immunotherapy.pdf (Accessed January 12, 2021).
55 Postow MA, Sidlow R, Hellmann MD. Immune-related adverse events associated with immune checkpoint blockade. N Engl J Med. 2018 Jan;378(2):158–168.
56 National Comprehensive Cancer Network. Management of immunotherapy-related toxicities (version 1.2020). https://www.nccn.org/professionals/physician_gls/pdf/immunotherapy.pdf (Accessed January 12, 2021).
57 Wolfe RM, Ang DC. Biologic therapies for autoimmune and connective tissue diseases. Immunol Allergy Clin North Am. 2017;37:283–299.
58 National Comprehensive Cancer Network. Management of immunotherapy-related toxicities (version 1.2020). https://www.nccn.org/professionals/physician_gls/pdf/immunotherapy.pdf (Accessed January 12, 2021).
59 National Comprehensive Cancer Network. Management of immunotherapy-related toxicities (version 1.2020). https://www.nccn.org/professionals/physician_gls/pdf/immunotherapy.pdf (Accessed January 12, 2021).
60 Fellner A, Makranz C, Lotem M, Bokstein F, Taliansky A, Rosenberg S, Blumenthal DT, Mandel J, Fichman S, Kogan E, Steiner I. Neurologic complications of immune checkpoint inhibitors. J Neurooncol. 2018;137(3):601–609.
61 Brahmer JR, Lacchetti C, Schneider BJ, Atkins MB, Brassil KJ, Caterino JM, Chau I, Ernstoff MS, Gardner JM, Ginex P, Hallmeyer S. Management of immune-related adverse events in patients treated with immune checkpoint inhibitor therapy: American Society of Clinical Oncology Clinical Practice guideline. J Clin Oncol. 2018;36(17):1714–1768.
62 Stroud CR, Hegde A, Cherry C, Naqash AR, Sharma N, Addepalli S, Cherukuri S, Parent T, Hardin J, Walker P. Tocilizumab for the management of immune mediated adverse events secondary to PD-1 blockade. J Oncol Pharm Pract. 2019;25(3):551–557.

63 National Comprehensive Cancer Network. Management of immunotherapy-related toxicities (version 1.2020). https://www.nccn.org/professionals/physician_gls/pdf/immunotherapy.pdf (Accessed January 12, 2021).
64 Stroud CR, Hegde A, Cherry C, Naqash AR, Sharma N, Addepalli S, Cherukuri S, Parent T, Hardin J, Walker P. Tocilizumab for the management of immune mediated adverse events secondary to PD-1 blockade. J Oncol Pharm Pract. 2019;25(3):551–557.
65 Naidoo J, Page DB, Li BT, Connell LC, Schindler K, Lacouture ME, Postow MA, Wolchok JD. Toxicities of the anti-PD-1 and anti-PD-L1 immune checkpoint antibodies [published correction appears in Ann Oncol. 2016 Jul;27(7):1362]. Ann Oncol. 2015;26(12):2375–2391. doi:10.1093/annonc/mdv383.
66 Howard SC, Jones DP, Pui C-H. The tumor lysis syndrome. N Engl J Med. 2011;364:1844–1854.
67 *Venclexta (Venetoclax)* [Prescribing Information]. North Chicago, IL: Abbvie Inc; November 2020.
68 Martasin v Hilton Head Health System. State of South Carolina: Court of appeals. Case Number 3984. https://www.sccourts.org/opinions/displayOpinion.cfm?caseNo=3984 (Accessed March 27, 2021).
69 FDA approves Elitek (rasburicase) for management of plasma uric acid levels in adults with leukemia, lymphoma, and solid tumors receiving anti-cancer therapy. Press Release. October 16, 2019. http://www.news.sanofi.us/press-releases?item=118501 (Accessed March 27, 2021).
70 Grigorian A, O'Brien CB. Hepatotoxicity secondary to chemotherapy. J Clin Transl Hepatol. 2014;2(2):95–102.
71 Cortes JE, de Lima M, Dombret H, Estey EH, Giralt SA, Montesinos P, Röllig C, Venditti A, Wang ES. Prevention, recognition, and management of adverse events associated with gemtuzumab ozogamicin use in acute myeloid leukemia. J Hematol Oncol. 2020;13:137.
72 Mohty M, Malard F, Abecassis M, Aerts E, Alaskar AS, Aljurf M, Arat M, Bader P, Baron F, Bazarbachi A, Blaise D. Sinusoidal obstruction syndrome/veno-occlusive disease: Current situation and perspectives-a position statement from the European Society for Blood and Marrow Transplantation (EBMT). Bone Marrow Transplant. 2015;50(6):781–789.
73 Dignan FL, Wynn RF, Hadzic N, Karani J, Quaglia A, Pagliuca A, Veys P, Potter MN; Haemato-Oncology Task Force of the British Committee for Standards in Haematology and the British Society for Blood and Marrow Transplantation. BCSH/BSBMT guideline: Diagnosis and management of veno-occlusive disease (sinusoidal obstruction syndrome) following haematopoietic stem cell transplantation. Br J Haematol. 2013;163(4):444–457.
74 Madden T, de Lima M, Thapar N, Nguyen J, Roberson S, Couriel D, Pierre B, Shpall EJ, Jones RB, Champlin RE, Andersson BS. Pharmacokinetics of once-daily IV busulfan as part of pretransplantation preparative regimens: A comparison with an every 6-hour dosing schedule. Biol Blood Marrow Transplant. 2007;13(1):56–64.
75 *Busulfex (Busulfan Injection)* [Prescribing Information]. Rockville, MD: Otsuka America Pharmaceutical, Inc; April 2020.
76 *Mylotarg (Gemtuzumab Ozogamicin)* [Prescribing Information]. Philadelphia, PA: Wyeth Pharmaceuticals Inc; June 2020.
77 *Bespona (Inotuzumab Ozogamicin)* [Prescribing Information]. Philadelphia, PA: Wyeth Pharmaceuticals Inc; March 2018.
78 Kantarjian HM, DeAngelo DJ, Stelljes M, Martinelli G, Liedtke M, Stock W, Gökbuget N, O'Brien S, Wang K, Wang T, Paccagnella ML. Inotuzumab ozogamicin versus standard therapy for acute lymphoblastic leukemia. N Engl J Med. 2016;375:740–753.
79 Kebriaei P, Cutler C, De Lima M, Giralt S, Lee SJ, Marks D, Merchant A, Stock W, Van Besien K, Stelljes M. Management of important adverse events associated with inotuzumab ozogamicin: Expert panel review. Bone Marrow Transplant. 2018;53:449–456.

17 Dangers of Opioids

Jennifer Splawski, James T. O'Donnell, and James J. O'Donnell III

SYNOPSIS

DOI: 10.1201/9781003615323-19

17.1 INTRODUCTION

17.1.1 Definitions

There are four chemical classes of opioids,[1] which are presented in Table 17.1.

Tramadol does not fit into one of these standard opioid classes. It is an atypical opioid that is structurally similar to codeine with central GABA, catecholamine, and serotonin activities.

17.1.2 History

A brief history of opium is presented in Table 17.2.

TABLE 17.1
Chemical Classes of Opioids

Class	Compound
Phenanthrenes	Morphine, codeine, hydromorphone, levorphanol, oxycodone, hydrocodone, oxymorphone, buprenorphine, nalbuphine, butorphanol
Benzomorphans	Pentazocine, dezocine
Phenylpiperidines	Fentanyl, alfentanil, sufentanil, meperidine
Diphenylheptanes	Propoxyphene, methadone

TABLE 17.2
Brief History of One of the Most Ancient and Powerful Drugs Known to Humankind[2]

Date	Event
3400 B.C.	The opium poppy is cultivated in lower Mesopotamia. The Sumerians refer to it as Hul Gil, the "joy plant."
1300 B.C.	Opium poppies are grown by ancient Egyptians in the capital city of Thebes.
460 B.C.	Acknowledged by Hippocrates, "the father of medicine."
1527 A.D.	Paracelsus recommends laudanum or black pills made from opium, as a pain killer in European medical literature.
1753	Linnaeus, the father of botany, first classifies the poppy, *Papaver somniferum*, as "sleep-inducing," in his book *Genera Plantarum*.
1803	Friedrich Sertürner of Paderborn, Germany, discovers morphine, by dissolving opium in acid and then neutralizing it with ammonia.
1827	E. Merck & Company of Darmstadt, Germany, begins commercial manufacturing of morphine.
1874	Heroin is first synthesized by English researcher C.R. Wright.
1895	The Bayer Company of Elberfeld, Germany, begins commercial manufacturing of heroin.

17.2 PHARMACOLOGY OF OPIOIDS

17.2.1 Effects

Effects of opioids include analgesia, drowsiness, mood changes, respiratory depression, nausea, vomiting, reduced gastrointestinal (GI) motility, and alteration of endocrine and autonomic nerve systems.[3] Analgesic effects are currently measured using subjective self-assessment pain scales, but more objective methods which correlate pain with brain activity and chemistry are being researched.[4]

17.2.2 Opioid Neural Receptors

17.2.2.1 Central Nervous System Receptors

Central nervous system (CNS) receptors and effects include the following:[1]

1. Mu (μ): analgesia, euphoria, respiratory depression, miosis
2. Kappa (K): analgesia, sedation, respiratory depression, miosis
3. Sigma (s): dysphoria, psychosis
4. Delta (Δ): euphoria, seizures

17.2.2.2 Peripheral Nervous System Receptors

Opioid peripheral nervous system receptors are expressed in the musculoskeletal system, the autonomic ganglia, the submucosal and myenteric plexus of the GI tract, and the adrenal medulla.[5] Importantly, they mediate constipation, a common side effect of opioids that works through opioids' regulation of the GI tract.

17.2.3 Routes of Administration

17.2.3.1 Oral

The oral route is the most common route of administration for opioid medications. The onset of pain relief is not as quick as the intravenous route due to first-pass metabolism.[6] Enteric-coated, sustained- or controlled-release tablets delay drugs from being released from the stomach and therefore are slower to be absorbed.

17.2.3.2 Intramuscular

Intramuscular injections are often given into the deltoid or vastus lateralis muscle and can be extremely painful.[7] This route presents less of an initial delay than oral administration, but the unpredictability of absorption and short peak effect restricts its use.

17.2.3.3 Subcutaneous

Subcutaneous injections are absorbed beneath the skin into the connective tissue. Subcutaneous injection of opioids has equivalent bioavailability to intravenous injections; however, this route of administration is associated with a delayed rise to maximum plasma concentration.[7] Subcutaneous administration may increase the time to analgesia and decrease the risk of bloodstream infections compared to the intravenous route.

17.2.3.4 Intravenous

Medications given via the intravenous route are given through a vein directedly into systemic circulation. This includes bolus injection, continuous infusion, and patient-controlled analgesia: the greater absorption and predictability of this route (compared to those previously mentioned) is offset by a greater risk of sudden allergic reaction and respiratory depression.[6]

17.2.3.5 Transdermal

Medications administered via the transdermal route allow the opioid to be absorbed through the skin. One transdermal medication is the fentanyl patch. The advantages of sustained constant release and ease of application are offset by a long initial delay to a steady state (~15 hours) and a long half-life after removal (~21 hours). This slow decay exacerbates the risk of respiratory depression and should only be used in patients who are opioid tolerant.[6]

17.2.3.6 Sublingual and Buccal

These methods avoid first-pass metabolism and increased onset of action of the medication. Sublingual administration is placing the medication underneath the tongue, whereas buccal administration is placing the medication inside the cheek to be absorbed.

17.2.3.7 Neuraxial

This route, which includes epidural and intrathecal administration, has the advantage of a strong effect and long duration with a relatively small dose. Medications are administered in the subarachnoid or epidural space to produce analgesia. Caution must be exercised to avoid synergistic effects with other opioids and drugs.[6] Anesthesia may also be administered via this route.

17.2.4 Metabolism

Many adverse effects and therapeutic effects are related to opioid metabolites. Most opioids are metabolized by glucuronidation or by the cytochrome P450 (CYP450) system in the liver. Metabolism is determined by genetic makeup, gender, age, as well as diet and concurrent medications and disease states.[1,8]

17.2.5 Excretion

Most opioids are excreted as metabolites via the kidneys.[1] Individuals with renal dysfunction may exhibit toxicity of accumulated active opioid metabolites.

17.3 TOXICITY OF OPIOIDS

17.3.1 Respiratory Depression

Respiratory depression, a potentially fatal condition, results from the presence of μ-opioid receptors in the ventrolateral medulla.[9] The μ-opioid receptors cause a medullary diminished response to hypercarbia and a decreased response to hypoxia. Therefore, there is a decreased stimulus to breathe by the patient, causing apnea.

17.3.2 Symptoms of Overdose

Symptoms of opioid overdose include the following:[10]

- Coma
- Miosis (pinpoint pupils)
- Respiratory depression, shallow breathing, hypopnea, and bradypnea
- Altered mental states, unresponsiveness
- Hypotension
- Pulmonary edema
- Fresh track marks
- Euphoria
- Nausea/vomiting

17.4 EPIDEMIOLOGY OF OPIOID ABUSE

In a 2012 National Health Interview study, 11.2% of adults reported having daily pain.[11] From 2007 to 2012, opioid prescriptions increased by 7.3% per capita. These rates were more common in family practice, general medicine, and internal medicine, compared to other specialties. Prescribers have become more cautious in their opioid prescribing practices. The overall opioid prescribing rate in the United States peaked and leveled off from 2010 to 2012 and has been declining since 2012, however the number of opioids in morphine milligram equivalents (MME) prescribed per person is still approximately the same and 16% of patients receiving >1-week opioid supply of drug. [12] For every 100 Americans, there are still almost 58 opioid prescriptions written in 2017. Per the Centers for Disease Control (CDC), higher-prescribing counties have the following characteristics: [13]

- Generally smaller cities or larger towns
- Higher percentage of white residents
- Higher number of dentists and primary care physicians per capita
- More people who are uninsured or unemployed
- More residents who have diabetes, arthritis, or a disability

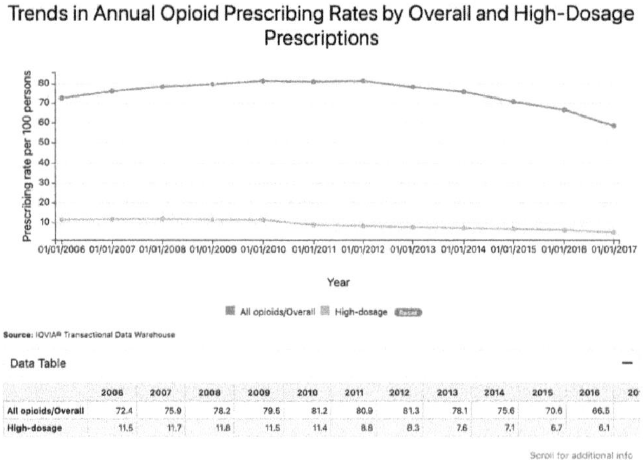

	2006	2007	2008	2009	2010	2011	2012	2013	2014	2015	2016	20
All opioids/Overall	72.4	75.9	78.2	79.5	81.2	80.9	81.3	78.1	75.6	70.6	66.5	
High-dosage	11.5	11.7	11.8	11.5	11.4	8.8	8.3	7.6	7.1	6.7	6.1	

FIGURE 17.1 Trends in Annual Opioid Prescribing Rates by Overall and High-Dosage Prescriptions.

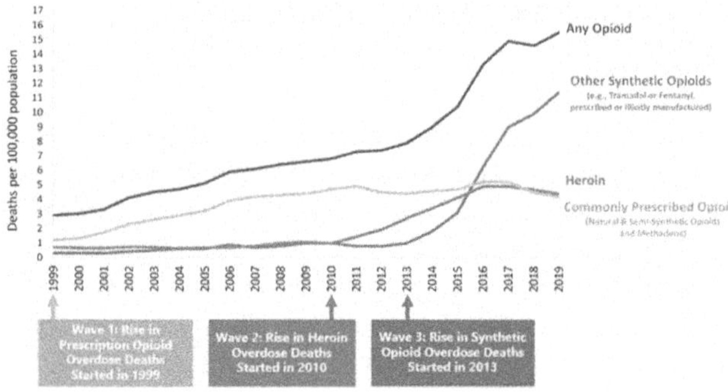

FIGURE 17.2 Three Waves of the Rise in Opioid Overdose Deaths.

Source: National Vital Statistics System Mortality File.

Deaths from drug overdose continue to be a public health burden in the United States. The age-adjusted rate of drug overdose deaths increased from 1999 through 2017.[14] The age-adjusted rate of drug overdose deaths in 2019 (21.6 per 100,000) was higher than in 2018 (20.7). Data from CDC's National Center for Health Statistics indicate that there were an estimated 100,306 drug overdose deaths in the United States during the 12-month period ending in April 2021, an increase of 28.5% from the 78,056 deaths during the same period the year before.[15] Figure 17.2 demonstrates the three waves of opioid overdose deaths.

17.4.1 Opioid Abuse in Adolescents and Young Adults

A retrospective analysis was completed on the prevalence of opioid use, misuse, use disorder, and additional substance use in adolescents and young adults (ages 12–25) from 2015 to 2016 by the National Survey on Drug Use and Health.[16] This study found that 32.8 million individuals (27.5% of the respondents) used prescription opioids in the previous year. The prevalence of opioid misuse was reported at 3.8% of adolescents and 7.8% of young adults. Individuals who reported misusing opioids received them free from a friend or relative or from a single prescriber. These individuals who reported misuse also reported a high prevalence of use of other substances such as cocaine, hallucinogens, inhalants, and heroin.

An extensive review article was published in 2020 outlining prescription opioid misuse in adolescents and emerging adults.[17] It found that the annual national prevalence of prescription opioid misuse ranges from 4.8% to 7.5% for adolescents and 7.6% to 13.2% for emerging adults. Although prevalence rates vary, the study reports that 1 in 20 adolescents and 1 in 10 emerging adults currently report misuse. The heightened risk for morbidity and mortality is reflected in the rise in deaths from opioid poisoning deaths among this population. Opioid poisoning hospitalizations related to suicide between the ages of 15 and 19 increased between 1997 and 2012.

17.4.2 Opioids in Pregnancy

A 2015 MMWR report focused on opioid birth defects, indicating that opioids may cause birth defects such as neural tube defects, gastroschisis, and congenital heart defects, especially in the first few weeks of pregnancy when the woman may not be aware she is pregnant.[18] Hence, greater care must be given to prescribing opioids to women of reproductive age. Additionally, variability in outpatient prescription claims across insurance type, race, and geographical location suggests that over-prescription of opioids may affect certain groups disproportionately. Between 2008 and 2012 opioid prescription rates were consistently higher in the Medicaid population (39.4%) compared to privately insured women (27.7%) ($p < 0.001$). This is alarming because 50% of births are to females on Medicaid. Additional variability that was observed was that among privately insured women, opioid prescriptions were highest in the south, and for Medicaid-enrolled women opioid claims were highest among non-Hispanic whites ($p < 0.001$). To avoid birth defects, it is recommended to prescribe alternative pain medications to women of reproductive age.

An MMWR report from 2018 showed that the prevalence of opioid use disorder (OUD) in the United States among pregnant women at hospital delivery was estimated to have increased from 1.5 to 6.5 cases per 1,000 deliveries from 1999 to 2014.[19] This trend was observed in all 28 states that provided data. These rates are consistent with the increase in neonatal abstinence syndrome and the rates of OUD across the country.

17.5 CONTRIBUTIONS TO THE OPIOID EPIDEMIC

17.5.1 Opiates Handed Out Like Candy to "Doped-Up" Veterans

In 2009, a Veteran's Affairs (VA) Hospital in Tomah, Wisconsin, was given the nickname "Candyland" due to the skyrocketing amount of opioid painkillers prescribed.[20] Dr. David Houlihan, a psychiatrist, was the chief of staff for over a decade and one of the top prescribers. Between 2004 and 2012, the number of opioids prescribed in the Tomah VA quintupled and was ignored by the federal government.

Police reports and court records detail that veterans were repeatedly caught with drugs on hospital grounds and were selling recently filled opioid prescriptions while addicts preyed on other patients and hospital workers. Employees at the Tomah VA were reported to have called the 911 emergency line >2,000 times in the past five years to ask police for help in cases involving battery and burglary, attempted kidnapping, and unexpected deaths.

Current and former employees also tried to raise complaints to superiors. Employees reached out to their congressmen and senators, filed whistleblower complaints, and sent emails directly with VA Secretary, Robert McDonald. When a nursing assistant raised complaints to Dr. Houlihan's boss, she was laughed at.

The problems at this rural medical center underscore the difficulty the VA had maintaining standards of quality patient care even after a national scandal forced VA Secretary Eric Shinseki to resign in May 2014.

17.5.2 United States Reaches $22 Million Settlement Agreement with CVS for Unlawful Distribution of Controlled Substances

In 2015, CVS Health agreed to pay $22 million to resolve allegations that two of its stores in Stanford, Florida, distributed controlled substances based on prescriptions that had not been issued for legitimate medical purposes by a healthcare provider acting in the usual course of professional practice.[21]

This settlement was part of the Drug Enforcement Agency's (DEA) crackdown on pill mills in Florida. Prescription drug addicts were traveling to Florida to access physicians and pharmacies that would fill prescriptions for controlled substances without regard to medical need. The DEA licenses of both stores were revoked in 2012.

This settlement illustrates the U.S. Attorney's Office's efforts to address the wrongdoing that occurred at the height of Florida's pill mill crisis.

17.5.3 Former Walmart Pharmacists Say Company Ignored Red Flags as Opioid Sales Boomed

In rural Michigan, Ashwani Sheoran, a pharmacist for Walmart, would see patients line up for opioid refills at his Walmart store prior to opening. He kept seeing what the DEA considers "red flags." Patients were driving long distances to buy their pills from Walmart. They could not explain why they needed such powerful opioid doses. As he moved from store to store, he would see other red flags—for example, prescriptions were not filled out properly or physician signatures sometimes appeared to be printed by a computer. When he tried to reach physicians to find out what was happening, he often couldn't get them on the phone. He would send emails to his supervisor in Michigan and headquarters in Arkansas, alerting them that Walmart was feeding into the black market of prescription opioid sales.

The pharmacist was told to keep quiet, and his employment was threatened. He was told not to report to the DEA. He did report this behavior to the local police as well as the DEA. He was later suspended from Walmart and ultimately fired.

On December 22, 2020, internal company documents were made public as part of a Justice Department lawsuit against Walmart, showing pharmacists all over the country warned Walmart executives about opioid sales that appeared unsafe. Former employees told National Public Radio that they were pressured into filling opioid prescriptions and to not ask many questions.

From 2006 to 2012, as the prescription opioid crisis exploded, Walmart's distribution network shipped more than five billion opioid pills for sale at Walmart and Sam's Club pharmacies. Walmart had the ability and the means to stop the diversion of opioid prescriptions and chose to not do so.

17.5.4 Federal Judge Approves Landmark $8.3 Billion Purdue Pharma Opioid Settlement

In November 2020, Purdue Pharma pleaded guilty to three felony counts of criminal wrongdoing during the opioid crisis.[22] This will lead to an $8.3 billion settlement, and any future profits from opioids will go to fund opioid addiction programs.

In the early 1990s Purdue Pharma aggressively and falsely marketed opioids, which fueled a deadly epidemic which we are still facing. Pharmaceutical representatives were guided to market OxyContin for "moderate to severe" chronic pain.[23] An OxyContin promotional video from 1989 advertised that these medications "don't wear out" and "don't have serious side effects" and encouraged prescribers to use these medications much more than they are now. Purdue Pharma chose physicians to target their marketing of OxyContin by analyzing data on which physicians treated chronic pain. When physicians were concerned about patient addiction, pharmaceutical representatives were told to state this was not a true addiction; it was "pseudo-addiction" or dependence, and the patient was in control. Pseudo-addiction was defined as patients exhibiting similar behaviors to addicts, but their pain was just not controlled. If the patient's pain was adequately controlled (i.e., doses were increased), the behaviors would decrease. Once, in 2007, Purdue pled guilty to this practice but then continued to aggressively market opioids to maximize its profits.[22] In the first four years (1996–2000), profits soared to a billion dollars and grew to three billion over the next decade.[23]

In February 2021, McKinsey & Company reached a $573 million agreement in their role in exacerbating the opioid crisis.[24] The consulting company worked with Purdue to drive high-dose opioid sales. Further, even when the drug maker pled guilty to wrongdoing in 2007, McKinsey advised on how to work together with other opioid manufacturers to ward off the Food and Drug Administration (FDA). In the agreement, $478 million will be used for opioid abuse treatment, prevention, and recovery programs.

17.6 COMBATING THE OPIOID EPIDEMIC

OUD has grown to epidemic proportions in the United States. This section will focus on several ways to battle the opioid epidemic. However, it is not an inclusive effort to review all efforts on how to combat the epidemic.

17.6.1 Prescription Monitoring Programs

A prescription monitoring program (PDMP) is an electronic database that tracks controlled substance prescription prescribing in a state.[25] PDMPs can provide information to healthcare providers about prescribing and patient behaviors that may contribute to the opioid epidemic. This system is useful only if healthcare providers check the system prior to prescribing or filling controlled substance medications. Some states have mandated prescribers to check the system prior to prescribing controlled substances. These databases are also accessed by health departments to track data and follow trends to help make meaningful interventions in the community.

Some states have shown success after the implementation of these systems, with decreases in controlled substance prescribing.[26] However, there are some criticisms of the program. These PDMPs can incorrectly target patients who use controlled substances over long periods of time for legitimate medical purposes. An emergency medicine provider described that he had a chronic pain patient who used a small dose of daily oxycodone to perform her activities of daily living. After switching to a new primary care physician, he reviewed the PDMP and stopped the prescription. The patient started buying oxycodone from friends and on the street and later transitioned to heroin. She ended up homeless, suicidal, and addicted to heroin.

The PDMP is a valuable tool and should be used with caution and in conjunction with a full patient interview and assessment. If the provider is concerned with opioid misuse disorder, this should be a conversation with the patient with proper referrals or treatment, if necessary. Opioids should not be abruptly stopped as this may potentially result in withdrawal and other deleterious outcomes.

17.6.2 Naloxone Dispensing

Naloxone (Narcan®) is an opioid antidote. It works by reversing the effects of opioids and temporarily restoring normal respirations by blocking μ-opioid receptors. Naloxone can be administered by several different routes of administration, including intramuscular, intranasal, intravenous, subcutaneous, endotracheal, and nebulization. Most commonly when distributed to the lay person, it is administered via intramuscular or intranasal route.

Naloxone distribution has helped combat the opioid epidemic and save lives. From 1996 through June 2014, organizations that provide community-based overdose prevention services, including the provision of naloxone to laypersons, recorded more than 26,000 opioid overdose reversals in the United States.[27] A naloxone distribution program in Massachusetts reduced opioid overdose deaths, without increasing opioid use, by an estimated 11% in the 19 communities that implemented the program.[28] Another study showed that states with naloxone access and/or Good Samaritan law showed that opioid overdose deaths decreased by 14% in states after they enacted naloxone access laws.[29]

From 2017 to 2018 naloxone prescriptions have nearly doubled (270,000 to 556,000); however, there is more work to be done. In 2018, Surgeon General Jerome Adams, MD,

MPH, issued an advisory to expand the availability of naloxone and urged more Americans to carry the drug.[30] Expanding awareness of the medication is a key part of the public health response; research shows that when communities are educated about overdose response, overdose deaths decrease in those areas.

The CDC and Health and Human Services recommend that naloxone be distributed in pharmacies via "standing order" such that a prescription is not required. The CDC also recommends that providers offer naloxone prescriptions or medications for those at risk for opioid overdose as a standard of care.

Most states have laws designed to protect healthcare professionals who prescribe and dispense naloxone from civil and criminal liabilities. Similarly, most states have Good Samaritan laws to protect people who administer naloxone or call for help during an opioid overdose emergency.[30,31]

17.6.3 Medication for OUD

Heroin, OxyContin, fentanyl, and other opioids bind to opioid receptors. When an opioid binds to the μ-opioid receptor, two effects are produced: pain relief and pleasure (reward). When a person administers heroin (aka diacetylmorphine), the drug is rapidly metabolized in the blood to 6-acetylmorphine (6-AM) via deacetylation; further metabolism slowly produces morphine. 6-AM and morphine activate the opioid receptors involved in the reward system of the brain. Stimulation of these receptors results in feelings of reward and activates the pleasure pathways due to greater amounts of dopamine. This induces a potent euphoric experience. The large amounts of dopamine and reward system stimulation can lead to addiction seen in heroin drug users.[32]

Medication for opioid use disorder (MOUD) is the substitution of longer-acting or partial agonist alternative opioids which bind to the same μ-opioid receptor but are useful in combating OUD. Two medications are currently being used for OUD: methadone and buprenorphine. This has been shown to save lives and increase recovery rates. These medications have been shown to cut overdose rates by two-thirds, lower HIV and hepatitis C infections, and reduce criminal behavior.[33,34] When using these medications, up to 70% of patients are still in treatment after one year, compared to 6% of patients without using these medications.

17.6.3.1 Buprenorphine

Buprenorphine is a schedule III medication indicated for opioid detoxification, opioid maintenance, and pain management. It can be prescribed for addiction by a qualified prescriber with a DEA license and DATA 2000 waiver. Per waiver requirements, a prescriber may treat 30 patients at one time using buprenorphine.[35]

Buprenorphine is a partial opioid agonist, which can be used in combination with naloxone or as a monotherapy.[36] It can produce mild euphoria or respiratory depression; however, these effects are lower than full agonists such as methadone and heroin. Buprenorphine can lower withdrawal symptoms, lower the potential for misuse, and increase safety in case of overdose.[35] When prescribed for outpatients, it is prescribed in combination with naloxone. If the medication is crushed and snorted or injected, the naloxone acts as an antagonist and blocks the opioid from binding the opioid receptor and thus stops it from triggering the reward system.

17.6.4 Pharmacokinetics

Buprenorphine has poor oral bioavailability and must be given buccally or sublingually to be effective. It is available in sublingual tablets and film strips. The mean time to peak plasma concentration following sublingual administration is one hour, ranging from 30 minutes to 3.5 hours. It is metabolized through the liver by CYP34A. Buprenorphine functions as an inhibitor of CYP2D6 and CYP3A4 and thus may increase the levels of drugs metabolized by either of those enzymes.[36,37]

17.6.5 Adverse Effects

Buprenorphine is well-tolerated and has been shown to have side effects similar to other opioids, however less severe.[35] The most common side effects include constipation, headache, nausea, and urinary retention. More serious adverse effects of buprenorphine include hepatic events. Effects range from elevated transaminase enzymes to hepatic failure. In studies where these adverse effects were shown, many patients had pre-existing liver dysfunction.[35,36] A large post-marketing liver safety study, however, yielded no evidence of liver toxicity.[37] It is still recommended to periodically assess liver function during treatment.

A black box warning for buprenorphine exists due to the potential for serious, life-threatening respiratory depression.[36] The reason for this warning is due to the self-injection of dissolved buprenorphine or the use of buprenorphine and benzodiazepines.[35,36] There have been no reports of significant buprenorphine overdoses when taken sublingually; however, this medication should be used cautiously with patients with concomitant benzodiazepine abuse.

17.6.6 Place in Therapy

Current evidence shows that buprenorphine is better tolerated than methadone but equal in treatment retention.[34,35]

In pregnant patients, the MOTHER trial compared methadone and buprenorphine to determine the relative safety of each in terms of maternal and neonatal outcomes. The trial found that buprenorphine was superior to methadone in terms of briefer length of neonatal abstinence syndrome after birth.[37] Per the 2017 ACOG position statement states that it is the preferred agent in treating OUD in pregnancy and is safer than methadone or medically supervised withdrawal.[34] If pregnant patients are already on methadone maintenance therapy, they should not switch to an alternative therapy,

Buprenorphine has been used for OUD since 1975 and has been shown to be an effective treatment modality for OUD.[37] Despite its longevity, patients across health systems are still not receiving effective medication treatment, and more effort is needed to disseminate knowledge on the treatment of OUD.

A case was highlighted in the *Journal of Hospital Medicine*, entitled "Things We Do for No Reason™: Discontinuing Buprenorphine When Treating Acute Pain."[38] A 40-year-old patient with OUD on buprenorphine/naloxone was admitted to the hospital for incision and drainage of an abscess. The patient reported severe pain after the procedure, and the provider orders a pain regimen including ibuprofen, oral hydromorphone, and intravenous hydromorphone and subsequently discontinues the patient's buprenorphine/naloxone so that her pain regimen could take effect.

One theory of why this is done is fear of "precipitated withdrawal." This can occur when buprenorphine/naloxone is first introduced to a patient. The patient should be in a period of abstinence prior to starting buprenorphine/naloxone. Buprenorphine has a higher affinity to the mu receptor than almost any other opioid. As a result, when a patient has a full agonist bound to the opioid receptor, buprenorphine can replace the full agonist opioid. Since buprenorphine is a partial agonist, replacing the full agonist with buprenorphine results in a lower level of activity, potentially precipitating withdrawal. This effect occurs only when initiating buprenorphine. In addition, patients receiving buprenorphine/naloxone can be exposed to other opioids without precipitated withdrawal from the naloxone component, as naloxone is not absorbed into the systemic circulation via sublingual or buccal administration. The naloxone is present only in the formulation to dissuade intravenous administration of the medication.

Despite buprenorphine's high affinity at the mu receptor, additional receptors remain available for other opioid agonists to bind and activate, providing effective pain relief even in patients using buprenorphine. Patients may need higher doses of opioids for pain control; however, it has been shown that they experience similar pain control, lengths of stay, and functional outcomes when compared to control groups.

A question of the Data 2000 or "X waiver" has come up in this case as well as throughout healthcare systems. If a provider would like to prescribe buprenorphine products for OUD in an outpatient setting an X waiver is needed. A waiver is not needed to prescribe buprenorphine products to hospitalized patients with a primary medical diagnosis.

This practice of holding a patient's buprenorphine/naloxone while hospitalized is not supported by any current practice models. Temporarily discontinuing the MOUD treatment can cause serious risks to the patient such as opioid withdrawal; this can further complicate their hospitalization and, worse, may lead them to relapse when discharged.

17.6.6.1 Methadone

In the 1960s, methadone replaced morphine as the preferred agent to treat heroin withdrawal.[39] Methadone is a long-lasting opioid analgesic which has been used to treat MOUD for 50 years. It prevents withdrawal for 24 to 36 hours, enabling a system where patients can come in for treatment once a day.

17.6.7 Pharmacokinetics

Methadone's distinct pharmacological characteristics necessitate higher precautionary measures than the other opioid therapies. It has both a slow onset of action and a long elimination half-life. The elimination half-life of methadone has a broad range—between 8 and 59 hours—and is longer than the duration of its analgesic action (four to eight hours).[40,41]

Deaths due to cardiac and respiratory threats from methadone have been reported during initiation (onset of treatment) and conversion of chronic pain patients to methadone treatment from treatment with other opioids such as OxyContin. It is important to consider the pharmacokinetics and pharmacodynamics of methadone before converting patients from other opioids to methadone. A degree of vigilance needs to be in place before the onset of treatment conversion to prevent harm to the patient.[42]

Methadone has a greater risk of respiratory depression due to its unique kinetics (long half-life) and efficacy (longer duration of analgesic action) compared to shorter half-life opioids. This means that at the beginning of methadone therapy, methadone can stay present in the body for 15 to 30 hours, and the patient may be taking the drug up to three times a day. In some fatal cases, significant respiratory depression occurred within 48 hours. Methadone also has a large volume of distribution (V_d), which means that it is distributed heavily to extravascular tissues such as the lung, brain, and fat stores. The accumulation in fat stores may cause inadequate analgesia. As dosing is increased for further pain relief, more methadone is distributed to the fat. Once the analgesia wears off and metabolism drives down drug concentration in the blood, the resultant concentration gradient causes methadone to be released from the fat stores and redistributes into the blood. This released methadone can induce a toxic reaction in the brain's respiratory center, representing a continued risk for respiratory depression even after cessation of the drug regimen.

17.6.8 Equianalgesic Dosing

If using methadone for pain, it is important to realize the usual equianalgesic dosing tables are only a guideline. When converting from morphine or oxycodone to methadone, it is likely to underestimate methadone's potency. Previous use of ineffective high doses of morphine sulfate may lead to overestimation of the correct replacement dose of methadone. There is a broad variation in individual responses when transitioning to methadone, and therefore each patient should be evaluated separately. The starting dose should be conservative and dose increments should not be made frequently. Until a stable pattern of effective dosing has been established, frequent monitoring of each patient undergoing a change to methadone is of vital importance.

17.6.9 Drug Interactions

The pharmacology of methadone differs greatly from person to person. The idiosyncrasies of an individual may result in a pharmacological effect that is too small, too strong, or too prolonged after the administration of the same dose of methadone. Methadone is mostly metabolized in the liver by CYP3A4 into an inactive metabolite.[41] The idiosyncratic effects mentioned earlier apply to the activity of CYP3A4 in which varied CYP3A4 enzymes result in differences in methadone bioavailability.

During methadone treatment, other medications may be necessary to treat the co-morbidities of patients with OUD and chronic pain patients. Patients taking combined drug treatments must therefore be carefully monitored. Some potential medication classes known to interact with methadone are antipsychotics, antibiotics, anticonvulsants, and antiretroviral drugs. As an example, antiretroviral medications are CYP3A4 inducers and therefore can decrease the levels of methadone, thereby causing withdrawal symptoms.[41] Patients taking this combination of medications must be carefully monitored, and methadone can be slowly increased as needed for possible withdrawal. However, if the antiretroviral is stopped, it is important to proactively decrease to methadone dose to avoid potential methadone overdose.[42]

Other than pharmacokinetic drug interactions, methadone's additive pharmacodynamic drug interactions result in an increased CNS depressive effect with drugs such as sedatives, benzodiazepines, and alcohol. These interactions result in respiratory depression and sedation. Because methadone can potentiate the effects of alcohol, the two drugs should never be co-administered.[43]

17.6.10 Cardiovascular Effects

QT interval prolongation and cardiac arrhythmias (torsades de pointes) have been observed in patients undergoing methadone treatment. Co-administration with other drugs such as haloperidol, amiodarone, and levofloxacin can increase the risk of these abnormal cardiac occurrences and cause sudden cardiac death. Many of these cases include chronic pain patients being treated with large, multiple doses per day; however, some cases involve patients undergoing treatment for OUD.[44] The FDA has reviewed a number of reports of death and serious side effects such as slowed breathing and dangerous alterations in heartbeat. This may be due to the buildup of methadone to a toxic level in the body if methadone is taken too often. High doses range between 400 and 1000 mg. In these patients, the QT prolongation can occur without any co-administered interacting drugs.[45]

17.6.11 Consequences of Ignorance of Proper Dosing of Methadone

The scientific and pharmacological literature documenting the adverse effects of methadone use is well-established. Figure 17.3, compiled with data extracted from the FDA MedWatch database, presents the outcomes of 4,031 methadone adverse events from Q1 2004 through Q1 2007.

According to the U.S. National Center for Health Statistics, medical examiners listed methadone as a contributor to 3,849 deaths in 2004.[40] That number was up from 790 in 1999. Approximately 82% of those were accidental deaths, and most deaths involved adverse drug interactions with methadone, especially benzodiazepines.

On November 29, 2006, the U.S. FDA issued a Public Health Advisory about methadone.[46] The advisory stated that the FDA had received several reports of death and serious side effects related to methadone use and that they occurred in patients beginning methadone for pain and in patients that had switched to methadone after other potent narcotic pain relievers. The Agency justifiably vocalized caution directed at physicians who were prescribing methadone to patients who are naïve to the drug, emphasizing that methadone should be taken exactly as directed. In many cases, the patient will deviate from the dosing regimen or may simply react poorly to the medication with proper doses. Therefore, as with any strong medication with the potential to be fatal in large doses, methadone must be taken properly and with due care. The accumulation of methadone could potentially reach a level of toxicity if the dose is too high or if the patient's metabolism of the drug is too slow (i.e., CYP3A4 inhibition). A patient who reacted normally after the first few doses could reach high, toxic levels of the drug in their body while taking no more than what was prescribed. For this reason, it is essential to ensure that when sent home, patients and their families are educated about the symptoms characteristic of opioid overdose.

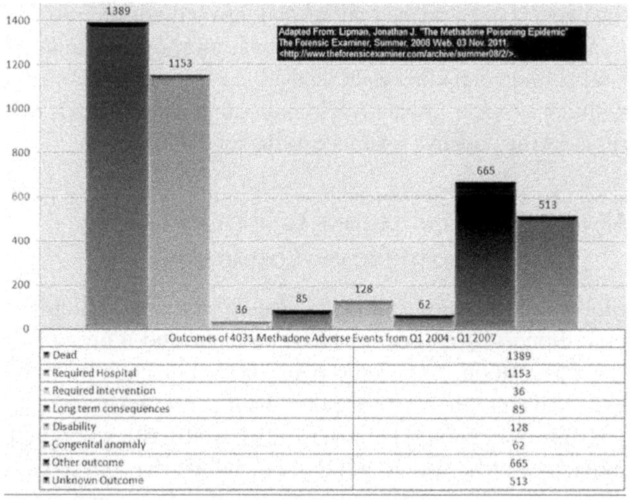

FIGURE 17.3 MedWatch Methadone Adverse Events.

17.6.12 Methadone Legal Case Examples Involving Patient Demise

Patient 1: A 35-year-old mother of two was being treated by a pain management physician in a Midwestern state. She had a long history of low back pain and a laminectomy a few years earlier, which did not seem to improve her condition. Her pain was maintained with OxyContin 20 mg every 12 hours. She complained to her physician that her husband lost his job, and they no longer had health insurance. Her physician then prescribed methadone, 10–15 mg every 8 hours, and the OxyContin was discontinued. The woman and her husband went to a local chain pharmacy to fill the prescription for methadone. He does not recall counseling about the danger of taking methadone and the risk of respiratory depression. She took 15 mg that night, two 10 mg in the morning, 10 mg mid-day, and 15 mg at bedtime. The husband found her unresponsive on the laundry room floor the following morning. EMS was called, and she was declared dead at the scene.

Patient 2: A 35-year-old divorced male schoolteacher and wrestling coach in a southwestern state was seen by a sports medicine specialist. He had complained of chronic lower back pain, and he had been taking hydrocodone/acetaminophen for the pain. The sports specialist was concerned about acetaminophen toxicity and prescribed "low dose" methadone, 10 mg twice daily, and discontinued the hydrocodone/acetaminophen. The next day, he stayed at his parent's home. He was very drowsy, sleeping on and off most of the day, and went to bed early. In the late morning of the third day, his mother was unable to awaken him. He was declared dead by EMS.

Findings from autopsy and toxicology studies conducted on both patients 1 and 2 found toxic levels of methadone. Methadone intoxication was noted by the medical examiners to be the cause of death in both cases.

Both physicians (and their practices—one a local hospital, the other a specialty group) were sued for wrongful death of these patients. Both testified that the dose of methadone used was "equivalent" to the prior opiates. They also considered the patients to be opioid tolerant and the methadone prescriptions to be safe. Neither physician was aware of the unusual (and cumulative) kinetics of methadone, nor the need to start with a low dose, gradually discontinue existing opioids and reassess the patient's tolerance to the methadone.

17.6.13 Applying Lessons Learned and Action for Institutional Committees

Methadone is a medication that should be made available to practitioners. It is used for OUD patients, and it provides a low-cost option for chronic pain patients, especially those who have lost their prescription drug health insurance. Its use, however, should be governed by well-written and promulgated prescription guidelines, informing physicians, pharmacists, and especially patients on the safe and effective use of methadone.

Clear warnings and usage data including adverse events are readily available for use in prescribing guideline development and in clinical staff member education of the risk management components of their clinical care. Examples of clinical staff members who would benefit from this education include but are not limited to physicians, nurses, and pharmacists.

Medical care delivery organizations (hospitals, clinics, or medical groups) and their clinical staff are not only at the forefront of patient care but also readily exposed to various malpractice claims, creating significant financial and negative reputation exposure for all parties in a legal suit. Individual practitioners, along with key institutional operating committees, such as P&T and Quality Improvement, share a need to protect both their patients and their organization from causing avoidable errors.[47]

17.7 CASE REPORTS: OPIOID TOXICITY CAUSING RESPIRATORY ARREST, BRAIN DAMAGE, AND DEATH

Several case reports follow that discuss the clinical course, drug treatment, toxicity, morbidity, and sometimes mortality following the clinical use of opioids.

17.7.1 Case Report: Respiratory Arrest and Brain Damage Following Morphine Overdose

The following case report describes an overdose in a clinical setting; a very high dose of morphine administered with a very short frequency, with no special monitoring by the nurses, in a patient with extrapulmonary risk factors, which resulted in respiratory arrest and brain damage.

This case involves the administration of morphine to Ms. Patient and an evaluation of excessive dosage, leading to acute respiratory failure and subsequent anoxic brain damage. Ms. Patient was 5′4″ and 263 lbs. She was considered morbidly obese (greater than 100% over the ideal body weight of 120 lbs.), which is an increased risk for respiratory depression, thus exacerbating the risk from morphine. Electroencephalographic impression showed diffuse slowing (of brain waves)—indicative of severe toxic metabolic encephalopathy. The patient was described to be in decerebrate posturing.

17.7.1.1 Opinions

In my opinion, with reasonable pharmacological certainty, Ms. Patient was prescribed and administered morphine sulfate at excessive dosages and insufficient time intervals. She had inadequate monitoring, diagnosis, and treatment of her obvious respiratory depression (8:20 am). Furthermore, the combination of overdosage, inadequate monitoring, and non-recognition of the severity of morphine toxicity was a proximate cause of her anoxic brain damage and permanent neurological deficits.

Finally, in my opinion, aggressive reversal of morphine at the first sign of overdose (8:00 am) would have prevented any permanent injury to this young lady. Pulse oximetry, arterial blood gases (ABGs), and intensive monitoring should have been executed at this point. When naloxone (an opioid antidote) was finally prescribed (10:20 am), inadequate doses were administered. Adequate and responsive naloxone administration would have shortened the time that this patient was experiencing narcosis and hypoxia. The following recitation of facts and background information regarding morphine pharmacology, toxicology, and requisite monitoring will serve as the basis for my opinions.

17.7.1.2 Bases for Opinions

The following physician orders, drug administration records, and patient chart notes are relevant in this case evaluation:

- Temazepam (Restoril) 15 mg po qHS PRN
- Meperidine (Demerol) 25 mg IV q 3H PRN severe pain
- Metoprolol (Lopressor) 50 mg po qHS
- Promethazine (Phenergan) 25 mg IV q6h PRN nausea.
  - 0210 25 mg
- Morphine sulfate 10 mg IV q 4–6 hours PRN Pain
  - 1810 10 mg
  - 2210 10 mg
  - 0030 10 mg
  - 0215 10 mg
- Change morphine 20 mg q 2H IV PRN pain (given at 5 A.M. and 7 A.M.)
  - (On the PRN chart, there is a strike out, changing q2 to q3–4)
- Life Flight note "20 mg MS at 0700"
- 0835 decrease morphine to 20 mg IV q 3–4 hours as needed. (Responsive only to pain, thought to be in mild overdose of narcotics, no signs of respiratory depression) Pt. sleeping, not able to arouse, had 40 mg MS in the last 2–3 hours. Hold the next dose until the patient is awake. The nurse's notes for 0830 note a focus on shallow respirations, and what appears to be a strike over originally written as 34/min and finally written at 24/min. (*These are clearly signs of respiratory distress.*)
- 1020 called to room, peripheral cyanosis (nail bed cyanosis), pulse oximetry 30, decerebrate posturing, poor response to 0.4 mg naloxone. Pupils were pinpointed and fixed bilaterally at 0800 m (these signs were actually at 0955, according to the nurse's notes)
  - Clinical Progress Note: Pt. sleeping, not able to arouse. Had 40 mg morphine sulfate in the last 2–3 hours
- 1020 Pulse ox ~30%, naloxone—no response
- 1050 Blood draw for ABGs

17.7.1.3 Case Discussion/Facts

The patient was admitted to the hospital for severe headache and was administered several doses of morphine and a single dose of promethazine and a single dose of temazepam. Diagnoses recorded at the subsequent hospital admission include anoxic brain damage, respiratory failure, hypothyroidism, obesity, hypertension, and tobacco use. An admission note of a possible iatrogenic morphine overdose is recorded. The history/present illness is relevant for the following entry: during the hospitalization, a total dose of 50 mg of morphine plus promethazine was administered. Early this morning, the patient became unresponsive and apneic. Upon arrival at the emergency room, 8 mg of naloxone was administered, and the patient became quite violent and agitated. (A later chart note indicates the patient received 60 mg of morphine sulfate within eight hours of IV overnight. Actually, the 60 mg of morphine was given between 0030 and 0655, precisely 6 hours and 25 minutes.) The final diagnostic impression of J. Physician MD is iatrogenic morphine overdose.

This patient had several factors that compromised her respiratory system. First, she had morbidly obese apnea. She had 60 mg of morphine administered in a little more than six hours. It is likely that obesity, the very large doses of morphine, and the lack of adequate monitoring and treatment measures contributed to respiratory arrest in this patient.

The physician and hospital settled the case with the patient's guardian, thus avoiding the need for a trial.

17.7.2 Case Report: Fentanyl Epidural Respiratory Arrest

This case went to trial in a midwestern city. The interesting part of this case is that the hospital had a policy requiring continuous pulse oximetry (a measure of oxygen saturation in the blood) for all fentanyl epidural patients. Unfortunately, the labor and delivery nursing staff elected not to follow the safety policy: "We don't do that (pulse oximetry) in L&D." The hospital settled the case during trial for $8 million. The pharmacologist case report (with fictitious names) is provided as follows:

I reviewed the following materials in this matter:

1. Complaint at law
2. Medical records comprised of 70 alphabetized file folders
3. Glasgow Coma Record Synopsis
4. 24 Hour Flowsheet Synopsis
5. Thirteen medical personnel depositions
6. Authoritative texts (Harrison's Internal Medicine On-Line, 2001, Goodman and Gilman, The Pharmacological Basis of Therapeutics, McGraw Hill, New York, 1995), and manufacturers' prescribing information (package inserts) describing the pharmacology and toxicology of fentanyl, lorazepam, trifluoperazine, carbamazepine, bupropion, and related drugs.

17.7.2.1 Facts of the Case and Summary of Testimony

Ms. Patient was admitted to a community hospital for a scheduled elective C-section and a tubal ligation. Her previous deliveries had been accompanied by postpartum depression, and she had been receiving psychiatric care for depression and bipolar disorder. She had also been seen by a postpartum depression group as an outpatient. Nurse K, RN, was her coordinator for the postpartum depression counseling clinic. Dr. K was the previous prescribing physician for the psychiatric medications. Dr. L was the psychiatrist at the hospital; K did not have the authority to prescribe at the hospital. The patient asked for and received a referral from an obstetrician, Dr. B, who admitted her for elective C-section on April 17, 1998.

The patient was received at the birthing room at the hospital at 6:00 am entered the birth center operating room at 7:30 am had the epidural fentanyl anesthesia started at 7:35 am and had the incision for the C-section at 8:25 am. Surgery ended at 9:20 am, and Ms. Patient left the operating room at 9:25 am (per the birth center data record), and a live baby boy was delivered at 8:31 am (anesthesia record). Her anesthesiologist, Dr. Moore, wrote the following orders for post-op continuous epidural infusion:

> Post-op orders: Fentanyl, 1,000 mcg in 100 ml normal saline, final concentration fentanyl 10 mcg/ml. Initial dose: none. Infusion: start at 6 cc per hour and increase in increments of 2 cc up to maximum of 14 cc per hour. Dr. M also wrote routine orders for diphenhydramine for severe itching and for naloxone as an antidote along with a bag-valve mask and oxygen set up.

Dr. M also wrote: No. 7 RR and sedation scale every hour when the patient is asleep and/or on bed rest. Also: continuous pulse oximetry for 24 hours and for 24 hours after any increase in dose.

Dr. M recalls that a nurse called who said that the patient was not relieved with 14 cc (fentanyl) so "I asked her to give her some Dalgan*." 16:30: Post-anesthesia note: "Patient being very well and comfortable with CLE and Dalgan."

**Dalgan (Dezocine) is a opioid pain reliver that was typically used for post-operative pain. It is a mixed agonist/antagonist and was noted to have stronger respiratory effect than morphine. It was discontinued in the United States in 2011.*

Although this patient was described as being in no acute distress, she was also described as drowsy, and wheezing was heard in both lungs. Her history included smoking, sleep apnea, and postpartum depression. Prescriptions originated by Dr. Ralph K, continued by Dr. L, and ordered by Dr. B include carbamazepine, lorazepam, bupropion, and trifluoperazine.

The patient's psychotropic drugs, namely, trifluoperazine 2 mg, lorazepam 2 mg, bupropion XL 150 mg, and carbamazepine 200 mg, per Dr. L's recommendation and Dr. B's postoperative major gynecology orders, were added to the patient's post-op medications and given at 22:00 on April 18. It should be noted that although Dr. B states in her deposition that she ordered the 2 mg dose because that is what Ms. Patient was taking, her adult health history done on 4/9/98 and her prenatal flow sheet (the last page of it) has Ms. Patient only taking a one 1 mg dose at a time. This differs from the birth center data, which appears to have a change in the dosage amount and time. At this time, the patient was receiving fentanyl at 14 cc per hour and had received Delgan at 16:30.

Nurse B's shift began at 23:00 and she received the patient from Nurse Jones who gave her a verbal report: Bence recalls that Jones told her the patient was post-C-section with a history of PP depression, that she had a carotid endarterectomy anesthesia (CEA) and IV and the basics of her medical condition. The first time that Nurse B checked on the patient, she found her at 23:54. "Patient found in bed unresponsive to verbal and tactile stimuli. The patient was found lying on the right side in the supine position. Color, cyanotic. Unable to obtain a pulse. No respirations. Code blue call. CPR in progress."

Although the post-anesthesiology orders required pulse oximeter monitoring for this patient (and other patients), according to the testimony of the nurses, these orders were routinely ignored per their training and no pulse oximeters were on the postpartum floor. The same post-anesthesiology orders called for frequent vital signs and evaluations which were admittedly not followed as well. The orders read as follows:

> *Monitor the patient and notify the anesthesiologist if any of this symptomatology occur such as respiratory rate less than 10 respirations per minute, pulse oximetry, that the oxygen level in the blood is less than 90, evidence of obstruction of the airway. Patient is drowsy, excessively somnolent, or unable to arouse. Pain relief is deemed inadequate.*

It was routine to ignore, per the nurse's training, this post-anesthesia order regarding pulse oximeter monitoring at that time. Nurse M says that the standard operating procedure for a floor admission post-C-section was a measurement of vital signs on admission, at two hours, then every four hours for 48 hours. This practice is contrary to Dr. M's orders recorded in the chart and the policy and procedures for that floor.

The patient's history of sleep apnea was not considered in evaluating fentanyl and other drug-induced respiratory depression. The patient had some wheezing and was listed as 245 pounds, but these were mistakenly considered normal for a term pregnancy.

Dr. P, a board-certified pulmonologist, was consulted on the night of the respiratory arrest. The arrest occurred around midnight from 4–17 to 4–18. She arrived around 3:00 A.M. on 4–18. She charted around 7:00 A.M.: cardiorespiratory arrest followed by seizures.

> Impression: history of postpartum depression and bipolar disorder; left lower lobe pneumonia; sleep apnea; history of smoking. Respiratory arrest may

have been caused by a combination of obstructive sleep apnea with upper airway obstruction, combined with the use of epidural fentanyl and possible drug interaction with psychiatric medications.

Laboratory toxicology samples were sent to outside laboratories—National Medical in Pennsylvania and MedTox in Minnesota. Neither fentanyl nor lorazepam were reported in these toxicology tests.

17.7.2.2 Opinions

I hold the following opinions with reasonable pharmacological certainty:

1. Ms. Patient suffered a respiratory arrest leading to a cardiac arrest because of the combined effects and interactions of fentanyl, lorazepam, trifluoperazine, bupropion, and carbamazepine. There is a strong temporal relationship between the administration of psychotropic medications and CEA. The interactive and synergistic toxicity of these medications with fentanyl (and other opioid analgesics) is well-known and cautioned in product information for all the drugs involved, as well as in authoritative literature. For purposes of this report and my opinions, fentanyl, trifluoperazine, and lorazepam will be discussed. Compared to bupropion and carbamazepine, trifluoperazine and lorazepam have the greatest effect on the CNS, thus exacerbating the respiratory depression of fentanyl.
2. The labor and delivery nurses were negligent in adequate monitoring and failed to follow the orders of the anesthesiologist, specifically the failure to monitor the oxygenation of the patient's hemoglobin through pulse oximetry. Naloxone, although ordered, was not administered, and should have been. These nurses should have considered the dangerous interactive potential of the CEA fentanyl and the psychotropic drugs which were prescribed. Systematically ignoring the safety policy, they demonstrated reckless disregard for the welfare of their patients.
3. The hospital nursing and hospital administration were negligent for failure to uniformly implement the safety policies for labor and delivery patients as it applies to the use of pulse oximetry for CEA patients on opioids such as fentanyl.
4. The postpartum psychiatric medications should not have been administered to this patient receiving the CEA fentanyl. The nurses and physicians should have considered the dangerous interactive potential of the CEA fentanyl and the psychotropic drugs which were prescribed.
5. Use of the pulse oximeter would have detected a drug-induced respiratory depression and oxygen deprivation and prevented the cardiorespiratory arrest. The pulse oximetry alarm, appropriate oxygenation, establishment of an airway, and reversal of opioids with naloxone would have precluded the hypoxic injury to Ms. Patient's brain.
6. The toxicology tests are limited by their design. Fentanyl was not detected; it was probably not part of the panel screen of the test, so therefore, it would not be reported. The clinical record supports that fentanyl was administered, and had a proper test been administered, it would have been detected. Benzodiazepines were negative. Since lorazepam was charted, it would be expected to be detected in the sample. Either the test result is erroneous (since it should be there), or the specific screen was not designed to detect the specific benzodiazepine lorazepam. Further investigation will be needed to fully address these toxicology testing issues.

The drugs: opioids (fentanyl) and respiratory depression, with and without additional CNS depressants.

17.7.2.3 Fentanyl

Fentanyl is a synthetic opioid, 100 times more potent than morphine. It is used as an anesthetic and analgesic, both intravenously and epidurally. It is a very short-acting analgesic, but it also demonstrates a bi-phasic kinetic profile, which has been reported to result in late toxicities (rebound) after the infusion is stopped. The following text is taken directly from the fentanyl manufacturer's package insert:

> Fentanyl citrate is a narcotic analgesic. A dose of 100 mcg (0.1 mg) is approximately equivalent in analgesic activity to 10 mg of morphine or 75 mg of meperidine. The principal actions of therapeutic value are analgesia and sedation. Alterations in respiratory rate and alveolar ventilation, associated with narcotic analgesics, may last longer than the analgesic effect. As the dose of narcotic is increased, the decrease in pulmonary exchange becomes greater. Large doses may produce apnea. Fentanyl appears to have less emetic activity than either morphine or meperidine. Histamine assays and skin wheal testing in man indicate that clinically significant histamine release rarely occurs with fentanyl. Recent assays in man show no clinically significant histamine release in dosages up to 50 mcg/kg. Fentanyl preserves cardiac stability and blunts stress-related hormonal changes at higher doses.

The onset of action of fentanyl is almost immediate when the drug is given intravenously; however, the maximal analgesic and respiratory depressant effects may not be noted for several minutes. The usual duration of action of the analgesic effect is 30 to 60 minutes after a single intravenous dose of up to 100 mcg. Following intramuscular administration, the onset of action is from seven to eight minutes, and the duration of action is one to two hours. As with longer-acting narcotic analgesics, the duration of the respiratory depressant effect of fentanyl may be longer than the analgesic effect. The following observations have been reported concerning altered respiratory response to carbon dioxide (CO_2) stimulation following the administration of fentanyl citrate:

> Diminished sensitivity to CO_2 stimulation may persist longer than depression of respiratory rate. (Altered sensitivity to CO_2 stimulation has been demonstrated for up to four hours following a single dose of 600 mcg fentanyl to healthy volunteers.) Fentanyl frequently slows the respiratory rate, duration and degree of respiratory depression being dose related. The peak respiratory depressant effect of a single intravenous dose of fentanyl citrate is noted 5 to 15 minutes following injection. See also WARNINGS and PRECAUTIONS concerning respiratory depression.

Serious respiratory depression can occur, even with proper doses, in vulnerable individuals. As with other potent anesthetic agents, fentanyl has been associated with cases of serious respiratory depression in individuals with respiratory disorders, cases of excessive or improper dosage, individuals with unsuspected abnormalities of absorption or metabolism of the drug, and in rare cases where no specific etiology can be identified. Fentanyl should be administered only in specifically monitored settings and by persons specifically trained in the use of anesthetics and the management of the respiratory effects of potent opioids, including establishment and maintenance of a patent airway and assisted ventilation (see also BOXED WARNING and PRECAUTIONS).

Respiratory depression caused by opioid analgesics can be reversed by opioid antagonists such as naloxone, also known as Narcan. Because the duration of respiratory depression produced by fentanyl may last longer than the duration of the opioid antagonist action, appropriate surveillance should be maintained. As with all potent opioids, profound analgesia is accompanied by respiratory depression and diminished sensitivity to CO_2 stimulation, which may persist into or recur in the postoperative period.

> Impaired Respiration: Fentanyl should be used with caution in patients with chronic obstructive pulmonary disease, patients with decreased respiratory reserve, and others with potentially compromised respiration. In such patients, narcotics may additionally decrease respiratory drive and increase airway resistance. During anesthesia, this can be managed by assisted or controlled respiration.

Because of the risk of hypoventilation, the lowest effective dose of oral fentanyl should be used, and it should be administered only in monitored settings and by persons specifically trained in the use of anesthetics and the management of the respiratory effects of potent opioids, including the establishment and maintenance of a patent airway and assisted ventilation.

> Drug Interactions: Other CNS depressant drugs (e.g., barbiturates, sedatives, narcotics, and general anesthetics) will have additive or potentiating effects with fentanyl. When patients have received such drugs, the dose of fentanyl required will be less than usual. Following the administration of fentanyl citrate, the dose of other CNS depressant drugs should be reduced.

17.7.2.4 Trifluoperazine (Stelazine®)

Selected text, relevant to this case, is excerpted from the manufacturer's prescribing information for trifluoperazine, a potent phenothiazine antipsychotic:

> If agents such as sedatives, narcotics, anesthetics, or alcohol are used either simultaneously or successively with the drug, the possibility of an undesirable additive depressant effect should be considered.

17.7.2.5 Lorazepam (Ativan®)

The following is an excerpt from the manufacturer's prescribing information:

> Lorazepam is an anti-anxiety drug, and a member of the benzodiazepine class. It is classed as a CNS depressant. Lorazepam is indicated for the management of anxiety disorders or for the short-term relief of the symptoms of anxiety or anxiety-associated with depressive symptoms. Anxiety or tension associated with the stress of everyday life usually does not require treatment with an anxiolytic.
>
> Lorazepam is not recommended for use in patients with a primary depressive disorder or psychosis. As with all patients on CNS-acting drugs, patients receiving lorazepam should be warned not to operate dangerous machinery or motor vehicles and that their tolerance for alcohol and other CNS depressants will be diminished.
>
> Clinically significant drug interactions: benzodiazepines, including lorazepam, produce CNS-depressant effects when administered with such medications as barbiturates or alcohol.
>
> Lorazepam produces depression of the CNS when administered with ethanol, phenothiazines, barbiturates, MAO inhibitors, and other antidepressants. Doses of other injectable CNS depressant drugs should ordinarily be reduced (see PRECAUTIONS).

17.7.2.6 Obesity-Hypoventilation Syndrome

Ms. Patient had additional risk factors for respiratory depression in addition to the combination of fentanyl and other CNS depressant drugs (trifluoperazine, lorazepam, carbamazepine, bupropion). These risk factors include wheezing and dyspnea as noted in Dr. A's anesthesia evaluation and obesity.

17.7.2.7 Summary and Conclusions

In my opinion, Ms. Patient's respiratory arrest was caused by the fentanyl and other medications she was administered. The gross negligence of the labor and delivery nursing staff at the hospital allowed this tragedy to occur, which would have been prevented had the staff exercised reasonable and prudent judgment and care and followed the policies and procedures which were in place to protect patients undergoing therapy with predictably dangerous analgesics. The use of the psychotropics for postpartum depression enhanced the fentanyl respiratory toxicity and must therefore be considered at least additive and probably was not needed/should have been avoided until the patient was off the fentanyl. The resuscitation efforts, once the patient was discovered as unresponsive (Code Blue), were inadequate in that naloxone was not administered and the bag-valve mask giving the patient oxygen was not administered until seven minutes after Ms. Patient was found.

17.7.3 Case Report: Fentanyl (Duragesic®) Death in Discharged Patient

I reviewed the medical center records, the death certificate, autopsy, and toxicology reports, and the Certificate of Merit by Dr. Anesthesiologist. I also reviewed authoritative pharmacology, toxicology, and prescribing information for fentanyl.

Mr. Decedent had ear nose and throat surgery related to tonsillar cancer by Dr. ENT Surgeon and was discharged home the next morning. He died the next day. An autopsy toxicology report found elevated tissue liver levels of fentanyl, a synthetic opioid, the active ingredient in the Duragesic patch. In addition to Duragesic, he was discharged on Vicodin (hydrocodone/acetaminophen—also a synthetic opioid) tablets crushed through a feeding gastroscopy tube.

While recovering from surgery, Mr. Decedent was treated with a morphine PCA (patient-controlled analgesia) pump as well as single morphine IV doses throughout that day ("D/C IV Morphine in 12 hours. May continue Vicodin II tab QID per G tube"). One week prior, Vicodin was initiated. Duragesic 75 mcg/hour was prescribed one week later. Mr. Decedent experienced significant respiratory depression. The following excerpts from the medical record are instructive:

> *Rec'd pt Lethargic pale w/d. Resp 16–18 with stridorous/congested respirations noted. Responds quickly to verbal/tactile stimuli but drifts back to sleep within a few seconds. Lips pink w/d; vss; D. H made aware of above. Suctioned with thick dark beige sputum noted. Respo. Clear . . . PO2—<60–70s 0900 Dr. Surgeon paged by D. Nurse made aware of above. Rec'd order for Narcan 0.4 mg in titrated doses. Narcan 0.13 mg IVP given—Pt. alert and responding verbally to questions within 1" of Narcan administered. Pt. then became alert and responded appropriately to questions and pulse ox(imetry) increased to 88%. Removed fentanyl 75 mcg. Successful reversal of narcotic effect. D. Nurse RN (Oncology CNS Note) and Narcan (naloxone-narcotic antagonist/antidote) was prescribed/administered (09:25 and 11:15) to reverse the effect of the Duragesic/fentanyl ("remove Fentanyl patch").*

Inexplicably, "change Fentanyl dose to 100 mcg d/t (due to) narcotic effect," a higher dose of fentanyl, was prescribed for home use. Oxygen was also prescribed for home use.

17.7.3.1 Fentanyl (Duragesic®)

The prescribing information (package insert) for Duragesic® states:

> Serious respiratory depression can occur, even with proper doses, in vulnerable individuals as with other potent anesthetic agents, fentanyl has been associated with cases of serious respiratory depression in individuals with respiratory disorders, cases of excessive or improper dosage, in individuals with unsuspected abnormalities of absorption or metabolism of the drug, and in rare cases where no specific etiology can be identified. Fentanyl should be administered only in specifically monitored settings and by persons specifically trained in the use of anesthetics and the management of the respiratory effects of potent opioids, including establishment and maintenance of a patent airway and assisted ventilation (see also BOXED WARNING and PRECAUTIONS).
>
> Hypoventilation (respiratory depression): Hypoventilation may occur at any time during the use of fentanyl. Because significant amounts of fentanyl are absorbed from the skin for 17 hours or more after the system is removed, hypoventilation may persist beyond the removal of fentanyl. Consequently, patients with hypoventilation should be carefully observed for degree of sedation and their respiratory rate monitored until respiration has stabilized.
>
> The use of concomitant CNS active drugs requires special patient care and observation. See WARNINGS.

17.7.3.2 Dosage and Administration

With all opioids, the safety of patients using the products is dependent on healthcare practitioners prescribing them in strict conformity with their approved labeling with respect to patient selection, dosing, and proper conditions for use.

As with all opioids, dosage should be individualized. The most important factor to be considered in determining the appropriate dose is the extent of preexisting opioid tolerance. (See BOXED WARNING and CONTRAINDICATIONS.) Initial doses should be reduced in elderly or debilitated patients (see PRECAUTIONS).

17.7.3.3 Dose Selection

Doses must be individualized based on the status of each patient and should be assessed at regular intervals after fentanyl application. Reduced doses of fentanyl are suggested for the elderly and other groups discussed in precautions.

17.7.3.4 Opinions

1. Mr. Decedent died from the respiratory toxicity of fentanyl, which may or may not have been used in combination with Vicodin.
2. Mr. Decedent experienced significant respiratory toxicity from fentanyl in the hospital, hours prior to his discharge, following an attempt to treat his pain with a Duragesic 75 mcg/hr patch. He had been treated with morphine 4 mg/hour as well as Vicodin. The clinical record clearly shows that the Duragesic dose of 75 mcg/hr was too much for him, as evidenced by the administration of Narcan to reverse narcotic effects.

3. Once started on the Duragesic patch, the patient should be monitored for at least 24 hours in a controlled environment to determine the patient's ability to tolerate the "patch." This delay is necessary because it takes some time for the patch to reach peak efficacy, and early release may occur before the peak, therefore leaving the patient at risk.
4. Mr. Decedent was clearly toxic on a 75 mcg/hr dose strength patch. It is inexplicable why a higher dose, that is, 100 mcg/hr patch was ordered, in view of this known and demonstrated toxicity.
5. In my opinion, the prescribing physicians, attending nurses, and home-health nurses demonstrated incompetence and ignorance in their negligent use of the Duragesic patch, resulting in the death of Mr. Decedent from acute fentanyl overdose. The inappropriate prescribing, administering, and monitoring represent a departure from the standard of reasonable care upheld by healthcare professionals in the United States.
6. In this matter, the standard of care would have prevented the escalation of the dose of the Duragesic patch from 75 to 100 mcg/hr in the face of fentanyl toxicity. The standard of care would have dictated that Mr. Decedent would have been safely stabilized on an effective analgesic before being discharged home.

17.7.4 Case Report: High-Dose Fentanyl Patch Prescribed in Opiate-Naïve Patient—Death

17.7.4.1 Facts of the Case

Ralph Charles (pseudonym), a 42-year-old man with severe heart disease, implanted with an implantable cardioverter defibrillator, and a candidate for an orthotopic heart transplant, complained to Dr. H of pain. Dr. H prescribed fentanyl transdermal system (FTS), 100 mcg/hr patches, #5, apply one patch to the chest wall every 72 hours. The prescription was picked up by Mr. Charles' sister-in-law, at Dr. H's office and taken to a local pharmacy where it was filled. The completed prescription was picked up by Mr. Charles's wife. A single patch was applied to Mr. Charles's chest that evening. The next morning, his wife noted that Mr. Charles was still sleeping, and, indeed, was snoring. Mr. Charles was found dead in bed later that day. 911 was called, EMS arrived, and determined that CPR was futile, he was cold, stiff, and unresponsive. An autopsy was conducted; toxicology tests were ordered, but the toxicology test results were lost in the chaos associated with a hurricane in the region.

Dr. H testified at his deposition that he considered Mr. Charles a drug user, dependent, and opioid tolerant, and he ordered the highest dose out of "compassionate care," admittedly ignoring the dosing guidelines described in the prescribing information. Dr. H denied prescribing based on a phone call and insisted that Mr. Charles came to his office and was despondent, crying, and felt like he was dying.

The records described multiple prescription medications currently. The most recent opiate prescription was for 60 Darvocet 100 mg, prescribed in June 2005. A history of meperidine and hydrocodone/acetaminophen is noted earlier in May and June during the prior year.

17.7.4.2 Opinions and Basis of Opinions

All the following opinions are expressed with reasonable pharmacological certainty and by a preponderance of the evidence.

1. Mr. Charles' death was caused by an overdose of fentanyl, a potent synthetic opiate (an opioid) 100 times more potent than morphine. Mr. Charles' heart condition increased his risk of succumbing to the fentanyl overdose, but he would have died absent any cardiac disease. While Mr. Charles did have serious heart disease, his death was not imminent (testimony of Dr. H).
2. The dose prescribed, 100 mcg/hr, is the equivalent of ~360 mg oral morphine (package insert).
3. The onset of action and time to peak actions are consistent with the onset of sleep, the appearance of snoring (respiratory depression), and his death.
4. Mr. Charles was not opiate tolerant; indeed, even if he were still consuming the prescribed amounts of Darvocet, he was still not a candidate for the highest dose of FTS, that is, 100 mcg/hr. The use of meperidine and hydrocodone/acetaminophen 15 months earlier would not render Mr. Charles opiate tolerant or dependent.
5. The use of FTS at any dose in this patient at that was contraindicated. Contraindication, as noted in the black box warning for the FTS, means that the FTS should not have been used. FTS is indicated for opioid-tolerant patients requiring continuous high-dose opiates for a prolonged period. The high dose of FTS would only be justified by a titration up from lower doses. The lowest dose of FTS is 25 mcg/hr. The use of the 25 mcg/hr FTS would also have been contraindicated in Charles.

The FDA and manufacturers of FTS have frequently issued warnings and guidelines for the safe use of fentanyl patches. The following was issued shortly (July 2005) before Mr. Charles' death:

> FDA Public Health Advisory: Safety Warnings Regarding Use of Fentanyl Transdermal (Skin) Patches
>
> FDA is investigating reports of death and other serious side effects from overdoses of fentanyl in patients using fentanyl transdermal (skin) patches for pain control. Deaths and overdoses have occurred in patients using both the brand name product Duragesic and the generic product. The directions for using the fentanyl skin patch must be followed exactly to prevent death or other serious side effects from overdosing with fentanyl. These directions are provided in the product label and patient package insert.

MedWatch—The FDA Safety Information and Adverse Event Reporting Program issued an update that highlights important information on appropriate prescribing, dose selection, and the safe use of the FTS (patch). The FDA previously issued a Public Health Advisory and Information for Healthcare Professionals addressing the appropriate and safe use of the transdermal system. However, the agency continues to receive reports of death and life-threatening adverse events related to fentanyl overdose that have occurred when the fentanyl patch was used to treat pain in opioid-naïve patients and when opioid-tolerant patients have applied more patches than prescribed, changed the patch too frequently, or exposed the patch to a heat source. The fentanyl patch is only indicated for use in patients with persistent, moderate to severe chronic pain who have been taking a regular, daily, around-the-clock narcotic pain medicine for longer than a week and are opioid tolerant. Patients must avoid exposing the patch to excessive heat as this promotes the release of fentanyl from the patch and increases the absorption of fentanyl through the skin which can result in fatal overdose. Directions for prescribing and using the fentanyl patch must be followed exactly to prevent death or other serious side effects from fentanyl overdose.

Dr. H denies prescribing based on a phone call. The FTS would have been contraindicated even if he had seen Mr. Charles in his office previously. The use of FTS 100 mcg/hr would cause death in any opioid-naïve or slightly tolerant person.

17.7.4.3 Summary and Conclusion

Mr. Charles died because of the use of the prescribed FTS 100 mcg/hr patch. The prescription of the patch, considering the facts of the case, was contraindicated, and should not have occurred.

17.7.5 Case Report: Heroin and Other Opioids

Widespread abuse of heroin and other opioids (e.g., OxyContin) will predictably result in criminal and civil litigants who were charged as being "under the influence" as a result of evidence of opioid use. The following report was filed in civil cases where the issue of heroin use was considered.

17.7.5.1 Facts of the Case

The defendant was observed by Miami Police Officers at a "drug house" on the West Side of Chicago. As the defendant drove away, he was followed by police officers, who executed a stop, at which time, the defendant fled the police. During the "chase," the defendant narrowly missed colliding head-on with another Chicago Police Department vehicle; the crash was avoided by the officer, and then the defendant crashed the 1995 Mustang into a viaduct on Elm Street. An ambulance was called at the time of the crash; the officer anticipated that there would be injuries. The defendant exited his vehicle and resisted several officers who were attempting to arrest him, and he was handcuffed. Shortly after he was subdued and handcuffed, he complained of difficulty breathing. The police officers took the handcuffs off and again requested an ambulance. When the paramedics arrived, the defendant was in full arrest. He was taken to the hospital where he was pronounced dead.

The family and friends reported that the defendant was taking multiple medications for heart disease and blood pressure, which caused the defendant to be drowsy. The defendant's wife reported that he did not abuse alcohol or drugs.

The toxicology report identified morphine, 70 ng/ml in the postmortem testing. The postmortem examination noted a weight of 322 pounds. The medical examiner indicated that opiate intoxication contributed to the defendant's death.

A police dog examined the Mustang for the presence of drugs. The dog sensed drugs, but none were found.

17.7.5.2 Opinions

In my opinion, within a reasonable degree of pharmacological certainty, the defendant used heroin shortly before he was observed by the police and the pursuit began. A blood test of 70 ng/ml of morphine indicates a recent and high dose of an opiate. Based on the defendant's weight and height, I estimate that he consumed a dose of ~15–20 mg of heroin. The opiates responsible include heroin and morphine, as heroin is rapidly metabolized to morphine in the blood. Since morphine is generally not available on the street, and heroin is, it is probable that heroin was used by the defendant within a period of an hour or two before the crash. His subsequent actions and behavior, in my opinion, were impaired by heroin. He acted erratically and with poor judgment (fleeing police; attempting to collide with another police car; resisting arrest). After he was subdued, he complained of difficulty breathing and chest pain. In my opinion, the presence and actions of heroin on the respiratory center (breathing) probably contributed to the defendant's breathing difficulty, which preceded his cardiac arrest and death.

The records and statements indicate that the decedent was diagnosed with multiple medical conditions and treated with multiple medications. Those same statements indicate a concern that his medications caused drowsiness. Many medications may interact with and increase the toxicity of heroin and morphine.

17.7.5.3 Bases for Opinions

Intoxication and impairments by heroin, an illegal narcotic (opiate) CNS depressant, causes brain and behavioral toxicity, including lethargy, euphoria, dysphoria, mental clouding, hallucinations, depression, cognitive impairment, and paranoia.

Morphine and related opioids produce their major effects on the CNS. The effects are remarkably diverse and include analgesia, drowsiness, changes in mood, respiratory depression, decreased GI motility, nausea, vomiting, and alterations of the endocrine and autonomic nervous systems.

Morphine-like opioids depress respiration, at least in part by virtue of a direct effect on the brainstem respiratory centers. The respiratory depression is discernible even with doses too small to disturb consciousness and increases progressively as the dose is increased. In human beings, death from morphine poisoning is nearly always due to respiratory arrest. Therapeutic doses of morphine depress all phases of respiratory activity (rate, minute volume, and tidal exchange) and may also produce irregular breathing. The diminished respiratory volume is due primarily to a slower rate of breathing, and with toxic amount the rate may fall to three or four breaths per minute. Although respiratory effects can be documented readily with standard doses of morphine, respiratory depression is rarely a problem clinically in the absence of underlying pulmonary dysfunction. However, the combination of opiates with other medications, such as general anesthetics, tranquilizers, alcohol, or sedative-hypnotics, may present a greater risk of respiratory depression. Maximal respiratory depression occurs within five to ten minutes after intravenous administration of morphine or within 30 to 90 minutes following intramuscular or subcutaneous administration, respectively. Maximal depressant effects occur more rapidly with more lipid-soluble agents. Following therapeutic doses, respiratory minute volume may be reduced for as long as four to five hours. The primary mechanism of respiratory depression by opioids involves a reduction in the responsiveness of the brainstem respiratory centers to carbon dioxide. Opioids also depress the pontine and medullary centers involved in regulating respiratory rhythmicity and the responsiveness of medullary respiratory centers to electrical stimulation.

17.7.5.4 Conclusion

The defendant/decedent was intoxicated and impaired by heroin when he resisted arrest and fought with the police, and the presence, action, and toxicity of the heroin probably impaired his ability to breathe. The toxicity of heroin and morphine is greater in a naïve or occasional user. (His wife told police that her husband did not abuse drugs.) The peak action of heroin/morphine is 10–15 minutes. Respiratory depression can occur at therapeutic doses without significant mental and motor depression. This intoxication and impairment are also consistent with the abnormal behavior manifested by the decedent.

17.7.6 Case Report: Hydromorphone (Dilaudid®) Respiratory Arrest

17.7.6.1 Facts of the Case

Ruth T. was an elderly woman admitted to a local hospital from the emergency department (ED) for a complaint of left flank pain radiating down to the left lower abdomen. She was found to have a kidney stone. In the ED, Ms. T's oxygen saturation initially was 98% on room air. In the ER, she received two injections of hydromorphone: 2 mg IV (intravenous) at 7:00 pm and at 2:00 am and 11:00 am on the next morning. Shortly thereafter, she was admitted to the fourth floor and was treated by staff nurses and nurse's aides.

At 12:25 pm, she had a nursing assessment that revealed a respiratory rate of 24, pulse 114, and an oxygen saturation was 81% on room air. Oxygen by nasal cannula was administered, and her oxygen saturation went up to 95%. An ABG was ordered and performed at 1:00 pm that revealed a pH of 7.29, $pCO_2 = 53$, pO_2 175. HCO_3 26. The blood gas showed acute respiratory acidosis. Later that day, Ms. T's oxygen was removed when she was eating, and her oxygen saturation deteriorated to below 88%. Nurse notations indicate that her pupils were constricted. Other than the standard vital sign (VS) equipment and pulse oximetry, no cardiac monitoring with telemetry was available on this floor and the nurses observed standard assessments once per shift.

A pulmonary consult was ordered for shortness of breath (SOB). The pulmonary consultant, Dr. C, saw the patient, and ordered a bronchodilator treatment as needed; he did not note any concern or relationship to her abnormal oxygen and blood gas status to the hydromorphone either in the chart or in his deposition.

At 1:35 pm a routine pharmacy note reduced the levofloxacin antibiotic order from 500 to 250 mg, due to a decreased glomerular filtration rate (GFR—a measure of kidney perfusion and function affecting the clearance of medications from the body), per hospital protocol.

Dr. A testified that the hypoventilation was secondary to pain, not respiratory depression due to Dilaudid. Ms. T received an additional 2 mg of hydromorphone at 4:00 am on the next morning. When Dr. A first saw Ms. Tighe before 7:30 am that morning, she was complaining of nausea and vomiting with liquids, and he questioned whether this was due to her kidney stone or the hydromorphone. Ketorolac, a parenteral NSAID, was ordered as an additional pain medication, in the hope of reducing the hydromorphone or not increasing it. He did, however, increase the frequency of the hydromorphone from 2 mg every four hours to 2 mg every two hours. Later that day, she received 2 mg of hydromorphone at 11:15 am, 5:00 pm, and 9:45 pm.

Several of the nurses who treated this patient have testified that they were not aware of the risk of giving hydromorphone at all. Some did not know that it had a risk of causing respiratory depression and did not know the risk was greater in the elderly. The night shift nurse assessed the patient around midnight but did not record her assessment until 3:30 am. She was medicated with hydromorphone 2 mg IV by the nurse at 1:25 am.

That nurse testified that she would usually check on each patient hourly but would not awaken them if sleeping comfortably. She had no recollection of these checks. She had no recollection of finding the patient in any distress until 6:15 am when the patient was unresponsive and without a pulse. A code was called. The patient expired at 6:50 am. No autopsy was done; no toxicology was tested.

17.7.6.2 Opinions

In my opinion, with reasonable pharmacological certainty, Ruth T suffered a respiratory arrest that progressed to a cardiac arrest directly resulting from the effect of hydromorphone. Any pre-existing cardiac disease would increase her risk of hydromorphone respiratory depression.

17.7.6.3 Bases for Opinions

1. Ms. T was a small woman with impaired GFR, who had two documented episodes of decreased oxygen saturation following the initiation of hydromorphone. The respiratory toxicity was further documented by ABG analysis indicating respiratory acidosis and hypercapnia (elevated CO_2), which is evidence of narcotic-induced respiratory depression. These documented respiratory warnings are compelling.
2. Her clinical signs are consistent with hydromorphone effects and toxicity: constricted pupils, pain relieved, urinary incontinence, SOB, nausea and vomiting, unresponsiveness
3. Opiates cause respiratory depression at therapeutic doses.
4. The defense experts suggest that the timing of the hydromorphone administration and Ms. T's death makes it unlikely that respiratory issues contributed to her death. I disagree. The elderly are particularly sensitive to the effects of opiates, especially respiratory depression. Clearance of opiates may be decreased in geriatric patients, resulting in a longer duration of action. Care should be exercised, and appropriate dosage adjustments (e.g., lower initial doses and longer dosing intervals) should be considered. Hydromorphone is a particularly potent opiate, seven times more potent than morphine. The half-life and thus the blood levels and toxicity are enhanced with decreased renal function. The half-life of hydromorphone in the elderly is up to four hours, bringing the maximum effects (in the first half-life) after the 1:25 am dose during the period in which no vital signs were taken. She was only observed as resting comfortably. The nurse's observations would not be able to discern compromised breathing function, changes in respiratory rate or depth of respirations, and increasing risk of narcosis—until she was noted to be unresponsive at ~6:15 am.
5. Renal function is depressed by opioids. It is believed that in humans this is chiefly due to a decreased renal plasma flow. Opioids can decrease systemic blood pressure and GFR. Opiate agonists (hydromorphone) may have a prolonged duration and cumulative effect in patients with hepatic or renal dysfunction. Care should be exercised, and the initial dosage of the opiate should be reduced in patients who have renal insufficiency. Recall that the calculated GFR in Ms. T was low, precipitating a reduction of the dose of the levofloxacin.
6. The half-life of hydromorphone is 1.5–3.8 hours. The metabolite, hydromorphone-3-glucuronide, appears to have significant pharmacological activity and lasts longer than the active ingredient, contributing to cumulative and prolonged activity. The use of hydromorphone may result in muscle flaccidity (urinary incontinence).
7. The defense experts suggest that because Ms. T did not have obvious changes in mental status on January 18 and January 19, hydromorphone did not contribute to her demise. I disagree. Standard methods for assessing the level of consciousness may not detect respiratory depression. Even though patients can be aroused for a brief period and may in fact be able to speak, they may immediately fall back into a state of over-sedation when the stimulus is removed. In addition, an overly sedated patient's respiratory rate may improve with stimulation but quickly decreases when the stimulation is removed.

17.8 INVESTIGATION AND PROSECUTION OF PAIN CLINICS BY THE DEPARTMENT OF JUSTICE

Aside from aggressive nationwide lawsuits against opioid pharmaceutical manufacturers, distributors, and national pharmacy companies, the Department of Justice (DOJ) has initiated several investigations of pain clinics prescribing practices, ostensibly for overprescribing and not monitoring pain patients prescribed various and sometimes quite high doses of opiates. One such investigation of a Pain Clinic resulted in a report being issued by one of the authors of this chapter (JTOD) in defense of the clinic's practice.

17.8.1 Report in Defense of Pain Clinic Practices

17.8.1.1 Assignment

Comment on the medical, pharmacological, scientific, regulatory, and legal implications of limiting analgesic dosing of opiates to 90 MME or less per day (guideline for general practitioners); and whether a chronic pain patient's prescription dose may exceed that recommendation within reasonable medical and pharmacological standards, and whether it is medically appropriate to compare the two. Also, to render opinions on reasonable and prudent controlled substance prescribing practices regarding the prescriptions for the 40 (GROUP I-14, GROUP II-18, GROUP III-8) patient files (AUSA selected).

17.8.1.1.1 Materials Reviewed

1. Assistant U.S. Attorney (AUSA) requested patient file table/data summary
2. Explanatory memo and statistics—Pain Clinic (PC)

3. Patient files (listed in #1); cursory review for organization; audits for starting dose(s), prior medical records, PMP reports, Pharmacy records, compliance drug testing, imaging, communication with other providers, dismissal for pain contract violations
4. PC Patient Data.xlsx (Denial or dismissal tabulation; 962 entries)
5. PC Policy and Procedure Manual
6. PC patient summary (statistics)
7. CDC (U.S. Public Health Service) "Guideline for Prescribing Opioids for Chronic Pain" *(https://www.cdc.gov/drugoverdose/prescribing/guideline.html)*
8. CDC Newsroom Some Policies attributed to the Guideline are inconsistent with its recommendations. *(https://www.cdc.gov/media/releases/2019/s0424-advises-misapplication-guideline-prescribing-opioids.html)*
9. Literature from Pain Management, Pharmacy, Anesthesia, Medicine, and other professional sources. I reviewed this literature to support my opinions and compare the prescriptive practices of the Pain Center to CDC, International Pain Society (IPS), University pain services, regulatory and legislative actions, and authoritative pain literature sources.

17.8.1.1.2 Statement of Opinions

There is no medical, pharmacological, scientific, regulatory, or legal bases for limiting the daily opioid dose to 90 MME nor applying (comparing) the 90 MME limit for primary care patients to chronic pain patients, particularly those treated in a pain management practice. The Pain Center complied with governmental (DEA, Board of Medicine, Board of Pharmacy), pain management specialty, medical, and pharmacologic standards, guidelines, and recommendations when treating the chronic pain patients subject to this audit. The details of this compliance are listed in Opinion #14.

I held this opinion prior to my engagement in this case.

17.8.1.1.3 Opinions and Bases of Opinions

These opinions are expressed with a reasonable degree of pharmacologic and pharmaceutical certainty.

1. The 90 MME limit is a CDC Guideline and it applies to primary care (general practice), not pain management specialists.[1,2] Indeed, the CDC recently issued a press release titled: "Some policies, practices attributed to the (CDC) Guideline are inconsistent with its recommendations."
2. A guideline does not carry the force of a regulation for law.
3. Patients with intractable pain may require doses in excess of 90 MME to adequately relieve their pain.[3,4]
4. Arbitrarily limiting chronic pain patients to < 90 MME dosing places them at risk for pain and suffering, and consequences associated with pain.[5,6,7]
5. Dismissing patients from a pain practice who require > 90 MME dosing per day may prompt patients to seek pain relief from clandestine, illegal, and risky/dangerous settings.[8]
6. States that have set 90 MME dosing limits direct patients requiring higher dosing to pain specialists. These states do NOT prohibit higher than 90 MME.[9,10] Two states set the threshold for 120; higher doses require a pain management consult.[11,12]
7. Conventional wisdom consensus describes NO UPPER LIMIT to an opioid dose,[13] due to the well-known and well-established phenomenon of tolerance that predictably develops in chronic opioid/opiate therapy.[14]
8. Chronic pain patients treated by pain specialists are safer than those treated by primary care of other non-pain specialist providers. As a result of the extra monitoring dictated by their (pain specialists') Standard of Care, CDC guidelines, and Pain Societies' guidelines, chronic pain patients are treated without the attendant risks associated with higher doses administered in an uncontrolled, less-monitored setting outside the Pain Management guidelines/standards of practice.[15] (See also the "Justification for Morphine Equivalent Opioid Dose above 90 mg" Table, appended to this report.)
9. Treatment with chronic opioids for opioid-tolerant patients in a controlled environment is a lesser risk of organic toxicity to the patient (renal, hepatic, neurological, hematological, dermatological, and GI).
10. All prescriptions for the audited patients had their prescriptions filled by a local pharmacy. This review includes an independent review of legitimate medical purpose by another licensed healthcare professional (pharmacist) who had a "corresponding responsibility"—a DEA term.
11. Chronic pain patients are difficult patients. They are in a difficult place in their life—living with pain is no picnic! Some patients had no violations and continued as patients. Many patients (a high percentage) violated the PC contract and were discharged from PC (illegal drug substances, multiple prescribers, criminal justice matters, drug abuse). A review of the patient records, particularly those of discharged patients, clearly proves that PC strictly enforced its drug testing policies. PC did not contribute nor was aware of any drug abuse by its patients, and, when PC became aware, patients were discharged from the clinic. PC educated patients on compliance rules and continued to provide pain management treatment to those patients who complied with the rules.

12. PC referred its patients, when needed, to specialists, including orthopedic, neurological, emergency, and psychological counseling.
13. PC monitored their patients' prescriptions with drug utilization reviews and DIs (drug interaction screens) and frequently attempted to lower the dose of opiates (MME) and other medications used to treat their patients' pain.
14. PC's practice, in general and in particular, for the 40 AUSA selected patients:

- Mirrors CDC and IPS and University of Utah Pain treatment guidelines
- Mirrors the PC Policy and Procedures (which mirror CDC, IPS, University of Utah)
- The Pain Center does not treat patients without reasonable pain diagnoses; the Pain Center requests and reviews prior records
- Dismisses (a high percentage of patients) patients who violate pain contracts (drug tests, pill counts, doctor shopping, pharmacy shopping)
- Accepted less than 20% of patients inquiring to be admitted as patients of the practice
- Most of the inherited and newly admitted patients (90%) were all on MME > 90 MME
- Most chronic pain patients receiving opiates exceed the 90 MME threshold limit for primary care practitioners (PCPs). For example, a patient with chronic pain receiving oxycodone 30 mg, #180 tablets/month, is prescribed six tablets per day, the tablets to be taken around the clock. While the 90 MME is clearly exceeded, the level of pain medication is dictated by the patient's pain and the patient's response (analgesia) and the development of tolerance (dose increased); both concepts are very well described in pain medicine. This patient can be safely treated by careful clinical assessment, verifying compliance and adherence, and lack of abuse or diversion, which are all stated and verified practices of the Pain Center.
- Monitors Prescription Monitoring Program (PMP)
- Implements MME reductions (13/40 patients—32.5%)
- Maintains MME dose (7/40 patients—17.5%)
- Combined dose maintenance or reduction of MME dose in 50% of patients
- Prescribes adjunctive analgesia (non-opioid) drugs (22/40 patients—55%)

Fortunately, after a long, detailed, and expensive legal defense of their practices, and after the submission of this expert report citing authorities in pain medicine, the DOJ dropped the investigation. Unfortunately, the Pain Center closed, leaving a void in pain medication services in the community it served.

17.9 CONCLUSIONS

Opiates and opioids have always been considered dangerous. The introduction and criminal marketing of OxyContin ~25 years ago made them more dangerous, creating the "opioid epidemic," which killed hundreds of thousands of Americans in that period. Other opioid manufacturers, "pill mills," excessive opioid prescribing by providers, and complicity by pharmacists certainly contributed to the epidemic. Opiate deaths again spiked in by the lockdown and depressing effects of the COVID-19 pandemic. Patients who need opioids have suffered great pain without them as a result of restrictive medical and pharmacy boards and aggressive investigation of legitimate pain clinics. Rational pain treatment prescribing, good faith dispensing, and cautious use by patients should help mitigate this opioid scourge. Hopefully, this epidemic will end soon and not be repeated.

NOTES

1 Bolen J. A Legal Interpretation of the CDC Opioid Prescribing Guideline. PPM – Practical Pain Management 9/13/17. Access 8/15/17

2 Utah Pain Management Slides 081518.pdf (at slide 36). Accessed 8/15/18.

3 Busse JW et al. Guideline for opioid therapy and chronic noncancer pain. CMAJ 2017 May 8;189:E659–66. doi: 10.1503/cmaj.170363

4 Morasco BJ et al. Clinical Characteristics of Veterans Prescribed High Doses of Opioid Medications for Chronic Non-Cancer Pain. Pain 2010 December; 151(3): 625–632.

5 https://www.npr.org/sections/health-shots/2018/07/08/622729300/patients-with-chronic-pain-feel-caught-in-an-opioid-prescribing-debate. Accessed 8/15/18

6 Serafini M. The Physicians' Quandary with Opioids: Pain versus Addiction. *New England J Med. Catalyst.* April 25, 2018.

7 Rosenblum A, Marsch LA, Joseph H, and Portenoy RK. Opioids and the Treatment of Chronic Pain: Controversies, Current Status, and Future Directions. Exp Clin Psychopharmacology. 2008 October; 16(5): 405–416.

8 Fields HL. The Doctor's Dilemma: opiate analgesics and chronic pain. Neuron. 2011 Feb. 24 2011; 69(4); 591–594.

9 Prescribing Policies: States Confront Opioid Overdose Epidemic. National Conference of State Legislature. www.ncsl.org/research/health/prescribing-policies-states-confront-opiod=overdose-epidemic.aspx. Access 8/15/18.

10 https://www.npr.org/sections/health-shots/2018/07/08/622729300/patients-with-chronic-pain-feel-caught-in-an-opioid-prescribing-debate

11 http://www.agencymeddirectors.wa.gov/Files/FY16-288SummaryAMDGOpioidGuideline_FINAL.pdf. Accessed 8/15/18.

12 Communication Department. State of Ohio. New Rules for Chronic Pain Prescriptions will help Patients and Prescribers Work to Prevent Addiction. Accessed 8/15/18.

13 Kobus AM et al. Correlates of Higher Dose Opioid Medication Use for Low Back Pain in Primary Care. *J Pain*. 2012 November; 13(11): 1131–1138.

14 Volkow ND and McLellan T. Opioid Abuse in Chronic Pain – Misconceptions and Mitigation Strategies. *New England J Med.* 374:13 March 31 2016. 1253–1263.

15 Nafziger AN and Barkin RL. Opioid Therapy in Acute and Chronic Pain. *J Clin Pharmacology.* 2018, 58(9): 1111–1122.

REFERENCES

1. Datta S, Trescot A, Lee M, Hansen H. Opioid pharmacology. *Pain Physician Journal.* 2008;11(2S).
2. Booth M. *Opium: A History.* 1st ed. Edited by St. Martin's Griffin. New York: St. Martin's Griffin; 1999.
3. Agin H, Çalkavur S, Özdemir D, Bak M. A case of opium intoxication mimicking nephrotic syndrome. *The Internet Journal of Pharmacology.* 2002;1(1):4.
4. Ulrich T. Putting a number on pain. 2014. https://medicalxpress.com/news/2014-07-pain.html, 2020.
5. North RA, Egan TM. Actions and distributions of opioid peptides in peripheral tissues. *British Medical Bulletin.* Jan 1983;39(1):71–75.
6. Lierz P, Punsmann P. Opioids in pain therapy. *The Internet Journal of Pharmacology.* 2000;1(1).
7. Stoner KL, Harder H, Fallowfield LJ, Jenkins VA. Intravenous versus subcutaneous drug administration: Which do patients prefer? A systematic review. *Patient.* Jul 2014.
8. Smith HS. Opioid metabolism. *Mayo Clinic Proceedings.* 2009;84(7):613–624.
9. McCrimmon DR, Alheid GF. On the opiate trail of respiratory depression. *American Journal of Physiology-Regulatory, Integrative and Comparative Physiology.* 2003;285(6):R1274–R1275.
10. Kaufman MS, Ganti L, Rusovici A. *First Aid for the Medicine Clerkship.* 3rd ed. New York: McGraw-Hill Medical; 2010.
11. Dowell D, Haegerich TM, Chou R. CDC guideline for prescribing opioids for chronic pain: United States, 2016. *JAMA.* 2016;315(15):1624–1645.
12. Prevention CfDCa. Prescribing practices. https://www.cdc.gov/drugoverdose/data/prescribing/prescribing-practices.html.
13. Shah A, Hayes CJ, Martin BC. Characteristics of initial prescription episodes and likelihood of long-term opioid use: United States, 2006–2015. *Morbidity and Mortality Weekly Report.* 2017;66(10):265–269.
14. Drug overdose deaths in the United States, 1999–2019. 2020. https://www.cdc.gov/nchs/products/databriefs/db394.htm, 2021.
15. Drug overdose deaths in the U.S. top 100,000 annually. 2021. https://www.cdc.gov/nchs/pressroom/nchs_press_releases/2021/20211117.htm. Accessed 27 December 2021.
16. Hudgins JD, Porter JJ, Monuteaux MC, Bourgeois FT. Prescription opioid use and misuse among adolescents and young adults in the United States: A national survey study. *PLoS Medicine.* 2019;16(11):e1002922.
17. Bonar EE, Coughlin L, Roche JS, Philyaw-Kotov ML, Bixler EA, Sinelnikov S, Kolosh A, Cihak MJ, Cunningham RM, Walton MA. Prescription opioid misuse among adolescents and emerging adults in the United States: A scoping review. *Preventive Medicine.* 2020;132:105972.
18. Ailes EC, Dawson AL, Lind JN, Gilboa SM, Frey MT, Broussard CS, Honein MA. Opioid prescription claims among women of reproductive age: United States, 2008–2012. *Morbidity and Mortality Weekly Report.* 2015;64(2):37–41.
19. Haight SC, Ko JY, Tong VT, Bohm MK, Callaghan WM. Opioid use disorder documented at delivery hospitalization: United States, 1999–2014. *Morbidity and Mortality Weekly Report.* Aug 10 2018;67(31): 845–849.
20. Glantz A. 'Candy Land' VA effects ripple through state. *Stevens Point Journal.* 2015.
21. Florida DoJUSAsOMDo. United States reaches $22 million settlement agreement with CVS for unlawful distribution of controlled substances. 2015.
22. Mann B. Federal judge approves landmark $8.3 billion purdue pharma opioid settlement. 2020. https://www.npr.org/2020/11/17/936022386/federal-judge-approves-landmark-8-3-billion-purdue-pharma-opioid-settlement. Accessed 1 October 2021.
23. Netflix. The business of drugs. Fox A, trans. *Opioids.* 2020;1. Netflix:40 min.
24. Forsythe M, Bogdanich W. McKinsey settles for nearly $600 million over role in opioid crisis. *The New York Times*, 2021.
25. Control CFD. Prescription drug monitoring programs (PDMPs). 2020. https://www.cdc.gov/drugoverdose/pdmp/states.html. Accessed 1 April 2021.
26. Wood SP. Prescription monitoring programs: Helpful or harmful? 2018. https://www.health.harvard.edu/blog/prescription-monitoring-programs-helpful-or-harmful-2018060814001. Accessed 1 April 2021.
27. Wheeler E, Jones TS, Gilbert MK, Davidson PJ. Opioid overdose prevention programs providing naloxone to laypersons: United States, 2014. *Morbidity and Mortality Weekly Report.* Jun 19 2015;64(23):631–635.
28. Walley AY, Xuan Z, Hackman HH, Quinn E, Doe-Simkins M, Sorensen-Alawad A, Ruiz S, Ozonoff A. Opioid overdose rates and implementation of overdose education and nasal naloxone distribution in Massachusetts: Interrupted time series analysis. *BMJ.* 2013;346:f174.
29. McClellan C, Lambdin BH, Ali MM, Mutter R, Davis CS, Wheeler E, Pemberton M, Kral AH. Opioid-overdose laws association with opioid use and overdose mortality. *Addiction Behavior.* Nov 2018;86:90–95.

30. General OotS. U.S. Surgeon General's advisory on naloxone and opioid overdose. 2018. https://www.hhs.gov/surgeongeneral/priorities/opioids-and-addiction/naloxone-advisory/index.html. Accessed 26 January 2021.
31. Control CfD. Reverse overdose to prevent death. 2020. https://www.cdc.gov/drugoverdose/prevention/reverse-od.html, 2021.
32. *Clinical Guidelines for Withdrawal Management and Treatment of Drug Dependence in Closed Settings*. Geneva: World Health Organization; 2009.
33. Foundation CH. Medication-assisted treatment for opioid use disorder. 2021. https://www.chcf.org/collection/medication-assisted-treatment-for-opioid-use-disorder/.
34. Velander JR. Suboxone: Rationale, science, misconceptions. *The Ochsner Journal.* Spring 2018;18(1): 23–29.
35. Welsh C, Valadez-Meltzer A. Buprenorphine: A (relatively) new treatment for opioid dependence. *Psychiatry (Edgmont (PA: Township)).* 2005;2(12):29–39.
36. Buprenorphine Package Insert. https://www.accessdata.fda.gov/drugsatfda_docs/label/2021/020732s024lbl.pdf
37. Shulman M, Wai JM, Nunes EV. Buprenorphine treatment for opioid use disorder: An overview. *CNS Drugs.* Jun 2019;33(6):567–580.
38. Haber LA, DeFries T, Martin M. Things we do for no reason™: Discontinuing buprenorphine when treating acute pain. *Journal of Hospital Medicine.* Oct 1 2019; 14(10):633–635.
39. Kleber HD. Methadone maintenance 4 decades later. *JAMA.* 2008;300(19):2303–2305.
40. Fingerhut LA. Increases in poisoning and methadone-related deaths: United States, 1999–2005, 2008.
41. https://www.drugs.com/drug-interactions/methadone.html
42. Ferrari A, Coccia CP, Bertolini A, Sternieri E. Methadone: Metabolism, pharmacokinetics and interactions. *Pharmacology Research.* Dec 2004;50(6):551–559.
43. *Drug and Human Performance Fact Sheet.* National Highway Traffic Safety Administration; 2004. https://rosap.ntl.bts.gov/view/dot/1759
44. DOLOPHINE. RXList; 2021. https://www.rxlist.com/methadone/generic-drug.htm
45. *Methadone Hydrochloride (marketed as Dolophine) Information.* Food and Drug Administration; 2015. https://www.fda.gov/drugs/postmarket-drug-safety-information-patients-and-providers/methadone-hydrochloride-marketed-dolophine-information
46. Group MMW. *Methadone.* Drug Enforcement Administration Office of Diversion Control; 2007.
47. O'Donnell J, Vogenberg FR. Applying legal risk management to the clinical use of methadone. *P & T: A Peer-Reviewed Journal for Formulary Management.* 2011;36(12):813–822.

18 Adverse Effects of Diabetic Drugs
Focus on Hypoglycemia

Gourang P. Patel and James T. O'Donnell

SYNOPSIS

18.1 DIABETES DEMOGRAPHICS AND EPIDEMIOLOGY

Millions of patients with diabetes are treated with insulin and sulfonylureas, oral drugs which lower blood sugar. Occasionally, patients receive either insulin or oral sugar-lowering drugs in error. In diabetic patients and in those patients who receive these drugs in error, the toxic effects may be devastating or fatal. The pharmacology of insulin and sulfonylureas are in themselves the topics of review articles and chapters. For the purposes of this chapter, these topics are briefly reviewed to assist in understanding the disease, and the use of agents that treat diabetes, along with the factors leading to hypoglycemia, is presented. Hypoglycemic injuries will be demonstrated by a thorough discussion of the pathophysiology and elucidated through case discussion from the literature and litigation files.

For a more comprehensive review, the reader is referred to references 1 through 6, which include several excellent reviews on these topics.

18.2 INSULIN

The first patient to receive the active extracts of the pancreas was prepared by Banting and Best in 1922 in Toronto. Insulin facilitates cells in the liver, skeletal muscles, and fat tissue to absorb glucose delivered from the blood, thus inducing a reduction in the abnormally high concentration and excretion of blood glucose (sugar). Daily injections were then begun, and there was immediate improvement. Thus, replacement therapy with the newly discovered

DOI: 10.1201/9781003615323-20

hormone, insulin, had interrupted what was clearly an otherwise fatal metabolic disorder.[1] Stable extracts were eventually obtained, and patients in many parts of North America were soon being treated with insulin.[2,3] The Nobel Prize in Medicine and Physiology was awarded to Banting and Macleod with remarkable rapidity in 1923.[4]

18.3 INSULIN PREPARATIONS

Insulin preparations available in the United States differ in concentration, time of onset and duration of action, purity, and species of origin. Clinically significant differences among them have been reviewed. Each of these factors plays a role in determining the type and dose of insulin that is best suited to an individual patient. Insulin U-100 (100 units/ml) is the most commonly used concentration. (The numeral following the "U" indicates the number of units of insulin per milliliter.) Although most diabetics today use U-100 insulin, U-40, U-200, and U-500 insulins are also available. U-40 syringes are color-coded "red"; U-100 products are color-coded "orange with black lettering."

Recombinant-engineered human-type insulin, primarily used in the U-100 concentration, has almost completely replaced natural beef and pork insulins and has, in turn, largely been replaced by bio-synthetic insulin analogs. These "engineered insulins" are claimed to cause less insulin resistance and less hypersensitivity risk and have more predictable pharmacokinetics. The downside is that additional insulin preparations increase the opportunity for medication errors. The insulin analog preparations that have been added to the market for use include three ultra-short-acting drugs (i.e., activity ranging from 5 to 15 minutes). Examples of ultra-short-acting insulin medications include lispro, aspart, and glulisine. Pre-mixed preparation of short- and medium-acting insulins and insulin analogs are also popular. There are also extended-action preparations now available such as glargine, degludec, and detemir[4] whose action is constant over a 24-hour period except when given intravenously—when they behave like ordinary insulin. It is essential, to reduce errors, that insulin analogs are referred to by their proper names at all times rather than referred to as simply as "insulin", especially when requesting assays for plasma "insulin".

18.4 CLINICAL USE OF INSULIN

Insulin and its bio-synthetic analogs are the mainstay for treatment of all patients with type 1 or post-pancreatectomy diabetes, as well as those with gestational diabetes and many type 2 diabetic patients, especially those who are not adequately controlled by diet and/or oral hypoglycemic agents.[5] Insulin is critical for the management of diabetic ketoacidosis (commonly abbreviated in medical documentation as DKA) and hyperglycemic, nonketotic coma (commonly abbreviated in medical documentation as HHNK) and the perioperative management of both type 1 and type 2 diabetic patients. Its popularity for the prevention of hyperglycemia in non-diabetic patients in intensive care units has declined as its association with increased morbidity and mortality has been appreciated. Long-term treatment with insulin or analogs relies on subcutaneous injection, but it can be administered intravenously or intramuscularly when necessary. In all cases, the goal is to mimic physiological insulin secretion to achieve normalization of blood glucose and all aspects of metabolism. An optimal treatment strategy requires a comprehensive approach to regulate diet, exercise, and insulin administration.

18.4.1 Dosing

There are a number of methods for dosing insulin. For hospitalized patients, many clinicians prefer a "sliding scale" approach. Blood glucose concentrations are ordered several times a day (e.g., every four hours, every six hours, or at specified times—7 A.M., 11 A.M., 4 A.M., and midnight) such that fasting values and values before meals are obtained. The concept of sliding scale has been adjusted in clinical practice as scheduled dosing three times daily based on meal consumption. Subcutaneously administered regular insulin is then ordered in an amount that increases corresponding to an increase in blood glucose. When the patient's insulin requirement has stabilized over two to three days, the number of units required during the previous 24 hours is totaled. The patient can then be given a single injection of intermediate-acting insulin; the beginning dose is two-thirds to three-fourths of the 24-hour regular insulin dose and is given 30 minutes before breakfast. The dose can then be "fine-tuned" and adjusted based on blood sugar values over the next several days.[6]

As the type 2 diabetic is usually not prone to ketoacidosis, there is less urgency to initiate aggressive therapy. Most patients can be started on diet and metformin, to which one or more of the other oral anti-diabetic agents may be added. Eventually, some 50 percent of patients with type 2 diabetes will require insulin or one of its analogs either alone or in combination with other drugs for adequate diabetic control. Patients should use the same preparation continuously to avoid a change in dosage requirement.

18.5 HYPOGLYCEMIA (LOW BLOOD SUGAR)

Far and away the most frequent causes of hypoglycemia are the administration of insulin and ingestion of oral anti-diabetic agents. Such agents are also responsible for factitious hypoglycemia in both diabetic and non-diabetic patients; these properties have been exploited for use as a poison by people with malevolent or homicidal intent.[7] A list of recognized causes of hypoglycemia is given in Table 18.1. Another risk factor for hypoglycemia is renal insufficiency. The kidney has a role in insulin secretion. Patients with kidney insufficiency impair insulin secretion, and the retained insulin can also contribute to low blood sugar and result in hypoglycemia.

18.5.1 Etiologies of Hypoglycemia

Alcohol consumption can induce hypoglycemia but is uncommon except in fasting malnourished individuals

TABLE 18.1
Etiologies of Hypoglycemia

Postprandial hypoglycemia	
Idiopathic	
Alimentary	
Early type 2 diabetes mellitus	
Leucine sensitivity	
Enzyme deficiencies	
Fasting hypoglycemia or underproductive glucose	
Hormone deficiencies	
	Hypopituitarism
	Adrenal insufficiency
	Catecholamine deficiency
	Glucagon deficiency
	Counter-regulatory hormone deficiency in diabetes mellitus
Enzyme defects	
	Glycogen storage disease
	Gluconeogenesis enzyme deficiency
Substrate deficiency	
	Ketotic hypoglycemia of infancy
	Severe malnutrition
	Exercise
	Uremia
	Pregnancy
Acquired liver disease	
Hepatic congestion (congestive heart failure)	
Hepatitis, hepatic necrosis	
Cirrhosis	
Drug-induced disease	
Inhibition of glycogenolysis of beta-blockers	
Fasting hypoglycemia or overuse of glucose	
Hyperinsulinism	
	Insulinoma
	Exogenous insulin administration
	Administration of sulfonylureas
	Immune disease with insulin antibodies
	Abrupt discontinuation of total parenteral nutrition
Appropriate insulin levels	
	Extrapancreatic tumors
	Cachexia with fat depletion
	Carnitine deficiency

and children.[8] Hepatic metabolism of ethyl alcohol blunts gluconeogenesis, causing blood glucose levels to decline gradually into the symptomatic hypoglycemic range. Characteristically, alcohol-induced fasting hypoglycemia occurs within 6–36 hours after the conclusion of drinking and carries much higher mortality than insulin-induced hypoglycemia. The combination of alcohol and insulin overdose is especially dangerous. Alcohol also accentuates the propensity to produce reactive hypoglycemia in response to the ingestion of a sugary solution on an empty stomach,[1] giving rise to the aptly named "gin and tonic hypoglycemia".

An unusually severe type of reactive hypoglycemia occurs in a condition known as autoimmune insulin syndrome (AIS) in which the plasma contains very high titers of insulin auto-antibodies whose kinetic characteristics resemble those of antibodies induced by insulin in insulin-treated diabetics. Common in Japan and East Asia, and associated with the use of thiol-based drugs, AIS is rare in the United States and most other Western countries. Glucose tolerance is frequently impaired, and AIS may be difficult to differentiate from malicious insulin-induced hypoglycemia unless insulin auto-antibodies are specifically assayed and excluded.

Whether late afternoon fatigue, mood changes, depression, and anxiety—the "five o'clock dwindles"—are related to blood glucose levels has been argued in the lay press and some medical publications. Most data do not support a correlation but suggest that such manifestations are purely emotional in origin or are derivative perversions of the hunger drive. In a very small number of individuals, however, glucose levels do drop to symptomatically low concentrations following a meal rich in rapidly absorbed carbohydrates and is appropriately described as reactive hypoglycemia.[9]

18.5.2 Insulin-Induced Hypoglycemia

Though not the only one, hypoglycemia is easily the most common adverse reaction to insulin and its analogs. This may result from an inappropriately large dose, from a mismatch between the time of peak delivery of "insulin" into the circulation and food intake, or from the superimposition of additional factors that increase sensitivity to insulin (adrenal insufficiency, pituitary insufficiency), or that increase insulin-independent glucose uptake (of which exercise is the most important). Hypoglycemia is the major risk that must be weighed against any benefits of intensive therapy. The more vigorous the attempt to achieve constantly normal blood glucose levels—usually described as "good diabetes control"—as determined by a near-normal hemoglobin A1c (HbA1c) level, the more likely the patient is to experience hypoglycemia, especially that unaccompanied by symptoms so-called "hypoglycemia unawareness". Mild, but significant, hypoglycemic episodes are much more common than severe reactions—defined as requiring third-party assistance—and their frequency also increases with intensive therapy. Careful investigation of a patient's insulin therapy is necessary to ensure insulin preparations have not been mistakenly taken and/or incorrectly filled by the pharmacy, as there are many different insulin preparations available for patient therapy.

18.6 PATHOPHYSIOLOGY AND CLINICAL SYMPTOMS OF HYPOGLYCEMIA

Since brain tissue depends on glucose as its primary fuel, hypoglycemia, or a low blood glucose level, has a marked impact on brain metabolism. Alterations of brain function are responsible for the characteristic symptoms of hypoglycemia even though they are manifested throughout the body. As blood glucose levels fall, characteristic signs and symptoms appear—though not invariable. In normal volunteers given infusions of insulin, hypoglycemic symptoms occur when their glucose falls to about 45 mg/dl (2.5 mol/l); however, symptoms quite often occur at higher blood glucose concentrations, especially in diabetic patients whose diabetes is poorly controlled, depending on the rate and magnitude of the change.

The commonest symptoms both in diabetic patients and in volunteers are sweating, anxiety, a sense of inner trembling and a pounding heart, fatigue and muscular weakness, light-headedness, blurred and double vision, and hunger. Nausea is quite common but vomiting from insulin-induced hypoglycemia is virtually unknown—except in children in whom it is common—and its occurrence in the adult should always lead to suspicion as to the cause of the hypoglycemia.

Many of the prodromal symptoms are attributed to the activation of the sympathetic and parasympathetic nervous systems and are accompanied by objective signs of tachycardia, coldness of the skin, and pallor. As blood glucose levels decline further, cerebration becomes impaired, leading to confusion, abnormalities in decision-making processes, the appearance of a glassy-eyed stare, aberrant behavior, and occasionally overt hostility and aggression. If glucose levels fall gradually, especially in diabetic patients who are trying to achieve "good diabetic control" the prodromal syndrome—often referred to as "warning symptoms"—may be entirely lacking; and the patient is totally unaware of any problem. Instead, they may progress directly into a confusional state and unconsciousness or, very rarely, a state of "neuroglycopenic automatism" during which habitual tasks may be carried out in an automaton-like manner and of which the patient has no recollection of being restored to normal. Hypoglycemia may lead to convulsions in children, but this is rare in adults. If the hypoglycemia is severe and prolonged—usually as a result of deliberate suicidal overdosing with "insulin"—irreversible brain damage and even death may ensue.[10–12]

The correlation between a measured blood glucose concentration and its effect on cerebral function is poor. This is as true for the more subtle manifestations of neuroglycopenia as for those resulting from stimulation of the autonomic nervous system that, when experienced by patients receiving treatment with insulin or sulfonylureas, are often referred to as "warning symptoms". They are so named because they are used by patients on anti-diabetic therapy to warn of impending severe mental and physical disability unless aborted by taking readily available carbohydrates by mouth. By the time a patient gets "warning symptoms" they will, however, probably already have suffered some degree of cognitive impairment of which they themselves are unaware. This can often be recognized by a close relative as an early sign of impending, severe brain malfunction and lead them to suggest remedial action. Sometimes "warning symptoms" never develop,[1] as in the condition called "sub-acute neuroglycopenia" when it occurs in cases of "spontaneous hypoglycemia". It is more graphically described as "hypoglycemia unawareness" when it occurs in patients treated with anti-diabetic drugs who had previously experienced and appreciated the significance of "warning symptoms".

Confusion, inability to concentrate, clouding of consciousness, irritability and irrational behavior or anger, stupor, and coma are among the many manifestations of neuroglycopenia whether they are preceded by autonomic symptoms or not. And it is these neuroglycopenic features that bring patients with hypoglycemia into conflict with the law, not the more obvious autonomic or warning symptoms, of which sweating, anxiety, tremors, and pounding heartbeat are the most common, and which are known to every diabetic patient treated with insulin and many treated with a sulfonylurea. It is a common defense to claim never to have been told by one's medical team the clinical significance of warning symptoms although this is now usually and easily refuted. Obstinacy amounting to bloody-mindedness (hemodementia) is a characteristic and particularly dangerous symptom as it may prevent a patient from taking the corrective action they would otherwise take instinctively.

The essential biochemical trigger is a blood sugar level of less than 25–30 mg/100 ml. It does not usually lead to permanent brain damage until it has lasted some six hours in adults. Coma used to be thought to be caused by lack of fuel but is now believed to be due, largely, if not exclusively, to the release of excitogenic aminoacids such as glutamate in the brain. Any part of the brain may be affected but the cerebellum is usually spared. Characteristically the hippocampus and dentate nuclei are affected and may serve to distinguish hypoglycemic from anoxic brain damage. The cerebral cortex may suffer major damage; cortical nerve cells degenerate and are replaced by microgliocytes and astrocytes.[13–15]

Another issue that is of concern is whether or not a diabetic patient has an appropriate physiologic response to hypoglycemia. The mechanisms of hypoglycemia unawareness in diabetic patients are multi-factorial and can include a combination of any of the following: chronic low blood sugar, recurrent severe hypoglycemia, and failure of counter-regulatory hormones. Previous hypoglycemia can blunt or decrease the physiologic response of our endogenous catecholamines, which should help identify the clinical episode. In addition, during recurrent hypoglycemia, the blood flow to the brain is significantly reduced which would naturally lead to less activation of vital neurons in the brain as well. Since glucose is a vital substrate for fuel and energy for the brain, the changes can be very impactful. Some researchers have also discovered that recurrent episodes actually increase a critical neurotransmitter in the brain (i.e., GABA) which functions normally as an inhibitor, so this physiologic change further complicates the way a diabetic patient can respond to recurrent hypoglycemia episodes.

18.7 INCIDENCE

Clinically documented hypoglycemia occurs most frequently in the insulin-requiring diabetic. Other organic causes of hypoglycemia such as islet cell tumors; insulin-like growth factor (IGF-2)-secreting tumors; hepatic, renal, and cardiac failure; infections; and alcohol intake also deserve consideration in the symptomatic individual. The issue of animal versus human insulin-induced hypoglycemic reactions has now largely disappeared and has been replaced by an interest in insulin analogs.[11] It is now generally accepted that the increased incidence of "hypoglycemia unawareness" in patients treated with human-type insulin and insulin analogs is closely related to the tightness of diabetic control and that its prevention by raising the target level for HbA1c in insulin, and sulfonylurea-treated diabetic patients is remarkably successful. Pharmacists should not substitute insulin preparations without the approval of the prescribing physician or without informing the patient of the type of insulin change to be made.[12]

18.8 PATHOPHYSIOLOGY AND BIOCHEMISTRY OF HYPOGLYCEMIA

Glucose normally furnishes 98–100 percent of the brain's energy needs but can, under special circumstances, be replaced by the "ketone", beta-hydroxybutyrate. Glucose is actively conveyed from the blood plasma into the nerve cells largely through the mediation of the glucose transporter protein GLUT 1. [14]A genetic deficiency of this transporter leads to brain malfunction associated with "normoglycemic neuroglycopenia". Downregulation of GLUT1 in chronic hyperglycemic states is believed to account for the onset of neuroglycopenic symptoms at higher blood glucose levels in diabetics than in healthy subjects. The minimum glucose level needed to maintain glucose transport across the blood–brain barrier and into brain cells is undefined and varies. Some individuals adapt to ambient blood glucose levels as low as 30–40 mg/100 ml,[16–18] and a few retain consciousness at blood glucose levels of 20 mg/100 ml or below. Conversely, an insulin-dependent diabetic may experience a "hypoglycemic" reaction at a blood glucose value of 100 mg/100 ml if the blood glucose had been rapidly lowered from a previous level of 300 mg/100 ml or so. Thus, the level of circulating glucose is imprecisely correlated with the brain's substrate requirements. Consequently, it is often difficult to assess the significance of symptoms, especially those with alleged reactive hypoglycemia. We have therefore distinguished hypoglycemia, an arbitrarily defined measured blood glucose concentration, from the neuroglycopenic symptoms to which it gives rise, and which are specifically relieved by glucose. Insulin-dependent diabetics may also have defective counter-regulatory mechanisms and thus may be exceptionally vulnerable to hypoglycemia.

18.9 ADVERSE REACTIONS INVOLVING HYPOGLYCEMIA

Clinically, one of the most important situations in which severe hypoglycemia develops is accidental or deliberate overdosing with insulin. The following cases demonstrate this type of occurrence.

18.9.1 Insulin Damages Baby's Brain; Pharmacist Error Suggested

In this case, a hospital pharmacist and technicians violated their own policies and procedures regarding operations in the laminar flow hood and IV additive room. As a result of the pharmacist's negligence in preparing sterile admixtures, a Fairfax, Virginia neonate became brain damaged, following insulin-induced hypoglycemic encephalopathy. After several seizures, the child's physicians suspected hypoglycemia and searched for a cause, initially suspecting that insulin was added to the total parenteral nutrition (TPN) bag by the pharmacist. Although none was ordered, insulin was assayed in the suspect TPN bag, confirming the suspicion of insulin-induced hypoglycemia. Others in the hospital, including the risk manager and the pharmacists involved, insisted that the insulin was not added to the pharmacy. The police were called in to look for an interloper. Hospital spokesmen argued that someone must have added the insulin to the bag while it was hanging at the patient's incubator's side in the busy ICU. Shades of Beverley Allitt—a British nurse who murdered four children and attempted murder of nine other victims using insulin in the 1990s. The child suffered irreversible brain damage and required admission to a home for brain-damaged children. Glucose levels as low as 14 mg/100 ml were detected during periods of seizure, tremulousness, hypotonia, and pallor—all classical signs of hypoglycemia and insulin shock.

In the opinion of the pharmacist expert (JTOD) in the case, the insulin was accidentally added to the baby's TPN bags while in the pharmacy, resulting in severe hypoglycemia and irreversible brain damage. Negligence was apparent in the pharmacy, policies and procedures were ignored, and this was the most probable cause for the accident to happen. Opportunities for risk were ignored or overlooked. After a series of legal battles and unfavorable rulings regarding document requests by a malpractice panel and trial judge, the Fairfax Hospital settled the case for the statutory limit of $1 million shortly before the trial was scheduled to begin.[19,20] Coincidentally, on the same day the infant suffered hypoglycemic-induced seizures, another infant received an overdose of insulin in a neonatal TPN bag in the neonatal ICU. The other neonate died following a severe brain-damaging insulin hypoglycemic reaction. The second family also filed a medical malpractice suit that was resolved.

Shortly after the settlement, the first family sued the Fairfax Hospital, and its insurance company and its lawyers requested $60 million in compensatory and punitive damages.[21] The plaintiffs charge that Fairfax Hospital breached its duty to the parents to honestly and expeditiously communicate to the parents all relevant information pertaining to the infant's health care, including all relevant information.

According to the court complaint, at the time the neonates were treated, it was known to the hospital that another patient at a prior time had received unauthorized administration of insulin, causing that patient's death. The lawsuit charged that the defendants engaged in a deliberate cover-up and a pattern of withholding information, which was motivated by a fear of negative publicity and a potential loss of revenue. The defendant placed these considerations ahead of the hospital's duty to communicate honestly and fully the circumstances of the injury.

After the hypoglycemic incidents occurred, an investigative team composed of the hospital risk manager and legal affairs director immediately interviewed pharmacists, nurses, physicians, and others involved in the care of the two injured neonates. They caused testing to be made of the contents of the infant's TPN bags and notified the police about the incidents. The police interviewed several individuals, but they were never invited to interview the pharmacists involved in the preparation of the TPNs. The plaintiffs charged that key investigative information concerning the problems uncovered in the pharmacy was not provided to the police. One defense expert who concluded that the error occurred in the pharmacy was told to tear up his notes. The matter was not referred to a regular Morbidity and Mortality committee or similar peer review committee as would normally be done for such a medical misadventure. The investigation quickly disclosed that the insulin was detected in the two neonates' TPN bags, which would not be possible under ordinary clinical circumstances. Insulin, if used in NICU, was diluted first and then only added to the intravenous tubing, never the IV bag. Both bags were supposed to contain heparin; neither did, a fact concealed in the investigation and subsequent litigation discovery, until the risk manager admitted this fact close to the time of trial. This was a critical point since it explains how the insulin could have been placed in the bags, accidentally replacing the ordered heparin.

At the time following the first neonate injury, the family was not informed of the similar insulin toxicity experienced by the Smith child, nor of the previous insulin death. They were informed that both the hospital and the police investigation had determined that the injury was conclusively the result of an unknown third party's intentional act and not any fault on the part of the hospital. The lawsuit charged that the defendants, to deflect liability for the hospital's malfeasance, concocted the explanation that a third-party interloper entered the NICU without being seen, entered two different rooms, and injected insulin into the IV bags of both neonates, an explanation which is contradicted by the findings of the hospital's own investigation. When contacted, the public relations department of the Hospital declined to discuss any remedial changes implemented by the pharmacy at the hospital, stating that to admit that changes had taken place was tantamount to an admission that the errors had occurred, and the hospital maintained that the insulin was placed in the bag(s) by a criminal interloper, not negligently by the pharmacy. Such a deference is in our experience common in similar cases. The hospital representative hastened to add that the settlement in the underlying suit does not assume an admission of guilt or liability. According to Philip Hirschkop, the Alexandria, Virginia plaintiff's attorney, all of the defendants (hospital, attorneys, and insurance company) refused to answer any discovery in the case pending outcome of demurrers that say that the complaint does not, as a matter of law, state sufficient claims upon which claims can be granted. The trial judge in the case forced the defense to turn over work product notes.[22] The resolution of the concealment case is unknown.

18.10 END PRODUCT TESTING RECOMMENDED

In a related case with a newborn, *Hospital Pharmacy Report* correspondent Gebhart reports that the Good Samaritan Hospital of West Palm Beach, Florida, agreed to a $1.5 million settlement in what appeared to be a pharmacy error in which a TPN bag contained no glucose. After nearly a week on TPN, the child started having seizures. Medical staff suspected infection, but no evidence of sepsis could be found. They did notice, however, that bolus doses of glucose seemed to calm the seizures. It took several hours to discover that the real problem was hypoglycemia. The resulting hypoglycemia caused irreversible brain damage to the neonate. The mother of the infant, an intensive care nurse, campaigned for a change in pharmacy and nursing practice standards to prevent a recurrence, calling for testing of all TPN solutions before administration to detect such errors.[22]

This plea for absolute certainty has also come from within pharmacy editorial circles as well. Neil Davis, a recognized medication error specialist, in an editorial, suggested a final check of admixtures formulated with automatic compounders using a refractometer, providing an instantaneous reading of the approximate concentration of dextrose present.[23] Some compounders are now manufactured with such refractometers; however, the device is optional. Refractometry is important in pharmacy because it can be used as an aid in (1) identifying a pure substance, (2) establishing the purity of some substances, (3) determining the concentrations of some simple solutions, and (4) quickly determining the uniformity of final compounded preparations. Refractometry is a simple technique used for both qualitative and quantitative analysis.[24] Refractometry (glucose concentration testing) is now a requirement of <USP797>.[25] On January 1, 2004, *USP* chapter 797, Pharmaceutical Compounding—Sterile Preparations, became official. The change from a chapter numbered above 1000 to a chapter below 1000 transitioned from an advisory standard to an enforceable one. *USP* chapter 797 has since been revised several times. The National Association of Boards of Pharmacy supports the inclusion of compounding regulations into state pharmacy practice legislation by drafting such wording in the association's Model Rules and Model State Pharmacy Act. Pharmacy state boards should be consulted to determine the current status of sterile compounding regulations and guidelines.[26]

18.11 INSULIN MURDERS

Murder using insulin is not new to the scientific, forensic, or lay press. In the first edition of *Drug Injury* (2000), the Claus von Bulow story was described. It was publicized widely as a criminal trial, then a book, then a made-for-TV movie, and finally a second trial at which he was completely exonerated. He was accused of criminally administering insulin shots to his wife, resulting in her lapsing into a prolonged coma from which she never recovered, dying some 30 years later. At the second trial, it was demonstrated that Martha von Bulow had experienced spontaneous hypoglycemia on each of two occasions, separated by a year. There was nothing to suggest insulin as their cause apart from what turned out to be a false accusation by Martha von Bulow's maid that she had seen a vial of insulin in Von Bulow's possession and failure by the prosecution to consider the actual cause: sepsis on one occasion; alcohol on the other. The subject of insulin murders and other forensic aspects of hypoglycemia are dealt with in greater detail in the Forensic Criminal Applications of Diabetic Drugs chapter by Vincent Marks in chapter 21 of the Fourth Edition of the *Drug Injury* book series.

18.12 HYPOGLYCEMIA FROM THE SULFONYLUREA DERIVATIVES

Early anti-bacterial sulfa drugs used to treat soldiers in France were serendipitously discovered to lower blood sugar, some with serious and fatal results. Some sulfa substances, specifically the sulfonylureas, were subsequently proved effective in treating some diabetic patients. Carbutamide was the precursor of today's sulfonylureas but was withdrawn because it caused bone marrow depression. Sulfonylureas continue to be used to treat type 2 diabetics throughout the world in conjunction with diet, exercise, and usually at least one other anti-diabetic medicine. Sulfonylureas lower plasma glucose by stimulating β-cells to secrete insulin, which they can do regardless of the concentration of glucose in the blood perfusing them. Thus, the normal mechanism by which insulin secretion is regulated by the blood glucose concentration no longer applies, and hypoglycemia is a common and predictable adverse reaction to them.[27] Sulfonylureas and other insulin secretagogues are gradually being replaced by glucagon-like peptide-1 (GLP-1) mimetics, which are much less prone to produce hypoglycemia if indeed they do at all.[28] GLP-1 receptor agonists activate the GLP-1 receptor. This drug class is used in the treatment of type 2 diabetes. Adverse effects of the GLP-1 mimetics will be discussed later in this chapter.

18.13 ADVERSE EFFECTS OF THE SULFONYLUREAS

Adverse reactions to sulfonylurea range from relatively mild complaints of gastrointestinal upset to life-threatening hypoglycemia. The overall risk of an adverse reaction is said to be 5 percent, and less than 2 percent of people taking sulfonylurea need to discontinue it because of side effects.[29] Hypoglycemia can occur with any sulfonylurea. Seltzer reported a case series and noted that hypoglycemic reactions from sulfonylureas had a morbidity rate of 3 percent and were lethal in 10 percent of patients reporting this side effect.[30] Factors that predispose patients to sulfonylurea hypoglycemia include the use of high doses, age greater than 60 years old, decreased renal function, decreased hepatic function, dehydration, and decreased food intake. Sulfonylureas that pose the greatest threat include those with longer half-lives (glyburide) and were a major factor in the market withdrawal of chlorpropamide as a treatment for diabetes.

Hypoglycemia is a predictable adverse effect of sulfonylureas in those who use it as prescribed or deliberately to produce harm as well as in those who receive it accidentally, such as in the case described here:

> MF, a 76-year-old woman had undergone cardiac surgery for mitral valve replacement 3 years earlier. She was currently suffering from heart failure and had been housebound for the last eight to nine months. She was receiving regular treatment with digoxin, a cardiac stimulant, furosemide, and several other medicines. Her doctor wrote a prescription for 56 tablets of furosemide, 40mg, to be taken twice a day as instructed. The prescription was "cashed" at a local pharmacy by her husband. Three days later MF collapsed at home and her husband called the doctor immediately made his way to her home to find her apparently suffering from a stroke. He phoned the doctor who came to the home immediately and diagnosed a stroke. He phoned for an ambulance but after doing so he looked at the packaging of the tablets Mr F had given his wife. They were for (glyburide) glibenclamide and not the furosemide that had been prescribed. A POCT (point of care test) glucose was low and glucagon was administered. By the time MF arrived at the hospital, she was conscious. During the next 20–24 hours her blood glucose level was monitored at hourly intervals while receiving an intravenous glucose infusion, but she became hypoglycemic at least once and possibly more. During one such episode she convulsed. Despite continuing normoglycemia, MF became increasingly dyspneic and despite emergency treatment with intravenous furosemide she died 36 hours after her initial collapse.

The coroner heard that the furosemide and glibenclamide were stocked by the pharmacy near one another and came from the same supplier. They were color-coded in identical packaging differing only in the name of the medicine they contained. The pharmacist mistakenly gave the husband the wrong drug which he, being illiterate, did not appreciate and so gave his wife glibenclamide instead of the prescribed furosemide. Exactly how much of the wrong drug she consumed could not be stated with certainty as back calculation from the concentration of glibenclamide measured in her blood was unreliable. Although seven tablets were missing from the prescription pack, the husband was adamant that he gave his wife only three 5 mg tablets shortly before she collapsed with hypoglycemia.

Campbell and Dahlen reported that, in diabetic patients, symptomatic hypoglycemia caused by sulfonylurea is common, especially in those receiving insulin supplements though far less often than in those receiving insulin alone. Many patients have minor episodes that are relieved by food, but coma is rare with legitimate use.[31,32] Reactions have occurred after one dose, after several days of treatment, or after months of drug administration. Most reactions are observed in patients over 50 years of age, and they are more likely to occur in patients with impaired hepatic or renal function. Overdose or inadequate/irregular food intake may initiate hypoglycemia.

Some patients develop profound, refractory, and sometimes fatal hypoglycemia from sulfonylureas usually when taken deliberately in overdose. The propensity for hypoglycemia usually persists for several days even without overdose, so if intravenous glucose administration is required, it is usually for several days,[16–18] unlike hypoglycemia caused by therapeutic insulin use, which is usually instantaneous and short-lived. Treatment is facilitated by co-administration of diazoxide, a sulfonylurea antagonist, or more appropriately treatment with octreotide, a more potent inhibitor of glucagon and insulin.

The Pharmacist Mutual Insurance Company (*www.phmic.com*), which specializes in insuring pharmacies, reports oral hypoglycemics are among the top-ten drug class most frequently involved in litigation, usually resulting from some prescription error resulting in serious injury or death. The American Society for Pharmacy Law related a hypoglycemic reaction report that was almost exact from a report in the *White Sheet*. The case was originally reported by Scala-Barnett in 1986.[33]

On discharge from the hospital, a prescription was written for a patient for acetaminophen with codeine #3, one to two every four hours as needed for pain. The patient had the prescription filled at a community pharmacy. In a diary she kept, it was documented that she took the medication as directed but experienced no relief. A grocery delivery boy who saw the patient during this time related that she was stumbling in what appeared to be a drunken stupor. On the third day following discharge, concerned neighbors forced their way into her apartment and found her unconscious. Near her unconscious body were found two vials of medicine labeled Tylenol #3 and Panadol. Eight days later she died. Although initially thought to be suicide, it was discovered that the pharmacist accidentally filled her prescription with chlorpropamide (Diabenese, Pfizer, New York) instead of the prescribed acetaminophen with codeine #3. The error was discovered by Emergency Department personnel, who discovered that one of the medicine vials by the patient's body contained blue, D-shaped chlorpropamide tablets—distinctly different than the round, white acetaminophen with codeine #3 for which the vial was labeled.

Another case of hypoglycemia-induced brain injury is reported by Kalimo. While at a small local hospital as a convalescent after infection, the patient, due to an accidental exchange of medicine, received 10 mg glibenclamide and 50 mg phenformin at 4 P.M. one day. The following night the patient became comatose because of severe hypoglycemia. He received repeated injections of glucose intravenously starting at about 6 A.M. He awoke somewhat but after a seizure became comatose again, and the blood glucose was not measurable at 2:15 P.M., almost 24 hours after the medication error. The patient was transferred to a larger hospital where his blood glucose was normalized. On arrival, the patient's skin was cold and clammy, and he did not react to any stimuli. The patient remained unresponsive until he died three months later with signs of pulmonary edema and bronchopneumonia.

Several examples come to mind in the author's own consulting experience (O'Donnell). A 60-year-old Michigan woman has erroneously dispensed a prescription for Dymelor (acetohexamide) in place of Dynapen, an antibiotic, resulting in a coma and some residual neurologic sequelae. A 65-year-old Hawaiian woman was erroneously given Dymelor in place of a prescription for Diamox, resulting in a coma, deterioration of her general health, and death shortly thereafter. The pharmacy company in Hawaii settled the wrongful death case for $400,000.

18.13.1 Case Report

A case in the Midwest deserves discussion. A middle-aged man was required by his prescription drug insurance plan to obtain his chronic medications from a mail service pharmacy. He did this for several years without incident. However, after receiving his "Xanax" prescription, he suffered a series of inexplicable serious and life-threatening hypoglycemic reactions—inexplicable until the pills in his "Xanax" bottle were identified as glimepiride (Amaryl), an oral sulfonylurea hypoglycemic agent. This was identified as a prescription mis fill (error) by physicians at Mayo Clinic as well as by the patient's primary care physician. At the Mayo Clinic, the patient was evaluated by a psychiatrist and found not to be exhibiting factitious behavior, that is, fabricating the error and that he was not, nor he had been suicidal (taking a lethal dose of drugs FOUR times). The patient injured his left leg during his first hypoglycemic coma event (trapped his leg under his body for several hours), and he continues to suffer pain and neurological deficit (sciatica, neuropathy, regional pain syndrome—left lower extremity from that insult. He tried working after the series of hospitalizations but was unable to work and has had IME and FCE and neurology rulings of disability. His ability to work is limited to sedentary work—incompatible with his work as a mortician.

Three mail service pharmacy employees. At least one employee of the three admits that errors in filling prescriptions have occurred. However, all three pharmacy employees testified that the "system" cannot make mistakes, and checking computer records "proves" that alprazolam—not glimepiride—was in the patient's Xanax prescription bottle in August 2010 and therefore denies any mistake by the mail service pharmacy.

My opinions (JTOD), who served as a pharmacist expert, are expressed with reasonable pharmaceutical certainty.

1. More likely than not, glimepiride, not alprazolam, was in the bottle delivered in August 2010, and, thus, the mail service pharmacy and its pharmacists provided the wrong drug, was mislabeled, contained the wrong fill date, and in doing so were negligent and departed from the standard of care of reasonable and prudent pharmacists.
2. All pharmacies, unfortunately, commit errors, even with good systems. The most frequent pharmacy error is dispensation of the wrong drug.[34,35]
3. If glimepiride, not alprazolam, was in the bottle delivered, then the pharmacy and its pharmacists provided the wrong drug, mislabeled it, and provided the wrong fill date; in doing so, they were negligent and departed from the standard of care of reasonable and prudent pharmacists.
4. Glimepiride, a second-generation oral sulfonylurea agent, given to a euglycemic patient, will lower blood sugar and, if the blood sugar is lowered too much, may lead to dangerously low blood sugar levels, with resultant metabolic and encephalopathy and other neurological sequelae.[36]
5. The pharmacy error is the proximate cause of several life-threatening experiences, a permanent disability to the patient's (left leg), and cognitive deficits.

18.13.2 Bases for Opinions

Pharmacists have a duty to dispense the correct drug, label the prescription container, identify the prescriber and the patient, and note the date that the prescription is filled on the prescription label and receipt. These are universal requirements throughout the United States. To provide the wrong drug, wrong instructions, wrong fill date, wrong name, and so on is a violation of pharmacy practice acts and is negligence. When an incorrectly dispensed drug is taken by a patient and the patient is injured, the pharmacist's error/negligence is proximately related to the injury.

The patient's hypoglycemia documented in several hospitalizations was caused by his unintentional and accidental consumption of glimepiride. His chronic sciatic neuropathy is traced to an injury to his leg when he nearly died following the first hypoglycemic injury. Other experts have evaluated and found him disabled, having limited work capacity, and cognitively impaired, all related to his initial hypoglycemic reactions.

Sulfonylureas clearly make up the majority of community pharmacy-related hypoglycemia adverse events and therefore should command the respect and diligence of each pharmacist handling and dispensing these products.[37] Sulfonylureas have been used in criminal activities on very few occasions, but their use to produce self-harm is far from rare. The major laboratory findings in such cases, namely, hypoglycemia associated with inappropriately high insulin and appropriately high C-peptide levels are indistinguishable from those of insulin-secreting tumors of the pancreas. Consequently, factitious sulfonylurea-induced hypoglycemia will be wrongly diagnosed as an insulinoma unless a screening test for sulfonylureas of sufficient sensitivity to detect therapeutic concentrations is carried out in all cases of endogenous hyperinsulinism. This can lead to untold misery as well as to litigation.

18.14 DRUG INTERACTIONS WITH SULFONYLUREAS

Drug interactions with the sulfonylureas, as with all drugs, can be characterized as being either pharmacokinetic or pharmacodynamic. Pharmacokinetic interactions are those drug interactions that affect the absorption, distribution, metabolism, or excretion of a drug. Pharmacodynamic drug interactions affect the pharmacologic effect of the drug. Primary examples of pharmacokinetic interactions with the sulfonylureas include displacement interactions and induced or inhibited hepatic clearance. Drugs that have pharmacodynamic interactions with sulfonylureas include all medications that may increase or decrease blood glucose. The most common of these include glucocorticoids and thiazides. Pharmacodynamic interactions are also listed in Table 18.2. Included in these drug interaction tables are

TABLE 18.2
Drug Interactions with the Sulfonylurea Agents

Decrease Blood Glucose	Increase Blood Glucose
Pharmacokinetic	
Displacement from Plasma Binding Sites	**Enzyme Induction**
Clofibrate	Alcohol (chronic use)
Phenylbutazone	Phenobarbital
Salicylates	Rifampin
Sulfonamides	
Decrease Hepatic Clearance	
Dicumarol	
Chloramphenicol	
Cimetidine	
MAO inhibitors	
Methyldopa	
Phenylbutazone	
Decreased Excretion	
Probenecid	
Phenylbutazone	
Salicylates	
Sulfonamides	
Pharmacodynamic	
Increase Hypoglycemic Effect	**Impair Insulin/Increase Hepatic Glucose Production**
Alcohol	L-Asparaginase
Anabolic steroids	Caffeine
Disopyramide	Corticosteroids
Guanethidine	Diazoxide
Propranolol	Diuretics
Salicylates	Estrogens
Indomethacin	Isoniazid
Lithium	Nicotinic acid (high doses)
Pentamidine	Phenytoin
Propranolol	Sympathomimetics

some nonprescription product ingredients that should also be screened for in the diabetic patient who is having difficulty controlling her or his blood glucose.

18.15 THE GLIPTIN CLASS NEW DRUGS FOR DIABETES TREATMENT TYPE 2 DIABETES

The late 20th and early 21st centuries have seen the introduction of several entirely new classes of drugs for the treatment of type 2 diabetes. Some such as the GLP-1 mimetics work by inhibiting glucagon secretion and stimulating insulin secretion—unlike the sulfonylureas—only in the presence of hyperglycemia. Hence, they do not cause "fasting" hypoglycemia. A health-scare linking GLP-1 mimetics to pancreatic cancer has not withstood critical scrutiny, but a parallel association with acute pancreatitis is still ongoing. Nevertheless, they are now gaining popularity for the treatment of type 2 diabetes when treatment with metformin alone fails. Other insulin secretagogues such as the meglitinides also stimulate insulin only in the presence of hyperglycemia. Consequently, they only very rarely produce clinically significant hypoglycemia even in overdose.

Most of the other classes of anti-diabetic drugs currently in use do not stimulate insulin secretion, nor do they cause hypoglycemia when used alone but may accentuate the hypoglycemic effects of insulin and sulfonylureas. They may, however, cause problems in other ways. Examples are given in the following section.

18.16 THIAZOLIDINEDIONES

18.16.1 Hepatic Failure

This class of drugs works by stimulating peroxisome proliferator-activated receptors to improve insulin sensitivity. They also affect the kidney's sodium (Na) channels, which increases the absorption of salt and water, causing water retention and edema as a side effect common to all members of the class. The FDA recognized this adverse drug reaction and issued a warning to prescribing clinicians.[38–40] Routine monitoring can ensure that should it occur in any particular patient, the drug can be discontinued.

18.16.2 Bladder Cancer

Subsequently, another member of the class, Pioglitazone, was temporarily withdrawn because of its association with bladder cancer, which, while heavily disputed, nonetheless is part of the manufacturer package insert warning.[41]

> Bladder cancer: Preclinical and clinical trial data, and results from an observational study suggest an increased risk of bladder cancer in pioglitazone users. The observational data further suggest that the risk increases with duration of use. Do not use in patients with active bladder cancer. Use caution when using in patients with a prior history of bladder cancer.

Thiazolidinedione (TZDs) increases the risk of bladder cancer, according to a study published in the *Journal of the National Cancer Institute*.[42] Patients taking TZD drugs have a two- to three-fold increased odd for the development of bladder cancer than those who took other common drugs for diabetes. Among patients taking TZDs, 170 patients per 100,000 are estimated to develop bladder cancer. In contrast, an estimated 60 per 100,000 patients treated with sulfonylurea drugs (e.g., glipizide) are estimated to develop bladder cancer.

This isn't the first time the drug has been associated with heightened odds of bladder cancer. A study published in *BMJ* found that taking Actos for two years can double the risk. Azoulay said it's not clear yet *how* Actos might raise the risk of bladder cancer, but he said some animal studies suggested that the drug may cause the development of crystals in the bladder causing irritation, a potential precursor in the development of bladder cancer. Johnson added that it's important to keep in mind that bladder cancer is a relatively rare cancer, and even with the increased risk, any one person's risk of bladder cancer "is pretty small".[43]

Numerous lawsuits have ensued, and some cases have gone to trial. *Takeda & Eli Lilly Fail to Overturn $9 Billion Actos Award.*[44] In April 2014, one of the largest damage verdicts in US history was imposed on Indianapolis-based Eli Lilly and their Japanese partner company *Takeda.* The jury ordered Takeda and Lilly to pay $6 and $3 billion, respectively, over the drug Actos and its link to cancer risks. Takeda and Lilly have just failed to have the judge throw out the verdict. Evidence presented in the case—tried in Lafayette, Louisiana, and presided over by US District Judge Rebecca Doherty—was compelling and convincing enough to prove to the jury that Takeda and Lilly were both aware of the possible cancer risks associated with the diabetes drug. Further, the jury was convinced that neither company took the necessary precautions in warning patients and healthcare providers of the risks associated with using Actos.

Shortly after the $9 billion verdict, US District Judge Rebecca Doherty in Lafayette, Louisiana, reduced the verdict by 99 percent in a punitive damages award. Jurors found that officials of Osaka (Japan)-based Takeda and Indianapolis-based Lilly intentionally hid the health risks of the drug and were ordered to pay punitive damages. "The panel's decision to order Takeda to pay $6 billion and Lilly $3 billion was excessive and should be reduced to a total of $36.8 million", she said.

18.17 SUMMARY AND CONCLUSIONS

Insulins and oral sulfonylureas provide life-sustaining therapeutic effects but frequently cause serious, severe, and sometimes irreversible and fatal outcomes. These are mostly accidental or negligent but occasionally malicious with murderous intent. Differentiation of hypoglycemia secondary to underlying disease from that induced by medication may be extremely difficult or impossible if appropriate investigations are not carried out at the time of the incident. A thorough review of their proper indications, requisite monitoring, patient education, and avoidance of interactive risks provide caregivers with a clinical challenge each time these agents are used by them or their patients. Attorneys and law enforcement officers dealing with a case of suspected wrongful death or injury should consult a knowledgeable expert as soon as possible to help determine the cause for injury or death early on and to preserve objective evidence, such as needles, IV bags, and drug containers, as well as contemporaneous eye-witness statements from relevant persons.

NOTE

1 Oba-Yamamoto C, Takeuchi J, Nakamura A, Takikawa R, Ozaki A, Nomoto H, Kameda H, Cho KY, Atsumi T, Miyoshi H. Combination of alcohol and glucose consumption as a risk to induce reactive hypoglycemia. J Diabetes Investig. 2021 Apr;12(4):651–657.

REFERENCES

1. Banting FG, Best CH, Collip JB, Campbell WR, Fletcher AA. Pancreatic extracts in the treatment of diabetes mellitus. Can. Med. Assoc. J. 12:141–146 (1922).
2. Schwinghammer TL. Diabetes mellitus. In *Pharmacotherapy Handbook*, Barbara Wells, et al., eds. 7th ed. New York: McGraw-Hill Medical Pub. Division, 2009;19:210–227.
3. Miyahara RK. Pharmacotherapy of oral hypoglycemic agents. J. Pharm. Pract. V(5):271–279 (1992).
4. Bliss M. *The Discovery of Insulin*. University of Chicago Press, 1982
5. Crasto W, Jarvis J, Khunti K, Davies MJ. New Insulins and new Insulin regimens: A review of their role in improving glycaemic control in patients with diabetes. Postgrad. Med. J. 85:257–267 (2009).
6. Cryer PE, Davis SN, Shamoon H. Hypoglycemia in diabetes. Diabetes Care. 26:1902–1912 (2003).
7. Kearney T, Dang C. Diabetic and endocrine emergencies. Postgrad. Med. J. 83:79–86 (2007).
8. O'Donnel JT. Alcohol: Gastrointestinal and other toxicites. J. Pharm. Prac. 7(4):196–208 (1994).
9. Castro W, Jarvis J, Khunti K, Davies MJ. New insulins and new insulin regimens: A review of their role in improving glycaemic control in patients with diabetes. Postgrad. Med. J. 85:257–267 (2009).
10. Kalimo H, Olsson Y. Effects of severe hypoglycemia on the human brain: Neuropathological case reports. Act Neurol. Scand. 62:345–356 (1980).
11. Teuscher A, Berger WG. Hypoglycemia unawareness in diabetics transferred from beef/porcine insulin to human insulin. Lancet. 15;2(8555):382–385 (1987).
12. American Diabetes Association (ADA). Insulin administration: "Position statement." Diabetes Care. 14(Suppl 2):30 (1991).
13. Hepburn DA, Frier BM. Hypoglycemic unawareness and human insulin (letter). Lancet: 1393 (June, Vol 17;1., 1989).
14. Cahill GF, Arky RA, Perlman AJ. Diabetes mellitus in metabolism. In *Scientific American Medicine*. New York: Scientific American, 1987.
15. Powers AC. Diabetes mellitus. In *Harrisonís Principles of Internal Medicine*, AS Fauci, et al., eds. 17th ed. New York: McGraw-Hill Medical, 2008:338.
16. Cryer PE, Davis SN, Shamoon H. Hypoglycemia in diabetes. Diabetes Care. 26:1902–1912 (2003).
17. Kearney T, Dang C. Diabetic and endocrine emergencies. Postgrad. Med. J. 83:79–86 (2007).
18. Kwon KT, Tsai VW. Metabolic emergencies. Emerg. Med. Clin. N. Am. 25:1041–1060 (2007).
19. American Medical Association (AMA). Parenteral and enteral nutrition chapter update. In *Drug Evaluations Annual 1992*. Chicago: American Medical Association, 1991:2045.
20. O'Donnell JT. Pharmacist error suggested in baby's brain damage. Drug Topics Suppl. Hospital Pharmacy Report, September, 1991:1, 26–27.
21. Meyer GE, Novelli KA, Smith JE. Use of a refractive index measurement for quality assurance of pediatric parenteral nutrient solutions. Am. J. Hosp. Pharm. 44:1617–1620 (1987).
22. Gebhart F. Test hyperal solutions? Fla. mom says yes. Drug Topics Suppl. Hospital Pharmacy Report, February 1992:35.
23. Davis NM. Unprecedented procedural safeguards needed with the use of automated IV compounders (editorial). Hosp. Pharm. 27:488 (1992).
24. Martin-Timon I, Canizo-Gomez FJ. Mechanisms of hypoglycemia unawareness and implications in diabetic patients. World J Diabetes. 2015;6:912–926.
25. Allen LA. Quality control: Refractive index I: Parenteral nutrition solution. Int. J. Pharmaceut. Compound. 3(11) (2014).
26. ASHP guidelines on compounding sterile preparations. Am. L. Health-Syst. Pharm. 71:145–146 (2014).
27. Seltzer HS. Severe drug-induced hypoglycemia: A review. Comp. Ther. 5:21–29 (1979).
28. Standards of medical care in diabetes: 2012. Diabetes Care. 35(Suppl 1):S11–S63 (2012). DOI: 10.2337/dc12-s011.PMC 3632172. PMID 22187469.
29. Campbell IW. Metformin and the sulfonylureas: Comparative risks. Horm. Metab. Res. 15(Suppl):105–111 (1985).
30. Davis NM. Unprecedented procedural safeguards needed with the use of automated IV compounders (editorial). Hosp. Pharm. 27:488 (1992).
31. Scala-Barnett DM, Donoghue ER. Dispensing error causing fatal chlorpropamide intoxication in a nondiabetic. J. Forensic Sci. 31(1):293–295 (1986).
32. O'Donnell JT, Benjamin DM. Pharmacist malpractice. In *Legal Medicine*, 8th ed., American College of Legal Medicine; Chicago.2010.
33. Alsahli M, Gerich JE. Hypoglycemia, chronic kidney disease, and diabetes mellitus. Mayo Clin. Proc. 11:1564–1571 (2014).
34. O'Donnell JT, Benjamin DM. Pharmacist malpractice. In *Legal Medicine*, 7th ed., American College of Legal Medicine; Chicago 2007.
35. Patel G, O'Donnell JT. Adverse effects of diabetic drugs. In *Drug Injury: Liability, Analysis, and Prevention*, JT O'Donnell, ed. 3rd ed. Tucson, AZ: Lawyers & Judges Publishers, 2012.
36. O'Donnell JT. Hypoglycemic injuries. *Legal Medicine*, November 1994.
37. FDA MedWatch. Avandia (rosiglitazone): Ongoing review of cardiovascular safety, February 2010.

38. Juurlink DN, Gomes T, Lipscombe LL, Austin PC, Hux JE, Mamdani MM. Adverse cardiovascular events during treatment with pioglitazone and rosiglitazone: Population based cohort study. BMJ. 1–6 [online first] (2009).
39. Khanderia U, Pop-Busui R, Eagle KA. Thiazolidinedione in type 2 diabetes: A cardiology perspective. Ann. Pharmacother. 42:1466–1474 (2008).
40. http://www.takeda.us/products/.
41. Mamtani R, Haynes K, Bilker WB, Vaughn DJ, Strom B, Glanz K, and Lewis JD. Association Between Longer Therapy With Thiazolidinediones and Risk of Bladder Cancer: A Cohort Study, *JNCI: Journal of the National Cancer Institute*, Volume 104, Issue 18, 19 September 2012, Pages 1411–1421
42. Azoulay L, Yin H, Filion KB, Assayag J, Majdan A, Pollak MN, Suissa S. The use of pioglitazone and the risk of bladder cancer in people with type 2 diabetes: Nested case-control study. *BMJ*. 2012, 344:e3645.
43. http://www.drugdangers.com/news/09/11/2014/takeda-eli-lilly-fail-to-overturn-9-billion-actos-award.
44. http://www.bloomberg.com/news/articles/2014-10-27/takeda-lilly-get-9-billion-actos-award-cut-99-percent.

19 Parenteral Nutrition-Related Errors and Complications

Erica M. Fernandez

SYNOPSIS

19.1 INTRODUCTION

The Institute of Safe Medication Practices (ISMP) lists parenteral nutrition (PN) as a high-alert medication used in acute care settings.[1] High-alert medications may cause significant harm in the event of an error.[1] In their "Top 10 Medication Errors and Hazards for 2020" news release, ISMP listed a PN near miss that previously led to the death of an infant ten years earlier, demonstrating the need for clinicians and administrators to review the systems used for PN provision.[2–4] Vigilance is required in avoiding PN-related errors because of its prevalent use; the American Society of Parenteral and Enteral Nutrition (ASPEN) estimates over 300,000 Americans receive PN per year in the acute care setting.[5]

A multidisciplinary, multistep approach is required to safely provide PN, creating many opportunities for human error. The chapter focuses on the stages of preparation, predictable complications, and the effects of medication shortages on PN-related errors and harms. It introduces foundational knowledge of PN-related medication errors. The topics discussed will assist with evaluating possible gaps in systems currently in place within an institution or health-system. The discussion of all areas for gap analysis and review is beyond the scope of the chapter.

19.2 BASIC PRINCIPLES OF PN

PN is the provision of nutritional requirements in intravenous form for patients with significant gastrointestinal compromise for ages ranging from premature neonates up to elderly adults.[6] It includes all macronutrients such as protein, carbohydrates, and fat, as well as vitamins, minerals, and electrolytes.[7] These components should be balanced to meet the specific needs of each patient, considering their comorbidities, baseline nutrition status, and nutritional goals.

Protein, carbohydrates, and fat are provided as amino acids, dextrose, and lipid emulsions, respectively.[6] Vitamins and minerals are commonly referred to as micronutrients.[8] Vitamins are provided using multivitamin injection (MVI) with the necessary fat and water-soluble vitamins or through individual injectable vitamin products.[6] Minerals are also referred to as trace elements and are provided through a product containing multiple trace elements or individual injectable trace elements (e.g. zinc, selenium).[8]

19.3 PN PROVISION CATEGORIES

ASPEN and ISMP group recommendations for PN provision and adverse drug events into several categories.[9] Each area of PN provision has several recommendations for mitigating errors; however, many errors may have contributing factors from more than one category.

DOI: 10.1201/9781003615323-21

19.3.1 Prescribing

Prescribing errors may go unrecognized when organizations do not utilize nutrition support-trained pharmacists for PN order reviews such as appropriate indication and dosing of macro- and micronutrients for the indicated conditions.[10] A 2012 study reviewing PN orders in the NICU and PICU found a 3.9% prescribing error rate with a majority of errors related to concentration ranges for micronutrients or electrolytes recognized by a pharmacist review.[11]

Lack of institutional standard order sets or order forms, standard units of measure for each component, and properly trained personnel may lead to patient harm. Prescribing errors can be decreased by standardizing systems and adhering to the ASPEN safe practice recommendations for this stage of PN management, as well as through decision support implementation in computerized physician order entry systems.[9] Setting evidence-based limitations or "guard rails" for the various components utilized in PN directly in the ordering template mitigates the likelihood of prescribing errors reaching the patient. Prescribing order forms should also match the units used for compounding PN prescriptions to prevent further unintended errors.[12]

With the reported undertraining of physicians in nutrition support, other disciplines have moved into the role of leaders in managing this complex medication including pharmacists, dietitians, and nurses.[7] In a 2013 gap analysis, approximately two-thirds of PN prescribing was performed by the primary service followed by members of the nutrition support service including pharmacists, dietitians, advanced practice nurses, and physician assistants in descending order.[10] This pattern was consistent across all hospital types. Board certification and certificate programs are available for pharmacists wishing to specialize or improve their skills in nutrition support. Dietitians, nurses, physicians' assistants, as well as physicians and other healthcare providers may become certified nutrition support clinicians through the National Board of Nutrition Support Certification established by ASPEN.

Due to the likelihood of decreasing prescribing errors pursuant to targeted education programs, ASPEN recommends all team members involved in prescribing PN have training or education as well as annual competency in the provision of PN.[13,14] Standardized competencies are available from ASPEN to ensure comprehensive training of all healthcare providers involved in PN management.[15–17] Additional safety recommendations include limiting the ordering of PN during hours when properly trained personnel are available for prescribing and reviewing new orders, as well as directing healthcare organizations in the appropriate training and credentialing of personnel responsible for writing PN orders.[13,14]

19.3.2 Transcribing and Verification

Prescriber orders are reviewed in the transcription and verification stage of medication provision. Many PN-related events causing patient harm originated from errors occurring during this step.[3,4,12] PN orders may need to be entered into a separate pharmacy order program, the compounding software programs, or outside compounding pharmacy software. The transcription of the order also requires several steps of verification prior to being dispensed from the pharmacy, including an initial order review and checks during the compounding process.

Examples of errors in this stage of PN provision that cause harm are often due to dosing with incorrect units of measure and miscalculations. A 16-year-old boy received a hypotonic solution of PN due to a transcription error involving the units of order for sodium.[12] The electrolyte was ordered in milliequivalents per kilogram but transcribed to milliequivalents per day due to pharmacy systems not matching the provider order entry template. No harm came to the child in this case; however, other errors in sodium concentrations have led to deaths. A six-week-old infant died after the incorrect amount of sodium was entered into the software for the automated compounder and the supervising pharmacist did not recognize the error prior to dispensing.[18] In another case, a preterm infant received a 1000-fold overdose of zinc after a correct conversion of the prescribed concentration was erroneously entered into the pharmacy system as milligrams instead of micrograms.[4] Despite early recognition of the error and administration of an antidote, the error resulted in the death of the neonate.

In all these cases, there was an opportunity to make an error due to a template mismatch between the provider order entry or order form and the available pharmacy programs. Standardization of prescribing templates is essential for reducing prescribing errors; however, errors in transcription and verification stages may occur without built-in redundancies in the ordering systems.[14] In instances where the order is not automatically transcribed into the pharmacy systems in use, every effort should be made to ensure the units of order in the pharmacy systems are identical to the prescribing system. This standardization may have avoided the tragic death of the neonate from the zinc overdose.

Several recommendations for reducing transcription-related errors have been issued by professional societies. The ASPEN 2014 PN safety guidelines recommend osmolarity calculations, calcium and phosphorus solubility review, and independent double-checks for any orders that require transcription from one program to another.[14] This includes transcription into a pharmacy order program or third-party compounder software. The error that occurred with the hypotonic solution provided to the pediatric patient reported previously may have been avoided through the implementation of these review modalities.[12] Standardization of units system-wide between the prescribing and pharmacy systems, required osmolarity calculations, or built-in automated guard rails for osmolarity could have alerted pharmacists to the low osmolarity of the product prior to verification.

Ultimately, verification of the PN order should occur in multiple places in the order review and compounding process. At a minimum, verification procedures should be implemented at the point of PN order entry, prior to any injection of additives into the PN, as well as a final review of the product prior to dispensing.[9]

19.3.3 Compounding

Compounding of PN occurs in hospital pharmacies, outsourced sterile compounding pharmacies, as well as in patients' homes.[14] The latter of these may not involve comprehensive compounding, but rather additions of MVI to a premixed bag of macronutrients by patients or their caregivers.[19] Errors that occur during the compounding phase of PN provision often have multiple root causes. These errors can be associated with process breakdowns in compounding resulting in suboptimal sterility, solution compatibility problems, or dosing errors.

A 2011 outbreak of *Serratia marcescens* from PN solutions highlights the necessity of recognized standards in sterile compounding.[20] The United States Pharmacopeia (USP) is a non-profit, non-governmental organization recognized by the Food and Drug Administration for the standards it sets in many areas including sterile compounding. In 2011, 19 adults developed bacteremia after exposure to *S. marcescens*-contaminated PN products.[20] Nine of those patients died at six different hospitals in Alabama. The pharmacy had moved to high-risk compounding of amino acid 15% solution from bulk powder.[21] Investigations uncovered several practices that did not follow USP standards. These included improperly filtered solutions with excess particulate matter, the extended time the solution was left to dissolve, and the repeated sterilization filter replacement. The pharmacy used improperly filtered tap water, likely adding particulate matter to the solution. Additionally, the solution was allowed to remain without any sterility filtering for one to two days at a time, and employees of the pharmacy commented that the solution often required several sterilization filter changes due to filter clogging. USP standards at the time recommended sterilization of such products within six hours of compounding. The investigators concluded that the *S. marcescens* likely originated from the faucet that provided the tap water, grew during the period it remained unfiltered, and contaminated the final product because of the numerous sterilization filter changes performed due to clogging. ISMP and FDA recommended further pharmacy board and Joint Commission oversight of pharmacy USP 797 compliance as a result of this deadly error, and two pharmacists pleaded guilty to federal charges in this case.[22]

In addition to solution sterility, solution compatibility is equally important for a safe PN product. For PN solutions containing phosphorus salts and calcium, the formation of calcium phosphate crystals is of greatest concern. These crystals can deposit in organ tissue, for example, the lungs, which may lead to pulmonary emboli and respiratory arrest.[23] While infusing PN using an in-line filter is an important tool to prevent this adverse event (further discussed in Section 3.D., Administration), an appropriate review of compatibility at the point of prescribing and compounding can mitigate the formation of crystals.[13] In addition to calcium and phosphate concentrations, other factors influencing the solubility of salts include the amino acid concentration, form of calcium salt, pH of the final solution, dextrose concentration, temperature, and order of mixing (see Table 19.1).[24] Compatibility curves, which are graphic representations of expected calcium and phosphate solubilities for specific concentrations of macronutrient solutions, is available for many commercial products; however, the curves are validated only under specific parameters. Therefore, clinicians should use multiple strategies for reducing the risk of calcium phosphate crystal formation instead of relying solely on these curves. Additionally, ACDs may have predictive models provided by the manufacturer to guide compatibility decisions when using their product.[23]

PN preparations are provided as two-in-one and three-in-one solutions; the two and three refer to how many macronutrients are included in the bag. The two-in-one preparations contain amino acids and dextrose components, electrolytes, and micronutrients with the lipid component infused separately.[9] The three-in-one solutions contain dextrose, amino acids, and lipids in one infusion. Some advantages of the three-in-one formulations include less risk of contamination due to fewer manipulations required at the point of administration and possible improved fat clearance with the infusion administered over longer than 12 hours.[25] However, the stability of the overall product is more sensitive to varying concentrations of dextrose, amino acids, and electrolytes as well as pH than the two-in-one formulations.

Compounding PN can be performed via manual manipulation or by using an automated compounding device

TABLE 19.1
Characteristics Affecting Calcium/Phosphorus Compatibility

Parameter	Effect on Calcium/Phosphorus Compatibility[24]
pH of formulation	Lower pH decreases the risk of crystal formation.
Calcium phosphate concentration	The product of the calcium and phosphorus contents should never be used alone and should be used in combination with predictive solubility curve models.
Amino acid concentration	Higher amino acid concentrations result in lower pH.
Calcium salt form	Calcium chloride should never be used in a solution containing phosphorus due to its propensity to dissociate.
Dextrose Concentration	Higher concentrations result in lower pH.
Order of mixing additives	When adding electrolytes, inject phosphorus first. Vigorously agitate the solution after each additive is injected. Calcium gluconate should be the last electrolyte added.
Temperature	Increased temperature results in increased crystal formation

(ACD).[25] Manual compounding is performed by mixing the base dextrose and amino acid solutions by hand or gravimetric compounder or by using commercially available premixed solutions.[9] All additive doses are individually prepared in syringes with manual verification of the products prior to injection into the final PN compound. Of note, the "pull-back" method is not recommended as a safe process for reviewing accuracy, as this occurs after compounding has been performed. The pharmacist reviews syringes in this method after the pharmacy technician measures the additive, injects it into the product, and then pulls the plunger back on the empty syringe to indicate the amount of additive injected. ACDs decrease the risk of human contamination by decreasing the physical contact with the components through automated methods for compounding PN.[25] The system requires the technician or pharmacist to enter the required amounts of each component, and the ACD will precisely add the components in a validated order to ensure compatibility.[9] However, there are instances where manual injection of components may still be required. Manual additive injection should follow a standardized and validated order, while the method using the ACD should follow the manufacturer's recommendations.[25]

While the ACD leads to more precision and a decreased potential for contamination, standard practices around their use should be implemented to avoid dosing errors.[9] As previously discussed, failure to have dose limit warnings programmed into the ACD or matching entry templates to others at the facility, and lacking standard processes for verification of components led to errors and in some cases death.[3,12,18] Following these errors, ISMP recommended the utilization of the programming software in the ACDs including dose limit warnings. ASPEN recommended verification processes for database changes to the ACD, independent double-check requirements for ACD setup, and refilling of ingredients with barcoding requirements.[13] An additional safety step included presenting vials during the pharmacist's final verification when multiple vials are used for one ingredient in the compounding of a single PN prescription.

As described in the previous sections, the provision of PN should be limited to the hours when appropriately trained staff are available, including compounding personnel. In the case of the neonate that died due to a 1000-fold zinc overdose, the prescribing and transcription process was the source of the error; however, the compounding technician and verifying pharmacist failed to recognize the inordinate volume of zinc required to complete the prescription.[4] The error was discovered after an experienced pharmacy technician learned of the volume used from the previous shift and notified a pharmacist. These errors further support the crucial role every member of the multidisciplinary team has with PN management.

19.3.4 Administration

There is a higher risk of error during the administration of PN due to it being the point of contact with the patient and no proceeding steps in the process to identify additional errors.[9] Common administration errors include infusion rate errors and complications resulting from infusing PN without an in-line filter.[9,23]

An ASPEN review of the ISMP Medication Errors Reporting Program found that administration errors are the second-most common type of errors reported involving PN.[26] Infusion rate errors can cause life-threatening metabolic disturbances including electrolyte-induced arrhythmias, hyperglycemia, and fat overload syndrome.[27] Infusion rate errors may occur more often when intravenous fat emulsions are infused separately given the need to program two infusion pumps.

The omission of in-line filters is another common error made during the administration phase of PN provision.[23] Historically, in-line filters were commonly used for many intravenous infusions as a theoretical method of preventing line-related infections by filtering contaminants and endotoxins.[28] In 2002, the CDC recommended against the continued use of these filters as evidence did not support the theoretical benefits and frequent filter use increased the risk of infection due to line manipulations. In 2020, an ASPEN position paper hypothesized this change may have led to the inadvertent decline in the use of in-line filters due to a misunderstanding of their indication in PN.[23]

Increased awareness of the dangers of particulate matter in PN started from an FDA safety alert in 1994 reporting four patients with respiratory distress due to microvascular pulmonary emboli presumed to be from calcium phosphate crystal deposits.[29] Two of the four patients expired. Intravenous lipid emulsion (ILE) product recalls due to particulate matter in 2016 resulted in a change to manufacturer labeling for all ILE products to be infused with a 1.2-micron filter.[23] Incorrect 0.22-micron filter use with ILE leads to instability of the emulsion due to compression within the filter. ASPEN, FDA, Infusion Nurses Society, and the European Society of Enteral and Parenteral Nutrition, as well as manufacturer labeling support the use of in-line filters with PN. Despite this support, errors resulting from incorrect use of in-line filters continue to be reported.

Case reports of particulate-related injury or death continued after the 1994 safety alert. Symptoms ranged widely; however, the most dangerous and common complication was respiratory distress from crystalline deposits in the lungs.[23] Dr. James T. O'Donnell recently consulted on a case where the improper provision and use of in-line filters contributed to the death of a young woman who suffered from respiratory complications. Particulate-related injury is most likely to affect neonatal, pediatric, critically ill patients, or those requiring long-term infusions.[23] Adult and neonatal pulmonary capillary diameters are approximately the same (~6.3 microns) with neonates having an overall smaller number of capillaries and vessel size. A review of neonatal PN by Puntis et al. attributed 80% of particulate matter to the ILE component of the PN formula.[30] Oie et al. found that PN formulations containing additives, such as electrolytes, had statistically more particulates greater than 1.2 microns 24 hours after compounding, indicating particulate matter increases with time.[31]

ASPEN has endorsed the use of in-line filters since 2004 with variable strength of recommendations.[6,9] Generally, the recommendation was to utilize a 0.22-micron filter for two-in-one mixtures and 1.2-micron filters for mixtures containing ILE. Despite these recommendations, a 2016 national survey showed in neonatal, pediatric, and adult populations, 18.6% to 20.6% of respondents did not use an in-line filter for three-in-one formulations (not applicable in neonates), 1% to 7.2% of respondents did not use an in-line filter in two-in-one formulations, and 9.7% to 19.4% of respondents used no filter for separate ILE.[32] The variability of practice was attributed to a misunderstanding of the indication for in-line filtration, associated cost, and complexity of line setup with two filters. The ASPEN recommendation for administering all PN products with a single filter size infusion set using a 1.2-micron filter and eliminating the 0.22-micron filter requirement is designed to address these barriers.[23] Caveats with the recommendation include a careful review of product component compatibility, parameters for filter priming modalities and replacement, and discontinuation of use of a product if the high-pressure alarms on the infusion pumps continue to alert during administration. Clinicians should also consider patient-specific factors including expected length of therapy, resources available for home infusions, and patient competency if therapy is self-administered.

Evidence-based strategies to mitigate administration errors should be included in institutional policies.[17] Common strategies reported include independent double-check validation of the PN bag and intravenous pump settings, staff competency at orientation and with technology changes, as well as education as part of continuous quality improvement processes.[25]

19.4 MONITORING AND COMPLICATIONS

Monitoring of PN is critical because of the potential for rapid physiologic changes in response to therapy. ASPEN recommends monitoring frequencies for different laboratory parameters based on patient comorbidities and condition stability.[25] Laboratory findings are used to assist with the identification and management of potential complications from PN. Complications including hyperglycemia, refeeding syndrome, pulmonary and hepatic complications, essential fatty acid deficiency, as well as vitamin and micronutrient deficiencies are possible with the provision of PN.[7] Generally, newly started PN patients, acutely ill, critically ill, or patients with recent surgeries are monitored at least daily, stable patients with no changes in formula for one week are monitored at least every two to seven days, and those without formula changes for greater than one week are monitored every one to four weeks.[9]

Inappropriate blood draws have the potential to cause patient harm due to the complications from the therapeutic interventions undertaken in response to inaccurate lab results. Blood drawn from the venous access device may easily be contaminated with some of the PN solution, resulting in false values for glucose and electrolytes on the basic metabolic panel. Two independent studies reviewed the effects of spurious labs and found several incidents of patient harm, resulting from the treatment of falsely elevated results.[33,34] This treatment commonly causes hypoglycemia and hypokalemia. ASPEN recommends avoiding blood sampling from the patient venous access device to minimize the risk of microbial contamination of the line as well as spurious laboratory results.[9]

Consistent monitoring of symptoms, nutrition status, and laboratory parameters are essential steps in safe PN management. Reviewing trends and patterns may prevent or mitigate some of the common complications of PN therapy.

19.4.1 Glycemic Control

Hyperglycemia during PN therapy in adult patients has been associated with increased complications such as pneumonia, infection, and in-hospital mortality.[35,36] ASPEN guidelines recommend maintaining a glucose goal of 140–180 mg/dL.[37] Several conditions predispose patients to hyperglycemia during PN, including increased body mass index, concurrent steroid use, hyperglycemia prior to PN initiation, and excess carbohydrate administration.[25,38] Insulin-resistant hyperglycemia may also be due to a chromium deficiency.[25] Nutrition support specialists should anticipate hyperglycemia and consider management with insulin or other pharmacotherapy modifications (e.g., steroid dose reduction), as appropriate.

There is no consensus on the type or route of insulin administration for patients with PN-induced hyperglycemia. Regular insulin is often utilized in the PN formula to infuse simultaneously with the carbohydrate.[25] Recent studies have compared this method with various strategies using subcutaneous insulin alone, as well as a strategy using insulin glargine in combination with nutritional regular insulin in the PN infusion.[39–42] Most found varying differences in glycemic control depending on the population studied with a trend toward more hypoglycemic events in regimens utilizing subcutaneous insulin administration. In patients on cycled PN (infused for 8–20 hours/day instead of a continuous 24-hour infusion), there is a risk for rebound hypoglycemia after the completion of the infusion.[43,44] Providers should consider tapering down the infusion for the last one to two hours of the cycle, as well as measuring capillary blood glucose 30 minutes to an hour post-infusion to identify rebound hypoglycemia.[25] Hyperglycemia in combination with electrolyte disturbances in the early course of PN management may indicate the patient is experiencing refeeding syndrome and may require additional therapeutic interventions.

19.4.2 Refeeding Syndrome

The introduction of calories from either enteral or parenteral routes in patients with prolonged malnutrition has led to adverse events, including metabolic derangements, cardiac arrhythmias, respiratory failure, and death.[45] This response by the body to the reintroduction of calories is termed "refeeding syndrome." The refeeding syndrome was first identified in World War II after prisoners of war and victims of concentration camps experienced higher incidences of sudden cardiac arrest following the reintroduction of nutrition. Patient populations at risk for refeeding syndrome include those with anorexia nervosa, mental health disorders, alcohol, and substance use disorders, those with a history of bariatric surgeries or bowel resections or malabsorptive disorders such as celiac disease, and patients with malignancies. Cases have also been reported in children who suffer from child abuse and starvation, as well as young adults under physical stress such as military recruits or athletes. Refeeding syndrome diagnostic criteria per the ASPEN 2020 guidelines are defined as a decrease in any or multiple electrolytes including potassium, magnesium, or phosphorus within five days of initiating or significantly increasing calorie provision. The severity of the refeeding syndrome is determined by the percent decrease of the electrolyte levels. A 30% change in electrolyte levels, organ dysfunction due to electrolyte changes, or thiamine deficiency is categorized as severe refeeding syndrome.

Nutrition support providers should carefully assess patients for comorbidities or nutrition histories, which may put their patients at higher risk for refeeding syndrome. The calculation of provided calories includes any calories from medications or maintenance intravenous fluids the patient is receiving. Clinicians should consider initiating no more than 10–20 kcal/kg in adults or a maximum of 40–50% of the goal in pediatric patients at risk of refeeding syndrome.[45] Despite conservative calorie initiation, patients may still have significant electrolyte abnormalities.[46–49] Nutrition advancement considerations, laboratory monitoring frequency, and treatment with thiamine are essential for the appropriate management of a patient at risk of refeeding syndrome.[45]

19.4.3 Hepatobiliary Complications

As a patient continues on PN therapy, their likelihood of developing PN-associated liver disease (PNALD) increases significantly.[50] The duration of PN therapy is a risk factor for all age groups for the development of PNALD. Steatosis, cholestasis, and gallbladder stasis are the most common PN-related hepatobiliary complications. Steatosis is most common in adults, while PN-associated cholestasis (PNAC) is more likely to occur in children, especially infants.[51,52] Gallbladder stasis occurs in both populations and is typically related to the lack of enteral stimulation.[50] PNAC may lead to liver cirrhosis and liver failure if PN is not discontinued promptly after early identification.[25]

Identifying PNALD utilizes liver function test analysis and the exclusion of medication- or disease-induced liver dysfunction such as essential fatty acid deficiency (further discussed in Section 19.5).[50] Steatosis is relatively benign, presenting with elevated aminotransferase levels, whereas PNAC presents with elevated alkaline phosphatase, elevated gamma-glutamyl transferase, and elevated conjugated bilirubin with or without jaundice.[53]

There are interventions nutrition support specialists may implement to decrease the severity or prevalence of PNALD, although none are likely to eliminate the risk entirely. The first is appropriately feeding the patient, taking care to provide a balanced intravenous formula with 70–80% of calories from carbohydrates and 15–30% as fat.[6] Carbohydrate content should not exceed 25–40 kcal/kg/day to remain below the reported 50–60 kcal/kg/day calories from dextrose correlated with steatosis.[54] Infusion of lipids at rates >1 g/kg/day is correlated with an increased risk of cholestasis. Second, cycling PN may stabilize or reverse some elevated liver enzymes and bilirubin.[43] Reducing the daily time of continuous infusion may prevent some of the hepatobiliary complications. This technique provides a patient's daily calories in an abbreviated duration, commonly over 8–20 hours.[43,44] The duration of the cycle is highly dependent on the patient's caloric needs and tolerance; however, all cycled PN should initiate with one to two hours of a lower infusion rate followed by the goal hourly infusion rate and finish with one to two hours at a tapered rate.[25] This technique for up-titration and tapering the infusion reduces the risk of hyperglycemia and rebound hypoglycemia, respectively. Clinicians should carefully monitor for signs of hepatobiliary complications and proactively address aspects of the PN therapy that may be increasing the patient's risk for these complications.

19.4.4 Complications Involving Micronutrients

The effects of micronutrient toxicities or deficiencies have been described in the literature for decades. A thorough review of adverse events relating to the various micronutrients provided in PN is beyond the scope of the chapter; thus, the discussion will focus on related cases involving PN. Reversible symptomatic deficiencies of zinc and chromium were reported early after the provision of intravenous nutrition began in the 1960s.[8] Complications from the exclusion of thiamine in PN products have led to cardiac complications and death[55] (see Section 19.5). In 1980, an adult patient experienced night blindness due to vitamin A deficiency despite the PN prescription providing an appropriate dose of the vitamin.[56] Investigations revealed multiple home PN patients with low vitamin A levels. At the time, the pharmacy was compounding all of the components of the PN prescription on a weekly basis. The bags were protected from light and stored at 4°C. Further evaluation of the solutions affirmed a substantial dose of the vitamin A was adsorbed into the plastic bags over time, and the patients were subsequently receiving very little or no vitamin A. After the patients were instructed to inject the MVI into the PN immediately prior to administration, no further deficiencies were noted. Presently, most home PN patients will add the MVI themselves immediately prior to starting the infusion.[19]

In a 2012 position paper by ASPEN, MVI formulations and trace elements were reviewed and recommendations for changes were made.[55] This included decreased dose of copper and manganese for pediatric and adult MVI injections, as well as an option to provide chromium-free trace elements in adults. These changes were proposed because available evidence indicated excessive chromium may lead to renal toxicity, hypermanganesemia may lead to neurotoxicities (mostly in infants with cholestasis), and copper organ deposits may occur in patients with hepatic dysfunction. Proper care should be made to monitor patients for micronutrient deficiencies or toxicities through clinical symptoms and laboratory findings when appropriate.

19.5 PN COMPONENT SHORTAGES AND ADVERSE EVENTS

Medication shortages have become commonplace in the United States. This is an ongoing complication of managing PN. Reports of patient harm from PN due to medication shortages date back to the 1980s, with 12 cases reported in that decade related to MVI shortages.[57] Three adults out of 59 treated with PN at a large university medical center died from thiamine-related lactic acidosis after MVI was omitted from the PN due to a market shortage in 1988. At the time ASPEN sent letters to its members advising of the risk of thiamine deficiency; however, in the 1990s, another three patients were reported to have suffered from thiamine-related lactic acidosis during that MVI shortage.[58] In response to this event, ASPEN created a task force to recommend strategies for management of the shortage as well as a thorough dissemination of the information to other healthcare practitioners in addition to its members.[59] During the most recent era of severe medication shortages, the number of injectable products affected peaked at 183 in 2011, with the FDA reportedly averting an additional 165 products from going into shortage during that same year.[60]

During the late 2000s and early 2010s, many reports of patient harm directly resulting from changes in practice due to injectable product shortages were published. This occurred despite a robust response from ASPEN with open-access recommendations available on their website.

Symptomatic thiamine deficiency may present with neurological deficits (dry beriberi, Wernicke's encephalopathy), cardiac abnormalities (wet beriberi), and hematologic conditions such as anemia, thrombocytopenia, and neutropenia.[61] Most commonly, however, patients experience lactic acidosis due to the conversion of pyruvate to lactate in the absence of thiamine. In a case reported by Ramsi et al. in 2014, a 16-year-old boy received PN for three weeks without MVI or thiamine supplementation because it was excluded due to a shortage.[62] The child required intubation for respiratory failure due to severe lactic acidosis and decompensated shock attributed to thiamine deficiency and subsequently recovered following thiamine supplementation. In a case reviewed by Dr. James T. O'Donnell, an adult patient developed neurological effects consistent with Wernicke's encephalopathy following weeks of PN administration deficient in thiamine due to an injectable MVI shortage. Undertrained pharmacists and lack of interdisciplinary communication led to the omission of thiamine and the subsequent harm to the patient. The patient has residual and likely permanent neurological toxicity, including gereralized weakness. She struggles with her thinking, occasionally feels "cloudy." She also reports some occasional gait disturbance or possible ataxia. Another case reported in 2014 highlighted a 21-year-old patient on home PN presenting to the ED in respiratory distress also requiring intubation.[61] His home PN regimen included the ASPEN recommendation of 50% MVI provision during shortages.[61,63] Current thiamine recommendations for adults are 6 mg/day or the equivalent of 42 mg/week. The conservation strategy provided 18–24 mg/week. This case highlighted the limitations of conservation strategies with authors advocating for a thorough review of the patient's baseline status prior to initiating a strategy.

Trace element shortages have led to several reports of zinc and selenium deficiencies. Seven infants were reported to experience zinc deficiency in Washington, DC, and Houston, Texas, between 2012 and 2013 after zinc supplies were exhausted.[64] Six of the seven infants had dermatologic manifestations of zinc deficiency. The trace elements available were not used to supplement zinc due to the risk of chromium or manganese toxicity.

Cases from Japan have previously highlighted the effects of selenium deficiencies including cardiomyopathy, alopecia, growth stunting, vision loss, slurred speech, and depigmentation of hair, eyebrows, and eyelashes.[65–67] Selenium deficiencies were reported in multiple cases involving neonates and pediatric patients during the shortages from 2010 to 2016. Their symptoms ranged from scaly skin to hair texture change and growth abnormalities.[67–69] A three-year-old girl in Brazil requiring PN due to ultra-short bowel syndrome from complications after birth and subsequent surgeries was treated for severe hypothyroidism before selenium deficiency was recognized by clinicians.[69] The multiple trace elements available in Brazil at the time contained zinc, copper, chromium, and manganese, but selenium (selenious acid) was on shortage during the initiation of PN. Following discharge and the resolution of the shortage, selenium (selenious acid) was never introduced into her formula. After three years of PN supplementation, she presented with strabismus, regression of motor development and new dysarthria, pseudoalbinism, growth stunting, anemia, and an undetectable selenium level. She was diagnosed with myxedema, encephalopathy, and metabolic bone disease resulting from severe chronic selenium deficiency. Many symptoms resolved with selenium supplementation; however, the child remains with a bone age significantly lower than her actual age and requires ongoing physical and occupational therapy. Chen et al. conducted a retrospective review of infants on PN at their institution during shortage and non-shortage periods to compare their biochemical markers for selenium deficiency.[70] All infant selenium levels were below the recommended range; however, those treated during shortage had higher magnitudes of deficiency. This study and the cases described may indicate that current supplementation recommendations are inadequate. As with the conservation strategies used for thiamine, patients requiring long-term PN with conservation strategies for selenium supplementation should be monitored closely given that clinical signs of selenium deficiency may take months to years to manifest.

ISMP conducted a safety survey in 2011 at the height of the drug shortage crisis in the early 2010s. Twenty percent of respondents reported having witnessed events that caused patient harm due to a medication shortage.[71] As discussed in the chapter, providing PN without the added complexity of shortage management has many places for potential error and patient harm. The introduction of multiple electrolyte shortages in addition to the vitamin and trace element shortage, alternative products from outside of the United States, as well as premixed PN solutions significantly complicates the process for all members of the healthcare team. Deficiencies in the acetate salts of sodium and potassium could lead to formulas with excess chloride and non-anion gap acidosis, shortages in calcium gluconate create opportunities for inappropriate calcium chloride substitution and significant precipitation, and inadequate phosphorus salts increase the risk of adverse events in refeeding patients.[63,71–74] Macronutrient shortages have led to periods of unintentional starvation or emergence of essential fatty acid deficiency as well as significant mortality.[75–77] The amino acid compounding error previously discussed resulting in harm to 19 patients including 9 deaths was ultimately due to an amino acid shortage.[21] As a result of the shortage, the pharmacy was forced to bulk compound the product. The shortage of sterile ethanol injection caused unexpected harm to home PN patients.[78] Corrigan et al. published a case series of six patients in their care with insufficient supplies to continue the sterile ethanol central line locks. Within one month, five of the six patients had presented with a central line associated infection. At the time of the study publication, none of the patients had a recurrence of infection after resuming the ethanol locks.

These events highlight the severity of the shortages, limitations of conservation strategies, and the importance of involving nutrition support-trained clinicians in the review and provision of PN as well as early involvement in hospital shortage strategy management. In 2012 over 19 sterile injectables used for PN compounding were on shortage simultaneously.[72] At the time of the writing of this chapter, 14 sterile injectables used in PN are on national shortage including adult and pediatric MVI, sodium chloride and acetate preparations, magnesium sulfate, potassium and phosphate salts, and amino acids.[79,80]

19.6 SUMMARY AND CONCLUSION

PN is a life-sustaining medication that is equally harmful if used inappropriately or mismanaged. Errors can occur in many steps of the process, and all members of the healthcare team, including administrators, have responsibilities for ensuring PN is provided as safely as possible. Health systems should have robust processes in place to mitigate the frequency of errors, easily accessible medication error systems to report and review PN errors, and established strategies to minimize the risk of future errors.

Additional resources regarding PN provision, as well as peer-reviewed checklists for each step in this process, can be found at http://www.nutritioncare.org/pnresources/.

REFERENCES

1. *ISMP List of High-Alert Medications in Acute Care Settings.* ISMP; 2018. Accessed February 23, 2021. https://www.ismp.org/sites/default/files/attachments/2018-10/highAlert2018new-Oct2018-v1.pdf
2. Start the new year off right by preventing these top 10 medication errors and hazards. Accessed January 8, 2021. https://www.ismp.org/resources/start-new-year-right-preventing-these-top-10-medication-errors-and-hazards
3. *Too Close for Comfort: Fatal Zinc Overdose Narrowly Avoided.* Institute of Safe Medication Practices (ISMP). Accessed January 20, 2021. https://www.ismp.org/resources/too-close-comfort-fatal-zinc-overdose-narrowly-avoided
4. *Fatal 1,000-Fold Overdoses Can Occur, Particularly in Neonates, by Transposing mcg and mg.* Institute of Safe Medication Practices (ISMP). Accessed January 20, 2021. https://www.ismp.org/resources/fatal-1000-fold-overdoses-can-occur-particularly-neonates-transposing-mcg-and-mg
5. *Nutrition Support Patient Data.* ASPEN. Accessed February 23, 2021. http://www.nutritioncare.org/about_clinical_nutrition/nutrition_support_patient_data_fact_sheet/
6. Mirtallo J, Johnson D, Kumpf V. Safe practices for parenteral nutrition. *J Parenter Enteral Nutr.* 2004;28(6):S39–S70. doi:10.1177/0148607104028006s39
7. Mundi MS, Nystrom EM, Hurley DL, McMahon MM. Management of parenteral nutrition in hospitalized adult patients [formula: See text]. *JPEN J Parenter Enteral Nutr.* 2017;41(4):535–549. doi:10.1177/0148607116667060
8. Blaauw R, Osland E, Sriram K, Ali A, Allard JP, Ball P, Chan LN, Jurewitsch B, Logan Coughlin K, Manzanares W, Menéndez AM. Parenteral provision of micronutrients to adult patients: An expert consensus paper. *JPEN J Parenter Enteral Nutr.* 2019;43 Suppl 1:S5–S23. doi:10.1002/jpen.1525
9. Ayers P, Adams S, Boullata J, Gervasio J, Holcombe B, Kraft MD, Marshall N, Neal A, Sacks G, Seres DS, Worthington P. A.S.P.E.N. parenteral nutrition safety consensus recommendations. *J Parenter Enteral Nutr.* 2014;38(3):296–333. doi:10.1177/0148607113511992
10. Boullata JI, Guenter P, Mirtallo JM. A parenteral nutrition use survey with gap analysis. *JPEN J Parenter Enteral Nutr.* Mar 2013;37(2):212–222. doi:10.1177/0148607112464781
11. Hermanspann T, Schoberer M, Robel-Tillig E, Härtel C, Goelz R, Orlikowsky T, Eisert A. Incidence and severity of prescribing errors in parenteral nutrition for pediatric inpatients at a neonatal and pediatric intensive care unit. *Front Pediatr.* 2017;5:149. doi:10.3389/fped.2017.00149
12. *Mismatched Prescribing and Pharmacy Templates for Parenteral Nutrition (PN) Lead to Data Entry Errors.* Institute of Safe Medication Practices (ISMP). Accessed December 30, 2020. https://www.ismp.org/resources/mismatched-prescribing-and-pharmacy-templates-parenteral-nutrition-pn-lead-data-entry

13. Boullata JI, Gilbert K, Sacks G, Labossiere RJ, Crill C, Goday P, Kumpf VJ, Mattox TW, Plogsted S, Holcombe B, American Society for Parenteral and Enteral Nutrition. A.S.P.E.N. clinical guidelines: Parenteral nutrition ordering, order review, compounding, labeling, and dispensing. *JPEN J Parenter Enteral Nutr.* Mar–Apr 2014;38(3):334–377. doi:10.1177/0148607114521833
14. Ayers P, Adams S, Boullata J, Gervasio J, Holcombe B, Kraft MD, Marshall N, Neal A, Sacks G, Seres DS, Worthington P. A.S.P.E.N. parenteral nutrition safety consensus recommendations. *JPEN J Parenter Enteral Nutr.* Mar–Apr 2014;38(3):296–333. doi:10.1177/0148607113511992
15. Boullata JI, Holcombe B, Sacks G, Gervasio J, Adams SC, Christensen M, Durfee S, Ayers P, Marshall N, Guenter P, Parenteral Nutrition Safety Committee, American Society for Parenteral and Enteral Nutrition. Standardized competencies for parenteral nutrition order review and parenteral nutrition preparation, including compounding: The ASPEN model. *Nutr Clin Pract.* Aug 2016;31(4):548–555. doi:10.1177/0884533616653833
16. Guenter P, Boullata JI, Ayers P, Gervasio J, Malone A, Raymond E, Holcombe B, Kraft M, Sacks G, Seres D, Parenteral Nutrition Safety Task Force, American Society for Parenteral and Enteral Nutrition (ASPEN). Standardized competencies for parenteral nutrition prescribing: The American Society for parenteral and enteral nutrition model. *Nutr Clin Pract.* Aug 2015;30(4):570–576. doi:10.1177/0884533615591167
17. Guenter P, Worthington P, Ayers P, Boullata JI, Gura KM, Marshall N, Holcombe B, Richardson DS, Parenteral Nutrition Safety Committee, American Society for Parenteral and Enteral Nutrition. Standardized competencies for parenteral nutrition administration: The ASPEN model. *Nutr Clin Pract.* 2018;33(2):295–304. doi:10.1002/ncp.10055
18. *Another Tragic Parenteral Nutrition Compounding Error.* Institute for Safe Medication Practices (ISMP). Accessed December 30, 2020. https://www.ismp.org/resources/another-tragic-parenteral-nutrition-compounding-error
19. Fuhrman MP. Micronutrient assessment in long-term home parenteral nutrition patients. *Nutr Clin Pract.* 2006;21(6):566–575. doi:10.1177/0115426506021006566
20. *TPN-Related Deaths Call for FDA Guidance and Pharmacy Board Oversight of USP Chapter <797>.* Institute for Safe Medication Practices (ISMP). Accessed December 30, 2020. https://www.ismp.org/resources/tpn-related-deaths-call-fda-guidance-and-pharmacy-board-oversight-usp-chapter
21. Gupta N, Hocevar SN, Moulton-Meissner HA, Stevens KM, McIntyre MG, Jensen B, Kuhar DT, Noble-Wang JA, Schnatz RG, Becker SC, Kastango ES. Outbreak of *Serratia marcescens* bloodstream infections in patients receiving parenteral nutrition prepared by a compounding pharmacy. *Clin Infect Dis.* Jul 2014;59(1):1–8. doi:10.1093/cid/ciu218
22. January 28, 2016: Federal criminal charges filed against two pharmacists for adulteration of drugs in connection with Alabama-based compounding pharmacy, 2016. https://www.fda.gov/inspections-compliance-enforcement-and-criminal-investigations/press-releases/january-28-2016-federal-criminal-charges-filed-against-two-pharmacists-adulteration-drugs-connection
23. Worthington P, Gura KM, Kraft MD, Nishikawa R, Guenter P, Sacks GS, ASPEN PN Safety Committee. Update on the use of filters for parenteral nutrition: An ASPEN position paper. *Nutr Clin Pract.* Feb 2021;36(1):29–39. doi:10.1002/ncp.10587
24. Newton DW, Driscoll DF. Calcium and phosphate compatibility: Revisited again. *Am J Health Syst Pharm.* Jan 2008;65(1):73–80. doi:10.2146/ajhp070138
25. Ayers P, Bobo E, Hurt R, Mays A, Worthington P. *ASPEN Parenteral Nutrition Handbook.* 3rd edition. American Society for Parenteral and Enteral Nutrition; 2020.
26. Guenter P, Ayers P, Boullata JI, Gura KM, Holcombe B, Sacks GS. Parenteral nutrition errors and potential errors reported over the past 10 years. *Nutr Clin Pract.* 2017;32(6):826–830. doi:10.1177/0884533617715868
27. Ayers P, Adams S, Boullata J, Gervasio J, Holcomb B, Kraft MD, Marshall N, Neal A, Sacks G, Seres DS, Worthington P. A.S.P.E.N. parenteral nutrition safety consensus recommendations: Translation into practice. *Nutr Clin Pract.* Jun 2014;29(3):277–282. doi:10.1177/0884533614531294
28. Guidelines for the prevention of intravascular catheter-related infections. *CDC.gov*, 2021.
29. McKinnon BT. FDA safety alert: Hazards of precipitation associated with parenteral nutrition. *Nutr Clin Pract.* Apr 1996;11(2):59–65. doi:10.1177/011542659601100259
30. Puntis JW, Wilkins KM, Ball PA, Rushton DI, Booth IW. Hazards of parenteral treatment: Do particles count? *Arch Dis Childhood.* 1992;67(12):1475–1477. doi:10.1136/adc.67.12.1475
31. Oie S, Kamiya A. Particulate and microbial contamination in in-use admixed parenteral nutrition solutions. *Biol Pharm Bull.* Dec 2005;28(12):2268–2270. doi:10.1248/bpb.28.2268
32. Christensen ML, Ayers P, Boullata JI, Guenter P, Gura KM, Holcombe B, Seres DS, Sacks GS, ASPEN PN Safety Committee. Lipid injectable emulsion survey with gap analysis. *Nutr Clin Pract.* 2017;32(5):694–702. doi:10.1177/0884533617719671
33. Fairholm L, Saqui O, Baun M, Yeung M, Fernandes G, Allard JP. Monitoring parenteral nutrition in hospitalized patients: Issues related to spurious bloodwork. *Nutr Clin Pract.* Dec 2011;26(6):700–707. doi:10.1177/0884533611427041
34. Binkley JF, Mills B, Roy MA, Diaz JJ, Jensen GL. Spurious laboratory values from improper sampling of blood containing parenteral nutrition. *Nutr Clin Pract.* Oct 2004;19(5):540–541. doi:10.1177/0115426504019005540
35. Pasquel FJ, Spiegelman R, McCauley M, Smiley D, Umpierrez D, Johnson R, Rhee M, Gatcliffe C, Lin E, Umpierrez E, Peng L. Hyperglycemia during total parenteral nutrition: An important marker of poor outcome and mortality in hospitalized patients. *Diabetes Care.* Apr 2010;33(4):739–741. doi:10.2337/dc09-1748
36. Olveira G, Tapia MJ, Ocón J, Cabrejas-Gómez C, Ballesteros-Pomar MD, Vidal-Casariego A, Arraiza-Irigoyen C, Olivares J, Conde-García MC, García-Manzanares Á, Botella-Romero F. Hypoglycemia in noncritically ill patients receiving total parenteral nutrition: A multicenter study (Study group on the problem of hyperglycemia in parenteral nutrition; Nutrition area of the Spanish Society of Endocrinology and Nutrition). *Nutrition.* Jan 2015;31(1):58–63. doi:10.1016/j.nut.2014.04.023
37. McMahon MM, Nystrom E, Braunschweig C, Miles J, Compher C, American Society for Parenteral and Enteral Nutrition (ASPEN) Board of Directors. A.S.P.E.N. clinical guidelines: Nutrition support of adult patients with hyperglycemia. *JPEN J Parenter Enteral Nutr.* Jan 2013;37(1):23–36. doi:10.1177/0148607112452001
38. Alchaer M, Khasawneh R, Heuberger R, Hewlings S. Prevalence and risk factors of total parenteral nutrition induced hyperglycemia at a single institution: Retrospective study. *Metab Syndr Relat Disord.* 2020;18(5):267–273. doi:10.1089/met.2019.0040

39 Hakeam HA, Mulia HA, Azzam A, Amin T. Glargine insulin use versus continuous regular insulin in diabetic surgical noncritically ill patients receiving parenteral nutrition: Randomized controlled study. *J Parenter Enteral Nutr.* 2017;41(7):1110–1118. doi:10.1177/0148607116644710
40. Olveira G, Abuín J, López R, Herranz S, García-Almeida JM, García-Malpartida K, Ferrer M, Cancer E, Luengo-Perez LM, Alvarez J, Aragon C. Regular insulin added to total parenteral nutrition vs subcutaneous glargine in non-critically ill diabetic inpatients, a multicenter randomized clinical trial: INSUPAR trial. *Clin Nutr.* 39(2):388–394. doi:10.1016/j.clnu.2019.02.036
41. Truong S, Park A, Kamalay S, Hung N, Meyer JG, Nguyen N, Momenzadeh A. Glycemic control in adult surgical patients receiving regular insulin added to parenteral nutrition vs insulin glargine: A retrospective chart review. *Nutr Clin Pract.* Oct 2019;34(5):775–782. doi:10.1002/ncp.10252
42. Neff K, Donegan D, MacMahon J, O'Hanlon C, Keane N, Agha A, Thompson C, Smith D. Management of parenteral nutrition associated hyperglycaemia: A comparison of subcutaneous and intravenous insulin regimen. *Ir Med J.* May 2014;107(5):141–143.
43. Stout SM, Cober MP. Metabolic effects of cyclic parenteral nutrition infusion in adults and children. *Nutr Clin Pract.* Jun 2010;25(3):277–281. doi:10.1177/0884533610368701
44. Austhof SI, DeChicco R, Cresci G, Corrigan ML, Lopez R, Steiger E, Kirby DF. Expediting transition to home parenteral nutrition with fast-track cycling. *J Parenter Enteral Nutr.* 2017;41(3):446–454. doi:10.1177/0148607115595620
45. da Silva JS, Seres DS, Sabino K, Adams SC, Berdahl GJ, Citty SW, Cober MP, Evans DC, Greaves JR, Gura KM, Michalski A. ASPEN consensus recommendations for refeeding syndrome. *Nutr Clin Pract.* Apr 2020;35(2): 178–195. doi:10.1002/ncp.10474
46 Cormack BE, Jiang Y, Harding JE, Crowther CA, Bloomfield FH, Group PT. Neonatal refeeding syndrome and clinical outcome in extremely low-birth-weight babies: Secondary cohort analysis from the ProVIDe trial. *JPEN J Parenter Enteral Nutr.* Jan 2021;45(1):65–78. doi:10.1002/jpen.1934
47. Pantoja F, Fragkos KC, Patel PS, Keane N, Samaan MA, Barnova I, Di Caro S, Mehta SJ, Rahman F. Refeeding syndrome in adults receiving total parenteral nutrition: An audit of practice at a tertiary UK centre. *Clin Nutr.* 2019;38(3):1457–1463. doi:10.1016/j.clnu.2018.06.967
48. Miller SJ. Death resulting from overzealous total parenteral nutrition: The refeeding syndrome revisited. *Nutr Clin Pract.* Apr–May 2008;23(2):166–171. doi:10.1177/0884533608314538
49. Fernandes VPI, Lomazi da Costa Pinto EA, de Fatima Santana Ferreira Boin I, Nogueira RJN. Phosphorus levels during infusion of parenteral nutrition with calorie-based phosphorus concentration: A case series. *e-SPEN Eur e-J Clin Nutr Metab.* 2009;4(5):e252–e256. doi:10.1016/j.eclnm.2009.08.001
50. Kumpf VJ. Parenteral nutrition-associated liver disease in adult and pediatric patients. *Nutr Clin Pract.* 2006;21(3):279–290. doi:10.1177/0115426506021003279
51. Peyret B, Collardeau S, Touzet S, Loras-Duclaux I, Yantren H, Michalski MC, Chaix J, Restier-Miron L, Bouvier R, Lachaux A, Peretti N. Prevalence of liver complications in children receiving long-term parenteral nutrition. *Eur J Clin Nutr.* Jun 2011;65(6):743–749. doi:10.1038/ejcn.2011.26
52. Btaiche IF, Khalidi N. Parenteral nutrition-associated liver complications in children. *Pharmacotherapy.* Feb 2002;22(2):188–211. doi:10.1592/phco.22.3.188.33553
53. Angelico M, Guardia PD. Review article: Hepatobiliary complications associated with total parenteral nutrition. *Aliment Pharmacol Therapeut.* 2000;14(Suppl. 2):54–57. doi:10.1046/j.1365-2036.2000.014s2054.x
54. Montalvo-Jave EE, Zarraga JL, Sarr MG. Specific topics and complications of parenteral nutrition. *Langenbeck's Arch Surg.* 2007;392(2):119–126. doi:10.1007/s00423-006-0133-6
55. Vanek VW, Borum P, Buchman A, Fessler TA, Howard L, Jeejeebhoy K, Kochevar M, Shenkin A, Valentine CJ, Novel Nutrient Task Force, Parenteral Multi-Vitamin and Multi–Trace Element Working Group, American Society for Parenteral and Enteral Nutrition (ASPEN) Board of Directors. A.S.P.E.N. position paper: Recommendations for changes in commercially available parenteral multivitamin and multi-trace element products. *Nutr Clin Pract.* Aug 2012;27(4):440–491. doi:10.1177/0884533612446706
56. Howard L, Chu R, Feman S, Mintz H, Ovesen L, Wolf B. Vitamin A deficiency from long-term parenteral nutrition. *Ann Intern Med.* Oct 1980;93(4):576–577. doi:10.7326/0003-4819-93-4-576
57. Deaths associated with thiamine-deficient total parenteral nutrition. *MMWR Wkly.* 1989;38(3):43–46.
58. Hahn JS, Berquist W, Alcorn DM, Chamberlain L, Bass D. Wernicke encephalopathy and beriberi during total parenteral nutrition attributable to multivitamin infusion shortage. *Pediatrics.* Jan 1998;101(1):E10. doi:10.1542/peds.101.1.e10
59. Mirtallo JM, Holcombe B, Kochevar M, Guenter P. Parenteral nutrition product shortages: The A.S.P.E.N. strategy. *Nutr Clin Pract.* Jun 2012;27(3):385–391. doi:10.1177/0884533612444538
60. Drug shortages infographic. *FDA.gov.* Accessed February 15, 2021. https://www.fda.gov/drugs/drug-shortages/drug-shortages-infographic
61. Da Silva YS, Horvat CM, Dezfulian C. Thiamin deficiency as a cause of persistent hyperlactatemia in a parenteral nutrition-dependent patient. *J Parenter Enteral Nutr.* 2015;39(5):604–606. doi:10.1177/0148607114545128
62. Ramsi M, Mowbray C, Hartman G, Pageler N. Severe lactic acidosis and multiorgan failure due to thiamine deficiency during total parenteral nutrition. *BMJ Case Rep.* Jun 2014. doi:10.1136/bcr-2014-205264
63. Plogsted S, Adams SC, Allen K, Cober MP, Greaves J, Mogensen KM, Ralph A, Ward C, Ybarra J, Holcombe B, Product CP. Parenteral nutrition multivitamin product shortage considerations. *Nutr Clin Pract.* Aug 2016;31(4): 556–559. doi:10.1177/0884533616647718
64. Ruktanonchai D, Lowe M, Norton S, Garrett T, Soghier L. Zinc deficiency-associated dermatitis in infants during a nationwide shortage of injectable zinc—Washington, DC, and Houston, Texas, 2012–2013. *MMWR Wkly.* 2014;63(2):35–37.
65. Masumoto K, Nagata K, Higashi M, Nakatsuji T, Uesugi T, Takahashi Y, Nishimoto Y, Kitajima J, Hikino S, Hara T, Nakashima K. Clinical features of selenium deficiency in infants receiving long-term nutritional support. *Nutrition.* Nov–Dec 2007;23(11–12):782–787. doi:10.1016/j.nut.2007.08.001
66. Oguri T, Hattori M, Yamawaki T, Tanida S, Sasaki M, Joh T, Matsukawa N, Ojika K. Neurological deficits in a patient with selenium deficiency due to long-term total parenteral nutrition. *J Neurol.* Aug 2012;259(8):1734–1735. doi:10.1007/s00415-012-6427-4
67. Davis C, Javid PJ, Horslen S. Selenium deficiency in pediatric patients with intestinal failure as a consequence of drug shortage. *JPEN J Parenter Enteral Nutr.* Jan 2014;38(1):115–118. doi:10.1177/0148607113486005

68. Hanson C, Thoene M, Wagner J, Collier D, Lecci K, Anderson-Berry A. Parenteral nutrition additive shortages: The short-term, long-term and potential epigenetic implications in premature and hospitalized infants. *Nutrients.* 2012;4(12):1977–1988. doi:10.3390/nu4121977
69. Uchoa KMCB, Evangelista NMA, Carvalho de Camargo MF, Leite HP. Severe hypothyroidism in a child receiving long-term home parenteral nutrition without selenium. *JPEN J Parenter Enteral Nutr.* 2020;44(5):944–947. doi:10.1002/jpen.1807
70. Chen CH, Harris MB, Partipilo ML, Welch KB, Teitelbaum DH, Blackmer AB. Impact of the nationwide intravenous selenium product shortage on the development of selenium deficiency in infants dependent on long-term parenteral nutrition. *JPEN J Parenter Enteral Nutr.* 2016;40(6): 851–859. doi:10.1177/0148607115572834
71. Holcombe B. Parenteral nutrition product shortages: Impact on safety. *JPEN J Parenter Enteral Nutr.* Mar 2012;36(2 Suppl):44S–47S. doi:10.1177/0148607111434777
72. Hassig TB, McKinzie BP, Fortier CR, Taber D. Clinical management strategies and implications for parenteral nutrition drug shortages in adult patients. *Pharmacotherapy.* Jan 2014;34(1):72–84. doi:10.1002/phar.1350
73. Curtis CS, Busch RA, Crass RL, Webb AP, Kudsk KA. Use of premixed parenteral nutrition during a phosphate shortage in a non-critically ill population. *Nutr Clin Pract.* Apr 2016;31(2):218–222. doi:10.1177/0884533615583093
74. Plogsted S, Adams SC, Allen K, Breen HB, Cober MP, Greaves J, Mogensen KM, Ralph A, Ward C, Ybarra J, Holcombe B. Parenteral nutrition electrolyte and mineral product shortage considerations. *Nutr Clin Pract.* Feb 2016;31(1):132–134. doi:10.1177/0884533615621550
75. Gramlich L, Meddings L, Alberda C, Wichansawakun S, Robbins S, Driscoll D, Bistrian B. Essential fatty acid deficiency in 2015. *J Parenter Enteral Nutr.* 2015;39(1_suppl): 61S–66S. doi:10.1177/0148607115595977
76. Duerksen D, Mccurdy K. Essential fatty acid deficiency in a severely malnourished patient receiving parenteral nutrition. *Digest Dis Sci.* 2005;50(12):2386–2388. doi:10.1007/s10620-005-3068-9
77. Roongpisuthipong W, Phanachet P, Roongpisuthipong C, Rajatanavin N. Essential fatty acid deficiency while a patient receiving fat regimen total parenteral nutrition. *BMJ Case Rep.* Jun 2012. doi:10.1136/bcr.07.2011.4475
78. Corrigan M, Kirby DF. Impact of a national shortage of sterile ethanol on a home parenteral nutrition practice: A case series. *JPEN J Parenter Enteral Nutr.* Jul 2012;36(4):476–480. doi:10.1177/0148607111428453
79. Service UoUDI. *Current Drug Shortages.* ASHP. Accessed February 22, 2021. https://www.ashp.org/Drug-Shortages/Current-Shortages?loginreturnUrl=SSOCheckOnly
80. Drug Shortages. *FDA.gov.* Accessed February 22, 2021. https://www.fda.gov/drugs/drug-safety-and-availability/drug-shortages

20 Antidepressants
Clinical Use and Litigation

Henry Cohen and Michael Liu

SYNOPSIS

20.1 MAJOR DEPRESSIVE DISORDERS

Approximately 18 percent of the U.S. population will suffer from a major depressive disorder at least once in their lifetime, and 6.7 to 7.6 percent have had a depressive episode in the past 12 months.[1] Depression is nearly 1.5 to 3 times more common in women than it is in men.[2] The average onset of a major depressive disorder varies with age, with the highest prevalence in adults aged 20 and 30 years old at 20 percent, while the prevalence in youth aged 12 to 17 years, adults aged 40 to 59 years, and adults 60 years and older are 5.7, 10, and 5.4 percent, respectively. The duration of these episodes

DOI: 10.1201/9781003615323-22

is between six months and two years when left untreated. Eighty percent of untreated patients have recurrent episodes.

Seventy-five percent of patients who have suffered from depression also suffer from another psychiatric disorder. The primary additional disorders include:

- Posttraumatic stress (19.5 percent);
- Generalized anxiety (17.2 percent);
- Social phobia (27.1 percent);
- Panic (9.9 percent); and
- Alcohol dependence (23.5 percent).

In this chapter, we discuss several scenarios involving antidepressants and the possible basis for litigation in those scenarios.

20.2 ANTIDEPRESSANT PHARMACOLOGY

The high incidence of depression in the United States is consistent with the high use of antidepressants; with antidepressants being the third most commonly taken prescription medication during 2009–2012; and with 9 percent of the population filling at least one prescription in the past 30 days.[3] Nevertheless, about 40 percent of non-institutionalized adults with severe depressive symptoms go untreated.[4] Antidepressants are the primary treatment in the management of depression.

The first antidepressant drug, Tofranil (imipramine hydrochloride, Novartis), was introduced in the late 1940s. Currently, antidepressants are classified as tricyclic antidepressant (TCA) agents or first-generation antidepressants, such as Tofranil or Elavil (amitriptyline, Merck), or second-generation agents, such as Serzone (nefazodone hydrochloride, Bristol-Myers Squibb). Second-generation antidepressants include selective serotonin reuptake inhibitors (SSRIs), such as Prozac, Zoloft, Paxil, Lexapro, and Celexa, and the serotonin/norepinephrine reuptake inhibitors (SNRIs) such as Effexor, Pristiq, and Cymbalta. The term *cyclic antidepressant* can refer to either first- or second-generation antidepressants. Table 20.1 provides a list of the entire class of cyclic antidepressants.

TABLE 20.1
Generic and Brand Names of Tricyclic and Second-Generation Antidepressants

Generic Name	Brand Name
Tricyclic Antidepressants	
amitriptyline	Elavil
amoxapine	Asendin
clomipramine	Anafranil
desipramine	Norpramin
doxepin	Sinequan
imipramine	Tofranil
nortriptyline	Aventyl, Pamelor
protriptyline	Vivactil
trimipramine	Surmontil
Second-Generation, Non-Tricyclic Antidepressants	
bupropion	Wellbutrin,[a] Zyban
desvenlafaxine	Pristiq
duloxetine	Cymbalta
maprotiline	Ludiomil
mirtazapine	Remeron[b]
nefazodone	Serzone
trazodone	Desyrel
venlafaxine	Effexor[c]
Second-Generation, Selective Serotonin Reuptake Inhibitors, Antidepressants	
citalopram	Celexa
escitalopram	Lexapro
fluoxetine	Prozac[d]
fluvoxamine	Luvox
paroxetine	Paxil[e]
sertraline	Zoloft

[a] Also available in sustained-release formulations (Wellbutrin SR, Wellbutrin XL, Budeprion SR, Budeprion XL).
[b] Also available in orally disintegrating tablets.
[c] Also available in extended-release formulation (Effexor XR).
[d] Also available in weekly dosage form (Prozac weekly).
[e] Also available in controlled-release formulation (Paxil CR).

TCAs can often cause a range of adverse effects:[5]

- Peripheral antimuscarinic effects (dry mouth, blurred vision, constipation, urinary retention, rapid heart rate, increased blood pressure, increased body temperature, and mydriasis);
- Central antimuscarinic effects (agitation, hallucinations, confusion, sedation, coma, and seizures);
- Antihistaminic effects (sedation, drowsiness, dizziness, and weight gain);
- Anti-adrenergic effects (low blood pressure and subsequent fainting spells);
- Heart rhythm and rate disturbances; and
- Seizures.

SSRIs have supplanted TCAs as the first-line treatment for depressive disorders primarily because their adverse effect profiles are better. The SSRIs do not generally produce antimuscarinic, antihistaminic, or adrenergic adverse effects, and they are less cardiotoxic or seizuregenic.[5] Because SSRIs have fewer adverse effects, patients tolerate them better and comply better with their prescription regimen. SSRIs also appear to be safer in patients with suicidal ideation. The SNRI's neurohormonal effects are more similar to TCAs because they affect both norepinephrine and serotonin. The SNRIs generally produce less antimuscarinic, antihistaminic, or anti-adrenergic adverse effects, and they are less cardiotoxic or epileptogenic than TCAs but slightly greater than the SSRIs. In 2019, the Federal Drug Administration (FDA) approved esketamine for the treatment of treatment-resistant depression, defined as patients with major depressive disorder that have not responded to at least two antidepressant treatments given at both adequate doses and duration for their present depressive episode. Esketamine is a *N*-methyl-D-aspartate receptor antagonist, and its exact antidepressant effects are unknown, although based on its mechanism it may be due to the suppression of excitatory neurotransmitters such as glutamate. Because of the risk for acute sedation, dissociation, and hypertension for up to two hours upon administration, esketamine is a schedule 3 controlled substance that may only be dispensed and administered in a certified doctor's office or clinic and under the direct supervision of a healthcare provider.[6]

20.3 ANTIDEPRESSANT OVERDOSE

Despite the distinct pharmacological advantages of SSRIs, TCAs are still widely prescribed, which may be because TCAs have less-expensive generic equivalents. The American Association of Poison Control Centers recently reported that antidepressants are among the top 5 pharmaceutical exposures associated with fatalities. SSRIs are noted as being the most commonly reported antidepressant in multi-substance exposure fatalities, and TCA is the most common of the antidepressant class in single-substance exposure fatalities.[7]

In the early 1990s, the annual incidence of TCA overdose in the United States was approximately 500,000.[8] Cyclic antidepressants (tricyclics, bicyclics, and monocyclics) are among the most common causes of self-poisoning. Morbidity has also been associated with SSRIs, however, but with less frequency. More than 100,000 antidepressant exposures annually have been reported to poison control centers throughout the United States.[7]

20.3.1 Trazodone and Permanent Neurologic Sequelae

Dr. Carvey describes a case of a patient who developed a permanent neurologic deficit after the pharmacy had dispensed trazodone 300 mg twice a day instead of labetalol (Trandate) as intended by the patient's physician.[9] The total daily dose of 600 mg exceeds the maximum outpatient daily dose of 400 mg and equivalent to the maximum daily dose of 600 mg as a monitored inpatient. The prescription was filled immediately prior to the vacation, and during the trip the patient complained of numerous typical signs and symptoms of high-dose trazodone including excessive sleepiness, lethargy, upset stomach, and a clouded mental state. He continued on the trazodone for one month and was then informed of the error by the prescribing physician.

Almost three years following exposure, the patient continues to demonstrate abnormal behaviors, anxiety, reduced self-esteem, and word-finding difficulties atypical for a man his age. Based on interviews conducted by Dr. Carvey with family and friends as well as colleagues at work (documented in the vocational assessment and neuropsychological evaluation), his activities of daily living have markedly changed, his work productivity has deteriorated significantly, and his quality of life has diminished. He was due for a significant promotion that would have doubled his salary, but, following the trazodone exposure, his bonuses were reduced to zero and he did not receive the promotion. His company has been carrying him but may have to let him go. Thus, the patient was a reasonably healthy, normal individual aside from hypertension, chronic sinusitis, knee surgery, and a minor cardiac event who was a high-functioning individual destined for promotion. However, he now is an individual with low self-esteem and a documented anxiety disorder following exposure to trazodone, and is at significant risk of losing his job. A reasonable pharmacological conclusion is that trazodone as the cause of his new problems, as permanent disorders may arise from drug exposure, including psychotropic drugs.

20.4 ANTIDEPRESSANTS AND THE PATIENT WITH SUICIDAL IDEATION

Depressive disorders and suicides tend to cluster in families and first-degree relatives of patients. Females are two to three times more likely to attempt suicide than males. Males, however, succeed three times more often.[10] All depressed patients should be assessed for suicidal ideation. Myths regarding suicide include:

- Suicide attempts are just a call for attention,
- Suicidal people are crazy or insane, and
- If you ask someone who is considering committing suicide about their intentions, they will be more likely to follow through with the suicide attempt.

When suicidal ideation is suspected, patients should be asked about their desire to harm or kill themselves. Patients often attempt suicide by using prescription drugs. Adults tend to poison themselves with several different drugs at once. Combinations of antidepressants—benzodiazepines, barbiturates, alcohol, and over-the-counter pain relievers—are commonly used in suicidal attempts. Prescribing antidepressants to patients with suicidal ideation must be done carefully.

TCA overdose is often fatal when the adverse effects are pronounced and simultaneous. Symptoms of a TCA overdose include drowsiness, lethargy, cardiac arrhythmias, hypotension, and seizures. In hospital emergency rooms, life-threatening effects from TCA overdose usually begin within two to six hours of the patient's arrival at the hospital. Antidotes are unavailable for TCA overdose: gastric decontamination, activated charcoal, sodium bicarbonate, and supportive care are the usual treatment. To minimize the risk of overdose, doctors should prescribe no more than a one-week supply of a TCA and no more than 1 gram of the drug at any one time.[3] If refills are allowed, the pharmacist must not dispense them prematurely. Larger drug quantities through mail-order pharmacies should be prohibited.

In patients with suicidal ideation, prescribing a less-toxic antidepressant is critical: SSRIs or Desyrel (trazodone hydrochloride, Apothecon) are preferred. Although these second-generation agents are generally safer, overdose fatalities have also been reported using them. In most instances, the doses taken were many times greater than the usual therapeutic dose. Another factor that increases a depressed patient's risk of suicide is the slow therapeutic onset of cyclic antidepressants—generally about two to four weeks. The frustrated, depressed patient may double or triple their dose in an attempt to increase the efficacy.

SSRIs should be favored over TCAs for depressed patients with suicidal ideation. If a TCA must be used (such as for a patient with a history of SSRI failure), only small doses, not exceeding 1 gram, should be prescribed and dispensed. Furthermore, family members of patients with suicidal ideation should be notified, psychiatric care should be sought, and hospital admission should be considered.

20.4.1 Prozac and Suicidal Ideation

Eli Lilly & Co. first marketed Prozac in 1987. Since then, the drug has been accused of causing patients to commit violent crimes and become suicidal. In the early 1990s, several lawsuits were filed against Eli Lilly, including a suit by Abbie Hoffman and another by the rock star Del Shannon.[11] Epidemiological studies have since demonstrated that Prozac was not associated with more incidents of violent crimes or suicidal behavior. The behavior was, instead, a consequence of an affective or mood disorder.

A comprehensive meta-analysis of clinical data was undertaken to assess a possible association between fluoxetine and suicidal acts or ideation.[12] The incidence of suicidal acts did not differ significantly between fluoxetine and placebo or between fluoxetine and TCAs. A marginally significant drop in suicidal ideation was found with fluoxetine when compared with a placebo, and a slightly larger gap was found between fluoxetine and TCAs. No worsening of suicidal ideation was found between fluoxetine and a placebo or between fluoxetine and TCAs. Nevertheless, Prozac's package insert, and the inserts of all other antidepressants such as paroxetine, has the following precautionary statement:

> Depression and other psychiatric disorders are independently associated with increased risk of suicide. This affects patients of all ages who are started on antidepressant therapy and thus, all patients should be monitored appropriately and observed for clinical symptoms for suicidality, or abnormal changes in behavior. Families and caregivers should be informed and provide close observation and communication with the patient and prescriber.[13]

20.4.1.1 *Woulfe v. Eli Lilly & Co*

In *Woulfe v. Eli Lilly & Co.* the plaintiff Daniel Clinton Woulfe was the father of Jack Wayne Woulfe, who committed suicide by hanging on February 1, 1991.[14] Woulfe brought action against Eli Lilly & Co., claiming that its failure to warn about the risk of suicide from Prozac caused or contributed to Woulfe's death and suffering. In particular, the plaintiff claimed that the warnings provided in the package insert for Prozac sold in the United States were deficient when compared with the language used in the package insert for the German market. The German insert advised prescribing physicians that:

- Prozac did not have a general sedative effect on the central nervous system (CNS);
- Patients, for their safety, had to be sufficiently observed until the antidepressive effect of Prozac set in; and
- The use of an additional sedative might be necessary in some cases.

The deceased was prescribed Prozac by his physician on January 4, 1991. The doctor believed that the warnings Eli Lilly provided about Prozac were adequate and that any additional warnings about its use would not have changed his decision to prescribe the antidepressant to the deceased. Jack Wayne Woulfe did not exhibit or have a history of anger, anxiety, agitation, impulsivity, agitated ruminating, or volatile outbursts that might have suggested to the physician the need for additional treatment or referral to a psychiatrist.

Under Oklahoma law, Eli Lilly did not have the duty to personally warn Jack Wayne Woulfe of the possible risks associated with the use of Prozac. Under this "learned intermediary doctrine," the manufacturer of a prescription drug is shielded from liability if it adequately warns prescribing physicians of the dangers associated with the drug. Based on that argument, Eli Lilly's motion for summary judgment on the plaintiff's "failure to warn" claim was granted, and the case was dismissed.

20.4.1.2 *Espinoza v. Eli Lilly & Co*

In *Espinoza v. Eli Lilly & Co.* the surviving family of Vera Espinoza claimed that she shot and killed her two children and immediately thereafter committed suicide as a result of her ingestion of Prozac.[15] She was diagnosed with major depression and dependent personality disorder. Espinoza was treated with Prozac for several years before her death, and during the last three months of her life, her dosage was increased from 20 to 40 mg. The deceased, however, was known to adjust her dosage as she saw fit, and it is uncertain how much Prozac she was taking when she died. Autopsy results revealed concentrations of Prozac and its metabolite norfluoxetine at ten times the approved therapeutic concentration.

In the days before her death, Espinoza was calm. She began giving away possessions, suggesting that she planned her suicide. She was not exhibiting symptoms of akathisia (restlessness), a mixed state (mania and depression), mania, or hypomania at that time. The family members offered a psychiatrist and suicidology expert as their sole expert in determining the cause of these homicides and suicide. The psychiatrist concluded that Prozac was a contributing cause of Espinoza's suicide because the medication disinhibited her, limiting her self-control, increasing her impulsivity, and making it difficult for her to control her aggression.

The court noted a controversy within the psychiatric community in determining whether the observed association—between ingestion of certain types of antidepressants and suicidal or violent behavior—was causal. The expert's opinion on causation relied on an article that showed a causal connection between Prozac and akathisia and an association between akathisia and suicidal ideation. The court held, however, that the expert's opinion did not "fit" the facts of this case because Espinoza did not suffer from akathisia. Without expert testimony that the drug caused the deaths, it was not possible to show that any inadequacy in the drug's warnings was a substantial factor in bringing about the deaths. As a result, Eli Lilly's motion for summary judgment was granted on the grounds that the plaintiffs lacked admissible expert testimony and a proximate cause.

20.4.1.3 *Cassidy v. Eli Lilly & Co*

Diane Cassidy took Prozac for weight loss. Ms. Cassidy became partially paralyzed and mentally impaired after a failed suicide attempt. Eli Lilly & Co. settled with the plaintiff.[16]

20.4.2 Paxil and Suicidal Ideation

20.4.2.1 *Dolin v. GlaxoSmithKline*

In *Dolin v. GlaxoSmithKline (GSK).* the plaintiff Wendy Dolin was the wife of Stewart Dolin, who at 57 years old committed suicide by jumping in front of an oncoming commuter train in 2010.[17] Dolin brought action against GSK and the generic company Mylan in 2012, claiming that their failure to warn about the risk of suicide from paroxetine, the generic of Paxil, in patients 24 years of age and older caused or contributed to Steward's suicide. Mr. Stewart was prescribed paroxetine for depression and anxiety. Six days after filling the prescription, he committed suicide, and blood tests confirmed the presence of paroxetine in his system. Since the generic company had limited influence on the contents of the drug labels as they followed the labeling from the brand manufacturer, the generic company was dismissed from the lawsuit in 2014. In 2021, the federal court jury awarded the plaintiff $3 million from GSK. However, the Seventh Circuit reversed the district court decision, since federal law prevented GSK from adding the warning about the alleged association between paroxetine and suicides in older adults.

20.4.3 Antidepressant and Increased Suicidality in Pediatrics

In recent years there has been much debate over whether use of antidepressant medication in pediatric patients may increase suicidal thinking and behavior. In October 2004 the FDA required that manufacturers of all antidepressants add a black box warning of increased risk of suicidality and in May 2007 extended this warning to those up to the age of 24.[18,19] In June 2004 GSK settled a lawsuit for $2.5 million on the basis that GSK had hidden research that showed children that had taken Paxil had increased risk of suicidality.[16] Again in 2008 GSK paid out another $40 million in settlement in regard to its medication Paxil and children. GSK also reimbursed health insurance companies that paid for Paxil, as GSK was purported to have suppressed studies that showed the medication was ineffective and may increase suicidality in this population.[17]

20.4.3.1 *Schilf v. Eli Lilly & Co*

In *Schilf v. Eli Lilly & Co* the plaintiffs were the parents of Peter Schilf, who committed suicide on December 24, 2004. Schilf brought suit against Eli Lilly & Co., claiming their failure to warn led to the death of their son. On November 26, 2004, Peter Schilf, 16 years old, went to his family practitioner, Dr. Briggs. At this visit the doctor diagnosed Peter with depression and gave him samples of the medication Cymbalta. Dr. Briggs decided to prescribe Cymbalta over Prozac, as at the time he believed it was less linked with suicide, as it was not included in the pooled data that the FDA based its suicidality warning. It came out during the trial that Dr. Briggs was unaware of the five suicides that were completed during Cymbalta's clinical trials. Within a day of getting the samples, Peter along with his father researched Cymbalta and went to the medication website. Mr. Schilf noted that he did not see any warning for suicidality on the Cymbalta website and if he did he would have not let his son take the medication. Peter on December 24, 2004, committed suicide. Cymbalta literature was updated a month later to include the mandated black box warning.[20]

At first the court granted summary judgment against the plaintiffs, as Dr. Briggs had testified at his deposition that he would have still prescribed Cymbalta even with adequate warning. This decision was overturned on appeal as noted from Dr. Briggs's testimony and based on his behavior that if he had known about the link between Cymbalta and suicidality and previous suicides that occurred during Cymbalta clinical trials he may have not prescribed the medication to Peter.[20] A month before the jury trial was to start Eli Lilly & Co. settled for an undisclosed amount with the Schilfs.[21]

20.5 BROKEN HEART SYNDROME: TAKO TSUBO CARDIOMYOPATHY ASSOCIATED WITH USE OF ANTIDEPRESSANTS

Broken heart syndrome, which was first described in the early 1990s, is also known as "Tako Tsubo" (meaning "octopus trap" in Japanese) cardiomyopathy. It is a reversible condition that mimics an acute myocardial infarction or heart attack. It is primarily diagnosed in postmenopausal women following abrupt emotional or physical stress.[22,23] Patients present with chest pain and shortness of breath, which appear within hours of the event. The left ventricle of the heart enlarges; an electrocardiogram depicting the beating of the heart shows abnormal heart contractions, and, overall, there is not enough oxygenated blood in the body, since the heart is failing. However, the heart arteries are not blocked and patients are not experiencing a heart attack.[24] Although the exact cause of this condition remains unclear, it is believed to be the result of increased catecholamines such as serotonin and norepinephrine. Since antidepressants exert their efficacy by enhancing the concentrations of serotonin and norepinephrine, dosages above those therapeutically recommended may be associated with Tako Tsubo cardiomyopathy. This condition is treated by discontinuation of the offending agent(s) and management of symptoms. The mortality rate is less than 8 percent and patients experience full recovery within six to eight weeks.

Christoph et al. describe the case of a 43-year-old woman who developed Tako Tsubo cardiomyopathy after an accidental overdose of venlafaxine, which increases serotonin and norepinephrine concentrations.[2] A 24-hour urine collection showed increased concentrations of norepinephrine. The serum levels of venlafaxine and its active metabolite desmethylvenlafaxine were elevated above the therapeutic range. Upon discontinuation of the antidepressant and management of the heart symptoms, the patient fully recovered in six weeks.

Perry et al. describe the case of a 60-year-old female who presented to the emergency department with chest pain, lightheadedness, nausea, and diaphoresis. At home, the patient was taking the antidepressant, duloxetine, for the management of peripheral neuropathy (nerve pain).[25] While taking the antidepressant, she developed a urinary tract infection and was prescribed the antibiotic ciprofloxacin. This antibiotic has the ability to inhibit the metabolism of duloxetine, leading to supratherapeutic concentrations of the antidepressant. At the hospital, further workup ruled out the diagnosis of a heart attack, and the patient was eventually found to have Tako Tsubo cardiomyopathy, which may have been the result of increased duloxetine concentrations. The antidepressant was discontinued, and the patient's heart symptoms were managed. Full recovery was observed in about six weeks.

Since all antidepressants exert their efficacy by increasing the concentrations of norepinephrine and serotonin, doses above those therapeutically recommended can potentially lead to Tako Tsubo cardiomyopathy. Importantly, the co-administration of medications that can dangerously increase the concentrations of antidepressants can potentially cause this heart condition, which when left untreated can be fatal.

20.6 THE ADVERSE EFFECTS OF ANTIDEPRESSANTS AND THE DUTY TO WARN

TCAs are associated with many more adverse effects than SSRIs. SSRIs, however, cause a higher incidence of gastrointestinal side effects, such as nausea, vomiting, diarrhea, and erectile dysfunction. Pharmaceutical manufacturers have a duty to inform prescribers and pharmacists of all indications, contraindications, allergies, adverse effects, cautions, precautions, drug–drug and drug–food interactions, and dosing schedules. Both the prescriber and the pharmacist are responsible for monitoring a drug for its efficacy and toxicity and counseling the patient about the therapy. Is there, however, a duty to warn someone for whom a drug was not prescribed? If so, who would be responsible for performing that duty—the pharmaceutical manufacturer, the physician, or the pharmacist?

20.6.1 *Docken v. Ciba-Geigy*

In *Docken v. Ciba-Geigy*, the court was asked to determine whether the manufacturer, the physician, or the pharmacist owed a "duty of care" to warn someone who was not prescribed a drug.[26] In 1979, a physician prescribed the TCA Tofranil, manufactured by Ciba-Geigy and dispensed by a hospital pharmacy, for the plaintiff's son Tim. A hospital pharmacist dispensed it. In 1983, the plaintiff's other son Terry ingested several Tofranil tablets, hoping that it would remedy the same enuresis (bedwetting) problem that his brother had. Terry died as a result of ingesting the Tofranil. The plaintiff filed a lawsuit against the pharmaceutical manufacturer, physician, and pharmacist. The plaintiff's product liability theory alleged that the drug was dangerous and defective because of its inadequate labeling. Specifically, the plaintiffs said the defendants:

- Failed to label Tofranil in a manner adequate to ensure its safe use;
- Failed to warn that Tofranil must be taken and administered with extreme caution because of the potentially fatal effect of excessive dose;
- Failed to warn that Tofranil must be disposed of properly after use because of the potential fatal effect of an overdose;
- Failed to warn that Tofranil must be stored safely, away from children;
- Failed to warn that Tofranil does not quickly leave a person's body, resulting in potentially fatal drug accumulation; and
- Failed to warn that an excessive dose of Tofranil can result in death, especially in children.

The plaintiff alleged that the defendants were negligent by failing to warn of these dangers. The plaintiff failed to allege that the physician and the hospital pharmacy were in the business of selling drugs, so the plaintiff's complaint was missing an important element, failing to state a cause of action based on strict product liability. Therefore, Ciba-Geigy was the only defendant left to face liability claims regarding negligence and failure to warn. Had this case been presented differently and had the plaintiff proved that the physician and pharmacist did not warn the patient, it is plausible that one or both of them might have been held liable as well.

20.6.2 Stebbins v. Concord Wrigley Drugs, Inc. et al

In *Stebbins v. Concord Wrigley Drugs, Inc. et al.* the plaintiff Bonnie Stebbins had been seriously injured when a car driven by Joseph Zagone struck her automobile.[27] A psychiatrist had prescribed Tofranil for Zagone's psychiatric illness. Concord Discount Drugs dispensed the drug to Zagone. After eating breakfast one day, Zagone got in his car and ran a red light, hitting Stebbins' automobile and seriously injuring her. Stebbins filed a lawsuit against Zagone, his physician, the pharmacy, and the pharmacist, claiming that they had failed to warn the motorist of the adverse effects and hazards of Tofranil. Stebbins alleged that Zagone should have been told not to drive while receiving Tofranil therapy. Zagone subsequently settled out of court with Stebbins.

The physician claimed that he had told Zagone to use Tofranil at bedtime. Zagone had been taking 75 mg of Tofranil at bedtime for some time without any adverse effects or daytime drowsiness. Zagone was confused, however, about whether he took Tofranil at bedtime or in the morning on the day of the accident. The court granted the physician's motion for summary judgment, concluding that he had given due warning. At the time in 1987, the court ruled that the pharmacist had no duty to warn the patient of possible side effects when the prescription was proper and when neither the physician nor the manufacturer had required the pharmacist to warn the patient. However, the Omnibus Budget Reconciliation Act (OBRA) enacted in 1990 required pharmacists to counsel all patients about adverse effects, drug interactions, and drug doses.[28] So, if the case was tried today, the pharmacist may have assumed some liability.

20.6.3 Morgan et al. v. Wal-Mart Stores, Inc.

In *Morgan et al. v. Wal-Mart Stores, Inc.*, Jacquelyn Morgan and Charles Pettus, the parents of Cameron Pettus, alleged that their son's death in August 1993 was caused by an adverse reaction to desipramine.[29] In 1989, Cameron Pettus was diagnosed with attention deficit hyperactivity disorder. He also experienced mood swings, so desipramine was prescribed to control them. Cameron did not start taking the antidepressant until April 1991. Some months later and on various occasions, he complained of chest pains, and his mother took him to a hospital emergency room. No healthcare professional attributed Cameron's chest pains to desipramine. Until the time of her son's death, no pharmacist ever counseled Cameron's mother about the medication's adverse events when she picked up the prescription.

Cameron was later prescribed an antibiotic to heal a lymph node infection, thought to be the result of a mosquito bite. In the following weeks, Cameron's lymph node remained swollen, and he continued to experience chest pains. Finally, he was diagnosed with hyper-eosinophilic syndrome, a disorder that consists of a high number of eosinophils in the blood and bone marrow, which can damage the heart, lungs, liver, and other internal organs. A few days later, Cameron slipped into a coma, was declared brain dead, and was eventually removed from life support. The medical staff concluded that Cameron's death was the result of a hyper-eosinophilic syndrome caused by a reaction to the desipramine. Wal-Mart was alleged to be negligent in the sale of desipramine "by failing to properly warn intended users of the hazards and harms associated with the use of the product." The jury assigned 14 percent responsibility to Wal-Mart and the rest was assigned to Cameron's physicians and the other pharmacies from which Cameron's desipramine was purchased.

On appeal, the court ruled that "pharmacists have no generalized duty to warn patients of potential adverse reactions to prescription drugs . . . pharmacists are not legally obligated to do so." The judgment of the trial court was reversed in favor of Wal-Mart. The interesting part of this case is that the Wal-Mart pharmacist testified that, although the standard of practice required patient counseling and warnings, the law did not require them, so she did not warn the patient.

20.6.4 Kampmann v. Mason

In *Kampmann v. Mason*, the plaintiff made claims that the pharmacist and physician did not meet standards of care by failing to warn the plaintiff of the side effects of the medication that he was prescribed.

In August 1998 the plaintiff went to West Jefferson Mental Health Clinic for the treatment of depression. Dr. Mason saw the plaintiff on August 20, 1998, and prescribed him sertraline and trazodone. The plaintiff filled his prescriptions at the health clinic pharmacy that evening. Neither the doctor nor the pharmacist had informed the plaintiff that priapism was a possible side effect of trazodone on his visit.

On September 1, 1998, Mr. Kampmann woke up with an erection that did not go away and by the next day required him to be hospitalized for treatment of trazodone-induced priapism. The plaintiff ended up being hospitalized for 13 days and requiring four procedures.

In March 1999 the plaintiff filed a complaint with the Patient Compensation Fund against the prescriber and pharmacist who filled the trazodone prescription requesting a medical review panel. In February 2003 the medical review panel concluded that neither the prescriber nor the pharmacist had failed to meet the standard of care. In March 2003 the plaintiff filed suit against both the prescriber and the pharmacist who dispensed the trazodone for medical malpractice and negligence. In August 2003 the plaintiff also filed suit to add Sidmak, the manufacturer the plaintiff believed manufactured the trazodone he had taken, as a codefendant to the current malpractice suit. The suit claimed that Sidmark failed to inform prescribers and pharmacists of the side effects of trazodone despite its knowledge and that the manufacture should update its package insert to have a warning on priapism.[30]

Originally the court dismissed that case versus the manufacturer based on the "learned intermediary doctrine" defense. In 2006 the court reversed this decision stating that "We are not inclined to hold that a drug manufacturer fulfills its duty under the Louisiana Products Liability Law to use reasonable means to notify the user of the product by a mere warning to the wholesalers."[31] In May, 2007 Sidmak filed a motion for dismissal as it was not the manufacturer of the Trazadone that the plaintiff consumed. In June 2007 the plaintiff filed a supplemental and amending petition to replace Mutual in place of Sidmak Laboratories. Mutual in November 2007 was dismissed from the case as noted the plaintiff only had until October 2003 to file suit against any joint tortfeaso

For the claim filed against the pharmacy and the pharmacist, the court ruled in a summary judgment that the "Pharmacist has no duty to warn of potential adverse effects" under any of the cited Louisiana jurisprudence. Instead, the law places that duty on the prescribing physician because he is the "informed intermediary between the manufacturer and the patient." [32]

20.6.5 *Cottam v. CVS*

In *Cottam v CVS,* the plaintiff claims CVS and the prescriber were negligent in failing to warn him of the side effects of trazodone. This case looks at whether a pharmacy has a duty to warn patients it dispenses medication to of potential side effects, and how in-depth.[33]

CVS pharmacy implemented a computer system that would provide written information about the side effects of medication to customers in May 1994. It was available in two forms: a long form and a short form. On filling a prescription, the short form automatically would print out, but the company required on any new prescription that the long form would be provided to the patient. In March 1994 the plaintiff was admitted to the hospital for treatment of depression, for which he was prescribed trazodone. Upon discharge from the hospital, the plaintiff went to CVS to have the trazodone filled in August 1994. During the trial, the plaintiff noted that with his prescription he was only given the short form of the medication print and the pharmacist counseled the plaintiff that the medication could cause drowsiness.

The plaintiff took the first dose of trazodone that night before bed and woke with an erection that continued through the day. The plaintiff did not contact his doctor as he already had an appointment the next day with his primary care doctor and decided to wait till the next day. The plaintiff took another dose of trazodone that night before bed. When the plaintiff saw his primary care provider, he was sent to see a urologist immediately who admitted the plaintiff to the hospital for emergency surgery for priapism. The surgery left him permanently impotent. Mr. Cottam claims that if he had been aware that priapism was a side effect of the trazodone he would have sought medical attention sooner. He sued the prescribing physician, therapist, and pharmacy that dispensed the medication.[33]

The plaintiff settled with the other two defendants but the case with CVS proceeded to trial. CVS was found 51 percent negligent and the plaintiff 49 percent. The plaintiff was awarded $357,000. CVS appealed the decision, but the original judgment was affirmed as the pharmacy neglected to meet the voluntary standards it had set for itself. The patient only received the short-form patient hand out, which did not have information about priapism. As the form only contains a single warning, it would be reasonable to believe that the plaintiff would have believed that all side effects were included on this form.[33,34]

20.7 ANTIDEPRESSANTS AND ALCOHOL

The TCAs and several of the second-generation antidepressants possess potent CNS-depressant effects and should not be taken with alcohol, which is also a CNS depressant. The combination of alcohol and a cyclic antidepressant can lead to additive or synergistic CNS-depressant effects, including drowsiness, dizziness, confusion, and impaired motor activity. Operating heavy machinery, such as driving a vehicle or flying a plane, should be avoided. Patients with a known history of alcohol abuse should not be treated with CNS-depressing antidepressants. Some agents, such as Prozac, do not cause CNS depression but instead cause CNS excitation. CNS excitation manifests as tremors, nervousness, anxiety, and dizziness, so similar warnings regarding the operation of heavy machinery apply. Perhaps the agent least likely to cause CNS depression or excitation is the SSRI Zoloft. Paxil may also be a safer option; however, there have been several reports of Paxil-induced drowsiness.

It is the duty of the pharmaceutical manufacturer to provide warnings and information to healthcare providers about the effects of antidepressants and alcohol combinations. Both the prescriber and the pharmacist must counsel the patient regarding this interaction. Patients should be told that alcohol is contraindicated while using antidepressants. Because of the long half-life of many antidepressant agents, residual blood concentrations and pharmacologic effects can remain after discontinuing the therapy. Therefore, alcohol should be avoided for at least 24 to 96 hours after the last dose of an antidepressant. To minimize CNS depression, antidepressants are usually taken at bedtime. Some antidepressants cause insomnia. To limit the CNS excitation and sleep disturbances of Prozac, for example, it is recommended to take the medication by 2:00 P.M. Patients with suicidal ideation might also combine alcohol with their antidepressant, so a safer agent, such as Prozac, Zoloft, or Paxil, might be a more prudent prescription choice.

20.7.1 *Kirk v. Michael Reese Hospital*

In *Kirk v. Michael Reese Hospital*, the issue was whether a hospital and its physicians have a duty to warn a patient before his discharge that the drugs given at the hospital might impair physical abilities.[35,36] A passenger injured in a car accident sued Michael Reese Hospital, two psychiatrists, and two drug companies for failing to warn the car driver about the danger of his drinking alcohol in combination with the psychotropic drugs—Prolixin (fluphenazine hydrochloride) and Thorazine (chlorpromazine)—he had been given. Both of the psychotropics possess a pharmacological adverse effect profile similar to TCAs. The driver received a Prolixin injection and oral Thorazine on the day of his discharge from the hospital. He also consumed alcohol that day as well. The patient later lost control of his car and smashed into a tree.

The plaintiff alleged that the two drugs diminished the patient's mental and physical abilities, impairing his driving skills, and causing him to get into the accident. The plaintiff further alleged that the pharmaceutical manufacturers had failed to provide adequate warnings, and the physicians and hospital had failed to warn the patient before discharge that the medications could impair his motor skills and should not be taken with alcohol. The court first addressed the foreseeability of the plaintiff's injury. The court held that the injury was sufficiently foreseeable to the pharmaceutical manufacturers, physicians, and hospitals. The court further ruled that the failure to warn of the adverse effects and interactions of the drugs could result in injury to the plaintiff or to other members of the public. The court noted that the defendants had a duty to warn, rather than a duty to control or to prevent.

The hospital argued that it could not be liable for negligence because the administration of these drugs was within the purview of the physician. The physicians were neither employed nor controlled by the hospital. The court concluded that the hospital's negligence was for failure to warn and not because the treatment was inappropriate. Hospitals plainly do far more than merely furnish an edifice for treatment. They regularly employ on a salaried basis a staff of physicians, nurses, and pharmacists; the cost for these personnel is factored into the amount that patients are then charged by the hospital for their visit. It follows that hospitals must assume certain responsibility for the care and treatment of their patients.

The court concluded that if the hospital knows, or should have known, that medications administered in the hospital can have adverse effects that might impair a patient's motor skills, or if mixing those agents with foods or beverages, such as alcohol, could intensify those adverse effects, they must warn the patient.[35]

Two years later, the Illinois Supreme Court reversed the appellate court decision because the plaintiff had failed to establish the existence of a legal duty.[36] The court recognized that there was a duty to warn and that such a duty may extend to those outside the purchasing chain. That duty, however, extends only to conduct that is reasonably foreseeable. The pharmaceutical manufacturers could not control physicians or hospitals that dispensed their drugs without warnings. The court reasoned that holding a hospital responsible for the harmful acts committed by its patients would place an unreasonable burden on hospitals. Additionally, the court took notice that the state was attempting to decrease the burden on healthcare providers from overzealous plaintiffs suing for medical malpractice. The physicians did have a duty to warn; that duty, however, is to warn the patient and does not extend to unknown non-patients in the public. Evidently, a hospital and physicians might have been liable if the driver—who was administered the Prolixin and Thorazine but not warned about their side effects or their interaction with alcohol—had pursued this case.

20.7.2 *Hand v. Krakowski*

In *Hand v. Krakowski*, the issue of whether a pharmacist has a duty to warn an alcoholic of the possible dangers of concurrent administration of psychotropic drugs was evaluated.[37] The executor of the estate of a known alcoholic brought a lawsuit. For more than six years, the employees of the defendant pharmacy had dispensed various psychotropics prescribed by the patient's physicians. The pharmacist knew that the patient was an alcoholic. In the six months preceding the patient's death, the pharmacy dispensed 728 units of psychotropic drugs, even though it was known that these agents included opiates that were contraindicated with concurrent alcohol use. The autopsy report revealed that the cause of death was pancreatitis secondary to severe hepatic cirrhosis. The hepatic cirrhosis may have resulted from concurrent use of psychotropics, opiates, pain relievers (acetaminophen), and alcohol. Alcohol abuse may have predisposed the patient to hepatic disease induced by alcohol, psychotropics, opiates, and pain relievers.

The pharmacy moved for summary judgment, and the motion was granted. The executor of the estate appealed, and the summary judgment was reversed. The court found that the pharmacist had a duty to warn the decedent of the adverse sequelae incurred when combining psychotropic drugs, including opiates, with alcohol. The court stated that "the rule of ordinary care as applied to the business of a druggist means the highest practical degree of prudence, thoughtfulness, and vigilance commensurate with the dangers involved and the consequences which may attend inattention."

The court concluded that dispensing psychotropic drugs to a known alcoholic is a breach of a pharmacist's duty of ordinary care by knowingly ignoring the danger and consequences of an alcoholic's ingestion of medications for which alcohol is known to be contraindicated. However, the court was not willing to dismiss the notion that in certain settings and with appropriate monitoring and dosing adjustments, it is plausible to administer contraindicated psychotropics to a known alcoholic. The issue in this case was whether the pharmacist breached the standard of care required, rather than the pharmacist's duty to warn the patient. Nevertheless, the pharmacist was found liable.

20.8 SSRIS AND THE SEROTONIN SYNDROME

When the SSRIs Prozac, Zoloft, and Paxil are combined with serotonergic agents (see Table 20.2 for a list of selected serotonergic agents), serotonin levels in the CNS can become abnormally high, which can produce the *serotonin syndrome*.[5] The serotonin syndrome is a constellation of mental status changes and nervous system and neuromuscular effects that result from an excess of serotonin. A diagnosis of serotonin syndrome can be made when three of the following effects develop in the presence of high serotonin levels: agitation, diaphoresis, diarrhea, fever, hyperreflexia, incoordination, mental status changes, myoclonus, shivering, or tremor. Other manifestations include seizures and muscle rigidity. The onset of serotonin syndrome symptoms usually takes place within minutes or hours, and so does the resolution. Management consists of gastric decontamination, activated charcoal, and supportive care, which may require ventilator support or admission to an intensive care unit. There is no antidote for the serotonin syndrome. Anecdotally, however, serotonin antagonists such as methysergide, cyproheptadine, and propranolol have been of some success.

Combinations of meperidine and the popular cough suppressant dextromethorphan—both serotonin reuptake inhibitors that can significantly increase serotonin concentrations within the neuronal synapses—can potentially produce a severe serotonin syndrome that can be deadly. Any combination of serotonergic agents or a high dose of a single serotonergic agent can predispose a client to the dangerous serotonin syndrome. Healthcare providers must counsel patients on the dangers of using over-the-counter products such as l-tryptophan with an SSRI. L-Tryptophan, used for the management of depression and as a sedative-hypnotic, decarboxylates into serotonin, increasing serotonin synthesis. Furthermore, the popular alternative-medicine product, St. John's wort, possesses serotonin reuptake or releasing properties and should not be administered with SSRIs.

20.9 HEPATIC CYTOCHROME P450 DRUG INTERACTIONS AND CYCLIC ANTIDEPRESSANTS

The SSRIs Prozac, Paxil, and Zoloft are potent inhibitors of the hepatic cytochrome (CY) P450-2D6 isoenzyme system. Therefore, when meperidine, a popular analgesic, is administered, an SSRI can inhibit its hepatic metabolism and cause elevated meperidine levels. Elevated meperidine concentrations can result in severe CNS depression and seizures. Additionally, both meperidine and SSRIs may increase serotonin concentrations, increasing the risk of the serotonin syndrome. The combination of SSRIs and CYP450-2D6 substrates should be avoided to diminish the possibility of an exaggerated substrate effect and subsequent toxicity.

The SSRIs can be ranked by the strength with which they inhibit CYP450-2D6 in this order from greatest inhibition to weakest:

- Prozac
- Paxil
- Zoloft
- Celexa

Despite Zoloft's weaker inhibitory properties, it is associated with significant increases in substrate blood concentrations. Celexa and Lexapro are considered weak inhibitors of CYP450-2D6 and would be good alternatives to avoid a significant drug interaction. Drug–drug interactions can also affect several other hepatic CYP450 enzymes such as 3A4, 1A2, 2C9, and 2C19. Pharmacists must screen for

TABLE 20.2
A List of Selected Serotonergic Categories and Agents

Increase Synthesis	Serotonin Reuptake Inhibitors	Inhibit Serotonin Metabolism	Serotonin Agonists	Increase Serotonin Release
L-Tryptophan	Amphetamines	Phenelzine	Buspirone	Amphetamines
	Citalopram	Selegiline	LSD	Cocaine
	Cocaine	Linezolid	Lithium	Fenfluramine
	Dextromethorphan	St. John's Wort	Mescaline	Mirtazapine
	Escitalopram		Sumatriptan	
	Fluoxetine		Rizatriptan	
	Fluvoxamine		Naratriptan	
	Meperidine		Zolmitriptan	
	Paroxetine			
	Pentazocine			
	Sertraline			
	TCAs			
	Venlafaxine			

antidepressant drug interactions, notify prescribers, and recommend safer alternatives that do not interact.

20.10 ANTIDEPRESSANTS AND HERBAL AGENTS DRUG INTERACTIONS

Herbal agents such as Ginkgo, Ginseng, Kava-Kava, Licorice, Ma Huang, Saw palmetto, St. John's wort, and Valerian are usually depicted as benign since they are not prescription medications and are readily available over-the-counter to be purchased at pharmacies, health food stores, supermarkets, and even grocery stores. In fact, the FDA does not strictly regulate herbals and supplements, and, hence, there is no guarantee of the purity of the product and most herbals have not been thoroughly tested for drug interactions.[38,39] However, published literature has shown that herbals can mimic, increase, decrease, or antagonize the effects of prescription drugs. Herbal–drug interactions are as common as drug–drug and drug–food interactions. In a study by Taylor et al., it was found that 71 percent of patients who used herbal agents never informed their healthcare provider of such use because they were either never asked about it; did not deem it important to let their physician know about it; herbals are not drugs; or expected their physician to disapprove of the use of the herbal.[40] In the same study, 15 potential drug–herbal interactions were identified in 9 patients and an astounding number of 97 theoretical potential interactions in 51 patients.

St. John's wort (*Hypericum perforatum*) is a popular herbal agent that is being marketed for multiple indications including depression, anxiety, and seasonal affective disorder.[41] It is common for patients suffering from depression to start taking St. John's wort thinking that it will complement the efficacy of the prescription medication. However, St. John's wort shares the pharmacology of SSRIs, and its concomitant use with prescription antidepressants can lead to increased serotonin levels, ultimately resulting in serotonin syndrome (discussed previously in this chapter). Such cases have been reported with the concomitant use of St. John's wort and sertraline and nefazodone. Lethargy and grogginess have been reported in a patient taking the herbal with paroxetine. A few isolated case reports have documented serotonin syndrome with the use of St. John's wort alone. St. John's wort may also have the ability to increase the metabolism of amitriptyline and nortriptyline, potentially leading to treatment failure.[38–42]

Ginkgo (*Ginkgo biloba*) is an herbal agent marketed for the treatment of dementia, peripheral vascular diseases, and tinnitus (ringing in the ears).[39] There has been one case report of an 80-year-old woman who was prescribed Ginkgo and a low dose of trazodone after treatment failures for the management of dementia.[43] After three days of taking the herbal agent and the prescription medication together, she fell into a coma. Subsequently, she was taken to the hospital where she was quickly managed with an intravenous medication and awoke immediately. Ginkgo and trazodone were never restarted and two months later, the patient remained stable. It is hypothesized that Ginkgo may have increased the metabolism of trazodone via CYP3A4 and, hence, increased the production of the antidepressant's active metabolite, a potent hypnotic agent.

Herbal–drug interactions are common and far from benign. Patients and healthcare providers should be educated on their use, toxicities, and interactions, and discussion should be encouraged to avoid harmful combinations.

20.11 SERZONE AND LIVER DISEASE

Serzone is a second-generation non-TCA that has been associated with severe liver disease (hepatotoxicity).[44–46] The incidence of hepatic injury associated with Serzone is 29 cases per 100,000 patient-years.[47] In 2002, the FDA required a "black box warning" concerning the hepatotoxicity risk for patients taking Serzone.[48] The manufacturer (Bristol-Myers Squibb) also sent out "Dear Doctor" letters that described several instances of liver failure—some of which were fatal or required a liver transplant—with a reported rate in the United States of one case per 250,000 to 300,000 patient-years.[49] The Canadian Adverse Drug Reaction Monitoring Program database identified 32 cases of liver injury due to Serzone, of which 81 percent were classified as severe.[44] Out of those 32 cases, 11 patients were taking only Serzone, and liver injury developed in 88 percent of the cases within the first six months of therapy. Interestingly, 70 percent of the 32 cases of liver injury were women, which is consistent with the greater incidence of depression among women.[50]

Current recommendations suggest caution in prescribing Serzone to any patient taking other drugs metabolized by the hepatic cytochrome P450-3A4 isoenzyme system. This precaution is to avoid drug interaction with Serzone, which is a substrate and an inhibitor of that metabolic pathway. A warning is also issued *not* to prescribe Serzone to any patient with preexisting liver disease. In addition, it is recommended that liver enzyme tests be monitored periodically (the time to liver injury generally ranges from two weeks to six months). Patients should also be advised about the signs and symptoms of liver injury (such as nausea, vomiting, abdominal pain, and yellow discoloration of the skin) so that the drug can be stopped if they occur, and patients can be evaluated. Serzone should be stopped in patients who experience liver enzyme elevations of more than three times the upper limit of normal.

20.12 HIGH BLOOD PRESSURE ASSOCIATED WITH VENLAFAXINE USE

Venlafaxine, a second-generation non-TCA, was approved in 1994 as the first agent to inhibit both norepinephrine and serotonin. It is FDA-approved for the management of generalized anxiety disorder, panic disorder with or without agoraphobia (the fear of being in public places), and social phobia.[51,52] It has been observed that 0.4 to 13 percent of patients taking venlafaxine experience persistent increases in blood pressure, also known as hypertension. However, the incidence of hypertension varies depending on the dose and dosage form prescribed. Venlafaxine is available as immediate-release tablets and extended-release tablets and capsules. The immediate-release tablets are dosed at least twice daily and the extended-release formulations are only once daily. The incidence of hypertension with the immediate-release tablets is 3 to 7 percent (at doses between 100 and 300 mg daily) to 13 percent (at doses of 300 mg or greater daily). The incidence of high blood pressure with the extended-release formulations is much less at 0.4 to 3 percent.[51,53]

Venlafaxine-induced hypertension is a dose-dependent effect that results from its pharmacologic mechanism of action. At doses above 150 mg per day, venlafaxine increases only the concentrations of norepinephrine, a catecholamine known to increase blood pressure. In addition, the risk of hypertension while taking venlafaxine is hypothesized to be more likely in patients who are at risk for high blood pressure (pre-hypertensives) and in those already diagnosed with hypertension than in patients with normal blood pressure (normotensives).[54] Therefore, it is vital that patients monitor their blood pressure daily while taking venlafaxine, especially with dose escalations and if they are already at risk for high blood pressure.

Khurana et al. describe the case of a 37-year-old woman who developed a hypertensive crisis, a condition where blood pressure is so high that it is considered a medical emergency, while taking venlafaxine 75 mg once daily.[55] After nine days of taking the antidepressant, the patient developed blurry vision which progressed to cotton wool spots in the eyes, right arm and leg numbness, and headache. Upon hospital admission, a hypertensive crisis was diagnosed and all of her medications were withheld. The patient was successfully treated with intravenous medications. In this case, the patient was taking a low dose of venlafaxine; however, when the antidepressant was prescribed, the patient was already taking disulfiram for anxiety. Disulfiram has the ability to inhibit the metabolism of venlafaxine and, hence, increase venlafaxine's concentrations and its potential to increase blood pressure. Physicians should be cognizant that even at low doses, venlafaxine has the ability to increase blood pressure when it is co-administered with medications that can inhibit its metabolism.

20.13 SSRI USE AND BIRTH DEFECTS

Anywhere from 14 to 23 percent of pregnant women will have symptoms of depression. Negative outcomes for the infant have been associated with both maternal depression and its treatment during pregnancy, namely antidepressants. The American College of Obstetricians and Gynecologists and the American Psychiatric Association came out with a joint report in 2009 that made recommendations for the management of women planning on getting pregnant to those who are pregnant with depression. Depending on the patients' specific comorbid conditions, past medical history, severity, preferences, and presentation, antidepressants are one option that is recommended.[56]

Birth defects caused by prenatal use of SSRIs have been an area of interest recently. In May 2015, a study was published examining if there is an association between SSRIs (citalopram, escitalopram, fluoxetine, paroxetine, or sertraline) and birth defects. An association was seen with an increased risk of 2 to 3.5 times more frequent birth defects with the use of fluoxetine and paroxetine early in pregnancy and a slight association was seen for increased neural tube defects with citalopram.[57]

In July 2010, it was noted that GSK paid more than $1 billion to settle over 800 cases relating to Paxil-caused birth defects. This settlement came after the Kilker family was awarded $2.5 million in damages from GSK as Lyam Kilker's mother took Paxil prenatally and, he was born with a heart defect. The case brought against GSK claimed they failed to warn Lyam's mother's provider of the risk of taking Paxil.[58] In 2017, GSK also reached a settlement of $6.2 million in a class action lawsuit brought forth by Faith Gibson, who was on Paxil throughout her pregnancy when her daughter was born in 2005 with a heart defect, with nearly 50 other Canadian mothers joined in on the class action.[59] In April 2015 and June 2015, similar cases brought against Pfizer for its antidepressant sertraline were dismissed.[60,61] It was noted in the most recent trial that the jury found in favor of Pfizer as they concluded that sertraline's label had adequate warning of the risks versus benefits of using sertraline in pregnancy.[62]

20.14 BUPROPION XL AND SEIZURES

All antidepressants are associated with an increased risk of seizure or lower seizure threshold, although the risk for seizures is lower with SSRIs and SNRIs than with TCAs.[5] Bupropion, a weak neuronal uptake inhibitor of norepinephrine and dopamine, exhibits dose-dependent seizure risk. The two-year seizure risk with the medication is 0.1 percent with a daily dose of 300 mg, and the risk increases to 0.35–0.44 percent with a daily dose of 450 mg.[63]

Dr. O'Donnell describes a case of a patient who expired due to probable seizure disorder by the medical examiner while on bupropion XL 300 mg daily.[64] The patient had no history of seizures and was initially prescribed bupropion XL 150 mg daily for major depressive disorder, with the dose subsequently increased to 300 mg approximately three months later. Two months after the dose increased, the patient experienced a ruptured ovarian cyst, and about a week later she developed a fatal seizure event. The patient's post-mortem peripheral blood reported a bupropion level of 470 ng/mL, hydroxybupropion of 550 ng/mL, and codeine of 22 ng/mL. While the bupropion level is two-fold higher than what would be expected in a living individual consuming the same dose, levels post-mortem are typically inaccurate as a result of post-mortem redistribution. In addition, the presence of hydroxybupropion suggests the patient had normal liver metabolism and therefore prevented the accumulation of bupropion. Based on the available information, the only certainty that may be drawn from the blood level is the deceased had bupropion in her system, and any other attempt to rely on the blood level for any other confirmation would be purely speculative.

20.15 THE PHARMACIST'S ROLE

Pharmacists are the healthcare professionals most qualified to help consumers make the best use of their medications. Pharmaceutical education before 2000 required a minimum of five years of education and training leading to a B.S. degree in pharmacy. Since 2000, graduating pharmacists in the United States hold entry-level doctor of pharmacy (Pharm.D.) degrees. This degree requires a minimum of two to four years of pre-pharmacy training, followed by a four-year pharmacy program. The Pharm.D. program is rigorous and specialized and concentrates on pharmacotherapy and the application of pharmaceutical care. A number of Pharm.D. graduates choose to continue their training for an additional one to two years of post-graduate pharmacy residency training, or fellowships. Pharmacy residents are intensely trained to develop, hone, and maximize pharmacotherapy skills. They receive comprehensive, intense, individualized training in all aspects of pharmacotherapy.

Pharmacists are experts on the thousands of medications available today, how each works in the body, and the ways to use each safely. The public should be aware that the pharmacist is obligated by law to provide pharmaceutical care. Pharmaceutical care requires that the pharmacist review the client's prescribed drug regimen, intervene and adjust medication regimens as necessary, and educate the patient, to maximize patient care to ensure a positive outcome. The pharmacist's role is vital to patient care. It is paramount that the consumer seek out an effective pharmacist willing to provide pharmaceutical care services.

20.16 THE OMNIBUS BUDGET RECONCILIATION ACT

OBRA[28] requires pharmacists in all states to ensure appropriate answers to the following questions for every prescription filled:

- Is the medication prescribed indicated?
- Does the patient have any contraindications to the medication prescribed?
- Is the dosing schedule and route of administration appropriate?
- Are there existing or potential problems with drug side effects, drug–drug interactions, drug–nutrient interactions, or adverse drug reactions?
- What recommendations can be made to minimize adverse effects while maximizing therapeutic efficacy?

For a pharmacist to maximize the positive benefit and outcome of medication therapy, she must be a good pharmaceutical historian and take a thorough history from the client. The client must inform the pharmacist of all adverse events experienced with any medication; any allergies; dietary regimens followed; vaccination schedules; and all medications used, including over-the-counter drugs, homeopathic agents, and home remedies.

Under the OBRA of 1990, pharmacists are also required to perform prospective and retrospective drug utilization reviews (DURs). DURs contain explicit criteria for drug indications, drug contraindications, drug interactions, adverse reaction detection, monitoring parameters, tailored drug regimens, and expected outcomes. A prospective DUR ensures the appropriate use of a drug with every prescription. A retrospective DUR studies trends and adverse outcomes to detect inappropriate prescribing patterns.

20.17 HOW SAFE IS IT TO BUY PRESCRIPTION MEDICATIONS OVER THE INTERNET?

With the proliferation of the Internet, it has become very easy for patients to buy their medications at a minimum cost online. Multiple advertisements for less-expensive prescription medications are e-mailed to millions of consumers daily. But how safe is it to buy prescription medications online?

On February 16, 2007, the FDA alerted consumers of unsafe, misrepresented drugs purchased over the Internet.[65] A number of patients who purchased, among other medications, citalopram over the Internet, received instead a product that contained haloperidol, a potent antipsychotic medication used to treat schizophrenia. Many of the patients ended up in the hospital with difficulty breathing, muscle spasms, and stiffness, all of which are symptoms of haloperidol toxicity. The consumers named multiple websites where the products were purchased; however, it is difficult to identify the vendors due to the deceptive practices of many commercial outlets over the Internet.

One of the FDA's website links is devoted to warning patients about the possible dangers of buying medications over the Internet.[66] Even though there are many legitimate websites that operate legally, there are many more that offer to sell medications that have not been reviewed for safety and efficacy. In fact, some of the products sold on illegal websites may contain too much or too little of the active ingredient or may contain dangerous ingredients. Signs of a legitimate online pharmacy include the following: located in the USA; licensed by the state board of pharmacy; a licensed pharmacist available to answer questions; requires a prescription; provides contact information and allows you to talk to a person. Another way is to look for the National Association Boards of Pharmacy's Verified Internet Pharmacy Practice Sites Seal, also known as VIPPS® Seal.

20.18 IN A PERFECT WORLD

The ideal scenario for a patient starting and receiving drug therapy would be for a client and pharmacist to be able to spend 15 to 30 minutes in an office-based counseling session. Today most pharmacies have a private consultation area because pharmacies that do not have them cannot provide clients with the privacy conducive to effective counseling. No client wants his health profile and medication recommendations discussed within the confines of a noisy, cluttered area, with a crowd of customers and clerks and a busy cash register. Preferably, caregivers would attend the counseling sessions to maximize patient compliance. With the occurrence of the coronavirus disease 2019 (COVID-19) pandemic, telepharmacy, or pharmacist-supervised remote dispensing via HIPAA-compliant two-way audio and visual technology, has expanded significantly and as of 2021 an accepted practice in 25 states.[67] Telepharmacy in both small community hospitals without 24-hour pharmacy services and health is associated with increased weekly documented pharmacist interventions, cost savings per hospital, and improved nursing job satisfaction, while in health system it is also associated with shorter medication order-processing time.[68,69]

Failure to use the services pharmacists are trained for can be life-threatening. Having a prescription filled by a non-pharmacist health professional prevents the crucial quality checks that detect and prevent harmful drug interactions, reactions, and mistakes. Most healthcare professionals are not familiar with all the pharmacological effects of a drug, the potential side effects, or the drug's interactions. All healthcare professionals must familiarize themselves with their client's prescribed regimen and thoroughly review each drug's pharmacology. Cross-checking by pharmacists, nurses, physicians, and other healthcare professionals helps to minimize drug toxicity and maximize therapeutic efficacy. In addition, clients must be encouraged to choose one pharmacy for all their medications. Most clients will see several physicians concurrently, increasing the risk of drug interactions and contraindications. Patients who choose one pharmacy enable a pharmacist to maintain an accurate medication profile and to detect any potentially harmful drug combinations.

20.19 SUMMARY AND CONCLUSIONS

It is obvious that appropriate prescriptions and counseling are critical in minimizing a patient's risks of an adverse outcome. The pharmacist plays a vital role in protecting the patient and the prescriber by using their pharmacotherapy knowledge and offering appropriate counseling and monitoring a patient's therapy. It is the duty of the pharmaceutical manufacturers to provide adequate and current information to the medical community. It is the responsibility of the hospital or medical institution to ensure that its healthcare providers are knowledgeable and skilled in their disciplines and to provide the resources for them to practice safely. Almost every state mandates continuing education for physicians and pharmacists, and quality assurance ensures the upkeep of that continuing education. Finally, it is evident that when prescribing antidepressants, the SSRIs are generally a safer alternative to TCAs.

REFERENCES

1. American Psychological Association. Clinical practice guideline for the treatment of depression across three age cohorts. Updated February 16, 2019. Accessed May 9, 2021. https://www.apa.org/depression-guideline/guideline.pdf.
2. Li, L. Chapter 39: Mood disorders. In: Amthor, F.R., Theibert, A.B., Standaert, D.G., and Roberson, E.D., eds. *Essentials of Modern Neuroscience*. 1st ed. Mc-Graw Hill Lange; 2020:605–618.
3. National Center for Health Statistics. *Health, United States, 2015: With Special Feature on Racial and Ethnic Health Disparities*. Table 80: Selected Prescription Drug Classes Used in the Past 30 Days, by Sex and Age: United States, Selected Years 1988–1994 Through 2009–2012. Hyattsville, MD; 2016.
4. Shim, R., Baltrus P., Ye J., and Rust G. Prevalence, treatment and control of depressive symptoms in the United States: Results from the National Health and Nutrition Examination Survey, 2005–2008. J. Am. Board Fam. Med. 24(1):33–38 (2011).
5. Cohen, H., Hoffman, R.S., and Howland, M.A. Antidepressant poisoning and treatment: A review and case illustration. J. Pharm. Pract. 10(4):249–270 (1997).
6. FDA. FDA approves new nasal spray medication for treatment-resistant depression; available only at a certified doctor's office or clinic. Accessed May 9, 2021. https://www.fda.gov/news-events/press-announcements/fda-approves-new-nasal-spray-medication-treatment-resistant-depression-available-only-certified.
7. Gummin, D.D., Mowry, J.B., Beuhler, M.C., Spyker, D.A., Brooks, D.E., Dibert, K.W., Rivers, L.J., Pham, N.P., and Ryan, M.L. 2019 Annual report of the American Association of poison control centers'. Clin. Toxicol. 58:1360–1541 (2020).
8. Nicholson, D.P. The immediate management of overdose. Med. Clin. North Am. 67:461–498 (1991).
9. Case of patient/trazodone error with residual neurological deficits by P.M. Carvey, PhD (email communication, April 2021).
10. Vaillant, G.E., and Blumenthal, S.J. Risk factors and life span development. In: Blumenthal, S.J., and Kupfer, D.J., eds. *Suicide Over the Life Cycle*. Washington, DC: American Psychiatric Press; 1990:1–16.
11. Neuman, S.M., and Borja, A. Prozac: A question of which came first, the chicken or the egg? In: Moch, J.W., Borja, A., and O'Donnell, J., eds. *Pharmacy Law: Litigating Pharmaceutical Cases*. Tucson, AZ: Lawyers and Judges Publishing Co; 1995:121–131.
12. Beasley, C.M., Dornseif, B.E., Bosomworth, J.C., Sayler, M.E., Rampey, A.H., Heiligenstein, J.H., Thompson, V.L., Murphy, D.J., and Masica, D.N. Fluoxetine and suicide: A meta-analysis of controlled trials of treatment of depression. BMJ. 21:685–692 (1991).

13. Suicidality and antidepressant drugs. Last Accessed September 10, 2015. http://www.fda.gov/downloads/Drugs/DrugSafety/InformationbyDrugClass/UCM173233.pdf.
14. *Woulfe v. Eli Lilly & Co.*, 965 F. Supp. 1478 (ED Okla, 1997).
15. *Espinoza v. Eli Lilly & Co.*, 207 F.Supp. 2d 308 (2002); Lexis 16740 Case No. 2:00-cv-256 consolidated with case no. 2:00-cv-393.
16. Chronology of psychotropic drug lawsuits. Last Modified 2009 Citizens Communion of Human Rights. www.cchr.org. Last Accessed September 7, 2015.
17. *Dolin v. GlaxoSmithKline*. Appeal from the United States District Court for the Northern District of Illinois, Eastern Division. Case No. 12-cv-6403.
18. FDA launches a multi-pronged strategy to strengthen safeguards for children treated with antidepressant medications. Last Modified April 2013. Accessed August 31, 2015. http://www.fda.gov/NewsEvents/Newsroom/PressAnnouncements/2004/ucm108363.htm.
19. FDA proposes new warnings about suicidal thinking, behavior in young adults who take antidepressant medications. Last Modified April 2013. Accessed August 31, 2015. http://www.fda.gov/NewsEvents/Newsroom/PressAnnouncements/2007/ucm108905.htm.
20. *Schiff v. Eli Lilly and Co.*, 687 F.3d 947 (8th Cir. 2012).
21. Swiatek, Jeff. Eli Lilly and Co. settles wrongful death lawsuit: April 9, 2013. Accessed August 16, 2015. http://ssristories.org/eli-lilly-co-settles-wrongful-death-lawsuit-indy-star/.
22. Hanson, T. Takotsubo cardiomyopathy: A case study of stress induced transient left ventricular apical ballooning syndrome. Internet J. Adv. Nurs. Pract. 10(2) (2009).
23. Christoph, M., Ebner, B., Stolte, D., Ibrahim, K., Kolschmann, S., Strasser, R.H., and Schön, S. Broken heart syndrome: Tako Tsubo cardiomyopathy associated with an overdose of the serotonin-norepinephrine reuptake inhibitor Venlafaxine. Eur. Neuropsychopharmacol. Article in Press. Available online May 7, 2010.
24. Bybee, K.A., Kara, T., Prasad, A., Lerman, A., Barsness, G.W., Wright, R.S., Rihal, C.S. Systematic review: Transient left ventricular apical ballooning: A syndrome that mimics ST-segment elevation myocardial infarction. Ann. Intern. Med. 141:858–865 (2004).
25. Perry, R. Duloxetine-induced takotsubo cardiomyopathy: A case report. College of psychiatric and neurologic pharmacists award finalists for the 2008 poster abstracts. J. Pharm. Pract. 2008;21:60–61.
26. *Docken v. Ciba-Geigy*, 739 P.2d 591 (Ore. Ct. App. 1987).
27. *Stebbins v. Concord Wrigley Drugs, Inc. et al.*, 416 N.W.2d 381 (Mich. App. 1987).
28. Omnibus Budget Reconciliation Act of 1990. Public Law 101–508. Section 4401. 101st Cong., 2d sess. (Nov. 5, 1990).
29. *Morgan et al. v. Wal-Mart Stores, Inc.*, 30 S.W.3d 455 (Tex. App. 2000).
30. *Kampmann v. Mason*, 7 So. 3d 675 (5th Circuit 2009).
31. *Kampmann v. Mason*, 921 So. 2d 1093 (5th Circuit 2006).
32. *Kampmann v. Mason*, 42 So. 3d 411 (5th Circuit 2010).
33. *Cottam v. CVS Pharmacy*, 436 Mass. 316 (Mass: Supreme Judicial Court 2002).
34. Somonsmeier, Larry. Pharmacy sued for failing to warn of priapism. Last Modified September 1, 2005. Accessed July 15, 2015. http://www.pharmacytimes.com/publications/issue/2005/2005-09/2005-09-9847.
35. *Kirk v. Michael Reese Hospital*, 483 N.E.2d 906 (Ill. App. 1 Dist. 1985).
36. *Kirk v. Michael Reese Hospital* 513 N.E. 2d 387 (Ill. S.Ct. 1987).
37. *Hand v. Krakowski*, 453 NYS.2d 121 (NY App. 1982).
38. Natural Standard Research Collaboration. Drugs & supplements: St. John's wort (Hypericum perforatum L.) (2009). Accessed March 29, 2012. www.nlm.nih.gov/medlineplus/druginfo/natural/patient-stjohnswort.html.
39. Wood, A.J.J. Herbal remedies. N. Engl. J. Med. 347:2046–2056 (2002).
40. Taylor, D.M., Walsham, N., Taylor, S.E., and Wong, L. Potential interactions between prescription drugs and complementary and alternative medicines among patients in the emergency department. Pharmacotherapy. 26:634–640 (2006).
41. "St. John's Wort" drug monograph. *Micromedex(R) 2.0.* Thompson Reuters; 2010.
42. University of Michigan Health System Drug Information Service. Selected herb-drug interactions (2010). Accessed March 29, 2012. www.personal,umich.edu/~mschlafer/Lectures/herbdrug.pdf.
43. Galluzzi, S., Zanetti, O., Binetti, G., Trabucchi, M., and Frisoni, G.B. Coma in a patient with Alzheimer's disease taking low dose trazodone and gingko biloba. Letter to the Editor. J. Neurol. Neurosurg. Psychiatry. 68:679–680 (2000).
44. Novak, D., and Lewis, J.H. Drug-induced liver disease. Curr. Opin. Gastroenterol. 19:203–215 (2003).
45. Health Canada. Hepatotoxicity associated with Nefazodone (serzone). Can. Med. Assoc. J. 161(1):74–75 (July 1999).
46. Aranda-Michel, J., Koehler, A., Bejarano, P.A., Poulos, J.E., Luxon, B.A., Mobin Khan, C., Ee, L.C., Balistreri, W.F., and Weber, F.L., Jr. Nefazodone-induced liver failure: Report of three cases. Ann. Intern. Med. 130(4):285–288 (1999)
47. Garcia-Pando, A.C., del Pozo, J.G., Sánchez, A.S., Martin, A.V., de Castro, A.R., and Lucena, M.I. Hepatotoxicity associated with the new antidepressants. J. Clin. Psychiatry. 63:135–137 (2002).
48 Katz, R. *Letter to Bristol Myers Squibb Company Re: Black Box Warning Required for Serzone.* NDA 20-152/S-028. Rockville, MD: FDA; December 7, 2001.
49. Jody, D.M. *Letter to Health Care Professional Re: Important Drug Warning Including Black Box Information.* Princeton, NJ: Bristol Myers-Squibb Company; June 2001.
50. Stewart, D.E. Hepatic adverse reactions associated with nefazodone. Can. J. Psychiatry. 47:375–377 (2002).
51. Eisendrath, S.J., Cole, S.A., Christensen, J.F., Gutnick, D., Cole, M.R., and Feldman, M.D. Depression. In: Feldman, M.D., and Christensen, J.F., eds. *Behavioral Medicine in Primary Care: A Practice Guide.* 3rd ed. McGraw-Hill Medical Companies; 2008:199–226.
52. *Effexor XR(R) (Venlafaxine Hydrochloride) Extended Release Capsules: Package Insert.* Philadelphia, PA: Wyeth Pharmaceuticals Inc.; 2017.
53. Thase, M.E. Effects of venlafaxine on blood pressure: A meta-analysis of original data from 3744 depressed patients. J. Clin. Psychiatry. 59:502–508 (1998).
54. Feighner, J.P. Cardiovascular safety in depressed patients: Focus on venlafaxine. J. Clin. Psychiatry. 56:574–579 (1995).
55. Khurana, R.N., and Baudendistel, T.E. Hypertensive crisis associated with venlafaxine. Letter to the Editor. Am. J. Med. 115:676 (2003).

56. American College of Obstetrics and Gynecology. Depression during pregnancy: Treatment recommendations. Last Updated August 21, 2009. Accessed August 30, 2015. http://www.acog.org/About-ACOG/News-Room/News-Releases/2009/Depression-During-Pregnancy
57. Reefhuis, J., Devine, O., Friedman, J.M., Louik, C., and Honein, M.A. Specific SSRIs and birth defects: Bayesian analysis to interpret new data in the context of previous reports. BMJ. 351:h3190 (2015).
58. Feeley, J., and Kelley, T. Glaxo said to have paid $1 billion over paxil suits. July 10, 2012. Last Accessed September 7, 2015. http://www.bloomberg.com/news/articles/2010-07-20/glaxo-said-to-have-paid-1-billion-to-resolve-paxil-birth-defect-lawsuits
59. Fraser, K. Moms reach $6.2 settlement over claims that anti-depressant caused kids' heart problems. *The Province*, March 1, 2017. Accessed May 10, 2021.
60. Dye, J. Pfizer wins first U.S. trial over Zoloft birth-defect risk. April 17, 2015. Last Accessed September 7, 2015. http://www.reuters.com/article/2015/04/17/us-pfizer-zoloft-idUSKBN0N82HY20150417.
61. Feeley, J. Pfizer wins second trial over zoloft and birth defects link. June 11, 2015. Last Accessed September 7, 2015. http://www.bloomberg.com/news/articles/2015-06-11/pfizer-wins-trial-over-claims-zoloft-caused-birth-defects.
62. Dye, J. U.S. jury clears Pfizer in second trial alleging Zoloft birth defects. June 11, 2015. Last Accessed September 7, 2015. http://www.reuters.com/article/2015/06/11/us-pfizer-zoloft-verdict-idUSKBN0OR2HL20150611.
63. Davidson, J. Seizures and bupropion: A review. J. Clin. Psychiatry. 50:256–261 (1989).
64. Case of patient/casuation of bupropion XL with seizures by J.T. O'Donnell, Pharm.D., MS (email communication, March 2021).
65. U.S. Food and Drug Administration (FDA) (2007). www.fda.gov/NewsEvents/Newsroom/PressAnnouncements/2007/ucm108846.htm Accessed March 29, 2012.
66. U.S. Food and Drug Administration. The possible dangers of buying medicines over the Internet. *FDA Consumer Information*, March 1–3, 2010.
67. Gebhart, F. Scaling up telepharmacy for the future. *Drug Topic*, April 5, 2021. https://www.drugtopics.com/view/scaling-up-telepharmacy-for-the-future. Accessed May 10, 2021.
68. Schneider, P.J. Evaluating the impact of telepharmacy. Am. J. Health Syst. Pharm. 70(23):2130–2135 (2013).
69. Garrelts, J.C., Gagnon, M., Eisenberg, C., Moerer, J., and Carrithers, J. Impact of telepharmacy in a multihospital health system. Am. J. Health Syst. Pharm. 67(17): 1456–1462 (2010).

21 Contrast Media Neurotoxicity Following Myelography

Stephanie E. Tedford and James T. O'Donnell

SYNOPSIS

21.1 INTRODUCTION

The administration of contrast media agents is relatively safe and rarely causes systemic toxicity in the course of routine imaging studies. While the incidence of serious toxicity is low, these drugs usually have fatal effects after central nervous system (CNS) exposure, when contraindicated, in routes of administration allowing CNS or spinal cord entry, and in doses that exceed user recommendations. Most patients do not survive overdose effects, and, therefore, limited information exists on long-term sequelae following such incidents. We provide evidence for the acute and chronic effects of exposure to contrast media overdose in two patient cases. We report findings from inadvertent overdose following administration of iopamidol and iothalamate resulting in the manifestation of serious and persistent adverse effects. Expertise in assessing adverse drug reaction reports is an essential and required responsibility of drug developers and regulators.

Myelography is a type of radiographic imaging used to assess the integrity of the spinal canal. A myelogram test provides insights into abnormalities of the spinal cord that may be underlying clinical deficits. This assessment is useful for visualizing bones, herniated discs, and other soft tissues surrounding the spinal canal that may be compressing the nerves and/or spinal cord. Contrast agents are administered prior to imaging to enhance structure resolution. A number of different contrast media agents with various toxicities are used in myelography.[1,2] Iodinated contrast agents are commonly employed and are considered to be generally safe and effective when administered correctly. Iodinated contrast agents are most frequently administered through intravascular injection, but due to the pharmacokinetic properties of the compound, the agent quickly redistributes to the extravascular space.[1,3] However, rare, contrast-induced toxicity can result in serious complications that can be life-threatening.[4–9] Dosing and administrative errors contribute to increased risk for toxicity. Contrast toxicity may present in a variety of ways. While not fully understood, each manifestation often has several likely underlying mechanisms. There is scant information detailing outcomes and side effects of contrast agent overdose other than death since most patients do not survive. In this report, we provide evidence from two patient cases on the acute and chronic effects of exposure to contrast media overdose.

21.2 CASE REPORTS

21.2.1 Case I Intrathecal Iopamidol

A 62-year-old woman was inadvertently administered an intrathecal overdose of iopamidol (Isovue-M), an iodinated contrast agent, while undergoing a total columnar myelogram. The manufacturers recommend a 10 ml injection of iopamidol (300 mg/ml iodine) for a dosing range of 2,000–3,000 mg iodine in adults. The patient was administered 22 ml of Isovue-M for a total administered dose of 6,600 mg iodine. The dose administered was two to three times the recommended maximum dose for the myelogram procedure. Following the procedure, the patient developed altered cognitive function, memory loss, and seizure activity within several hours during her hospitalization and upon discharge was released with ongoing medical problems including "altered mental status", "contrast-induced seizures", and "status epilepticus". A head CT performed

DOI: 10.1201/9781003615323-23

18 hours post-procedure showed iopamidol in the subarachnoid spaces, and CT density readings of the cerebral spinal fluid (CSF) were 829, which is over 200 times higher than normal CSF CT density scores. Moderately high iodine contrast content in CSF was still observed in the aspirate two days later. Following the procedure, the patient experienced mental disorientation and memory loss within five to six hours. The patient developed seizure activity during her hospitalization, which was treated and did not recur after discharge from the initial hospitalization.

Prior to the patient's unintentional exposure to iopamidol, she was neurologically intact with no reports of the deficits described following the event. Following the overdose, the patient continued to experience significant medical complications including cognitive deficits, seizures, impairments in memory function, and significant hearing loss.

21.2.2 Case II Intrathecal Iothalamate

A 45-year-old man was inadvertently administered an intrathecal dose of iothalamate (Conray contrast product), an iodinated contrast media agent, while undergoing a myelogram procedure. The procedure was conducted as part of a workup for paroxysmal vertigo, which may have been related to a left Meckel's Cave cyst previously identified by MRI. Following administration, the patient immediately exhibited signs of contrast-induced neurotoxicity including lower limb disturbances, seizure activity, cognitive dysfunction, and memory loss. He also presented with peripheral paresthesia, bilateral lower extremity tingling, and spasms. It was quickly determined that he had been administered the incorrect contrast product for intrathecal use in myelography; iothalamate is never to be administered intrathecally and is contraindicated for use in myelography. A CSF lavage with 100 cc of saline, in addition to a lumbar drain, was initiated to remove the contrast product from circulation. The patient was also treated transiently with Keppra to control his seizure activity. The patient was released four days following the procedure.

Prior to the patient's unintentional exposure to iothalamate, he was a neurologically sound individual whose primary complaint was symptoms of vertigo. Following the overdose event, the patient continued to experience persistent cognitive impairment, including the inability to concentrate, inability to multitask, dull tension-like headaches, and blurriness of vision. He also exhibits neuromuscular impairments such as diffuse hyperreflexia, dizziness, vibratory paresthesia, unsteadiness, generalized weakness, and intermittent muscle spasms.

21.3 DISCUSSION

A pharmacologist who reviewed the cases opined that both patients suffered an overdose of their respective iodinated contrast agents and the symptoms experienced were caused by contrast-induced toxicity. The chronic effects experienced by both patients stemming from this overdose can be attributed to sustained damage to various tissues exposed to the contrast agent. Both product inserts for iopamidol and iothalamate warn against the entry of a large or concentrated amount of the contrast medium into the brain, which can increase the risk of neurotoxicity. The medication errors that occurred in both cases resulted in the CNS being exposed to excessive amounts of contrast agents. The pathological underpinnings that drive these adverse effects are uncertain. We provide potential support for the posed underpinnings below.

21.3.1 Mechanisms for Cerebral (Neurotoxic) Injury

The exact mechanisms underlying cerebral insult following contrast agent administration remain uncertain. Several mechanisms of cellular neurotoxicity on selected regions of the brain affecting cognition, memory, hearing, and vision are described. Entry of the contrast agent into the brain parenchyma is attributed to the breakdown of the blood–brain barrier (BBB). BBB disruption can be explained by the hyperosmolarity and chemotoxicity of iodinated contrast agents.[6] Experimentally, the BBB will open upon exposure to hypertonic solutions.[10] Contrast agents generally possess significantly higher osmolarity than plasma, blood, and CSF; this may contribute to increased permeability of the BBB. The hypertonic contrast solution attracts water out of the endothelial cells of brain vessels, causing cellular dehydration, shrinkage, and subsequent uncoupling of tight junctions and enhanced endothelial pinocytosis, thereby allowing for entry of the contrast agent. Alternate theories include prolonged exposure of the contrast agent with the endothelium associated with extended bolus transit time.

The severity of the barrier dysfunction is proportional to the relative chemotoxic action of the respective contrast agent. Upon entry of the contrast medium into the cranial subarachnoid space, it permeates the extracellular space by passive diffusion through the pia mater. Exposure of high doses of iodine to brain tissue can induce severe disruption in cellular functions including changes in neural transmission and cell death. Altered neuronal membrane permeability and depolarization properties of neurons may contribute to dysfunctional neuronal communication. Changes in neurological activity such as the development of seizures, amnesia, and cortical ocular/auditory deficits occur when nonionic contrast products penetrate the brain. Entry of the contrast agent into the brain can result in profound neurotoxicity and serious complications. Contrast media neurotoxicity can mimic subarachnoid hemorrhage in a variety of imaging procedures.[11–13] The neurotoxic effects are generally considered self-limiting and reversible; however, case reports exist that detail prolonged neurological deficits similar to the patient cases in the present report.[14]

Contrast-induced adverse reactions are categorized as chemotoxic or idiosyncratic reactions. Chemotoxic reactions are related to the physicochemical properties of the contrast medium and dosing parameters. Pharmacodynamic properties of the contrast agent on tissue are included in this category. The incidence of electroencephalographic (EEG) changes by virtue of the intrinsic properties of the compound molecule underlies the neurotoxic effects of these agents. The brain is a homeostatic organ, and changes in osmolarity due to the hypertonicity of the contrast product may not only disrupt the BBB but in severe instances may cause widespread osmotic changes in the brain sufficient to induce global cell death. There are many case studies that detail contrast agent-mediated complications. A review conducted by Spina et al. found 52 reports of contrast-induced encephalopathy (CIE) following cardiac catheterization.[5] Encephalopathy, motor, sensory and visual disturbances, ophthalmoplegia, aphasia, and seizures were most commonly reported. Cortical blindness is the most commonly reported neurological syndrome, occurring in almost 50% of cases.

One case study reports fatal brain edema in a patient who experienced a contrast agent overdose following aortography. Generalized seizures began after the contrast agent was injected, and a CT scan performed 22 hours post-injection showed the contrast agent in the arteries at the basal brain. Imaging from the CT also revealed increased density in the cerebral cortex, basal ganglia, and thalamus consistent with the localization of the existing intracerebral agent. The patient succumbed to the cerebral insult 48 hours post-contrast injection. A CT confirmed that high concentrations of the contrast agent were still present in the patient at the time of death. In addition, four hours post-mortem an iodine assay by fluorescence excitation revealed extremely high iodine concentrations throughout the brain. The concentrations observed in the cortical, thalamic, and hippocampal regions were significant. Exposure to these levels of iodine would completely disrupt cellular function. An autopsy reported diffuse edema within the cerebrum and the cerebellum and subarachnoid hemorrhage. The authors report that the doses administered to this patient were grossly excessive and exceeded the maximum recommended dose.[7] Similarly, another patient who underwent aortography developed seizures, cortical blindness, and renal failure following contrast agent administration within a recommended dosing protocol. A follow-up CT revealed high iodine concentrations in the cortex and mild brain edema.[8] This report demonstrates the potential of serious contrast-induced disturbances even within a normal dosing protocol.

Therefore, significant changes in the osmolarity of the brain may contribute to leakage of the contrast product across the BBB. In addition, profound changes can induce considerable brain edema which may be detrimental to brain function. In patient case 1, the BBB was bypassed by an intentional direct intrathecal injection. The overdose and the maneuver to move the contrast media to the cervical vertebrae caused the brain to be showered with neurotoxic, chemotoxic, and hyperosmolar chemicals—poisonous to brain tissue.

21.3.2 Contrast-Induced Neurological and Cognitive Deficits

Both patients from Cases 1 and 2 immediately developed prolonged seizure activity along with acute and sustained deficits in cognition and memory function. A review of the US FDA MedWatch reporting database (conducted in September 2016) lists 676 cases of adverse reactions related to cognitive impairment, seizures, and amnesia with non-ionic radiographic contrast agents. There is substantial evidence for the development of seizures following the administration of iodinated contrast agents. Although epileptic seizures are a rare occurrence (typically observed in <1%), they are a well-documented complication. The development of seizure activity is a serious adverse event, and patients with a history of epilepsy are restricted from the use of contrast agents. Epileptic seizures generally occur within 10 hours following the injection of the contrast product and are self-limited. It is widely accepted that the injection of the contrast product is directly related to the appearance of seizures or seizure-like activity. Compelling clinical evidence from CT reports following contrast-induced seizures shows high levels of remaining contrast in the brain and enhancement in cortical brain regions.[15] Preclinical studies report that the administration of contrast agents is epileptogenic when directly exposed to brain tissue in rabbits and rats.[16,17] Contrast agent iopamidol slows EEG activity, increases the appearance of slow brain waves and seizures, and induces a shift in energy toward slower brain frequencies (0.5–3.5Hz).[18] While the precise mechanisms underlying seizure induction are not known, it has been suggested that contrast-mediated changes in neural activity within subcortical circuits induce seizures at the thalamic level and cause disruptions in thalamocortical communication.[18] The neural circuits involved in seizures are acutely and may be permanently altered structurally and functionally following a seizure episode. Englot and Blumenfeld's theory states that focal seizures spread to the thalamus and disrupt corticothalamic connectivity. These changes can underlie subsequent cognitive impairment commonly witnessed in epileptic patients. Acute presentation of altered cognitive abilities and memory loss can develop following seizures.[19]

In the CNS, long-term potentiation (LTP) and depression are two cellular events believed to underlie neuroplasticity, the functional readout for learning and memory processes. Disruptions in LTP are observed following pharmacologically induced seizures. For example, animals with ten flurothyl-induced seizures demonstrate reduced hippocampal LTP and behavioral deficits in spatial learning and memory tasks.[20] Mice treated with repeated systemic administration of SKF81297 to induce kindled seizures display hyperactivation of the mTOR signaling pathway in the hippocampus, disrupted LTP in the dentate gyrus, and altered recognition memories.[21] Electrically induced convulsive seizures disrupt spatial learning and also reduce LTP processes in the hippocampus.[22] In humans, reductions in LTP are observed in epileptic focal regions located in the hippocampus.[23] The accumulated evidence suggests that seizures can impact neural substrates within critical cortical and subcortical structures to induce cognitive and memory disturbances. Acute and permanent presentation of altered cognitive abilities and memory loss can develop following seizures. However, given the contraindicated dosing and toxic exposure, it is likely that persistent deficits exhibited in both of these case reports are due to damaged neurological substrates induced by the contrast agent.

The brain's mesial temporal structures are critically involved in the epileptogenic network but are also recognized as key structures involved in memory function. The process by which specific aspects of an event are encoded and stored in the brain continues to be elucidated. These processes include memory formation, storage, retrieval, and modification. The internal representation of an object consists of a diffuse network of cortical neurons that are activated by external stimuli. The variety of learned information and subsequent memory may not all be processed and stored by the same neural hardware in the brain. Thus, there is no single region of the brain that can be identified as the location for these events. Neural plastic changes in the brain are marked at the cellular level as a putative locale for memory. Changes in neuroplasticity occur throughout the CNS, and, therefore, it is generally accepted that memory storage occurs diffusely within the brain and even the periphery, may be dependent on the type of memory, and may coincide with the experience associated with the information. Furthermore, the context in which a memory is initially stored may be modified over time.

Cognitive deficits, such as global amnesia, described as the "abrupt onset of disorientation due to loss of immediate and recent memory, retention of alertness and responsiveness, and ability to perform fairly complicated menta tasks," have been described in patients treated with iodinated contrast agents.[17,24] Reports of amnesia associated with contrast agents dates back to the 1950s.[25] These effects can be permanent or transient and typically appear in the onset within hours of contrast agent injection. The US FDA MedWatch reporting database (conducted in September 2016) lists 98 reports of memory dysfunction including amnesia, global amnesia, and memory impairment associated with the use of nonionic radiographic contrast agents. Damage to the brain's mesial temporal lobe structures is a recognized substrate for permanent amnesia.[26] Adults with a diagnosis of temporal lobe epilepsy display deficits in memory function.[27] Indeed, episodic memory dysfunction is considered a significant feature of temporal lobe epilepsy. During temporal lobe seizures, abnormal neural excitation in the hippocampus indirectly reduces the excitation of neocortical structures. Of note, the lowest seizure thresholds within the brain are located in the hippocampus underscoring the relevance of this brain structure in seizure and memory dysfunction. Abnormalities in hippocampal function have long been studied and documented for their relevance in memory. Experimentally, permanent global amnesia is reported following bilateral lesions to the hippocampus.[28] More specifically, CA1 neurons located within the hippocampus are critical for the retrieval of both short and long-term memory.[29] Contrast agents induce excitatory changes in neurons and dose-dependent obliteration of recorded electrical activity in rat hippocampal slices.[17]

Additional cognitive effects include various forms of mental symptoms like difficulty planning, deficits in organizational skills, reduced motivational drives, and depression. One study subjected patients to psychometric testing following myelogram procedures with contrast agents metrizamide and iopamidol. Mild mental deficits were observed following metrizamide administration. The severity of cognitive impairment was dependent on the quantity of contrast medium diffusion delivered into the intracranial space, suggesting dose-related neurotoxicity.[30] Contrast-related effects targeted to the frontal lobe may be responsible for cognitive impairments. The frontal lobes are critical for executive functioning, also known as cognitive control. Altogether, altered patterns of hippocampal–neocortical interactions are suggested to underlie memory and other cognitive deficits. Thus, neurotoxicity in the frontal and temporal lobe structures (e.g., the hippocampus) following contrast agent injection likely contributes to altered cognition and memory function.

Alternately, it has been proposed that amnesia and cognitive deficits following injection of contrast agents may be related to subsequent ischemia in bilateral limbic structures. Cerebral ischemia, or loss of blood flow and oxygenation in the brain, can lead to significant cell damage and death. There is preclinical evidence that cerebral ischemia disturbs object recognition in rats, a process commonly associated with medial temporal brain structures (i.e., hippocampus).[31] Hippocampal neurons are at higher risk for degeneration following ischemia; however, neuronal degeneration is also observed in the entorhinal cortex and perirhinal cortex, medial dorsal thalamic nucleus, and cingulate cortex.[32] Ischemia-induced damage to neural structures may contribute to the symptoms exhibited by both patients following contrast agent overdose.

21.3.3 Contrast-Induced Visual and Auditory Impairment: Further Evidence for Cerebral Insult to Cortical Brain Structures

Cortical blindness refers to visual impairment or total visual loss caused by bilateral destruction of the visual cortex (occipital cortex). Cortical blindness is a rare but well-documented complication of contrast agent administration and can be transient or permanent. The US FDA MedWatch database (conducted in September 2016) reports a minimum of 66 adverse events associated with ocular disturbances including reductions in visual acuity and blindness following the injection of contrast agents. Spina et al. report that transient cortical blindness is the most commonly reported neurological syndrome in patients who experience CIE, occurring in approximately 50% of cases.[5] Significant changes to vision following contrast agent overdose probably reflect damage to brain structures involved in ocular processes.

Cortical blindness is suggested to occur from the osmotic disruption of the BBB in the visual cortex subsequent to the injection of contrast product.[33] Toxicity localized to the occipital lobes accounts for deficits in vision. Additional symptoms that may accompany cortical blindness include dysphasia, headache, seizure, and memory loss.[34] The most compelling evidence for contrast-induced insult to the visual cortex is imaging work conducted within close temporal ranges to symptom manifestation using both CT and MRI. MRI imaging shows high signal intensities in occipital lobes 12 hours following contrast agent injection in a cerebral angiography procedure in a patient who developed subsequent cortical blindness. A repeat MRI conducted three days later did not illustrate these abnormalities, and cortical blindness was resolved. The authors concluded that cortical blindness was a direct complication of the contrast agent.[35] These reports are consistent with a review published on four cases of cortical blindness induced by contrast products following cerebral angiography. CT imaging was conducted in all four patients within one hour of contrast injection, and all patients demonstrated abnormal contrast enhancement in the occipital lobes of the brain. In addition, MRI imaging was conducted on two of the patients and revealed abnormal high signal intensity in the occipital lobes.[36]

Visual impairment may also occur with occipital seizures as an ictal or post-ictal phenomenon. Hadjikoutis and colleagues describe a patient who presented with headache, vomiting, and bilateral visual loss. Persistent spike discharge was observed in the occipital lobes by EEG, suggesting occipital seizures.[37] It is also known that iodine itself is a retinotoxic compound. High doses of iodate administered intravenously are toxic to the retina. Ocular toxicity is reported after exposure to doses ranging between 600 and 1,200 mg.[38] It is possible that leakage of contrast agent to the retina could directly impair vision.[39]

Cortical deafness is also a rare complication that has been associated with contrast agents. It refers to sensorineural hearing loss (partial or complete) caused by damage to the primary auditory cortex. Cortical deafness is rare, and published reports are limited to case studies linking the symptom to the injection of contrast agents. For example, severe bilateral sensorineural hearing loss following injection of iopamidol was observed following angiography. The patient did not respond to the nurse during the procedure, and an auditory brainstem response test revealed no response in either ear even after click intensity was raised to 105 dB.[40] Similarly, another report describes sensorineural deafness in a patient following aortic angiography with iopamidol.[41] Experimentally, induced sensorineural hearing loss in gerbils demonstrates altered neuronal membrane potential, increased input resistance, higher instances of sustained neuronal firing, and elevated thalamocortical and intracortical evoked excitatory synaptic responses.[42] It is possible that exposure to high levels of contrast medium in the auditory cortex, located within the superior temporal gyrus of the temporal lobe, could damage neural tissue in this region, thus leading to deficits in hearing.

21.4 SUMMARY AND CONCLUSIONS

The patient case reports and relevant literature detail the serious acute and residual toxicity following an overdose of contrast agents used for myelogram procedures. The damage to neurological functions (e.g., cognition, memory, motor, vision, and hearing) likely originates from contrast-induced damage to brain structures involved in these processes, that is, mesial temporal, occipital, and temporal cortical structures. It is established that contrast agents are chemotoxic due to their intrinsic chemical nature and significant hyperosmolarity. Given the chemotoxicity of the contrast agents, contraindicated route of administration, excessive dose, and penetration of the agent into the CNS during these procedures, it is highly probable that the adverse reactions experienced by the patients in the case reports are contrast-induced chemotoxic reactions. Both patients were essentially neurologically intact before the contrast agent overdose. While commonly employed in imaging procedures, extreme caution should be taken to avoid medication errors with contrast agents to avoid toxicity.

REFERENCES

1. Pomerantz SR. Myelography: Modern technique and indications. *Handb Clin Neurol.* 2016;135:193–208. doi:10.1016/b978-0-444-53485-9.00010-6
2. Price DB, Ortiz AO. Myelography: From lipid-based to gadolinium-based contrast agents. *Magn Reson Imaging Clin N Am.* 2017 Nov;25(4):713–24. doi:10.1016/j.mric.2017.06.005
3. Ozdoba C, Gralla J, Rieke A, Binggeli R, Schroth G. Myelography in the age of MRI: Why we do it, and how we do it. *Radiol Res Pract.* 2011;2011:329017. doi:10.1155/2011/329017
4. Kariyanna PT, Aurora L, Jayarangaiah A, et al. Neurotoxicity associated with radiological contrast agents used during coronary angiography: A systematic review. *Am J Med Case Rep.* 2020;8(2):60–6. doi:10.12691/ajmcr-8-2-6
5. Spina R, Simon N, Markus R, Muller DW, Kathir K. Contrast-induced encephalopathy following cardiac catheterization. *Catheter Cardiovasc Interv.* 2017 Aug 1;90(2):257–68. doi:10.1002/ccd.26871
6. Uchiyama Y, Abe T, Hirohata M, et al. Blood brain-barrier disruption of nonionic iodinated contrast medium following coil embolization of a ruptured intracerebral aneurysm. *AJNR Am J Neuroradiol.* 2004 Nov–Dec;25(10):1783–6.
7. Junck L, Marshall WH. Fatal brain edema after contrast-agent overdose. *AJNR Am J Neuroradiol.* 1986 May–Jun; 7(3):522–5.

8. Studdard WE, Davis DO, Young SW. Cortical blindness after cerebral angiography: Case report. *J Neurosurg*. 1981 Feb;54(2):240–4. doi:10.3171/jns.1981.54.2.0240
9. Medication errors resulting in CNS damage from contrast agent overdose. *Rxisk*, 2020. https://rxisk.org/medication-errors-resulting-in-cns-damage-from-contrast-agent-overdose/
10. Rapoport SI, Hori M, Klatzo I. Reversible osmotic opening of the blood-brain barrier. *Science*. 1971 Sept 10;173(4001):1026–8. doi:10.1126/science.173.4001.1026
11. Pokersnik JA, Liu L, Simon EL. Contrast-induced encephalopathy presenting as acute subarachnoid hemorrhage. *Am J Emerg Med*. 2018 Jun;36(6):1122.e3–2.e4. doi:10.1016/j.ajem.2018.03.005
12. Taydas O, Ogul H, Ozcan H, Kantarci M. Gadolinium-based contrast agent extravasation mimicking subarachnoid hemorrhage after electroconvulsive therapy. *World Neurosurg*. 2018 Jun;114:130–3. doi:10.1016/j.wneu.2018.03.063
13. Huda SA, Ahmed M, Sampat PJ, Ibeche B, Sharma B. Contrast extravasation mimicking subarachnoid hemorrhage after cardiac catheterization. *Cureus*. 2020 Jul 15;12(7):e9212. doi:10.7759/cureus.9212
14. Leong S, Fanning NF. Persistent neurological deficit from iodinated contrast encephalopathy following intracranial aneurysm coiling. A case report and review of the literature. *Interv Neuroradiol*. 2012 Mar;18(1):33–41. doi:10.1177/159101991201800105
15. Numaguchi Y, Fleming MS, Hasuo K, Puyau FA, Nice CM Jr. Blood-brain barrier disruption due to cerebral arteriography: CT findings. *J Comput Assist Tomogr*. 1984 Oct;8(5):936–9. doi:10.1097/00004728-198410000-00024
16. Rapoport SI, Thompson HK, Bidinger JM. Equi-osmolal opening of the blood-brain barrier in the rabbit by different contrast media. *Acta Radiol Diagn (Stockh)*. 1974 Jan;15(1):21–32. doi:10.1177/028418517401500103
17. Giang DW, Kido DK. Transient global amnesia associated with cerebral angiography performed with use of iopamidol. *Radiology*. 1989 Jul;172(1):195–6. doi:10.1148/radiology.172.1.2633769
18. Caillé JM, Gioux M, Arné P, Paty J. Neurotoxicity of nonionic iodinated water-soluble contrast media in myelography: Experimental study. *AJNR Am J Neuroradiol*. 1983 Nov–Dec;4(6):1185–9.
19. Englot DJ, Blumenfeld H. Consciousness and epilepsy: Why are complex-partial seizures complex? *Prog Brain Res*. 2009;177:147–70. doi:10.1016/s0079-6123(09)17711-7
20. Zhou JL, Shatskikh TN, Liu X, Holmes GL. Impaired single cell firing and long-term potentiation parallels memory impairment following recurrent seizures. *Eur J Neurosci*. 2007 Jun;25(12):3667–77. doi:10.1111/j.1460-9568.2007.05598.x
21. Gangarossa G, Ceolin L, Paucard A, et al. Repeated stimulation of dopamine D1-like receptor and hyperactivation of mTOR signaling lead to generalized seizures, altered dentate gyrus plasticity, and memory deficits. *Hippocampus*. 2014 Dec;24(12):1466–81. doi:10.1002/hipo.22327
22. Reid IC, Stewart CA. Seizures, memory and synaptic plasticity. *Seizure*. 1997 Oct;6(5):351–9. doi:10.1016/s1059-1311(97)80034-9
23. Beck H, Goussakov IV, Lie A, Helmstaedter C, Elger CE. Synaptic plasticity in the human dentate gyrus. *J Neurosci*. 2000 Sep 15;20(18):7080–6. doi:10.1523/jneurosci.20-18-07080.2000
24. Fisher CM, Adams RD. Transient global amnesia. *Acta Neurol Scand Suppl*. 1964;40(Suppl 9):1–83.
25. Hauge T. Catheter vertebral angiography. *Acta Radiol Suppl*. 1954;109:1–219.
26. Helmstaedter C, Elger CE. Chronic temporal lobe epilepsy: A neurodevelopmental or progressively dementing disease? *Brain*. 2009 Oct;132(Pt 10):2822–30. doi:10.1093/brain/awp182
27. Bell B, Lin JJ, Seidenberg M, Hermann B. The neurobiology of cognitive disorders in temporal lobe epilepsy. *Nat Rev Neurol*. 2011 Mar;7(3):154–64. doi:10.1038/nrneurol.2011.3
28. Arnetoli G, Caffarra P, Paganini M, Zappoli F, Nencioni L, Parma M. Amnesia permanente da lesione bilaterale dell'ippocampo: Descrizione di un caso clinico. [Permanent amnesia as a result of a bilateral lesion of the hippocampus: Description of a clinical case]. *Riv Patol Nerv Ment*. 1983 Jul–Aug;104(4):151–7.
29. Izquierdo LA, Barros DM, Ardenghi PG, et al. Different hippocampal molecular requirements for short- and long-term retrieval of one-trial avoidance learning. *Behav Brain Res*. 15 Jun 2000;111(1–2):93–8. doi:10.1016/s0166-4328(00)00137-6
30. Galle G, Huk W, Arnold K. Psychopathometric demonstration and quantification of mental disturbances following myelography with metrizamide and iopamidol. *Neuroradiology*. 1984;26(3):229–33. doi:10.1007/bf00342419
31. Wood ER, Mumby DG, Pinel JP, Phillips AG. Impaired object recognition memory in rats following ischemia-induced damage to the hippocampus. *Behav Neurosci*. 1993 Feb;107(1):51–62. doi:10.1037//0735-7044.107.1.51
32. Bachevalier J, Meunier M. Cerebral ischemia: Are the memory deficits associated with hippocampal cell loss? *Hippocampus*. 1996;6(5):553–60. doi:10.1002/(sici)1098-1063(1996)6:5<553::Aid-hipo8>3.0.Co;2-j
33. Mentzel HJ, Neumann T, Fitzek C, Sauner D, Reichenbach JR, Kaiser WA. MR imaging in wegener granulomatosis of the spinal cord. *AJNR Am J Neuroradiol*. 2003 Jan;24(1):18–21.
34. Boyes LA, Tew K. Cortical blindness after subclavian arteriography. *Australas Radiol*. 2000 Aug;44(3):315–7. doi:10.1046/j.1440-1673.2000.00819.x
35. Suri V, Agarwal R, Jadhao N, Ahuja GK. Cortical blindness after contrast-enhanced CT scan in a patient of sarcoidosis: Is it related to posterior reversible encephalopathy syndrome? *Ann Indian Acad Neurol*. 2011 Oct;14(4):298–300. doi:10.4103/0972-2327.91956
36. Lantos G. Cortical blindness due to osmotic disruption of the blood-brain barrier by angiographic contrast material: CT and MRI studies. *Neurology*. 1989 Apr;39(4):567–71. doi:10.1212/wnl.39.4.567
37. Hadjikoutis S, Sawhney IM. Occipital seizures presenting with bilateral visual loss. *Neurol India*. 2003 Mar;51(1):115–6.
38. Bürgi H, Schaffner TH, Seiler JP. The toxicology of iodate: A review of the literature. *Thyroid*. 2001 May;11(5):449–56. doi:10.1089/105072501300176408
39. Lee AG, Hayman LA, Ross AW. Neuroimaging contrast agents in ophthalmology. *Surv Ophthalmol*. 2000 Nov–Dec;45(3):237–53. doi:10.1016/s0039-6257(00)00152-1

40. Matsuoka A, Shitara T, Okamoto M, Sano H. Transient deafness with iopamidol following angiography. *Acta Otolaryngol Suppl.* 1994;514:78–80. doi:10.3109/00016489409127566
41. Karim MR, Balsam L, Rubinstein S. Permanent hearing loss with iopamidol following aortic angiography in a hemodialysis patient: A case report and review of the literature. *Am J Kidney Dis.* 2010 Apr;55(4):712–6. doi:10.1053/j.ajkd.2009.08.016
42. Kotak VC, Fujisawa S, Lee FA, Karthikeyan O, Aoki C, Sanes DH. Hearing loss raises excitability in the auditory cortex. *J Neurosci.* 2005 Apr 13;25(15):3908–18. doi:10.1523/jneurosci.5169-04.2005

22 Fetal Drug Exposure

Damani Parran, James T. O'Donnell, and James J. O'Donnell III

SYNOPSIS

DOI: 10.1201/9781003615323-24

22.1 INTRODUCTION

The term "developmental toxicology" covers any detrimental effect produced by exposure to agents or conditions during embryonic and fetal stages that lead to abnormal development. Such lesions can be either irreversible or reversible including structural malformations, growth retardation, functional impairment and death of the organism.[1] Conditions that result in the death of the conceptus (embryo-lethal) result in resorption, spontaneous abortion or stillbirth. In the situation where the offspring survives, irreversible lesions may result in structural or functional abnormalities and are referred to as *teratogenic*. Persistent lesions that cause overall growth retardation or delayed growth of specific organ systems are generally referred to as *embryotoxic*. For an agent to be labeled a teratogen, it must significantly increase the occurrence of structural or functional abnormalities in offspring after it is administered to either the parent before conception, to the female during pregnancy or directly to the developing organism.

Birth defects have been depicted throughout time. As far back as 6500 B.C., a sculpture from the southern regions of Turkey depicts conjoined twins.[2] In around 3000 B.C., Egyptian wall paintings depicting cleft palate and achondroplasia were documented. By 300 B.C., early theories that maternal stress can lead to deleterious effects on the developing organism started to emerge.[3] This theory was expanded in 1649 by Ambrois Pare who stated that narrowness of the uterus, the faulty posture of the pregnant woman and physical trauma could lead to birth defects. Around this time, the early age of biological science emerged giving rise to scientifically based theories on the causes of birth defects including the theory of developmental arrest.[4] This theory states that malformations result from incomplete development of an organ or structure. The theory of developmental arrest was solidified in the early 20th century with several experiments showing that by chemical and physical manipulation of the growth medium, developmental malformation of minnow embryos was produced.[5] In addition, the nature of the malformation depended on the developmental stage and was explained that all non-hereditary malformations stem from developmental arrest. From the early 19th century through the middle of the 20th century, a variety of environmental conditions (temperature, microbial toxins, drugs) and physical trauma (jarring, inversion, pricking) were found to perturb development in several animal species, including avian, reptile, fish and amphibians.[4] The first documentation of birth defects in mammals as a result of nutritional stress was published in 1935.[6] As a result of maternal nutritional deficiency of vitamin A, swine offspring showed such malformations as anophthalmia and cleft palates. Numerous studies by Warkany and coworkers demonstrated that in addition to maternal dietary deficiencies chemical and physical agents such as nitrogen mustard, trypan blue, hormones, alkylating agents and x-rays were clearly shown to cause malformations in mammals.[7]

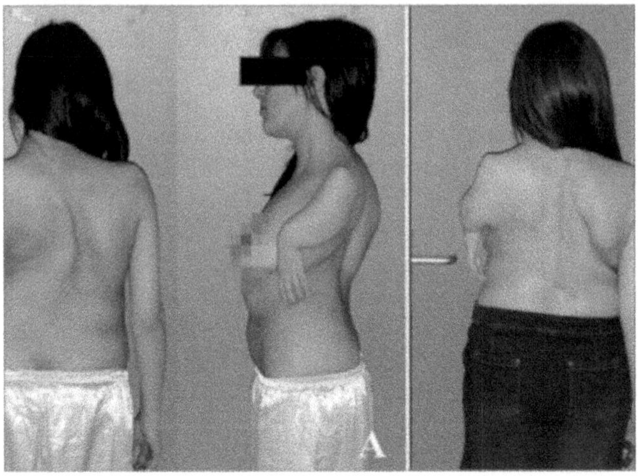

FIGURE 22.1 Phocomelia Patient.

The first truly documented human malformation epidemic occurred in the early 1940s, where a link between rubella viral infection and elevated incidences of eye, heart and ear malformations along with mental retardation was established.[8] Infection with the rubella virus in the first two months of pregnancy was associated with malformations in the heart and eye. By the third month, if infection occurs, elevated occurrences of hearing and speech defects and mental retardation were observed. In 1960 and 1961, a sharp increase in newborns born with exceedingly rare limb malformations was evident. The affected newborns had amelia (absence of the limbs) or various degrees of phocomelia (reduction of the long bones of the limbs); this usually affected the arms more than the legs and usually involved both the left and right sides, although to differing degrees. The unusual nature of the malformations was a key to unraveling the epidemic and in 1961, two separate research groups identified the sedative thalidomide as the causative agent.[9]

By this time, Wilson[10] (1959) proposed the basic principles of abnormal development, which have stood the test of time and remain an excellent guideline. Wilson stated that:

- Susceptibility to abnormal development depends on the genotype of the conceptus and the manner in which its genetic composition interacts with the environment.
- Agents that cause abnormal development vary with the developmental stage at the time of exposure.
- Teratogenic agents act in specific ways (mechanism) on developing cells and tissues to initiate abnormal embryogenesis (pathogenesis).
- The final manifestations of abnormal development are death, malformation, growth retardation and functional disorders.
- The access of adverse environmental influences to developing tissues depends on the nature of the influences (agents).
- Manifestations of deviant development increase in degree as dosage increases, from no effect to a totally lethal effect.

Many studies have validated these principles, with malformations as gross structural deficits being the main focus.[11] It has been demonstrated that any agent administered under appropriate dosing conditions and during specific developmental timepoints will lead to lesions in embryonic development.

22.2 CRITICAL PERIODS OF HUMAN DEVELOPMENT AND SUSCEPTIBILITY

As Wilson mentioned in his basic principles of abnormal development, the effect of an agent varies greatly depending on the developmental time of exposure.[10] Periods of human development during pregnancy are measured in trimesters, each being about three months. The most sensitive period for teratogenesis, the production of congenital defects, is during organogenesis (first trimester) in the embryonic stage.[12] Later during the fetal stage, the environment provided by the mother affects the baby's size, behavior, intelligence and health, rather than the formation of organs and limbs.[13] The timing of some key developmental events in human development is presented in Table 22.1. It should be made clear, however, that development is a continuum and that these stages are used for descriptive purposes and do not necessarily represent discrete developmental events.

Now, we will discuss each stage of human development in more detail and the possible outcomes following toxicological insults.

Following fertilization, the zygote undergoes cleavage, a series of mitotic divisions without accompanying cell growth and cavitation of the embryo to form fluid-filled blastocoels. While traversing the oviduct toward the uterus, the conceptus is surrounded by the zona pellucid, an acellular, polysaccharide-containing coating that prevents premature implantation.

TABLE 22.1
Timing of Key Developmental Events in Humans

Developmental Event	Developmental Age (Days of Gestation)
Blastocyst formation	4–6
Implantation	6–7
Primitive streak	16–18
Neural plate	18–20
First somite	20–21
First pharyngeal arch	20
Organogenesis	21–56
Ten somites	25–26
Upper limb buds	29–30
Lower limb buds	31–32
Forepaw rays	35
Testes differentiation	43
Heart septation	46–47
Palate closure	56–58
Length of gestation	267

Exposure to toxicants immediately after fertilization has been demonstrated to result in malformed fetuses for a number of agents, including ethylene oxide, ethyl methanesulfonate, ethylnitrosourea and triethylene melamine.[14]

The conceptus enters the uterus at gestational days 3–4, when it has developed into a solid cluster of 16 cells called a marula. The marula becomes a blastocyst by growing up to over 100 cells and developing a fluid-filled cavity between gestational days 4 and 5. The blastocyte contains two major types of cells, the inner cell mass and the trophoblast. The inner cell mass develops into the embryo, while the trophoblast makes up the outer layer of cells which develops into the chorion and the placenta. The fates of the cells in the early embryo stage are not completely determined at this stage. The relatively undifferentiated preimplantation embryo has great restorative growth potential.[15] This was exemplified by an experiment where eight-cell rabbit embryos were capable of producing normal offspring.[16] By gestational day 5, the blastocyte leaves the zona pellucid and can now directly interact with the endometrium. This begins the implantation stage of development.

Toxicity during preimplantation is largely thought to result in no effect or a slight effect on growth due to regulative growth. Death of the pre-implanted embryo is another result if it is overwhelmed by damage or failure to implant. Agents including DDT, nicotine and ethyl methanesulfonate can cause defects in body and brain weights and embryo death in the absence of malformations.[17]

Other agents including methylnitrosourea,[18] cyproterone acetate and medroxyprogesterone acetate,[19] can induce fetal malformations when administered at specific gestational timepoints. Specifically, malformations include neural tube defects and cleft palate. It is expected that agents that target DNA synthesis or microtubule assembly will be particularly toxic due to the rapid mitoses that occur during the preimplantation period.

Implantation occurs between six and seven days after fertilization in humans. At this point, the embryo undergoes gastrulation, where the three primary germ layers start to form: the ectoderm, mesoderm and endoderm. The ectoderm becomes the central nervous system. The mesoderm becomes the muscles, skeleton, circulatory system and internal organs. The endoderm becomes the digestive system, lungs, urinary tract and glands. The outer membrane of the blastocyte becomes the amnion, which encloses the developing zygote in the amniotic fluid. The foundation for the human uteroplacental circulation system starts to develop at gestation day 9, when vacuoles called trophoblastic lacunae emerge with the syncytiotrophoblast and maternal capillaries expand to form maternal sinusoids that anastomose with the trophoblastic lacunae.[20] Anastomosis is the connection between the blood vessels or between other tubular structures.[21,22] By gestational day 16, the extraembryonic mesoderm proliferates and invades the centers of the primary stem villi, forming secondary stem villi. By gestational day 21, the mesodermal tissue differentiates into connective tissue and blood vessels, forming the tertiary stem villi. Therefore, materials diffusing between maternal and fetal tissues must pass from the maternal blood in the lacunae, through the trophoblast layer, the connective tissue in the core of the villus and the endothelium of the embryonic villus capillaries.[20] It is well-known that toxic agents given during gastrulation can produce malformations in the eye, brain and face. This is indicative of damage to the anterior neural plate.

The formation of the neural plate in the ectoderm marks the onset of organogenesis, where most of the body structures and organs are established. Individual organ systems possess highly specific periods of susceptibility to teratogenic damage during organogenesis. Table 22.2 depicts the sensitive periods of the major human embryonic body systems and structures. At gestational day 21, the human conceptus is in most ways indistinguishable from other vertebrate embryos. By gestational day 56, the conceptus, which can now be termed a fetus, has a form clearly recognizable as human. The rapid changes in organogenesis require cell proliferation, cell migration, cell–cell interactions and morphogenetic tissue remodeling. These processes are exemplified by the neural crest cells, which originate at the border of the neural plate and migrate to form a wide variety of embryonic structures. Within organogenesis, there are periods of maximum susceptibility for each organ system and structure. Several animal studies demonstrated that malformations observed following carefully timed developmental exposures coincide with the timing of key developmental events in these structures.[21–23]

TABLE 22.2
Sensitive Periods of Body Systems During Human Embryonic Development

Body System	Especially Sensitive (weeks)	Development up to . . . (weeks)
Central Nervous System/brain	4th to 8th	Postnatal, through to adulthood
Heart	5th to 9th	12th
Upper limbs	6th to 10th	12th
Eyes	6th to 10th	Term
Lower limbs	6th to 10th	12th
Teeth	9th to 11th	Term
Palate	9th to 11th	16th
External genitalia	9th to 11th	Term
Ears	6th to 11th	13th

The end of organogenesis marks the beginning of the fetal period (gestation days 56–58), which is characterized by palate closure, tissue differentiation, growth and physiological maturation. This does not mean that the development of the organs is complete. However, most of the organs are present and grossly recognizable. Further maturation of organs occurs, including fine structural morphogenesis and biochemical maturation.

Insult at this relatively late stage of development leads to a broad spectrum of effects that generally manifest as growth retardation or as functional disorders and transplacental carcinogenesis. The fetus is more resistant to lethal effects than the embryo, but the incidence of stillbirth is still measurable. The functional manifestations are not immediately apparent prenatally and require very precise postnatal observation, testing and biomonitoring.[24] Such postnatal functional manifestations can be sensitive indicators of in utero toxicity. Recent reviews of the postnatal effects of the immune system,[25] the respiratory system,[26] the reproductive system,[27] the central nervous system[28,29] and heart and endocrine glands[30] are available. Major structural alterations can occur during the fetal period, but these changes generally result from deformations, which are disruptions of previously normal structures versus malformations. Development does not stop at birth and special susceptibilities exist in the neonatal, childhood and adolescent years.[31]

22.3 SPECIAL CONSIDERATIONS OF DRUG EXPOSURE DURING PREGNANCY

A pregnant mother's exposure to toxic agents and external insults represents a unique scenario both in managing a potential poisoning of the mother and direct/indirect effects on the developing embryo/fetus. The maternal, placental and embryonic compartments constitute independent yet interacting systems that undergo profound changes throughout the course of pregnancy. As a normal pregnancy progresses, specific hemodynamic and cardiovascular changes occur in the mother. The following general physiological changes are observed during normal pregnancy:[32]

A. Cardiac output can increase as much as 40% above normal nonpregnant levels during the first trimester and thus can be considered a natural state of volume overload. In a third trimester pregnant female, approximately 10% of cardiac output goes to the uteroplacental unit. Normally, uterine blood flow is directly related to maternal cardiac output. As pregnancy progresses, other adjustments occur that are necessary for fetal development. Cardiac output is increased largely because of an increase in stroke volume, with a normal or slightly increased heart rate. The altered hemodynamic status of the pregnant woman is often not recognized because of the large cardiovascular reserve found in the normal healthy system.
B. Increased tidal volume, resulting in a resting pCO_2 lower than normal.
C. Increased potential for regurgitation and aspiration, due to pressure on hollow abdominal viscera.
D. Inability to concentrate urine.
E. Decreased serum albumin.
F. Relative anemia.
G. Changes in absorption due to decreased gut motility, changes in hepatic metabolism or changes in excretion due to increased glomerular filtration rate.

Some of the physiological changes that occur in the mother during the course of pregnancy are summarized in Table 22.3.

For practical purposes, the fetus is exposed to most chemicals to which the mother is exposed, and the greater the dosage to the mother, the greater will be the exposure for the fetus. Although the placenta is a barrier for many purposes, it should not be considered a toxicological barrier with respect to many common drugs in use. The lipid membranes of the placenta are relatively permeable to substances having a molecular weight of less than 1,000 Daltons, although several large molecules have been identified as reaching the fetus. The passage of substances across the placenta increases with increased placental blood flow. A role for metabolism by the placenta has not been identified. However, due to differences in fetal circulation and metabolism at different stages of development, toxic exposure in a fetus may exhibit different levels of that agent during the exposure, equilibration and elimination phases of its kinetics.

Factors such as (but not limited to) variations in pH gradients between maternal and conceptual compartments, differences in maternal and conceptual fluid protein binding of chemicals and active transporters in the placenta may play important roles in regulating embryonic drug exposure.[33] The pH gradients between maternal blood and the embryonic fluid/cells influence the disposition of basic and acidic compounds from maternal blood to the embryo. This difference in pH may lead to the accumulation of some acidic or basic compounds in embryos due to ion trapping.[34,35] Ion trapping involves the net movement of protonated weak acids into a compartment with a relatively higher pH. Weak acids become ionized and can no longer diffuse back across the compartment membrane. This has been documented in

TABLE 22.3
Physiological Changes During Pregnancy

		Pregnant		
	Nonpregnant	First Trimester	Second Trimester	Third Trimester
Cardiac output (l/min)	4–6	Increasing	6–7	6–7
Heart rate (beats/min)	60–80	Increasing	Increasing	80–95
Systolic BP (mm Hg)	90–120	Decreasing 0–15	Decreasing 0–15	Normal
Diastolic BP (mm Hg)	60–90	Decreasing 10–20	Decreasing 10–20	Normal
HCT (%)	37–47	38	34–39	34–39
Peripheral WBC (m3)	4.7–10.6	5–12	12–18	12–18
Polymorphonuclears	55	66	69	60
Sed. rate (mm/hr)	20	Increasing	Increasing	Increasing
Fibrinogen (mg/dl)	200–400	200–286	286–315	353–410
BUN (mg/dl)	10–16	7–10	7–10	7–10
Creatinine (mg/dl)	0.5–1.5	0.4–0.8	0.4–0.8	0.4–0.8
Systemic vascular resistance (dynes/cm³)	1,743	979	1,277	1,224
Blood volume (ml)	2,600	3,150	3,850	3,950

a number of animal studies, with compounds including valproic acid, methoxyacetic acid, butyric acid, propionic acid and glycolic acid.[33,36] In these studies, embryonic and/or exocoelomic fluid concentrations of the agents were two to four times higher than those of maternal blood. In humans, the pH of the coelomic fluid is 0.2 pH units lower than that of maternal blood, while amniotic fluid pH is similar to maternal pH until 10 weeks of gestation, but then decreases between gestation weeks 11–14.[37] If embryonic dosimetry were based solely on these pH gradients, one would expect weak bases to accumulate in early human embryos. However, many other factors that influence embryo dosimetry are in play and may be more influential than ion trapping.

Another factor is protein binding. Extensive protein binding in the maternal circulation would decrease the amount of unbound, free chemicals from crossing the placenta and thus decrease embryonic exposure. In general, plasma protein binding occurs to a lesser extent in experimental animal models than in humans. The total protein concentration of maternal blood tends to decrease with advancing gestation. Factors that may influence the extent of protein binding include co-administration of other drugs, hormones, nutrition and stress.[34] In humans, the concentration of protein in coelomic fluid is reportedly 18-fold lower than in maternal blood.[37]

An additional means of crossing the placenta is through active transport by carrier systems for pyrimidine, amino acids and other nutrients. Active transport is the movement of material against the concentration gradient, and it requires energy. Since it is carrier-mediated, active transport is also governed by the laws of competitive inhibition. Besides essential materials, there are a number of drugs that are moved by active transport into cells including fluorouracil and alpha-methyldopa.[38] The presence or absence of a particular transporter could influence the bioavailability and perhaps the toxicity of particular chemicals to the embryo.

22.4 HISTORICAL HUMAN DEVELOPMENTAL TOXICANTS

It has been estimated that more than 3,300 agents have been tested for teratogenic potential.[39] Approximately 63% of these agents were not considered a teratogen, 7% were teratogenic in more than one species, 21% were teratogenic in most species tested and 9% produced equivocal experiment results. The following are several human developmental toxicants which provide both a historical view of the field of development toxicology and an illustration of Wilson's[40] key principles of teratology.

22.4.1 Thalidomide

Thalidomide was introduced in 1956 by Chemie Grunenthal as a sedative/hypnotic and was used throughout the world as a sleep aid. In addition, thalidomide was used to ameliorate nausea and vomiting during pregnancy. It had no apparent toxicity or addictive properties in humans or adult animals at therapeutic doses (50 to 200 mg/day). In 1960, a significant increase in newborns with extremely rare limb malformations started to emerge. The affected individuals had an absence of limbs (amelia) or various degrees of long bone reduction (phocomelia), which usually affected the arms more than the legs and involved both the left and right sides. Limb reduction anomalies of this nature are exceedingly rare. For example, there were no cases of phocomelia in Germany before 1959.[41] In 1959, there was one case and the following year, there were 30 cases. By 1961, there were 154 cases of phocomelia in Germany. In addition to the limb malformations, congenital heart disease, ocular, intestinal, external ear and renal anomalies were observed. The unusual nature of the malformations was a key to solving this epidemic. Two separate research teams determined that this sedative/sleep aid was the causative agent.[42–44] Once this association was established, thalidomide was removed from the market and case reports ended in mid-1962. Over 5,800 malformed infants were born worldwide.[45] As a result of this catastrophe, many countries began developing regulations requiring the evaluation of the effects of drugs on pregnancy outcomes.

Thalidomide continues to be a topic of discussion. Since July 16, 1998, thalidomide has been licensed for use in the United States in treating complications related to leprosy.[46] Also, since October 26, 2006, it has been authorized in cases of multiple myeloma.[47,48] Since August 4, 2010, Canada also authorized the use of thalidomide in the treatment of patients with multiple myeloma who are 65 years of age or older.[49] With the recent licensing of thalidomide, a recent scientific study indicates that thalidomide is still causing birth defects around the world. In Brazil, there have been claims that thalidomide was given to people suffering from leprosy to treat the symptoms, including women, who have taken this drug unaware of the risks they may cause during pregnancy.[50,51] In Brazil, thalidomide was re-licensed in 1965 as a treatment for skin lesions, a complication of leprosy. Researchers now say that over 100 Brazilian children have injuries exactly like those caused by thalidomide.

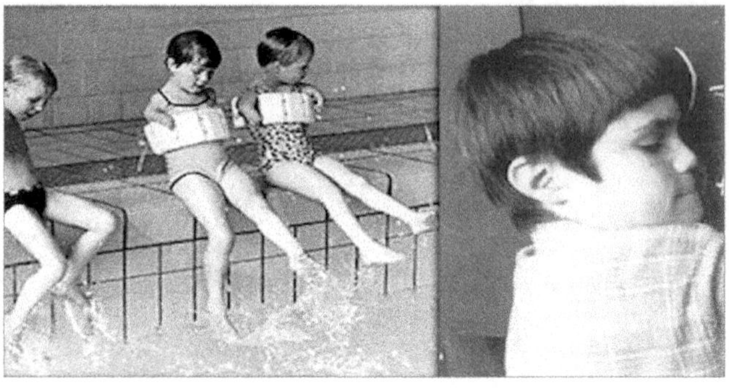

FIGURE 22.2 Thalidomide Birth Defect.

22.4.2 Ethanol

The developmental toxicity of ethanol has been recognized throughout time but it was not until the early 1970s when Jones and Smith[52] described fetal alcohol syndrome (FAS) that a clear pattern of its development effect was accepted. FAS refers to a distinct cluster of congenital abnormalities observed in the offspring of alcoholic mothers.[53] Prolonged exposure to ethanol during gestation and lactation is correlated with a pattern of abnormal development in newborns. The spectrum of alcohol's teratogenic effects spans a wide continuum that includes central nervous system dysfunction, optical abnormalities, craniofacial anomalies, growth deficiency and pathologic organ and skeletal conditions. The mechanisms by which ethanol exerts its teratogenic effects are not understood, but excess cell death in sensitive cell populations appears to be a common finding.[54]

Dittmer and Lentz-Kapua[54] describe the following neurodevelopment abnormalities associated with FAS: microcephaly, corpus callosum agenesis or hypoplasia, developmental delay, intellectual impairment (mild to moderate retardation), low intelligence quotient (IQ 65–70), hypotonia, poor coordination, cognitive impairment, irritability in infancy and hyperactivity in childhood or attention-deficit hyperactivity disorder (ADHD), language impairment, sleep/wake cycle disturbances, seizure disorder, delayed or deficient myelination, electroencephalogram hypersynchrony, echolalia and cerebral palsy.[55] Several aspects of the developmental program are involved in the alcohol-induced malformations of the brain.[56] Among them, the most striking abnormalities appear to involve the impairment of neuronal cell migration.[57,58] FAS patients show a wide spectrum of neuroanatomical abnormalities at different ages which include white matter lesions.[59–63] White matter abnormalities have been documented in the optic nerves, hippocampus, basal ganglia, corpus callosum, cerebellar vermis and temporal, parietal and occipital lobes. Lesions in the temporal, parietal and occipital white matter were described by Archibald et al. (2001),[61] where a decrease in white matter volume in these structures was observed in the brains of children with a history of prenatal alcohol exposure. A common abnormality was a leptomeningeal neurological neuroglial[64] heterotopias that assumes the form of a sheet of aberrant neuronal and glial cells covering portions of the cerebral, cerebellar and brainstem surfaces.[65] Aberrations of brainstem and cerebellar development have also been especially frequent along with the migrational disturbances of schizencephaly and polymicrogyria.[66] Disordered midline prosencephalic formation, for example, agenesis of the corpus callosum, septo-optic dysplasia and incomplete holoprosencephaly, has also been documented.[67] Thus it appears that multiple aspects of central nervous system development can be affected, including neurulation, canalization and retrogressive differentiation, prosencephalic development, neuronal proliferation, neuronal migration and neuronal differentiation and synapse formation.[68] Several animal studies have also demonstrated that even a single administration of a high level of alcohol during a period of pregnancy can cause serious effects on the migration of immature neurons.[68] Microcephaly is also present in nearly all cases and this manifestation of disturbed brain growth is accompanied by delayed neurologic development in approximately 90% of cases.[69]

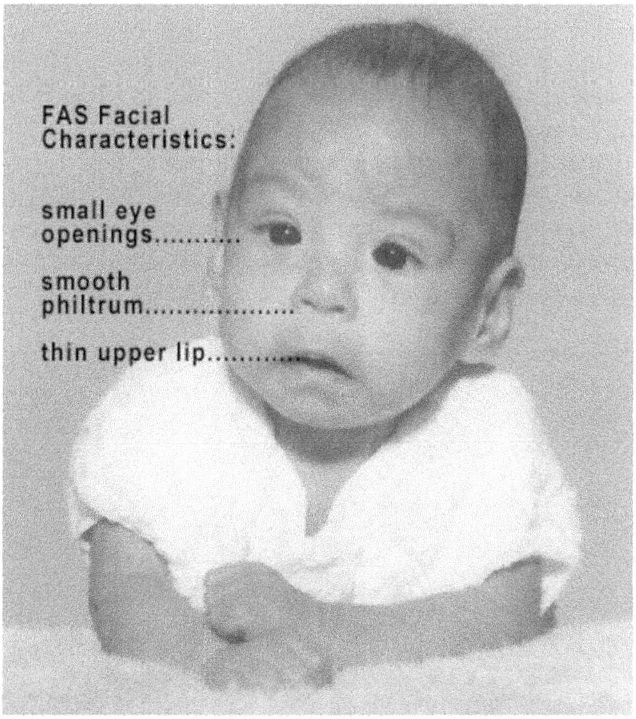

FIGURE 22.3 Fetal Alcohol Syndrome.

The eyes and vision have also been shown to be damaged by maternal alcohol misuse during pregnancy.[70–73] Up to 90% of the children whose mothers have misused alcohol in pregnancy may show ocular manifestations.[73] Several studies report that one of the greatest areas of white matter lesioning is in optic radiation. Clinically, many FAS patients show ocular and visual abnormalities, with up to 76% showing optic nerve hypoplasia.[73] All parts of the eye can be affected, from the periocular facial region to the intraocular structures and the optic nerve. Children with FAS may show a spectrum of eye abnormalities, ranging from extensive malformations, such as microphthalmus, buphthalmus (enlarged eye), coloboma of the iris and uvea (abnormal closure of choroidal embryonic eye fissure), persistent hyperplastic primary vitreous body or a severely malformed retina, to minor anomalies.[73,74] Microphthalmia has frequently been observed among children with FAS[73,74] and was included in the criteria for a diagnosis of FAS set by the Fetal Alcohol Study Group of the US Research Society on Alcoholism.[75] Retinal abnormalities in FAS are wide ranging and may include discrete lesions of the optic disc up to serious retinal malformations. The most frequent abnormalities are optic nerve hypoplasia and increased tortuosity of the retinal vessels.[73,74,76] Hypoplasia of the optic nerve head is characterized by subnormal vision and a subnormal number of optic nerve axons, showing morphological signs such as small size, pallor, irregular margins and an abnormal retinal vascular pattern of the optic disk. Optic nerve hypoplasia was found in a group of children with FAS and morphometrically assessed by retinal fundus photographs. The analysis showed that 48% of the optic discs were hypoplastic in these patients.[73]

22.4.3 Diethylstilbestrol

Diethylstilbestrol (DES) is a synthetic nonsteroidal estrogen that was first synthesized in 1938 and was made available in the 1940s through the 1970s in the United States as a drug to prevent miscarriages. DES gained notoriety in 1971 when several young women between the ages of 14 and 22 were diagnosed with clear cell adenocarcinoma of the vagina. This type of tumor had never been seen before in patients under the age of 30. Following an epidemiological study, an association between DES exposure during the first trimester and the development of clear cell adenocarcinoma was established.[77] Specifically, DES exposure before gestation day 126 appeared to increase the risk of developing this tumor by 40-fold. DES is considered an established human carcinogen and is the only transplacental carcinogen known in humans. In addition to clear cell adenocarcinoma, developmental DES exposure was linked to other abnormalities of the reproductive tract, including vaginal epithelial changes, increased cervical transformation zone and uterine abnormalities. Females born following in utero exposure to DES may also have a slightly increased risk of breast cancer after the age of 40. A 2006 study (Palmer et al.)[78] in the United States, suggested that overall breast cancer risk is not increased, but after the age of 40, the exposed female offspring had approximately twice the risk of breast cancer as unexposed women of the same age and with similar risk factors. However, a 2010 study from Europe found no difference in breast cancer risk between DES-exposed and unexposed women and no difference in overall cancer risk (Verloop J 2010).[79] A 2011 study found that about 2% of a large cohort of DES-exposed women had developed breast cancer due to their exposure (Hoover RN 2011).[80] In male offspring of exposed pregnancies, a high incidence of epididymal cysts, hypotrophic testes and capsular induration was observed.[81]

22.4.4 Retinoids

Retinoids are a class of chemical compounds that are related to vitamin A. When taken in excess, retinoids can induce widespread development effects, including malformations of the face, limbs, heart, central nervous system and skeleton. Retinol from the diet is transformed by the body's diet and stored in the liver as retinyl esters. Esters are acidic compounds condensed with alcohols. Retinyl esters are transformed through hydrolysis into retinol, which is transported into the bloodstream throughout the body. Retinol is converted to retinoic acid, its metabolite, through two enzymes: retinol dehydrogenases (ROLDH) and retinal dehydrogenases (RALDH). Enzyme ROLDH converts retinol to retinaldehyde whereas enzyme RALDH converts retinaldehyde into retinoic acid. In the cell nucleus, retinoic acid binds to activate two families of transcriptional factors. These include retinoic acid receptors and retinoid X receptors. Studies with mammalian models show that retinoids act directly on the embryo, causing the embryo to develop abnormally. Developing organs depend in part on the amount of active retinoid that accumulates over time during the different stages of organ development. All trans-retinoic acids and the 13-cis isomer produce congenital malformations in all mammalian species test, with varying ranges of sensitivity. The 13-cis retinoid acid is an active compound in the recalcitrant cystic acne drug Accutane.

Despite clear warnings against the use of Accutane during pregnancy on the label of this prescription drug, an extensive physician and patient education program and restrictive requirements for prescription to women of childbearing age; infants with malformations of the ears, heart, brain and thymus began to be reported.[82,83] It has also been shown that the risk of premature delivery doubles if the developing embryo is exposed to the 13-cis retinoic isomer during the first trimester.[83]

The Food and Drug Administration (FDA) placed strict risk management protocols upon retinoids (e.g., isotretinoin and etretinate) to prevent the manifestation of their teratogenic effects. Isotretinoin was the first retinoid approved for use in the United States to treat severe acne. The FDA classified isotretinoin as a Category X drug—the most severe category during pregnancy assigned by the FDA. Category X includes drugs where preclinical and clinical studies show fetal abnormalities and where the drug risks by pregnant women outweigh any potential benefits. In the United States, patients cannot take isotretinoin unless they are enrolled in *iPLEDGE*—a comprehensive risk management program designed to prevent fetal exposure to isotretinoin and to inform about the serious risks of taking the drug. Patients, doctors and pharmacists are all required by

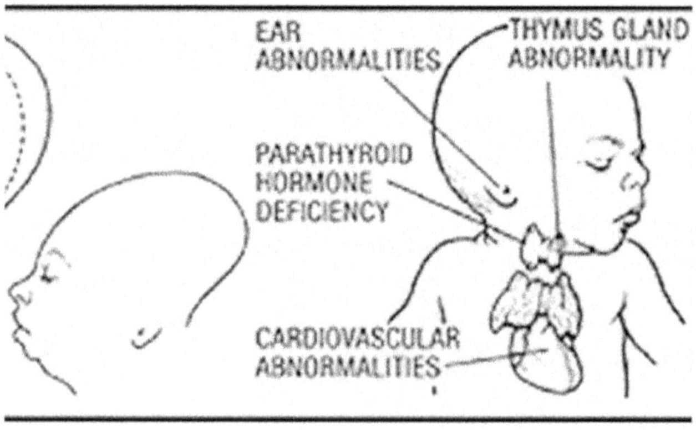

FIGURE 22.4 Accutane Birth Defect.

the FDA to register and use *iPLEDGE* to receive, prescribe or dispense isotretinoin. The program has been criticized because it has not reduced the exposure of pregnant people to the drug. Specifically, the program has been criticized for being overly complicated and difficult for users to navigate successfully. For example, if there is a problem with the data a patient or prescriber enters, the patient may be locked out of the system and thus unable to obtain the drug for that 30-day cycle. Additionally, if a patient who can become pregnant misses their seven-day prescription pickup timeframe, they must meet with their prescriber again for another pregnancy test before being able to receive the drug. This return visit to the doctor can be inconvenient and costly.

Another disparagement of the *iPLEDGE* program involves the registration requirements for transgender patients. There is the potential for transgender men taking testosterone treatments to develop acne as a side effect. This can be treated using isotretinoin. Since trans men have female reproductive organs, they have the potential to become pregnant whether they are on testosterone or not. Under the previous patient classification model, *iPLEDGE* required that transgender patients register based on their assigned at-birth gender. This meant that the *iPLEDGE* program required trans men be misgendered as female to receive isotretinoin in the United States. A proposed solution was for *iPLEDGE* to make their classifications of patients gender-neutral, instead focusing on the potential to become pregnant. The new approach was intended to make the *iPLEDGE* program more inclusive to transgender patients by reducing the three risk categories (1) females of reproductive potential, (2) females not of reproductive potential and (3) males to just two: (a) those capable of getting pregnant and (b) those not capable.

Acitretin (trade names Soriatane and Neotigason) is a second-generation retinoid. Acitretin is an oral agent that is commonly used for the treatment of severe resistant psoriasis. It is usually reserved for treatment-resistant severe psoriasis cases due to the potential for significant side effects. Acitretin is highly teratogenic and associated with severe birth defects. Acitretin must not be used by pregnant females or those who intend to become pregnant during therapy or at any time for the following three years of drug discontinuation. This drug requires females to use reliable contraception while undergoing treatment and for the three years following drug discontinuation. Acitretin is a metabolite of the compound etretinate (trade name: Tegison). Both drugs are linked to major human fetal abnormalities. Clinically, ingestion of acitretin and ethanol combined may cause the formation of etretinate, which has a significantly longer elimination half-life than acitretin. The longer elimination half-life of etretinate increases the duration of teratogenic potential. Therefore, ethanol must not be ingested by female patients during treatment with Soriatane or for two months after drug discontinuation. This delay accounts for the full elimination of acitretin, thus removing the substrate for transesterification to etretinate. The precise mechanisms for the conversion of acitretin to etretinate are not fully elucidated. Preclinical evidence shows that acitretin induces embryotoxic and/or teratogenic effects in rabbits, mice and rats. Doses tested in animals are up to three times the maximum recommended therapeutic dose in humans. Major human fetal abnormalities associated with acitretin and/or etretinate treatment include decreased cranial volume, cardiovascular malformation, meningomyelocele, meningoencephalocele, multiple synostoses, facial dysmorphia, malformations of hip, ankle and forearm, syndactyly, absence of terminal phalanges, low-set ears, high palate and alterations of the skull and cervical vertebrae.

Etretinate was approved by the FDA in 1986 as a synthetic retinoid used to treat severe psoriasis. Due to its high incidence of teratogenic effects, etretinate was removed from the US market in December 2002.

22.4.5 Cocaine

Cocaine, a plant alkaloid derived from coca, is a local anesthetic with vasoconstrictor properties. Pharmacologically, cocaine disrupts neural transmission by blocking fast sodium channels and neuronal uptake of catecholamines and 5-hydroxytryptamine (serotonin).[84–86] Researchers have studied women who have (1) used cocaine only; (2) used cocaine plus other narcotics; (3) used narcotics in the past and were maintained on methadone during pregnancy; and 4) drug-free. Women who use cocaine had a significantly higher rate of spontaneous abortion. Infants that were exposed to cocaine during development had depression of interactive behavior with poor organization response to environmental stimuli. This observation was similar to that found in infants delivered to methadone-maintained women,[85] women addicted to pentazocine, tripelennamine and phencyclidine during pregnancy.[85,87] Increased fetal activity and premature labor were observed within minutes of using cocaine. A variety of other adverse effects have been reported, including abruption placentae, premature delivery, microcephaly, altered prosencephalic development, decreased birth weight, abnormal sleep, tremor, poor feeding, irritability, occasional seizures and sudden infant death syndrome (SIDS). Congenital malformations of the genitourinary tract have also been reported.[88] Both vasoconstriction, which could inhibit placental transport and function, and the pharmacological effect have been implicated as causes of altered embryo development.

22.5 DEVELOPMENTAL TOXICITY OF PRESCRIPTION DRUGS

Ideally, the pregnant woman should not take any medications during pregnancy, other than those associated with routine prenatal care. However, there are situations that may require active pharmaceutical intervention including seizures, thrombotic disorders and anxiety. The pathophysiological consequences of maternal seizures are a major risk for the fetus. Maternal grand mal seizures associated with apnea can lead to acidosis and transient hypoxia in the fetus.[89] Prompt control of breakthrough seizure activity is of utmost importance to minimize the effects of oxygen deprivation on the fetus. Obstruction of blood flow through the circulatory system, specifically to the fetus can also pose a major concern and may require pharmaceutical intervention with the use of anticoagulants. The mental well-being of the pregnant mother may require the need to prescribe sedative and antipsychotic drugs. Maternal disorders and the following treatment of these disorders during pregnancy may present an increased risk to the fetus and the newborn infant. The long-term cognitive function of the offspring of pregnant women taking the following prescription drugs is also a concern.

22.5.1 Serotonin Reuptake Inhibitors and Serotonin-Noradrenalin Reuptake Inhibitors

Depression is a common mental disorder with a lifetime prevalence rate of approximately 16% (Kessler RC 2003).[90] Women, especially during their childbearing age, are at increased risk for first onset of major depression and have a lifetime rate of major depression 1.7–2.7 times greater than men (Burt VK 2002).[91] During pregnancy, prevalence rates vary widely from 1% to 20% depending on the classification used (Sie 2012).[92] Besides maternal morbidity and mortality, untreated or undertreated depression is associated with perinatal complications like cesarean delivery, prematurity and low birth weight, lower-quality interactions between mother and child and higher levels of psychiatric disturbances among children (Sie et al. 2012).[92] Given the potentially serious consequences of perinatal depression for both mother and child, adequate treatment is essential. Treatment of depression consists of non-pharmacological strategies, including psychotherapy and pharmacological treatment with antidepressants. Two of the most commonly prescribed antidepressant classes are selective serotonin reuptake inhibitors (SSRIs) and serotonin-norepinephrine reuptake inhibitors (SNRIs). As SSRIs and SNRIs are frequently used during pregnancy, the association between maternal use during pregnancy and birth defects in infants has been the topic of much discussion.

Serotonin is a neurotransmitter released from serotonergic neurons, and dysregulation of serotonergic activity may lead to mood and behavior problems. SSRIs selectively inhibit the reuptake of serotonin into the presynaptic neuron, leading to increased levels of serotonin in the synaptic cleft. Another increasingly used antidepressant is venlafaxine, an SNRI. Differences are observed with respect to the pharmacokinetic properties among SSRIs.[92,93] Furthermore, the drug effect is affected by enzyme polymorphism and individual drug metabolism. Side effects of SSRIs and SNRIs tend to be similar and include gastrointestinal symptoms, headache, insomnia and agitation. Tremors, excessive sweating and weight changes are also reported. Somnolence is seen in patients using mirtazapine, due to its antihistaminergic effect. After initial reports of an association between paroxetine and heart defects, the FDA published an advisory warning of this potential association in 2005.[94] The available clinical data for specific antidepressants vary widely. Fluoxetine, paroxetine, citalopram and citalopram are the most studied SSRIs (more than 5,000 subjects), compared with fluvoxamine, escitalopram and the SNRI venlafaxine (around 1,300 subjects). Currently, there is no association between major congenital malformations and the use of venlafaxine.[92,95,96]

A variety of symptoms have been reported after prenatal exposure to SSRIs and to a lesser extent to SNRIs. These symptoms include tremors, jitteriness, irritability, muscle tone regulation disorders, excessive crying, sleep disturbances, tachypnea and feeding problems less frequently, lethargy, weak cry and convulsions have been reported. Symptoms generally occur within two days after birth. These SSRI/SNRI-related symptoms occur in approximately 30% of in utero exposed infants.[92] Several additional factors, like maternal dose and metabolism, the specific SSRI and SNRI used, the individual, drug clearance and possibly genetic predisposition may be needed for symptoms to develop.[97]

Although the analysis supports the validity of the associations that were observed, the increase in the absolute risks is small. The two strongest analyses point to maternal paroxetine treatment and anencephaly or right ventricular outflow tract obstruction cardiac defects in the infant.[97] Assuming a causal association, absolute risks in the children of women who are treated with paroxetine early in pregnancy would increase for anencephaly from 2 per 10,000 to 7 per 10,000; for right ventricular outflow tract obstruction cardiac defects increase from 10 per 1,000,025 to 24 per 10,000.[97] The absolute risks for birth defects were still low. This analysis highlights the need for further research to evaluate the association between specific SSRIs and birth defects rather than comparing entire drug classes or a heterogeneous group of birth defects. Although SSRIs may be classified into the same group pharmacologically, there are many drugs that differ chemically with selectivity and indirect effects on receptor systems. SSRIs differences pharmacologically may contribute to differences in teratogenic activity, whether or not the mechanism involves inhibition of serotonin receptors.[97]

22.5.2 Valproic Acid

Valproic acid (2-propylpentanoic acid) was approved in 1978 in the United States for the treatment of epilepsy. In 1982, a surveillance study in Lyon, France, revealed that in 146 cases of spina bifida aperta, nine of the mothers had taken valproate during the first trimester.[98,99] The estimated risk of a valproate-exposed woman having a child with spina bifida was calculated to be about 1.2%. This risk level was similar to that of a woman whose previous child was born with a neural tube defect.[100] More recent cohort studies of more than 1,700 babies exposed to monotherapy with valproic acid showed an associative relative risk of 2.59 for major malformations (95% confidence interval [CI] 2.11 to 3.17) when compared with monotherapy using other anticonvulsant drugs.[101–110] When compared to untreated epileptic patients, the relative risk was 3.16 (95% CI 2.17 to 4.60).[106–109,111,112]

When compared to the general population of healthy control subjects the relative risk of major congenital malformations among patients receiving monotherapy with valproic acid was 3.77 (95% CI 2.18 to 6.52).[113] This means that women exposed to valproic acid monotherapy during embryogenesis have more than 2.5 times the risk of having babies with malformations and that this trend is highly significant ($p < 0.001$).[114]

When valproic acid was administered as part of an anticonvulsant polytherapy, the relative risk also increased significantly over that of other anticonvulsant drugs (1.84 [95% CI] 1.34 to 2.52), untreated epilepsy (3.24 [95% CI] 2.06 to 5.08) and healthy control subjects (3.35[95% CI] 1.87 to 6.01).[104–109,115–117]

The experimental animal work by Nau and colleagues was very important in establishing that valproic acid caused the development of neural tube defects.[118] These authors introduced the relationship between teratogenicity and embryonic pH, where 8 of 11 chemicals known to produce congenital anomalies is humans were acids and that none were bases. They also noted that valpromide produced only one exencephalic fetus among 116 implants in the mouse compared to 61 affected fetuses among 136 implants after exposure to the more acidic sodium valproate. Valproic acid concentrations in the mouse embryo were at least twice as high as in maternal plasma; whereas valpromide concentrations were similar in the two compartments. This is consistent with the theory that ion trapping would be greater for more acidic compounds. Even though valproic acid concentrations were higher in the umbilical cord blood than maternal plasma concentrations, the theory of ion trapping may not completely explain this difference in humans and other mammalian models. The fetal pH is lower than maternal pH in humans[119] and sheep.[120] The differences in maternal and fetal concentrations are better explained by the extent of protein binding for valproic acid. As gestation advances, fetal albumin concentration increases and free valproic acid decreases.[121]

Due to the large number of serious and possibly fatal side effects, the FDA has placed several warnings and advisories on valproic acid products. The label carries black box warnings for the following: (1) pancreatitis in children and adults; (2) liver failure (hepatotoxicity); and

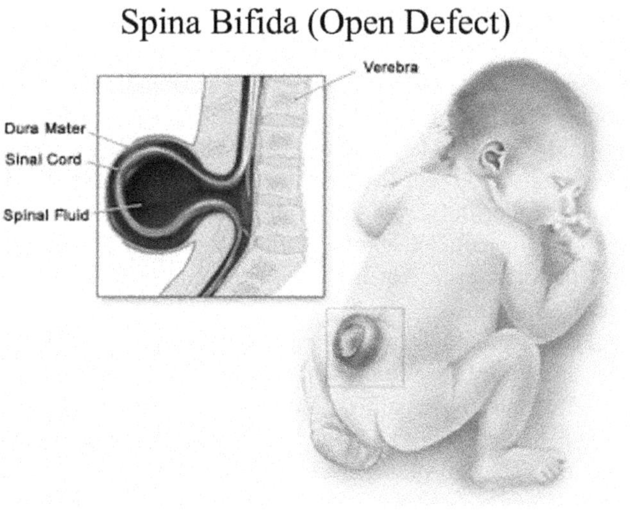

FIGURE 22.5 Spina Bifida Birth Defect.

(3) birth defects, including spina bifida. The FDA classifies Depakote, a highly prescribed valproic acid derivative, as a class D drug, which means it has been shown to cause harm to human fetuses and should only be taken during pregnancy if no other medications can be used to treat a condition.

In the past several years, Abbott Laboratories has been charged with numerous fines regarding Depakote. In May 2012, Abbott was ordered to pay $1.6 billion over the company's illegal marketing of the drug.[122] In the four-year investigation, the Justice Department found that Abbott violated federal FDA regulations and state and federal laws in marketing the drug to promote off-label uses, including schizophrenia, depression and anxiety.

In July 2012, 27 victims filed suit against Abbott in an Illinois federal court. The plaintiffs, all women, said they took Depakote early in their pregnancies to control migraines and epilepsy symptoms. They alleged their children were born with Depakote-induced birth defects, including developmental delays, spina bifida, cleft palate and bodily malformations.[122]

22.5.3 Phenytoin

Phenytoin was first introduced for the treatment of partial and generalized tonic-clonic seizures in 1938. Rapidly it became one of the most commonly used drugs for the control of epileptic seizures because it had no sedative side effects.[123] A number of antiepileptic drugs, including phenytoin, interfere with maternal folate metabolism.[124,125] Patients taking phenytoin may therefore become deficient in folate, leading to the development of macrocytic anemia and possible complications during pregnancy. It has become widely accepted that maternal deficiency in folate is associated with neural tube defects in the fetus (American Academy of Pediatrics Committee on Genetics).[126] Because the neural tube develops between 18 and 30 days after conception, many women do not know that they are pregnant when these defects are occurring. Research indicates that phenytoin causes a decreased plasma concentration of folate by depleting total hepatic folate.[127] Therapy recommendations suggest that women begin taking folic acid supplements throughout the first trimester to reduce the risk of neural tube defects. Additionally, phenytoin therapy may increase the metabolism of vitamin D, leading to a decrease in vitamin D levels that can in turn cause alterations in calcium homeostasis.[127]

Fetal hydantoin syndrome is a rare disorder that is caused by exposure to phenytoin. Major signs of this disorder include abnormalities of the skull and facial features, growth deficiencies and underdeveloped nails on the fingers and toes. The full-blown syndrome is estimated to occur in approximately 5–10% of newborns exposed to phenytoin in utero.[128] The teratogenic mechanism of phenytoin may also be related to an accumulation of epoxides, which are highly reactive oxidative metabolites of phenytoin.[129]

Phenytoin was the most commonly implicated antiepilepsy drug in several large-scale studies.[129,130] In these studies, approximately 2% of infants born to women with epilepsy who were taking antiepilepsy drugs experienced congenital heart disease and/or had cleft lip or cleft palate. These rates are 4-fold greater than the rates in the general population for congenital heart disease and 10-fold greater than the rates for cleft lip or cleft palate.[127]

The effect of maternal epilepsy on cognitive function in the offspring has been studied. Small head sizes can occur in neonates prenatally exposed to antiepilepsy drugs.[128] Infants with fetal hydantoin syndrome may have cognitive impairments, but whether these impairments are permanent or disappear over time is unclear.[131] There is evidence that small head size is a common observation in infants prenatally exposed to multiple antiepilepsy drugs versus a single antiepileptic exposure. Persistent learning disorders in approximately 12% of phenytoin-exposed infants were also observed compared to only 1% of the general population.[132]

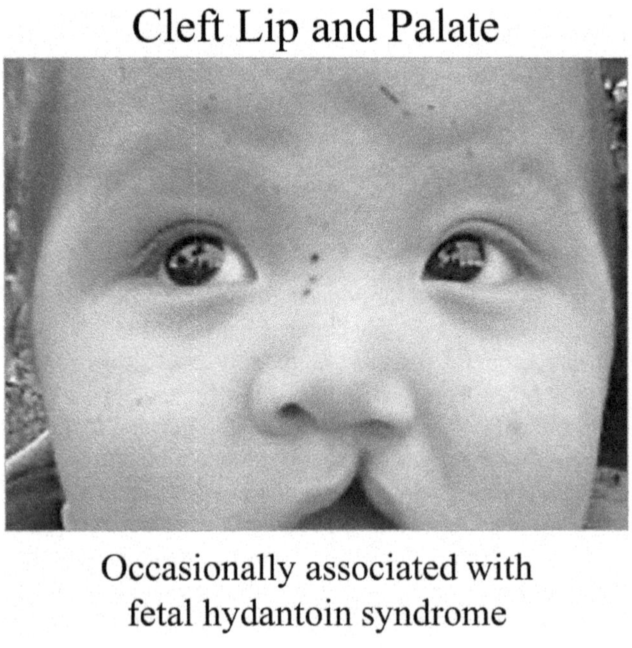

FIGURE 22.6 Cleft Lip or Palate Birth Defect.

22.5.4 Warfarin

Warfarin is an oral anticoagulant that inhibits the synthesis of vitamin K-dependent clotting factors including factors II, VII, IX and X and the anticoagulant proteins C and S.[133] Warfarin is a synthetic derivative of dicoumarol, a 4-hydroxycoumarin-derived mycotoxin and coagulant found in spoiled clover-based animal feeds. Coumarin derivative exposure in the first trimester of pregnancy results in a specific malformation syndrome known as warfarin embryopathy, which is characterized by nasal hypoplasia and punctate stippled calcifications of the laryngeal cartilage, head of the ribs, transverse process of the vertebrae or epiphyses.[134–137] Ophthalmologic abnormalities are frequently observed[135] and include optic atrophy, microphthalmia, lens opacities and large prominent eyes. Also, use of warfarin during the second and third trimesters has been associated sporadically with central nervous system abnormalities, including mental retardation, microcephaly and blindness.[138–141] Overall risk of central nervous system defects is about 3%.

In the late third trimester, exposure to coumarin anticoagulants may result in late prenatal, perinatal or postnatal hemorrhages.[142,143] One study reported 418 cases of warfarin exposure from conception to 38 weeks after birth.[144] About 16% of all pregnancies ended in spontaneous abortions or stillbirths, and another 15% resulted in babies with abnormalities at birth. The abnormalities included skeletal malformations (e.g., stippling of cervical vertebrae, sacrum and femurs; kyphoscoliosis; and nasal hypoplasia), deafness, focal cerebral atrophy, respiratory distress, seizures and bilateral optic atrophy leading to blindness.

In another study, a report on 128 babies exposed to warfarin therapy from 0 to 38 weeks' gestation observed that about 8% of the 38 live-born infants displayed teratogenic effects of warfarin at birth, including nasal hypoplasia, choanal stenosis and stippled epiphyses.[145] When compared with 68 pregnancies where women's warfarin therapy had been replaced with 1 g of acetylsalicylic acid and 400 mg of dipyridamole daily at the onset of pregnancy, it was clear that the rate of spontaneous abortions was significantly higher in the warfarin group (28% vs 10%). The rate of neonatal deaths was also higher in the warfarin group (2.3% vs 0). The rate of stillbirths was approximately 7% in both groups. Warfarin dose was adjusted for a target prothrombin time of 2 to 2.5 times control in most women.

In summary, coumarin derivative use or abuse by mothers during gestation results in one-sixth of pregnancies ending with abnormal live-born infants, one-sixth ending in abortion or stillbirth, and about two-thirds ending with a relatively normal outcome.

Warfarin has been assigned to pregnancy Category X by the FDA. Problems associated with perinatal administration of warfarin have included central nervous system defects, spontaneous abortion, stillbirth, prematurity, hemorrhage and ocular defects when given anytime during pregnancy and a fetal warfarin syndrome when given during the first trimester. Warfarin is considered contraindicated during pregnancy.

22.5.5 Benzodiazepines

Benzodiazepines are a group of psychoactive drugs whose core chemical structure is the fusion of a benzene ring and a diazepine ring. There are numerous benzodiazepines marketed in the United States, and these differ primarily in their pharmacokinetic properties.[146] Exposure to benzodiazepines, assessed by calls to American poison control centers, represents half of all exposures to sedative-hypnotic and antipsychotic drugs. Benzodiazepines are among the drugs most frequently prescribed to women of reproductive age and to pregnant women for reducing anxiety and managing preeclampsia or eclampsia in the latter part of pregnancy.[147]

Benzodiazepines are divided into three categories on the basis of elimination half-life ($t_{1/2}$): 1) short-acting ($t_{1/2}$ < 10 hours); 2) intermediate-acting ($t_{1/2}$ = 10–24 hours) and; 3) long-acting ($t_{1/2}$ > 24 hours).

The following are common short-, intermediate- and long-acting benzodiazepines:

- Short-acting: Midazolam (Versed), Temazepam (Restoril), Triazolam (Halcion)
- Intermediate-acting: Alprazolam (Xanax), Lorazepam (Ativan), Oxazepam (Serax)
- Long-acting: Diazepam (Valium), Chlordiazepoxide (Librium), Chlorazepate (Tranxene), Flurazepam (Dalmane), Prazepam (Centrex)

Short- and intermediate-acting benzodiazepines are generally used to treat insomnia, while long-acting benzodiazepines are used to treat anxiety. In general, benzodiazepines are relatively safe drugs even in overdose because of the rapid body adaptations to high blood levels. There is controversy concerning the safety of benzodiazepines in pregnancy, specifically their association with cleft palate and neuro-behavioral disorders as a result of prenatal exposure.[148] The FDA classifies benzodiazepines as either a D- or X-category drug, which means that the potential for harm in the newborn has been demonstrated.[149]

All major classes of benzodiazepine compounds can be assumed to be excreted into the breast milk and diffuse readily across the placenta to the fetus. This depends on the characteristics of the particular drug-plasma protein binding, ionization, the degree of lipophilicity, molecular weight, half-life, maternal blood concentrations, oral bioavailability and pharmacokinetics.[150] Among anxiolytic agents, only diazepam has been systematically studied among pregnant women. Until the early 1980s, diazepam was the most prescribed benzodiazepine in the United States and worldwide. Diazepam and its major metabolite, N-desmethyldiazepam, are both pharmacologically active and freely cross the human placenta during early pregnancy as a result of their high lipid solubility.[151–158] Natural processes during pregnancy have been shown to facilitate the transport of diazepam across the placenta and both diazepam and N-desmethyldiazepam extensively bind to fetal plasma proteins and do so to a higher degree than to maternal plasma proteins.[159–161] Available data from various epidemiological studies are inconsistent in showing the risk of congenital malformations among children born to women who took diazepam during pregnancy. Several studies found that the use of diazepam during the first trimester of pregnancy was significantly greater among mothers of children born with oral clefts. Aarskog found that 6.3% of 30 infants born with cleft palate in the United States between 1967 and 1971 had been exposed to diazepam in the first trimester, compared with 1.1% of control infants.[162] This rate of exposure to diazepam (6.2%) among the children with cleft palate was similar to another study.[163] Safra and Oakley reported that mothers of infants with cleft lip, cleft palate or both had used diazepam four times more frequently than mothers of control infants.[164] However, in another article these same authors pointed out that a fourfold increase in oral clefts, if confirmed, implies only a 0.4% risk of cleft lip with or without cleft palate and a 0.2% risk of cleft palate.[165] A review of 599 oral clefts by Saxen and Saxen showed a significant association ($p < 0.05$) between ingestion of anxiolytics, mostly diazepam, during the first trimester of pregnancy.[165] Many other epidemiological studies have shown an association between the use of diazepam in the first trimester and oral clefts.[166–170] However, these studies were followed by prospective and retrospective studies that did not show a greater risk of congenital malformations.[170–174] Also, there has been a large increase in the use of diazepam over the past several years, without a concomitant increase in the occurrence of cleft lip or cleft palate.

Chlordiazepoxide, another long-acting benzodiazepine, has been associated with congenital malformations following exposure during early pregnancy.[175] An analysis of over 19,000 live births revealed that several congenital anomalies were present including spastic diplegia, microcephaly, duodenal atresia and mental deficiency. These anomalies were more prevalent among infants of mothers who took chlordiazepoxide during the first 42 days of pregnancy than among infants of mothers who took other drugs or no drugs (11.4 per 100 compared with 4.6 per 100 and 2.6 per 100, respectively). Fetal death rates were also higher in the chlordiazepoxide group. In another study of more than 50,000 pregnancies, malformations were identified in approximately 6.5% of the offspring before their first birthday.[176]

22.6 ADDITIONAL PRENATAL ENVIRONMENTAL INFLUENCES

22.6.1 Malnutrition

Women who begin pregnancy underweight, eat poorly during pregnancy and consequently do not gain at least 3–4 pounds per month in the second and third trimesters run a much higher risk of having low-birth-weight babies.[177] Research indicates that obese women should gain 15 to 24 pounds during pregnancy; normal-weight women 24 to 35 pounds; and underweight women even more. Beyond overall weight, certain nutrients defend against low birth weight, including zinc, iron and folic acid. Indeed, malnutrition (not age) is the primary reason young teenagers tend to have small babies. They tend to eat sporadically and unhealthily, and because their own bodies are still developing their diet is inadequate to support the growth of two. If the baby is malnourished, there is serious damage to the central nervous system (CNS), seen in lower brain weight. It will also affect other organ system development, especially the immune system, resulting in frequent illness. Lack of folic acid particularly affects neural tube formation, showing up as anencephaly or spina bifida.

22.6.2 Poverty

Compared with women of higher socioeconomic status, pregnant women at the bottom of the economic ladder are more likely to be ill, malnourished, teenaged and stressed.[178] They often receive late or inadequate prenatal care, breathe polluted air, live in overcrowded conditions, move from place to place and ingest unhealthy substances. Poor women have less access to family planning services, and they live in communities that encourage higher birth rates, partly because these communities have higher death rates. In this way, the social context may underlie many of the biological causes of low birth weight.

- Of the more than 25 million low-birth-weight infants born worldwide each year, the overwhelming majority are in developing countries.
- Developing countries in the same geographic region, with similar ethnic populations, have markedly different low-birth-weight rates when they have different average incomes.
- Within nations, differences in low-birth-weight rates among ethnic groups follow socioeconomic differences among those groups.
- Within the United States, low birth rates in the poorest states are almost twice those in wealthier states.

22.6.3 Emotional State

The mother's stress can be transmitted to the fetus. When a pregnant woman experiences intense fears, anxieties and other emotions, physiological changes occur in the fetus. These include changes in respiration and glandular secretions. For example, producing adrenaline in response to fear restricts blood flow to the uterine area and may deprive the fetus of adequate oxygen. Also, reassuring the mother of fetal well-being has positive outcomes for the infants in the study.[178] Stress also relates to miscarriage, prematurity, low birth weight and baby irritability and GI tract problems. In addition, stress is related to cleft palate and pyloric stenosis, which affects nutritional intake.

22.6.4 Mother's Age

Two time periods are of special interest: adolescence and the thirties and beyond. Infants born to adolescents are often premature. The mortality rate of infants born to mothers who are adolescents is twice as high compared to infants born to mothers in their twenties. Down syndrome, a form of mental retardation, is associated with increased age of the mother. By the age of 40, the probability of having a child with down syndrome is ~ 1 in 100. By age 50, it increases to ~ 1 in 10. This risk is also higher if the mother is younger than 18. In general, women also have more difficulty in becoming pregnant after the age of 30.[178]

22.6.5 Infections and Diseases

Maternal diseases and infections can produce defects by crossing the placental barrier. For example, the greatest damage to the fetus from the mother contracting German measles occurs during the third and fourth weeks of pregnancy. Syphilis is more damaging later in prenatal development, four months or more after conception. Rather than affecting organ development as rubella does, syphilis damages organs after they have formed. The importance of the mother's health to the health of her offspring is nowhere better exemplified than when the mother is infected with HIV.[160] HIV and AIDS is passed to a fetus 20–30% of the time. It causes weight loss, diarrhea, respiratory illness and brain damage. Most babies survive only five to eight months once symptoms appear. If the mother uses AZT, it reduces transmission to the baby 95% of the time.

22.7 PREGNANCY CATEGORIES FOR PRESCRIPTION DRUG LABELING—PAST AND PRESENT

More than 80% of all drugs approved and on the market are not officially approved by the FDA for use during pregnancy.[179] Although there is much animal and human research undertaken to determine teratogenicity, an FDA statement that a substance is safe for use during pregnancy is usually won after long empiric experience and is not often granted.

Until June 2015, the prescription drug labeling for newly approved drugs contained one of five required pregnancy categories (A, B, C, D and X) as one of the items in the "Precautions" section of the package insert and other labeling. This follows an FDA regulation that became effective on December 26, 1979.[179] All prescription drugs absorbed systemically or known to have a potential for harm to the fetus came under this rule as part of the FDA labeling revision on November 1, 1980.

- Category A: Controlled studies in women failed to demonstrate a risk to the fetus in the first trimester and there is no evidence of a risk in later trimesters. The possibility of fetal harm appears remote.
- Category B: Either studies of animal reproduction have not demonstrated a fetal risk but there are no controlled studies in pregnant women or studies of animal reproduction have shown an adverse effect (other than a decrease in fertility) that was not confirmed in controlled studies in women in the first trimester (and there is no evidence of a risk in later trimesters).
- Category C: Either studies in animals have revealed adverse effects on the fetus (teratogenic or embryocidal effects or other), and there are no controlled studies in women or studies in women and animals are not available. Drugs should be given only if the potential benefit justifies the potential risk to the fetus.
- Category D: There is positive evidence of human fetal risk, but the benefits from use in pregnant women may be acceptable despite the risk (e.g., if the drug is needed in a life-threatening situation or for a serious disease for which safer drugs cannot be used or are ineffective). There will be an appropriate statement in the "Warnings" section of the labeling.
- Category X: Studies in animals or humans have demonstrated fetal abnormalities or there is evidence of fetal risk based on human experience, or both, and the risk of the use of the drug in pregnant women clearly outweighs any possible benefit. The drug is contraindicated in women who are or may become pregnant. There will be an appropriate statement in the "Contraindications" section of the labeling.

Twenty-five years later, and seven years since the proposed Pregnancy Rule was published in the Federal Register, FDA issued a Final Rule for Pregnancy and Lactation labeling, described in an FDA release.[180]

The US FDA published a final rule today that sets standards for how information about using medicines during pregnancy and breastfeeding is presented in the labeling of prescription drugs and biological products. The new content and formatting requirements will provide a more consistent way to include relevant information about the risks and benefits of prescription drugs and biological products used during pregnancy and breastfeeding. The final rule replaces the current product letter categories—A, B, C, D and X—used to classify the risks of using prescription drugs during pregnancy with three detailed subsections that describe risks within the real-world context of caring for pregnant women who may need medication.

"Prescribing decisions during pregnancy and lactation are individualized and involve complex maternal, fetal and infant risk–benefit considerations. The letter category system was overly simplistic and was misinterpreted as a grading system, which gave an oversimplified view of the product risk," said Sandra Kweder, M.D., deputy director of the Office of New Drugs in the FDA's Center for Drug Evaluation and Research. "The new labeling rule provides for explanations, based on available information, about the potential benefits and risks for the mother, the fetus and the breastfeeding child."

The final rule requires the use of three subsections in the labeling titled "Pregnancy," "Lactation" and "Females and Males of Reproductive Potential" that provide details about the use of the drug or biological product. The detailed subsections must include a summary of the risks of using a drug during pregnancy and breastfeeding, a discussion of the data supporting the summary and relevant information to help health care providers make prescribing and counseling decisions.

The Pregnancy subsection will provide information relevant to the use of the drug in pregnant women, such as dosing and potential risks to the developing fetus, and will require information about whether there is a registry that collects and maintains data on how pregnant women are affected when they use the drug or biological product. Information in drug labeling about the existence of any pregnancy registries has been previously recommended but not required until now.

The Lactation subsection will provide information about using the drug while breastfeeding, such as the amount of drug in breast milk and potential effects on the breastfed child. The Females and Males of Reproductive Potential subsection will include information about pregnancy testing, contraception and infertility as it relates to the drug. This information has been included in labeling, but there has been no consistent placement for it until now.

The "Pregnancy" and "Lactation" subsections will also include three subheadings: "risk summary," "clinical considerations" and "data." These subheadings will provide more detailed information regarding, for example, human and animal data on the use of the drug and specific adverse reactions of concern for pregnant or breastfeeding women.

There are over six million pregnancies in the United States every year, and pregnant women take an average of three to five prescription drugs during pregnancy. Women with preexisting medical conditions, such as asthma or high blood pressure, may need to continue to use prescription drugs to treat those conditions during pregnancy and breastfeeding. Women may also need to take medications for new or acute conditions that may occur during pregnancy or breastfeeding. The new labeling format and requirements reorganize information and are structured to help inform healthcare professionals' prescribing decisions and the counseling of patients using prescription drugs.

The final rule is part of a broad effort by the agency, which began with the Physician Labeling Rule, to improve the content and format of prescription drug labeling. The rule finalizes many of the provisions in the proposed rule that the FDA issued in May 2008 and will be in effect as of June 30, 2015. Once the final rule is in effect, newly approved drug and biological product applications will be required to use the new format immediately, while the new labeling content and format requirements for previously approved products subject to the Physician Labeling Rule will be phased in gradually.

22.8 CASE REPORTS FROM LITIGATION

When births occur with difficulty and residual effects present in children exposed to drugs in utero or in the perinatal period and problems are encountered, litigation frequently occurs. Drug exposure may be therapeutic or recreational. With some drug classes, the risk is well-known (i.e., teratogens, presented earlier in this chapter) while for others it is not so well-known.

Pharmacologists are frequently retained to assess the case, determine the extent and (trimester) of fetal exposure, identify mechanisms of fetal or perinatal toxicity and determine/opine what contribution, if any, the exposure(s) is or can be attributed to that exposure.

Injury is a risk/complication of any drug therapy and more damaging to the patient and the caregiver if the drug was selected, administered, dispensed or monitored negligently, contributing greatly to the injury. Although injury itself does not establish malpractice or negligence, drug injury litigation is common and is the second most common reason for medical malpractice suits.

For purposes of this forensic or deeper dive into drug injury, focus on this risk group to illustrate the variety and basic trend(s) that can be seen. Obstetrical patients (and fetus/newborn) are at even greater risk, given the paucity of data concerning the teratologic and embryo-fetal toxicity of many drugs given during pregnancy and the perinatal period.

22.8.1 Analysis of Fetal/Neonatal Drug Injuries

Nine (9) cases from the consulting practice of Drs. James T and James J O'Donnell provide the reader with an application of drug causation principles and methodology to rule in or rule out causation in the vulnerable population of the fetus and perinatal infant.

Most cases are confidential and are not disclosable as resolutions were confidential, or cases were dropped upon thorough analysis.

22.8.2 Fatal Electrolyte Disturbance in Hyperemesis Gravidum

Diagnosed in office as constipated based on history of no bowel movement in seven days and no eating in seven days; seen in obstetrician office; nausea and vomiting for three weeks; 14 lb weight loss; and clinical dehydration. Patient was sent from office to hospital; labs "stat"; soap suds enema (SSE) ordered and administered. Labs of significance were potassium (K+) 1.8; sodium (Na+) 121; 20 mEq potassium (KCL) in dextrose 5% normal saline at 50ml/hour ordered; and patient admitted to labor & delivery unit. A second lab panel showed K of 1.5 mEq. However, patient experience a cardiac arrest 60″ after admission and staff were unable to resuscitate.

Case findings showed critical K+ & Na+ levels that required immediate attention with careful and aggressive replenishment in an intensive care setting or "ICU." There was slow "clinical" electrolyte replenishment, insufficient for treatment of acute/chronic severe deficiency. The severe hypokalemia created a significant risk for a fatal arrhythmia. The severe hyponatremia created a significant risk for seizures. Ultimately too little, too late and too slow a response by healthcare professionals.

Case resolution/legal outcome was that the Ob/Gyn and hospital were sued for malpractice; insufficient clinical monitoring and care; inadequate urgency and treatment at hospital and "standard of care." The plaintiff's OB/Gyn expert testified the defendants "violated standard of care." As a result, the case settled on eve of trial with agreed contribution by both OB/Gyn and hospital defendants.

22.8.3 Renal Embryotoxicity Following Angiotensin II Receptor Blocker Inhibitor in Pregnant Woman

Valsartan (an angiotensin II receptor blocker—ARB) was prescribed for hypertension in a 30-year-old woman and was filled at an outpatient/community pharmacy. The drug was prescribed by a general practitioner physician. A prenatal vitamin prescription was listed on the pharmacy profile; however, the pharmacist did not inquire or warn about the use of valsartan during pregnancy. This prescription was discovered later in the pregnancy and was discontinued. However, oligoamnios (deficiency in amniotic fluid) was viewed on ultrasound examination at that time.

Fetal urine production is the major source of amniotic fluid production in the second and third trimesters. If blood pressure drops, angiotensin II maintains kidney perfusion and thus glomerular filtration rate due to autoregulation. Late pregnancy usage of angiotensin-converting enzyme inhibitors (ACEI) and ARB may cause severe oligohydramnios due to fetal renal impairment (second and third trimesters). There is a BLACK BOX Warning(s)—*May cause fetal and neonatal morbidity and mortality if used during Pregnancy. ACE inhibitors also may increase the risk of major congenital malformations when administered during the first trimester of pregnancy.* ACEIs and ARBs are listed as: Teratogenic Effects: Pregnancy Category D (see the FDA Pregnancy classifications earlier in this chapter).

Resolution/legal outcome from this case: The neonate recovered without long-term renal toxicity. Pharmacist claimed—"doesn't inquire about pregnancy to not embarrass patient"; Prenatal vitamins "used for other things." The pharmacist was sued for violation of the standard of care. The pharmacist should have inquired and advised both physicians of the prescription for the ARB. This case was settled by the pharmacy out of court.

22.8.4 Deformed Skull in Newborn Following Opiate Therapy During Pregnancy

The legal complaint stated that opiates caused the fetus to decrease movement and were the cause of skull deformity. Reports of severe chronic pain that mom and doctors knew of opiate use. A lawsuit against the obstetrician (OB) was filed.

There are multiple causes of deformed cranium identified in the literature and in antiquity and even some postpartum causes in floppy babies due to inactivity in a crib. There was no literature support for opiate-induced in utero flaccidity or decreased movement to cause cranial deformity. The resolution of this case was that the plaintiff's case was dismissed after the defense pharmacologist's opinion/report disclosed a lack of a clear causation for the claimed injury.

22.8.5 "Off-Label" Tocolytics and Beta-Blockers in a Hypertensive Premature Labor Resulting in Fetal Loss

The plaintiff was a 33-week gestation woman with uterine contractions and 149/92 blood pressure (BP) who was admitted for tocolysis. Antihypertensives (calcium-channel blocker—nifedipine) and tocolytic (terbutaline) were prescribed; BP was controlled, contractions stopped; and the patient was discharged from the hospital. The patient was found unresponsive eight days later at home with a suspected eclamptic seizure. An ultrasound in the hospital showed fetal demise (both twins) along with placental blood clot—abruption. The mother continued hemorrhaging and required a hysterectomy.

According to a plaintiff Obstetrics expert, the twins should have been delivered earlier, and, if so, no bad outcome would have been expected. The maternal-fetal medicine (MFM) MD "should have discontinued the antihypertensives to get true pressure readings." The drug "Procardia (nifedipine) is known to mask hypertension therefore the standard of care (SOC) required the doctor to get true blood pressure readings"

There was conflicting literature as to a direct cause:

1. Saudan P, Billieux MH, Pechere A, Irion O, Savoldelli G, Boulvain M. OS014. Which firstline drug to control severe hypertension in pregnancy? A pilot study. *Pregnancy Hypertens.* 2012 Jul;2(3):
2. King JF, Flenady VJ, Papatsonis DN, Dekker GA, Carbonne B. Oral antihypertensive therapy for severe hypertension in pregnancy and postpartum: A systematic review. *Cochrane Database Syst Rev.* 2002;(2):CD002255.
3. Flenady V, Wojcieszek AM, Papatsonis DNM, Stock OM, Murray L, Jardine LA, Carbonne B Calcium channel blockers for inhibiting preterm labour and birth (Review) http://www.thecochranelibrary.com. Copyright © 2014 The Cochrane Collaboration. Published by John Wiley & Sons, Ltd.
4. Yamasato K, Burlingame J, Kaneshiro B. Hemodynamic effects of nifedipine tocolysis. J Obstet Gynaecol Res. 2015 Jan;41(1):1722. doi: 10.1111/jog.12478. Epub 2014 Aug 27

When a pregnant patient is treated, it does not mask hypertension—it treats hypertension by lowering blood pressure and thus eliminates/controls hypertension. The defense pharmacologist expert stated, "Under the circumstances the use of nifedipine in this case is completely appropriate—the best drug choice for treatment." As a result, the MFM and hospital refused to settle. Prior to trial, the parties agreed upon a nuisance settlement.

22.8.6 False-Positive Morphine Meconium in Neonate Resulting in Action by Child Protective Services

An admitted heroin user—last used in the first trimester—"when I learned I was pregnant, I stopped." Her obstetrician continued the use of Xanax (alprazolam) to lessen the risk of heroin use. Alprazolam use continued through labor and after delivery. The neonate's meconium test was positive for morphine (screening), confirmed with GCMS (confirmatory testing). No benzodiazepines were detected in the meconium.

The kinetics of meconium drug disposition and meconium drug detectability became a key issue in this case. It was determined that the estimation of time of use detected in amniotic fluid—8 weeks and the timing of meconium formation (12 weeks). Thus, the residence of drugs (morphine) in meconium × detectability—20 weeks (range). Were the toxicology results expected? Morphine (from heroin) was present—long interval from last use to birth, but possible. Xanax (alprazolam)—no benzodiazepines present. Benzo should have been present. There is "Something wrong with this picture!"

A pharmacologist expert for the mother provided an opinion—"Sample must be from another patient." Since hospitals do not document the chain of custody in the fashion seen in criminal cases, there was no way to verify the chain of custody. With continuous use of benzodiazepines, the meconium test should have been positive for benzodiazepines (Xanax). Since the test was benzodiazepine test was negative, it created significant doubt as to the chain of custody of the meconium tested at the confirmation level. "Test cannot be accurate." Incidentally, the testing laboratory brochure describing the test (ARUP labs) stated: "not for forensic purposes" (https://www.aruplab.com/). Resolution: The child protective agency dropped the action against the mother due to the questionable identity of the meconium-positive morphine test.

22.8.7 Negligent Epidural Infusion of Magnesium Sulfate in a Woman in Labor

Magnesium sulfate (MgSO4) is the most common medication used for the treatment of eclampsia and prophylaxis of eclampsia in patients with severe pre-eclampsia. It is usually given by either the intramuscular or intravenous routes. A concentration of 1.8 to 3.0 mmol/L has been suggested for the treatment of eclamptic convulsions.

What happens with epidural administration?

In this case, a nursing student erroneously obtained a MgSO4 IV bag from a Pyxis (drug storage cabinet) instead of lidocaine and connected the MgSO4 to an epidural catheter. The patient complained of increased pain, burning and paralysis of her lower extremities. Examination led to the discovery of the medication error. The patient was monitored for several days. Fortunately, she made a full recovery, with no residual neurotoxicity. The newborn was examined and monitored and found to have no signs of magnesium toxicity or elevated magnesium serum levels.

The obstetrical and anesthesia literature is replete with reports of magnesium administration errors in labor. A reported case example may be found at Dror A, Henriksen E. Accidental epidural magnesium sulfate injection. Aneth Analg. 1987 ct;66(10): 1020–1.

The hospital was sued. The hospital blamed the nursing school for inadequate supervision of its students. The plaintiff's pharmacist expert criticized hospital access to the $MgSO_4$ and lack of supervision of nursing students, as well as verification of the $MgSO_4$ fluid connection. Resolution of the case: the hospital paid a settlement for pain and suffering.

22.8.8 Opioid Toxicity and Maternal Death in an Unmonitored Woman in Labor

Post C-section, a patient received a fentanyl epidural. Her history included the use of antipsychotics, anxiolytics and antihistamines. Her lung findings showed wheezing bilateral She was also morbidly obese. Her pre-operative drugs were re-ordered and administered post-partum to help relieve post-partum depression.

No pulse oximetry was used by the Labor and Delivery nurses post-partum. It is well-known that opioids cause respiratory depression at therapeutic doses. CNS depressants add to the respiratory depressant effect of opioids. Sleep apnea, morbid obesity, respiratory compromise and abdominal surgery increase the risk of opioid respiratory depression. The only effective means of monitoring are frequent vital signs, pulse oximetry and/or capnography. The patient arrested 16 hours post-op was resuscitated; however, she developed hypoxic encephalopathy and permanent brain damage.

The hospital had a pulse oximetry policy in place, and anesthesia ordered pulse oximetry for this patient. Inexplicably, the Labor and Delivery nurses testified: "We don't use pulse ox in Labor and Delivery" (!)

The case was tried by a Jury and resulted in a $16,000,000 verdict against the hospital. The hospital subsequently negotiated a $8,000,000 cash settlement, which was accepted by the family to avoid appeal (*Oladanie v Good Samaritan Hospital*, Cook County, IL 2002. Case Citation Analyses of Litigated Cases Alleging Fetal Drug Injury).

22.8.8.1 Effects of Methadone and Smoking in Pregnancy

One case recently reviewed in litigation involved high-dose methadone treatment throughout pregnancy as well as smoking (tobacco) by a mother who gave birth. The methadone was part of medication-assisted treatment (MAT) for the mother, who was previously addicted to intravenous heroin. Allegations of malpractice were made against the obstetrician, MFM specialists, anesthesiologist treating the baby at birth and the hospital. The child presented with respiratory depression, hypotension, hypoglycemia, metabolic acidosis and shock liver after a cesarean section birth. The child was later diagnosed with speech and language developmental delay, behavioral disturbances and ADHD.

Any drug-induced injury causation assessment requires an evaluation utilizing accepted methodologies. While fetal toxicity was well-recognized as being associated with smoking while pregnant, methadone was not.

The methodology used by the consulting pharmacologist (James T. O'Donnell) was as follows:

1. Review medical treatment and diagnoses of the mother and her male child. Document prior heroin use, methadone and nicotine (smoking) use prior to, during and after the mother's cesarean delivery of the infant.
2. Review authoritative and peer review clinical and preclinical literature on the effects on the fetus in utero and after birth in a setting of opioid and smoking (nicotine) use by parents.
3. Documentation of biological plausibility of claimed toxicity resulting from the exposures.

4. Identify the documented causes of the child's residual developmental and behavioral deficits.
5. Identify developmental delays, behavioral deficits and diagnoses existent in the child and also identified in the literature in children born to opioid- and nicotine-exposed mothers during pregnancy.
6. Summarize the child's existing developmental delays and behavioral deficits that are known to be associated with exposure to opioids and smoking during pregnancy.

22.8.8.1.1 *Scope of Review*

The review of the literature and medical, obstetrical, anesthesia and pediatric record materials was limited to an inquiry into the effects of opiates and opioids as well as tobacco (cigarettes) on the fetus in utero and to document any residual effects on development and behavior in children born to women who use these substances during pregnancy.

22.8.8.1.2 *Opioid Fetal Toxicity Summary*

Most commonly, opioids are used medicinally to alleviate severe and chronic pain associated with ongoing illness or due to an injury. All opioids are controlled substances ranking from Schedule I through Schedule V depending on their prescribed medical indication, the risk for abuse and the risk for the development of physical dependence. Opioids also include heroin, which is an illegal substance used for its euphoric effects.

While used most for analgesic properties, opioids also activate reward neurocircuitry in the brain to produce a hedonic ("rewarding") effect that underlies the misuse and abuse of these drugs. Opioids are among the most widely abused substances in America today. When abused, opioids cause dependence, addiction, overdose and even death.

22.8.8.1.3 *Opioid Mechanism of Action*

Opioids bind to multiple receptors in the CNS including the mu, kappa and delta receptors. Subtypes demonstrate varying effects, but, in general, all receptors induce analgesia. The Mu and Kappa receptors are responsible for euphoric and psychomimetic effects, respiratory depression and physical dependence. The analgesic effects are propagated through the activation of opioid receptors located on nociceptive C and A delta fibers which indirectly inhibit calcium channels, decreasing cAMP levels and blocking the release of neurotransmitters that relay pain signals, such as glutamate, substance P and calcitonin gene-related peptide. The hedonic effects of opioids relate to the activation of opioid receptors expressed in limbic structures of the brain such as the nucleus accumbens, ventral tegmental area and ventral pallidum. Activation of mu and possibly delta opioid receptors located within the mesolimbic dopamine system is considered a key mechanism underlying the abuse liability of these drugs. Indirect increases of dopamine in these critical reward structures in the brain are responsible for the rewarding properties of these drugs.

22.8.8.1.4 *Opioid Toxicity*

The use of opioids in pregnancy is not contraindicated; however, their use during pregnancy can have serious consequences for the mother and the infant. Current opioid guidelines with respect to pregnancy are based on limited evidence. Pregnant patients who use opioids represent a distinct group; it is important to differentiate between opioid use as it relates to medical care, opioid abuse and untreated opioid use disorder (OUD). Methadone (and to a lesser extent, buprenorphine) has been referred to as the "gold standard" for opioid treatment in pregnant women who have a history of OUD. Neither methadone nor buprenorphine have been approved by the FDA for use in pregnant women. The FDA classifies both drugs as Teratogenic-Pregnancy Category C, which indicates that studies in animal reproduction have revealed an adverse effect on the fetus and that there are no well-controlled studies in humans, but potential benefits may warrant the use of the drug in pregnant women despite the potential risk.

The package insert for methadone states, "Methadone should be used during pregnancy only if the potential benefit justifies the potential risk to the fetus."

Elucidating the direct interaction between fetal toxicity and opioid exposure is complicated by confounding factors, logistics and methodology caveats. Most compelling is the direct evidence from controlled clinical studies; however, research with patients who are currently engaging or have a history of drug abuse presents many uncontrolled factors that need to be considered. These factors include the pharmacological purity of substances ingested, dosing, other drug intake and the accuracy of reporting from the patient on their patterns of drug use. In addition, data collected postnatally may be impacted by other factors such as maternal and infant malnutrition, health care accessibility, infant exposure to toxins, exposure of infants to drugs postnatally and suboptimal child-rearing environments in families with drug abuse. Despite these caveats, clinical data is essential to evaluate the impact of fetal opioid exposure.

22.8.8.1.5 *Maternal Transfer of Opioids to Fetus*

Opioid drugs pass from the mother to the fetus in utero with varying pharmacokinetic properties. Following infusion of methadone, peak transfer and concentration is observed in the umbilical vein within two minutes. An umbilical venous–arterial gradient is present for 10–15 minutes indicating transfer and uptake of methadone to the fetal tissue. The transfer of opioids from mother to fetus is incomplete, with approximately two to five times lower concentrations in the fetus compared to the mother. Methadone is rapidly distributed to the fetus from the mother, but concentrations remain lower than maternal concentrations. In comparison to morphine, methadone is cleared from the mother to fetus about 15 times faster and the fetal nonplacental clearance of methadone is also higher than that of morphine.

22.8.8.1.6 *In utero Effect of Opioid Exposure on the Fetus*

Several studies demonstrate that in utero exposure to opioids has physiological effects on the fetus. Fetal monitoring conducted at various time points during gestation demonstrates that buprenorphine-exposed fetuses have higher levels of fetal heart rate variability, more accelerations in fetal heart rate and greater coupling between fetal heart rate and fetal movement. Group differences were found for the number of fetal heart rate accelerations, nonreactive nonstress test (NST) and biophysical profile scores for methadone and buprenorphine-exposed fetuses. Significant decreases occur following methadone and buprenorphine for mean fetal heart rate, fetal heart rate accelerations, reactive NST and fetal movement. Reductions in accelerations and reactive NST were significant only in methadone-exposed fetuses, and this resulted in a lower likelihood of a reactive NST. When comparing buprenorphine to methadone, less suppression of mean fetal heart rate, fetal heart rate reactivity and the biophysical profile score after drug delivery is observed. Methadone-maintained pregnancies are significantly associated with a higher incidence of nonreactive NST, longer intervals to achieve reactive NSTs and lower NST scores compared to controls. This may reflect methadone-induced changes in the fetal CNS neurotransmitters and fetal behavior. Overall, these studies demonstrate that in utero, the delivery of opioids exerts direct effects on the fetus which can be detected using fetal monitoring.

22.8.8.1.7 *Clinical Evidence for Opioid Fetal Toxicity*

Ideally, complete abstinence from opioids during pregnancy is the safest for both mother and fetus; however, opioid discontinuation during pregnancy is not recommended. Repeated cycles of opioid use and cessation are associated with fetal distress that can cause placental insufficiency and subsequent pregnancy loss, intrauterine growth restriction, preterm labor and premature birth. Pregnant mothers with OUDs are commonly placed on long-acting opioid agonist MAT (i.e., methadone or buprenorphine) to prevent potential relapse and overdose. Treatment with methadone and buprenorphine maintains opioid blood levels that reduce maternal drug craving and thus improve pregnancy outcomes in the context of untreated opioid use or opioid withdrawal. Investigations into the relationship between exposure to opioids in utero, including methadone and buprenorphine, are ongoing.

A systemic and meta-analysis review of in utero effects of buprenorphine and methadone on the fetus and child shows potential for spontaneous fetal death, fetal/congenital anomalies, reduced growth outcomes, increased risk of preterm birth, lower birth weight, abnormalities in neurodevelopment and lower head circumference. Several studies evaluated malformations or other defects at birth or pregnancy loss and identified chromosomal defects and cardiovascular, CNS, craniofacial and musculoskeletal malformations.

22.8.8.1.8 *Physical Development*

Numerous studies report reductions in various parameters of growth and physical development. Low birth weight and head circumference are observed following in utero exposure to opioids. The proportion of infants with low birth weights (i.e., <2,500 grams at birth) averages 45% for heroin-exposed infants, 25% for methadone-exposed infants and 15% for unexposed infants. Lowered birth weights of methadone-exposed infants were not related to preterm birth and appear to be related to fetal growth retardation. Lower birth weights are noted in heroin-exposed infants versus methadone. This is likely due to better prenatal care and medical oversight for mothers enrolled in methadone programs. Other parameters of fetal growth include head circumference size and height. Multiple reports demonstrate a reduction of 0.5 to 2.0 cm in opioid-exposed neonates. It is suggested that low birth weight and reduced head circumference are related to symmetric growth retardation as a result of an insult during pregnancy. Indeed, Naeye et al. report low birth weight and brain weight related to a reduced cell number in heroin-exposed fetuses evaluated at a mean gestational age of 30 weeks. Higher proportions of methadone-exposed children are below targeted percentiles for height. Overall, evidence suggests that opioid exposure is at least one contributor to reduced growth in exposed children. Reduced birth weight and head circumference are attributed to intrauterine growth retardation and potential deficits in growth hormone release or reduced uterine/placental blood flow.

22.8.8.1.9 *Behavioral development*

Behavioral deficits are noted in both infants and children following opioid exposure. Clinical and laboratory findings support abnormal neonatal behaviors following in utero exposure to opioid drugs. Infants are hyperresponsive and easily aroused. This pattern may be related to withdrawal; however, neurobehavioral development after the neonatal period also shows abnormal patterns. Rosen et al. showed a greater incidence of neurological abnormalities in methadone-exposed children. These included nystagmus, strabismus, tone and coordination. One study showed behavioral disturbances (hyperactivity, brief attention span, temper outburst) identified in 50% of infants observed one year or longer with 14% also showing neurological abnormalities.

Children born to methadone-maintained mothers have higher predictors of developmental difficulties including delayed motor development, greater vulnerability of males to adverse environmental conditions and behavioral abnormalities. Infants exposed to opioids in utero generally have poor motor coordination, hyperactivity and poor attention spans. Abnormal attentional functioning tends to appear later on (>1 year) and may be an indicator of a permanent neurobehavioral syndrome and related to ADHD.

Studies which have followed opioid-exposed children into early childhood show reduced function in auditory memory and perceptual performance. Johnson et al.

report a higher incidence of abnormal neurological findings in methadone-exposed infants. They report that 45% of methadone-exposed children showed deficits in tone, gross and fine motor coordination, balance and hyperactivity compared to only 20% of unexposed children. Subjective ratings from parents describe opioid-exposed children (ages 3–6 years) as having greater challenges with areas of self-adjustment, social adjustment and physical adjustment. Children were also scored with higher impulsiveness, uncontrolled tempers, poor self-confidence, aggressiveness and difficulty with socializing.

Olofsson et al. evaluated 89 opioid-exposed children at follow-ups ranging from one to ten years and reported only 25% of children with normal physical, mental and behavioral growth. A total of 62% of the children were hyperactive and aggressive with a lack of concentration and social inhibition. Follow-up of children (aged two months to two years, eight months) with drug-addicted mothers showed a small percentage (3/15) exhibiting delayed speech development.

Wilson et al. followed 40 heroin-exposed children through elementary grade levels. Children were between first and fifth grade at the time of assessment. Wilson reports that 65% of opioid-exposed children required special educational services or were withheld from progressing to the next levels of education. Approximately 66% of the children displayed problem behaviors, 50% showed problems with inattention and poor self-discipline and 33% showed low self-confidence, poor peer relations and failure to participate. Behavioral issues in school-aged and adolescents exposed to opioids prenatally emerge strongly during this developmental time frame.

Overall, there is ample evidence suggesting abnormalities in the development of children exposed to opioids prenatally. Physical and behavioral deficits are most notable in the literature. The neurological underpinnings are assumed; however, no studies to date have shown evidence for specific neurological structures affected by opioid exposure in utero.

22.8.8.1.10 *Preclinical Literature*

While clinical data provides the most compelling evidence for opioid-induced fetal toxicity, preclinical studies also provide valuable insights and supporting information. Animal studies suggest that in utero delivery of opioids results in structural and functional changes in the brain and altered behavioral outputs. Methadone-treated offspring show delayed growth, reduced brain weight and length, cerebral width and cerebellar weight and width. Exposure to morphine in utero alters adult hypothalamic norepinephrine levels in male and female rats. Following morphine exposure, norepinephrine content was increased to 95% in the hypothalamus of male rats, whereas in the hypothalamus of female rats, it was decreased by 57% relative to controls. One study demonstrated reduced brain weight and slowing of synaptogenesis and biochemical development of the brain in methadone-exposed pups. Results indicated, in part, that general growth deficits seen in perinatally addicted pups were related to maternal undernutrition, but that delays in central synaptogenesis or in the pattern of biochemical maturation of the brain are independent of nutritional deficit. Furthermore, methadone-exposed pups display a delay in cellular maturation in the brain leading to generalized deficits in critical neural development such as synaptogenesis and synaptic function, involving multiple transmitter systems. Fetal and neonatal methadone exposure results in increased stillbirths among prenatal methadone litters. Long-lasting growth retardation and less emotionality and activity were noted in pups exposed pre- and postnatally to methadone. Rats demonstrate hyper-responsiveness (i.e., more avoidances, escapes and intertrial shuttles) when tested in a massed-trial avoidance procedure following methadone exposure. Behavior was attributed to subtle but lasting changes in limbic dopamine functions as a consequence of fetal exposure to methadone.

22.8.8.1.11 *Nicotine (Smoking) Fetal Toxicity Summary*

While the negative impact of tobacco use has widely been studied and shared through public warnings, tobacco use during pregnancy is estimated in approximately 6.4–7.2% of pregnancies in the United States. An evaluation of 25 million pregnancies reports nearly 9.4% of women smoking before pregnancy and 7.1% during pregnancy, both at high and low intensities. Of interest in this report is the association of prenatal exposure to tobacco smoke and the subsequent effects on the development of the fetus in utero and beyond. A wealth of research and thorough reviews exist detailing the consequences of prenatal nicotine exposure. The evidence is compelling and leaves no doubt that nicotine exposure in utero is responsible for detrimental effects on fetal development across multiple organ systems.

22.8.8.1.12 *Nicotine Mechanism of Action*

The biological effects of nicotine are wide ranging and extend to most organ systems with a higher impact on cardiovascular, respiratory, renal and reproductive systems. Nicotinic acetylcholine receptors (nAChRs) are located throughout the central and peripheral nervous system. These receptors are transmembrane-gated ion channels that respond to ligand binding, facilitating fast synaptic transmission. The neurotransmitter acetylcholine (ACh) is the primary endogenous ligand for nAChRs; however, nicotine can also bind and activate these receptors with high affinity. Nicotine works to produce physiological and pathological effects through three major mechanisms: ganglionic transmission, nAChRs on chromaffin cells via catecholamines and CNS stimulation of nAChRs. The hedonic effects of nicotine are related to the binding of nAChRs and the subsequent release of dopamine in the mesolimbic reward pathway. Nicotine also activates the endogenous opioid system through α-7 nAChRs binding and indirectly alters other neurotransmitter release including norepinephrine, ACh, serotonin, g-aminobutyric acid and glutamate.

Nicotine exposure can cause abnormal activity of nAChRs during critical periods of neural development. Nicotinic acetylcholine receptors are expressed in the first trimester in humans and by the second gestational week in rodents and thus are susceptible to the effects of maternal exposure. Maternal smoking not only has direct nicotinic effects on the fetus but also exposes the fetus to other toxic smoke constituents, such as carbon monoxide and hydrogen cyanide.

22.8.8.1.13 Regulatory Position on Nicotine Use During Pregnancy

The use of nicotine in pregnancy is not recommended and can have serious consequences for the mother and the infant. Under FDA regulation, 21 CFR 1141.10(a), a required warning must be included on tobacco products with (1) a textual warning label statement and (2) a color graphic to accompany the textual warning label statement.

The textual warning label statements are as follows:

- WARNING: Tobacco smoke can harm your children.
- WARNING: Smoking during pregnancy stunts fetal growth.
- WARNING: Tobacco smoke causes fatal lung disease in nonsmokers.
- WARNING: Smoking causes type 2 diabetes, which raises blood sugar.
- WARNING: Smoking reduces blood flow to the limbs, which can require amputation.
- WARNING: Smoking causes cataracts, which can lead to blindness.
- WARNING: Smoking causes bladder cancer, which can lead to bloody urine.
- WARNING: Smoking reduces blood flow, which can cause erectile dysfunction.
- WARNING: Smoking causes head and neck cancer.
- WARNING: Smoking can cause heart disease and strokes by clogging arteries.
- WARNING: Smoking causes COPD, a lung disease that can be fatal.

22.8.8.1.14 Maternal Transfer of Nicotine to Fetus

Nicotine, and its primary metabolite cotinine, readily passes through the placenta to gain access to the fetus. Following maternal exposure, nicotine concentrates in fetal blood, amniotic fluid and breastmilk. Fetal concentrations demonstrate higher (~15%) concentrations than those achieved initially in the mother. Cotinine has a half-life of 15–20 hours and serum concentrations that are approximately ten-fold higher than nicotine concentrations in the bloodstream. A controlled, cross-sectional study conducted in 125 women (62 smokers) identified cotinine and polycyclic aromatic hydrocarbons (PAHs) in the urine and amniotic fluid of pregnant smokers and the umbilical cord blood of their fetuses. The cotinine concentrations in pregnant smokers were approximately six times higher in the urine, 25 times higher in the amniotic fluid and 2.6 times higher in the cord blood when compared to nonsmokers. Additionally, increased fetal exposure to 1-hydroxypyrene was detected, a known carcinogenic substance. Preclinical studies likewise show the passing of nicotine through the placenta into the fetal bloodstream and subsequent activation of fetal nAChRs.

22.8.8.1.15 Effect of Nicotine on Fetal Development

The effect of a toxin during fetal development (e.g., nicotine) depends on the dose and timing of the exposure. Differing developmental processes are at play throughout gestation. Therefore, acute exposure to nicotine may have a more specific impact on select functions developing during that precise timeframe during gestation, whereas chronic exposure will affect many different functions and processes in the developing fetus.

During fetal development, neurotransmitter activation of specific receptors, coupled with cellular differentiation processes, drives the fate of the cell. Overlapping influence during the developmental stage results in the dual involvement of neurotransmitters and receptor types on cellular replication, termination of replication and initiation of differentiation, cell growth, apoptosis and determination of the innate functionality of cellular responses to future stimuli. Nicotinic acetylcholine receptors are expressed during the first trimester in humans, by the time the neural tube is being formed. In the context of nervous system development, ACh plays a critical role in cellular proliferation, maturation and differentiation of multiple types of brain cells. Nicotine activates a specific population of cholinergic targets influencing the multifaceted roles of ACh as a neurotrophic factor. Surplus activity due to in utero nicotine exposure at these receptors can be expected to elicit abnormalities in normal developmental processes. The effect of nicotine through direct or indirect associations with multiple transmitter pathways influences synaptogenesis, neuronal migration, neurotransmitter release and a multitude of other molecular and functional outcomes. Nicotinic cholinergic receptors are major drivers of catecholaminergic function in the CNS, and, as such, the association among other transmitter systems, namely, noradrenergic and dopaminergic synaptic transmissions, is also affected adversely by fetal nicotine exposure. Accordingly, defects may appear after a prolonged period, presenting as in a myriad of cognitive and behavioral defects that appear in childhood or adolescence.

Fetal nicotine exposure upregulates nicotinic receptor binding sites resulting in supersensitive cholinergic trophic responses to target cells. This effect continues through early synaptogenesis, when cholinergic input is critical for structural and functional development in the brain. These effects are likely attributed, at least in part, to cell loss as well as synaptic abnormalities observed following neonatal exposure to nicotine. Deficits in postsynaptic signaling mechanisms are well-recognized and in turn likely contribute to adverse behavioral outcomes. In addition to the altered cholinergic stimulatory response, fetal nicotine exposure alters the ontogeny of cholinergic tone. Developmental disruption by nicotine impacts a variety of cellular outputs ranging from outright cell loss to specific alterations of neural activity, to mis-programming of signaling molecules. Therefore, underlying defects in synaptic function can be identified readily to account for behavioral disruption by fetal nicotine exposure.

Additionally, the detection of PAHs and their metabolites in the fetus following exposure to tobacco smoke also raises concerns regarding the direct effects of PAHs on fetal development. PAHs are responsible for the generation of reactive oxygen species, which generate oxidative stress, lipid peroxidation, protein modifications and DNA damage. Evidence suggests that exposures to certain carcinogenic PAHs during pregnancy may damage fetal DNA through histone modification, potentially resulting in chromosomal abnormalities. PAH-DNA adducts, representative of a critical step in the carcinogenic pathway, are detected in the umbilical cord and maternal blood supply after exposure to ambient air PAHs and dispose the fetus to abnormalities in the cord blood. Critical fetal developmental periods, when the rates of DNA synthesis are high and DNA methylation patterns are being established, may be particularly vulnerable to the negative impact of PAH exposure resulting in epigenetic dysregulation.

22.8.8.1.16 *Clinical Evidence for Nicotine Fetal Toxicity*

Decades of epidemiological studies link prenatal nicotine exposure to spontaneous abortion, neonatal intensive care unit admission, perinatal death, death from SIDS, increased risk of learning disabilities, behavioral abnormalities and ADHD.

22.8.8.1.17 *Physical Development*

A meta-analysis of 20 prospective studies of over 100,000 women found that smoking during pregnancy increased preterm births by approximately 25%. A recent study found that maternal smoking during pregnancy was associated with an increased risk of preterm delivery. Liu et al. performed a dose–response analysis of 25 million mother–infant pairs and found approximately 9.9% of mothers smoked before pregnancy, 7.4% smoked during the first trimester and 6.4% smoked during the second trimester. Of the births, 2,378,398 (9.3%) were preterm births. Low-intensity cigarette consumption that occurred during the first or second trimester of pregnancy (e.g., as low as one to two cigarettes per day), was linked to an increased risk of preterm birth. Smokers who quit before pregnancy, regardless of smoking intensity, showed a comparable risk of preterm birth with nonsmokers.

At birth, nicotine-exposed infants are more likely to have smaller body weights, height and head circumference (effects suggestive of third and possible second-trimester nicotine exposure) and these effects appear to follow a dose–response relationship. Nicotine-exposed children are more likely to have chronic health conditions including impaired function of the endocrine, reproductive, respiratory, cardiovascular and neurologic systems. Multiple studies have shown increased lower respiratory illness in infants born to mothers who smoke. In a study evaluating 12,743 children, increased incidence of bronchitis and hospital admissions for lower respiratory illness during the first five years of life were reported in children with smoking mothers. One study reports that prenatal, but not postnatal, exposure to nicotine was linked with increased lower respiratory illness in children. Large cohort studies have further supported the association between prenatal smoke exposure and reduced respiratory health outcomes. A pooled analysis of 21,000 children showed maternal smoking during pregnancy was associated with an increased likelihood of wheezing and asthma in children at four to six years of age. A longitudinal study conducted over 10 years in 6,000 children demonstrated that in utero smoke exposure was independently associated with asthma. Developmental deficits in offspring lung function and health include increased hospitalization for respiratory infections, increased prevalence of childhood wheeze and asthma, decreases in forced expiratory flows and decreased passive respiratory compliance. Low birth weight and premature birth are also important risk factors for altered lung development.

Nicotine is also linked to the increased likelihood of birth defects (e.g., limb reduction and oral clefts). Maternal smoking is associated with reduced head size, abdominal circumference and femur length. Furthermore, higher-intensity maternal cigarette use was associated with a lower head size compared to lower-intensity use. A meta-analysis of 24 studies estimated that mothers who smoked during pregnancy had a 1.3-fold increased risk of having a baby with cleft lip with or without cleft palate and a 1.2-fold risk of cleft palate alone.

Findings for cardiovascular and metabolic influences of fetal smoke exposure are suggestive and varied. One review found that maternal smoking during pregnancy is associated with higher blood pressure, obesity, adverse cardiovascular diseases and type 2 diabetes in children and adults.

22.8.8.1.18 *Behavioral Development*

In utero exposure to tobacco smoke has been related to numerous adverse behavioral effects in newborns, infants, children, adolescents and adults. Behavioral effects range from poor academic performance to significant behavioral disruptions, including ADHD, aggressive behaviors and future substance abuse.

Newborns exposed in utero to nicotine are more irritable and have poorer attention spans than unexposed infants and often exhibit hypertonicity, increased tremors and startle responses and deficient speech processing. Exposed infants also show signs of poor self-regulation and require more handling by caregivers. Newborns demonstrate an attenuated response to auditory stimuli, an effect that notably contributes to deficits in language and learning function later in life.

A review of observational studies conducted between 2000 and 2011 on the association between prenatal nicotine exposure and cognitive outcomes in children found that the most consistent results were observed for reduced academic achievement and impaired intellectual abilities. Children aged six and younger show increased risk of language impairment, decreased receptive language skills and poor performance on language tasks which can contribute to language comprehension deficits. Exposed children also show poorer academic performance and cognitive scores and impaired reading performance.

A small, controlled study evaluated children exposed prenatally to tobacco in a working memory task combined with fMRI. Children exposed to tobacco show greater activation in inferior parietal regions of the brain, whereas unexposed children showed greater activation in inferior frontal regions. The differential activation of various brain regions was observed following correct responses, suggesting that abnormalities exist in neural circuitry between exposed and unexposed children. Another fMRI study found differences in regional brain morphometry and impulsivity in adolescents who were exposed prenatally to tobacco. In adolescents, pallidum volume was reduced and increased impulsivity was correlated with thalamic volume following prenatal tobacco exposure, further demonstrating differences in structural brain maturation during adolescence.

Prenatal exposure to nicotine appears to be a primary contributor to attention disorders. Evidence suggests that children as young as six years old show attentional deficits, including a clinical diagnosis of ADHD. Smoking exposure during the second and third trimesters have been correlated to attention problems. In preschool-aged children, increases in scores on Oppositional Behavior, Immaturity, Emotional Instability, Physical Aggression and Activity scales were related to prenatal tobacco exposure. Oppositional behavior was correlated to third-trimester nicotine exposure. Similar behavioral issues, including aggression, oppositional defiance and delinquency, have been noted in older children (6–16 years old).

22.8.8.19 Nicotine, Perinatal Mortality and SIDS

Fetal development is also influenced by nicotinic actions outside of the CNS. Evidence suggests that deficits in neonatal cardiovascular and/or respiratory function underlie SIDS, a condition where cardiorespiratory failure occurs during the presentation of a hypoxic episode (predictably from an airway obstruction or sleep apnea). Survival during fetal or neonatal hypoxia requires cellular responses that relate to the autonomous secretion of adrenal catecholamines and appropriate adrenergic receptor populations in the myocardium. Maternal smoking during pregnancy is considered a risk factor for SIDS. Nicotine exposure results in a diminished or absence of the adrenomedullary response to hypoxia, presenting a significant deficiency in normal autonomic functioning. The fetal and neonatal heart are not fully developed with incomplete neural connections and therefore are dependent on circulating catecholamines for stimulation. The loss of adrenal responsiveness is correlated with SIDS in infants with prenatal exposure to nicotine.

22.8.8.1.20 Preclinical Literature Support for Nicotine/Smoking Fetotoxicity

Preclinically, nicotine exposure in utero is associated with abnormal respiratory, myocardium and catecholamine response. Animals exposed prenatally to nicotine also lack the autonomous adrenomedullary secretory response. This occurs in conjunction with a reduction in stimulatory beta-adrenergic receptors in the myocardium and a reduced cardiac response to adrenergic stimulation. Mice exposed in utero to nicotine develop abnormal respiratory responses to hypoxia and depressed responses to intermittent hypoxia. Additionally, mice lacking functional nAChRs demonstrate similar respiratory responses as nicotine-exposed pups. Nicotine administration to pregnant baboons results in offspring with altered serotonergic and nAChR binding in the medulla, a critical area responsible for the regulation of cardiorespiratory output. In normal functioning animals, exposure to hypoxic environments results in the secretion of approximately 40% of the entire catecholamine content of the adrenal, whereas animals exposed to nicotine secrete little to no catecholamines. The resulting cardiac consequence presents as an immediate decline in heart rate in a low-oxygen environment and increased mortality in animals following an extended period of hypoxia.

In vitro and in vivo preclinical studies provide compelling evidence for adverse effects in the nervous, respiratory, immune and cardiovascular systems, following nicotine exposure, particularly when exposure occurs during critical developmental periods of gestation. Injections of nicotine into pregnant rats throughout gestation result in cell damage to the fetal brain, including abnormal development of neurotransmitter systems, that is, neuronal cell loss, increased glia, decreases in cell size, changes to spine density, dendritic length and dendritic branching. These neural alterations impact development and contribute to the functional deficits observed later in life. Continuous infusion of nicotine via osmotic minipumps further shows detrimental effects including fetal resorption and neurological damage. Some studies suggest that acute exposure to nicotine initiates a change in long-term cell development with long-lasting effects on cell loss. Overexpression of c-fos, a proto-oncogene, is observed in postnatal brain regions following prenatal nicotine exposure. It is suggested that apoptosis contributes to brain cell loss caused by fetal nicotine exposure and that neuronal loss is irreversible.

Consistent with clinical reports, multiple rodent studies show reductions in fetal weight following nicotine exposure. Animal models of learning, memory and sensory processing also detect deficits in these processes following nicotine exposure. Rodents exposed in utero to nicotine show performance deficits on associated tests of learning, memory and sensory functions, including the radial arm maze, Morris water maze and two-way active avoidance. These findings further support clinical evidence that prenatal nicotine exposure alters long-term learning, memory and sensory function through development. Deficits were largely attributed to abnormalities in nicotinic acetylcholine receptors and related disruptions in neural transmission processes.

22.8.8.1.21 Conclusions

A clear relationship exists between the use of opioids and nicotine exposure in utero and the acute and long-lasting impact on infant and child development. There is no question that opioids and/or nicotine ingested by the mother are transferred to the fetus and can cause extensive damage. In utero opioid and nicotine exposure produces developmental disruption at the cellular level. These developmental abnormalities are likely to involve associated transmitter systems involved in neural development. Opioid and nicotine exposure impacts the fetal brain at critical stages of gestation in pregnant women. The subsequent effects at the cellular levels with regard to neural development likely account for the cognitive, emotional and behavioral problems observed in these children.

An abundance of literature suggests that opioid exposure in utero may have an acute and long-lasting impact on infant and child development. There is no question that maternal ingestion of opioids results in transfer to the fetus with direct actions that are detectable in utero. Perinatal opioid exposure delays physical growth and interferes with normal behavioral outcomes, likely due to the augmented development of the nervous system. The majority of reports show behavioral and motor complications: hyper-responsiveness, impulsivity, reduced self-control, poor motor coordination and poor attentional focus. While the underlying mechanisms are unclear, preclinical evidence supports reductions in neural development which produces generalized deficits in synaptogenesis and synaptic function and the involvement of multiple transmitter systems. These neural effects could play a causal role in the behavioral deficits observed in opioid fetal toxicity.

22.8.8.2 Expert Pharmacologist Opinions Related to the Child's Fetal Exposure and Residual Effects From In Utero Exposure

Many of the child's current diagnoses are documented to be associated with in utero exposure to maternal use of opiates and smoking/nicotine. These include cognitive impairment, developmental delays, behavior notable for marked inattention, impulsivity, behavioral disturbances and ADHD. Methadone and nicotine exposures in utero must be considered as contributory to these deficits. Based on all of the reports in the clinical and preclinical literature, the documented mechanisms of fetal neurotoxicity and the documented in utero exposure of the child, it is my opinion that methadone and nicotine contributed to the child's current and ongoing neurological deficits.

22.8.9 Effects of Lisinopril on Fetus—Defense of Causation

22.8.9.1 Materials Reviewed

1. Medical, obstetrical, pediatric and pharmacy records for the mother and child.
2. Published scientific and clinical literature on the pregnancy exposure effects of ACEIs and ARBs on fetal development and post-partum effects cited as endnotes.
3. Published literature on the determination of causation of adverse drug effects as well as Pregnancy Classifications (as discussed in the report), which I reviewed to aid in the development of my professional opinions of the issues in this case.
4. Standards of Practice for the Profession of Pharmacy.

22.8.9.2 Facts of the Case

Ms. Patient is an R.N. with a diagnosis of Type II diabetes since age 16 with a known family history of diabetes (father, maternal grandfather, paternal grandmother). From what I reviewed in the medical records, the patient's blood sugar was not well-controlled with a reading above 200 mg/dl and an A1C of 14.4 (which is more than twice normal) in 2016. I also reviewed notes of diabetic noncompliance—February 2016 recommendation for follow-up with endocrinology which was not followed—see August notes of a medical assistant with her obstetrician's office.

At age 28, additional past medical history included long-standing hypertension and hypothyroidism. Medications which I noted in her records included lisinopril, metformin and Synthroid. At the age of 32, Ms. Patient experienced a spontaneous abortion. The medical records for that time period again note the past medical history of Type II diabetes, hypertension with a blood pressure of 156/104 and hypothyroidism. Medications were Lantus and again, lisinopril, metformin and Synthroid.

In the first MFM office visit in August 2016, Ms. Patient was determined to be at five weeks' gestation, with a due date of April 23, 2017. During that office visit, she had a blood pressure of 155/104 and serial blood pressures were 155/104 and 178/105 and she was started on labetalol 200 mg b.i.d. in place of lisinopril.

The above visit was with a nurse practitioner, who documented thatPregestational diabetes complicating pregnancy is associated with an increased risk of maternal, fetal and neonatal complications including miscarriage, congenital anomalies, fetal growth abnormalities, amniotic fluid imbalances, maternal and fetal birth trauma, NICU admission, preeclampsia and still birth. These complications were discussed with the patient today. Risks of these complications are significantly decreased by achieving optimal glycemic control prior to and during pregnancy. Glycemic goals in pregnancy include fasting/pre-meal blood sugars of 70–90 mg/di and one-hour postprandial blood sugars of < 135 mg/di.

A fetal ultrasound was also performed that day and interpreted by Orion Rust, M.D., who documented, Singleton IUP 6 weeks and 0 days by this ultrasound (EDD = APR 25 2017).

Ms. Patient was seen by an endocrinologist in late August. He updated her diabetes diagnosis to Type II diabetes. During this visit, the patient was noted to have significant gestational edema and 2+ pitting edema with weight gain of close to 20 lbs. Blood pressure was improved at 144/88, but the patient's blood sugar remained elevated despite counseling—HGBA1C on 8/18/16 was 14.4.

During this office visit, the endocrinologist documented, "I discussed the risk of congenital malformations and miscarriage give her high initial A1c. I reviewed goal ranges for optimal glycemic control. Start bid Lantus and Novolog was adjusted–see instructions. Fu 4 wks. with repeat A1c."

On 8/30/16, there was a pregnancy diabetic counseling session documented with a dietitian with the MFM practice. The patient was instructed on monitoring and evaluation for:

1. Carbohydrate intake, fat/cholesterol intake, protein intake
2. Weight body composition
3. Glucose monitoring

During the next MFM office visit on 9/7/16, the patient was seen and evaluated by a nurse practitioner. Initial BP today was 180/100, and on recheck it was 156/84. The provider documented, "She is following her meal plan most of the time but is very active and busy at work and does not get much time to inject insulin/eat on schedule." The patient was instructed—increase Procardia *(nifedipine)* to 60 mg QD and will check her BP at work Friday and email the results. Blood glucose logs continued to show elevated glucose, 120s to 190s.

9/13.16, she was six weeks and three days gestation by ultrasound findings and due date. Amniotic fluid volume was normal. Blood pressures were 162/82 and 158/84. Weight was 166 pounds for a total weight gain of 23 pounds. With 4+ pitting edema in the mid-thigh and ongoing elevated systolic blood pressures, the record indicates that an MFM physician documented by way of history for systolic blood pressure control, the patient had been started on Lisinopril in the past for renal protection, not really for HTN. Had been off that for many years. Had seen her family doctor a few times this year with elevated BPs but not formally given the diagnosis and was not on any meds. BPs very elevated at initial visit—was initially started on labetalol—the day she stared labetalol, she started having significant SOB and CP. EKG and echo were normal. Labetalol was switched to Procardia XL and her CP and SOB resolved, although her BPs are still high. The physician intended to add 25 mg of hydrochlorothiazide to her medication regimen. Inadvertently, hydrochlorothiazide with benazepril was checked in the EMR (Lotensin HCT), resulting in the issuance of a prescription for Lotensin HCT *(benazepril and hydrochlorothiazide combination)*.

On September 13, 2016, an ultrasound was performed which estimated a then-current gestational age of eight weeks four days. The LMP of this 32-year-old, gravida 2, para 0, patient was July 17, 2016, giving her an EDD of APR 23, 2017, and a current gestational age of eight weeks two days by dates.

Blood pressure on 10/13/16 was 134/78 and swelling had improved. Ultrasound at that time showed normal amniotic fluid volume and growth. In the next endocrine examination, blood pressure again edged up at 130/78 and aspirin was started for preeclampsia prophylaxis. The patient also had vision problems that were noted around this time period and was diagnosed with diabetic retinopathy.

The patient took Lotensin HCT from 9/13/16 at 8w2d until 11/10/16 at 14+ weeks gestation when the medication error was noted. At that time, an ultrasound was performed which revealed anhydramnios and the Lotensin HCT was immediately discontinued and replaced by Procardia XL) 30mg 24 hr. tablet. The patient was directed to drink plenty of fluids and amniotic fluid increased and the infant measured nine days behind in growth. Throughout the remainder of the pregnancy with serial ultrasounds, the fluid levels improved.

The first trimester is generally considered to end at 13 6/7 weeks, with the second trimester starting at 14 0/7 weeks, as defined by LMP. The LMP of this 32-year-old, gravida 2, para 0, patient was on July 17, 2016, giving her an EDD of APR 23, 2017. The patient entered the second trimester on 10/24/16—she was at 14 0/7 weeks on 10/23/16. Lotensin HCT was administered for eight weeks and two days starting on 9/13/16 in the first trimester until 11/10/16. Therefore, the patient took Lotensin for only 16 days of the second trimester.

The mother's blood pressure remained controlled on Procardia until late February 2017, but the record reflects that glucose levels remained high. On February 28, after elevated blood pressure readings at home, the patient reported to a local hospital for evaluation with chronic hypertension with superimposed preeclampsia at 32 weeks gestation.

This patient's medical and obstetric history is referenced to demonstrate pregnancy risk factors and relevant treatment and findings:

1. Longstanding hypertension, Type II diabetes (since age 16) with a known family history of diabetes—father, maternal grandfather, paternal grandmother and hypothyroidism. Although the past medical records indicate that lisinopril, metformin and Synthroid were prescribed, reviewing the Wegman's Pharmacy records that cover the

period from 1/1/09 to 1/7/19 indicates that none of these medications were ever filled.

2. During a 2/22/16 office visit, when she first tested positive for pregnancy (resulting in spontaneous abortion), she was counseled to follow-up with an endocrinologist because her glucose levels were fluctuating and she had not seen an endocrinologist in years. The record indicates that she was going to follow-up with an endocrinologist, but the records show that she never did and the pharmacy records show no medications for diabetes control.
3. From 2012 through 2016, the patient's blood pressure from the records indicates 150s to 160s over 100. Thus, it appears that the patient, a registered nurse, despite knowing the effects of uncontrolled diabetes and hypertension, took no steps to control or treat either condition before attempting to get pregnant. In August of 2016, when she called into the Medical Clinic about a positive pregnancy test, her hemoglobin A1c was 14.4 and her blood pressure continued to run high in the 150s/100. She was five weeks pregnant at that point. At that point, she was already 1 month into her pregnancy.
4. The patient saw an endocrinologist on 8/30/16. During this visit, blood pressure was recorded at 144/88 and there was a significant weight gain of 18.5 pounds (140 pre-pregnancy weight to 158.5 pounds) with 2+ pitting edema. The endocrinologist documented a discussion regarding the profoundly elevated hemoglobin A1c (14.4%) and the increased risk of congenital malformations as well as miscarriage from hypertension and diabetes.
5. The physician had difficulty controlling the patient's continued high blood pressure. The MFM physician (a defendant in the case) intended to prescribe hydrochlorothiazide (HCTZ) as prior prescriptions of labetalol 20 mg and Procardia 30 mg and then Procardia 60 mg. were ineffective. When the MFM physician entered the prescription for HCTZ into the EPIC record, she inadvertently clicked the prescription for Lotensin HCT. The patient took Lotensin HCT for 8 weeks from 9/13/16 at 8w2d until 11/10/16, at 15 weeks gestation 7 weeks during the first trimester and only 16 days during the second trimester. Angiotensin-converting enzyme inhibitors are not recommended in the second and third trimesters only. It should be recognized that vesicoureteral reflux (VUR) is not causally caused by Lotensin usage—here 16 days is a limited exposure and the exposure for the entire second and third trimesters does not cause VUR or heart congenital defects or premature birth or prolonged development; however, diabetes and hypertension do result in premature birth or prolonged development. The mother's blood pressure remained controlled on Procardia until late February 2017. On February 28, after elevated blood pressure readings at home, the patient reported to the local hospital for evaluation with chronic hypertension with superimposed preeclampsia at 32 weeks gestation.
6. When the patient underwent an ultrasound on 11/10/16, anhydramnios was noted. The prior ultrasound on 10/18/16 revealed normal amniotic fluid and normal growth. This is when the Lotensin was discontinued and the mother was instructed to drink plenty of fluids. On the next ultrasound on 11/12/16, amniotic fluid was improved—mild oligohydramnios and normal thereafter. Fetal growth by ultrasound appeared normal by 11/22/16. If there was any connection, it was minimal and quickly returned to normal.
7. On 2/28/17 (32+1 weeks), blood pressure again increased—to 140–150/90 and the patient was instructed to come in for triage. She was admitted with blood pressures running 109–179/59–101 and the baby was in breach position. The child was delivered by C-section on March 3, 2017, at 32 weeks and five days due to a breech presentation. APGAR scores were 7 and 8, and the child weighed 3 lbs. 3 oz. at birth and was admitted to the NICU.

According to my review of the legal pleading in this matter, the parents, on behalf of the child have brought a claim alleging that the child has a number of diagnoses/medical conditions, which they claim resulted from the limited exposure to Lotensin HCT, specifically VUR, congenital cardiac issue, premature birth and developmental delay.

The child was seen in consultation on October 27, 2018, by a urologist at a university-affiliated children's hospital. He reported that the child is a 19-month-old female with a history of febrile urinary tract infections and VUR. An initial diagnosis of VUR was in May 2017, which followed a pyelonephritis infection in March 2017. One urologist's diagnosis was Grade 3 VUR; a second urologist's diagnosis was Grade 2. On review of the VCUG (voiding cystourethrography), he felt that the patient had a Grade 2 VUR and not a grade 3. The child had been treated with Bactrim prophylaxis with the last urinary tract infection on July 19, 2018. The university urologist did not recommend surgical intervention but recommended a DMSA (dimercapto succinic acid)—a renal scan to evaluate for scarring. Surgery was not felt to be necessary as the child grows.

A renal ultrasound was performed on February 5, 2020, which was reported as totally normal. On the same date, a voiding cystourethrogram was performed and was interpreted as a bilateral grade 3 VUR, which differs from the diagnosis of a grade 2 VUR.

With regard to the allegation of a congenital heart defect, I also reviewed an echocardiogram dated August 15, 2019, which was totally normal.

As indicated earlier, the plaintiff's complaint alleges complications of bilateral VUR (Grade 2 or Grade 3)—

differing diagnoses by two different urologists, congenital heart defect, resolved; gastroesophageal reflux which appears to have resolved; external rotation of the right foot and developmental delay (communication, physical skills, weight <1%). None of these conditions, in my professional pharmacologic opinion to a reasonable degree of medical certainty, are related to or caused by the maternal use of Lotensin. Previously diagnosed patent ductus arteriosus (PDA) and ventricular septal defect (VSD) have resolved/closed, as evidenced by an ECHO on August 19, 2019.

22.8.9.3 Assignment

You have asked that I review and evaluate the medical records of care and the pharmacologic features of the antihypertensive medications administered in this matter as well as their potential side effects and provide my expert pharmacologic opinions on the effects of the administration of Lotensin HCT generally and specifically in this case during the first versus second trimester, as well as describe the effects of non-ACE inhibitors (other drugs used to treat hypertension), hypertension and diabetes (drugs and disease) on the same periods and fetal outcomes. I have specifically focused my pharmacologic opinions on any causation and risk exposure links to provide opinions on the relationship between any medical diagnoses of the child including VUR as well as the fetal exposure to the Benazapril-HCTZ and any downstream effects of that medication.

22.8.9.4 Opinions

All of my opinions are based upon my education, training, experience and relevant scientific literature (cited as endnotes) and expressed with reasonable medical, pharmacological and pharmaceutical certainty.

1. Lotensin usage during the limited exposure in this case (16 days into the second trimester) did not cause any of the conditions that the child was diagnosed with—VUR, heart congenital defect—resolved, premature birth and delayed development. Lotensin usage has no adverse effects when used during the first trimester and is not known to and did not cause these conditions when used as it was for 16 days of the second trimester. There is *no* scientific or clinical evidence supporting any relationship between the fetal exposure of Lotensin HCT (benazepril-HCT) and any of the conditions alleged. More specifically, the VUR currently experienced by the child is specifically unrelated to fetal exposure to Lotensin HCT (benazepril-HCT). This opinion is based upon my experience and my review of the evidence of fetotoxicity of ACE and ARB, which is devoid of any mention of VUR, as well as the literature describing the epidemiology (cause) of VUR, as detailed in the BASES FOR OPINIONS section of this report.
2. VUR is a common condition in premature female children.
3. Premature birth is known to occur from diabetes and hypertension. Developmental delay is known to be associated with high-risk pregnancy. The infant is the product of a high-risk pregnancy with pre-treatment uncontrolled diabetes and high blood pressure. These conditions are well-known to cause intraocular hemorrhage, prematurity and small for gestational age. External rotation of the right foot and developmental delay are not related in any way to Lotensin exposure. While there is sparse literature suggesting structural cardiac effects following ACEI and ARBs in the second trimester, the PDA and VSD that were originally identified have resolved—closed. Frankly, these cardiac findings are present absent any risk factors in a large percentage of newborns. Moreover, the cardiac condition appears to have resolved as evidenced by the normal ECG referenced earlier.
4. Ms. Patient, an R.N., was warned by a caution label affixed on the prescription vial of benazepril-HCTZ that it is not to be taken while pregnant.

—DO NOT USE IF YOU ARE PREGNANT—

5. The prescription vial contained a printed warning: **Do not use if you become pregnant**. Also, pharmacies routinely provide patient information with prescriptions that would have contained a similar warning not to take if pregnant.
6. The local pharmacy would and should have provided Ms. Patient with a MEDICATION GUIDE) which warns in red box letters:

IMPORTANT WARNING:

Do not take benazepril if you are pregnant. If you become pregnant while taking benazepril, call your doctor immediately. Benazepril may harm the fetus.

7. The pharmacist dispensing the benazepril-HCTZ prescription to Ms. Patient would and should have inquired/advised regarding Ms. Patient's pregnancy status and, upon learning thereof, contacted the MFM physician immediately to advise of the risk of benazepril during pregnancy. The prescription would have identified the prescriber as a Maternal—Fetal Medicine/OBGYN physician, which in and of itself would have alerted the pharmacist to the likelihood of Ms. Patient being pregnant, the need for pharmacist intervention and the potential risk to the fetus.
8. The mother is identified as an ICU Nurse. She certainly would have had the training and awareness of the risks of medications in general, a realization/appreciation of the need to read labels and

instructions and to heed cautions and the ability to research the pregnancy risk of any drugs prescribed to her, and if indeed she was cautioned by the pharmacist/vial label, known not to take the drug without first contacting her (defendant) physician.

22.8.9.5 Bases for Opinions

A cautionary warning of fetal toxicity is included in the FDA-approved Lotensin HCT (benazepril with hydrochlorothiazide) labeling (Package Insert) which states):

Fetal toxicity
Pregnancy

The use of drugs that act on the renin-angiotensin system *during the second and third trimesters* of pregnancy reduces fetal renal function and increases fetal and neonatal morbidity and death. Resulting oligohydramnios can be associated with fetal lung hypoplasia and skeletal deformations. Potential neonatal adverse effects include skull hypoplasia, anuria, hypotension, renal failure and death. When pregnancy is detected, discontinue Lotensin HCT as soon as possible. These adverse outcomes are usually associated with the use of these drugs in the second and third trimesters of pregnancy. Most epidemiologic studies examining fetal abnormalities after exposure to antihypertensive use in the first trimester have not distinguished drugs affecting the renin-angiotensin system from other antihypertensive agents. Appropriate management of maternal hypertension during pregnancy is important to optimize outcomes for both mother and fetus.

22.8.9.6 Mechanism of Action

Benazepril and benazepril inhibit ACE in human subjects and in animals. ACE is a peptidyl dipeptidase that catalyzes the conversion of angiotensin I to the vasoconstrictor substance, angiotensin II. Angiotensin II also stimulates aldosterone secretion by the adrenal cortex. Inhibition of ACE results in decreased plasma angiotensin II, which leads to decreased vasopressor activity and decreased aldosterone secretion. The latter decrease may result in a small increase in serum potassium. Hydrochlorothiazide is a thiazide diuretic. Thiazides affect the renal tubular mechanisms of electrolyte reabsorption, directly increasing the excretion of sodium and chloride in approximately equivalent amounts. Indirectly, the diuretic action of hydrochlorothiazide reduces plasma volume, with consequent increases in plasma renin activity, increases in aldosterone secretion, increases in urinary potassium loss and decreases in serum potassium. Intrauterine exposure to thiazide diuretics is associated with fetal or neonatal jaundice, thrombocytopenia and possibly other adverse reactions that have occurred in adults.

NOTE: VUR is not recognized as a risk of taking or causally related to Lotensin usage and is not noted in the warning.

22.8.9.7 Preclinical Toxicology Literature

No teratogenic effects were seen when benazepril and hydrochlorothiazide were administered to pregnant rats at a dose ratio of 4:5. On a mg/kg basis, the doses used were up to 167 times the maximum recommended human dose. Similarly, no teratogenic effects were seen when benazepril and hydrochlorothiazide were administered to pregnant mice at total doses up to 160 mg/kg/day, with benazepril/hydrochlorothiazide ratios of 15:1. When hydrochlorothiazide was orally administered without benazepril to pregnant mice and rats during their respective periods of major organogenesis, at doses up to 3,000 and 1,000 mg/kg/day respectively, there was no evidence of harm to the fetus. Similarly, no teratogenic effects of benazepril were seen in studies of pregnant rats, mice and rabbits; on a mg/kg basis, the doses used in these studies were 300 times (in rats), 90 times (in mice) and more than three times (in rabbits) the maximum recommended human dose.

FDA Pregnancy categories have been published from 1980 until revised in 2015. These are excerpted and presented earlier in this chapter.

ACE inhibitors (Lotensin) are classified as *Category C* for the first trimester and *Category D* for the second and third trimesters.

22.8.9.8 Methodology of Determining Causation

The evaluation (methodology) of drug-induced adverse effects is well established and has application to understanding a lack of proven causal relation between the very short period of second-trimester exposure of the Rinaldi child in utero and her current conditions and claims in this matter. My opinion that VUR is *not* related to Lotensin HCT exposure is supported by presenting the evidence of results of studies and testing of fetotoxicity of ACE and ARB, which is devoid of any mention of VUR, premature birth or developmental delay; this conclusion is also supported by the literature describing the epidemiology (cause) of VUR, which is also devoid of any mention of ACEI, ARB, fetal exposure to drugs or oligoamnios. Relevant scientific literature is cited as endnotes. The full text of each cited article is provided with this report.

The ACE inhibitors are warned against during pregnancy, especially during the late second and third trimesters, unless the patient's hypertension cannot be controlled by other therapies.

No evidence exists supporting Lotensin's (ACEI) negative effects during the first trimester of pregnancy. First-trimester effects were suggested by one study but have not been confirmed in other studies. According to Reprotox, first-trimester pregnancy exposure to ACE inhibitors was studied largely by combining exposures to all agents of the ACE inhibitor group, and the studies therefore referenced are not directly on point or reliable. They report that available data is not sufficient to conclude that first-trimester use of ACE inhibitors alters the risk of congenital defects. Reprotox cites several case studies, but none were conclusive or reliable enough to establish a direct causal link between ACE inhibitor usage during the first trimester and birth defects. I have chosen to identify in this report, *a meta-analysis that referenced a number of the case studies and concluded that exposure to ACE Inhibitors during the first trimester did not increase the risk for malformations than exposure to any other* antihypertensives. According to my review of the literature, beginning in 1992, the US FDA required a warning on all ACEI fetotoxic effects when used during the second and third trimesters.

According to Reprotox, administration of ACEI during these precautioned periods (second and third trimesters) is associated with renal damage, cranial ossification defects, oligohydramnios and delayed intrauterine growth. Fetal damage may be mediated by the hypotension caused by the drug rather than by a direct action of the drug. The inhibitors of angiotensin II (ARB), more recently in use, have shown the same effects as the ACE inhibitors; therefore, even their use is warned against during pregnancy. Lotensin exposure in the second trimester here was so limited with a quick return to normal amniotic fluid within one week of discontinuance, and fetal growth was normal by ultrasound dated 11/22/16.

At present, the drug of choice for hypertension during pregnancy is alpha-methyldopa. Drugs of second choice would be beta-blockers or calcium antagonists. Ms. Patient had been treated before her pregnancy with a beta blocker—labetalol, but it caused an adverse effect (significant blood pressure drop—hypotension) and was discontinued. A calcium-channel blocker was prescribed when the Lotensin was discontinued. Incidentally, the oligoamnios was discovered following a period of severe and symptomatic hypotension (BP 80/50), which in and of itself can cause the oligoamnios by decreasing renal perfusion and thus formation of amniotic fluid.

An abundance of literature describes known fetotoxic and post-partum residual toxicities to fetal exposure to ACE inhibitors and ARBs. Benazepril is an ACEI. For purposes of this report, both ACEI and ARB drugs are considered to impart the same fetotoxic risks. The literature is cited hereafter as endnotes; each is provided in full text as well. Human kidney development begins in the first trimester. During *the late second and third trimesters, there is an exponential increase in nephrons between 18 and 32 weeks.* Nephron development is complete between 32 and 36 weeks. Fetal urine becomes a major contributor to amniotic fluid at about 20 weeks. After term birth, no new nephrons are formed. The growth of the kidney to adult size is solely based on hypertropia.

As presented in the case details, Lotensin exposure started in the first trimester (LMP to 13 6/7 weeks) at 8 weeks gestation and lasted almost 14 weeks gestation, based upon time from LMP. Thus, there is an extremely limited actual time of Lotensin fetal exposure and as indicated, amniotic fluid development, which is a direct measure of fetal renal function, quickly returned to normal within 1 week of the discontinuance of Lotensin, and fetal growth was normalized by November 22, 12 days after Lotensin was discontinued. Again, in my experience and opinion, Lotensin usage during the first trimester and 16 days of the second trimester had no causal connection to the VUR and growth restriction and developmental delay alleged in this matter.

22.8.9.9 ACE Inhibitors and ARBs

Renal toxicity of fetal exposure to ACEIs or ARBs (ATI antagonists) during the mid- to late second and/or third trimester is not debated. It results in renal tubular dysgenesis (absence or poor development of proximal tubules), fetal anuria leading to oligohydramnios and the Potter sequence of facial dysmorphia, limb-positioning defect and lung hypoplasia associated with skull ossification defect. The syndrome has been named fetal renin-angiotensin-system blockade syndrome. Clinical evolution is variable, from in utero death to postnatal survival with persistent renal symptoms or to complete recovery but always with short follow-up data. None of these findings were present or claimed to be caused by the Lotensin exposure in the Rinaldi child and there was no Lotensin exposure during the mid- to late second trimester through the third trimester.

22.8.9.10 Mechanism of ACEI Fetotoxicity

The mechanism of toxicity is as follows. Fetal urine production and kidney function start at the end of the first trimester. ACEs appear at about 26 weeks gestation. ACE inhibitors reduce the tonus of kidney vessels and, therefore, urine production is reduced. This is followed by oligohydramnios. Beyond the sixteenth gestational week, fetal urine production is the main source of the amniotic fluid. Similar developmental disturbances were observed in experimental animal studies with high doses of ACE inhibitors. The period of time of ingestion of Lotensin by Ms. Rinaldi here is from the 8th to the 14th+ week and temporarily is unrelated.

22.8.9.10.1 Oligohydramnios

The case summary states that on November 17, 2016, during an office visit, the patient was diagnosed with oligohydramnios. Oligohydramnios is a deficiency of amniotic fluid. Urine production in the fetus is related to the regulation of the amniotic fluid volume. Amniotic fluid provides some protection from pathogenic bacteria during fetal life. The amniotic fluid compartment provides the fetus space to grow, move about and develop. Without this space, the uterus can constrain the fetus and restrict development. Potter syndrome is a condition caused by oligohydramnios where the affected fetus develops pulmonary hypoplasia, limb deformities and characteristic facies. Agenesis of the fetal kidneys is the most common cause which is due to the lack of fetal urine. Oligohydramnios is associated with drug exposure, including ACE inhibitors. None of these abnormalities are diagnosed in the Rinaldi child nor are they claimed to be caused by the Lotensin exposure.

22.8.9.11 Definition and Occurrence and Epidemiology of VUR

VUR is the only documented urinary tract finding; it is not associated with ACEI fetal exposure, and there are no other findings associated with ACEI fetal exposure. *Importantly, no association between fetal drug exposure, including ACEI and ARB or anhydromnios or oligoamnios are discussed, considered or identified as being causative for post-natal VUR*. The prevalence of vesicoureteric reflux in the general population is 1% to 2% of children; it is the most common congenital urological anomaly and is increased in certain risk groups, such as children with symptomatic urinary tract infection, schoolgirls with asymptomatic bacteriuria, first-degree relatives of patients with reflux and children with prenatal dilatation of their upper urinary tract. VUR may be present in 0.4–1.8% of normal healthy children, with the lower figure probably being more accurate.

One investigator performed ultrasonography on 3,856 fetuses after 28 weeks of gestation. When anomalies were identified the newborns and babies were evaluated at 6 days and 6 weeks of age. VUR was identified in 14 children. The incidence of VUR was estimated to be 3.6 per 1,000 births. Another research group, Najmaldin et al., presented the results from routine obstetric ultrasonography carried out between 28 and 39 weeks of gestation and discussed their findings relative to prenatal ultrasound and post-natal VUR and UTI. When anomalies were identified the newborns and babies were evaluated at 6 days and 6 weeks of age.

None of these reviews on the epidemiology/causation of VUR mention or refer to ACEIs.

Nino et al. reviewed the genetics of VUR (*Current Genomics*, 2016, 17, 79–79). They identified VUR as a complex genetic developmental disorder, the result of a shortened intravesical ureter with an enlarged or mal-positioned ureteric orifice. Previous studies show a heterogeneous genetic pattern of VUR. No single major locus or gene for primary VUR has been identified. Mutations in genes that are critical for urinary tract morphogenesis are associated with a multitude of congenital syndromes, of which most show VUR as a feature. Importantly, this review article does not mention any role of ACE inhibitor drugs as causative for VUR, either directly or by interference with genetic functions in the development of the kidney and urinary tract.

22.8.9.12 Conclusion

My opinion in this case is that the presence of VUR in this child was not caused by her in utero exposure to Lotensin. While there is a temporal relationship, she was exposed and her exposure was limited and was primarily in the first trimester, with only 16 days in the second trimester to the 14th week. Once Lotensin was discontinued on 11/10/16, amniotic fluid returned to normal within one week, which is a direct measurement of fetal renal performance and intrauterine growth normalized by the 22nd. In my opinion, a competing cause for the oligoamnios was the hypotension that preceded the finding of the diminished amniotic fluid. One urologist advised a wait-and-see approach—she may grow out of it. Other unmet criteria include a lack of biological plausibility—no mechanisms of ACEI-induced VUR are described, a documentation of a lack of literature precedence. The literature does, however, describe VUR development as a very common condition, especially in young girl infants, unrelated to the use of antihypertensives.

Lotensin HCT contains an ACE inhibitor (benazepril) and is associated with fetal toxicities. Consequently, it should only be prescribed in pregnancy, especially in the second or third trimester, when no other agent(s) can be used. The toxicities are related to physiologic changes, in contrast to teratologic changes. Two methodologic approaches in evaluating causation were utilized in this matter: (1) what is known about the disease (VUR), and (2) what is known about the drug? Both approaches fail to identify any link. No reports, suggestions, analysis, relationship or claims supporting the post-partum development of VUR and fetal exposure to benazepril (or any other ACEI or ARB) are found in the scientific literature. There was at least one warning (prescription vial) to Ms. Patient not to use during pregnancy, and additional warnings would have and should have been provided by the pharmacist to the patient and to the prescribing physician. If called as a witness at trial, I would testify that the VUR in this child, the premature birth and the developmental delay, as well as the cardiac condition alleged (resolved) are not related to the benazepril pregnancy exposure and the other opinions expressed in this report.

22.9 SUMMARY AND CONCLUSIONS

Pregnancy and the physiological milieu of pregnancy and the interaction of this environment are quite complex and not fully understood. The same can be said about the effects of fetal drug exposure—indeed, perhaps even less is known.

REFERENCES

1. R.D. Hood. Developmental and reproductive toxicology, a practical approach, 2nd ed. Boca Raton: Taylor & Francis, 2006.
2. J. Warkany. Teratology: Spectrum of a science. In H. Kalter (ed.) Issues and reviews in teratology. New York: Plenum Press, 1983, Vol. 1, pp. 19–31.
3. N. Chernoff, J.M. Rogers, A.J. Alles, R.M. Zucker, K.H. Elstein, E.J. Massaro, K.K. Sulik. Cell cycle alterations and cell death in cyclophosphamide teratogenesis. Teratogenesis Carcino Mutagen (1989) 9: 199–209.
4. J.M. Rogers, R.J. Kavlock. Developmental toxicology. In C.D. Klaassen (ed.) Toxicology: The basic science of poisons, 5th ed. New York, NY: McGraw-Hill, 1996, pp. 301–331.

5. C. R. Stockard. Developmental rate and structural expression: An experimental study of twins, "double monsters," and single deformities, and the interaction among embryonic organs during their origin and development. Am J Anat (1921) 28: 115–277.
6. F. Hale. Pigs born without eyeballs. J Hered (1935) 27: 105–106.
7. J. Warkany, R.C. Nelson. Appearance of skeletal abnormalities in the offspring of rats reared on a deficient diet. Science (1940) 92: 383–384.
8. N.M. Gregg. Conenital cataract following German measles in the mother. Tr Ophthalmol Soc Aust (1941) 3: 35–40.
9. W.G. McBride. Thalidomide and congenital anomalies. Lancet (1961) 2: 1358.
10. J.G. Wilson. Experimental studies on congenital malformations. J Chronic Dis (1959) 10: 111–130.
11. T.W. Sadler, E.S. Hunter. Principles of abnormal development: Past, present and future. In C.A. Kimmel, J. Buelke-Sam (eds.) Developmental toxicology, 2nd ed. New York: Raven Press, 1994, pp. 53–63.
12. W. Lenz. Time plan of human organogenesis as a standard in the assessment of teratogenic effects. Fortschr Med (1969) 87: 520–526.
13. D. Bernstein, P. Nash. Human Development. In D. Bernstein, P. Nash (eds.) Essentials of psychology, 2nd ed. Boston: Houghton Mifflin Company, 2008, pp. 341–388.
14. W.M. Generoso, J.C. Rutledge, K.T. Cain, L.A. Hughes, P.W. Braden. Exposure of female mice to ethylene oxide within hours after mating leads to fetal malformations and death. Mutat Res (1987) 176: 269–274; and W.M. Generoso, J.C. Rutledge, K.T. Cain, L.A. Hughes, D.J. Downing. Mutagen-induced fetal anomalies and death following treatment of females within hours after mating. Mut Res (1988) 199: 175–181.
15. M.H. Snow, P.P. Tam. Is compensatory growth a complicating factor in mouse teratology? Nature (1979) 3: 461–480.
16. N.W. Moore, C.E. Adams, L.E. Rowson. Development potential of single blastomeres of the rabbit egg. J Reprod Fertil (1968) 17: 527–531.
17. S. Fabro. Passage of drugs and other chemicals into the uterine fluids and preimplantation blastocyst. In L. Boreus (ed.) Fetal pharmacology. New York: Raven Press, 1973, pp. 443–461; and S. Fabro, J.A. McLachlan, N.M. Dames. Chemical exposure of embryos during the preimplantation stages of pregnancy: Mortality rate and intrauterine development. Am J Obstet Gynecol (1984) 148: 929–938.
18. I.K. Takeuchi. Teratogenic effects of methylnitrosourea on pregnant mice before implantation. Experienta (1984) 40: 879–881.
19. H.G. Eibs, H. Speilman, and M. Hagele. Teratogenic effects of cyproterone acetate and medroxyprogesterone treatment during the pre- and postimplantation period of mouse embryos. Teratology (1982) 25: 27–36.
20. A.C. Enders. Anatomy of the placenta and its relationship to function. Mead Johnson Symp Perinat Dev Med (1981)18: 3–7.
21. R.E. Shenefelt. Morphogenesis of malformations in hamsters caused by retinoic acid: Relation to dose and stage of treatment. Teratology (1972) 5: 103–118.
22. J.M. Rogers, B.D. Barbee, B.F. Rehnberg. Critical periods of sensitivity for the developmental toxicity of inhaled methanol. Teratology (1993) 47: 395.
23. D. Neubert, P. Zens, A. Rothenwallner, H.-J. Merker. A survey of the embryotoxic effects of TCDD in mammalian species. Environ Health Perspect (1973) 5: 63–79.
24. L.L. Needham, A.M. Calafat, D.B. Barr. Assessing the developmental toxicant exposures via biomonitoring. Basic Clin Pharmacol Toxicol (2008) 102: 100–108.
25. S.D. Holladay, R.J. Smialowicz. Development of the murine and human immune system: Differential effects of immunotoxicants depend on time of exposure. Environ Health Perspect (2000) 108(Suppl 3): 463–475.
26. K.E. Pinkerton, J.P. Joad. The mammalian respiratory system and critical windows of exposure for children's health. Environ Health Perspect (2000) 108(Suppl 3): 457–462.
27. J.L. Pryor, C. Hughes, W. Foster, B.F. Hales, B. Robaire. Critical windows of exposure for children's health: The reproductive system in animals and humans. Environ Health Perspect (2000) 108(Suppl 3): 491–504.
28. D. Rice, S. Barone Jr. Critical periods of vulnerability for the developing nervous system: Evidence from human and animal models. Environ Health Perspect (2000) 108(Suppl 3): 511–533.
29. P.M. Rodier. Vulnerable periods and processes during central nervous system development. Environ Health Perspect (1994) 102(Suppl 2): 121–124.
30. T.W. Sadler. Susceptible periods during embryogenesis of the heart and endocrine glands. Environ Health Perspect (2000) 108(Suppl 3): 555–562.
31. P.S. Guzelian, C.J. Henry, S.S. Olin (eds.). Similarities and differences between children and adults: Implications for risk assessment. Washington DC: ILSI Press, 1992.
32. J.L. Margulies. Special considerations in pregnancy. In P. Viccellio (ed.) Handbook of medical toxicology. Boston: Little, Brown and Company, 1993, pp. 128–135.
33. E.W. Carney, A.B. Liberacki, B. Tornesi, D.A. Markham, K.K. Weitz, T.M. Luders, K.G. Studniski, J.C. Blessing, R.A. Gies, R.A. Corley. Ethylene glycol kinetics in pregnant rats: Differences between slow and fast dose-rate exposures. Toxicologist (2002) 66(Suppl 1): 139.
34. H. Nau, W.J. Scott Jr. Weak acids my act as teratogens by accumulating in the basic milieu of the early mammalian embryo. Nature (1986) 323: 276–278.
35. M. Srivastava, M.D. Collins, W.J. Scott Jr, W.H. Nau. Transplacental distribution of weak acids in mice: Acumulation in compartments of high pH. Teratology (1991) 43: 325–329.
36. N. Brown. Teratogenicity of carboxylic acids: Distribution studies in whole embryo culture. In H. Nau, W.J. Scott Jr (eds.) Pharmacokinetics in teratogenesis. Boca Raton: CRC Press, 1987, Vol. II, pp. 154–163.
37. E. Jauniaux, B. Gulbis. Fluid compartments of the embryonic environment. Hum Reprod (2000) 6: 268–278.
38. H.P. Kuemmerle. The diaplacental kinetics of drugs. Int J Clin Pharmacol (1974) 9: 298–304.
39. J.L. Schardein. Chemically induced birth defects, 2nd ed. New York: Marcel Dekker, 1993.
40. J.G. Wilson. Experimental studies on congenital malformations. J Chronic Dis (1959) 10: 111–130.
41. H.B. Taussig. A study of the German outbreak of phocomelia: The thalidomide syndrome. JAMA (1962) 180: 1106.
42. W.G. McBride. Thalidomide and congenital anomalies. Lancet (1961) 2: 1358.
43. W. Lenz. Kindliche Missbildungen nach Medikament-Einnahme während der gravidität? Dtsch Med Wochenschr (1961) 86: 2555–2556.
44. W. Lenz. Das thalidomide-syndrom. Fortschr Med (1963) 81: 148–153
45. W. Lenz. A short history of thalidomide embryopathy. Teratology (1988) 38: 203–215.

46. S.G. Stolberg. Thalidomide approved to treat leprosy. With other uses seen. *New York Times* (1998).
47. D.R. Bielenberg, P.A. D'Amore. Judah Folkman's contribution to the inhibition of angiogenesis. Lymphat Res Biol (2008) 6(3–4): 203–207.
48. National Cancer Institute (NCI). FDA approval for thalidomide (2013).
49. Medicines and Healthcare Products Regulatory Agency. Thalidomide: Risk of second primary malignancies, 2013.
50. F.J. Paumgortten, I. Chadoud. Thalidomide embryopathy cases in Brazil after 1965. Reprod Toxicol (2006) 22(1): 1–2.
51. A. Crawford. Brazil's new generation of thalidomide babies. *BBC News* (2013).
52. K.L. Jones, D.W. Smith. Recognition of the fetal alcohol syndrome in early infancy. Lancet (1973) 2: 999–1001.
53. H.L. Rosett, L. Weiner. Alcohol and the fetus: A clinical perspective. New York: Oxford University Press, 1984.
54. L.E. Kotch, K.K. Sulik. Experimental fetal alcohol syndrome: Proposed pathogenic basis for a variety of associated facial and brain anomalies. Am J Med Genet (1992) 44: 168–176.
55. C.D. Dittmer, S.L. Lentz-Kapua. Fetal alcohol syndrome. http://www.emedicine.com/PED/topic767.htm (2006).
56. C. Guerri. Mechanisms involved in central nervous system dysfunction induced by prenatal ethanol exposure. Neurotox Res (2002) 4: 327–335.
57. M.W. Miller. Effects of alcohol on the generation and migration of cerebral cortical neurons. Science (1986) 233: 1308–1311.
58. M.W. Miller. Migration of cortical neurons is altered by gestational exposure to ethanol. Alcohol Clin Exp Res (1993) 17: 304–314.
59. T.M. Roebuck, S.N. Mattison, E.P. Riley. A review of the neuroanatomical findings in children with fetal alcohol syndrome or prenatal exposure to alcohol. Alcohol Clin Exp Res (1998) 22: 339–344.
60. E.R. Sowell, P.M. Thompson, S.N. Mattison, K.D. Tessner, T.L. Jernigan, E.P. Riley, A.W. Toga. Voxel-based morphometric analyses of the brain in children and adolescents prenatally exposed to alcohol. Neuroreport (2001) 12: 515–523.
61. S.L. Archibald, C. Fennema-Notestine, A. Gamst, E.P. Riley, S.N. Mattison, T.L. Jernigan. Brain dysmorpholgy in individuals with severe prenatal alcohol exposure. Dev Med Child Neurol (2001) 43: 148–154.
62. National Institute on Alcohol Abuse and Alcoholism. Prenatal exposure to alcohol. Alcohol Res Health (2000) 24: 32–41.
63. S.K. Clarren, E.C. Alvord Jr, S.M. Sumi, A.P. Streissguth, D.W. Smith. Brain malformations related to prenatal exposure to ethanol. J Pediatr (1978) 92: 64–67.
64. E.R. Sowell, P.M. Thompson, S.N. Mattison, K.D. Tessner, T.L. Jernigan, E.P. Riley, A.W. Toga. Voxel-based morphometric analyses of the brain in children and adolescents prenatally exposed to alcohol. Neuroreport (2001) 12: 515–523.
65. S.K. Clarren, E.C. Alvord Jr, S.M. Sumi, A.P. Streissguth, D.W. Smith. Brain malformations related to prenatal exposure to ethanol. J Pediatr (1978) 92: 64–67.
66. J. Peiffer, F. Majewski, H. Fishbach, J.R. Bierich, B. Volk. Alcohol embryo and fetopathy. J Neurol Sci (1979) 41: 125–137.
67. C.L. Coulter, R.W. Leech, G.B. Schaefer, B.W. Scheithauer, R.A. Brumback. Midline cerebral dysgenesis, dysfunction of the hypothalamic–pituitary axid and fetal alcohol effects. Arch Neurol (1993) 50: 771–775.
68. T. Kumada, Y. Jiang, D.B. Cameron, H. Komuro. How does alcohol impair neuronal migration? J Neurosci Res (2007) 85: 465–470.
69. J.C. Marcus. Neurological findings in the fetal alcohol syndrome. Neuropediatrics (1987) 18: 158–160.
70. B. Altman. Fetal alcohol syndrome. J Pediatric Ophthal (1976) 13: 255–258.
71. T. Chan, R. Bowell, M. O'Keefe, B. Lanigan. Ocular manifestations in fetal alcohol syndrome. Br J Ophthal (1991) 75: 524–526.
72. M.T. Miller, J. Israel, J. Cuttone. Fetal alcohol syndrome. J Pediatr Opththal (1981) 18: 6–15.
73. K. Stromland. Ocular abnormalities in the fetal alcohol syndrome. Acta Ophthalmol Scand (1985) 63(Suppl 171): 369–392.
74. T. Chan, R. Bowell, M. O'Keefe, B. Lanigan. Ocular manifestations in fetal alcohol syndrome. Br J Ophthalmol (1991) 75: 524–526.
75. H. Rosett. Guest editorial. A clinical perspective of fetal alcohol syndrome. Alcoholism (1980) 4: 119–122.
76. K. Stromland. Ocular abnormalities in the fetal alcohol syndrome. Acta Ophthalmol Scand (1985) 63(Suppl 171): 369–392.
77. A.L. Herbst, P. Cole, T. Colton, S.J. Robboy, R.E. Scully. Age-incidence and risk of diethylstilbestrol-related clear cell adenocarcinoma of the vagina and cervix. Am J Obstet Gynecol (1977) 128: 43–50.
78. J.R. Palmer, L.A. Wise, E.E. Hatch, R. Troisi, L. Titus-Ernstoff, W. Strohsnitter, R. Kaufman, A.L. Herbst, K.L. Noller, M. Hyer, R.N. Hoover. Prenatal diethylstilbestrol exposure and risk of breast cancer. Cancer Epidemiol Biomark Prevent (2006) 15(8): 1509–1514.
79. J. Verloop, F.E. van Leeuwen, T.J. Helmerhorst, H.H. van Boven, M.A. Rookus. Cancer risk in DES daughters. Cancer Causes Control (2010) 21(7): 999–1007.
80. R.N. Hoover, M. Hyer, R.M. Pfeiffer, E. Adam, B. Bond, A.L. Cheville, T. Colton, P. Hartge, E.E. Hatch, A.L. Herbst, B.Y. Karlan, R. Kaufman, K.L. Noller, J.R. Palmer, S.J. Robboy, R.C. Saal, W. Strohsnitter, L. Titus-Ernstoff, R. Troisi. Adverse health outcomes in women exposed in utero to diethylstilbestrol. New Engl J Med (2011) 365: 1304–1314.
81. M. Bibbo, W. Gill, F. Aziz, R. Blough, V.S. Fang, R.L. Rosenfield, G.F. Schumacher, K. Sleeper, M.G. Sonek, G.L. Wied. Follow-up study of male and female offspring of DES-exposed mothers. Obstet Gynecol (1977) 49: 1–8.
82. F.W. Rosa. Teratogenicity of isotretinoin. Lancet (1983) 2: 513.
83. E.J. Lamner, D.T. Chen, R.M. Hoar, N.D. Agnish, P.J. Benke, J.T. Braun, C.J. Curry, P.M. Fernhoff, A.W. Grix Jr, I.T. Lott, J.M. Richard, S.C. Sun. Retinoic acid induced embryopathy. New Engl J Med (1985) 313: 837–841.
84. J. Shin, C.T. Cheetham, L. Wong, F. Niu, E. Kass, M.A. Yoshinaga, M. Sorel, J.S. McCombs, S. Sidney. The impact of the iPLEDGE program on isotretinoin fetal exposure in an integrated health care system. J Am Acad Dermatol (2011) 65(6): 1117–1125.
85. N. Prevost, J.C. English. Isotretinoin: Update on controversial issues. J Pediatr Adolesc Gynecol (2013) 26(5): 290–293.

86. I. Torjesen. Managing acne female-to-male transgender persons. *Dermatology Times* (2018) (Retrieved 2021–03–20).
87. K. Dolheny. iPledge rollout: As frustration mounts, FDA agrees to help solve issues. Medscape Pharmacist. Medical News (2021).
88. P.M. Zito, T. Mazzoni. Acritretin. StatPearls. Treasure Island, FL: StatPearls Publishing, 2021.
89. Soriatane (Acitretin). Stiefel Label. https://www.accessdata.fda.gov/drugsatfda_docs/label/2011/019821s018lbl.pdf.
90. I.J. Chasnoff, R.P. Hatcher, W.J. Burns. Polydrug and methadone addicted newborns: A continuum of impairment? Pediatrics (1982) 70: 210–213.
91. I.J. Chasnoff, R.P. Hatcher, W.J. Burns, S.H. Schnoll. Pentazocine and tripelennamine ("t's and blue's") effects on the fetus and neonate. Dev Pharmacol Ther (1983a) 6: 162–169; and. I.J. Chasnoff, W.J. Burns, R.P. Hatcher, K.A. Burns. Phencyclidine effects on the fetus and neonate. Dev Pharmacol Ther (1983b) 6: 404–408.
92. I.J. Chasnoff, W.J. Burns, S.H. Schnoll, K.A. Burns. Cocaine use in pregnancy. New Engl J Med (1985) 313: 666–669.
93. I.J. Chasnoff, W.J. Burns, R.P. Hatcher, K.A. Burns. Phencyclidine effects on the fetus and neonate. Dev Pharmacol Ther (1983b) 6: 404–408.
94. B. Lutiger, K. Graham, T.R. Einarson, G. Koren. Relationship between gestational cocaine use and pregnancy outcome: A meta-analysis. Teratology (1991) 44: 405–414.
95. J.O. Donaldson. Neurologic complications. In G.N. Burrow, T.P. Duffy (eds.) Medical complications during pregnancy, 5th ed. Philadelphia, PA: WB Saunders Co, 1999, pp. 410–412.
96. R.C Kessler, P. Berglund, O. Demler, R. Jin, D. Koretz, K.R. Merikangas, A.J. Rush, E.E. Walters, P.S. Wang, National Comorbidity Survey Replication. The epidemiology of major depressive disorder: Results from the National Comorbidity Survey Replication (NCS-R). JAMA (2003) 289: 3095–3105.
97. V.K. Burt, K. Stein. Epidemiology of depression throughout the female life cycle. J Clin Psychiatry (2002) **63**(Suppl 7): 9–15.
98. S.D. Sie, J.M.B Wennink, J.J. van Driel, A.G.W te Winkel, K. Boer, G. Casteelen M.M. van Weissenruch. Maternal use of SSRIs, SNRIs and NaSSAs: Practical recommendations during pregnancy and lactation. Arch Dis Child Fetal Neonatal Ed (2012) 97: F472–F476.
99. C. Hiemke, S. Härtter. Pharmacokinetics of selective serotonin reuptake inhibitors. Pharmacol Ther (2000) 85: 11–28.
100. FDA. FDA advising of risk of birth defects with Paxil. www.fda.gov/NewsEvents/Newsroom/PressAnnouncements/2005/ucm108527.htm (2005).
101. M. Reis, B. Källén. Delivery outcome after maternal use of antidepressant drugs in pregnancy: An update using Swedish data. Psychol Med (2010) 40: 1723–1733.
102. T.F. Oberlander, W. Warburton, S. Misri, W. Riggs, J. Aghajanian, C. Hertzman. Major congenital malformations following prenatal exposure to serotonin reuptake inhibitors and benzodiazepines using population-based health data. Birth Defects Res B Dev Reprod Toxicol (2008) 83: 68–76.
103. T.F. Oberlander, M. Papsdorfm, U.M. Brain, S. Misri, C. Ross, R.E. Grunau. Prenatal effects of selective serotonin reuptake inhibitor antidepressants, serotonin transporter promoter genotype (SLC6A4), and maternal mood on child behavior at 3 years of age. Arch Pediatr Adolesc Med (2010) 164: 444–451.
104. D. Lindhout, D. Schmidt. In utero exposure to valproate and neural tube defects. Lancet (1986) 1: 1392–1393.
105. Centers for Disease Control. Valproic acid and spina bifida: A preliminary report—France. MMWR (1982) 31(42): 565–566.
106. Centers for Disease Control. Valproate: A new cause of birth defects—Report from Italy and follow up from France. MMWR (1983) 32(33): 438–439.
107. E.B. Samren, C.M. van Duijn, S. Koch, V.K. Hiilesmaa, H. Klepel, A.H. Bardy, G.B. Mannagetta, A.W. Deichl, E. Gaily, M.L. Granström, H. Meinardi, D.E. Grobbee, A. Hofman, D. Janz, D. Lindhout. Maternal use of antiepileptic drugs and the risk of major congenital malformations: A joint European prospective study of human teratogenesis associated with maternal epilepsy. Epilepsia (1997) 38: 981–990.
108. E.B. Samren, C.M. van Duijn, G.C. Christiaens, A Hofman, D. Lindhout. Antiepileptic drug regimens and major congenital abnormalities in the offspring. Ann Neurol (1999) 46: 739–746.
109. R. Canger, D. Battino, M.P. Canevini, C. Fumarola, L. Guidolin, A. Vignoli, D. Mamoli, C. Palmieri, F. Molteni, T. Granata, P. Hassibi, P. Zamperini, G. Pardi, G. Avanzini. Malformations in offspring of women with epilepsy: A prospective study. Epilepsia (1999) 40: 1231–1236.
110. S. Kaneko, D. Battino, E. Andermann, K. Wada, R. Kan, A. Takeda, Y. Nakane, Y. Ogawa, G. Avanzini, C. Fumarola, T. Granata, F. Molteni, G. Pardi, L. Minotti, R. Canger, L. Dansky, M. Oguni, I. Lopes-Cendas, A. Sherwin, F. Andermann, M.H. Seni, M. Okada, T. Teranishi. Congenital malformations due to antiepileptic drugs. Epilepsy Res (1999) 33: 145–158.
111. G. Mawer, J. Clayton-Smith, H. Coyle, U. Kini. Outcome of pregnancy in women attending an outpatient epilepsy clinic: Adverse features associated with higher doses of sodium valproate. Seizure (2002) 11: 512–518.
112. R. Meischenguiser, C.H. D'Giano, S.M. Ferraro. Oxcarbazepine in pregnancy: Clinical experience in Argentina. Epilepsy Behav (2004) 5: 163–167.
113. K. Wide, B. Winbladh, B. Kallen. Major malformations in infants exposed to antiepileptic drugs in utero, with emphasis on carbamazepine and valproic acid: A nationwide, population-based register study. Acta Paediatr (2004) 93: 174–176.
114. M. Artama, A. Auvinen, T. Raudaskoski, I. Isojarvi, J. Isojarvi. Antiepileptic drug use of women with epilepsy and congenital malformations in offspring. Neurology (2005) 64: 1874–1878.
115. J. Morrow, A. Russell, E. Guthrie, L. Parsons, I. Robertson, R. Waddell, B. Irwin, R.C. McGivern, P.J. Morrison, J. Craig. Malformation risks of antiepileptic drugs in pregnancy: A prospective study from the UK Epilepsy and Pregnancy Register. J Neurol Neurosurg Psychiatry (2006) 77: 193–198.
116. D.F. Wyszynski, M. Nambisan, T. Surve, R.M. Alsdorf, C.R. Smith, L.B. Holmes. Increased rate of major malformations in offspring exposed to valproate during pregnancy. Neurology (2005) 64: 961–965.
117. E. Kaaja, R. Kaaja, V. Hiilesmaa. Major malformations in offspring of women with epilepsy. Neurology (2003) 60: 575–579.

118. N. Adab, U. Kini, J. Vinten, J. Ayres, G. Baker, J. Clayton-Smith, H. Coyle, A. Fryer, J. Gorry, J. Gregg, G. Mawer, P. Nicolaides, L. Pickering, L. Tunnicliffe, D.W. Chadwick. The longer term outcome of children born to mothers with epilepsy. J Neurol Neurosurg Psychiatry (2004) 75: 1575–1583.
119. E.B. Samren, C.M. van Duijn, S. Koch, V.K. Hiilesmaa, H. Klepel, A.H. Bardy, G.B. Mannagetta, A.W. Deichl, E. Gaily, M.L. Granström, H. Meinardi, D.E. Grobbee, A. Hofman, D. Janz, D. Lindhout. Maternal use of antiepileptic drugs and the risk of major congenital malformations: A joint European prospective study of human teratogenesis associated with maternal epilepsy. Epilepsia (1997) 38: 981–990.
120. G. Koren, A.A. Nava-Ocampo, M.E. Moretti, R. Sussman, I. Nulman. Motherisk Update: Major malformations with valproic acid. Canadian Family Physician (2006) 52: 441–447.
121. P. Tanganelli, G. Regesta. Epilepsy, pregnancy, and major birth anomalies: An Italian prospective, controlled study. Neurology (1992) 42(4 Suppl 5): 89–93.
122. E.B. Samren, C.M. van Duijn, G.C. Christiaens, A Hofman, D. Lindhout. Antiepileptic drug regimens and major congenital abnormalities in the offspring. Ann Neurol (1999) 46: 739–746.
123. S. Kaneko, D. Battino, E. Andermann, K. Wada, R. Kan, A. Takeda, Y. Nakane, Y. Ogawa, G. Avanzini, C. Fumarola, T. Granata, F. Molteni, G. Pardi, L. Minotti, R. Canger, L. Dansky, M. Oguni, I. Lopes-Cendas, A. Sherwin, F. Andermann, M.H. Seni, M. Okada, T. Teranishi. Congenital malformations due to antiepileptic drugs. Epilepsy Res (1999) 33: 145–158.
124. H. Nau, R. Zierer, H. Spielmann, D. Neubert, C.A. Gansau. A new model for embryotoxicity testing: Teratogenicity and pharmacokinetics of valproic acid following constant-rate administration in the mouse using human therapeutic drug and metabolite concentrations. Life Sci (1981) 29: 2803–2814.
125. D.W. Fowler, M.J. Eadie, R.G. Dickinson. Transplacental transfer and biotransformation studies of valproic acid and its glucuronide(s) in the perfused human placenta. J Pharmacol Exp Ther (1989) 249: 318–323.
126. S. Kumar, H. Wong, S.A. Yeung, K.W. Riggs, F.S. Abbott, D.W. Rurak. Disposition of valproic acid in maternal, fetal and new borm sheep. I: Placental transfer; plasma protein bind and clearance. Drug Metab Dispos (2000) 28: 845–856.
127. H. Nau, B Krauer. Serum protein binding of valproic acid in fetus-mother pairs throughout pregnancy: Correlation with oxytocin administration and albumin and free fatty acid concentrations. J Clin Pharmacol (1986) 26: 215–221.
128. N.C. Aizenman. Abbot laboratories to pay $1.6 billion over illegal marketing of Depakote. *Washington Post* (2012).
129. B.K. Alldredge. Seizure disorders. In E.T. Herfindal, D.R. Gourley (eds.) Textbook of therapeutics: Drug and disease management, 7th ed. Philadelphia, PA: Lippincott Williams & Wilkins, 2000, pp. 1118–11120.
130. M.L. Netzloff, R.R. Streiff, J.L. Frias, O.M. Rennert. Folate antagonism following teratogenic exposure to diphenylhydantoin. Teratology (1979) 19: 45–50.
131. D.K. Hansen, R.E. Billings. Phenytoin teratogenicity and effects on embryonic and maternal folate metabolism. Teratology (1985) 31: 363–371.
132. American Academy of Pediatrics Committee (AAPC) on Genetics. Folic acid for the prevention of neural tube defects. Pediatrics (1999) 104: 325–327.
133. J.M. Brewer, P.A. Wattman. Epilepsy and pregnancy: Maternal and fetal effects of phenytoin. Crit Care Nurse (2003) 23: 93–98.
134. J.J. Volpe. Teratogenic effects of drugs and passive addiction. In Neurology of the newborn, 4th ed. Philadelphia, PA: WB Saunders Co., 2001, pp. 859–898.
135. R.H. Finnell, B.A. Buchler, B.M. Kerr, P.L. Ager, R.H. Levy. Clinical and experimental studies linking oxidative metabolism to phenytoin-induced teratogenesis. Neurology (1992) 42(Suppl 4): 25–31.
136. M. Ogun, L. Dansky, E. Andermann, A. Sherwin, F. Andermann. Improved pregnancy outcome in epileptic women in the last decade: Relationship of maternal anticonvulsant therapy. Brain Dev (1992) 14: 371–380.
137. M.S. Yerby, A. Leavitt, D.M. Erickson, K.B. McCormick, R.B. Loewenson, C.J. Sells, T.J. Benedetti. Antiepileptics and the development of congenital anomalies. Neurology (1992) 42: 132–140.
138. A.B. Dessens, P.T. Cohen-Kettenis, G.J. Mellenbergh, J.G. Koppe, N.E. van De Poll, K. Boer. Association of prenatal Phenobarbital and phenytoin exposure with small head size at birth and with learning problems. Acta Paediatr (2000) 89: 533–554.
139. J. Koch-Wesser, E.M. Sellers. Drug interactions with coumarin anticoagulants. New Engl J Med (1971) 285: 487–498.
140. P.J Disaia. Pregnancy and delivery of a patient with a Starr-Edwards mitral valve prosthesis. Obste Gynecol (1966) 28: 469–472.
141. W.L. Shaul, J.G. Hall. Multiple congenital anomalies associated with oral anticoagulants. Am J Obstet Gynecol (1977) 127. 191–198.
142. R.M. Pauli, J.G. Hal, K.M. Wilson. Risks of anticoagulation during pregnancy. Am Heart J (1980) 100: 761–762.
143. M.J. Robinson, J. Pash, J. Grimwade, J. Campbell. Fetal warfarin syndrome. Med J Aust (1978) 1: 157.
144. W. Holzgreve, J.C. Carey, B.D. Hall. Warfarin-induced fetal abnormalities. Lancet (1976) 2: 914–915.
145. D. Born, E.E. Martinez, P.A. Almeida, D.V. Santos, A.C. Carvalho, A.F. Moron, C.H. Miyasaki, S.D. Moraes, J.A. Ambrose. Pregnancy in patients with prosthetic heart valves: The effects of anticoagulation on mother, fetus, and neonate. Am Heart J (1992) 124: 413–417.
146. P. Sareli, M.J. England, M.R. Berk, R.H. Marcus, M. Epstein, J. Driscoll, T. Meyer, J. McIntyre, C. van Gelderen. Maternal and fetal sequelae of anticoagulation during pregnancy in patients with mechanical heart valve prosthesis. Am J Cardiol (1989) 63: 1462–1465.
147. P.I. Pillans, E.J. Coetzee. Anticoagulation during pregnancy. S Afr Med J (1986) 69: 469.
148. G. Quenneville, B. Barton, E. McDevitt, I.S. Wright. The use of anticoagulants for thrombo-phlebitis during pregnancy. Am J Obstet Gynecol (1959) 77: 1135–1149.
149. U. Villasanta. Thromboembolic disease in pregnancy. Am J. Obstet Gynecol (1965) 93: 142–160.
150. J.G. Hall, R.M. Pauli, K.M. Wilson. Maternal and fetal sequelae of anticoagulation during pregnancy. Am J Med (1980) 68: 122–140.
151. E. Salazar, A. Zajamas, N. Gutierrez, I. Hurbe. The problem of cardiac valve prostheses, anticoagulants, and pregnancy. Circulation (1984) 70(Suppl 1): 169–177.

152. N. Sussman. The benzodiapines: Selection and use in treating anxiety insomnia and other disorders. Hosp Formul (1984) 20: 298–305.
153. M.B. Bracken, T.R. Holford. Exposure to prescribed drugs in pregnancy and association with congenital malformations. Obstet Gynecol (1981) 58: 336–344.
154. American College of Obstetricians and Gynecologist Committee on Practice Buletins—Obstetrics. ACOG Practice Bulletin no. 92: "Use of psychiatric medications during pregnancy and lactation." Obstet Gynecol (2008) 111(4): 1001–1020.
155. S.S. Roach, S.M. Ford. Sedatives and hypnotics. Introductory clinical pharmacology, 8th ed. Lippincott Williams & Wilkens, 2006, p. 236.
156. M.M. Iqgal, T. Sobhan, T. Ryals. Effects of commonly used benzodiazepines on the fetus, the neonate and the nursing infants. Psychiatr Serv (2002) 53: 39–49.
157. W. Kuhnz, H. Nau. Differences in in vitro binding of diazepam and N-desmethyldiazepam to maternal and fetal plasma proteins at birth: Relation to free fatty acid concentration and other parameters. Clin Pharmacol Therapeut (1983) 34: 220–226.
158. M. Mandelli, P.L. Morselli, S. Nordio, G. Pardi, N. Principi, F. Sereni, G. Tognoni. Placental transfer of diazepam and its disposition in the newborn. Clin Pharmacol Therapeut (1975) 17: 564–572.
159. O.M. Bakke, K. Haram, T. Lygre, G. Wallem. Comparison of the placental transfer of thiopental and diazepam in caesarian section. Eur J Clin Pharmacol (1981) 21: 221–227.
160. C. Gillberg. "Floppy infant syndrome" and maternal diazepam. Lancet (1977) 2: 244.
161. E. Mazzi. Possible neonatal diazepam withdrawal: A case report. Am J Obst Gynecol (1977) 129: 586–587.
162. J.E. Cree, J. Meyer, D.M. Hailey. Diazepam in labour: Its metabolism and effect on the clinical condition and thermogenesis of the newborn. Br Med J (1973) 4: 251–255.
163. R.W. Shannon, G.P. Fraser, R.G. Aitken, J.R. Harper. Diazepam in preeclamptic toxemia with special reference to its effect on the newborn infant. Br J Clin Pract (1972) 26: 271–275.
164. E. Van der Kleijn. Protein binding and lipophilic nature of ataractics of the metrobamate and diazapime group. Arch Int Pharmacodyn Ther (1969) 179: 225–250.
165. M.D. Allen, D.J. Greenblatt. Comparative protein binding of diazepam and desmethyldiazepam. J Clin Pharmacol (1981) 21: 219–223.
166. W.A. Colburn, M. Gibaldi. Plasma protein binding of diazepam after a single dose of sodium oleate. J Pharm Sci (1978) 67: 891–892.
167. J. Krasner, S.J. Yaffe. Drug-protein binding in the neonate. In P.L. Morselli, S. Garattini, F. Sereni (eds.) Basic and therapeutic aspects of perinatal pharmacology. New York: Raven, 1975.
168. D. Aarskog. Association between maternal intake of diazepam and oral clefts [letter]. Lancet (1975) 2: 921.
169. I. Saxen. Associations between oral clefts and drugs taken during pregnancy. Int J Epidemiol (1975) 4: 37–44.
170. M.D. Safra, G.P. Oakley. Association between cleft lip with or without cleft palate and prenatal exposure to diazepam. Lancet (1975) 2: 478–480.
171. I. Saxen, L. Saxen. Association between maternal intake of diazepam and oral clefts. Lancet (1975) 2: 498.
172. L. Rosenberg, A.A. Mitchell, J.L. Parsells, H. Pashayan, C. Louik, S. Shapiro. Lack of relation of oral clefts to diazepam use during pregnancy. New Engl J Med (1983) 309: 1282–1285.
173. S.S. Entman, W.K. Vaughn. Lack of relation of oral clefts to diazepam use in pregnancy [letter]. New Engl J Med (1984) 310: 1121–1122.
174. A. Czeizel. Diazepam, phenytoin, and aetiology of cleft lip and/or cleft palate [letter]. Lancet (1976) 1: 810.
175. I. Saxen. Epidemiology of cleft lip and palate: An attempt to rule out chance correlations. Br J Prevent Soc Med (1975) 29: 103–110.
176. A. Czeizel, A. Lendvay. In utero exposure to benzodiazepines [letter]. Lancet (1987) 1: 628.
177. P.H. Shino, J.L. Mills. Oral clefts and diazepam use during pregnancy. New Engl J Med (1984) 311: 919–920.
178. A. Czeizel. Endpoints of reproductive dysfunction in an experimental epidemiological model: Self-poisoned pregnant women. In P.L. Chambers, P. Gehring, F. Sakai (eds.) New concepts and developments in toxicology. Amsterdam: Elsevier, 1986, p. 34.
179. A. Czeizel, A. Pazsy, J. Pusztai, M. Nagy. Aetiological monitor of congenital abnormalities: A case-control surveillance system. Acta Paediatr Hung (1983) 24: 91–99.
180. A.J. Gelenberg. Diazepam: Not a teratogen? Massachusetts General Hospital Newsletter (1984) 7(2).

23 Geriatric Medication Misadventures[1]

Rodney G. Richmond and James C. Norris

SYNOPSIS

23.1 INTRODUCTION

Adults aged 65 years and older represent 14.9% of the US population but account for 34% of prescription medications and 50% of over-the-counter medications.[1–3] According to the *National Health and Nutrition Examination Survey* conducted by the CDC, it was found that, during the period of 2015–18, approximately 90% of the people aged 65 and older used at least 1 prescription drug each month, 67% used 3 or more each month, and 42% used 5 or more each month.[4] Another survey of 17,000 Medicare beneficiaries found similar results in that two out of five patients reported taking more than five prescription medications.[5] The frail elderly consume the largest number of medications, along with hospitalized elderly and residents of long-term care facilities.[6]

Unfortunately, greater medication use in the elderly is associated with an increased risk of preventable drug misadventures (e.g., adverse drug events (ADEs), medication errors) and related morbidity, mortality, and economic costs. Various factors contribute to the increased risk of medication-related problems including age-related physiologic changes that can alter the pharmacokinetic and pharmacodynamic properties of drugs. In turn, these altered properties affect the handling of and response to specific drugs, polypharmacy, multiple comorbidities, transitions of care, inadequate monitoring, inappropriate medication use, and medication nonadherence. Further, drug misadventures are more common in the elderly across clinical care settings, regardless of whether they are cared for in the ambulatory setting, are hospitalized, or reside in long-term care facilities.[7]

23.1.1 Outpatient Medication Use

A population-based survey of community dwelling persons found that 37% of men and 36% of women between the ages of 75 and 85 years took at least five prescription drugs, the most common of which included diuretics, statins, beta-blockers, antihypertensives, hypoglycemics, and levothyroxine. Among this same group, 47% reported using an over the counter (OTC) product and 54% a dietary supplement.[3] Another study that evaluated unnecessary drug use in an elderly male outpatient population found that 59% took one or more unnecessary prescription drugs (e.g., central nervous system (CNS), gastrointestinal (GI), and vitamins).[8]

Adverse Drug Events: Adverse drug events in the outpatient setting have been evaluated in a number of studies.

1. Pharmacy Residents Chassidy Seward, PharmD, and Pranav Amin, PharmD.

DOI: 10.1201/9781003615323-25

A study in 30,000+ Medicare enrollees, who by rule are aged 65 or over, found that 5% suffered an adverse drug event during the 1-year study period. The same study showed that of all reported adverse events, one-third were categorized as serious, life-threatening, or fatal and that 42% of these serious events were preventable.[9] Factors that have been identified as increasing the risk of an adverse drug event in the elderly include multiple comorbidities, multiple prescribers, age ≥85 years, dementia, regular use of alcohol, decreased renal function, history of a prior adverse drug event, and recent hospitalization.[10–12] Adverse drug events have also been shown to be an important cause of morbidity in individuals more than 65 years that lead to emergency department visits. A two-year *National Electronic Injury Surveillance System—Cooperative Adverse Drug Event Surveillance* project produced annual estimates that individuals more than 65 years were more likely than younger individuals to both sustain an adverse drug event and require hospitalization.[13] It has been estimated that adverse drug events in the elderly increase the probability of an emergency department visit by two- to three-fold,[14] accounting for 25% of all emergency department visits, and increase the hospitalization by seven-fold,[14] approximating one-half of all hospitalizations being due to an adverse event occurring in the elderly.[15]

While it is known that specific types of medications are more harmful than beneficial in elderly patients (e.g., benzodiazepines), most ADEs result from commonly used medications that have known risks but offer significant benefits when used properly. These include antiplatelet agents (such as aspirin and clopidogrel), antidiabetic agents (e.g., insulin), oral anticoagulants (e.g., warfarin), and opioid pain medications. Collectively, these medications account for over 50% of emergency department visits for ADEs in Medicare patients.[16]

Medication Errors: Medication errors were separately assessed in the outpatient setting as a sub-analysis of the 30,000+ Medicare cohort previously described. The majority of errors that led to an adverse event occurred when the medication was administered (32%), the regimen was modified (42%), or when clinical advice about medications was not followed (22%). The drug classes most often involved included hypoglycemics (29%), cardiovascular medications (22%), anticoagulants (19%), and diuretics (10%). The odds ratio did not differ on the basis of age or gender but significantly increased as the number of medications increased.[17] A home health population of 6,718 patients of more than 65 years who took a median of five drugs revealed a 19% medication error rate over a two-year period.[18]

23.1.2 Hospital Medication Use

There is a paucity of studies that have evaluated the extent of medication use in the elderly in the hospitalized setting. One multicenter study in 384 frail, elderly veterans found that 21% were taking one to four drugs, 41% took at least five to eight medications, and 37% were taking more than nine medications. They also reported that 59% of the patients took more than one unnecessary prescription drug, the most common of which included GI and CNS drugs, and therapeutic nutrients/minerals.[19] A European multicenter study conducted in 1,332 inpatients ≥65 years found that on admission, 52% of patients were taking more than five medications with an average of five diagnoses, and by discharge, this rate increased to 67% of patients taking an average of six medications with six diagnoses. The most common drug classes being taken at discharge included GI, diuretics, ACE inhibitors, beta-blockers, lipid-lowering agents, hypoglycemics, digoxin, and antithrombotics.[20]

Adverse Drug Events: It has been estimated that 243,000 seniors are hospitalized each year due to reactions between prescription and OTC drugs.[2] A large US study conducted in a representative sample of hospitals, excluding psychiatric and Veterans Administration hospitals, evaluated 15,000 patients after discharge. Their findings indicated that patients more than 65 years had a higher incidence of preventable adverse drug events (0.63%), attributable to the clinical complexity of their care rather than age.[21] The Harvard medical practice study supported these findings which found that elderly patients had a higher incidence of adverse drug events.[22] Another study reported the incidence of adverse drug events to be as high as 53% in an elderly hospitalized population.[14] Risk factors for the occurrence of an adverse drug event in the elderly during hospitalization have been shown to include renal failure, greater number of medications, inappropriate medications, and more than 75 years of age.[23,24]

Medication Errors: Medication errors in the elderly have been evaluated in the hospital setting. One retrospective study evaluated medication errors in geriatric patients that occurred during 10,187 hospitalizations at a Midwest teaching hospital over a 3.5-year period. Using a voluntary incident reporting system, 861 medication errors were reported, 96% of which may have been preventable. Most were errors of omission (49%) involving administration (54%) or transcription (38%) errors. Variables associated with medication errors included polypharmacy, select drugs, nursing staffing changes, medical and nursing interventions, and patient gender and race.[25] A number of studies have evaluated the frequency and nature of medication errors in the elderly during transitions of care. A Swedish study found that elderly patients had on average two medication errors each time they transferred from hospital to primary care.[26] Other studies have demonstrated that medication errors are common both upon admission to and discharge from the hospital.[27–31]

23.1.3 Long-Term Care Medication Use

Generally, it is held that residents of long-term care facilities receive more medications than older adults in the outpatient or acute-care setting.[32] While long-term care residents on average receive seven to eight medications,[6] drug use in this setting reached such heights that the Center for Medicare and Medicaid Services (CMS) implemented a polypharmacy quality indicator to target residents taking more than nine medications. Based on data from the 2004 National Nursing Home Survey, approximately 40% of the 13,403 long-term care residents evaluated were receiving more than medications. Among these residents, the most frequently reported drugs included GI agents, CNS drugs, and nonnarcotic analgesics.[33] In comparison, a study of 64,395 Canadian nursing home patients revealed that 16% were receiving more than nine medications[34] compared to 24% who were taking ≥ ten medications in European countries.[35]

Adverse Drug Events: Adverse drug events in elderly residents are described as the most common drug-related problems in long-term care facilities.[36,37] Expressed in economic terms, for every $1.00 spent on medications in long-term care, another $1.33 is consumed in healthcare resources to treat drug-related morbidity.[38] Risk factors that have been identified for the occurrence of an adverse drug event in nursing home residents include polypharmacy, defined as the use of more than seven medications or more than three cardiac medications and the use of high-risk drugs.[39]

Medication Errors: Medication errors in long-term care are surprisingly common.[40] The Institute of Medicine reports that approximately 800,000 preventable drug-related injuries occur each year in Medicare recipients in the long-term care setting and that $887 million is spent annually to treat these errors.[41] A study in two large academic long-term care facilities indicated that one out of every ten nursing home residents suffers a medication-related injury and that 73% of the most severe injuries were preventable.[42] A multicenter study reporting on 2,731 discrete errors over a 1-year period found that errors occurred most commonly during medication administration with the most common type of errors being: omission of dose (32%), overdose (14%), underdose (7%), wrong patient (6%), wrong product (6%), and wrong drug strength (6%). Seven drugs were implicated in 28% of all errors: Lorazepam, oxycodone, warfarin, furosemide, hydrocodone, insulin, and fentanyl.[43] Polypharmacy and inappropriate medication use are major risk factors for medication errors in long-term care.[44]

23.2 ALTERED CLINICAL RESPONSE TO DRUGS

While the sheer volume of medication use in the elderly no doubt directly contributes to the higher incidence of adverse drug events and medication errors, there are age-related factors that play a role in contributing to the higher risk of negative medication outcomes. An elderly individual's clinical response to a drug is the sum of a number of complex factors, including age-related physiologic changes, underlying comorbidities, concomitant medications, and frailty among others. These changes do not occur abruptly but rather progress gradually over time.[11] Age-related physiologic changes can result in an alteration of pharmacokinetics (i.e., what the body does to the drug), including absorption, distribution, metabolism, and elimination. Changes in homeostatic mechanisms and drug receptor sensitivity can have an effect on a drug's pharmacodynamics (what the drug does to the body). While these factors cannot be controlled, their impact on drug therapy must be considered as a means of understanding and preventing adverse drug events and medication errors in the elderly. The following is a description of how some of these changes can often predictably result in an altered clinical response to drugs in the elderly. Additionally, the tables provide tools from the published literature that can be used to evaluate causation in a malpractice or negligence case brought against a caregiver, hospital, or long-term care facility.

23.2.1 PHARMACOKINETICS

Absorption: Some physiologic changes that occur with advancing age include elevated gastric pH, slowed gastric emptying, and reduced small bowel surface area. For most oral drugs that are absorbed passively, these changes may decrease the rate of absorption but generally have no significant effect on the extent of absorption.[45] Some nutrients from vitamins (e.g., vitamin B_{12}, iron, calcium, and magnesium) that undergo absorption by active transport may have impaired absorption.[46] For drugs that require an acidic environment for absorption (e.g., calcium carbonate), there may be reduced extent of absorption. Increases in gastric pH might also alter absorption from enteric-coated dosage forms due to an early release.[47] Drugs that undergo first-pass metabolism (e.g., propranolol, labetalol) may demonstrate an increased bioavailability, while pro-drugs (e.g. enalapril, codeine) may show a decreased bioavailability. Drug–food interactions, concurrent medication use, and comorbidities impacting gastrointestinal function must still be considered.[48] Transdermal drug administration is becoming more popular for some medications for the elderly, and skin changes can affect drug absorption of hydrophilic drugs (e.g., acetylsalicylic acid) and, to a lesser extent, lipophilic drugs (e.g., estradiol).[49] Such changes in absorption may help predict or explain an enhanced or diminished effect of certain drugs in an elderly patient.

Distribution: There are a number of age-related changes that can alter drug distribution in the body. Body composition changes include reduced total body water and lean mass which can result in higher concentration of drugs (e.g., lithium, digoxin) if the dose is unadjusted. Conversely, total body fat increases with age which can result in an

TABLE 23.1
Drugs Requiring Dosage Adjustment in Hepatic Impairment*.

Acetaminophen	Fenofibrate	Omeprazole
Alprazolam †	Fentanyl	Ondansetron
Amiodarone	Finasteride	Oxycodone
Amlodipine	Flecainide	Paroxetine
Anastrozole	Fluoxetine	Phenytoin
Atorvastatin	Glipizide	Pravastatin
Bisoprolol	Glyburide	Propranolol
Bumetanide	Hydrocodone	Risperidone
Bupropion	Hydroxychloroquine	Rivaroxaban
Buspirone	Ibuprofen	Rivastigmine
Carvedilol	Lamotrigine	Rosuvastatin
Celecoxib	Lansoprazole	Simvastatin
Citalopram	Levetiracetam	Solifenacin
Colchicine	Lidocaine †	Telmisartan
Cyclobenzaprine	Lorazepam	Tizanidine
Desipramine †	Losartan	Tramadol
Diazepam	Meperidine	Trazodone
Diclofenac	Metformin	Triamterene
Diltiazem	Methotrexate	Triazolam †
Doxazosin	Metronidazole	Venlafaxine
Duloxetine	Morphine	Verapamil
Escitalopram	Naproxen	Warfarin
Esomeprazole	Nebivolol	Zolpidem
Ezetimibe	Nifedipine	
Felodipine	Nortriptyline	

*Source: *Based on drugs listed in the Top 200 Medicare Part D drugs commonly used by seniors in 2015 on Aetna and Coventry Individual Medicare formularies.*[53] *† These medications have demonstrated a decreased hepatic metabolism in men but not in women.*[47]

increased volume of distribution, accumulation, and prolonged elimination half-life with chronic use of highly lipophilic drugs (e.g., diazepam).[45,48] Factors potentially impacting plasma protein binding include an age-related increase in α1-acid glycoprotein and a decrease in serum albumin. The clinical effect of these changes on serum drug binding is unclear except for drugs that are highly protein-bound. However, acute illness, concomitant drugs, and malnutrition can further decrease albumin, a protein that is a major drug-binding site, resulting in enhanced effects of some drugs (e.g., phenytoin, warfarin).[49] Decreased blood flow due to a decreased cardiac output can result in a slowed distribution of drugs to their sites of action in muscle or fat.[48] Permeability of the blood–brain barrier may also be altered in aging due to decreased P-glycoprotein activity which can affect the distribution of drugs into the CNS and potentially result in exposure to higher drug levels[49] (http://accesspharmacy.mhmedical.com/content.aspx?bookid=689&sectionid=48811433–57521318).

Metabolism: Liver metabolism is dependent upon liver blood perfusion and metabolic capacity, both of which are altered by the aging process.[50] Drugs with high hepatic-extraction ratios are dependent on liver blood flow (i.e., perfusion) which can be reduced in the elderly by as much as 20–50%. This results in decreased hepatic metabolism of drugs like amitriptyline, diltiazem, verapamil, nitrates, barbiturates, lidocaine, morphine, metoprolol, and propranolol.[51] The elderly are reported to have reduced liver size and enzyme content, but interpreting the effect aging has on capacity-limited drug metabolism is more complex as it depends on the unbound fraction of drug in blood and the intrinsic hepatic clearance.[11] Generally, the hepatic metabolism of many drugs by phase I reactions (oxidative cytochrome P450 enzyme system, reduction, hydrolysis) is more likely to be decreased with age. However, age does not greatly affect the clearance of drugs metabolized through phase II pathways (conjugation, acetylation, sulfonation, glucuronidation) except in frail older adults.[47] Reduction of the metabolism rate and thus clearance of a drug result in elevated drug concentrations, potentially resulting in toxic effects. Table 23.1 summarizes examples of frequently used drugs for which there are recommended dosage adjustments in liver impairment.

Elimination: Kidneys are the primary route of elimination for many drugs and their metabolites. As such, one of the most important age-related pharmacokinetic changes is decreased renal elimination of drugs due to reduced renal plasma flow, glomerular filtration rate, and tubular secretion.[47,50] As a result of such changes, the half-life of a number of renally excreted drugs can be prolonged. Decreased renal drug clearance may increase the concentration of renally cleared drugs to potentially high levels if the dosing regimens are based on the normal renal excretion rates of young, healthy individuals. Consequently, decreased renal clearance results in more adverse drug events than any other age-related physiological change. However, the actual clinical implications will depend on the extent to which renal elimination contributes to total body elimination. Creatinine clearance, whether measured or estimated using the Cockcroft–Gault equation (see Equation 23.1),[52] can serve as an indication of renal function and can be used to guide dosage adjustments for drugs that heavily rely on renal elimination. The Cockcroft–Gault equation can be used to estimate creatinine clearance in adults with stable renal function whose actual body weight is within 30% of ideal. Age is expressed in years, weight in kg, and serum creatinine in mg/dL. The resulting creatinine clearance is in units of mL/min. For women, multiply this result by 0.85. Table 23.2 summarizes examples of frequently used drugs for which there are recommended dosage adjustments for reduced renal function in older adults. It should be recognized that some drugs which are metabolized by the liver can produce active metabolites (e.g., normeperidine, morphine-6-glucuronide) that are also eliminated by the kidneys and can accumulate with advancing age because of reduced renal function.

Equation 23.1 shows Cockcroft–Gault equation for estimating creatinine clearance.

$$\textit{Creatinine clearance} = \frac{(140 - Age)(Actual\ body\ weight)}{72(Serum\ creatinine\ concentration)} \quad (23.1)$$

23.2.2 Pharmacodynamics

Separate from age-related physiologic changes that can alter the way an older patient handles the absorption, distribution, metabolism, and elimination of a drug, aging can also alter the type, intensity, and duration of drug effect. Unfortunately, the effects that aging can have on the pharmacodynamic response to a drug are multifactorial and therefore are often variable. While there is a general trend of increased sensitivity to drug effect with aging (e.g., benzodiazepines), a diminished response can also be seen (e.g., beta-blockers) with the end result ranging from treatment failure to major drug toxicity. Examples of the effect aging can have on the pharmacologic action of select drugs or drug classes are given in Table 23.3. A number of mechanisms have been suggested to explain this altered drug response, including changes in the number of drug receptor sites, changes in drug–receptor binding; changes in drug concentration at the receptor; altered sensitivity to a given drug concentration; pathologic organ changes due to disease and/or aging; depletion of neurotransmitters; and impairment of homeostatic mechanisms.[54–57]

To date, most of the work in which age-related pharmacodynamic differences have been evaluated has focused on the CNS and cardiovascular system. As it relates to CNS drug effect, brain atrophy, decreased cerebral blood flow, decreased oxygen consumption, increased cerebrovascular resistance, increased permeability of the blood–brain barrier, decreases in numbers of neurons and receptors, increased monoamine oxidase activity, and decreased levels of neurotransmitters (e.g. acetylcholine, dopamine, and serotonin) have all been described with advanced age.[11,49,56,57] The elderly are particularly sensitive to anticholinergic effects of drugs, especially patients with cognitive impairment (e.g., Alzheimer's disease). Anticholinergic drugs (see Table 23.4), even when taken in low doses, commonly cause increased sedation, confusion, memory loss,

TABLE 23.2
Drugs Requiring Dosage Adjustment in Renal Impairment*.

Acyclovir	Dorzolamide/Timolol	Meloxicam	Probenecid †
ACE Inhibitors	Duloxetine	Memantine	Risperidone
Bisphosphonates	Escitalopram	Meperidine †	Rivaroxaban
Allopurinol	Esomeprazole	Metformin	Rivastigmine
Amantadine	Fenofibrate	Methotrexate	Ropinirole
Atenolol	Fentanyl	Metronidazole	Rosuvastatin
Bisoprolol	Flecainide	Morphine	Simvastatin
Bumetanide	Fluconazole	Nabumetone	Sitagliptin
Bupropion	Gabapentin	Nadolol	Solifenacin
Buspirone	Gemfibrozil	Naproxen	Sotalol
Celecoxib	Glimepiride	Nebivolol	Spironolactone †
Cephalexin	Glipizide	Nitrofurantoin †	Tamsulosin
Ciprofloxacin	Glyburide †	Olmesartan	Thiazides
Citalopram	H_2 Receptor Antagonists	Oxycodone	Tizanidine
Clonidine	Hydralazine	Paroxetine	Topiramate
Codeine	Hydrocodone	Penicillins	Tramadol
Colchicine †	Hydroxychloroquine	Pramipexole	Triamterene †
Cotrimoxazole †	Lamotrigine	Pravastatin	Valacyclovir
Dabigatran	Levetiracetam	Prednisone	Valsartan
Diclofenac	Levofloxacin	Pregabalin	Venlafaxine
Digoxin	Lovastatin	Primidone	Verapamil

**Source:* Based on drugs listed in the Top 200 Medicare Part D drugs commonly used by seniors in 2015 on Aetna and Coventry Individual Medicare formularies.[53] † These medications should be avoided in elderly patients with a creatinine clearance <30 ml/min, based on consensus guidelines for oral dosing of primarily renally cleared medications in older adults.[52]*

TABLE 23.3
Effects of Aging on Drug Pharmacodynamics.

Drug/Drug Class	Pharmacologic Effect	Effect of Aging[55–59]
ACE inhibitors	Hypotensive effect	↑
Albuterol	Bronchodilation	↓
Anesthetic agents	Increased sensitivity	↑
Angiotensin receptor blockers	Hypotensive effect	↑
Antidepressants, SSRI	Hyponatremia	↑
Antidepressants, tricyclic	Anticholinergic effects	↑
Antihistamines, first-generation	Anticholinergic effects, sedation	↑
Antipsychotics	Extrapyramidal effects, hypotension	↑
Antispasmodics, GI	Anticholinergic effects	↑
Antispasmodics, urinary	Anticholinergic effects	↑
Barbiturates	Psychomotor effects, sedation	↑
Benzodiazepines, long-acting	Psychomotor effects, sedation	↑
Benztropine	Anticholinergic effects	↑
Beta-blockers	Hypotensive, chronotropic effects	↓
Calcium-channel blockers	Hypotensive effect, constipation	↑
Diuretics	Diuresis	↓
Heparin	Bleeding risk	↑
Insulin	Insulin sensitivity	↓
Iron supplements	Constipation	↑
Isoproterenol	Inotropic, chronotropic effects	↓
Lithium	Risk of toxicity	↑
Metoclopramide	Extrapyramidal symptoms, sedation	↑
NSAIDS	Bleeding risk	↑
Opiates	Analgesia	↑
Skeletal muscle relaxants	Anticholinergic effects, sedation	↑
Theophylline	Bronchodilation	↓
Thrombolytics	Bleeding risk	↑
Warfarin	Bleeding risk	↑

blurred vision, urinary retention, dry mouth, constipation, and orthostatic hypotension.[60] Generally speaking, drugs with anticholinergic effects should be avoided in the elderly, and an alternative drug should be used when possible. From a cardiovascular perspective, examples of age-related changes that may result in an altered pharmacodynamic drug response include impaired baroreceptor response to blood pressure changes increasing the risk of orthostatic hypotension, decreased cardiac output, increased systemic vascular resistance, decreased heart rate, and decreased responsiveness of beta-adrenergic receptors.[57]

Although not strictly a pharmacodynamic issue, the elderly may demonstrate a supratherapeutic drug response because of a lack of pharmacokinetic or pharmacodynamic data to guide proper dosing. In essence, because of their reduced ability to tolerate usual adult doses, some elderly patients may receive a relative overdose. This is because historically the elderly have been underrepresented in clinical trials. While older patients take more medications, drug studies sponsored by the pharmaceutical industry are primarily conducted in the younger adult population. Further, if a drug is evaluated in the elderly, it is usually a "healthy" geriatric population, and the frail or aged population with multi-morbidity and polypharmacy is excluded. This is likely due to difficulties associated with patient selection and reporting of clinical trial results when assessing age-related differences in drugs.[61] Similarly, because of the exclusion from or a paucity of clinical trial data in the elderly, there can be an underestimation of benefits and an overestimation of risk which can lead to underutilization of pharmacotherapy. Clearly, the extrapolation of dosage regimens and potential adverse effects for use in the geriatric population is not optimal, and there is a need for drug data in various cohorts of the elderly population.

23.2.3 Multiple Comorbidities

Based on a the CDC's report entitled *The State of Aging and Health in America 2013*, there has been a major shift occurring over the past century in the leading causes of death for all age groups from acute conditions to chronic diseases and degenerative illnesses.[62] While heart disease and cancer continue to pose the greatest risk as people age, two out of every three older adults have multiple chronic conditions including diabetes, stroke, hypertension, arthritis, chronic lower respiratory diseases, and Alzheimer's

TABLE 23.4
Commonly Used Drugs with Anticholinergic Properties.

High			
Amitriptyline	Cyproheptadine	Hydroxyzine	Protriptyline
Amoxapine	Darifenacin	Hyoscyamine	Pyrilamine
Atropine	Desipramine	Imipramine	Scopolamine
Belladonna	Dicyclomine	Ipratropium	Solifenacin
Benztropine	Dimenhydrinate	Maprotiline	Thioridazine
Brompheniramine	Diphenhydramine	Meclizine	Thiothixene
Carbinoxamine	Doxepin	Nortriptyline	Tizanidine
Carisoprodol	Doxylamine	Orphenadrine	Tolterodine
Chlorpheniramine	Fesoterodine	Oxybutynin	Trifluoperazine
Chlorpromazine	Flavoxate	Perphenazine	Trihexyphenidyl
Clomipramine	Fluphenazine	Promethazine	Trimipramine
Clozapine	Homatropine	Propantheline	Trospium
Moderate			
Baclofen	Cyclobenzaprine	Methadone	Pimozide
Carbamazepine	Fexofenadine	Olanzapine	Prochlorperazine
Cetirizine	Hydrocodone	Oxcarbazepine	Pseudoephedrine
Cimetidine	Meperidine	Paroxetine	Tramadol
Low			
Alprazolam	Cycloserine	Iloperidone	Phenelzine
Amantadine	Cyclosporine	Isosorbide	Phenobarbital
Ampicillin	Desloratadine	Ketorolac	Piperacillin
Aripiprazole	Dexamethasone	Ketotifen	Pramipexole
Asenapine	Dextromethorphan	Levocetirizine	Prednisolone
Atenolol	Diazepam	Lithium	Prednisone
Azathioprine	Digoxin	Loperamide	Quetiapine
Benazepril	Diltiazem	Loratadine	Quinidine
Betaxolol	Dipyridamole	Lorazepam	Ranitidine
Bisacodyl	Disopyramide	Metformin	Risperidone
Bupropion	Divalproex	Methocarbamol	Selegiline
Captopril	Domperidone	Methotrexate	Sertraline
Carbidopa	Entacapone	Methylprednisolone	Sumatriptan
Cefoxitin	Escitalopram	Metoclopramide	Temazepam
Celecoxib	Estazolam	Metoprolol	Theophylline
Cephalothin	Famotidine	Midazolam	Trandolapril
Chlordiazepoxide	Fentanyl	Mirtazapine	Trazodone
Chlorthalidone	Fluoxetine	Morphine	Triamcinolone
Citalopram	Flurazepam	Naratriptan	Triamterene
Clidinium	Fluvoxamine	Nefazodone	Triazolam
Clindamycin	Furosemide	Nifedipine	Valproic acid
Clonazepam	Gentamicin	Nizatidine	Vancomycin
Clorazepate	Guaifenesin	Oxazepam	Venlafaxine
Codeine	Haloperidol	Oxycodone	Warfarin
Colchicine	Hydralazine	Paliperidone	Ziprasidone
Cortisone	Hydrocortisone	Pancuronium	Zolmitriptan

Source: Adapted with permission from Salahudeen MS, Duffull SB, Nishtala PS. Anticholinergic burden quantified by anticholinergic risk scales and adverse outcomes in older people: a systematic review. BMC Geriatr. 2015 Mar 25; 15:31 (Open Access, BioMed Central).[60]

disease. Another source indicates that 20% of Medicare beneficiaries have more than five chronic conditions.[63]

The challenge in geriatrics is in providing optimal care for patients with multiple comorbidities. Treatment guidelines are often used to direct the clinical care of patients, including pharmacologic management, but most guidelines focus on the management of a single disease. The application of multiple treatment guidelines to a patient population with multiple comorbidities contributes to the proliferation of polypharmacy and associated drug-related problems including adverse effects, drug interactions, and geriatric syndromes (e.g., falls, gait disorders, dizziness, syncope, weakness, appetite disorders, weight loss, fecal/urinary incontinence, functional decline, sensory deficit, cognitive impairment, and delirium).[64,65]

A variety of strategies have been employed, but the optimal approach to managing the cumulative effects of chronic diseases and syndromes while streamlining the drug regimen to prevent polypharmacy and potential drug-related morbidity remains unclear.[66]

23.2.4 Drug Interactions

Another common cause of adverse drug events in elderly patients is drug interactions. In an interrelated fashion, the vicious cycle of multiple comorbidities that require an increased medication burden coupled with age-related pharmacokinetic and pharmacodynamic changes predisposes older adults to drug interactions. A number of studies have established a direct correlation between the number of medications taken and the risk of an adverse drug event due to a drug interaction.[67–72]

On an outpatient basis, a retrospective analysis of more than 70,000 outpatient visits by patients more than 65 years in the *National Ambulatory Medical Care Survey* and the *National Hospital Ambulatory Medical Care Survey* found there was at least one inappropriate drug–drug combination in 0.74% of visits involving more than 2 prescriptions, and one or more inappropriate drug–disease combinations were found in 2.58% of visits involving at least 1 prescription.[73] A study of a group of 1,601 elderly individuals from across 6 European countries who were living at home revealed that 46% had at least one drug combination that posed a potential drug–drug interaction.[74] A Brazilian study reported the risk of drug interactions increased as the number of medications consumed increased from two to three (39%) to four to five (89%) to six to seven (100%).[75] In patients receiving a statin in combination with a fibrate, macrolide, or protease inhibitor, the risk of myopathy is increased.[76]

In the hospital setting, drug–drug interactions are also a frequent cause of preventable medication-related hospitalizations.[9] A prospective study of 275 patients more than 65 years who were consecutively admitted to a community hospital with more than 5 medications found that the prevalence of a potential cytochrome-mediated drug-drug interactions was 80%. The probability of a drug–drug interaction increased as the number of medications increased from 5–9 drugs (50%) to 10–14 drugs (81%) to 15–19 drugs (92%) to more than 20 drugs (100%), with the addition of each medication to the 5-drug regimen conferring a 12% increased risk.[77] A seven-year Canadian study evaluated hospitalizations related to toxicity in a population of older patients for three common drug therapies including glyburide, digoxin, or an ACE inhibitor. In patients receiving a glyburide–cotrimoxazole combination, the risk of hospitalization for hypoglycemia was six times greater. In patients receiving a digoxin–clarithromycin combination, the risk of hospitalization for digoxin toxicity was 12 times greater. In patients receiving an ACE inhibitor–potassium-sparing diuretic combination, the risk of hospitalization for hyperkalemia was 20 times greater.[78]

Studies in frail elderly veterans have shown the risk of drug–disease interactions to increase as the number of medications increased, with one or more interactions occurring 15–40% of the time.[79,80] Clearly, the potential for clinically significant drug–drug or drug–disease interactions in the elderly must be considered when more than one medication is being prescribed and with the addition of each new medication.

23.3 PREVENTABLE DRUG-RELATED PROBLEMS

As pointed out in the previous discussion, physiologic changes in the elderly are uncontrollable, but an ongoing assessment of their potential impact on drug therapy is an important part of the standard of care. In addition to patient-related factors, elderly patients often suffer from suboptimal drug utilization (e.g., overuse, underuse, misuse) that results from practice-related issues. Medication-use practices that are known to be problematic include polypharmacy, inadequate drug monitoring, use of potentially inappropriate medications, and mismanagement of drug therapy through transitions of care. Such practices have been shown to significantly contribute to drug misadventures in the elderly. An ongoing review process should be employed that focuses both on the initial drug regimen selection as well as on enhanced monitoring so that drug misadventures in the elderly can be avoided or minimized. The following discussion is a description of practice-related problems that are often predictable and preventable, and how they can result in an unintended negative drug therapy outcome. As in the previous section, tools are provided from the published literature that can be used in a legal case to evaluate whether steps were taken to minimize or prevent an adverse drug event or medication error.

23.3.1 Polypharmacy

Polypharmacy, frequently but somewhat arbitrarily defined as taking more than five medications, is common in the elderly.[81,82] Polypharmacy has been further characterized as simply either the use of multiple medications or as the use of more medications than are medically necessary. As described previously, polypharmacy is a common finding across a variety of practice settings, and there are a number of factors that contribute to the problem. It is important to remember when assessing the overall polypharmacy burden that the uses of prescription drugs, OTC products, herbal remedies, dietary supplements, minerals, and multivitamins all be considered. The use of evidence-based treatment guidelines in the pharmacologic management of each individual chronic condition in the elderly contributes to polypharmacy, even though evidence for applying such guidelines to this patient population is generally lacking.[62] Prescribing cascades also directly contribute to polypharmacy.[83] Side effects of drugs often masquerade as a new medical problem, and when this occurs, sometimes a new drug is prescribed to treat the problem. Similarly, this new drug may also be associated with a side effect that is again interpreted as a new medical problem, and a prescribing cascade is perpetuated. An example of drug use that might precipitate a prescribing cascade is the use of an OTC sleep-aid (e.g., diphenhydramine) that can cause symptoms of urinary retention. In an elderly male, this may be diagnosed as benign prostate hyperplasia and end up being treated with an alpha-blocker. The alpha-blocker then in turn can cause significant orthostatic hypotension which could result in a fall. Drug-induced disease should always be considered as a possibility in the elderly.

Studies have demonstrated that polypharmacy is associated with increased adverse drug events, drug interactions, as well as an increased risk for the use of potentially inappropriate medications. One study revealed that the risk increased for an outpatient or emergency department visit due to an adverse drug event as the number of medications taken increased (odds ratio (OR) = 1.4 for 3–4 medications; OR = 1.88 for >5 medications).[84] Another study evaluated the association between polypharmacy and drug–drug interactions in the elderly and found the risk for a drug–drug interaction increased as the number of medications taken increased (odds ratio (OR) = 1.9 for 6–10 medications; OR = 4.5 for >11 medications).[72] Finally, yet another study demonstrated in older adults that as the number of medications prescribed increased, the prevalence of potentially inappropriate medication also increased.[85] Studies have also shown that the likelihood of medication errors in the elderly increases when the total number of drugs being used is greater,[86] with the odds of a medication error increasing by 5% for each additional medication.[25] Other studies have demonstrated an association between polypharmacy and increased morbidity and mortality, increased cost, and decreased adherence.[20,66,81,82,87]

One way to combat the problem of polypharmacy is to identify unnecessary drug use. For example, in the long-term care setting, a drug regimen review process[88] is used to identify unnecessary drugs. Unnecessary drugs are defined as any medications that a resident may be receiving without an indication for use, in excessive dose or duration, with inadequate monitoring, or in the presence of any adverse consequences that indicate that the dose should be reduced or discontinued.[89] Through the drug regimen review process, which involves a review of the patient's medication list alongside appropriate portions of their clinical record, criteria that assess medication appropriateness can be applied to avoid unnecessary drugs. If there is no explicit indication for a drug, if a drug that is being prescribed is not effective in treating the condition, if there is unnecessary duplication of therapy with other drugs, or if the duration of therapy is excessive, the drug may not be needed.[90]

23.3.2 Transitions of Care

The elderly with multiple chronic illnesses commonly experience transitions in care, going from one care setting to another. The *National Transitions of Care Coalition* defines a transition of care as

> [T]he movement of patients between healthcare locations, providers, or different levels of care within the same location as their conditions and care needs change, [and] frequently involves multiple persons, including the patient, the family member or other caregivers, nurses, social workers, case managers, pharmacists, physicians, and other providers.[91]

In 2019, *The Journal of the American Medical Association* published a study that tracked adverse events in patients discharging from acute care settings back to nursing home facilities, which revealed that nearly 20% of subjects developed an adverse event related to medication. The same study indicated that most negative outcomes seen were preventable, estimating that nearly 70% could have been circumvented.[92] Every transition necessarily involves a coordination of care between healthcare providers (e.g., primary care, specialist care, assisted living facility, hospital, home health, skilled nursing facility, etc.) to ensure optimal care.

One element of coordination that is commonly employed across the continuum of care is medication reconciliation. According to the *Agency for Healthcare Research and Quality*, medication reconciliation is a process that works to decrease medication errors and avoid patient harm by helping to ensure the communication of information about a patient's drug regimen at each point of transition in the healthcare system.[93] According to the *Joint Commission*, the process involves obtaining, verifying, and documenting the patient's current drug regimen (e.g., prescription drugs, OTC drugs, supplements, herbals, vitamins, and topicals) including drug name, dose, frequency, and route of administration; comparing the resulting list against physician orders at the time of each admission, transfer, or discharge; making medical decisions based on the comparison; and communicating the intended drug regimen going forward to the patient, caregivers, and/or healthcare providers.[94]

Although medication reconciliation plays an integral role in reducing medication errors,[95–97] poor communication of medication information during transitions of care has been stated to cause up to 60% of all medication errors.[91,98] Further, while the aim of the medication reconciliation is to reduce medication errors, errors can occur in or be created by the reconciliation process. Factors present in the elderly population that have been shown to contribute to reconciliation errors include advanced age, presence of multiple comorbidities, and polypharmacy.[99] Several studies have documented discrepancies during the medication reconciliation process during transitions of care.

In the hospital setting, one study of 651 patients found that 85% percent of the patients had errors that originated from their medication histories, almost 50% of which were medication omissions. Another 36% experienced discrepancies resulting in changes of physicians' orders, 52% of which were rated as potentially requiring increased monitoring or intervention to preclude harm, and 12% were rated as potentially harmful.[100] Another prospective study of 151 inpatients who were taking at least 4 prescription medications reported that 81 patients (54%) had at least one unintended discrepancy. The most common error (46%) was the omission of a routine medication, and 39% of the discrepancies had the potential to cause moderate-to-severe discomfort or clinical deterioration.91

Studies in long-term care facilities have demonstrated similar results. In a study involving patients transitioning from a hospital to a skilled-nursing facility, at least one medication discrepancy was identified in 142 (71%) of a total of 199 admissions. Of the 2,319 medications reviewed on admission, 495 (21%) had a medication discrepancy. The discharge summary and patient care referral form did not match for 104 of the 199 patients (52%), accounting for 307 (62%) of all medication discrepancies. Anti-infective, cardiovascular, neuropsychiatric, and diabetes medications along with high-alert drugs including opioids and anticoagulants accounted for more than 50% of all medication discrepancies.[101] Another study in long-term care examined actual harm that was caused by medication discrepancies during 122 transfers between acute and long-term care facilities. A mean of 3.1 and 1.4 medication orders were altered (drug discontinuation, dosage changes, class substitutions) during transfer from nursing facility to hospital and from hospital to nursing facility, respectively. Adverse drug events attributable to medication changes occurred in 20% of transfers.[102] In addition to medication errors and adverse drug events, failure to employ safeguards within medication reconciliation at transitions of care can further lead to confusion about a patient's condition, duplicate tests, inadequate patient monitoring, lack of follow-up, and rehospitalization, among others.[103–106]

23.3.3 Inadequate Monitoring

Once drug therapy has been initiated in an older adult, it is necessary to continually and systematically reassess their drug regimen, because appropriate monitoring of drug therapy helps to guide therapeutic decision-making and identify opportunities for improvement in care. Unfortunately, inadequate monitoring increases the risk of therapeutic failure and adverse drug events. It has been reported that medications requiring regular monitoring are the root cause of more than 50% of elderly admissions to the hospital and that upon discharge, adverse drug events due to monitoring errors are more common than those due to prescribing errors.[9,13,107] A systematic review of published studies on the incidence and characteristics of preventable adverse drug events in ambulatory care resulting in hospitalization noted that 45% of adverse drug events were caused by inadequate monitoring, and 16% were due to ignoring a clinical or laboratory result and, when considered together, were 1.4 times more common than adverse events resulting from an inappropriate drug, dose, or frequency.[71,108] Studies that looked at elements of patient complaints have found that prescribers frequently fail to solicit complaints about drug-related side effects and that when patients did offer complaints about drug-related symptoms, prescribers failed to respond appropriately 63% of the time.[109–111] Physicians' failure to change therapy in another study resulted in 65% of the applicable patients experiencing an ameliorable adverse drug event.[112] Related to laboratory monitoring, many physicians (56–59%) expressed dissatisfaction with systems they use to track and review test results due to delays in accessing the data, but yet another study documented that 37% of preventable adverse drug events were due to failure to act on available clinical or laboratory information.[9,113,114] Other documented monitoring-related problems have included failure to recognize a symptom or abnormal lab test as being drug-related or recognizing a connection between an abnormal lab or symptom and a drug but failing to reduce the dose or discontinue the offending drug.[115,116]

These findings both exemplify how suboptimal monitoring can result in a high rate of preventable adverse drug events, and why emphasis must be placed on a monitoring approach that prospectively anticipates such problems. While various approaches have been taken,[71,117,118] an effective framework for periodically monitoring current drug therapy, in view of the patient's clinical status and therapeutic goals, at a minimum should include assessing effectiveness and adherence to the regimen, discontinuing any unnecessary medications, adjusting to use the lowest possible effective dose, and considering safer alternative medications or non-pharmacologic strategies. Monitoring must also be aimed at detecting adverse effects, drug interactions, or unintended responses to a drug. A consensus list of select drug–lab combinations (Table 23.5) has been identified as signals that can be used to detect potential adverse drug events.[119] Finally, laboratory tests, vital signs, or other appropriate objective measures should be used to monitor efficacy and toxicity for each medication. Table 23.6 lists recommendations for laboratory monitoring intervals for chronic medications used in long-term care facilities.[120]

23.3.4 Potentially Inappropriate Medication Use

Because of, or in addition to, the altered clinical response to drugs that can be brought on by age-related changes in pharmacokinetics and pharmacodynamics and multiple comorbidities, there are some drugs or drug classes that pose special concern in the elderly. While some drugs should be avoided altogether, others may only need to be avoided in certain circumstances, and yet others can still be used but with caution. The phrase *potentially inappropriate medications* have been coined to describe such drugs which simply mean medications that are inappropriate if their potential for harm is greater than their potential for benefit.[121]

TABLE 23.5
Laboratory–Medication Combination Signals for Detecting ADRs in the Nursing Home Setting.

Laboratory/Medication Combination Signals	Mean Score*	95% CI
Hypoglycemia (as indicated by a low or decreasing glucose concentration) is found in an individual taking a drug that may cause or worsen hypoglycemia	4.6	4.4–4.8
Supratherapeutic (above upper limit of normal range) international normalized ratio (INR) is found in an individual taking warfarin	4.6	4.4–4.8
Clostridium difficile toxin is found in an individual taking a drug that may cause pseudomembranous colitis	4.5	4.3–4.7
Hyperkalemia (as indicated by a high or increasing potassium concentration) is found in an individual taking a drug that may cause or worsen hyperkalemia	4.5	4.3–4.7
Hypokalemia (as indicated by a low or decreasing potassium concentration) is found in an individual taking a drug that may cause or worsen hypokalemia	4.5	4.3–4.7
Thrombocytopenia (as indicated by a low or decreasing platelet count) is found in an individual taking a drug that may cause or worsen thrombocytopenia	4.5	4.3–4.7
Supratherapeutic activated partial thromboplastin time (PTT) is found in an individual taking heparin	4.4	4.2–4.7
Subtherapeutic concentration (below lower limit of normal range) of thyroid-stimulating hormone (TSH) or elevated concentration of thyroxine (T4) is found in an individual taking a drug that may cause hyperthyroidism	4.4	4.2–4.6
Hyponatremia (as indicated by a low or decreasing sodium concentration) is found in an individual taking a drug that may cause or worsen hyponatremia	4.4	4.2–4.5
Leukopenia (as indicated by a low or decreasing white blood cell count) is found in an individual taking a drug that may cause or worsen leukopenia	4.3	4.1–4.6
Elevated alanine aminotransferase (ALT) or aspartate aminotransferase (AST) concentration is found in an individual taking a drug that may cause hepatocellular toxicity	4.3	4.1–4.5
Elevated creatinine or blood urea nitrogen (BUN) concentration is found in an individual taking a drug that may increase creatinine or BUN	4.3	4.1–4.5
Supratherapeutic concentration of TSH or decreased concentration of T4 is found in an individual taking a drug that may cause hypothyroidism	4.3	4.1–4.4
Agranulocytosis or neutropenia (as indicated by a low or decreasing neutrophil count) is found in an individual taking a drug that may cause or worsen agranulocytosis or neutropenia	4.2	4.1–4.3
Elevated creatine phosphokinase (CPK) concentration is found in an individual taking a drug that may increase CPK	4.2	4.0–4.4

Source: *Each item was rated on a 5-point Likert scale, with 5 indicating strong agreement with the likelihood that the item signaled an adverse drug reaction. The mean likelihood score and 95% confidence interval (CI) were calculated for each item. Consensus was indicated by a lower-limit 95% CI of ≥4.0. Reprinted with permission from Handler SM, Hanlon JT, Perera S, Roumani YF, Nace DA, Fridsma DB, Saul MI, Castle NG, Studenski SA. Consensus list of signals to detect potential adverse drug reactions in nursing homes. J Am Geriatr Soc. 2008 May; 56(5):808–15. (Copyright © 2008, John Wiley and Sons).[119]*

TABLE 23.6
Recommended Laboratory Monitoring Intervals for Chronic Medications.

Drug or Drug Class	Monitoring Parameter	Interval (months)
ACE inhibitors	Serum potassium	6
Acetaminophen (>4 gm/day)	Liver function tests	*
Amiodarone	Liver function tests, TSH level, baseline chest X-ray	6
Antipsychotics	Blood glucose (fasting), hemoglobin A1c, lipid panel, AIMS test	6
ARB blockers	Serum potassium	6
Carbamazepine	Therapeutic drug monitoring	3 – 6
Cyclosporine	Therapeutic drug monitoring	3
Digoxin	Serum creatinine, BUN, therapeutic drug monitoring	6
Disopyramide	Therapeutic drug monitoring	†
Diuretics	Serum sodium and potassium levels	3
Erythropoiesis stimulants	CBC	1

(Continued)

TABLE 23.6
Continued

Drug or Drug Class	Monitoring Parameter	Interval (months)
Fibrates	Liver function tests, CBC	6
Glucocorticoids	Blood glucose (fasting), hemoglobin A1c	3
Hypoglycemics	Blood glucose (fasting), hemoglobin A1c	6
Lithium	Therapeutic drug monitoring	3
Metformin	Serum creatinine, BUN	6
Niacin	Blood glucose (fasting), hemoglobin A1c, liver function tests	6
Phenobarbital	Therapeutic drug monitoring	3 – 6
Phenytoin	Therapeutic drug monitoring	3 – 6
Primidone	Therapeutic drug monitoring	3 – 6
Procainamide	Therapeutic drug monitoring	6
Quinidine	Therapeutic drug monitoring	6
Salicylates	Therapeutic drug monitoring	6
Statins	Liver function tests, lipid panel	6
Theophylline	Therapeutic drug monitoring	3
Thyroid replacement	TSH level	6
Ticlopidine	CBC	3
Tricyclic antidepressants	Therapeutic drug monitoring	12
Valproic acid	Therapeutic drug monitoring	3 – 6
Warfarin	PT/INR	1

Source: **There was no agreement about interval but recommendations ranged from every 1 to 6 months*
† There was no agreement about interval, but recommendations ranged from every 3 to 12 months
Adapted from Handler SM, Shirts BH, Perera S, Becich MJ, Castle NG, Hanlon JT. Frequency of laboratory monitoring of chronic medications administered to nursing facility residents: results of a national Internet-based study. Consult Pharm. 2008 May; 23(5):387–95 with permission of the American Society of Consultant Pharmacists, Alexandria, Virginia, www.ascp.com. All rights reserved.[120]

Despite the development of explicit drug-use criteria, potentially inappropriate medication use remains high in the elderly. In a study published in the *Journal of American Geriatric Society*, Fralick and colleagues estimated that between 2014 and 2018, 43 billion inappropriate doses were distributed, equating to over 25 billion in drug cost.[122] On average, based on explicit criteria, it has been estimated that 20–65% of older adults take potentially inappropriate medications, although this varies considerably between care settings.[86] Studies in ambulatory, community-dwelling older adults have revealed a rate of preventable inappropriate medication use ranging between 15 and 28%,[9,80,123–125] while residents in long-term care are nearly double that rate at 25–42%.[42,126–131] Adverse effects of potentially inappropriate medications have also been shown to cause emergency hospitalization in 7% of patients ≥65 years with two-thirds being due to just four drugs—insulin, oral antiplatelet drugs, warfarin, and oral hypoglycemic agents.[132] Once hospitalized, this number can balloon to 92% of older inpatients receiving at least one potentially inappropriate medication.[133]

Several sets of comprehensive criteria, either explicit or implicit, have been developed by expert panels to aid in identifying potentially inappropriate medications, including overprescribing and misprescribing. While the most well known are the Beers' and STOPP/START criteria, others include *Medication Appropriateness Index* (1992), *Prescribing Appropriateness Index* (1998), *Assessment of Underutilization of Medication Tool* (1999), *Improved Prescribing in the Elderly Tool* (2000), Zhan's criteria (2001), Rancourt's Canadian criteria (2004), *Drug Burden Index* (2007), French Consensus Panel List (2007), *Australian Prescribing Indicators Tool* (2008), Thailand criteria (2008), *Fit FOR The Aged* list (2009), Norwegian General Practice criteria (2009), German Priscus list (2010), and the annually updated *Healthcare Effectiveness Data and Information Set* of high-risk medications in older adults.[134,135] The following is an outline of the Beers' and STOPP/START criteria.

Beers' Criteria: The Beers' criteria, which get their name from the noted geriatrician who led the development of the criteria, were initially developed in 1991 to target nursing home residents.[136] The Beers' criteria have undergone five revisions in 1997, 2003, 2012, 2015, and most recently in 2019, and have been broadened to encompass potentially inappropriate medications for the senior population regardless of where they reside or receive care.[121,137–140]

Developed by an interdisciplinary consensus panel of US experts based on the published literature, the Beers' criteria address 53 potentially inappropriate medications or medication classes. The criteria are divided into drugs that should be avoided in the elderly (Table 23.7), drugs that should be avoided in certain diseases and syndromes, and drugs that should be used with caution in the elderly. These criteria may be useful for identifying medications where risks may outweigh the potential benefits in the elderly. Identifying medications included in the criteria may help prevent adverse effects, poor outcomes, and increased costs in older patients.[66,121]

The most recent update to the Beers' criteria in 2015 was the result of a review of over "6,700 clinical trials and research studies from a pool of over 20,000 articles" over the time span from 2011 to 2014. New to the Beers' criteria are lists of drugs which should be dose-adjusted for kidney

TABLE 23.7
Beers' Criteria for Potentially Inappropriate Medication Use in Older Adults.

Organ System or Therapeutic Category or Drug	Rationale	Recommendation	Quality of Evidence	Strength of Recommendation
Anticholinergics (excludes tricyclic antidepressants)				
First-Generation Antihistamines (as single agent or as part of combination products) Brompheniramine Carbinoxamine Chlorpheniramine Clemastine Cyproheptadine Dexbrompheniramine Dexchlorpheniramine Diphenhydramine (oral) Doxylamine Hydroxyzine Promethazine Triprolidine	Highly anticholinergic; clearance reduced with advanced age, and tolerance develops when used as hypnotic; greater risk of confusion, dry mouth, constipation, and other anticholinergic effects and toxicity. Use of diphenhydramine in special situations such as acute treatment of severe allergic reaction may be appropriate	Avoid	Hydroxyzine and promethazine: High All others: Moderate	Strong
Antiparkinson Agents Benztropine (oral) Trihexyphenidyl	Not recommended for the prevention of extra-pyramidal symptoms with antipsychotics; more-effective agents available for the treatment of Parkinson's disease	Avoid	Moderate	Strong
Antispasmodics Dicyclomine Hyoscyamine Propantheline Scopolamine Belladonna alkaloids Clidinium-chlordiazepoxide	Highly anticholinergic, uncertain effectiveness	Avoid except in short-term palliative care to decrease oral secretions	Moderate	Strong
Antithrombotics				
Dipyridamole (oral short acting; does not apply to extended-release combination with aspirin)	May cause orthostatic hypotension; more effective alternatives available; intravenous form acceptable for use in cardiac stress testing	Avoid	Moderate	Strong
Ticlopidine	Safer effective alternatives available	Avoid	Moderate	Strong
Anti-infective				
Nitrofurantoin	Potential for pulmonary toxicity; safer alternatives available; lack of efficacy in patients with CrCl < 60 mL/min due to inadequate drug concentration in the urine	Avoid for long-term suppression; avoid in patients with CrCl <60 mL/min	Moderate	Strong

(Continued)

TABLE 23.7
Continued

Organ System or Therapeutic Category or Drug	Rationale	Recommendation	Quality of Evidence	Strength of Recommendation
Cardiovascular				
Alpha1 Blockers Doxazosin Prazosin Terazosin	High risk of orthostatic hypotension; not recommended as routine treatment for hypertension; alternative agents have superior risk/benefit profile	Avoid use as an antihypertensive	Moderate	Strong
Alpha Agonists, Central Clonidine Guanabenz Guanfacine Methyldopa Reserpine (>0.1 mg/d)	High risk of adverse central nervous system effects; may cause bradycardia and orthostatic hypotension; not recommended as routine treatment for hypertension	Avoid clonidine as a first-line antihypertensive; avoid others as listed	Low	Strong
Antiarrhythmics (Class Ia, Ic, III) Amiodarone Dofetilide Dronedarone Flecainide Ibutilide Procainamide Propafenone Quinidine Sotalol	Data suggest that rate control yields better balance of benefits and harms than rhythm control for most older adults. Amiodarone is associated with multiple toxicities, including thyroid disease, pulmonary disorders, and QT-interval prolongation	Avoid anti-arrhythmic drugs as first-line treatment of atrial fibrillation	High	Strong
Disopyramide	Disopyramide is a potent negative inotrope and therefore may induce heart failure in older adults; strongly anticholinergic; other antiarrhythmic drugs preferred	Avoid	Low	Strong
Dronedarone	Worse outcomes have been reported in patients taking dronedarone, who have permanent atrial fibrillation or heart failure. In general, rate control is preferred over rhythm control for atrial Fibrillation	Avoid in patients with permanent atrial fibrillation or heart failure	Moderate	Strong
Digoxin >0.125 mg/d	In heart failure, higher dosages are associated with no additional benefit and may increase risk of toxicity; slow renal clearance may lead to risk of toxic effects	Avoid	Moderate	Strong
Nifedipine (immediate release)	Potential for hypotension; risk of precipitating myocardial ischemia	Avoid	High	Strong
Spironolactone (>25 mg/d)	In heart failure, the risk of hyperkalemia is higher in older adults especially if taking >25 mg/d or taking concomitant NSAID, angiotensin converting-enzyme inhibitor, angiotensin receptor blocker, or potassium supplement	Avoid in patients with heart failure or with a CrCl <30 mL/min	Moderate	Strong
Central Nervous System				
Tertiary Tricyclic Antidepressants (alone or in combination) Amitriptyline Imipramine Clomipramine Trimipramine Doxepin >6 mg/d	Highly anticholinergic, sedating, and cause orthostatic hypotension; safety profile of low-dose doxepin (<6 mg/d) is comparable with that of placebo	Avoid	High	Strong

(Continued)

TABLE 23.7
Continued

Organ System or Therapeutic Category or Drug	Rationale	Recommendation	Quality of Evidence	Strength of Recommendation
Antipsychotics First generation, Conventional Chlorpromazine Fluphenazine Haloperidol Loxapine Molindone Perphenazine Pimozide Promazine Thioridazine Thiothixene Trifluoperazine Triflupromazine Second Generation, Atypical Aripiprazole Asenapine Clozapine Iloperidone Lurasidone Olanzapine Paliperidone Quetiapine Risperidone Ziprasidone	Increased risk of cerebrovascular accident (stroke) and mortality in persons with dementia	Avoid in behavioral problems of dementia unless nonpharmacologic options have failed and patient is threat to self or others	Moderate	Strong
Thioridazine Mesoridazine	Highly anticholinergic and risk of QT-interval prolongation	Avoid	Moderate	Strong
Barbiturates Amobarbital Butabarbital Butalbital Mephobarbital Pentobarbital Phenobarbital Secobarbital	High rate of physical dependence; tolerance to sleep benefits; risk of overdose at low dosages	Avoid	High	Strong
Chloral hydrate	Tolerance occurs within ten days, and risks outweigh benefits in light of overdose with doses only three times the recommended dose	Avoid	Low	Strong
Meprobamate	High rate of physical dependence; very sedating	Avoid	Moderate	Strong
Benzodiazepines Short and intermediate acting Alprazolam Estazolam Lorazepam Oxazepam Temazepam Triazolam Long acting Clorazepate Chlordiazepoxide Clonazepam Diazepam Flurazepam Quazepam	Older adults have an increased sensitivity to benzodiazepines and slower metabolism of long-acting agents. In general, all benzodiazepines increase risk of cognitive impairment, delirium, falls, fractures, and motor vehicle accidents in older adults. May be appropriate for seizure disorders, rapid eye movement sleep disorders, benzodiazepine withdrawal, ethanol withdrawal, severe generalized anxiety disorder, periprocedural anesthesia, end-of-life care	Avoid benzodiazepines for any type for treatment of insomnia, agitation, or delirium	High	Strong

(Continued)

TABLE 23.7
Continued

Organ System or Therapeutic Category or Drug	Rationale	Recommendation	Quality of Evidence	Strength of Recommendation
Non-Benzodiazepine Hypnotics Eszopiclone Zolpidem Zaleplon	Benzodiazepine-receptor agonists that have adverse events similar to those of benzodiazepines in older adults (e.g., delirium, fractures, falls); minimal improvement in sleep latency and duration	Avoid chronic use (>90 days)	Moderate	Strong
Ergot mesylates Isoxsuprine	Lack of efficacy	Avoid	High	Strong
Endocrine				
Androgens Methyltestosterone Testosterone	Potential for cardiac problems and contraindicated in men with prostate cancer	Avoid unless indicated for moderate-to-severe hypogonadism	Moderate	Weak
Desiccated thyroid	Concerns about cardiac effects; safer alternatives available	Avoid	Low	Strong
Estrogens (with or without progestins)	Evidence of carcinogenic potential (breast and endometrium); lack of cardioprotective effect and cognitive protection in older women. Evidence that vaginal estrogens for the treatment of vaginal dryness are safe and effective in women with breast cancer, especially at dosages of estradiol <25 mcg twice weekly	Avoid oral and topical patch. Topical vaginal cream: Acceptable to use low-dose intra-vaginal estrogen for the management of dyspareunia, lower urinary tract infections, and other vaginal symptoms.	High: Oral and patch Moderate: Topical	Strong: Oral and patch Weak: Topical
Growth hormone	Effect on body composition is small; associated with edema, arthralgia, carpal tunnel syndrome, gynecomastia, impaired fasting glucose	Avoid, except as hormone replacement after pituitary gland removal	High	Strong
Insulin (sliding scale)	Higher risk of hypoglycemia without any improvement in hyperglycemia management regardless of care setting	Avoid	Moderate	Strong
Megestrol	Minimal effect on weight; increases the risk of thrombotic events and possibly death in older adults	Avoid	Moderate	Strong
Sulfonylureas (long duration) Chlorpropamide Glyburide	Chlorpropamide: Prolonged half-life in older adults; can cause prolonged hypoglycemia; causes syndrome of inappropriate antidiuretic hormone secretion. Glyburide: Greater risk of severe prolonged hypoglycemia in older adults	Avoid	High	Strong
Gastrointestinal				
Metoclopramide	Can cause extrapyramidal effects including tardive dyskinesia; risk may be even greater in frail older adults	Avoid, unless for gastroparesis	Moderate	Strong
Mineral oil (oral)	Potential for aspiration and adverse effects; safer alternatives available	Avoid	Moderate	Strong
Trimethobenzamide	One of the least effective antiemetic drugs; can cause extrapyramidal adverse effects	Avoid	Moderate	Strong

(Continued)

TABLE 23.7
Continued

Organ System or Therapeutic Category or Drug	Rationale	Recommendation	Quality of Evidence	Strength of Recommendation
Pain				
Meperidine	Not an effective oral analgesic in dosages commonly used; may cause neurotoxicity; safer alternatives available	Avoid	High	Strong
Non-COX-selective NSAIDs (oral) Diclofenac Diflunisal Etodolac Fenoprofen Ibuprofen Meclofenamate Ketoprofen Mefenamic acid Meloxicam Nabumetone Naproxen Oxaprozin Piroxicam Sulindac Tolmetin Aspirin >325 mg/d	Increases the risk of GI bleeding and peptic ulcer disease in high-risk groups, including those aged >75 or taking oral or parenteral corticosteroids, anticoagulants, or antiplatelet agents. Use of proton pump inhibitor or misoprostol reduces but does not eliminate risk. Upper GI ulcers, gross bleeding, or perforation caused by NSAIDs occur in approximately 1% of patients treated for 3–6 months and in approximately 2–4% of patients treated for 1 year. These trends continue with longer duration of use	Avoid chronic use unless other alternatives are not effective, and the patient can take gastroprotective agent (proton pump inhibitor or misoprostol)	Moderate	Strong
Indomethacin Ketorolac (oral and parenteral)	Increases the risk of GI bleeding and peptic ulcer disease in high-risk groups. (See Non COX selective NSAIDs.) Of all NSAIDs, indomethacin has most adverse effects.	Avoid	Indomethacin: Moderate Ketorolac: high	Strong
Pentazocine	Opioid analgesic that causes central nervous system adverse effects, including confusion and hallucinations, more commonly than other narcotic drugs; is also a mixed agonist and antagonist; safer alternatives available	Avoid	Low	Strong
Skeletal Muscle Relaxants Carisoprodol Cyclobenzaprine Chlorzoxazone Metaxalone Orphenadrine Methocarbamol	Most muscle relaxants are poorly tolerated by older adults because of anticholinergic adverse effects, sedation, risk of fracture; effectiveness at dosages tolerated by older adults is questionable	Avoid	Moderate	Strong

Source: *Reprinted with permission from American Geriatrics Society 2012 Beers Criteria Update Expert Panel. American Geriatrics Society updated Beers Criteria for potentially inappropriate medication use in older adults. J Am Geriatr Soc. 2012; 60(4):616–31. (Copyright © 2012, John Wiley and Sons).*[121]

impairment and drug–drug interactions that are associated with harm in older adults. Amendments to the list of Potentially Inappropriate Medications (PIMs) in this latest revision include:

1. Anti-infective nitrofurantoin can be used in individuals with a creatinine clearance of 30 mL/min or greater (previous cut-off was 60 mL/min). Long-term use of this drug is still avoided due to multiple toxicities. New to the Beers' criteria list is a list of drugs which should be avoided or dose-adjusted because of kidney impairment.
2. Blanket "Recommendation to avoid all antiarrhythmic drugs (Classes 1a, 1c, III) as first-line treatment for atrial fibrillation has been removed." However, some of the members of these drug

classes still have restrictions (amiodarone, dronedarone, disopyramide, digoxin).

3. Avoid nonbenzodiazepine drugs that are agonists for the benzodiazepine receptor (eszopiclone, zaleplon, zolpidem). These drugs are particularly dangerous for cognitively impaired patients.
4. Unless there is a compelling reason, avoid using proton-pump inhibitors beyond eight weeks (infection, bone loss, and fractures).
5. Nocturnal polyuria drug desmopressin is to be avoided because of hyponatremia risk.
6. Avoid opioids in patients with history of falls or fractures.
7. Do not use antipsychotics as a first-line treatment for delirium.

The Beers' criteria have not been without controversy with concerns that the criteria might be universally applied to all geriatric patients without individual consideration of a patient's response to a particular medication.[140] Further, studies employing the Beers' criteria have shown conflicting results. While some studies have linked higher numbers of potentially inappropriate medications with adverse drug-related outcomes, there are others that found no association between potentially inappropriate medications on the Beers' list and adverse outcomes. Beers' drugs only accounted for about 7% of hospitalizations due to adverse drug events, most of which involved digoxin.[66] Regardless, the Beers' criteria have achieved broad application and have been used by healthcare providers, regulators, and researchers alike. For instance, the Beers' criteria have been incorporated into the CMS *Interpretive Guidelines for Long-Term Care Facilities* to evaluate nursing homes' compliance with medication-related regulations.[141]

While the Beers' criteria can prove useful when designing a geriatric pharmacotherapeutic regimen, in light of the controversy and conflicting results, some key principles to consider include: (1) Medications listed are potentially and not definitely inappropriate for elderly patients, (2) the recommendations provide guidance and are accompanied by exceptions to the recommendations, (3) prescribing should take into account why a drug is included in the criteria, (4) safer drug and non-drug alternatives are available, and (5) the criteria provide a beginning point from which a comprehensive process to improve medication appropriateness can be derived.[139]

STOPP/START Criteria: Another commonly used tool referred to as STOPP (Screening Tool of Older Person's Prescriptions) and START (Screening Tool to Alert doctors to Right Treatment) has been developed by an interdisciplinary consensus expert panel from academic centers in Ireland and the United Kingdom. The STOPP/START criteria were originally developed in 2008 and underwent one revision in 2015.[142–144] Utilizing evidence-based literature and clinical experience, the STOPP/START criteria are arranged according to physiological system (see Table 23.8) and can be used to identify inappropriate drug use. There are 80 STOPP criteria which focus on problems associated with drugs commonly prescribed to elderly patients (e.g., dose, duration of therapy, indication, avoidance of drugs and drug combinations in certain disease states, and need for additional therapy). There are also 34 evidence-based START criteria for common diseases in older adults.

STOPP and Beers' criteria overlap in some ways, but somewhat of a competition has developed between the criteria. In two studies, the use of STOPP criteria identified a higher proportion of elderly patients who required hospitalization due to a drug-induced adverse event than did the Beers' criteria. Use of STOPP/START criteria has been associated with improved prescribing as measured by the *Medication Appropriateness Index* and the *Assessment of Underutilization of Medication Tool.* No studies have reported a link between health outcomes and improvements in prescribing by applying the STOPP/START criteria.[144,145]

High-Alert Drugs: Collectively, for the reasons set forth in this chapter, the elderly constitute a high-risk or high-alert patient population. In the same way that high-alert medications are handled, geriatric pharmacotherapy must be targeted specifically for adverse event avoidance and error reduction interventions. In addition to adverse events or medication errors being more common in the elderly, their consequences can be more devastating. All geriatric drug regimens, including all dosages of high-alert medications as well as monitoring for potentially inappropriate medications, should be checked independently by at least two practitioners. Dosage limits should be established for high-alert drugs. If a prescribed regimen exceeds these established limits, a review process should be initiated to evaluate the safety of the regimen before it is given to the patient.[146] Solving the problem of inappropriate use in the elderly requires more than avoiding a short list of drugs and noting drug categories of concern. A patient's entire drug regimen should also be assessed regularly to determine potential benefit versus harm.[83]

23.4 LEGAL CASES' APPLICATION

Consequences of medication-related error can be devastating and costly. According to the benchmark report published by the Risk Management Foundation of Harvard Medical Institutions, medication-related malpractice is more likely to result in harm, as well as greater monetary compensation when compared to other forms of malpractice. Within the report, an analysis of 3,067 cases revealed that analgesics, anticoagulants, and antimicrobial and cardiovascular medications contribute to approximately half of medication-related cases. While these are the most common, many others are considered high risk and are frequently associated with medication error or adverse events.[147] The following is a collection of cases in elderly individuals that demonstrate plaintiff allegations of failures to properly prescribe, dispense, administer, or monitor treatment outcomes and factors related to causation in drug-related injury.

TABLE 23.8
Screening Tool of Older Persons' Potentially Inappropriate Prescriptions (STOPP Criteria).

System	Drug or Drug Class	Conditions and Concerns (in Italics)
Cardiovascular	Aspirin	• In combination with warfarin without a histamine type 2 receptor antagonist (except cimetidine due to warfarin interaction) or PPI due to high risk of GI bleeding. • With a past history of PUD without a histamine type 2 receptor antagonist due to the risk of bleeding. • In doses exceeding 150 mg/day due to increased bleeding risk and lack of evidence for increased efficacy. • With no history of coronary, cerebral, or peripheral vascular symptoms or occlusive event as aspirin is not indicated. • To treat dizziness not clearly attributable to cerebrovascular disease as aspirin is not indicated. • With concurrent bleeding disorder due to high risk of bleeding.
	B-Blockers	• With COPD due *to the risk of increased bronchospasm.* • In combination with verapamil due to the *increased risk of symptomatic heart block.*
	Calcium channel blockers	• Use of verapamil or diltiazem in patients with NYHA class III or IV heart failure due to an *increased risk of toxicity.* • With chronic constipation as this *may exacerbate constipation.*
	Clopidogrel	• With concurrent bleeding disorder due to *high risk of bleeding.*
	Digoxin	• For long-term use in doses >125 mcg/day with impaired renal function (GFR <50 ml/min) due to an *increased risk of toxicity.*
	Dipyridamole	• As monotherapy for cardiovascular secondary prevention due to *lack of evidence.* • With concurrent bleeding disorder due to *high risk of bleeding.*
	Loop diuretics	• For dependent ankle edema only (i.e., no clinical signs of heart failure) due to *lack of evidence* and compression *hosiery usually more appropriate.*
	Thiazide diuretics	• With a history of gout as this *may exacerbate gout.*
	Warfarin	• In combination with aspirin without a histamine type 2 receptor antagonist (except cimetidine due to warfarin interaction) or PPI due to *high risk of GI bleeding.* • For 1st uncomplicated pulmonary embolism for longer than 12 months' duration due to *lack of proven benefit.* • With concurrent bleeding disorder due to *high risk of bleeding.*
Central Nervous System	Anticholinergics	• To treat extra-pyramidal side effects of neuroleptic medications due to *risk of anticholinergic toxicity.*
	Antihistamines (first generation) Diphenhydramine Cyclizine Chlorpheniramine Promethazine	• Prolonged use (>1 week) due to *risk of sedation and anticholinergic side effects.*
	Benzodiazepines (long-acting) Chlordiazepoxide Flurazepam Nitrazepam Chlorazepate	• Avoid due to *high risk of prolonged sedation, confusion, impaired balance, and falls.*
	Benzodiazepines (long metabolites) Diazepam	• Avoid due to *high risk of prolonged sedation, confusion, impaired balance, and falls.*
	Neuroleptics	• With long-term (> 1 month) use due to *high risk of confusion, hypotension, extra-pyramidal side effects, and falls.* • With long-term (> 1month) use in patients with Parkinson's disease due to *risk worsening, extra-pyramidal symptoms.*
	Phenothiazines	• In patients with epilepsy as phenothiazines may *lower seizure threshold.*
	Selective serotonin reuptake inhibitors	• With a history of clinically significant hyponatremia defined as non-iatrogenic sodium <130 mEq/L within the previous two months.
	Tricyclic antidepressants	• With dementia due to the *risk of worsening cognitive impairment.* • With glaucoma as tricyclic antidepressants may *exacerbate glaucoma.* • With cardiac conduction abnormalities due to tricyclic antidepressants' *pro-arrhythmic effects.* • With constipation as tricyclic antidepressants may *worsen constipation.* • With opiate or calcium channel blockers as tricyclic antidepressants *may worsen constipation.* • With prostatism or prior history of urinary retention due to *increased risk of urinary retention.*

(Continued)

TABLE 23.8
Continued

System	Drug or Drug Class	Conditions and Concerns (in Italics)
Gastrointestinal	Anticholinergic antispasmodics	• With chronic constipation due to *risk of constipation exacerbation.*
	Diphenoxylate, loperamide, or codeine	• For the treatment of diarrhea of unknown cause due to the *risk of delayed diagnosis, possible exacerbation of constipation with overflow diarrhea, precipitation of toxic megacolon in inflammatory bowel disease, and delayed recovery in unrecognized gastroenteritis.* • For the treatment of severe infective gastroenteritis (i.e., bloody diarrhea, high fever, or severe systemic toxicity) due to the *risk of exacerbation or protraction of infection.*
	Prochlorperazine, metoclopramide	• With Parkinsonism due to the *risk of exacerbating Parkinsonism.*
	Proton pump inhibitors	• For PUD at full therapeutic dosage for >8 weeks.
Respiratory	Corticosteroids (systemic)	• For maintenance therapy in moderate-to-severe COPD instead of inhaled corticosteroids due to *unnecessary exposure to long-term side effects of systemic steroids.*
	Ipratropium (nebulized)	• In patients with glaucoma due to *possible glaucoma exacerbation.*
	Theophylline	• As monotherapy for COPD as *more safe and effective alternatives exist and for the risk of adverse effects due to narrow therapeutic index.*
Musculoskeletal	NSAIDs	• With a history of PUD or GI bleeding, unless with concurrent histamine type 2 receptor blocker, PPI, or misoprostol due to the *risk of PUD relapse.* • With moderate (160/100–179/109 mmHg) or severe (>180/110 mmHg) hypertension due to the *risk of exacerbation of hypertension.* • With heart failure due to the *risk of heart failure exacerbation.* • With warfarin concomitantly due to the *risk of GI bleeding.* • With chronic renal failure (GFR 20–50 ml/min) due to the *risk of deterioration in renal function.* • With long-term use (>3 months) for relief of mild joint pain due to risk of the above adverse effects. In osteoarthritis as *analgesics preferable and usually as effective for pain relief.*
	Colchicine	• For chronic treatment of gout where there is no contraindication to allopurinol *as allopurinol is considered first choice for prophylaxis in gout.*
	Corticosteroids	• For chronic treatment of gout where there is no contraindication to allopurinol *as allopurinol is considered the first choice for prophylaxis in gout.* • As long-term (>3 months) monotherapy for rheumatoid arthritis or osteoarthritis due *to the risk of major systemic corticosteroid side effects.*
Urogenital	Antimuscarinics	• With dementia due to the risk of *increased confusion and agitation.* • With chronic glaucoma due to the *risk of acute exacerbation of glaucoma.* • With chronic constipation due to the *risk of exacerbation of constipation.* • With chronic prostatism due to the *risk of urinary retention.*
	α-Blockers	• In males with frequent incontinence (i.e., one or more episodes of incontinence daily) due to *risk of urinary frequency and worsening incontinence.* • With long-term urinary catheter in situ (i.e. more than two months) as *drug is not indicated.*
Endocrine	Chlorpropamide or glyburide	• With type 2 diabetes due to the *risk of prolonged hypoglycemia.*
	β-Blockers	• In those with diabetes mellitus and frequent hypoglycemic episodes (i.e. >1 episodes/month) due to the *risk of masking hypoglycemic symptoms.*
	Estrogen	• With a history of breast cancer or venous thromboembolism due to an *increased risk of recurrence.* • Without progestin in patients with intact uterus due to the *risk of endometrial cancer.*
Drug Issues		
Analgesic drugs	Opiates	• Use of long-term power opiates (i.e., morphine or fentanyl) as first-line therapy for mild–moderate pain *as WHO analgesic ladder is not observed.* • Regular use for more than two weeks in those with chronic constipation without use of laxatives due to the *risk of severe constipation.* • Long-term use in those with dementia unless indicated for palliative care or management of moderate–severe chronic pain syndrome due to the *risk of exacerbation of cognitive impairment.*

(Continued)

TABLE 23.8
Continued

System	Drug or Drug Class	Conditions and Concerns (in Italics)
Duplicate drug class	ACE inhibitors Loop diuretics NSAIDS Opiates Selective serotonin reuptake inhibitors	• Use of any two concurrent duplicate medications as *optimization of monotherapy within a single drug class should be observed prior to considering a new drug class.*
Drugs adversely impacting elderly pone to falls	Antihistamines (first generation)	• *May cause sedation and impair sensorium.*
	Benzodiazepines	• *May cause sedation and impair sensorium.*
	Neuroleptics	• *May cause gait dyspraxia and Parkinsonism.*
	Opiates	• Long-term use in those with recurrent falls due to the *risk of drowsiness, postural hypotension, and vertigo.*
	Vasodilators (known to cause hypotension)	• In those with persistent postural hypotension (i.e. recurrent >20 mmHg drop in systolic blood pressure) due to the *risk of syncope and falls.*

Source: *ACE = angiotensin-converting enzyme; COPD = chronic obstructive pulmonary disease; NYHA = New York Heart Association; NSAID = nonsteroidal anti-inflammatory drug; PPI = proton pump inhibitor; PUD = peptic ulcer disease; WHO = World Health Organization. Reprinted with permission from Page RL 2nd, Linnebur SA, Bryant LL, Ruscin JM. Inappropriate prescribing in the hospitalized elderly patient: defining the problem, evaluation tools, and possible solutions. Clin Interv Aging. 2010 Apr; 5:75–87. (Open Access, Dove Medical Press Ltd.).*[152]

Amiodarone: Cardiovascular drugs are among the classes most commonly involved in geriatric medication errors. Amiodarone is a high-risk drug with unique pharmacokinetics (extremely long half-life, 56 days) and potentially serious adverse effects. It also has a unique history related to its journey toward FDA approval. Originally, amiodarone was developed in Belgium in 1962 as a potent coronary vasodilator and antianginal agent. Initial investigations from European trials demonstrated effectiveness in treating atrial and ventricular arrhythmias, but the FDA was not convinced. Nonetheless, these clinical trial results led to more common use in the United States as physicians acquired the drug from Europe and Canada to treat their patients. Prior to FDA approval, the use of amiodarone was sanctioned on a limited basis as one of the first-treatment INDs. Over time, demand grew with "positive" clinical experience, and although the FDA was reluctant to officially approve the drug, amiodarone was one of the few drugs approved by the FDA without rigorous clinical trials.

Amiodarone was approved in 1985 to treat life-threatening recurrent ventricular arrhythmias that are nonresponsive to other agents. A common off-label indication is atrial fibrillation, but literature suggests that rate control and anticoagulation are equally effective and less toxic. Safe use of amiodarone requires the use of the lowest possible dose for the shortest possible duration and familiarity with monitoring recommendations. A retrospective analysis of five amiodarone-related malpractice claims in elderly patients (65–80 years), all being treated for atrial fibrillation, identified causes of toxicity and potential error sources. Drug toxicities deemed probable based on scores determined using the Naranjo scale (see Table 23.9),[148] a tool that is reasonably reliable in assessing the probability of an adverse drug reaction, included pulmonary fibrosis or pneumonitis (60%, two resulting in death), neuropathies (40%), and hepatotoxicity (20%). Toxicity was associated with failure to monitor therapy (chest x-ray, liver function tests). Duties related to clinical judgment were determined to contribute to toxicity and included incorrect loading dose, maintenance dose titration during transitions of care (80%), and, in one case, failure to counsel. While physician-related issues played a role in each case, elements of pharmacists' clinical judgment were identified including improper drug regimen review and patient counseling.[149]

Amitriptyline: Amitriptyline is a tertiary tricyclic antidepressant that is sedating, highly anticholinergic, and can cause orthostatic hypotension. For these reasons, it is considered a potentially inappropriate medication in both the Beers' and STOPP criteria. In *Haycraft v. Walgreens (Jefferson County Circuit Court, KY, 2008),* the plaintiff was a 75-year-old male with multiple comorbid conditions including cardiovascular disease and polypharmacy (>11 medications). He was prescribed "Clinoril 150 mg," a nonsteroidal anti-inflammatory drug to be taken twice daily, but when the pharmacy filled the prescription, it was misinterpreted as "Elavil 150 mg" to be taken twice daily. A couple of days after beginning the prescription, the plaintiff presented via ambulance to the ER with a chief complaint of syncope and orthostatic hypotension. Other symptoms included psychosis, hallucinations, a decreased level of consciousness, confusion, fine tremors, shakiness,

TABLE 23.9
Naranjo Adverse Drug Reaction Probability Assessment Algorithm.

Question	No	No	Do Not Know	Score
1. Are there previous conclusive reports on this reaction?	+1	0	0	
2. Did the adverse event appear after the suspected drug was administered?	+2	-1	0	
3. Did the adverse reaction improve when the drug was discontinued, or a specific antagonist was administered?	+1	0	0	
4. Did the adverse reaction reappear when the drug was readministered?	+2	-1	0	
5. Are there alternative causes (other than the drug) that could on their own have caused the reaction?	-1	+2	0	
6. Did the reaction reappear when a placebo was given?	-1	+1	0	
7. Was the drug detected in the blood (or other fluids) in concentrations known to be toxic?	+1	0	0	
8. Was the reaction more severe when the dose was increased or less severe when the dose was decreased?	+1	0	0	
9. Did the patient have a similar reaction to the same or similar drugs in any previous exposure?	+1	0	0	
10. Was the adverse event confirmed by objective evidence?	+1	0	0	
Total Score:				

Source: *Interpretation of Scores: Score >9 (Definite): The reaction (1) followed a reasonable temporal sequence after a drug or in which a toxic drug level had been established in body fluids or tissues, (2) followed a recognized response to the suspected drug, and (3) was confirmed by improvement on withdrawing the drug and reappeared on re-exposure. Score = 5 to 8 (Probable): The reaction (1) followed a reasonable temporal sequence after a drug, (2) followed a recognized response to the suspected drug, (3) was confirmed by withdrawal but not by exposure to the drug, and (4) could not be reasonably explained by the known characteristics of the patient's clinical state. Score = 1 to 4 (Possible): The reaction (1) followed a temporal sequence after a drug, (2) possibly followed a recognized pattern to the suspected drug, and (3) could be explained by characteristics of the patient's disease. Score ≤0 (Doubtful): The reaction was likely related to factors other than a drug. Reprinted with permission from Naranjo CA, Busto U, Sellers EM, Sandor P, Ruiz I, Roberts EA, Janecek E, Domeco C, and Greenblatt DJ. A reliable method for estimating the probability of adverse drug reactions. Clin Pharmac Ther, 1981; (30):239–245. (Copyright © 2012, John Wiley and Sons).*[148]

anxiety, fidgeting, loss of coordination, gait disturbances, and seven episodes of falling. The plaintiff was admitted to the hospital, and eventually it was discovered that the pharmacy had dispensed the wrong medication. The symptoms experienced during his hospitalization were attributed to the erroneously dispensed amitriptyline. For several weeks after his hospitalization, the plaintiff required Risperdal® therapy for continuing psychiatric symptoms. While this case revolved around a dispensing error that could occur in the elderly and non-elderly alike, it demonstrates the profound CNS effects and related sequelae that can occur with the tricyclic antidepressants.

Colchicine: Colchicine is an alkaloid that is commonly used to treat gout, but its narrow therapeutic index has been the source of several fatalities due to inadvertent overdoses. In *Phillips v. Larry's Drive-In Pharm., Inc. (Supreme Court of Appeals, WV, 2007)*, the plaintiff visited his doctor complaining of pain and swelling in his left foot. The doctor diagnosed the plaintiff as suffering from acute gouty arthritis and wrote a prescription for colchicine. The plaintiff was also told to use the medication if the symptoms appeared in the future. The plaintiff went to Larry's Drive-In Pharmacy and presented the prescription. The pharmacy filled the colchicine prescription, and the instructions printed on the bottle by the pharmacy matched exactly those written on the prescription by the doctor: "take 1 tablet every hour until pain stops or diarrhea or nausea starts." Neither the doctor's prescription nor the pharmacy's printed instructions stated an upper limit on the number of tablets that the plaintiff could take during any given time period. The plaintiff began taking colchicine and did so for three days in accordance with the instructions on the bottle. After three days, the plaintiff began to experience stroke-like symptoms and was taken to a hospital. Doctors determined that the plaintiff was suffering from colchicine toxicity that had severely and permanently damaged the plaintiff's kidneys and as a result required routine kidney dialysis for the remainder of his life. The plaintiff filed suit against the doctor alleging that colchicine had been negligently prescribed without specifying a limit on the number of tablets that could be taken during a defined time period. The plaintiff also filed suit against the pharmacy for negligently filling the prescription without clarifying the doctor's instructions to specify a maximum daily dosage and in failing to recognize the potential toxicity of the prescribed dose of colchicine. This case also involved elements of risk factors for toxicity including concomitant disease states, diminished renal function, and failure to provide adequate patient counseling. The doctor settled with the plaintiffs and was dismissed from the lawsuit with prejudice, and the plaintiff ultimately received compensation from the pharmacy defendant. However, the case against the pharmacy was certified to the West Virginia Supreme Court of Appeals to answer the question, "In a civil action filed against a defendant licensed pharmacy for allegedly having negligently dispensed medication, is the pharmacy a 'healthcare provider', as defined by West Virginia Code?" The review was based on the West Virginia Medical Professional Liability Act which specifically excluded pharmacists and pharmacies as healthcare providers. The court ruled, based on the Legislature's verbiage in the act, that pharmacies and pharmacists were not considered to be a healthcare provider.[150] Incidentally, colchicine has undergone significant regulatory changes and approved NDAs. The injectable form has been discontinued and withdrawn from the market, and the tablets' dosing recommendations have been significantly reduced, based upon clinical studies submitted supporting the NDAs. These approvals were based on extensive evaluation of studies and new data that permitted the refinement of dosing regimens and labeling. When used in accordance with the approved labeling, single-ingredient oral colchicine was found to be well-tolerated and safe when taken at therapeutic doses and with appropriate dose reductions in susceptible populations or with potentially interacting drugs.

Glimepiride: Oral hypoglycemic agents like glimepiride are considered to be high-alert drugs in both the acute and ambulatory care settings. *Maletteri v. Visiting Nurse Association of Greater Philadelphia, et al. (Philadelphia County Court of Common Pleas, PA, 2002)* involved an 80-year-old, frail, thin female with multiple comorbidities, polypharmacy, and cognitive impairment who was homebound and lived alone. She was started on prednisone 5 mg daily for COPD. She was not diabetic, but blood sugars and glycosylated hemoglobin (HbA1c) were being monitored due to prednisone which has the propensity to raise blood sugar. On the basis of two HbA1c labs, the highest of which was 7.9% (goal in the elderly: <7.5%), the patient was started on glimepiride 2 mg (Amaryl®), a hypoglycemic, to treat prednisone-induced hyperglycemia. It was known by the home care nurses that the patient was not eating well. Two weeks after starting glimepiride therapy, the patient was found on the floor of her home with an undetectable blood glucose level. She was admitted to the ICU of a local hospital. She died seven days later. In the lawsuit, the plaintiff alleged that the defendants inappropriately attempted to achieve tight glycemic control with an excessive dose of glimepiride in a patient of advanced age for what amounted to a preventable, drug-induced hyperglycemia. The physician admitted in his deposition that

> [I]n a homebound, frail population, especially if they're cognitively impaired, clinically we tend to let people run higher blood sugars, especially if they're not symptomatic. This is because the risk of becoming hypoglycemic is actually worse than the moderate risks of hyperglycemia over a long period of time.

This case required consideration of appropriate glycemic control in a frail elderly patient, alternative therapies to avoid prednisone-induced elevated blood sugars (e.g., inhaler-delivered steroid therapy), geriatric renal dosing of glimepiride, polypharmacy with associated drug–drug interactions, and comorbidities (e.g., poor dietary intake, cognitive impairment). (Two additional chapters in this book address iatrogenic as well as criminal hypoglycemic reactions involving hypoglycemic agents; Patel, O'Donnell, and Marks, as well as Marks V.)

Methotrexate: Oral methotrexate for non-oncologic use is considered to be a high-alert drug in both the acute and ambulatory care settings. Methotrexate use as an immunomodulator in rheumatoid arthritis and psoriasis involves once-weekly administration, a nontraditional regimen that frequently leads to inadvertent once-daily administration, high doses, toxicity, and death. A retrospective analysis of 11 methotrexate-related malpractice claims in elderly patients identified causes of toxicity and potential error sources. Six (55%) of the cases involved mix-ups of once-weekly versus once-daily orally administered regimens for the treatment of rheumatoid arthritis. The patients ranged between 65 and 86 years of age. The most frequent intended dose was 7.5 mg/day which was clinically appropriate for renal function, and all patients received appropriate monitoring. However, on average, the mix-up in directions resulted in patients erroneously receiving once-daily dosing for 12 days (range 7–19 days) at a cumulative dose of 95 mg (range 68–143 mg) from the time once-daily dosing started until the onset of toxicity. Predictably, all patients experienced systemic toxicity (e.g., pancytopenia, opportunistic infections, elevated SCr/BUN, breakdown of mucosal membranes, bleeding, etc.) within a mean of 12 days (range 7–19 days), and 4 patients in this subset died as a direct result of methotrexate toxicity. All errors involved the long-term care setting and most frequently occurred during the transition of care from a hospital. A root cause analysis revealed that: (a) The individual who most frequently initiated the error cascade was a nurse (50%), physician (33%), and pharmacist (17%), but multiple pharmacists were involved in the process who could have prevented the error; (b) mechanics or stages of the errors included prescribing, transcription, medication reconciliation, drug regimen review, order entry, dispensing, administration, and consultant chart review; and (c) a median of 7 stages (range 5–12) were confirmed along the medication use process where the error could have been detected but was not.[151]

Mixed-Drug Combination: In the case of the *Estate of Boote v Shivers (Marshall County Chancery Court, TN, 2002),* a mixed combination of drugs was administered during the period that immediately preceded the signing of an antenuptial agreement made for an inauspicious start to a ten-year marriage. Mr. Boote, an 83-year-old man whose premarital estate was valued at $9.3 million, and Ms. Lingner, a 74-year-old woman whose estate was valued at $1.4 million, decided to wed in 1990. Soon after the proposal, at the behest of his adult children who stood to inherit his estate, Mr. Boote met with counsel to discuss what effect the marriage would have on how his estate was distributed upon his death. Financial disclosures were made, and an antenuptial agreement was prepared. Unfortunately, on the same morning the antenuptial was prepared for signature and only 15 days prior to the wedding, Ms. Lingner fell down a flight of steps and broke both ankles. She was transported to the hospital by ambulance where surgery was performed to repair both ankles. The decision was made to not postpone the wedding, so just three days post operation, Mr. Boote and his attorney arrived at the hospital and presented the antenuptial agreement to Ms. Lingner for her signature. During the three-day post-operative period, Ms. Lingner was receiving repeated doses of meperidine (Demerol®) and hydroxyzine pamoate (Vistaril®) injections and oral propoxyphene with acetaminophen (Darvocet-N 100®) and was wearing a scopolamine patch (Trans-Derm Scop®). Meperidine and propoxyphene are opiates that are both high-alert drugs and inappropriate for use in the elderly according to the Beers' and STOPP criteria. Hydroxyzine and scopolamine, also considered inappropriate drugs under the Beers' and STOPP criteria, are highly anticholinergic, have reduced clearance with advanced age, and pose a risk of confusion and other anticholinergic effects and toxicity. Prior to signing the antenuptial agreement that was dated and time-stamped at 12:00 noon, Ms. Lingner had received meperidine and hydroxyzine between 2:00 and 3:00 AM, had taken two propoxyphene/acetaminophen tablets at 7:30 AM and again at 11:30 AM, and was still wearing the three-day scopolamine patch for nausea that had been placed behind her ear prior to the surgery. The marriage was a happy one and lasted until Mr. Boote's death over ten years later. By that time, his estate had grown to approximately $35 million, from which Ms. Boote was entitled to only $600,000. The antenuptial agreement was challenged on the basis that she signed it under duress while under the influence of meperidine, hydroxyzine, scopolamine, and propoxyphene. A bench trial ensued with much of the testimony coming from experts who testified regarding the effects the recent surgery, pain, and medications had or could have had on Ms. Boote's cognitive functioning when she signed the antenuptial agreement. Ms. Boote's experts testified that more likely than not she would have been sedated with some degree of cognitive impairment and, therefore, would have been less able than normal to understand or make complex decisions. This was on the basis of the individual and additive effects of the drugs and decreased clearance with increased CNS sensitivity to the drugs in an elderly patient. Alternatively, the opposing experts stated unequivocally that the medications Ms. Boote received from the time of her surgery through the day before she signed the antenuptial agreement could not have had any clinically significant effects on her cognitive functioning when she signed the antenuptial agreement. They opined that the drugs had relatively short half-lives and discounted accumulation due to repeated dosing. They also opined that propoxyphene, a drug that has since been removed from the market by the FDA for safety reasons, was a mild drug being only slightly stronger than Tylenol® and that it was commonly ingested while conducting business affairs. Further, they stated that the scopolamine patch had no clinically significant effect on Ms. Boote's cognitive functioning at the time of the signing. Her treating physician testified that in his view, something as important as an antenuptial agreement should be dealt with away from the hospital setting if possible. The trial court entered an order that the antenuptial agreement was unenforceable based on its findings because Ms. Boote had not entered into it knowledgeably and without duress. The court granted Ms. Boote's petition to dissent from the will and awarded her the full $35 million estate. Mr. Boote's daughters appealed the ruling, and lengthy litigation ensued. Ultimately, under alternate theories largely unrelated to alleged drug effect, the judgment was reversed, and the antenuptial agreement was upheld.[152]

Quetiapine: Quetiapine (Seroquel®) is an atypical antipsychotic and part of a drug class that bears a black box warning regarding increased mortality in elderly patients with dementia-related psychosis. In *Hess v. United States of America (US District Court, MD, 2011),* a 70-year-old male, veteran with an 8-year history of Parkinson's disease, was receiving care at a VA Medical Center. His Parkinson's disease required treatment with carbidopa/levodopa, and his condition was worsening in all aspects, including signs of a developing dementia as evidenced by progressive personality changes, depression, and frequent sleep terrors. As it relates to the case, the doctor made a notation that he was going to use Seroquel to treat sleep terrors, but the drug went unprescribed. At his next visit three months later, the sleep terrors were continuing, and the doctors decided to prescribe Seroquel XR (sustained release) on the premise that this formulation had "less extrapyramidal side effects." A 300-mg dose was ordered, and the VA pharmacy filled the prescription. The first dose was taken at bedtime as prescribed, and the following morning, the patient was found notably weaker than normal, "frozen" in bed being unable to ambulate or speak, and confused with hallucinations. The patient presented to a local ER where he was diagnosed with an exacerbation of his Parkinson's symptoms and drug-induced delirium secondary to the Seroquel. Following a 6-day inpatient stay, Seroquel was reinitiated appropriately at a lower dose of 12.5 mg at bedtime. This case required consideration of a drug–drug interaction between Seroquel® and carbidopa/levodopa, a drug–disease interaction between Parkinson's and Seroquel®, and proper dose initiation by both the doctor who prescribed Seroquel® and the pharmacist who dispensed the drug.

Zolpidem: Sedative hypnotics such as zolpidem (Ambien®) are potentially inappropriate medications that are included in both the Beers' and STOPP criteria as drugs that predictably increase the risk of adverse events (delirium, falls) in older people with minimal improvement in sleep. In *Estate of Eunice Aaron v. UPMC Passavant (Allegheny County Court of Common Pleas, PA, 2006),* an 81-year-old female who suffered from multiple comorbidities and polypharmacy was admitted to the hospital to rule out a myocardial infarction. Between 8 PM and 3 AM on the fifth day of her hospitalization preceding the drug administration at issue in the case, the patient was documented drowsy and sleeping with no changes to note. Then, for the first time, the patient was administered zolpidem (Ambien®) at a dose of 10 mg; there was no documentation available to explain the decision to medicate with zolpidem at that time. Two hours later around 5 AM, she was found on the floor having experienced a fall. A large hematoma was noted on the back of her head, she was confused with a decreased level of consciousness, and her pupils were slow to respond. A CT scan confirmed a large acute subdural hematoma and hemorrhage, and she was transferred to an outside hospital for possible hematoma evacuation. The patient's condition deteriorated, and she died; the cause of death was determined to be as a result of blunt-force trauma to the head. This case required the consideration of the use of a potentially inappropriate medication; lack of an indication for use and inappropriate timing of administration of a hypnotic, geriatric dosing of zolpidem; altered pharmacokinetic (prolonged half-life) and pharmacodynamic (increased sensitivity to hypnotics) parameters; polypharmacy with associated drug–drug interactions (diazepam which would have additive effects with a hypnotic and heparin which contributed to the bleed after the fall); and failure to employ fall precautions in an at-risk patient.

23.5 SUMMARY AND CONCLUSIONS

The geriatric population, by virtue of their increased use of medication due to their increased incidence of multiple chronic disease conditions, are prescribed more drugs than the younger adult population.[153] This multiple drug approach increases risk for individual drug toxicity and drug interactions, as well as system-based medication errors. Each of these considerations contribute to some very unique and complicated scenarios that sometimes are aired in legal proceedings and require the expertise of an experienced pharmacist to sort out all the causes and effects of drug toxicity in the elderly.

REFERENCES

1. U.S. Census Bureau. The population 65 years and older in the United States. 2018. https://www.census.gov/library/publications/2018/acs/acs-38.html. Accessed March 14, 2021.
2. Cost overdose: Growth in drug spending for the elderly, 1992–2010, families USA, July, 2000, p. 2.
3. Qato DM, Alexander GC, Conti RM, Johnson M, Schumm P, Lindau ST. Use of prescription and over-the-counter medications and dietary supplements among older adults in the United States. JAMA. 2008;300(24):2867–2878.
4. Centers for Disease Control and Prevention. National Center for Health Statistics. National Health and Nutrition Examination Survey. Prescription drug use in the past 30 days, by sex, age, race and Hispanic origin: United States, selected years 1988–1994 through 2015–2018. 2019. https://www.cdc.gov/nchs/hus/contents2019.htm#Table-039. Accessed March 14, 2021.

5. Wilson IR, Schoen C, Neuman P, Strollo MK, Rogers WH, Chang H, Safran DG. Physician-patient communication about prescription medication nonadherence: A 50-state study of America's seniors. J Gen Intern Med. 2007;22(1):6–12.
6. Ruscin JM, Linnebur SA. Introduction to drug therapy in the elderly. In: RS Porter, JL Kaplan (Eds) *The Merck Manual Online*. The Merck Manuals Online Medical Library Database. http://www.merckmanuals.com/professional/geriatrics/drug-therapy-in-the-elderly/introduction-to-drug-therapy-in-the-elderly. Accessed June 9, 2015.
7. Wittich CM, Burkle CM, Lanier WL. Medication errors: An overview for clinicians. Mayo Clin Proc. 2014;89(8):1116–1125.
8. Rossi MI, Young A, Maher R, Rodriguez KL, Appelt CJ, Perera S, Hajjar ER, Hanlon JT. Polypharmacy and health beliefs in older outpatients. Am J Geriatr Pharmacother. 2007;5:317–323.
9. Gurwitz JH, Field TS, Harrold LR, Rothschild J, Debellis K, Seger AC, Cadoret C, Fish LS, Garber L, Kelleher M, Bates DW. Incidence and preventability of adverse drug events among older persons in the ambulatory setting. JAMA. 2003;289(9):1107–1116.
10. Hajjar ER, Hanlon JT, Artz MB, Lindblad CI, Pieper CF, Sloane RJ, Ruby CM, Schmader KE. Adverse drug reaction risk factors in older outpatients. Am J Geriatr Pharmacother. 2003;1(2):82–89.
11. Hajjar ER, Gray SL, Slattum PW, Starner CI, Maher Jr RL, Hersh LR, Hanlon JT. Chapter 8. Geriatrics. In: JT DiPiro, RL Talbert, GC Yee, GR Matzke, BG Wells, L Posey (Eds) *Pharmacotherapy: A Pathophysiologic Approach (9th ed)*. New York, NY: McGraw-Hill, 2014. http://accesspharmacy.mhmedical.com/content.aspx?bookid=689&Sectionid=48811433. Accessed June 8, 2015.
12. Field TS, Gilman BH, Subramanian S, Fuller JC, Bates DW, Gurwitz JH. The costs associated with adverse drug events among older adults in the ambulatory setting. Med Care. 2005;43:1171–1176.
13. Budnitz DS, Pollock DA, Weidenbach KN, Mendelsohn AB, Schroeder TJ, Annest JL. National surveillance of emergency department visits for outpatient adverse drug events. JAMA. 2006;296(15):1858–1866.
14. US Department of Health and Human Services. National action plan for adverse drug event prevention. 2020. https://health.gov/sites/default/files/2019-09/ADE-Action-Plan-Introduction.pdf. Accessed on March 14, 2021.
15. Budnitz DS, Shehab N, Kegler SR, Richards CL. Medication use leading to emergency department visits for adverse drug events in older adults. Ann Intern Med. 2007;147(11):755–765.
16. Agency for Healthcare Research and Quality. Medication errors and adverse drug events. 2019. https://psnet.ahrq.gov/primer/medication-errors-and-adverse-drug-events. Accessed March 14, 2021.
17. Field TS, Mazor KM, Briesacher B, Debellis KR, Gurwitz JH. Adverse drug events resulting from patient errors in older adults. J Am Geriatr Soc. 2007;55(2):271–276.
18. Meredith S, Feldman PH, Frey D, Hall K, Arnold K, Brown NJ, Ray WA. Possible medication errors in home healthcare patients. J Am Geriatr Soc. 2001;49(6):719–724.
19. Hajjar E, Hanlon JT, Sloane RJ, Lindblad CI, Pieper CF, Ruby CM, Branch LC, Schmader KE. Unnecessary drug use in frail older people at hospital discharge. J Am Geriatr Soc. 2005;53:1518–1523.
20. Nobili A, Licata G, Salerno F, Pasina L, Tettamanti M, Franchi C, De Vittorio L, Marengoni A, Corrao S, Iorio A, Marcucci M, Mannucci PM, SIMI Investigators. Polypharmacy, length of hospital stay and inpatient mortality among elderly patients in internal medicine wards. The REPOSI study. Eur J Clin Pharmacol. 2011;67:507–519.
21. Thomas EJ, Brennan TA. Incidence and types of preventable adverse events in elderly patients: Population based review of medical records. BMJ. 2000;320(7237):741–744.
22. Leape LL, Brennan TA, Laird N, Lawthers AG, Localio AR, Barnes BA, Hebert L, Newhouse JP, Weiler PC, Hiatt H. The nature of adverse events in hospitalized patients. Results of the Harvard Medical Practice Study II. N Engl J Med. 1991;324(6):377–384.
23. Gray SL, Sager M, Lestico MR, Jalaluddin M. Adverse drug events in hospitalized elderly. J Gerontol A Biol Sci Med Sci. 1998;53(1):M59–63.
24. O'Connor MN, Gallagher P, O'Mahony D. Inappropriate prescribing: Criteria, detection and prevention. Drugs Aging. 2012;29(6):437–452.
25. Picone DM, Titler MG, Dochterman J, Shever L, Kim T, Abramowitz P, Kanak M, Qin R. Predictors of medication errors among elderly hospitalized patients. Am J Med Qual. 2008;23(2):115–127.
26. Midlöv P, Bergkvist A, Bondesson A, Eriksson T, Höglund P. Medication errors when transferring elderly patients between primary health care and hospital care. Pharm World Sci. 2005;27(2):116–120.
27. Midlöv P, Holmdahl L, Eriksson T, Bergkvist A, Ljungberg B, Widner H, Nerbrand C, Höglund P. Medication report reduces number of medication errors when elderly patients are discharged from hospital. Pharm World Sci. 2008;30(1):92–98.
28. Lau HS, Florax C, Porsius AJ, De Boer A. The completeness of medication histories in hospital medical records of patients admitted to general internal medicine wards. Br J Clin Pharmacol. 2000;49(6):597–603.
29. Gleason KM, Groszek JM, Sullivan C, Rooney CD, Barnard C, Noskin GA. Reconciliation of discrepancies in medication histories and admission orders of newly hospitalized patients. Am J Health Syst Pharm. 2004;61(16):1689–1695.
30. Wilson S, Ruscoe W, Chapman M, Miller R. General practitioner-hospital communications: A review of discharge summaries. J Qual Clin Pract, 2001;21(4):104–108.
31. Paulino EI, Bouvy ML, Gastelurrutia MA, Guerreiro M, Buurma H. Drug related problems identified by European community pharmacists in patients discharged from hospital. Pharm World Sci. 2004;26(6):353–360.
32. Avorn J, Gurwitz JH. Drug use in the nursing home. Ann Intern Med. 1995;123(3):195–204.
33. Dwyer L, Han B, Woodwell D, Rechtsteiner EA. Polypharmacy in nursing home residents in the United States: Results of the 2004 National Nursing Home Survey. Am J Geriatr Pharmacother. 2009;8:63–72.
34. Bronskill SE, Gill SS, Paterson JM, Bell CM, Anderson GM, Rochon PA. Exploring variation in rates of polypharmacy across long term care homes. J Am Med Dir Assoc. 2012;13(3):309, e315–321.
35. Onder G, Liperoti R, Fialova D, Topinkova E, Tosato M, Danese P, Gallo PF, Carpenter I, Finne-Soveri H, Gindin J, Bernabei R, Landi F, SHELTER Project. Polypharmacy in nursing home in Europe: Results from the SHELTER study. J Gerontol A Biol Sci Med Sci. 2012;67(6):698–704.

36. Gurwitz JH, Field TS, Avorn J, McCormick D, Jain S, Eckler M, Benser M, Edmondson AC, Bates DW. Incidence and preventability of adverse drug events in nursing homes. Am J Med. 2000;109:87–94.
37. Handler SM, Wright RM, Ruby CM, Hanlon JT. Epidemiology of medication-related adverse events in nursing homes. Am J Geriatr Pharmacother. 2006;4:264–272.
38. Bootman JL, Harrison DL, Cox E. The health care cost of drug-related morbidity and mortality in nursing facilities. Arch Intern Med. 1997;157(18):2089–2096.
39. Lapane KL, Hughes CM. Identifying nursing home residents at high risk for preventable adverse drug events: Modifying a tool for use in the Fleetwood Phase III study. Consult Pharm. 2004;19:533–537.
40. Gurwitz JH, Field TS, Avorn J, McCormick D, Jain S, Eckler M, Benser M, Edmondson AC, Bates DW. Incidence and preventability of adverse drug events in nursing homes. Am J Med. 2000;109(2):87–94.
41. Institute of Medicine. Institute of Medicine report: Preventing medication errors. Washington, DC: National Academies Press, 2006.
42. Gurwitz JH, Field TS, Judge J, Rochon P, Harrold LR, Cadoret C, Lee M, White K, LaPrino J, Erramuspe-Mainard J, DeFlorio M, Gavendo L, Auger J, Bates DW. The incidence of adverse drug events in two large academic long-term care facilities. Am J Med. 2005;118(3): 251–258.
43. Pierson S, Hansen R, Greene S, Williams C, Akers R, Jonsson M, Carey T. Preventing medication errors in long-term care: Results and evaluation of a large scale web-based error reporting system. Qual Saf Health Care. 2007;16(4):297–302.
44. Field TS, Gurwitz JH, Avorn J, McCormick D, Jain S, Eckler M, Benser M, Bates DW. Risk factors for adverse drug events among nursing home residents. Arch Intern Med. 2001;161:1629–1634.
45. Corsonello A, Pedone C, Incalzi RA. Age-related pharmacokinetic and pharmacodynamic changes and related risk of adverse drug reactions. Curr Med Chem. 2010;17:571–584.
46. Shi S, Klotz U. Age-related changes in pharmacokinetics. Curr Drug Metab 2011;12:601–610.
47. Ruscin JM, Linnebur SA. Pharmacokinetics in the elderly, In: RS Porter, JL Kaplan (Eds) *The Merck Manual Online*. The Merck Manuals Online Medical Library database. http://www.merckmanuals.com/professional/geriatrics/drug-therapy-in-the-elderly/introduction-to-drug-therapy-in-the-elderly. Accessed June 9, 2015.
48. Hilmer SN. ADME-tox issues for the elderly. Expert Opin Drug Metab Toxicol. 2008;4:1321–1331.
49. Kim J, Mak M. Chapter 102. Geriatric drug use. In: BK Alldredge, RL Corelli, ME Ernst, BJ Guglielmo, PA Jacobson, WA Kradjan, BR Williams (Eds) *Koda-Kimble and Young's Applied Therapeutics: The Clinical Use of Drugs* (10th ed). Philadelphia, PA: Lippincott Williams and Wilkins, 2013, pp. 2359–2374.
50. Vestal RE. Aging and pharmacokinetic: Impact of altered physiology in the elderly. Physiol Cell Biol Aging. 1979;8:198–209.
51. McLachlan AJ, Pont LG. Drug metabolism in older people—A key consideration in achieving optimal outcomes with medicines. J Gerontol A Biol Sci Med Sci. 2012;67A:175–180.
52. Cockcroft DW, Gault MH. Prediction of creatinine clearance from serum creatinine. Nephron. 1976;16:31–41.
53. Aetna. Top 200 medicare part D drugs on 2015 Aetna and Coventry Individual Medicare formularies. 2014, November 11. http://coventry-medicare. coventryhealthcare.com/web/groups/public/@cvty_medicare_coventrymedicare/documents/document/c134538.pdf.
54. Hanlon JT, Aspinall SL, Semla TP, Weisbord SD, Fried LF, Good CB, Fine MJ, Stone RA, Pugh MJV, Rossi MI, Handler SM. Consensus guidelines for oral dosing of primarily renally cleared medications in older adults. J Am Geriatr Soc. 2009;57:335–340.
55. Corsonello A, Pedone C, Incalzi RA. Age-related pharmacokinetic and pharmacodynamic changes and related risk of adverse drug reactions. Curr Med Chem. 2010;17:571–584.
56. Bowie MW, Slattum PW. Pharmacodynamics in older adults: A review. Am J Geriatr Pharmacother. 2007;5:263–303.
57. Trifior G, Spina E. Age-related changes in pharmacodynamics: Focus on drugs acting on central nervous and cardiovascular systems. Curr Drug Metab. 2011;12:611–620.
58. Ruscin JM, Linnebur SA. Pharmacodynamics in the elderly. In: RS Porter, JL Kaplan (Eds) *The Merck Manual Online*. The Merck Manuals Online Medical Library database. http://www.merckmanuals.com/professional/geriatrics/drug-therapy-in-the-elderly/pharmacodynamics-in-the-elderly. Accessed June 26, 2015.
59. Cusack BJ, Vestal RE. Clinical pharmacology: Special considerations in the elderly. In: E Calkins, PJ Davis, AB Ford (Eds) *Practice of Geriatric Medicine*. Philadelphia, PA: WB Saunders Company, 1986, pp. 115–136.
60. Salahudeen MS, Duffull SB, Nishtala PS. Anticholinergic burden quantified by anticholinergic risk scales and adverse outcomes in older people: A systematic review. BMC Geriatr. 2015;15:31.
61. Beyth RJ, Shorr RI. Principles of drug therapy in older patients: Rational drug prescribing. Clin Geriatr Med. 2002;18:577–692.
62. Centers for Disease Control and Prevention. The state of aging and health in America 2013. Atlanta, GA: Centers for Disease Control and Prevention, US Department of Health and Human Services. http://www.cdc.gov/aging/pdf/state-aging-health-in-america-2013.pdf.
63. Wallace J, Paauw DS. Appropriate prescribing and important drug interactions in older adults. Med Clin N Am. 2015;99(2):295–310.
64. Boyd CM, Darer J, Boult C, Fried LP, Boult L, Wu AW. Clinical practice guidelines and quality of care for older patients with multiple comorbid diseases: Implications for pay for performance. JAMA. 2005;294(6):716–724.
65. Tinetti ME, Bogardus ST Jr, Agostini JV. Potential pitfalls of disease-specific guidelines for patients with multiple conditions. N Engl J Med. 2004;351(27):2870–2874.
66. Patient-centered care for older adults with multiple chronic conditions: A stepwise approach from the American Geriatrics Society: American Geriatrics Society Expert Panel on the care of older adults with multimorbidity. J Am Geriatr Soc. 2012;60(10):1957–1968.
67. Mallet L, Spinewine A, Huang A. The challenge of managing drug interactions in elderly people. Lancet. 2007;370:185–191.
68. Routledge PA, O'Mahony MS, Woodhouse KW. Adverse drug reactions in elderly patients. *Br J Clin Pharmacol*. 2004;57:121–126.
69. Grattagliano I, Portincasa P, D'Ambrosio G, Palmieri VO, Palasciano G. Avoiding drug interactions: Here's help. *J Fam Pract*. 2010;59:322–329.

70. Lin P. Drug interactions and polypharmacy in the elderly. *Can Alzheimers Dis Rev.* 2003;6:10–14.
71. Steinman MA, Handler SM, Gurwitz JH, Schiff GD, Covinsky KE. Beyond the prescription: Medication monitoring and adverse drug events in older adults. *J Am Geriatr Soc.* 2011;59:1513–1520.
72. Kashyap M, D'Cruz S, Sachdev A, Tiwari P. Drug-drug interactions and their predictors: Results from Indian elderly inpatients. Pharm Pract. 2013;11(4):191–195.
73. Zhan C, Correa-de-Araujo R, Bierman AS, Sangl J, Miller MR, Wickizer SW, Stryer D. Suboptimal prescribing in elderly outpatients: Potentially harmful drug-drug and drug-disease combinations. J Am Geriatr Soc. 2005;53(2):262–267.
74. Bjorkman IK, Fastbom J, Schmidt IK, Bernsten CB, Pharmaceutical Care of the Elderly in Europe Research (PEER) Group. Drug-drug interactions in the elderly. Ann Pharmacother. 2002;36:1165–1171.
75. Mendes-Nett RS, Silva CQ, Oliveira Filho AD, Rocha CE, Lyra-Junior DP. Assessment of drug interactions in elderly patients of a family health care unit in Aracaju (Brazil): A pilot study. *Afr J Pharm Pharmacol.* 2011;5:812–818.
76. Shao H, Chen L-Q, Xu J. Treatment of dyslipidemia in the elderly. *J Geriatr Cardiol.* 2011;8(1):55–64. doi: *10.3724/SP.J.1263.2011.00055.*
77. Doan J, Zakrewski-Jakubiak H, Roy J, Turgeon J, Tannenbaum C. Prevalence and risk of potential cytochrome p450-mediated drug-drug interactions in older hospitalized patients with polypharmacy. Ann Pharmacother. 2013;47:324–332.
78. Juurlink DN, Mamdani M, Kopp A, Laupacis A, Redelmeier DA. Drug-drug interactions among elderly patients hospitalized for drug toxicity. JAMA. 2003;289:1652–1658.
79. Lindblad CI, Artz MB, Pieper CF, Sloane RJ, Hajjar ER, Ruby CM, Schmader KE, Hanlon JT. Potential drug-disease interactions in frail, hospitalized elderly veterans. Ann Pharmacother. 2005;39:412–417.
80. Lindblad CI, Hanlon JT, Gross CR, Sloane RJ, Pieper CF, Hajjar ER, Ruby CM, Schmader KE, Multidisciplinary Consensus Panel. Clinically important drug- disease interactions and their prevalence in older adults. Clin Ther. 2006;28:1133–1143.
81. Kojima G, Bell C, Tamura B, Inaba M, Lubimir K, Blanchette PL, Iwasaki W, Masaki K. Reducing cost by reducing polypharmacy: The polypharmacy outcomes project. J Am Med Dir Assoc. 2012;13(9):818.e11–15.
82. Maher RL, Hanlon J, Hajjar ER. Clinical consequences of polypharmacy in elderly. Expert Opin Drug Saf. 2014;13(1):57–65.
83. Ruscin JM, Linnebur SA. Drug-related problems in the elderly. In: RS Porter, JL Kaplan (Eds) *The Merck Manual Online.* The Merck Manuals Online Medical Library database. http://www.merckmanuals.com/professional/geriatrics/drug-therapy-in-the-elderly/pharmacodynamics-in-the-elderly. Accessed June 30, 2015.
84. Bourgeois FT, Shannon MW, Valim C, Mandl KD. Adverse drug events in the outpatient setting: An 11-year national analysis. Pharmacoepidemiol Drug Saf. 2010;19(9):901–910.
85. Meredith S, Feldman PH, Frey D, Hall K, Arnold K, Brown NJ, Ray WA. Possible medication errors in home healthcare patients. J Am Geriatr Soc. 2001;49(6):719–724.
86. Mannucci PM, Nobili A, REPOSI Investigators. Multimorbidity and polypharmacy in the elderly: Lessons from REPOSI. Intern Emerg Med. 2014;9(7):723–734.
87. Jyrkkä J, Enlund H, Korhonen MJ, Sulkava R, Hartikainen S. Polypharmacy status as an indicator of mortality in an elderly population. Drugs Aging. 2009;26(12):1039–1048.
88. U.S. National Archives and Records Administration. Code of federal regulations. 42 CFR 483.60(c)(1)&(2), F428, Drug Regimen Review. 2005. http://www.ecfr.gov/cgi-bin/retrieveECFR?gp=&SID=2ea1a9f177a10271fa8c2d3c99e6ef26&mc=true&n=sp42.5.483.b&r=SUBPART&ty=HTML#se42.5.483_160. Accessed July 2, 2015.
89. U.S. National Archives and Records Administration. Code of federal regulations. 42 CFR 483.25(l), F329, Unnecessary Medications. 2005. http://www.ecfr.gov/cgi-bin/text-idx?SID=3a66dbb4aa4356a3354ed88c245f2f45&node=se42.5.483_125&rgn=div8. Accessed July 2, 2015.
90. Hanlon JT, Schmader KE, Samsa GP, Weinberger M, Uttech KM, Lewis IK, Cohen HJ, Feussner JR. A method for assessing drug therapy appropriateness. J Clin Epidemiol. 1992;45:1045–1051.
91. National Transitions of Care Coalition. Improving transitions of care: Findings and considerations of the "Vision of the National Transitions of Care Coalition." http://www.ntocc.org/portals/0/pdf/resources/ntoccissuebriefs.pdf. Accessed July 1, 2015.
92. Kapoor A, Field T, Handler S, Fisher K, Saphirak C, Crawford S, Fouayzi H, Johnson F, Spenard A, Zhang N. Adverse events in long-term care residents transitioning from hospital back to nursing home. JAMA Intern Med. 2019;179(9):1254–1261.
93. Gleason KM, Brake H, Agramonte V Perfetti C. Medications at Transitions and Clinical Handoffs (MATCH) toolkit for medication reconciliation. (Prepared by the Island Peer Review Organization, Inc., under Contract No. HHSA2902009000 13C.) AHRQ Publication No. 11(12)-0059. Rockville, MD: Agency for Healthcare Research and Quality, December 2011.
94. American Pharmacists Association, American Society of Health-System Pharmacists, Steeb D, Webster L. Improving care transitions: Optimizing medication reconciliation. J Am Pharm Assoc. 2012;52(4):e43–52.
95. Cornish PL, Knowles SR, Marchesano R, Tam V, Shadowitz S, Juurlink DN, Etchells EE. Unintended medication discrepancies at the time of hospital admission. Arch Intern Med. 2005;165(4):424–429.
96. Pronovost P, Weast B, Schwarz M, Wyskiel RM, Prow D, Milanovich SN, Berenholtz S, Dorman T, Lipsett P. Medication reconciliation: A practical tool to reduce the risk of medication errors. J Crit Care. 2003;18(4):201–205.
97. Institute for Healthcare Improvement. Protecting 5 million lives from harm, how-to guide: Prevent adverse drug events (medication reconciliation). Cambridge, MA. http://www.ihi.org/resources/Pages/Tools/HowtoGuidePreventAdverseDrugEvents.aspx. Accessed on July 1, 2015.
98. Kirwin J, Canales AE, Bentley ML, Bungay K, Chan T, Dobson E, Holder RM, Johnson D, Lilliston A, Mohammad RA, Spinler SA. Process indicators of quality clinical pharmacy services during transitions of care. Pharmacotherapy. 2012;32(11):e338–347.
99. Durán-García E, Fernandez-Llamazares CM, Calleja-Hernández MA. Medication reconciliation: Passing phase or real need? Int J Clin Pharm. 2012;34(6):797–802.
100. Gleason KM, McDaniel MR, Feinglass J, Baker D, Lindquist L, Liss D, Noskin G. Results of the Medications at Transitions and Clinical Handoffs (MATCH) study: An analysis of medication reconciliation errors and risk factors at hospital admission. J Gen Intern Med. 2010;25:441–447.

101. Tija J, Bonner A, Briesacher BA, McGee S, Terrill E, Miller K. Medication discrepancies upon hospital to skilled nursing facility transitions. J Gen Intern Med. 2009;5:630–635.
102. Boockvar K, Fishman E, Kyriacou CK, Monias A, Gavi S, Cortes T. Adverse events due to discontinuations in drug use and dose changes in patients transferred between acute and long-term care facilities. Arch Intern Med. 2004;164:545–550.
103. Martin CM. Avoiding errors during transitions of care: Medication reconciliation. Consult Pharm. 2012;27(11): 764–769.
104. Johnson A, Guirguis E, Grace Y. Preventing medication errors in transitions of care: A patient case approach. J Am Pharm Assoc. 2015;55(2):e264–276.
105. Kitts NK, Reeve AR, Tsu L. Care transitions in elderly heart failure patients: Current practices and the pharmacist's role. Consult Pharm. 2014;29(3):179–190.
106. Garcia-Caballos M, Ramos-Diaz F, Jimenez-Moleon JJ, Bueno-Cavanillas A. Drug-related problems in older people after hospital discharge and interventions to reduce them. Age Ageing. 2010;39(4):430–438.
107. Forster AJ, Murff HJ, Peterson JF, Gandhi TK, Bates DW. Adverse drug events occurring following hospital discharge. J Gen Intern Med. 2005;20(4):317–323.
108. Thomsen LA, Winterstein AG, Sondergaard B, Haugbolle LS, Melander A. Systematic review of the incidence and characteristics of preventable adverse drug events in ambulatory care. Ann Pharmacother. 2007;41(9):1411–1426.
109. Richard C, Lussier MT. Nature and frequency of exchanges on medications during primary care encounters. Patient Educ Couns. 2006;64(1–3):207–216.
110. Sleath B, Roter D, Chewning B, Svarstad B. Asking questions about medication: Analysis of physician-patient interactions and physician perceptions. Med Care. 1999;37(11):1169–1173.
111. Gandhi TK, Weingart SN, Borus J, Seger AC, Peterson J, Burdick E, Seger DL, Shu K, Federico F, Leape LL, Bates DW. Adverse drug events in ambulatory care. N Engl J Med. 2003;348(16):1556–1564.
112. Weingart SN, Gandhi TK, Seger AC, Seger DL, Borus J, Burdick E, Leape LL, Bates DW. Patient-reported medication symptoms in primary care. Arch Intern Med. 2005;165(2):234–240.
113. Poon EG, Gandhi TK, Sequist TD, Murff HJ, Karson AS, Bates DW. "I wish I had seen this test result earlier!": Dissatisfaction with test result management systems in primary care. Arch Intern Med. 2004;164(20):2223–2228.
114. Shirts BH, Perera S, Hanlon JT, Roumani YF, Studenski SA, Nace DA, Becich MJ, Handler SM. Provider management of and satisfaction with laboratory testing in the nursing home setting: Results of a national internet-based survey. J Am Med Dir Assoc. 2009;10(3):161–166.
115. Gandhi TK, Burstin HR, Cook EF, Puopolo AL, Haas JS, Brennan TA, Bates DW. Drug complications in outpatients. J Gen Intern Med. 2000;15(3):149–154.
116. Rochon PA, Gurwitz JH. Optimising drug treatment for elderly people: The prescribing cascade. BMJ. 1997;315(7115):1096–1099.
117. Scott IA, Gray LC, Martin JH, Mitchell CA. Minimizing inappropriate medications in older populations: A 10-step conceptual framework. Am J Med. 2012;125(6):529.
118. Rochon PA. Drug prescribing for older adults. *UpToDate*, 2013. http://www.uptodate.com/contents/drug-prescribing-for-older-adults#H25. Accessed July 10, 2015.
119. Handler SM, Hanlon JT, Perera S, Roumani YF, Nace DA, Fridsma DB, Saul MI, Castle NG, Studenski SA. Consensus list of signals to detect potential adverse drug reactions in nursing homes. J Am Geriatr Soc. 2008;56(5): 808–815.
120. Handler SM, Shirts BH, Perera S, Becich MJ, Castle NG, Hanlon JT. Frequency of laboratory monitoring of chronic medications administered to nursing facility residents: Results of a national Internet-based study. Consult Pharm. 2008;23(5):387–395.
121. Reprinted with permission from American Geriatrics Society 2015 Beers Criteria Update Expert Panel. American Geriatrics Society 2015 updated beers criteria for potentially inappropriate medication use in older adults. J Am Geriatr Soc. 2015;63 (11):2227–2246. (Copyright © 1999–2021, John Wiley and Sons).
122. Fralick M, Bartsch E, Ritchie CS, Sacks CA. Estimating the use of potentially inappropriate medications among older adults in the United States. J Am Geriatr Soc. 2020;68(12):2927–2930.
123. Hanlon JT, Schmader KE, Boult C, Artz MB, Gross CR, Fillenbaum GG, Ruby CM, Garrard J. Use of inappropriate prescription drugs by older people. J Am Geriatr Soc. 2002;50:26–34.
124. Willcox SM, Himmelstein DU, Woolhandler S. Inappropriate drug prescribing for the community-dwelling elderly. *JAMA*. 1994;272:292–296.
125. Zhan C, Sangl J, Bierman AS, Miller MR, Friedman B, Wickizer SW, Meyer GS. Potentially inappropriate medication use in the community-dwelling elderly: Findings from the 1996 Medical Expenditure Panel Survey. *JAMA*. 2001;286:2823–2829.
126. Briesacher B, Limcangco R, Simoni-Wastila L, Doshi J, Gurwitz J. Evaluation of nationally mandated drug use reviews to improve patient safety in nursing homes: A natural experiment. J Am Geriatr Soc. 2005;53:991–996.
127. Lapane KL, Hughes CM, Quilliam BJ. Does incorporating medications in the surveyors' interpretive guidelines reduce the use of potentially inappropriate medications in nursing homes? J Am Geriatr Soc. 2007;55:666–673.
128. Spore DL, Mor V, Larrat P, Hawes C, Hiris J. Inappropriate drug prescriptions for elderly residents of board and care facilities. *Am J Publ Health* 1997;87:404–409.
129. Dhall J, Larrat EP, Lapane KL. Use of potentially inappropriate drugs in nursing homes. *Pharmacotherapy*. 2002;22:88–96.
130. Williams B, Betley C. Inappropriate use of nonpsychotropic medications in nursing homes. *J Am Geriatr Soc*. 1995;43:513–519.
131. Beers MH, Ouslander JG, Fingold SF, Morgenstern H, Reuben DB, Rogers W, Zeffren MJ, Beck JC. Inappropriate medication prescribing in skilled-nursing facilities. *Ann Intern Med*. 1992;117:684–689.
132. Budnitz DS, Lovegrove MC, Shehab N, Richards CL. Emergency hospitalizations for adverse drug events in older Americans. N Engl J Med. 2011;365(21):2002–2012.
133. Hanlon JT, Artz MB, Pieper CF, Lindblad CI, Sloane RJ, Ruby CM, Schmader KE. Inappropriate medication use among frail elderly inpatients. Ann Pharmacother. 2004;38:9–14.
134. O'Connor MN, Gallagher P, O'Mahony D. Inappropriate prescribing: Criteria, detection and prevention. Drugs Aging. 2012;29(6):437–452.

135. Healthcare Effectiveness Data and Information Set (HEDIS). Summary table of measures, product lines and changes. http://www.ncqa.org/Portals/0/HEDISQM/Hedis2015/List_of_ HEDIS_2015_Measures.pdf. Accessed July 15, 2015.
136. Beers MH, Ouslander JG, Rollingher I, Reuben DB, Brooks J, Beck JC. Explicit criteria for determining inappropriate medication use in nursing home residents. UCLA Division of Geriatric Medicine. Arch Intern Med. 1991;151:1825.
137. Beers MH. Explicit criteria for determining potentially inappropriate medication use by the elderly. An update. Arch Intern Med. 1997;157:1531.
138. Fick DM, Cooper JW, Wade WE, Waller JL, Maclean JR, Beers MH. Updating the Beers criteria for potentially inappropriate medication use in older adults: Results of a US consensus panel of experts. Arch Intern Med. 2003; 163:2716.
139. Louden K. Geriatrics society updates list of inappropriate drugs. www.medscape.com/viewarticle/846136. Accessed September 23, 2015.
140. By the 2019 American Geriatrics Society Beers Criteria® Update Expert Panel. American Geriatrics Society 2019 updated AGS Beers Criteria® for potentially inappropriate medication use in older adults. J Am Geriatr Soc. 2019;67(4):674–694.
141. Department of Health and Human Services, Centers for Medicare and Medicaid Services. Interpretive guidelines for long-term care facilities, appendices P and PP. www.cms.gov/Regulations-and-Guidance. Accessed September 23, 2015.
142. Gallagher P, Ryan C, Byrne S, Kennedy J, O'Mahony D. STOPP (Screening Tool of Older Person's Prescriptions) and START (Screening Tool to Alert doctors to Right Treatment). Consensus validation. Int J Clin Pharmacol Ther. 2008;46(2):72–83.
143. O'Mahony D, O'Sullivan D, Byrne S, O'Connor MN, Ryan C, Gallagher P. STOPP/START criteria for potentially inappropriate prescribing in older people: Version 2. Age Ageing. 2015;44(2):213–218.
144. Gallagher P, O'Mahony D. STOPP (Screening Tool of Older Persons' potentially inappropriate Prescriptions): Application to acutely ill elderly patients and comparison with Beers' criteria. Age Ageing. 2008;37:673.
145. Hamilton H, Gallagher P, Ryan C, Byrne S, O'Mahony D. Potentially inappropriate medications defined by STOPP criteria and the risk of adverse drug events in older hospitalized patients. Arch Intern Med. 2011;171:1013.
146. Cohen MR, Smetzer JL, Tuohy NR, Kilo CM. Chapter 14. High-Alert Medications: Safeguarding Against Errors. In: MR Cohen (Ed) *Medication Errors (2nd ed).* Washington, DC: American Pharmacists Association, 2007, p. 328.
147.Risk Management Foundation of Harvard Medical Institutions. Medication malpractice risks-CIRCO benchmark report. 2017. https://www.rmf.harvard.edu/Malpractice-Data/Annual-Benchmark-Reports/Medical-Malpractice-in-America.
148. Naranjo CA, Busto U, Sellers EM, Sandor P, Ruiz I, Roberts EA, Janecek E, Domeco C, and Greenblatt DJ. A reliable method for estimating the probability of adverse drug reactions. Clin Pharmac Ther. 1981;(30):239–245.
149. Richmond RG, Heard K, Patel D. Amiodarone Toxicity: A case series and review of the literature with a focus on pharmacist liability and risk management. Consult Pharm. 28(10):634;2013.
150. *Phillips v. Larry's Drive-In Pharm., Inc.*, No. 33194, Supreme Court of Appeals of West Virginia, 220 W. Va. 484;647 S.E.2d 920;2007 W. Va. LEXIS 58, March 13, 2007, Submitted, June 28, 2007, Filed.
151. Richmond RG, Patel D, Heard K, Dollins A. Methotrexate toxicity—A case series and review of the literature with a focus on pharmacist liability and risk management. Consult Pharm. 2013;28(10):634.
152. Martha M. Boote v. Helen Boote Shivers, et al. No. M2003-00560-COA-R3-CV, Court of Appeals of Tennessee, at Nashville. 198 S.W.3d 732; 2005 Tenn. App. LEXIS 661. January 7, 2004, Session, October 21, 2005, Filed. SUBSEQUENT HISTORY: In re Estate of Boote v. Shivers, 2006 Tenn. LEXIS 354 (Tenn., Apr. 24, 2006). PRIOR HISTORY: Tenn. R. App. P. 3 Appeal as of Right; Judgment of the Chancery Court Reversed and Remanded. Appeal from the Chancery Court for Marshall County. No. 12099. J. B. Cox, Chancellor. In re Estate of Boote, 198 S.W.3d 699, 2005 Tenn. App. LEXIS 663 (Tenn. Ct. App., 2005). In re Estate of Boote v. Shivers, 2005 Tenn. App. LEXIS 317 (Tenn. Ct. App., 27, 2005).
153. Reprinted with permission from O'Mahony D, O'Sullivan D, Byrne S, O'Conner MN, Ryan C, Gallagher P. STOPP/START criteria for potentially inappropriate prescribing in older people: Version 2. Age and Ageing. 2015;44(2):213–218. (Copyright © 2021, Oxford University Press).

24 Medication Errors

James T. O'Donnell and James J. O'Donnell III

SYNOPSIS

24.1 HISTORY AND OVERVIEW

Since the publication of the Institute of Medicine's (IOM) original medication-error report, *To Err is Human: Building a Safer Health System* in 1999,[1] healthcare professionals, legislators, attorneys, and the public have developed an increased awareness of medical error and the need to reduce avoidable morbidity and mortality. Despite increases in technology and the introduction of new medications into the physician's armamentarium, today's practice of medicine is still plagued by the human factor, which contributes to error.

A more recent (2006) IOM report called for all prescriptions to be written electronically by 2010. Unfortunately, at that time, only 3% of hospitals had adopted these systems, and only a few physicians actually prescribed drugs electronically. Even simple medication-safety recommendations—block printing on hand-written prescription forms, for example—were widely ignored, creating extra complexity to the system that creates the perfect environment for error.[2] In the hospital setting, a physician writing a medication order for a patient has to wait until that order has been transcribed, sent to the pharmacy, and brought back to the floor before that mediation can be administered to the patient. Lucien Leape (M.D.), one of the authors of the IOM study, estimated that there are up to 20 steps involved with the prescribing-transcribing-dispensing-administration process in a paper-based (non-computerized) hospital setting. With so many interim steps to traverse, it is no wonder that errors occur. Contrast that scenario to the one in which a physician writes a prescription for a patient in an outpatient setting. The patient takes the prescription to the pharmacy and the pharmacist fills it. Simplicity supports safety. The fewer steps involved in the process, the lower the likelihood for error.

Fortunately, with the mandate for Electronic Medical Records (EMR) and now almost 50% of ambulatory prescriptions generated by computerized physician order

DOI: 10.1201/9781003615323-26

entry (CPOE), handwritten prescriptions will continue to decrease, minimizing the risks associated with poor and ambiguous prescriptions. It is noteworthy, however, that new errors associated with the new technology are being reported with greater frequency as well.

In 2000, Barbara Starfield (MD, MPH) of the Johns Hopkins School of Hygiene and Public Health reported that medical errors may actually be the third leading cause of death in the United States. According to her research, there are 2,000 deaths per year from unnecessary surgeries; 7,000 deaths per year from medication errors in hospitals; 20,000 deaths per year from "other" errors in hospitals; 80,000 deaths per year from infections in hospitals; and 106,000 deaths per year from non-error, adverse effects of medications.[3]

A later study in 2010 yielded almost twice as many deaths, at 180,000 deaths per year. A more recent study from 2013 estimated that the numbers range from 210,000 to 440,000 deaths per year. The latest numbers would make medication errors the third leading cause of death after heart disease and cancer.[4] However, these numbers can only be estimated because medical records are often inaccurate, and providers might be reluctant to disclose mistakes.

24.2 MEDICATION ERRORS IN EPIDEMIC PROPORTIONS

What stands out in all of these studies is the large contribution of medication errors towards medical-error-based mortality. In fact, prescribing the wrong drug or administering the wrong dosage represents a significant percentage of medication errors, and that number is growing. The 2006 IOM report shows that medication errors harm 1.5 million patients and account for several thousand deaths per year, costing the nation at least $3.5 billion annually.[5]

Error has a different meaning to some healthcare practitioners. One physician, when told he was going to be sued for a medication error retorted, "How can they sue me, I didn't **intend** to give the patient the wrong medication?".

The Webster's New Collegiate Dictionary lists several definitions for "error"—the one that seems to be most appropriate in the context of "medication error" is defined as "an act that through ignorance, deficiency, or accident departs from or fails to achieve what should be done." The key word in the dictionary's definition of error is "departure," and the key word in the NCCMERP definition is "preventable." Intent is not relevant. The dictionary definition also mentions "ignorance" and "deficiency" as being causes of error—two factors also identified in the contemporary literature on medical and medication errors.

The National Coordinating Council for Medication Error Reporting and Prevention (NCCMERP) define a medication error as:

> Any preventable event that may cause or lead to inappropriate medication use or patient harm while the medication is in the control of the healthcare professional, patient, or consumer. Such events may be related to professional practice, healthcare products, procedures, and systems, including prescribing; order communication; product labeling, packaging, and nomenclature; compounding; dispensing; distribution; administration; education; monitoring; and use.[6]

It is vitally important that physicians have the knowledge they need about the medications they are prescribing, along with the information about the patient's allergies, concomitant medications, current hepatic and renal function, and secondary diagnoses. Deficiencies in the current systems that supply critical information to the physician must be reengineered to make errors more difficult to commit. Many risk management and patient-safety experts recommend the application of Failure Mode Effect Analysis (FMEA) to determine the parts of the information transmission system that failed.

The key tenet is that if it was an error, then it could have been prevented. Preventing future mistakes requires developing safer systems. Other major causes of medication errors are poor oral or written communications. Enhanced communication skills and better interactions among members of the healthcare team and the patient are essential to reduce errors.

The reduction in medication errors involves an ongoing process of quality improvement. Sloppy, hand-written medication orders should be replaced by CPOE, a very effective technique for reducing prescribing/ordering errors in hospitals fortunate enough to be able to afford costly software. For hospitals with fewer resources, a less expensive—yet effective—change could involve retraining physicians to write all drug orders in plain English and prohibiting the use of confusing short-hand abbreviations that are subject to misinterpretation, such as q.d. and q.o.d., which are among the unapproved abbreviations referred to by The Joint Commission for Accreditation of Healthcare Organization (TJC) in their 2005 National Patient Safety Goals. The ultimate goal is clear: Seamless, computerized, and integrated medication delivery instituted by fully informed healthcare professionals who are adequately trained to utilize such technological advances. The frequency of drug administration can also be problematic. In one reported incident, a physician wrote an order for "Uniphyl (theophylline) 400 mg q.d." for a patient being discharged from the hospital to a nursing home. At the nursing home, another physician mistakenly transcribed the order as "Uniphyl 400 mg q.i.d.," and it went unnoticed by the nurses and pharmacists. The patient received the medication incorrectly for a week, at which point she began complaining of nausea. The next day. she was found unresponsive and was readmitted to the hospital. Her theophylline level at admission was 61 mg per mL (normal range is 10–20 mg per mL). Even when a prescriber has legible handwriting, errors can occur. The loop of a cursive "q" that comes up between the "q" and the "d" or a period after the "q" can look like the letter "i" making the frequency look like "q.i.d.". The use of the abbreviation "q.o.d." (every other day) has also caused problems because it has been misinterpreted as "q.d." (every day) or "q.i.d." (four times daily) if the "o" is poorly written. In order to prevent confusion, write out the directions "daily" and "every other day," instead of using abbreviations that can be open to misinterpretation. Do not abbreviate. Problems can arise when drug names are abbreviated or truncated. For example, a physician wrote a prescription for AZT for a patient with HIV. Unfortunately, the dispensing pharmacist failed to realize that, in his computer, the unofficial abbreviation "AZT" was used for zidovudine (Retrovir—GlaxoSmithKline).[7]

An educational campaign in 2009 involving the joint effort of ISMP and FDA sought to eliminate the use of error-prone abbreviations. These error-prone lists are updated and promulgated periodically. It is said (almost verbatim) that nearly everyone in healthcare uses shortcuts such as abbreviations and symbols in an effort to conserve time—when handwriting, or even typing—words, phrases, or units of measure. However, these shortcuts often lead to errors. All too often, it is not until these medical abbreviations, symbols, or nonstandard dose designations lead to patient harm that action is taken to prevent future misunderstandings. To sum it up, mind your "p"s and "q"s.

24.3 TYPES OF MEDICATION ERRORS

Traditionally, medication errors have been collectively referred to as "The Five Wrongs." These include: Wrong drug, wrong dose, wrong route of administration, wrong time, and wrong patient. Failure to monitor and/or follow up is also frequently mentioned as a cause of medication errors. With the exception of failure-to-monitor, the "Five Wrongs" usually occur as a result of some vague or ambiguous form of verbal or written communication. When drug names look alike or sound alike (e.g., Enalapril® and eldepryl or Lamisil® and Lamictal®), there is an increased risk of misidentifying one drug for another, especially during an oral or telephone order. Recognizing "look-alike" drug names and storing them in different areas of the pharmacy and drug cabinets on the floors reduce the risk of dispensing or administering the wrong one. Writing both the brand and generic names on the medication order or prescription followed by the condition to be treated, e.g., Lamictal® (lamotrigine) for seizures, minimizes the likelihood of reported confusion with the similar sounding anti-fungal, Lamisil® (terbinafine). The United States Pharmacopeia (USP) has compiled a list of "paired drugs" that are commonly mistaken for one another. The list covers several pages and demonstrates that this problem is a source of great concern for quality improvement specialists, physicians, pharmacists, and nurses.

Failure to monitor is another common cause of adverse reactions to medications, especially narcotics. Patients who receive parenteral narcotics in the hospital frequently develop itching from histamine release, a well-known effect of most narcotics. To treat the itching, an antihistamine-like diphenhydramine (Benadryl®) may be prescribed. If the patient has already received promethazine (Phenergan®) or hydroxyzine to potentiate the analgesic effect of the narcotic, then the concomitant administration of another antihistamine may intensify the respiratory depressant effects of the other drugs and produce a respiratory arrest. In the evening, patients often receive a benzodiazepine or other hypnotic for sleep, which also may contribute to respiratory depression. Once the patient has been "tucked in" for the night, the nurse may not return to assess the patient or take vital signs until the patient's oxygen has already desaturated and the patient is found cyanotic or begins to fibrillate.

Failure to monitor in the outpatient setting has a different appearance. A typical scenario may look like this: A patient is discharged from the hospital with a new set of medications and/or several new prescriptions. The patient is elderly and does not walk or drive. The new prescriptions are never filled, and after the patient runs out of the medication he/she was given at discharge, the new medications are no longer taken, and the patient's health deteriorates, or the patient has to be readmitted to the hospital in urgent or critical condition. Unfortunately, this is an all-too-common situation.

In order to avoid medication errors of this type, The Joint Commission (TJC) listed among its 2015 National Patient Safety Goals the need to Reconcile Medication Across a Continuum of Care.[8] This means that a Joint Commission (TJC) accredited facility must ensure that upon admission and upon discharge, the changes in a patient's medication regimen are "reconciled" (listed) and mandate that changes in medications and dosages are correctly recorded and implemented. Some hospitals utilize nurses or pharmacists to call patients after discharge to verify that new prescriptions have been filled and that the patient is taking his/her medications according to the most recent orders of the prescribing physician. The Visiting Nurse Association (VNA) can also play a valuable role in helping to ensure that newly prescribed medications are taken as directed.

Most medical errors, including medication errors, fall into two major categories—those that result from failing to complete a planned action (errors of execution) and those that result from following an erroneous plan (errors of planning). Errors can be further classified as either errors of commission or omission. Errors of commission occur when an action performed is done incorrectly (when surgery is performed at the wrong site) or when a wrong plan of action is used to achieve an objective (the wrong drug is prescribed). Errors of omission occur when an action is not performed as it should be. Examples include failure to follow up on an abnormal Papanicolaou test result or omission of recommended vaccinations. Table 24.1 illustrates various errors of commission and omission. Extent of the Challenge**:** Approximately 400,000 hospitalized patients each year experience some type of preventable harm[9] (permission granted CCC 060622).

The November 2016 issue of *Risk Management Monthly* (Volume 10, Number 11) extracted highlights from The Emergency Medicine Closed Claims Study from The Doctors Company that evaluated a total of 332 closed claims in emergency medicine from the years 2007 to 2013[11,12].

TABLE 24.1
Errors in Ambulatory Care[10].

Errors of Commission

- Wrong diagnosis
- Improper management of correct diagnosis
- Lack of patient information
- Inaccessible medical record
- Incomplete patient history and/or physical examination
- Prescription errors
- Wrong drug
- Wrong dosage or duration of therapy
- Failure to recognize drug–drug interactions
- Illegible prescriptions
- Transcribing errors by office staff or pharmacist
- Failure to refill in timely fashion
- Failure to monitor drugs that require monitoring

Errors of Omissions

- Failure to follow up on test results
- Failure to notify patients of test results
- Lack of necessary follow-up with practitioner
- Failure to make new appointment after patient or practitioner cancellation
- Failure to follow up after patient fails to show for a scheduled appointment
- Failure to coordinate care with consultants
- Lack of timely evaluation
- Delay in the referral process
- Failure to communicate findings and recommendations after consultation
- Delay in diagnosis
- Failure to perform preventive care
- Failure to provide proven disease-specific care
- Failure in information transfer among covering practitioners or between inpatient and outpatient providers
- Failure to educate patients

Major findings included:[13]

1. Issues related to diagnosis constituted the majority of cases. These included failure to diagnose, delayed diagnosis, or an incorrect diagnosis. This could involve one or more of the following: Failure to establish a differential diagnosis, failure to order diagnostic tests, failure to address abnormal findings, failure to consider available clinical information. Other issues adversely influencing the diagnostic process were a failure to obtain a consult and a premature discharge from the ED. The most frequently misdiagnosed conditions included acute cerebral vascular accident, myocardial infarction, spinal epidural abscess, pulmonary embolism, necrotizing fasciitis, meningitis, testicular torsion, subarachnoid hemorrhage, septicemia, lung cancer, fractures, and appendicitis. The study identified specific factors that contributed to the patient injury.
2. Contributing factors in medical errors included failure to order appropriate tests and address abnormal results, and failure to use clinical information and establish the differential diagnosis. Patient characteristics such as obesity (led to skipping specific exam elements), nonadherence to treatment plans and follow-up appointments, and poor patient hygiene also contributed.
3. Communication issues among providers led to medical errors, and these included failure to communicate, failure to review the medical record, poor professional rapport, and communication between providers and the patient/family including not using qualified interpreters when applicable.
4. A summary of the study's tips for avoiding diagnostic error: Avoid first impression or intuition-based diagnoses, complete and document a thorough differential diagnosis for each patient, ensure that all specialists who are called to evaluate patients in the ED receive a comprehensive summary of the clinical picture, and practice effective handoffs. The handoff discussion should include clear delegation of the individual who has the responsibility for review and follow-up of all test results.

24.3.1 Enhancing Healthcare Team Outcomes

The rates of medical errors have considerably decreased from the past, although they still represent a significant problem. It is necessary that all healthcare professionals on the team (e.g., pharmacist, nurse, clinician) are informed that medical errors may not only cause patients harm but also may result in medical malpractice lawsuits. It is important that clinicians confirm their orders before submitting them. The pharmacist then is required to perform an interaction check and verify all dosing and drug information. The nurse then serves as a final safeguard before the administration of a drug to again confirm agent, dosing, drug information, and correct patient for treatment. Medical errors are the result of multiple causes. Hospitals have introduced safeguards and regulations to minimize these errors with a system of checks and balances which ultimately improve awareness by every member of the team with the goal to reduce errors.

24.3.2 Improving the Reporting of Medication Errors

A recent evaluation of medical errors estimates a significant contribution to an estimate of 251,000 deaths annually in the United States. This makes medical errors the third leading cause of death in the United States. Error rates are significantly higher in the United States compared to other developed countries; however, less than 10 percent of medical errors are reported. One study investigated the implementation of the MEDMARX Medication Error

Reporting system in 25 hospitals in Pennsylvania where data was collected from 17,000 errors reported by participating hospitals over a year-long period. Data analysis revealed that the reporting of errors by providers increased significantly at each quarter, but the proportion of corrective actions installed by the hospitals remained relatively constant. A simulation model then examined the effect of potential organizational changes resulting from error reporting using four interventions. The results suggest that improving patient safety outcomes requires more effort than voluntary reporting of medical errors. Organizational changes not only need to be implemented but should also be institutionalized.[14]

24.4 MEDICATION USE PROCESS

The Medication Use Process (MUP) encompasses all the individual components of prescribing, transcribing, dispensing, and administering medications and monitoring their effects on the patient. The process can be schematized as shown next:

Transcription

Ordering → Dispensing → Administering → Monitoring

Communtcation

Table 24.2 shows the results of studies conducted by the Agency for Healthcare Research and Quality (AHRQ) to determine at what stage in the MUP errors occurred. Up to 50% of errors occurred during the prescribing/ordering phase. Twenty-five to 38% of errors occurred during administration, followed by transcription errors and pharmacy dispensing errors.[15]

Avoiding medication errors requires the communication of the right drug, the right dose, the right route, and the right frequency of administration from one healthcare professional to another. Miscommunications like illegible medication orders, look-alike drug names, and confusion of brand and generic names all can and do lead to medication errors.

When an error is made in the prescribing/ordering phase of the process, it can permeate the MUP and result in an adverse experience for the patient. Because of the prevalence of errors during the prescribing/ordering phase of the MUP, much attention has been given to instituting new practices for prescribing, such as Computerized Physician Order Entry (CPOE). One study showed that in the hospital setting, CPOE decreased serious medication errors by 55% and potential Adverse Drug Events (ADEs) by 84%.[18]

Computerized systems are defined as computer programs that maintain patient drug profiles and generate prescription-fill or dispensing lists. They may also interface with laboratory and other hospital departments. Computerization assists in the initial monitoring of a patient's drug therapy and decreases the chance of drug interactions. Most of the systems used today have built-in programs to detect potential drug interactions. Computerization also decreases the likelihood of drug sensitivities (allergies) going unnoticed, decreases the chance of therapeutic duplications of medications, warns of high-dose/low-dose alerts, and, sometimes, includes drug/disease contraindications. All these enhancements improve medication safety medication documentation.

Substantial progress has been made. According to the Office of the National Coordinator for Health Information Technology (ONC), almost all hospitals (96%) currently utilize certified electronic heath record (EHR) technology and meet meaningful use requirements promoted by the Centers for Medicare and Medicaid Services. A complementary technology, personal electronic health records (PHRs), increases patient access to information, allowing the monitoring and sharing of data. As the healthcare field standardizes EHR technology, the ONC predicts escalating PHR use.[19]

Along with the ERH mandates for hospitals, a similar mandate applied to physician practices, with financial incentives for the implementation and the threats of fines if not. The National Center for Health Statistics (2017) reported that 86% of office-based physicians were using any EMR/HER (Health Electronic Record) system, and 79% were using a certified EMR/HER system.[20]

The progress of HER has improved residential care facilities as well, but not to the same extent as hospitals and physician practices. There was an increase in the percentage of residential care communities that used EHRs from 2012 and 2016 (i.e., 20% to 26%). This included an increase for all bed size categories, chain and nonchain affiliation, the majority of census divisions, profit and nonprofit ownership, and MSA and non-MSA status. Computerized support for health information exchange with physicians and pharmacies also increased between 2012 and 2016 (i.e., 47.2% to 55.0%) and among communities that had more than 100 beds, were chain affiliated, for profit, located in the East North and East South Central census divisions, and in both MSAs and non-MSAs.[21]

For those remaining hospitals that do not have computer-based risk-management tools, there are some basic teachings that can be employed to decrease the likelihood of a prescribing error in a paper-based prescribing system. For example, when writing a medication order or prescription for an integer or whole number dosage, a physician should never use a trailing zero. If the decimal point is lost during transcription, a 10-fold dosing error can occur. The correct

TABLE 24.2
Occurrence of Medication Errors in Studies of Hospitalized Patients.[16,17]

Physician ordering	39–49%
Nursing administration	26–38%
Transcription	11–12%
Pharmacy dispensing	11–14%

procedure is to write 1 mg, not 1.0 mg. On the other hand, when writing for a decimal amount, the doctor should always use a leading zero. For example, Lanoxin 0.25 mg daily. Notice that the word "daily" has been used rather than the abbreviation "q.d.", which could be mistaken for q.i.d. (four times per day) or q.o.d. (every other day). The mnemonic to remember is "ALWAYS lead and NEVER follow."

In addition to poor handwriting, legibly written prescriptions can still be misinterpreted if the instructions are ambiguous. Several years ago, the unnecessary death of health reporter Betsy Lehman at a prestigious Boston cancer treatment center made front page news when she and a second patient both received fatal overdoses of cyclophosphamide, which had been prescribed (by a resident) as part of an experimental protocol to determine if cimetidine could augment the tumor-killing effects of cyclophosphamide in the treatment of breast cancer. According to the IOM report which was cited in an ECRI publication,[22] the cyclosphosphamide order was written "4 g/sq m over four days." Did this mean 4 g /sq m per day or 1 g/sq m per day for 4 days? Unfortunately, it meant 1 g/sq m per day for 4 days, but the full 4 grams/sq m were given in one day. Allegedly, the error was discovered by a Drug Utilization Review (DUR) clerk who noticed that the price charged to the patient's bill was four times the cost of a single dose. "Over four days" is too ambiguous. The order should have been written, 1 gram/sq m for four days, and should have been reviewed or counter-signed by the attending physician. Making up "instructions" is truly a prescription for error.

Fortunately, with the mandate and implementation of HER in virtually all hospitals and a high percentage of physician practices, electronic prescribing is now technically possible and represents an overwhelming majority of ambulatory medication prescriptions. E-prescribing is mandated for Medicare recipients. On April 16, 2018, CMS published a final rule (CMS-4182-F) to adopt a new NCPDP SCRIPT Standard Version 2017071(2017071) and retirement of current NCPDP SCRIPT Version 10.6 (10.6) for use in the Medicare Prescription Drug Benefit Program (Part D) effective from January 1, 2020. On May 23, 2019, CMS published a final rule (CMS-4180-F) requiring that Part D plans adopt one or more real-time benefit tools (RTBTs) capable of giving prescribers clinically appropriate patient-specific real-time formulary and benefit information. This mandate was effective from January 1, 2021.[23]

Initially prohibited, the Drug Enforcement Administration (DEA) has published interim final rules allowing e-prescribing. The DEA published an interim final rule in the Federal Register (March 31, 2010) which provides practitioners with the option of writing prescriptions electronically for controlled substances. The DEA has since received clarification requests for issues concerning the implementation and requirements for process of electronic prescribing of controlled substances. The DEA has now reopened the interim final rule to solicit comments from the public on specific issues outlined next regarding the electronic prescribing of controlled substances in anticipation of providing an update to the final rule on these topics.[24]

DATES: DEA reopened a comment period for the interim final rule published on March 31, 2010, at 75 FR 16236, which became effective from June 1, 2010. Electronic comments must have been submitted or postmarked on or before June 22, 2020.[25] E-prescribing controlled substances was estimated to reach 38% by 2019.[26]

E-prescribing is a prescriber's ability to electronically send an accurate, error-free, and understandable prescription directly to a pharmacy from the point-of-care and is an important element in improving the quality of patient care. The inclusion of e-prescribing in the Medicare Modernization Act (MMA) of 2003 provided initial momentum to the process change. The July 2006 Institute of Medicine report confirmed that e-prescribing supported the reduction in medication errors and received widespread acknowledgement and aided in building awareness for the role of e-prescribing in the future for patient safety. Facilitation of e-prescribing is a key contributor to the government's plan to increase the adoption of EMR and build a national electronic health information infrastructure in the United States. With universal adoption, it is expected to see a continued decrease in handwritten prescriptions which will minimize the risks associated with inaccurate and unclear prescriptions. Of note, the association of new errors is expected with this technology, and they are being reported with greater frequency. Further discussion on this topic follows later in this chapter. Surprisingly, Michael Cohen, Founder and President-Emeritus of the Institute for Safe Medication Practices (ISMP), recently stated: "We are seeing more computer related errors than we ever saw with hand-written prescriptions." (ISMP and Just Culture Company webinar *Lessons Learned about Human Fallibility, System Design, and Justice in the Aftermath of a Fatal Error* on May 6, 2022.)

24.5 SYSTEM ERRORS

"System Errors" describes errors in the MUP that support error-prone practices rather than practices which cannot lead to or do not support errors. In his 1995 article, Leape and co-authors described 13 system errors which were identified as "Proximal Causes" of medication errors.[27] These system errors are summarized in Table 24.3.

Of the 13 "Proximal Causes" identified by Leape et al., the failure to provide prescribers with knowledge about drugs accounted for 29% of errors, and systems failures to provide physicians with critical information about the patient (e.g., laboratory test results) were associated with 18% of errors. These two categories alone led to 47% of errors including drug–drug interactions, overdosing patients with diminished renal function, and prescribing drugs to which the patients were allergic.

TABLE 24.3
"Proximal Causes" of Medication Errors[28].

Lack of knowledge about the drug
Lack of information about the patient
Rule violations
Slips and memory lapses
Transcription errors
Faulty drug identification
Faulty interaction with other services
Dosing errors
Infusion pump/Parenteral delivery error
Inadequate monitoring
Drug stocking or delivery problem
Preparation error
Lack of standardization

24.5.1 Contraindicated Intrathecal Vincristine

One settled case dramatically describes a systems failure resulting in significant injury. This case involves a patient who received intrathecal vincristine. He did not die, but he was permanently paralyzed as a result of this medical error. This case makes for a good study of systems design, of the value of systems, and of what happens when the system breaks down (i.e., when the system is not followed). The patient, a 69-year-old farmer, was scheduled to complete a successful methotrexate/vincristine treatment for lymphoma at a major university medical center. His prognosis was good. One fateful day in May, he arrived at the oncology clinic for his scheduled methotrexate intrathecal and vincristine intravenous treatment. The intrathecal injection must be injected under guided fluoroscopy, so the oncologist had reserved a radiology suite. No nurse was available to accompany or assist the oncologist who was to administer the injection. The oncologist, not wanting to miss the appointment, stopped at the clinic pharmacy and asked the pharmacist for the "methotrexate and flush (preservative-free NaCl)." The syringes for both the vincristine IV and the methotrexate intrathecal had already been prepared. The staff pharmacist on duty in the clinic pharmacy asked the oncologist: "Would you like the complete order?" The oncologist confirmed, and the pharmacist proceeded to place both the vincristine and the methotrexate syringes in the container, which the oncologist then took to the radiology suite. There the oncologist injected what he thought was methotrexate, followed by the vincristine syringe (which he assumed was preservative-free NaCl).

The patient was taken back to the clinic, where, the oncologist believed, he would receive the intravenous vincristine, but the vincristine could not be found. A call to the pharmacy led to the discovery that the vincristine had been given to the oncologist, who immediately went to radiology and retrieved the discarded syringes from the sharps container. To his horror, he realized that the vincristine had mistakenly been administered intrathecally in place of the saline flush. An emergency spinal-fluid dialysis/replacement was undertaken, saving the patient's life. Sadly, the patient was left completely paralyzed below the nipple line of his body. The oncologist, devastated over the event, quickly settled with the patient for $500,000 and took one year off of practice.

The system failed in a number of ways. Had the system been followed, this accident probably would never have occurred. First off, a nurse should have accompanied the oncologist who, while engaged in a delicate intrathecal injection, did not read the label of the syringe he was administering. Next, the pharmacy department had a policy in place for utilizing the vincristine manufacturer's (Eli Lilly and Company, Indianapolis, Ind.) syringe label, which read:

> "FATAL IF GIVEN INTRATHECALLY. FOR INTRAVENOUS USE ONLY,"

and the red-bordered syringe overwrap that warned:

> "FATAL IF GIVEN INTRATHECALLY. FOR IV USE ONLY. DO NOT REMOVE COVERING UNTIL MOMENT OF INJECTION,"

The oncology clinic pharmacy manager decided that these were unnecessary for adult patients, because the oncology-clinic staff was "competent and well-informed." The staff pharmacist, who knew about the policy in place in the main hospital's sterile-products-compounding room, followed this "unofficial" exemption. That same pharmacist, given a verbal order for the "methotrexate and the flush," gave both the methotrexate and the vincristine, thereby violating another system rule—never to place both the methotrexate and the vincristine in the same container. As many staff pharmacists rotated through the oncology-clinic pharmacy, it was common knowledge that the precautionary syringe label and overwrap were not being used.

A lawsuit was brought against the university hospital, the staff pharmacist, the oncology clinic pharmacy manager, and the director of pharmacy. The lawsuit alleged that the

> Hospital and its employees failed to properly promulgate and enforce appropriate policies, procedures and protocols relating to the ordering, packaging, delivery, dispensing, and administration of vincristine; that the Hospital and its employees failed to properly train and supervise employees, and that those failures were substantial factors in causing the plaintiffs' injuries and damages.

The lawyers for the hospital and the pharmacists argued that it was the oncologist who was to blame and that the pharmacists and the university were not negligent. While it was recognized that the oncologist was (admittedly) negligent, an overriding theme of the litigation was that this was a systems failure—that if adequate systems controls had been in place and enforced, the accident would not have happened.

This was an unnecessary error. After protracted mediation and settlement negotiations, an additional $1,600,000 was added to the settlement package—thus providing a $2.1 million settlement, which would almost cover all of the future medical expenses and economic losses. A few years after the settlement, the pharmacy manager of the Oncology Clinic was arrested for theft of narcotics; he admitted abusing meperidine for several years, including the period in which the safeguards for protecting against this type of error were ignored. One can only speculate whether his abuse of narcotics clouded his judgment. One also can wonder what the outcome would have been had the plaintiff discovered the narcotic abuse during the pendency of the lawsuit.

24.5.2 Allergy

Allergies are also commonly implicated in drug-injury cases. Drug allergies are the body's overreaction to a foreign substance, be it dust, pollen, or a medication. Histamine is released in response to what the body perceives as a threat, and the results can be deadly. Of course, the immune system is designed to protect the body from dangerous invaders, which are usually viruses and bacteria but can also be medications, upon occasion.[29]

Unfortunately, there is no way to predict with 100% accuracy who will develop an allergic reaction to a medication. Allergies may develop at any time, even when an agent has been taken in the past. Indeed, multiple exposures actually raise the odds of developing an allergy to a particular substance. Additionally, some allergies do not develop for days or weeks after ingestion of or injection with a medication, which can make the reaction difficult to trace to the substance. Because of these reasons, causation is almost impossible to prove.

Although some other adverse drug reactions (ADRs) are dependent upon the amount of the drug administered, this is not the case with a drug allergy. Even a tiny amount of the medication can trigger a life-threatening anaphylactic episode.

Some types of drugs induce allergic reactions more readily than others and result in a spectrum of symptoms that may affect a range of tissues and organs. Medications with larger drug molecules seem to be more likely to cause reactions than those with smaller drug molecules.

Some examples of medications comprising larger drug molecules include:

- Insulin
- Antiserum-containing antibodies
- Recombinant proteins produced by genetic engineering

Many other allergens have molecules too small to set off alarm bells for the immune system. For examples, antibiotic drugs are unable to induce an immune response unless combined with a carrier protein in the blood or body cell. Drug allergies often are linked to the breakdown products, or metabolites, of the primary drug instead of the drug itself. In some cases, the same drug (e.g., penicillin) is capable of inducing a multitude of allergic reactions.

The most common drug sensitivity is to aspirin (ASA). Nearly 1 million Americans, primarily adults, are sensitive to ASA. However, many medications, including ASA and other nonsteroidal anti-inflammatory drugs (NSAIDs) such as ibuprofen (e.g., Advil, Motrin, and others), can lead to an asthma attack in children.

It is estimated that up to 10% of all people develop allergies to penicillin or other antibiotics at some point in their lives. Individuals taking several medications or frequent courses of antibiotics are reported to be more at risk for developing drug allergies. A comprehensive review of drug allergy is provided elsewhere in this book in the Adverse Drug Reactions Allergy Focus chapter.

Advances such as EMR and reconciling medication use can be helpful in supplying information about the patient's allergies and pathophysiological status but will not provide the physician with knowledge about the medications he/she is prescribing. Updates on adverse effects of medications, precautions, and contraindications are best obtained from the product labeling or authoritative compendia like the *Drug Information* text of the American Hospital Formulary Service (AHFS).

24.6 WHICH DRUGS ARE MOST OFTEN INVOLVED IN MEDICATION ERRORS?

"High Risk" drugs are those that have a low "therapeutic index" or are intrinsically toxic. The therapeutic index is defined as the ratio of the toxic dose to the therapeutic dose. Such low therapeutic index drugs provide little margin for overdose. Drugs that are intrinsically toxic include narcotics, anticoagulants, digitalis, and chemotherapy. Table 24.4 provides a list of common "High Risk" drugs, based on their pharmacologic properties. One such "High Risk" drug class is the opiate drug class—morphine and its congeners.

TABLE 24.4
Identifying High-Risk Drugs.

Characteristic	Prototypes
Low therapeutic index	Digoxin, anti-coagulants
Inherent undesirable effect(s)	Steroids, chemo
Class of drugs which shares toxicity	NSAIDs, ACEIs
Narcotics—PCA	Morphine, all
Newly approved drugs	Temafloxacin
"Off-label" uses of Drugs	Fen-Phen
Pharmacokinetic drug interactions	SSRI

24.6.1 Case Report

An acute morphine toxicity was alleged as the cause of death of the patient in the following case. A 49-year-old patient was being treated for chronic back pain. He had been given morphine by a nurse practitioner. He called the nurse practitioner to let her know that the medication was not working; she allegedly told him that a mistake had been made in that she had given him the wrong dosage, having switched it for another patient's dose. She claimed that his dosage should have been stronger. She increased the dosage and told him to take it another 24 hours. Two days later, he was acting strangely, jerking around, seeing purple, and was incoherent. The patient was immediately transported to the Northeast Texas Healthcare System Emergency Room where he was pronounced dead. The autopsy report stated the cause for death was "acute morphine intoxication." The plaintiffs claimed that the nurse overdosed the decedent on morphine. The plaintiffs alleged that the amount of morphine prescribed by the nurse practitioner was 22 times greater than the clinically accepted dosage for postoperative pain. The defendant argued that the nurse prescribed morphine authorized by a physician, and it was to be taken every few hours as needed. The defendants denied that the decedent took the medication as prescribed. They also denied that the increased amount of morphine was a lethal dose. This action settled for $595,000. (Bonnie Tartaro, Anthony Tartaro Jr. Christine Tartaro, Individually and as Heirs of the Estate of Anthony F. Tartaro SR. v. USA acting through the Department of Veterans Affairs, Texas District Court, Case No. 200-cv-00032.[30])

Another classification of "High Risk" drugs has been compiled by the TJC from its Sentinel Event reporting system. Even though the original list was compiled in 1999, the same drugs have continued to be problematic for the past 15 years, with a few new drugs added to the list. This fact certainly demonstrates the failure of educators, regulators, and legislators to effectively rectify the problems associated with transferring information about drugs to the prescriber. Many of the same drugs in the 1999 report are discussed in a 2015 publication on the topic.[31]

Another high-risk class includes Coumadin (warfarin) and heparin, both anticoagulants. The following is a case report related to heparin.

24.6.2 Case Report 2

A 53-year-old man entered the hospital for a femoral bypass surgery. Before his surgical procedure, there was an inadequate preoperative cardiac workup performed. Twenty hours after the uneventful surgery, the patient's hemoglobin and hematocrit were low, indicative for possible bleeding. After the surgery, the doctor ordered 7,500 units of heparin to be administered over a 24-hour period or 2,500 units every 8 hours continuously. One hour after the order was written, the nursing staff misread the instructions. Instead of administering 2,500 units of heparin, they administered 25,000 units of heparin. This caused the patient to continuously bleed, causing his urine output to decline to zero and his heart rate to increase to over 130. Consultation with a nephrologist and cardiologist was ordered to see if they could determine the cause of the continuing abdominal pain and the renal failure. At no time did the doctor believe that his orders were not followed with respect to heparin administration. Finally, about eight hours after the first heparin infusion, the patient was taken back to surgery for an exploratory laparotomy. However, a nurse again prepared him with an additional (negligently misinterpreted) 25,000 units of heparin. Profound and serious bleeding was apparent, but the physician team had no idea what was causing the bleeding. The patient died from a coronary thrombus. The plaintiff claimed that the cause of death was the failure to adequately perform a preoperative cardiac workup as well as the negligent administration of toxic levels of heparin. The defendant hospital admitted liability regarding the actions of the nurse but denied that the actions of the nurse had anything to do with the patient's death. The matter settled for $2.5 million after the jury was selected. (*Marie Lenoure, Special Administrator for the Estate of Victor LePore v. Oak Pak Hospital*, Cook County (IL) Circuit Court, Case No. 98 L 7257.[32])

24.6.3 Case Report—Anticoagulant—Coumadin (Warfarin)

A complex and confusing order for Coumadin (warfarin) was a factor in a patient's stroke. The patient was hospitalized for heart-valve replacement. Her attending physician prescribed three milligrams daily of Coumadin. Because the drug was not available in one milligram tablets, the physician prescribed a "net-three" dosage, alternating two milligrams one day with four milligrams the next. After discharge, the patient was transferred to a rehabilitation center with a regimen of medications that included the three-mg dosage of Coumadin. When the physician wrote the transfer order, he prescribed the net-three dosage on a five-day schedule showing two mg one day. He intended for the patient to take Coumadin indefinitely, but the medical director stopped giving the Coumadin after five days. When the patient was sent home two-and-one half weeks later, her daughter noticed that Coumadin was not on her medication list and called the doctor, who directed that she begin taking the drug immediately.

She did, but she suffered a severe stroke the next morning. After the stroke, she needed assistance to walk, was rendered incontinent, did not recognize her grandchildren, and underwent a personality change that made her combative at times. She died of unrelated causes two years later. The jury awarded a verdict of $850,000 (*Estate of Doris Hall v. Mildred Sabo*, Ocean County (NJ) Superior Court[33]).

Antineoplastics always will occupy the High Risk Sentinel list, not due to the inherent toxicity associated with these cancer chemotherapy drugs, for it is extremely rare for litigation to arise following routine chemotherapy despite frequent devastating toxicity associated with chemotherapy. Litigation, however, arises when mistakes are made, with the wrong dose, frequency, or route of administration, often with devastating results, and this leads to litigation.

24.6.4 Case Report—Antineoplastic Drug

A patient with esophageal cancer was receiving his second round of chemotherapy via a portable infusion pump, which was supposed to deliver the medication over five days at a small continuous rate. Tragically, the nurse programmed the pump to deliver the five-day dose in a five-hour period. After the overdose, the clinic assured the patient that he would be "okay," even though it was probable that he would not survive once his immune system was severely compromised. The patient died suddenly when his immune system crashed nine days later, without having a chance to say goodbye or get his affairs in order. The jury awarded $3,022,000. (*Richard Whiteaker and Francis Whiteaker, Jr. Individually and as Co-Administrators of the Estate of Francis Perry Whiteaker et al. v. C central Texa*s Oncology Associates. PA d/b/a Southwest Regional Cancer Center et al., Travis County (TX) District Court, Case No. 98–11826.[34]) A comprehensive review of antineoplastic therapy is presented in a separate chapter elsewhere in this book.

24.6.5 Case Report—Phenergan (Promethazine) Extravasation Injury

A 63-year-old patient, Ms. Levine, sued Wyeth Pharmaceuticals over whether the maker of the drug, Phenergan for Injection (Wyeth), should have included in the label an explicit warning against the route of administration, which was an IV (intravenous) push into her arm. IV push is a more aggressive method of drug delivery that quickly sends the anti-nausea medication into the blood stream, but it also potentially causes gangrene when it misses the artery. The plaintiff, a Vermont musician, went to an emergency room with a migraine headache. She received Demerol (meperidine) for the headache and injectable Phenergan (promethazine) for the nausea. It was given once intramuscularly and the second time in an IV push. The gangrene that resulted caused her to lose her right arm below the elbow.

The drug label, approved by the Food and Drug Administration (FDA), had warned that "inadvertent intra-arterial injection" can result in "gangrene requiring amputation." But the label did not rule out administration of the drug by IV push. Levine says no one discussed the risks of an IV push method of administration with her. She had been told that an IV administration would deliver "more potent and expeditious anti-nausea relief," according to Wyeth's brief. Injectable Phenergan has since been "discontinued" by Wyeth; however, it remains available from generic manufacturers as promethazine for injection.

24.6.6 Case Report—Do Generic-Drug Manufacturers Have the Same Responsibilities as Manufacturers to Warn?

An appeals court in California declined to review a decision extending liability in a products liability suit to a manufacturer that played no role in making the product that caused the plaintiff's injury. The one-sentence order declining review was a setback for the Washington Legal Foundation (WLF), which filed a brief urging that review be granted.[35]

In its brief filed in Conte v. Wyeth, Inc., the Washington Legal Foundation (WLF) argued that a pharmaceutical manufacturer of Reglan (metoclopramide), a pro-motility drug, should not be held liable for injuries sustained by the user of a drug that was produced by a different manufacturer. In this case, the defendant initially developed the formula for the drug in question, but the drug taken by the plaintiff was manufactured by a generic drug company, not the defendant. WLF contended that the defendant is not liable under the "failure to warn" theory, as the manufacturer owes no duty to provide warnings to those that do not use their products. The California Court of Appeal ruled last fall, however, that the plaintiff can prevail if she can show that her doctor relied on warnings given previously by the defendant in connection with its sale of a brand-name version of the drug. There are several new appellate court opinions on this issue, most recently with generic Reglan and other generic drugs.

24.7 PREVALENCE OF MEDICATION ERRORS

A systematic review and meta-analysis were performed to estimate the accurate prevalence of medical errors. In an evaluation of 40 studies, the most reported type of error was medication errors (62% of studies, range of prevalence, 10–80%). The most frequently identified settings with medication errors included university or teaching hospitals (75% of studies) and internal/intensive care wards (25% of studies). Overall, the estimated prevalence of medical errors was 50%. Results indicate a wide variation in the prevalence of medical errors, type, and clinical setting.[36]

A descriptive direct-observational study of drug administration errors in a hospital setting evaluated error rates per observation, nurse, patient, and the association between error rates and potential risk factors. An assessment of 237 patients and 28 nurses revealed 2,090 drug administration observations. Overall, a total of 5,531 errors were observed with an average number of 2.67 errors. At least 85% of the drug administration observations had ≥ 1 errors, with an overall error rate of 37.68% (per hundred error opportunities). Higher error rates were detected in injections, more notably in the intravenous route (39.58%). The most frequently reported errors were wrong documentation (90.96%) and wrong technique (78.90%) errors. The leading contributors to medication errors were higher numbers of shifts taken by nurses per month, weekends, elderly patients, night shifts, and illiteracy.[37]

Pediatric populations are at a higher risk for medication errors due to weight-based dosing, limitations in FDA-approved drugs, and human calculation errors. To provide more information on error frequency, type, and severity, one prospective observational study reviewed the number and type of medication prescribing errors in critically ill children in a pediatric intensive care unit (PICU). A total of 1,129 medication orders were analyzed; these showed 151 prescribing errors, giving an overall error rate of 14%. The medication groups with the highest prescribing errors were antihypertensives (50%), antimycotics (50%), drugs for nasal preparation (50%), anti-asthmatic drugs (25%), antibiotics (15%) and analgesics (14%). A total of 104 errors (70%) were classified as errors which required interventions and/or resulted in patient harm before interventions occur.[38]

Another study assessed the frequency and type of resident-prescribing errors in a pediatric clinic and further compared error rates of residents among different subspecialty training programs. The analysis reviewed 2,941 prescriptions collected over a period of five months. An overall resident-prescribing error rate was 5.88% with variations among subspecialties: Pediatric resident (4%), family medicine (11%), internal medicine (8%), and medicine/pediatrics (7%). The most frequent medication error type was overdose, followed by unclear quantity. Among the medication classes, topical agents and antimicrobials were among the top medications prescribed. Overall, numerous types of medication errors can occur in a pediatric clinic, and prescribing errors happen across all medical trainees.[39]

In an attempt to understand the error prevention impact of a double check system by two nurses for high-alert medications, one study evaluated pairs of nurses on simulated patient care. Nurses were randomized into single- and double-check groups. Various medication errors were intentionally introduced into the simulation, and errors were recorded. In the single-check group, 9% of nurses detected weight-based dosage errors compared to 33% of nurses in the double-check group; 54% percent of nurses in the single-check group detected the wrong vial error compared with 100% of nurses in the double-check group. This study demonstrates the utility of a double-check system which increases certain error detection rates for some medication errors. Of note, both techniques missed many errors highlighting the continuing issues in error generation.[40]

Altogether, these studies demonstrate that medication errors represent a major problem in various hospital settings, across all patient populations, and among all practitioners. Identifying contributors of prescribing errors aids in the design of actionable strategies to better navigate medication errors.

24.8 VACCINE ERRORS

The Institute for Safe Medication Practices (ISMP)[41] and the California Department of Public Health developed a national vaccine-error reporting system. Data collected by the ISMP National Vaccine Errors Reporting Program (VERP) is sent to the FDA and Centers for Disease Control and Prevention's (CDC) Vaccine Adverse Event Reporting System (VAERS) to evaluate the side effects reported from vaccines. Approximately, 1,000 reports submitted to VERP were analyzed to determine vaccines involved in errors and the common factors that are linked to vaccine errors.

In ISMP's recent report, multiple recommendations are offered to help lower the risk of the top vaccine-related medication errors.[42]

1. Age-specific formulation errors
2. Confusion between siblings, leading to wrong patient errors
3. Missed opportunities to vaccinate
4. Errors in route of administration
5. Combination vaccines and diluent errors
6. Errors due to vaccine nomenclature
7. Errors due to labeling and packaging
8. Vaccine storage problems—CDC toolkit for vaccine storage and handling
9. Expired vaccines
10. Patient should be involved in the vaccination verification process

24.9 PHARMACOGENOMICS: HOW HAS MODERN RESEARCH IMPROVED THERAPEUTICS AND REDUCED DRUG-RELATED MORBIDITY

Contemporary research into the metabolism of drugs by the Cytochrome P-450 (CYP) enzymes of the liver has given rise to a more complete understanding of the genetic differences among individuals and the related variability in the capacity of patients to metabolize drugs to various degrees. In past decades, pharmacologists talked about "slow" and "fast" acetylators of hydralazine and procainamide and the bimodal distribution of drug-induced lupus-like symptoms associated with each genetic phenotype. It was determined that slow acetylators of hydralazine and procainamide were more likely to develop the lupus-like syndrome than fast acetylators.[43] thus indicating that the parent compounds, and not the acetylated metabolites, were responsible for producing the syndrome.

Today, instead of discussing the CYP microsomal-enzyme system as a whole, researchers in pharmacogenetics have studied how the interindividual variations in the DNA sequence of a gene responsible for producing a protein that is involved in the absorption, transport, or metabolism of a drug affect drug action (pharmacodynamics).[44]. More than 27 families of CYP enzymes have been identified, but only three families (CYP1, CYP2, and CYP3) are believed to be involved with the vast majority of human drug metabolism [45]. These CYP families share more than 40% of the amino acids in their primary sequence and can be further subdivided into subfamilies that share more than 55% of their amino acid sequence.[46] Often, two or more enzymes catalyze the metabolism of a drug, but clearly the most influential families are the CYP3A, of which the CYP3A4 is involved in the metabolism of over 50% of all drugs and the CYP2D6 is involved in the metabolism of approximately 25% of drugs.[47] However, variations in the expression of the CYP2C9 subfamily are responsible for the great variability in the anticoagulant effect of warfarin. Also, the CYP2E1 enzyme that contributes to the metabolism of ethanol in frequent drinkers can be induced by ethanol, phenobarbital, and phenytoin. This, in turn, can increase the formation of n-acetyl-p-benzoquinone (NAPQI), the hepatotoxic metabolite of acetaminophen, and increase the likelihood of liver failure from moderate doses of acetaminophen,[48,49] Nutritional factors involving the ingestion of the sulfur-containing amino acid cysteine, which contributes to endogenous glutathione production, are also significant factors, especially in children since they rely more on sulfation than conjugation with glucuronic acid. Children under 12 years of age should never receive adult-strength acetaminophen products.

With the application of the Human Genome Project to clinical practice, the science of pharmacogenomics has the potential to determine how alterations in gene expression influence both drug discovery and pharmacogenetic polymorphisms[50]. Some researchers predict that bedside testing for a patient's capacity to metabolize a drug will become a standard part of clinical practice within the next two decades.[51] Elucidation of a patient's particular genomic composition can greatly decrease drug-induced disease and provide critical information on not only interindividual pharmacogenetic polymorphism, but also interracial differences in drug-metabolizing capacities.

Another application of pharmacogenetics and pharmacogenomics will be their effect on public policy issues regarding the removal of drugs from the marketplace due to drug–drug interactions. Within the past two decades, several drugs have been removed from the marketplace because of intolerable side effects which were caused by drug–drug interactions. Two of the agents best known to millions of Americans were Seldane® (terfenadine) and Hismanal® (astemizole)—the first two nonsedating antihistamines. These agents were removed from the market, despite the fact that the Food and Drug Administration (FDA) required the manufacturers to include "Black Box" warnings in their product labeling, warning about potential cardiotoxic effects such as prolongation of the QT interval due to the inhibition of the CYP3A4 pathway by "conazole" antifungals and macrolide antibiotics.[52] A similar set of circumstances led to the same effect on the QT interval with the gastrointestinal motility-enhancing agent cisapride (Propulsid®). According to one study, the manufacturer withdrew this drug from the market in March 2000 because the inclusion of a "Black Box" warning and the issuance of a "Dear Doctor" letter to 800,000 healthcare professionals failed to modify physician-prescribing practices sufficiently to reduce the contraindicated use of cisapride and further cardiotoxic events. The authors also commented on the need to find more effective ways to provide prescribers with critical new safety information on the proper use of drugs.[53]

According to the FDA:[54]

> The inability of the FDA to effectively warn health care providers and patients about drug interactions and our inability to translate existing knowledge into changes in prescribing have resulted in huge economic consequences for the pharmaceutical industry and the loss from the marketplace of effective drugs, including terfenadine, mibefradil, astemizole, and cisapride.

In the last 20 years or so, awareness has been raised about the medication error problems stated in this chapter. As a result, creative solutions have begun to emerge, and they seem, so far, to be highly effective. Many solutions involve changing the shape or color of tablets and capsules or bar-coding hospital medications, patients, and nurses, and more. Additionally, checks and balances in pharmacy practice have cut errors significantly. Focus on the problem is slowly sinking in, and the results are positive. A monitoring calendar often facilitates this task in practice. Dates for follow-up laboratory studies are entered on a patient's monitoring calendar. If the results are not received by the due date, a staff member or the practitioner contacts the patient to ask if the test was performed and arranges for testing. Any follow-up monitoring is also entered on the calendar.

24.10 SYSTEMS FOR MEDICAL ERROR PREVENTION

Dr. Leape, acclaimed for showing leadership in medical error prevention, described the following five basic principles of systems redesign in medicine:

- Reduce reliance on memory
- Improve information access
- Strive for an error-proof system
- Standardize processes of care
- Emphasize error avoidance when training medical personnel

24.10.1 Electronic Prescribing (E-Prescribing)

Simple electronic prescription programs can eliminate errors caused by handwriting and transcription errors, assist with dosing, and provide quick access to drug information. More sophisticated programs can be integrated with laboratory test results or complete electronic medical records, and these programs have the potential to prevent drug–drug interactions, drug-disease interactions, and allergic reactions to medications and to assist with patient-specific dosing. The impact of e-prescribing in outpatients has not yet been specifically studied, but studies from the inpatient arena show impressive results. Bates and his colleagues found an 88% reduction in serious medication errors and an 81% reduction in all medication errors (excluding missed doses) at Brigham and Women's Hospital in Boston, Massachusetts, after the introduction of a sophisticated computerized order-entry system. Bar-coding and robotic pharmacy systems are being tested in hospitals and may have a role in ambulatory settings in the future. If an electronic entry and barcode verification before administration system, along with good old-fashioned reading of the drug label, had been used with the *Postscript* report (given at the end of this chapter) of a death following the erroneous administration of vecuronium for Versed, with administration verification with barcode technology, the error (and death) most likely would have been avoided.

The main challenge with electronic prescribing and computerized order-entry systems are their cost and the significant changes in practitioner workflow. In addition, their impact on errors and cost-of-care has yet to be fully elucidated in the ambulatory arena. Nonetheless, cost-effectiveness analyses suggest that electronic prescribing can be a good investment for some practices, particularly large ones.

24.10.2 When Electronic Prescribing Is Unavailable

Several simple steps can reduce the medication errors associated with handwritten prescriptions. Verbal orders are especially susceptible to error and should be avoided except in emergencies. An electronic prescription or a handwritten one that is sent by fax is nearly always preferable. If verbal orders must be given, spell the name of the drug, say each numeral of the dosage amounts (e.g. "five zero milligrams" not "fifty milligrams"), and always have the pharmacist read the entire prescription back to you for verification. Some guidelines:

Avoiding polypharmacy:

- Minimizing the number of medications a patient (particularly an elderly one) takes is another means of avoiding medication errors. The more prescriptions a patient has, the greater the risk of an Adverse Drug Event (ADE). For example, medications may be prescribed to treat a symptom that is an unrecognized side effect of another medication, a chain of events termed the *prescribing cascade*. With careful attention to changes in the patient's medical status, many drugs can safely be removed from the regimens of elderly patients without adverse events.
- Maintaining a complete and accurate patient medication list is critical to safe prescribing. As primary care practitioners, our pen is our scalpel. It is crucial to review patients' medications, including OTC medications and supplements, at every visit. Patients should carry a complete and up-to-date list of their medications, and if, for some reason, they are unable to do that, before each visit they should put all their medications including OTCs and herbals in a bag and bring them to the visit. Routine drug reviews help the practitioner remove duplicate drugs, reduce polypharmacy, and avoid drug–drug interactions.
- Paying particular attention to medication lists when patients are discharged from the hospital—research shows that this is the time when many errors occur. Patients are often confused by their medication changes and may duplicate medications by taking their "new" ones along with the identical ones that they already have at home. Give patients a complete medication list at the time of discharge and make sure that they understand any changes from their previous outpatient medication regimen.

24.10.3 Effective Drug Monitoring Systems

- Some form of monitoring is usually required for patients taking anticoagulants, ACE inhibitors, digoxin, insulin, oral hypoglycemics, lithium, thiazolidinediones, and anticonvulsant medications, among others. A monitoring calendar often facilitates this task in practice. Dates for follow-up laboratory studies are entered on a patient's monitoring calendar. If the results are not received by the due date, a staff member or the practitioner contacts the patient to ask if the test was performed and arranges for testing. Any follow-up monitoring is also entered on the calendar.
- It is possible to keep track of a large number of patients in this manner, but to ensure that a process is used properly, it must be standardized for your practice, and the tracking system must also be kept up-to-date. Patients taking anticoagulants should be referred to anticoagulation clinics if they are available, because these facilities have developed solid systems for following patients, and their programs have proven efficacy in improving therapeutic anticoagulation. Practitioners prescribing new medications for patients taking warfarin should always check for drug–drug interactions—relying on memory alone often leads to disasters.

24.10.4 The Importance of Continuing Education

New drugs are released every year. And every year, older drugs are found to have interactions and adverse effects in "the field" that studies were unable to identify. It is up to the physician and pharmacist to stay abreast of the latest findings. Considering the possible liability/malpractice ramifications of being out of touch, it behooves physicians and pharmacists to stay current.

24.10.5 Reporting All Adverse Drug Events

The Adverse Event Reporting System (AERS) is a computerized information database designed to support the FDA's post-marketing safety surveillance program for all approved drug and therapeutic biologic products. The FDA uses AERS to monitor for new adverse events and medication errors that might occur with these marketed products.

Reporting of adverse events from the point of care is voluntary in the United States. FDA receives some adverse event and medication error reports directly from healthcare professionals (such as physicians, pharmacists, nurses, and others) and consumers (such as patients, family members, lawyers, and others). Healthcare professionals and consumers may also report these events to the products' manufacturers. If a manufacturer receives an adverse-event report, it is required to send the report to FDA, as specified by regulations. The MedWatch site provides information about mandatory reporting.

AERS is a useful tool for FDA, which uses it for activities such as looking for new safety concerns that might be related to a marketed product, evaluating a manufacturer's compliance to reporting regulations, and responding to outside requests for information. The reports in AERS are evaluated by clinical reviewers in the Center for Drug Evaluation and Research (CDER) and the Center for Biologics Evaluation and Research (CBER) to monitor the safety of products after they are approved by FDA. Adverse Drug Event monitoring systems by FDA and RxISK are presented in separate chapters elsewhere in this book.[55]

24.11 SUMMARY AND CONCLUSIONS

The standard of care for acceptable medical practice is to exercise that degree of care which a reasonably prudent practitioner would exercise under the same or similar circumstances. Physicians, pharmacists, and nurses all must consult drug labeling and/or learned treatises which contain warnings, precautions, and contraindications to the use of medications they prescribe, dispense, or administer. The information is available, and the likelihood for morbidity and death is reasonably foreseeable. Failure to recognize the potential adverse effects and to take reasonable precautions to guard against preventable errors are deviations from the standard of care.

Moreover, it is time to recognize that healthcare is a team activity. Practicing medicine, nursing, and pharmacy is too complicated for healthcare professionals to be able to carry all required information in their heads. Electronic and computerized systems can help, but first, all healthcare professionals must acknowledge that a problem exists. Today's philosophy is to improve faulty systems through root cause analysis and redesign. Computerized physician order entry, bar coding drugs and patient identification bands, and hiring clinical pharmacists to make rounds with physicians can decrease costly errors. Every preventable medication error costs almost $5,000 in extended or rehospitalization expenses. The data are clear that preventing medication errors will pay for itself. One pharmacist in one unit recommended changes in medication orders to physicians and saved a hospital a projected $270,000 that year. Moreover, fewer errors will be committed, quality of care rises, patients will be safer and better served, and less litigation will ensue. There is no question that the price of quality improvement is less than the costs of medication errors.

PostScript: At the time the book manuscript was being finalized for submission to the publisher, ISMP broadcasted a webinar: *Tragedy in Tennessee.* The text as follows, from a PPT slide, describes the events and consequences on the patient, on the healthcare worker, and on the institution:

> Two days after Christmas in 2017, Charlene Murphey, a patient at Vanderbilt University Medical Center, died after receiving an IV medication in error. The medication was administered by RaDonda Vaught, an experienced registered nurse who had retrieved the wrong drug (vecuronium—a paralytic agent instead of Versed/midazolam—an anxiolytic) instead and subsequently failed to detect and correct her mistake. Standard safety norms and technologies used to prevent and detect the original error before it could reach the patient were absent or incompletely deployed. The nurse, attempting to accomplish multiple tasks simultaneously, did not perform standard visual checks that could have surfaced the error. In this tragic constellation of individual and system failures, patient Charlene Murphey lost her life. Her family lost a beloved mother and grandmother, and Ms. Murphey's community lost a treasured friend and engaged citizen. Eight days later, Vanderbilt University Medical Center fired RaDonda Vaught, citing her failure to adhere to the Five Rights of Medication Administration. In July 2021, the Tennessee State Board of Nursing revoked RaDonda Vaught's nursing license and on March 25, 2022, she was convicted on two criminal counts: criminally negligent homicide and gross neglect of an impaired adult. She was sentenced to probation on May 13, 2022, in Davidson County, TN State Court. She could have been sentenced for up to 12 years in prison.

NOTES

1 Institute of Medicine. To Err Is Human: Building a Safer Health System. Washington, DC: National Academy Press; 1999.

2 Institute of Medicine. To Err Is Human: Building a Safer Health System. Washington, DC: National Academy Press; 2006.

3 Starfield B. Is US Health Really the Best in the World? JAMA, July 26, 2000;284(4):483–485.

4 Carver N, Gupta V, Hipskind JE. Medical Error. [Updated July 9, 2021]. In: StatPearls [Internet]. Treasure Island (FL): StatPearls Publishing; 2021 January. https://www.ncbi.nlm.nih.gov/books/NBK430763/.

5 Institute of Medicine. To Err Is Human: Building a Safer Health System. Washington, DC: National Academy Press; 2006.
6 About Medication Errors. https://www.nccmerp.org/about-medication-errors/. Accessed December 21, 2021.
7 ISMP Error-Prone Abbreviations List. https://www.ismp.org/recommendations/error-prone-abbreviations-list/. Accessed December 21, 2021.
8 National Patient Safety Goals. http://www.jointcommission.org/standards_information/npsgs.aspx/. Accessed December 21, 2021.
9 Rodziewicz TL, Houseman B, Hipskind JE. Medical Error Reduction and Prevention. August 6, 2021. In: StatPearls [Internet]. Treasure Island (FL): StatPearls Publishing; 2021 January. PMID: 29763131.
10 Charney W, Ed. Epidemic of Medical Errors and Hospital-Acquired Infections: Systemic and Social Causes. Boca Raton, FL: CRC Press; 2012.
11 Carver N, Gupta V, Hipskind JE. Medical Error. [Updated July 9, 2021]. In: StatPearls [Internet]. Treasure Island (FL): StatPearls Publishing; 2021 January. https://www.ncbi.nlm.nih.gov/books/NBK430763/.
12 World Freedom Alliance, Medical Error. https://worldfreedomalliance.org/au/news/medical-error/. Accessed August 28, 2024.
13 World Freedom Alliance, Medical Error. https://worldfreedomalliance.org/au/news/medical-error/. Accessed August 28, 2024.
14 Anderson JG, Abrahamson K. Your Health Care May Kill You: Medical Errors. Stud Health Technol Inform. 2017;234:13–17.
15 Bates DW, Cullen DJ, Laird N, Petersen LA, Small SD, Servi D, Laffel G, Sweitzer BJ, Shea BF, Hallisey R, Vander Vliet M. Incidence of Adverse Drug Events and Potential Adverse Drug Events: Implications for Prevention. ADE Prevention Study Group. JAMA. July 5, 1995;274(1):29–34.
16 Bates DW, Cullen DJ, Laird N, Petersen LA, Small SD, Servi D, Laffel G, Sweitzer BJ, Shea BF, Hallisey R, Vander Vliet M. Incidence of Adverse Drug Events and Potential Adverse Drug Events: Implications for Prevention. JAMA. 1995;274(1):29–34.
17 Leape LL, Bates DW, Cullen DJ, Cooper J, Demonaco HJ, Gallivan T, Hallisey R, Ives J, Laird N, Laffel G, Nemeskal R. Systems Analysis of Adverse Drug Events. ADE Prevention Study Group. JAMA. 1995 Jul 5;274(1):35–43.
18 Benjamin DM. Reducing Medication Errors and Increasing Patient Safety Through Better Communication. Focus on Patient Safety. 2001;4:6–8.
19 U.S. Adoption of Electronic Health Records Nears 100 Percent. https://www.eweek.com/it-management/u.s.-adoption-of-electronic-health-records-nears-100-percent/. Accessed December 21, 2021.
20 NCHS, National Electronic Health Records Survey, 2017; Myrick KL, Ogburn DF, Ward BW. Table. Percentage of Office-Based Physicians Using Any Electronic Health Record (EHR)/Electronic Medical Record (EMR) System and Physicians That Have a Certified EHR/EMR System, by U.S. State: National Electronic Health Records Survey, 2017. National Center for Health Statistics; January 2019.
21 Caffrey C, Cairns C, Rome V. Trends in Electronic Health Record Use Among Residential Care Communities: United States, 2012, 2014, and 2016. National Health Statistics Reports. Number 140; March 3, 2020.
22 Bates DW, Leape LL, Cullen DJ, Laird N, Petersen LA, Teich JM, Burdick E, Hickey M, Kleefield S, Shea B, Vander Vliet M. Effect of Computerized Physician Order Entry and a Team Intervention on Prevention of Serious Medication Errors. JAMA. 1998;280(15):1311–1316.
23 E-Prescribing. https://www.cms.gov/Medicare/E-Health/Eprescribing. Accessed December 21, 2021.
24 Alston & Bird Health Care Week in Review, April 24, 2020. *News & Insights|Alston & Bird*. https://www.alston.com/en/insights/publications/2020/04/ab-healthcare-week-in-review-april-24-2020.
25 Electronic Prescriptions for Controlled Substances. https://www.deadiversion.usdoj.gov/fed_regs/rules/2020/fr0421_3.htm. Accessed December 21, 2021.
26 Rate of Electronic Prescriptions in the United States From 2017 to 2020. https://www.statista.com/statistics/864380/share-of-us-e-prescriptions/. Accessed December 21, 2021.
27 HRC Risk Analysis, Vol. 4, ECRI, Plymouth Meeting, PA, September 2000, p. 4. https://www.ecri.org/components/HRC/Pages/default.aspx. Accessed February 13, 2015.
28 Leape LL, Bates DW, Cullen DJ, Cooper J, Demonaco HJ, Gallivan T, Hallisey R, Ives J, Laird N, Laffel G, Nemeskal R. Systems Analysis of Adverse Drug Events. ADE Prevention Study Group. JAMA. 1995 Jul 5;274(1):35–43.
29 Leape LL, Bates DW, Cullen DJ, Cooper J, Demonaco HJ, Gallivan T, Hallisey R, Ives J, Laird N, Laffel G, Nemeskal R. Systems Analysis of Adverse Drug Events. ADE Prevention Study Group. JAMA. 1995 Jul 5;274(1):35–43.
30 http://www.answers.com/topic/drug-allergies-sensitivities. Accessed February 13, 2015.
31 Anderson P, Townsend T. Preventing High-Alert Medication Errors in Hospital Patients. Am Nurs Today. 2015;10(5).
32 Laska L. Nurse Gives Overdose of Morphine to Postoperative Patient. Medical Malpractice, Verdicts, Settlements and Experts, June, 2001, p. 27.
33 Laska L. Failure to Perform Preoperative Cardiac Work Up and Administration of Excessive Heparin Blamed for Man's Death Following Femoral Bypass Surgery. Medical Malpractice Verdicts, "Settlements and Experts," July 2002, p. 19.

34 Laska L. Failure to Properly Interpret and Administer Referring Surgeon's Coumadin Prescription. Medical Malpractice Verdicts, Settlements and Experts, May 2002, p. 30.
35 https://www.wlf.org/2014/01/02/wlf-legal-pulse/sixth-circuit-affirms-preemption-defense-in-suit-against-branded-and-generic-drug-companies/. Accessed July 7, 2022.
36 Vaziri S, Fakouri F, Mirzaei M, Afsharian M, Azizi M, Arab-Zozani M. Prevalence of Medical Errors in Iran: A Systematic Review and Meta-Analysis. BMC Health Serv Res. 2019 Sep 2;19(1):622.
37 Al Tehewy M, Fahim H, Gad NI, El Gafary M, Rahman SA. Medication Administration Errors in a University Hospital. J Patient Saf. 2016 Mar;12(1):34–39.
38 Glanzmann C, Frey B, Meier CR, Vonbach P. Analysis of Medication Prescribing Errors in Critically Ill Children. Eur J Pediatr. 2015 Oct;174(10):1347–1355.
39 Honey BL, Bray WM, Gomez MR, Condren M. Frequency of Prescribing Errors by Medical Residents in Various Training Programs. J Patient Saf. 2015 Jun;11(2):100–104.
40 Douglass AM, Elder J, Watson R, Kallay T, Kirsh D, Robb W, Kaji AH, Coil C. A Randomized Controlled Trial on the Effec of a Double Check on the Detection of Mediation Erors. Ann Emerg Med. 2018 Jan;71(1):74–82.e1.
41 Report an Error. www.ismp.org/orderforms/reporterrortoismp.asp. Accessed December 21, 2021.
42 https://www.cdc.gov/vaccines/hcp/admin/storage/toolkit/index.html. Accessed December 21, 2021.
43 Laska L. Negligent Administration of Chemotherapy Overdose. Medical Malpractice Verdicts, Settlements, and Experts, January 2001, p. 51.
44 The Pharmacological Basis of Therapeutics, 12th Edition, Brunton, Chabner, Knollman, Eds. New York: McGraw Hill; 2011.
45 Lawrence J Lesko, Ronald A Salerno, Brian B Spear, Donald C Anderson, Timothy Anderson, Celia Brazell, Jerry Collins, Andrew Dorner, David Essayan, Baltazar Gomez-Mancilla, Joseph Hackett, Shiew-Mei Huang, Susan Ide, Joanne Killinger, John Leighton, Elizabeth Mansfield, Robert Meyer, Stephen G Ryan, Virginia Schmith, Peter Shaw, Frank Sistare, Mark Watson, Alexandra Worobec. Pharmacogenetics and Pharmacogenomics in Drug Delivery and Regulatory Decision Making: Report of the First FDA-PWG-PhRMA-DruSafe Workshop J. Clin Pharmacol. 2003;43:342–358.
46 Wrighton SA, Stevens JC. The Human Hepatic Cytochromes P450 Involved in Drug Metabolism. Crit Rev Toxicol. 1992;22:1–21.
47 The Pharmacological Basis of Therapeutics, 12th Edition, Brunton, Chabner, Knollman, Eds. New York: McGraw Hill; 2011.
48 Higashi MK, Veenstra DL, Kondo LM, Wittkowsky AK, Srinouanprachanh SL, Farin FM, Rettie AE. Association Between CYP2C9 Genetic Variants and Anticoagulation-Related Outcomes During Warfarin Therapy. JAMA. 2002;287:1690–1698.
49 Medical Toxicology: Diagnosis and Treatment of Human Poisoning, Ellenhorn, MJ and Barceloux, DG, Eds. New York: Elsevier; 1997.
50 The Pharmacological Basis of Therapeutics, 12th Edition, Brunton, Chabner, Knollman, Eds. New York: McGraw Hill; 2011.
51 Phillips KA, Veenstra DL, Oren E, Lee JK, Sadee W. Potential Role of Pharmacogenomics in Reducing Adverse Drug Reactions: A Systematic Review. JAMA. 2001;286:2270–2279.
52 Smalley W, Shatin D, Wysowski DK, Gurwitz J, Andrade SE, Goodman M, Chan KA, Platt R, Schech SD, Ray WA. Contraindicated Use of Cisapride: Impact of Food and Drug Administration Regulatory Action. JAMA. 2000;284:3036–3039.
53 Lasser KE, Allen PD, Woolhandler SJ, Himmelstein DU, Wolfe SM, Bor DH. Timing of New Black Box Warnings and Withdrawals for Prescription Medications. JAMA. 2002;287:2215–2220.
54 Drug Interactions and Labeling. https://www.fda.gov/drugs/development-resources/drug-interactions-labeling: Accessed December 21, 2021.
55 Adverse Event Reporting System (AERS). https://webarchive.library.unt.edu/eot2008/20080918004205/http://www.fda.gov/cder/aers/default.htm: Accessed August 28, 2024.

25 Anticoagulants
Therapeutics, Risks, and Toxicities

James T. O'Donnell, James J. O'Donnell III, and Stephanie E. Tedford

SYNOPSIS

25.1 INTRODUCTION

The purpose of this chapter is to provide the reader with the mechanisms of action, requisite clinical and laboratory monitoring, toxicities, and examples of errors and complications leading to litigation involving pharmacists and other healthcare providers. A secondary objective is to address the current knowledge on heparin-induced thrombocytopenia (HIT), a serious, life-threatening complication that is recognized but not well understood.

The below illustrates the serious consequences of administering too much or too little anticoagulant:

1. Pharmacist dispenses two mg warfarin instead of five mg; patient's routine INR (International Normalized Ratio) is nontherapeutic. Hospital notification system fails. Woman has stroke and is permanently disabled.
2. Pharmacist dispenses warfarin instead of Cogentin; technician testifies that pharmacist does

DOI: 10.1201/9781003615323-27

not check her prescriptions. Patient dies of intracerebral bleed (this case is described in full detail later in this chapter).

3. Nursery infants administered 50 times overdose of heparin for catheter flush (the Dennis Quaid case). Babies develop bleeding. California Boards of Nursing and Pharmacy investigate hospital practices. Floor stocking with 5,000 unit/mL vials instead of 10 unit/mL or 100 unit/mL discovered.
4. Texas hospital reports heparin overdoses in several infants. Heparin syringes compounded in hospital pharmacy contained excessive amounts of heparin. Some infants died of heparin overdose.
5. Doctor mistakenly writes 10 mg instead of 1 mg dose of warfarin. Pharmacist does not question the very high (almost never chronic) dose. Patient has an intracranial bleed and dies.
6. Patient transferred from one hospital to another with heparin infusion. The first hospital uses 25,000 units in 500 mL, and the receiving hospital infuses a more concentrated infusion at the first hospital's infusion rate, resulting in massive hematoma, allegedly leading to sciatic nerve injury.
7. A pregnant woman with a history of pulmonary emboli is noncompliant for enoxaparin treatment. Baby is born with low birth weight. Placenta 25 percent infarcted. OBGYN sued—defense of noncompliance by patient.

25.2 SUMMARY OF ANTICOAGULANT THERAPY

25.2.1 Definition

Anticoagulant drugs are substances that prevent coagulation. They inhibit blood-clotting processes and are used in the treatment of thrombotic disorders.[1]

25.2.2 Use

25.2.2.1 Treatment of Coronary Heart Disease

Morbidity and mortality associated with an arterial or venous thrombotic event are very high.[2,3] Anticoagulant drugs are used for the prevention and treatment of cardioembolic events in addition to venous thrombosis.[4] The use of anticoagulants has increased for the management of cardiovascular indications due to advances in our understanding of thromboembolism.

25.2.2.2 Warfarin and Dabigatran

Warfarin, the most commonly used oral anticoagulant, certainly does not fit the image of an ideal medicine. With a narrow therapeutic index, routine monitoring, and the risk of bleeding, warfarin therapy can be time consuming and risky for the healthcare professional as well as for the patient. Ideally, anticoagulant treatment would include once daily regimen with limited or no drug interactions, low risk of bleeding, no routine laboratory monitoring, and minimal side effects. A recent market addition of the oral anticoagulant dabigatran provides some benefits not achievable by warfarin (standard twice daily dose and without the need of INR tests and constant dosage adjustment). It is currently indicated for patients with atrial fibrillation not caused by a heart valve problem.[5]

Thrombin remains a target for many new oral pharmacotherapies that are under development for prevention and treatment of embolic events. Thrombin remains an ideal target as it works on the pathways for coagulation.

25.2.2.3 Treatment of Thrombogenesis

Arterial thrombosis, the most common cause of myocardial infarction, stroke, and peripheral arterial disease, is caused mainly by platelet aggregation and fibrin, which stabilize the thrombus. Initially, an atherosclerotic plaque ruptures, exposing tissue factor (TF) to the blood. Once the site is exposed, platelets attach to the sub-endothelium, where they are activated and aggregate. Platelet and fibrin deposition can form an occlusive thrombus that blocks blood flow to the coronary, carotid, or peripheral arteries. Venous thrombosis, which can lead to pulmonary embolism, occurs under low shear states and usually consists of fibrin and red blood cells. The origin of venous thrombi is typically the muscular veins of the calf as well as the valve cusp pockets of the deep calf veins. Vascular trauma (in addition to venous stasis) is commonly a source for coagulation in the veins. Exposure of TF activates the coagulation cascade following vessel wall injury. This leads to thrombin generation (Figure 25.1). Platelets adhere to the injured areas of the vessel walls by platelet glycoprotein (GP) Ib/IX on the platelet membrane binding with von Willebrand factor. Once activated, platelet aggregation occurs by several mechanisms. Storage granules on activated platelets release adenosine diphosphate (ADP), which stimulates adjacent platelets. Clotting factors gather on the surface of activated platelets, and further triggers thrombin formation leading to enhanced platelet activation and coagulation. In addition, platelets are also stimulated by the release of thromboxane A2 from activated platelets. Thrombin plays a key role in several stages of thrombus formation. Thrombin promotes platelet aggregation, cleavage of fibrinogen to fibrin to form the fibrin clot, and activation of factors that stabilize fibrin clots. Through feedback mechanisms, thrombin can also activate its own production, furthering the coagulation process. For these reasons, the inhibition of thrombin generation or activity is the focus of many investigational treatment strategies. To add more complexity to the pathway, thrombin also has a role in the anticoagulation as it serves as a cofactor for Protein C and S activation via thrombomodulin (TM) and endothelial protein (EPRC).

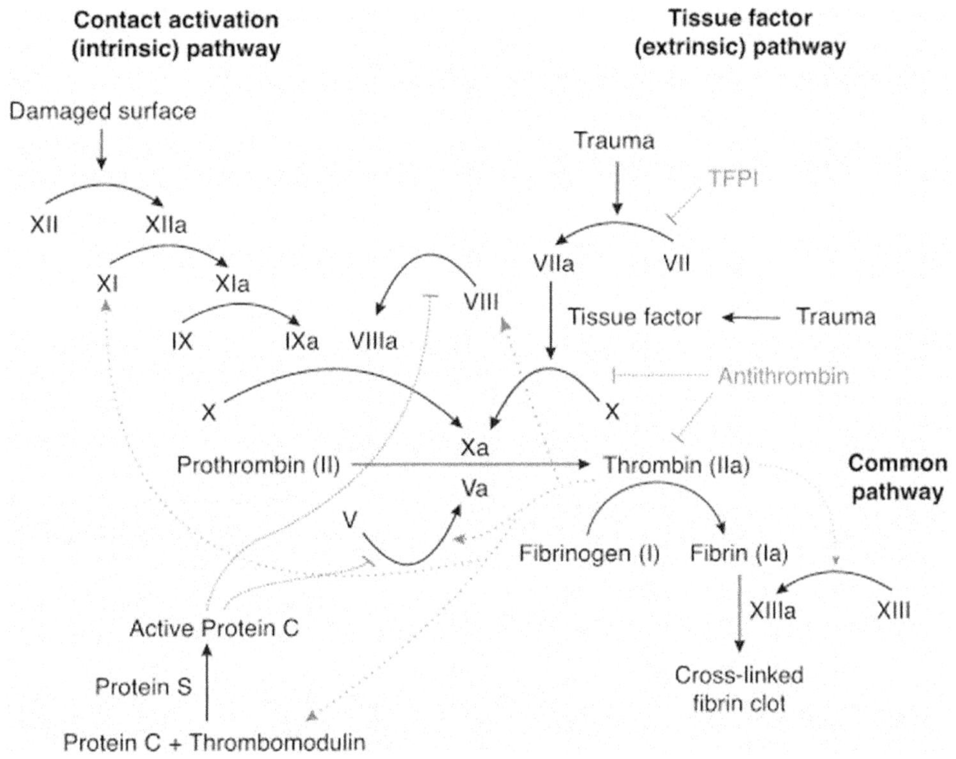

FIGURE 25.1 Coagulation Cascade of Secondary Hemostasis.

25.3 LIMITATIONS OF CURRENT THERAPY

All anticoagulants and fibrinolytic drugs have an increased bleeding risk as their principle toxicity, with intracranial hemorrhage (ICH) as the most severe example. Particularly serious episodes involve sites where irreversible damage may result from the compression of vital structures such as the pericardial, nerve sheath, or spinal cord, as well as massive internal blood loss that may not be diagnosed rapidly: Gastrointestinal, intraperitoneal, or retroperitoneal.

25.3.1 Heparin

Unfractionated heparin (UFH), while commonly used intravenously, is not orally bioavailable. UFH must be monitored closely due to the narrow therapeutic window and has a significant risk of bleeding. This risk can be decreased by scrupulous patient selection, careful control of dosage, and close monitoring. Heparin, an indirect thrombin inhibitor, increases endogenous antithrombin activity. Antithrombin normally inhibits factor Xa and thrombin. Heparin binding of antithrombin causes conformational changes in antithrombin, which expose its active site more, leading to a more rapid interaction with Factor Xa. Heparin's mechanism for enhancing thrombin inhibition is different. As (unfractionated) heparin binds both antithrombin and thrombin such that it places them in close proximity to each other, it acts as a catalytic template facilitating antithrombin–thrombin interaction.

Thrombin has three binding sites: An active site and two exosites. The first exosite is used for binding substrates such as fibrinogen in the correct orientation for cleavage to fibrin. Thrombin converts fibrinogen to fibrin, then remains bound to fibrin while continuing to activate platelets, enhancing thrombus formation. The second exosite (exosite 2) is used as the heparin-binding site. To inactivate thrombin, heparin must bind to antithrombin and exosite 2 on thrombin. If heparin binds to fibrin and exosite 2, thrombin is resistant to inactivation by the antithrombin/heparin complex, which enhances the thrombin/fibrin interaction and may lead to further thrombus formation. Once thrombin and fibrin are bound, heparin cannot inactivate thrombin.

Limitations of heparin use include heparin-induced thrombocytopenia (HIT). Studies show that HIT affects between 1 to 5 percent of patients receiving heparin, with up to 600,000 cases occurring yearly. It is important to recognize that HIT is generally underdiagnosed in patients with myeloproliferative syndromes because of high baseline platelet counts. Heparin can cause two types of HIT. Type 1, heparin-associated thrombocytopenia (HAT), occurs early (within 48 to 72 hours of administration), is a nonimmune cause of the disorder, and does not confer an increased risk of thrombosis. Platelet counts do not typically fall below 100,000 platelets per microliter (mcL) and return to normal limits within a few days, even with continued administration. Type 2, or HIT II, occurs within 5 to 10 days after initial heparin administration, with the platelet count usually falling to less than 100,000 platelets per mcL. Unlike HAT, HIT is associated with immune response and activation of platelets and has a high risk of thromboembolic events. Patients with HIT cannot receive heparin or low molecular weight heparin (LMWH). HIT patients need to be anticoagulated with agents such as direct thrombin inhibitors (DTI) to prevent thrombosis. DTIs should be continued until a sufficient number of platelets have been replenished.

25.3.2 Low Molecular Weight Heparin (LMWH)

Anticoagulant effects of LMWH are produced by the activation of antithrombin and consequent inactivation of factor Xa. Because LMWH is composed of smaller fragments than UFH, these fragments do not bind to thrombin. LMWH's binding to antithrombin only enhances binding to Factor Xa (through conformational changes); it does not affect thrombin binding to antithrombin. LMWH does not require routine monitoring like UFH and has a more predictable anticoagulant effect. Although LMWH can be used in the outpatient setting due to the lack of monitoring needed, its use is still restricted because of subcutaneous administration. Monitoring is, however, necessary for patients with extremes in weight (low/high or obesity) or renal failure. Pregnant patients requiring anticoagulation cannot use warfarin; LMWH is commonly used in this population instead of UFH. The incidence of HIT is lower with LMWH (less than 1 percent). However, the same problem exists with LMWH as with UFH; it cannot inactivate thrombin bound to fibrin.

25.3.3 Heparin-Induced Thrombocytopenia (HIT)

According to Priziola et al.,[6] anywhere from 15 to 58 percent of intensive care unit (ICU) patients are thought to experience thrombocytopenia, with an estimated 10 million persons per year having a drug-induced form of the disease.[3] Functionally, HIT occurs through bone marrow suppression, increased platelet destruction, or platelet sequestration, and should not be confused with pseudothrombocytopenia—an in-vitro clumping of platelets that does not carry the same clinical consequences.

Early descriptions of the clinical HIT syndrome delineated its emergence after 5 to 12 days of continuing heparin exposure, defining the disease in terms of a platelet count drop of around 50 percent.[7] This is the classic presentation, but in a patient exposed to heparin within the preceding three months, a preformed circulating antibody can lead to a rapid onset of HIT within hours or even minutes of reexposure. Some patients experience anaphylactic-like cardiorespiratory collapse upon reexposure.[8]

HIT results from autoimmune responses which lead to antibody generation targeted against platelet factor 4.[9] HIT should be diagnosed by combining its pretest probability with the quantitative result of a HIT-antibody assay. The treatment strategy for acute HIT development is the inhibition of thrombin generation through the use of non-heparin anticoagulant drugs. HIT patients can be reexposed to heparin due to the transient nature of HIT antibodies, provided that previous heparin treatment is remote and that anti-platelet factor 4/heparin antibodies are determined to be undetectable. Likewise, not all patients who develop antibodies against PF4/heparin complexes experience the platelet drop-off that would define them as having HIT.[10]

25.3.3.1 Pathogenesis of the Autoimmune Response

HIT is caused by the development of immunoglobulin G (IgG) antibodies that recognize a "self" protein, platelet factor 4 (PF4), bound to polyanions and forming PF4/heparin complexes.[6] PF4 is a positively charged protein of 70 amino acids belonging to the CXC subfamily of chemokines. It is synthesized by megakaryocytes and stored in α-granules in which it self-associates to form tetramers of approximately 31 kDa complexed with chondroitin sulfate. Upon platelet activation, PF4 is released, dissociates from chondroitin sulfate, and binds more anionic glycosaminoglycans (GAG) on cell surfaces, such as heparin sulfate. Unlike other cytokines that have clearly defined receptors, PF4 appears to function by this high-affinity cell-surface binding. It has been proposed that PF4 may be involved in several biological processes such as angiogenesis, immune response, thrombosis, and megakaryopoiesis.

Recent work has further investigated the molecular structure of PF4/heparin complexes, showing that conditions favoring the generation of anti-PF4/heparin antibodies differ from those required for intense platelet activation. Conceptually, the current working model of HIT immune pathogenesis implies the following aspects:

1. PF4 bound to anionic GAG expresses at least two immunogenic neoepitopes.
2. In-vivo PF4 bound to physiologic GAG forms antigenic complexes on cell surfaces.
3. Infusion of the more anionic heparin displaces PF4 from physiologic GAG, leading to the formation of PF4/heparin complexes.
4. PF4/heparin complexes carrying a net positive charge (i.e., those with a molar excess of PF4) are most immunogenic.
5. PF4/heparin complexes expressing neutral charges (i.e., those with a PF4–heparin molar ratio of about 1:1) are able to form the largest macromolecular complexes (more than 670 kDa), which are the most potent in mediating binding of HIT antibodies possibly by close approximation of PF4

tetramers and the inducement of heparin-dependent platelet activation.
6. Disruption of the PF4/heparin complexes by the infusion of excess heparin or protamine sulfate impairs their ability to bind anti-PF4/heparin antibodies and activate platelets.

This model, showing that PF4 bound in vivo to cell-surface GAG is immunogenic, could explain why healthy individuals are found to be positive for anti-PF4/heparin antibodies and why in HIT patients, anti-PF4/heparin antibodies of the IgG class are already detectable as early as five days after the initiation of heparin treatment. A second implication of this model, based on the different stoichiometries of PF4/heparin complexes, is that patients with higher degrees of surface-bound and circulating PF4 and lower (prophylactic) heparin concentrations would carry the highest risk of developing HIT. In fact, the incidence of HIT is higher among surgical than medical patients. Among surgical patients, it is higher in those with "traumatic" surgery such as orthopedics or cardiopulmonary bypass. Among medical patients, it is higher in those with peripheral arterial disease, cancer, or other inflammatory conditions promoting platelet activation and PF4 release. Moreover, the dissociation of conditions favoring the immune response from those necessary for platelet activation would explain why only a subset of patients who have developed anti-PF4/heparin antibodies progress to full-blown HIT.

Finally, it has been shown that PF4 is a modulator of T-cell activation, with opposite effects on regulatory versus non-regulatory T-cells, and that generation of anti-PF4/heparin antibodies is a T-cell-dependent process. Future research will have to delineate how PF4/heparin complexes initiate antigen presentation and modulate T-cell responses.

25.3.3.2 Pathogenesis of the Prothrombotic State

Ternary HIT-IgG/PF4/heparin complexes bind to cell surfaces. On platelets, the IgG Fc regions cross-link the low-affinity receptor for immune complexes, FcγRIIa (CD32), leading to platelet activation and the development of platelet-procoagulant activity. At the same time, HIT-IgG/PF4/heparin complexes are able to induce synthesis and expression of tissue factor on endothelial cells and monocytes.[11] All these events contribute to the development of unbalanced thrombin generation, which is central to the severe prothrombotic state peculiar to HIT.

In addition to the pro-coagulant state, other factors may increase the thrombotic risk in HIT. HIT antibodies may promote thrombosis through platelet adhesion to the vessel wall and formation of platelet–leukocyte aggregates.

25.3.3.3 Clinical Presentation of HIT

HIT is indicated by a severe decrease of platelet count (more than 50 percent drop or more than 150,000), sometimes with associated venous, arterial, and/or cutaneous thrombosis a week or two after the introduction of heparin (referred to as "typical onset").[12] Among patients who have previously been exposed to anti-PF4/heparin antibodies, HIT can present within hours after receiving heparin, with a drop of the platelet count, thrombosis, and symptoms such as flushing, hypotension, tachycardia, and dyspnea (this is referred to as "rapid-onset" HIT).[13] Finally, HIT can be diagnosed several days after heparin has been stopped ("delayed-onset" HIT). It is thus necessary to consider delayed-onset HIT as a possibility in order to be able to recognize and diagnose it. Bradner and Eikelboom (2001) found that "the presence of heparin-dependent antibodies in the blood was usually transient and did not always recur with subsequent heparin therapy."[14] This leads them to conclude that those with a history of heparin-induced thrombocytopenia should be reexposed to heparin only in extreme cases such as cardiac or vascular surgery, and then only if heparin-dependent antibodies cannot be detected.

A protocol useful for HIT detection includes:

1. Pre-op ELISA screening for all cardiac surgery patients.
2. Elimination of all unnecessary sources of heparin and availability of heparin-free products for all HIT-positive patients.
3. HIT precautions and testing for any cardiac surgery with thrombocytopenia.
4. Anticoagulant management of all post-operative ventricular assist device placement in patients with direct thrombin inhibitors.
5. Utilization of citrate for hemodialysis and CVVH.

While such practices do involve a minor increase in medication costs, this is more than made up for by the fact that they reduce costs associated with the failure to detect HIT.[15]

25.3.3.4 Diagnosis

It is common practice to institute alternative (i.e., non-heparin) anticoagulant treatment as soon as HIT is suspected as a possibility, as not doing so carries a far greater risk. However, alternative anticoagulants are extremely costly (estimated at $800–$1,000 per day) and potentially have life-threatening side effects such as major bleeding or anaphylactic reactions.[16] This suggests the need for the development of a rapid HIT diagnosis method to ensure proper action.

25.3.3.4.1 Dismissing HIT

The chance of a given patient experiencing HIT can be approximated through a clinical scoring system known as the "4T" in which patients are marked as having a low, intermediate, or high risk for the disease. Patients are scored between zero and eight, with scores less than three indicating a high negative predictive value for HIT. While this test does appear to be a reliable strategy to rule out HIT, combining pre-test clinical probability with rapid immunoassay results remains the most effective for excluding HIT.[17] Priziola et al. (2010) also indicate "this scoring system has not been validated in an ICU population."[18] An excellent and instructive figure "Use of the 4t's scoring system and results of PaGIA in the diagnosis of heparin-induced thrombocytopenia." may be viewed at *J. Thromb Haemost* 2007:5:1373–1370.

25.3.3.4.2 Diagnosing HIT

HIT cannot be diagnosed solely through clinical methods, but it must include a positive laboratory testing in the appropriate context. As such, it is critical here to consult a hematologist.

Tests for HIT antibodies include both immunological assays that detect PF4/heparin antibodies and functional platelet activation assays—such as the serotonin release assay—that work by detecting heparin-dependent antibodies. Functional assays have the advantage of very high specificity but are also technically demanding, have a long turn-around time, and are conducted by only a small fraction of laboratories. If a correctly performed functional assay produces positive results, then HIT can be definitively diagnosed with up to 99 percent certainty.[19] Unfortunately, platelet activation assays are not widely available for emergency testing, and it is possible that a patient may have HIT without testing positive.

The second group of methods for detecting HIT antibodies is immunoassays. Presently, there are three commercial enzyme-linked immunosorbent assays (ELISAs) (Asserachrom HPIA, GTI-PF4, Zymutest HIA) and a PaGIA (in-vitro diagnostic) called ID-Heparin/PF4—PaGIA are available to detect PF4 antibodies. All of these assays can detect IgG, IgM, and IgA antibodies and have a very high sensitivity, with a slightly better performance than the PaGIA, and are found to have operating characteristics in between the ELISA and functional assays. The drawback of these immunoassays is their relatively low specificity for pathogenic HIT antibodies, which in turn provides a risk of overdiagnosing HIT. This is especially problematic for the cardiovascular surgery population in which assay testing suggests that 25 to 50 percent of patients have heparin antibodies, while platelet-activating antibodies are actually found only in 15 to 20 percent of patients.[20]

25.3.3.4.3 Two Approaches: Class and Titer

One method against overdiagnosis uses immunoassays that only detect HIT antibodies of the IgG class. A second way to approach this problem is to consider the extent of the immunoassay result. Alberio (1998) has shown that

> [T]he absolute optical density values of two commercial ELISAs strongly correlate with the antibody titer obtained by the ID-H/PF4—PaGIA, and that the antibody titer independently correlates with a retrospective likelihood score for HIT, a positive functional platelet aggregation test, the prevalence of thromboembolic events during treatment with heparin, and the concentration of prothrombin fragments F1+2, thrombin—antithrombin complexes, and D-dimers.[21]

It is also worth noting that antigens besides PF4 may be a relevant factor in HIT pathogenesis, including interleukin 8 (IL-8) or neutrophil-activating peptide 2 (NAP-2), two PF4-related CXC chemokines with high affinity for heparin. A reasonable "gold standard" suggested by Alberio for diagnosing HIT is "either a positive functional assay or high-titer anti-PF4/heparin antibodies in the presence of a clinically-likely HIT."[22] Both plasma from sodium citrate or EDTA tubes and serum can be employed for detecting HIT antibodies by immunoassay.

25.3.3.5 Treatment of HIT

For patients suspected or known to have HIT, all heparin should be stopped without exception and replaced with alternative anticoagulation method by means of the direct thrombin inhibitors (DTIs) bivalirudin (half-life 30 min and dependent on renal clearance) or argatroban (half-life 45 minutes; hepatic metabolism; nonimmunogenic). The DTI danaparoid is not yet available in the United States.

HIT patients with or without thromboembolic complications require therapeutic anticoagulation. Platelet transfusions must also be discontinued, as they have been observed to potentiate thrombosis.[23]

Vitamin K antagonists (VKAs), such as warfarin, are ill-suited for cases of acute HIT because they fail to inhibit the marked hypercoagulability state of HIT, while at the same time they can cause a severe depletion of the vitamin K-dependent natural anticoagulant, protein C,[24] and VKAs increase the risk of microvascular thrombosis, especially venous limb gangrene.

25.3.3.5.1 Fondaparinux

Fondaparinux is a synthetic "pentasaccharide" anticoagulant, modeled after the antithrombin-binding sequence of heparin molecules. Interestingly, patients treated with fondaparinux develop anti-PF4/heparin antibodies with a frequency similar to those treated with low molecular weight heparin (LMWH), but fondaparinux-induced HIT appears to be exquisitely rare, although documented. This may be explained by the inability of fondaparinux to form large complexes with PF4, thus failing to activate platelets.[8] Recently, a few reports have suggested that fondaparinux may be useful in patients with acute HIT. This is an interesting option; however, prospective clinical studies should verify whether fondaparinux is able to control the strong procoagulant state of acute HIT. Moreover, several "unstable" HIT patients, such as those in ICU or those requiring surgical interventions, are not suited for treatment with a renally excreted anticoagulant with a long half-life and no antidote available. Finally, as fondaparinux can induce the formation of anti-PF4/heparin antibodies, one still has to be aware that a subsequent treatment with unfractionated heparin (UFH) or LMWH may precipitate HIT. The author's institution occasionally employs fondaparinux for prolonged anticoagulation after successful acute treatment with a DTI in those HIT patients who cannot be switched to VKA.

25.3.3.5.2 Reexposure with Heparin

There is a good rationale for short-term heparin re-exposure of patients with a history of HIT in order to permit surgery. In fact, HIT antibodies are transient, generally disappearing within four months, and patients with "rapid-onset" HIT have been shown to have circulating HIT antibodies. The feasibility of this option has been demonstrated for cardiovascular surgery. These publications clearly indicate that there is no anamnestic immune response in HIT. Moreover, the recent data on the stoichiometric requirements for the formation of immunogenic and platelet-activating PF4/heparin complexes would argue against an elevated recurrence risk as well.

25.3.3.6 Conclusion: HIT and HITT

Despite the decreasing use of UFH in favor of LMWH and fondaparinux, HIT still constitutes a clinically relevant challenge, based on difficulty in diagnoses, ubiquitous presence of heparin, high costs of alternative DTIs, and the life-threatening risk of HIT and heparin-induced thrombocytopenia and thrombosis (HITT). Advances in the understanding of pathogenic and clinically relevant issues will enable improvement in the treatment strategies for patients in this area.[25]

25.3.3.6.1 Anticoagulation Therapy for Atrial Fibrillation

Of interest for this report is the utilization of anticoagulation therapy to reduce the risk of stroke in patients with atrial fibrillation (AF). Atrial fibrillation is characterized by an irregular heartbeat that can cause clot-provoked strokes.

- A 2015 meta-analysis of 13 randomized trials involving more than 100,000 patients found DOACs associated with a 47% reduction in the risk of fatal bleeding compared with VKAs. Similarly, in a real-world study of more than 2,000 patients with anticoagulant-associated bleeding, the case-fatality rate was reduced with DOACs when compared to warfarin.
- The ARISTOTLE study evaluated the effect of apixaban (Eliquis)™ for the reduction of stroke and other thromboembolic events in AF and found a significantly reduced risk of stroke, major bleeding, and all-cause mortality when compared to warfarin. In patients with nonvalvular atrial fibrillation (NVAF), Eliquis 5 mg/twice daily significantly reduces the risk of stroke or systemic embolism by 21%, that of major bleeding by 31%, and that of death by 11% compared with warfarin. Furthermore, in treatment-resistant VKA patients or those unable to take VKA therapies, Eliquis reduces the risk of stroke or emic embolism by more than 50% compared with aspirin without a significant increase in the risk of major bleeding.[26],[27]

The management of patients who are taking a DOAC for AF and require elective surgery or an invasive procedure presents a common clinical scenario for which best practices are uncertain.

25.3.4 Warfarin

Warfarin is currently the standard for providing long-term oral anticoagulation for atrial fibrillation, prosthetic heart valves, venous thrombosis, and pulmonary embolism. Warfarin is an antagonist of vitamin K and interferes with hepatic synthesis of coagulation factors II, VII, IX, and X. Inhibition of the hepatic vitamin K conversion cycle causes the production of clotting factors with reduced coagulant activity. There are several shortcomings to warfarin therapy. As warfarin has a narrow therapeutic range and risk of bleeding, patients need to be frequently monitored. This can be difficult due to changes in dietary vitamin K consumption as well as the potential for drug interactions.[28] Individualized dosing plans must be specified for each patient to avoid thromboembolic events caused by subtherapeutic levels as well as supratherapeutic levels. High levels can cause an increased risk of bleeding. A therapeutic response to warfarin is not achieved for the first 12 hours after introduction and often takes between 3 and 5 days to become effective. This is because warfarin prevents the synthesis of coagulation factors but does not inhibit the action of existing factors. When rapid anticoagulant effect is needed, an additional form of anticoagulation such as heparin should be used, and warfarin should not be prescribed unless a patient's platelet count is above a minimum sustainable threshold. Finally, warfarin must *never* be administered during pregnancy (contraindicated: Pregnancy Category X) as it crosses the placenta readily and can cause a hemorrhagic disorder in the fetus.

If an excessive anticoagulant effect without bleeding occurs, the cessation of the drug responsible can often be enough. In the setting of severe bleeding, however, the warfarin effect can be rapidly reversed with the administration of prothrombin complex concentrates (PCCs) or rFVIIa coupled with intravenous vitamin K (though this carries a risk of anaphylaxis). Of note, due to the long half-life of warfarin, a single dose of vitamin K or rFVIIa may not be sufficient in all cases.[29] In addition, particular PCC products, like KCentra, have the FDA approval for bleeding associated with warfarin therapy.

Current therapy for prevention and treatment of thrombosis has been hindered by a lack of oral anticoagulants that are easily managed. There is a need for more effective anticoagulation treatments that utilize simplified dosing schedules, less monitoring, and less risk of bleeding complications to replace warfarin. Consistent oral bioavailability appears to be the key in developing the next oral anticoagulant. The new agents must be as effective as warfarin yet easier to monitor and, hopefully, safer, such as dabigatran as discussed next.

25.4 MONITORING ORAL ANTICOAGULATION

The number of indications for, as well as the number of patients on, oral anticoagulation (OAC) therapy has increased significantly. Primary indications for OAC therapy include venous thromboembolism, atrial fibrillation, cerebrovascular disease, heart valve prosthesis, peripheral vascular disease, and myocardial infarction. Evidence shows an exponential increase in the risk of thrombosis when international normalized ratio (INR) values fall below 2.0, and the risk of hemorrhage increases when INR values rise above 4.5. Thus, the maintenance of a close-target therapeutic range is a critical component of successful OAC therapy. Several drug- and patient-related factors make this task difficult to achieve, including a narrow therapeutic index of the drug, numerous drug–drug and drug–food interactions, and individual differences in dose–response to warfarin sodium. The aforementioned challenges make regular monitoring of patients' INR values and dosage adjustments an essential part of OAC therapy. The standard test is the plasma-based PT test, which was traditionally done in a laboratory. Point of Care (POC) testing eliminates the need of transporting blood specimens and enables the clinician to immediately assess the results and adjust the dosing of OAC therapy, if necessary. It has been suggested that the use of portable prothrombin time (PPT) monitors allows more convenient and thus more frequent testing, which may be translated to better control of OAC therapy. Patients requiring a long-term anticoagulant therapy are recommended to have their PT measured every one to four weeks. However, as PT values are dependent on the sensitivity of the thromboplastin reagent, INR is a better scale of measurement because it adjusts for this sensitivity factor:

$$INR = (\text{patient}\, PT \div mean\, normal\, PT) \times ISI \qquad (25.1)$$

Where ISI = the international sensitivity index.

Close supervision by a health professional remains an integral part of anticoagulant therapy.[30]

Indeed, Splawski and Minger, in Chapter 27, report the following regarding beneficial safety effects of pharmacists' monitoring of anticoagulant therapy:

> Several studies review the efficacy and safety of anticoagulation management when pharmacists are involved compared to physician-managed care. In 1995, Dager et al. compared a historical cohort of 60 consecutive pharmacist-managed warfarin patients randomly matched with 60 physician-managed patients in 1995. An anticoagulation pharmacist was assigned to review the patient's medical record and provide a written consult each day with dosing recommendations. The pharmacist used their clinical experience in addition to assessing the patients' INR trends, hemoglobin, hematocrit, liver function tests, platelets, albumin, concurrent medications and medical problems and previous warfarin dosing to assist with the dosing recommendations.
>
> Pharmacist management of warfarin therapy resulted in a significant decrease on patient length of stay compared to physician management from 9.5 + 5.6 days to 6.8 + 4.4 days ($p = 0.009$). Pharmacists significantly reduced supratherapeutic INR values (> 3.5 and > 6). Bleeding complications were less in the pharmacist group; however, this was not statistically significant. Lastly, only 6 patients in the pharmacist group received a drug with a major drug-drug interaction with warfarin, whereas 13 patients from the physician-managed group received a major interacting medication ($p = 0.02$). The benefits of pharmacist consultation in this case were in achieving treatment goals while reducing the length of stay.

25.5 DIRECT ORAL ANTICOAGULANTS—DOACS ALTERNATIVES TO WARFARIN

Warfarin has a well-defined safety profile with its noted drug interactions, is cost-effective, readily available, and partially reversible.[31] It is broadly indicated for a variety of conditions and is suitable for patients with mechanical valves. Despite these advantages, there are several recognized caveats of warfarin use, including a narrow therapeutic range, delayed drug–drug interactions, food–drug interactions, slow dose adjustment time, and genetic variability in the enzymes involved in its metabolism, all of which can affect INR.[32] Frequent patient monitoring is needed to assure that a therapeutic INR is maintained which can be cumbersome.[33] DOACs, which directly inhibit factor Xa (rivaroxaban, apixaban, and edoxaban) or thrombin (dabigatran), were developed to address some of the disadvantages of warfarin. DOACs have a predictable anticoagulant response, making regular laboratory monitoring unnecessary. Anticoagulation with DOACs is achieved quickly, reaching peak plasma concentrations in one to four hours following oral administration (with peak effect coinciding with peak concentration), in comparison with the delayed onset of warfarin. Half-lives of DOACs are shorter than that of warfarin and range from 5 to 15 hours. DOACs have fewer drug–drug and drug–food interactions than warfarin. Although rivaroxaban should be administered with food, the other DOACs can be administered without regard to food.[34]

Nonvitamin K antagonist (VKA) oral anticoagulants (DOACs) are at least as effective as warfarin for the prevention of stroke in AF and are associated with significantly decreased risks of intracranial hemorrhage.[9] Dabigatran, rivaroxaban, apixaban, and edoxaban have been approved for reducing the risk of stroke in patients with nonvalvular AF (NVAF).[35,36,37,38] The current guidelines (published prior to the approval of edoxaban) recommend the use of dabigatran, rivaroxaban, apixaban, and warfarin for cases of NVAF. Additionally, NOACs are recommended for patients who are not able to maintain therapeutic INR levels on warfarin.[39,40] Reasons include dietary restrictions, failure to routinely monitor and adjust doses when required, drug–drug interactions, missed doses, and genetic variability, all of which that can interfere with warfarin metabolism.[41]

25.5.1 Pradaxa (Dabigatran) versus Warfarin

Pradaxa (dabigatran) is a new medication designed to prevent clots that can be caused by atrial fibrillation. This drug has a few benefits not conferred by warfarin (Coumadin), including that it does not require frequent INR testing. Furthermore, dabigatran is less likely to adversely interact with other medications or with foods containing vitamin K (as warfarin does).

Warfarin still holds some advantages over Pradaxa, including its price, which is about one-third of the new drug. Also, warfarin requires only once-daily dosing, as opposed to dabigatran (twice-daily dosing).

Pradaxa may cause gastrointestinal side effects, especially when taken on an empty stomach.[42]

Dabigatran and other newer direct thrombin inhibitors (DTIs) had a disadvantage on market release. Unlike warfarin, there was no reversal agent, and patients who developed uncontrolled bleeding suffered significant morbidity, and many patients died. Recently, a new product, Idarucizumab, was released to "reverse" the effect of the DTI.

A recent Phase I study aimed to determine the safety, tolerability, and efficacy of increasing doses of idarucizumab in order to reverse the anticoagulant effects brought about by dabigatran. A total of 47 men were enrolled in the study, divided into groups to receive varying doses of idarucizumab plus oral dabigatran. According to the findings, dabigatran-induced anticoagulation was completely and immediately reversed in a dose-dependent manner. No serious adverse events were reported, and there were no adverse events that led to the treatment being discontinued. While further study is needed, the findings show that idarucizumab was associated with immediate and sustained reversal of dabigatran-induced anticoagulation in men. A *commentary* accompanying the study notes that while the findings are promising, "we must await the results of studies in real patients with bleeding to assess whether the antidotes are as effective in critically ill patients as they are in healthy young volunteers."[43]

Shortly after the completion of the clinical study, the FDA granted an accelerated approval to Praxbind (idarucizumab) for use in patients who are taking the anticoagulant Pradaxa (dabigatran) during emergency situations when there is a need to reverse Pradaxa's blood-thinning effects.

"The anticoagulant effects of Pradaxa are important and lifesaving for some patients, but there are situations where reversal of the drug's effects is medically necessary," said Richard Pazdur, M.D., director of the Office of Hematology and Oncology Products in the FDA's Center for Drug Evaluation and Research. "Today's approval offers the medical community an important tool for managing patients taking Pradaxa in emergency or life-threatening situations when bleeding can't be controlled."

25.5.2 Antiplatelet therapy

An "aspirin a day" is the oldest and a universal antiplatelet prescribed for patients who may be at risk for blood clots. Besides aspirin, there are a number of additional antiplatelet drugs used clinically. Patients on antiplatelet drugs must be closely monitored, as they are at increased risk for bleeding. The drugs, mechanisms, and safety/toxicity issues are discussed in this section.

1. *ASA*: Irreversible inhibition of COX in platelets which will lead to decreased activation. Used for prophylaxis for AMI and/or the first dose for the event. Dosing can be either low dose (i.e., 81 mg) or high dose (i.e., 325 mg) which is often given just once daily. The incidence of bleeding has often been associated with higher dosing of therapy and when combination agents are used (i.e., ADP antagonists, GPIIb/IIIa inhibitors, etc.)
2. *ADP inhibitors*: Blockade of the P2Y12 receptors on platelets to decrease their activation. Can be used for the treatment of AMI and/or after stent placement during PCI-cath lab and in unstable angina.

TABLE 25.1
Direct Oral Anticoagulants (DOACs).

Characteristic	Dabigatran	Rivaroxaban	Apixaban
Target	Thrombin	Xa	Xa
Prodrug	Yes	No	No
Bioavailability (%)	6	80	60
Dosing	Once or twice daily	Fixed, once daily	Fixed, twice daily
Half-life (hour)	14–17	7–11	12
Renal Cl (%)	80	66	25
Monitoring	None	None	None
Drug interactions	Potent inhibitor or P-gp	Potent inhibitor CYP450 3A4 and P-gp	Potent inhibitor of CYP450 3A4

Source: G. Patel, Rush Medical College. with permission

i. Drugs: Clopidogrel, prasugrel, and ticagrelor (metabolism via CYP3A4). The medications are listed in order, consistent with their onset of action from slowest to fastest on platelet activation inhibition when the loading doses are used. Agents are pro-drugs substrates of the CYP 2C19 enzyme system.
   1. Notable adverse reaction is with ticlopidine. The reaction is called thrombocytopenic purpura (TTP).

ii. Drug interaction: The drug interaction that can occur is with proton-pump inhibitors (PPI) used in gastric disorders or GERD. Since the PPIs are metabolized and serve as substrates via 2C19, there is scientific support for the idea that there is a competitive inhibition which could potentially result in lower concentrations of ADP antagonists, particularly ticlopidine and clopidogrel.

3. Glycoprotein (GP) IIb/IIIa receptor inhibitors: Inhibition of these receptors at more than 80% blockade would result in activity. The GP IIb/IIIa receptors are the final step in platelet–platelet aggregation. These drugs are either used for patients for medical management of acute coronary syndrome (ACS). For a very thorough explanation and an instructive figure on precise locations of action of these agents on the clotting cascade, see New Oral Anticoagulants for Thromboprophylaxis after Elective Total Hip and Knee Arthroplast by Friedman in *Thrombosis*, 2010: Jul 29: 280731.

iii. Drugs: Abciximab, eptifibatide, and tirofiban

iv. Abciximab: Indicated for cases during the PCI-Cath lab procedures. The drug involves hepatic metabolism and is given as intravenous bolus and infusion. In addition, the drug's metabolism occurs via the reticular endothelial system (RES) and dosing adjustment not needed for renal dysfunction.

v. Eptifibatide: Indicated for cases during the PCI-Cath lab and for medical management (i.e., no mechanical intervention). The drug is given as an intravenous bolus and infusion and requires dosing adjustment for renal dysfunction.

vi. Tirofiban: Indicated for cases during the PCI-Cath lab and for medical management. The drug is given as a bolus and intravenous infusion, and the infusion requires adjustment for renal dysfunction.

25.5.2.1 Anticoagulation Management with Surgical Procedures

Anticoagulation medication needs to be managed very carefully in the days prior, during, and following the surgical or invasive procedure.

Key contributors to significant risk during the procedural period include:

- The complex, individualized assessments that contribute to the comprehensive analysis of bleeding and thrombotic risks of the procedure and the patient.
- High transition of care turnover. Transitions of care are associated with increased patient vulnerability to medication discrepancies, therapeutic overlap, failure to resume anticoagulation, communication errors, and missed coordination of follow-up.
- Lack of familiarity with the differences in pharmacology of DOACs versus other anticoagulants, mainly warfarin. An understanding of the difference between DOACs and warfarin pharmacologic and treatment metrics is necessary as these medications have significantly different perioperative management approaches. It is not uncommon that DOAC patients are treated with periprocedural plans that have inappropriately prolonged hold times and/or overlapping therapy with low molecular weight heparin (LMWH), because providers manage these agents with an approach similar to that as they would use with warfarin.

25.5.2.2 Discontinuation Pre-Surgery or Invasive Procedure

The general consensus is more aligned to the discontinuation of DOACs, and specifically Eliquis, prior to surgery. A longer period of preoperative discontinuation, up to five days, can be considered for patients with renal or hepatic impairment or other conditions associated with decreased drug elimination.[44]

The American Society of Regional Anesthesia and Pain Medicine (ASRA) provides consensus guidelines updated regularly on anticoagulation therapy. Current ASRA guidelines (2018) recommend that DOACs be discontinued five half-lives prior to any medium- or high-risk pain procedure. After two, three, five, and six half-lives, 25%, 12.5%, 3.2%, and 1.6% of the drug remains in the blood, respectively.[45] In general, Eliquis should be discontinued two to three days prior to elective surgery or invasive procedures. In high-risk patients, an individualized approach is needed to minimize the period of subtherapeutic anticoagulation.[46]

25.5.2.3 Reinitiation of Anticoagulant Therapy

There is no exact timeframe for restarting Eliquis or other anticoagulants after surgery or an invasive procedure as individual factors including clotting and bleeding risks, the type of anticoagulant, and the type of procedure that was performed need to be considered. Therefore, the overseeing surgeon and attending physician should provide consensus as to when the patient is able to restart DOAC therapy after surgery.

Postoperative resumption of DOACs is again stratified on the basis of bleeding/thromboembolic risk and tend to vary among one another. For procedures with a low risk of postoperative bleeding, protocols recommend generally that DOACs can be continued at the earliest 24 hours postoperatively.[47,48] Patients who undergo operations with a higher risk for bleeding should be restarted 48–72 h postoperatively at the earliest.[49,50]

Reinitiation of Eliquis dosing should only resume once surgical hemostasis has been observed. Caution should be exercised with re-initiating Eliquis within the first 48 hours post-surgery. When there is a risk of postoperative venous thrombosis and the bleeding risk is also high, it may be suggested to consider a reduced dose (e.g., 2.5 mg BID—recommended prophylactic dose) for the immediate postoperative period.[51] Alternatively, in this scenario, you may go right to heparin bridge therapy for about three days, then the DOAC is reintroduced. This recommendation is made because the UFH (heparin) infusion is faster on/off with a known reversal agent (i.e., protamine) in cases of hemorrhage.[52]

A comprehensive review, covering literature through January 2022, on perioperative management of patients receiving anticoagulants provides guidance on restarting Eliquis postoperatively. Douketis et al. opine that Eliquis, at the same dose prescribed prior to surgery, be restarted once hemostasis has been achieved. The perceived bleeding risk will determine when Eliquis can be restarted. In general, Eliquis may be restarted within one day after a low/moderate-bleeding-risk procedure and two days after a high-bleeding-risk procedure.[53,54] Other reports suggest that most patients omit Eliquis for two total days for a low/moderate-bleeding-risk procedure and for four total days for a high-bleeding-risk procedure post-surgery.

The interim neuraxial ASRA guidelines recommend restarting DOACs no sooner than six hours after a neuraxial procedure or removal of an indwelling epidural catheter, while the interventional pain guidelines recommend waiting for 24 hours. However, if DOACs are held for a five half-life interval, ASRA recommends bridging patients who are at high risk for VTE. The decision regarding bridging should consider the bleeding risk, thromboembolic risk, and the withdrawal period for the DOAC regimen.[55]

25.5.2.4 Bridging Therapy

Bridging therapy refers to the administration of a short-acting anticoagulant, most commonly low-molecular-weight heparin (LMWH), during the interruption of a longer-acting anticoagulant. For outpatient setting, the most common would be LMWH, but for in-patient, the majority of the time it would be UFH infusion due to the ability of fast on/off and antidote availability in case of emergencies.

The goal of bridging anticoagulation is to reduce the patient risk for developing life-threatening blood clots; however, bridging may also increase the patient risk for developing potentially serious bleeding complications after surgery. Bridging anticoagulation may be necessary in patients at high risk for thromboembolism or in patients being treated for active VTE, but for most, it leads to excessive bleeding and poorer patient outcomes. Evidence suggests that the majority of atrial fibrillation (AF) patients are at risk of major bleeding from bridging therapy, with no reduction in the incidence of thromboembolism. The BRIDGE trial (a multicenter, randomized, double-blind placebo-controlled trial) showed that bridged AF patients with a CHADS score of 14 were at greater risk of major bleeding than thromboembolism when compared with no bridging. Discontinuation of oral antithrombotic agents and addition of low-dose heparin bridging therapy appear to be significantly associated with adverse events in the periprocedural period. Heparin bridging therapy was significantly associated with higher risk for both thromboembolic events and major bleeding in procedures with high bleeding risk.[56]

Bridging therapy is more common with patients on warfarin and generally not required for patients receiving oral direct thrombin inhibitor or Factor Xa inhibitor therapy. Warfarin has a slow onset and offset; DOACs are much quicker. Perioperative heparin bridging in DOAC-treated patients does not make pharmacologic sense, given the short half-lives, association with increased bleeding, and lack of efficacy. However, if the anticoagulant therapy of any type (warfarin or DOACs) is interrupted, then the risk versus benefit of using bridge therapy weighing risk versus benefit should be considered.

25.5.2.4.1 The MARK Study

The MARK study was a prospective, observational study to determine the management of antithrombotic agents during surgery or other medical procedures with bleeding risks.[57] The incidence of any thromboembolic event, major bleeding, and death was increased in the discontinuation group compared to the continuation group. In multivariate analysis, the discontinuation of anticoagulant agents was significantly associated with higher risk for both thromboembolic events and major bleeding in procedures with low bleeding risk. Discontinuation of anticoagulant agents was significantly associated with periprocedural TEs in low-bleeding-risk procedures. However, in high-bleeding-risk procedures, significant association was not observed between discontinuation of antithrombotic agents and TEs; however, heparin bridging therapy was significantly associated with higher risk for TEs.

25.5.2.5 Determination of Risk

While efforts have been made to standardize schema to categorize procedural risks relating to bleeding and thromboembolic event, variations exist across guidelines and within patient practice. Furthermore, each patient is unique, and recommendations based on comprehensive health analysis of the patient and the risk–benefit analysis of intervention may continuously change based on new information. In general, risk stratification may initially be categorized by multiple interventional techniques into low-risk, medium-risk, and high-risk categories. Risk class may be updated on the basis of other contributing factors.

25.5.2.5.1 Thromboembolic Risk Stratification

The three major pathological groups that have a known higher risk of thromboembolic events are those with AF, prosthetic heart valves, and previous/risk of thromboembolism. In AF, thromboembolic risk is estimated through clinical variables with the CHA2DS2VASc score.

The risk of thromboembolism is best determined by the overseeing physician. The CHADS2 score is used to estimate the annual risk of stroke in a patient with non-valvular AF when not on an anticoagulant.

The most common side effect or complication associated with all anticoagulation medications is bleeding. When evaluating bleeding risk, it is imperative to consider the type of surgery and clinical characteristics of the patient. Characteristics that contribute to patient bleeding risk include thrombocytopenia, renal dysfunction with uremia, significant hepatic impairment with baseline coagulopathy, history of bleeding, and concomitant medications such as antiplatelets or nonsteroidal anti-inflammatory drugs. Characteristics are objectively scored using the HAS-BLED (Hypertension, Abnormal liver or kidney function, Stroke, Bleeding history or predisposition, Labile International Normalized Ratio [INR], Elderly, Drugs, alcohol) score. A point is awarded for each positive item. A HAS-BLED score of more than 3 indicates a high bleeding risk. The BORDER study evaluated predictors of perioperative bleeding in patients undergoing invasive cardiac procedures. They found that the HAS-BLED score is a reliable predictor of perioperative bleeding.[58]

As a common guideline, the procedural bleeding risk can be divided into low risk (0–2% two-day risk of major bleeding) or high risk (2% to 4% two-day risk of major bleeding). Among the many types of surgical procedures, special consideration should be given to intracranial, cardiac, and neuraxial surgeries due to the locale of potential bleeding and poor patient prognosis outcomes that arise in the presence of these complications.[59]

TABLE 25.2
Classification of Risk for Thromboembolic Events.

Low	Medium	High
CHA_2DS_2-VASc 0–2	CHA_2DS_2-VASc 3–4	CHA_2DS_2-VASc 5–6
DVT > 12 months	DVT 3–12 months	DVT < 3 months
Double wing aortic	DVT in cancer patients	DVT with pulmonary embolism <12 months
Valve > 3 months with sinus rhythm	Recurring DVT	Stroke <3 months
	Double wing aortic valve with CHA_2DS_2-VASc > 0	Mitral valve replacement
	Biological heart valve with sinus rhythm	Older mechanical aortic valves
		Biological heart valve with atrial fibrillation
		Hereditary thrombophilias

TABLE 25.3
Procedural Bleeding Risk Related to Common Procedures.

Low Risk of Bleeding (Two-Day Risk of Major Bleed <2%)	High Risk of Bleeding (Two-Day Risk of Major Bleed 2–4%)
Cholecystectomy	Heart valve replacement
Hysterectomy	Coronary artery bypass
Gastrointestinal endoscopy +/- biopsy, stenting	Abdominal aortic aneurysm repair
Pacemaker and defibrillator insertion	Vascular surgery
Electrophysiological testing	Neurosurgery
Simple dental extractions	Urologic surgery
Carpal tunnel repair	Head and neck surgery
Single joint replacement	Abdominal surgery
Dilation and curettage	Breast cancer surgery
Skin cancer excision	Bilateral knee replacement
Abdominal hernia repair	Laminectomy
Hemorrhoid surgery	Transurethral prostate resection
Axillary node dissection	Kidney biopsy
Hydrocele repair	Polypectomy, variceal treatment
Ophthalmology procedures	Biliary sphincterotomy pneumatic dilation
Noncoronary angiography	PEG placement
Bronchoscopy +/- biopsy	Multiple tooth extractions
Central venous catheter removal	
Cutaneous biopsies	

Abbreviations: PEG = percutaneous endoscopic gastrostomy.

25.5.2.6 Interruption of Anticoagulant Therapy

Individuals receiving chronic anticoagulation often require interruptions due to a necessary surgery, invasive procedures, or other medical issues that require medication cessation for various durations. Surgical and invasive procedures have associated bleeding risks that may be increased by the actions of anticoagulant therapies. If the patient is at risk for bleeding from the surgery or procedure, the anticoagulant may need to be discontinued for a period of time to reduce the bleeding risk. However, the discontinuation of the anticoagulant increases thromboembolic risk. Thus, a balance must be reached between reducing the risk of thromboembolism and reducing the risk for excessive bleeding due to the surgery or procedure. An anticoagulant therapy interruption interval that is too long may increase thew thromboembolism risk, whereas an interruption interval that is too short may increase the bleeding risk which, in turn, delays anticoagulant resumption.

The following information is provided in the Eliquis Product Insert regarding temporary suspension of Eliquis:

> **Temporary Interruption for Surgery and Other Interventions**
>
> ELIQUIS should be discontinued at least 48 hours prior to elective surgery or invasive procedures with a moderate or high risk of unacceptable or clinically significant bleeding [see Warnings and Precautions (5.2)]. ELIQUIS should be discontinued at least 24 hours prior to elective surgery or invasive procedures with a low risk of bleeding or where the bleeding would be non-critical in location and easily controlled. Bridging anticoagulation during the 24 to 48 hours after stopping ELIQUIS and prior to the intervention is not generally required. Eliquis should be restarted after the surgical or other procedures as soon as adequate hemostasis has been established."[60]

Effective management of anticoagulation therapy requires balancing the prevention of blood clotting (anticoagulation) and the potential risk of bleeding due to the anticoagulation therapy.

25.6 FAILURE TO REINSTATE ANTICOAGULANTS AFTER SURGERY OR CARDIAC PROCEDURES

CASE REPORT

FACTS OF THE CASE

TM was diagnosed with obstructive uropathy and taken to surgery by the defendant urologist on 3/08/18. He had been prescribed and taking Eliquis for atrial fibrillation (AF) since November 29, 2018. His Eliquis was "held" on 3/6/2019 preoperatively. Intra- and postoperative assessments were without complications. His coagulation factors (HGB, HCT) were reported as being 12.3 and 38.5 on 3/9/2019. No clinical signs of bleeding were noted postoperatively. He was discharged home on 3/10/19 with an appointment to return to the urologist on 3/18/2019. Two days later (3/20/2019), TM suffered a thrombotic cerebral vascular accident (stroke). The prescribing information for apixaban (Eliquis) contained a **Black Box Warning (BBW)** regarding the increased risk of thrombotic events after premature discontinuation.

ASSIGNMENT

1. What does the pharmacologic and hematologic literature recommend regarding the resumption of apixaban and/or other anticoagulants following a surgical procedure?
2. What is the meaning of a **Black Box Warning**, and how have the Warnings evolved regarding the risk of premature discontinuation of apixaban?
3. To what extent are prescribers compliant with Black Box Warnings?
4. Was there any contraindication or increased bleeding risk associated with the resumption of apixaban within a period of two to four days (or anytime) following Mr. Moore's surgery?

OPINIONS

1. Direct Acting Oral Anticoagulants (DOACs) are indicated for the prevention of thrombotic events caused by AF.
2. The prescribing information states: Eliquis should be restarted after the surgical or other procedures as soon as adequate hemostasis has been established. The consensus in the literature recommends the resumption of apixaban after two to four days postoperatively.
3. **The Black Box Warning** for Eliquis states:
   a. WARNING (A) PREMATURE DISCONTINUATION OF ELIQUIS INCREASED THE RISK OF THROMBOTIC EVENTS. Premature discontinuation of any oral anticoagulant, including Eliquis, increased the risk of thrombotic events. If anticoagulation with Eliquis is discontinued for a reason other than pathological bleeding or completion of a course of therapy, consider coverage with another anticoagulant.

   The Package Insert (5.1) for Increased Risk of Thrombotic Events after Premature Discontinuation states:

Premature discontinuation of any oral anticoagulant, including Eliquis, in the absence of adequate alternative anticoagulation increases the risk of thrombotic events. An increase rate of stroke was observed during the transition from Eliquis to warfarin in clinical trials in atrial fibrillation patients. If Eliquis is discontinued for a reason other than pathological bleeding or completion of a course of therapy, consider coverage with another anticoagulant.

This warning was included in the initial approved package insert in 2012[61] and continues with the same wording in the 2021 package insert. Eliquis package inserts for this period are attached as Appendices to this report.

4. No pharmacological reason prohibited the resumption of apixaban after four days following his prostate surgery.
5. Failure to resume apixaban postoperatively increased Mr. Moore's risk of stroke.
6. Based on the pharmacokinetic and pharmacodynamic parameters of apixaban, resuming on March 18, 2019, ten days after surgery (the day he was examined by Dr. Bashey), the apixaban would have been providing full anticoagulation within four hours and achieve steady state in about two days. This cumulative pharmacodynamic action (decrease in clot formation) would have decreased Mr. Moore's risk of the stroke which occurred two days later on March 20, 2018.
7. Prescribers follow/heed warnings, especially **BLACK BOX WARNINGS**.

DISCUSSION

21 CFR 201.57 (4) (c)(1) *Boxed warning:* Certain contraindications or serious warnings, particularly those that may lead to death or serious injury, may be required by the FDA to be presented in a box. The boxed warning ordinarily must be based on clinical data, but serious animal toxicity may also be the basis of a boxed warning in the absence of clinical data. The box must contain, in uppercase letters, a heading inside the box that includes the word "WARNING" and conveys the general focus of the information in the box. The box must briefly explain the risk and refer to more detailed information in the "Contraindications" or "Warnings and Precautions" section, accompanied by the identifying number for the section or subsection containing the detailed information.

While it is true that physicians can prescribe drugs off-label or make their own decisions as to dosing, the Eliquis label establishes a different standard of care. The label is unambiguous in providing prescribing physicians with a clear directive on the risk of thrombotic events following premature discontinuation of apixaban.

The Defendant urologist's Counsel argued that the MARK study [xvi] provided justification to not reinstate the Eliquis after surgery, citing the findings of the MARK study:

Discontinuation of anticoagulant agents was significantly associated with peri-procedural thrombotic events (TEs) in low-bleeding-risk procedures. However, in high-bleeding-risk procedures, significant association was not observed between the discontinuation of antithrombotic agents and TEs; however, heparin bridging therapy was significantly associated with higher risk for TEs.

However, the MARK study only addressed perioperative period (without definition); further, it is silent on the resumption of anticoagulants postoperatively; its focus was risks of bleeding with heparin bridging (as indicated in the title). In other words, MARK study does not address the resumption or failure to resume anticoagulant therapy postop, thus, it should not apply as a defense in this case. Heparin bridging was not used in the TM case.

CONCLUSIONS

While general guidelines do exist, the re-initiation of Eliquis, or other DOACs after surgery or an invasive procedure, is dependent on expert opinion and individualized to the patient's unique bleeding and thromboembolic risk analysis. Typically, Eliquis is discontinued two to three days prior to the surgical event. For procedures with a low risk of postoperative bleeding, most protocols recommend a 24-hour delay in resuming DOAC anticoagulation after their procedure. In high-risk procedures, patients require an individualized approach to minimize the period of subtherapeutic anticoagulation while reducing complications from excessive bleeding. DOAC initiation is more subjective, but typical protocols suggest the reinitiation of two to four days post-surgery, pending the evidence of surgical hemostasis.

Apixaban was not resumed after surgery, even though hemostasis was established, and patient TM was free of bleeding complications. Failure to resume apixaban placed TM at risk for a stroke—a risk substantially greater than he would have had had the apixaban was resumed within two to four days after surgery. Given the rapid onset of action (3–4 hours) and steady state at 48 hours, resumption on postoperative day 10 (3/18/19) would have provided protection and decreased his risk of stroke brought on by the inexplicable failure to reinitiate apixaban therapy.

CASE REPORT

Plavix (clodiprogel) was omitted/overlooked post discharge from hospital. Myocardial Infarction secondary to thrombosis of coronary stents; heart failure, eventual death

FACTS OF THE CASE

This case is instructive for the application of the pharmacodynamics and pharmacokinetics of this important platelet inhibitor. JD, 73 years old, was admitted to a community hospital on October 9, 2013, complaining of chest pain and dyspnea on exertion and tested positive in a nuclear stress test. He was diagnosed with acute coronary syndrome and scheduled for a cardiac catheterization. Pre-cath medications included heparin infusion (an anticoagulant) and Integrilin (eptifibatide) (GPIIb/IIIa inhibitor) (bolus pre- and post-cath and infusion during the cath). Two coronary vessels (RCA, DIAG) were significantly occluded; each was stented with a DES—drug eluting stent. Plavix 300 mg oral was given post-cath (as a loading dose), followed by Plavix 75 mg every day. He also required a pacemaker installation. Coincidentally, he experienced a septic gouty infection in his lower extremity, was started on antibiotics, and discharged to a Nursing Rehab center on October 16, 2013 to complete the antibiotic treatment.

For some inexplicable reason, the discharging medical resident (MD) did not include Plavix on the discharge medication list. On admission, the assigned internist did not see the patient before his coronary event, which was expected, as he was listed as the Admitting Physician on the Rehab center records. No orders for Plavix were placed. Mr. D did not receive Plavix while at Rehab Center. A physiatrist was consulted for physical/occupational therapy. The physiatrist examined JD on the morning of October 22, 2013, sometime between 9 a.m. and 10:30 a.m. Around 11:30 a.m. to Noon that day, JD complained of significant chest pain and exhibited other symptoms which prompted a call to the assigned (internist) attending physician, and then to 911. EMS took JD to a nearby hospital arriving at 1:11 p.m. At the hospital, JD was started on high-dose heparin, and on 10/23/13, the next day, he underwent cardiac catheterization. A diagnosis of myocardial infarction and thrombosis of the stents is noted in the record.

The legal complaint lists "failure to write necessary and appropriate orders for continuation of Plavix". . . and "failed to consult with a physician from the discharging hospital concerning continuation of Plavix." Plaintiff's physiatry expert criticized the defendant physiatrist for not verifying that the transfer records were complete and not contacting the referring physician.

Plaintiff's cardiology expert opined:

1. JD's deterioration is a direct and proximate result of a deviation from the standard of care of (unnamed) caregivers who failed to administer dual antiplatelet therapy on time preceding his MI on October 22, 2015;
2. That the failure to administer Plavix at the Rehab Center was the cause of the thrombosis and myocardial infarction, admission, and treatment at the (next) hospital;
3. If JD had been given Plavix in a 300-mg loading dose 45 minutes to an hour before the thrombosis/MI, more likely than not, a clot(s) would not have formed that blocked the stent (s);
4. If he had received (Plavix) before October 22, 2015, and after October 20, 2015, with a loading dose of 300 mg at 75 mg a day, it would have prevented the myocardial infarction, and more likely than not he would not have had a myocardial infarction.

Examination of the Rehab Center records indicated their pharmacy was located 20 miles away.

OPINIONS

Even if Plavix had been administered in a "loading" dose of 300 mg at Rehab Center on the morning of 10/22/13, the outcome would have been the same. Absence of Plavix for five days removes any thrombosis protection and the stents were at high risk for thrombosis and the risk increases with each subsequent day. Without the administration of the Plavix, the platelet inhibition effect would return to baseline by day 5.[62] The risk of thrombosis/stent occlusion increases with each day no Plavix is administered. By 10/22/15, no platelet inhibition by Plavix would have remained. Plavix is not a "clot-buster"; it is a platelet inhibitor. It helps prevent the formation of a platelet plug (i.e., clot) directly where the recent coronary stents were inserted.[63]

There is a contradictory testimony by the plaintiff's expert cardiologist. His earlier statement that a loading dose of 300 mg within 45 minutes of the thrombosis/MI would, more likely than not, not have occurred. Contrarily, he stated that (paraphrase) at least three days, the administration of a loading dose of 300 mg Plavix on 10/20, followed by 75 mg Plavix on 10/21 and 75 mg Plavix on 10/22 would be needed to prevent the thrombosis which occurred.

Assuming, arguendo, that Plavix could provide *some* protection and lessen the risk of a myocardial infarction due to the thrombosis of the DES, there was insufficient time for the Plavix to work. Time requirements include:

a. Recognize the need (omission of a platelet inhibitor)
b. Contact the referring physician or the (internist) attending physician—uncertain turn around/response time.
c. Assuming an order was received, that order needs to be transferred by the Rehab Center nursing staff to the Pharmacy (electronic and telephonic notice describing the urgency). The Pharmacy is located 20 miles away, requiring at least 30 minutes driving time, assuming that some transport person/service was immediately available to deliver the Plavix to the Rehab Center.
d. Administration of a 300-mg Plavix on the morning of 10/22/15 would not have any appreciable clinical or pharmacologic effect on preventing the thrombosis of the stents. Once administered in a loading dose (300 mg), (some) platelet inhibition of only 30% (15–40% range) is achieved after 2 hours from the time of administration.[64 65] After single and repeated oral doses of 75 mg per day, clopidogrel is rapidly absorbed. Mean peak plasma levels of unchanged clopidogrel occurred approximately 45 minutes after dosing.[66] Once absorbed, the clopidogrel requires metabolism of the 2 oxo-clopidogrel intermediate metabolite (which) results in the formation of the active metabolite, a thiol derivative of clopidogrel. This metabolism takes further time beyond 45 minutes. The active thiol metabolite, which has been isolated *in vitro*, binds rapidly and irreversibly to platelet receptors, thus inhibiting platelet aggregation. At 45 minutes after a 300-mg dose, less than 15% (mean, range 10–30%) platelet inhibition is achieved. [iv] Dose-dependent platelet inhibition can be seen at two hours. [v] If a resumption of the previous 75 mg daily dose was ordered, 5 days are required to achieve adequate platelet inhibition and steady state effects.
e. The defendant physiatrist examined JD sometime between 9 am and 10:30 am, maybe later (deposition transcript). JD complained of chest pain at 11:30 a.m. to 12 noon.

Considering all the necessary steps described and the necessary time for the drug to be absorbed and work, it is logistically, pharmacokinetically, pharmacologically, and therapeutically impossible that this drug could have been administered and therapeutic effect (significant platelet inhibition) achieved that would have prevented the thromboses that occurred.

Plavix, given in a 300-mg loading dose, even if enough time would have allowed recognition, ordering, acquisition, and administration to Mr. Davis, would not have changed the outcome. The window of time available for the drug to be ordered, obtained, administered, absorbed, and start to work would exceed the available time interval, as described earlier.

The case was scheduled for trial in the Fall of 2022 at the time this chapter was completed.

25.7 SUMMARY AND CONCLUSIONS

The double-edged sword, caution applicable to any medication, is exemplified in anticoagulant therapy. These absolutely essential medications must be used for a variety of medical conditions; there are no substitutes. Pharmacists can better contribute to these patients' care by having a thorough understanding of the clinical pharmacology, indications, toxicity, and selection of anticoagulants to limit such toxicity. These efforts will predictably decrease claims of legal tort against pharmacists and other health workers (no injury/no lawsuit).

NOTES

1 Zehnder JL. Drugs Used in Disorders of Coagulation. In: Katzung BG, Vanderah TW. eds. Basic & Clinical Pharmacology, 15e. McGraw-Hill; 2021. Accessed April 08, 2025. https://accesspharmacy.mhmedical.com/content.aspx?bookid=2988&sectionid=250599717
2 A.M. Wendelboe, G.E. Raskob Global burden of thrombosis. Circ. Res., 118 (9) (2016), pp. 1340-1347
3 Vaqar S, Graber M. Thromboembolic Event. [Updated 2023 May 22]. In: StatPearls [Internet]. Treasure Island (FL): StatPearls Publishing; 2025 Jan-. Available from: https://www.ncbi.nlm.nih.gov/books/NBK549877/
4 Zehnder JL. Drugs Used in Disorders of Coagulation. In: Katzung BG, Vanderah TW. eds. Basic & Clinical Pharmacology, 15e. McGraw-Hill; 2021. Accessed April 08, 2025. https://accesspharmacy.mhmedical.com/content.aspx?bookid=2988&sectionid=250599717
5 Available from: www.pradaxa.com (official prescribing information).

6 Priziola JL, Smythe MA, and Dager WE. Drug-Induced Thrombycotpenia in Critically Ill Patients. Crit Care Med. 2010;39(6 Suppl): SI145–SI154.
7 Available from: www.pradaxa.com (official prescribing information).
8 Warkentin TE. Chapter 2: Clinical Picture of Heparin-Induced Thrombocytopenia. In Warkentin TE and Greinacher A, Eds. Heparin-Induced Thrombocytopenia, 4th Edition. Informa Healthcare, New York, 2007, p. 26.
9 Warkentin TE. Chapter 2: Clinical Picture of Heparin-Induced Thrombocytopenia. In Wakkentin TE and Greinacher A, Eds. Heparin-Induced Thrombocytopenia, 4th Edition. Informa Healthcare, New York, 2007, p. 21.
10 Warkentin TE. Chapter 2: Clinical Picture of Heparin-Induced Thrombocytopenia. In Warkentin TE and Greinacher A, Eds. Heparin-Induced Thrombocytopenia, 4th Edition. Informa Healthcare, New York, 2007, p. 26.
11 Warkentin TE. Chapter 2: Clinical Picture of Heparin-Induced Thrombocytopenia. In Warkentin TE and Greinacher A, Eds. Heparin-Induced Thrombocytopenia, 4th Edition. Informa Healthcare, New York, 2007, p. 21.
12 Alban S and Greinqacher A. Chapter 7: Role of Sulfated Polysaccharides in the Pathogenesis of Heparin-Induced Thrombocytopenia. In Warkentin TE and Greinacher A, Eds. Heparin-Induced Thrombocytopenia, 4th Edition. Informa Healthcare, New York, 2007, p. 172.
13 Alban S and Greinqacher A. Chapter 7: Role of Sulfated Polysaccharides in the Pathogenesis of Heparin-Induced Thrombocytopenia. In Warkentin TE and Greinacher A, Eds. Heparin-Induced Thrombocytopenia, 4th Edition. Informa Healthcare, New York, 2007, p. 172.
14 Bradner JE and Eikkelboom JW. Chapter 17: Emerging Anticoagulants and Heparin-Induced Thrombocytopenia: Indirect and Direct Factor Xa Inhibitors and oral Thrombin Inhibitors. In Wakkentin TE and Greinacher A, Eds. Heparin-Induced Thrombocytopenia, 4th Edition. Informa Healthcare, New York, 2007, p. 444.
15 Antiplatelet, Anticoagulant, and Fibrinolytic Drugs. In Fauci AS, Braunwald E, Kasper DL, Hauser SL, Oongo DL, et al. Eds. Harrison's Principles of Internal Medicine, 17th Edition.
16 Zehender JL. Drugs Used in Disorders of Coagulation. In Katung BG, Masters SB, and Trevor AJ, Eds. Basic and Clinical Pharmacology, 12th Edition. McGraw Hill, New York, 2012.
17 Pouplard C, Gueret P, Foussier M, Ternisien C, Trosssaert M, Regina S, and Gruel Y. Prospective Evaluation of the '4Ts' Score and Particle Gel Immunoassay Specific to Heparin/PF4 for the Diagnosis of Heparin-Induced Thrombocytopenia. J Thromb Haemostasis. July 2007;5(7):1373–1379.
18 NovoSeven® is recombinant human coagulation Factor VIIa (rFVIIa), intended for promoting hemostasis by activating the extrinsic pathway of the coagulation cascade. 1 NovoSeven (coagulation factor via recombinant) is a vitamin K-dependent glycoprotein consisting of 406 amino acid residues (MW 50 K Dalton). NovoSeven (coagulation factor via recombinant) is structurally similar to human plasma-derived Factor VIIa. Priziola JL, Smythe MA, and Dager WE. Drug-Induced Thrombycotpenia in Critically Ill Patients. Crit Care Med. 2010;39(6 Suppl): SI145–SI154.
19 Available from: www.pradaxa.com (official prescribing information).
20 Arepally, Gowthami M, and Ortel TL. Heparin-Induced Thrombocytopenia. N Engl J Med. 2006;355(24): 2598–2599. Print.
21 Alberio L. Heparin-Induced Thrombocytopenia: Some Working Hypotheses on Pathogenesis, Diagnostic Strategies and Treatment. Curr Opin Hematol. 2008;15(5):456–464.
22 Alberio L. Heparin-Induced Thrombocytopenia: Some Working Hypotheses on Pathogenesis, Diagnostic Strategies and Treatment. Curr Opin Hematol. 2008;15(5):456–464.
23 Refaai MA, Phipps RP, Spinelli SL, and Blumberg N. Platelet Transfusions: Impact on Hemostasis, Thrombosis, Inflammation and Clinical Outcomes. Thromb Res. 2011;127(4):287–291. Print.
24 Greinacher A and Warkentin TE. Chapter 12: Treatment of Heparin-Induced Thrombocytopenia: An Overview. In Wakkentin TE and Greinacher A, Eds. Heparin-Induced Thrombocytopenia, 4th Edition. Informa Healthcare, New York, 2007, p. 296.
25 Pouplard C, Gueret P, Foussier M, Ternisien C, Trosssaert M, Regina S, and Gruel Y. Prospective Evaluation of the '4Ts' Score and Particle Gel Immunoassay Specific to Heparin/PF4 for the Diagnosis of Heparin-Induced Thrombocytopenia. J Thromb Haemostasis. July 2007;5(7):1373–1379.
26 Granger CB, Alexander JH, McMurray JJ, Lopes RD, Hylek EM, Hanna M, Al-Khalidi HR, Ansell J, Atar D, Avezum A, and Bahit MC. Apixaban Versus Warfarin in Patients With Atrial Fibrillation. N Engl J Med. 2011;365(11):981–992.
27 Guimarães PO, Pokorney SD, Lopes RD, Wojdyla DM, Gersh BJ, Giczewska A, Carnicelli A, Lewis BS, Hanna M, Wallentin L, Vinereanu D, Alexander JH, and Granger CB. Efficacy and Safety of Apixaban Vs Warfarin in Patients With Atrial Fibrillation and Prior Bioprosthetic Valve Replacement or Valve Repair: Insights From the Aristotle Trial. Clin Cardiol. 2019 May;42(5):568-571. doi: 10.1002/clc.23178. Epub 2019 Apr 9. PMID: 30907005; PMCID: PMC6522998.

28 Zehender JL. Drugs Used in Disorders of Coagulation. In Katung BG, Masters SB, and Trevor AJ, Eds. Basic and Clinical Pharmacology, 12th Edition. McGraw Hill, New York, 2012.
29 NovoSeven® is recombinant human coagulation Factor VIIa (rFVIIa), intended for promoting hemostasis by activating the extrinsic pathway of the coagulation cascade. 1 NovoSeven (coagulation factor via recombinant) is a vitamin K-dependent glycoprotein consisting of 406 amino acid residues (MW 50 K Dalton). NovoSeven (coagulation factor via recombinant) is structurally similar to human plasma-derived Factor VIIa.
30 Refaai MA, Phipps RP, Spinelli SL, and Blumberg N. Platelet Transfusions: Impact on Hemostasis, Thrombosis, Inflammation and Clinical Outcomes. Thromb Res. 2011;127(4):287–291. Print.
31 Connolly SJ, Ezekowitz MD, Yusuf S, Eikelboom J, Oldgren J, Parekh A, Pogue J, Reilly PA, Themeles E, Varrone J, and Wang S; RE-LY Steering Committee and Investigators. Dabigatran Versus Warfarin in Patients With Atrial Fibrillation. N Engl J Med. 2009;361:1139–1151.
32 Refaai MA, Phipps RP, Spinelli SL, and Blumberg N. Platelet Transfusions: Impact on Hemostasis, Thrombosis, Inflammation and Clinical Outcomes. Thromb Res. 2011;127(4):287–291. Print.
33 Warkentin TE. Chapter 2: Clinical Picture of Heparin-Induced Thrombocytopenia. In Warkentin TE and Greinacher A, Eds. Heparin-Induced Thrombocytopenia, 4th Edition. Informa Healthcare, New York, 2007, p. 26.
34 Saliba W. Non-Vitamin K Antagonist Oral Anticoagulatns: New Choices for Patient Management in Atrial Fibrillation. Am J Cariovascular Drugs. 2015;15(5):323–335.
35 Zehender JL. Drugs Used in Disorders of Coagulation. In Katung BG, Masters SB, and Trevor AJ, Eds. Basic and Clinical Pharmacology, 12th Edition. McGraw Hill, New York, 2012.
36 NovoSeven® is recombinant human coagulation Factor VIIa (rFVIIa), intended for promoting hemostasis by activating the extrinsic pathway of the coagulation cascade. 1 NovoSeven (coagulation factor via recombinant) is a vitamin K-dependent glycoprotein consisting of 406 amino acid residues (MW 50 K Dalton). NovoSeven (coagulation factor via recombinant) is structurally similar to human plasma-derived Factor VIIa.
37 Available from: www.pradaxa.com (official prescribing information).
38 Arepally, Gowthami M, and Ortel TL. Heparin-Induced Thrombocytopenia. N Engl J Med. 2006;355(24):2598–2599. Print.
39 Warkentin TE. Chapter 2: Clinical Picture of Heparin-Induced Thrombocytopenia. In Warkentin TE and Greinacher A, Eds. Heparin-Induced Thrombocytopenia, 4th Edition. Informa Healthcare, New York, 2007, p. 26.
40 Alberio L. Heparin-Induced Thrombocytopenia: Some Working Hypotheses on Pathogenesis, Diagnostic Strategies and Treatment. Curr Opin Hematol. 2008;15(5):456–464.
41 Lip GY, Nieuwlaat R, Pisters R, Lane DA and Crijns HJ. Refining Clinical Risk Stratification for Predicting Stroke and Thromboembolism in Atrial Fibrillation Using a Novel Risk Factor-Based Approach: The Euro Heart Survey on Atrial Fibrillation. Chest. 2010;137(2):263–272.
42 Available from: www.pradaxa.com (official prescribing information).
43 Glund S, Stangier J, Schmohl M, et al. Idarucizumab Reverses the Anticoagulant Effect of Dabigatran in Healthy Men. The Lancet. 15 Jun 2015.
44 Ward C, Conner G, Donnan G, Gallus A and McRae S. Practical Management of Patients on Apixaban: A Consensus Guide. Thrombosis J. 2013;11:27. doi: 10.1186/1477-9560-11-27.
45 Horlocker TT, Vandermeulen E, Kopp SL, Gogarten W, Leffert LR and Benzon HT. Regional Anesthesia in the Patient Receiving Antithrombotic or Thrombolytic Therapy: American Society of Regional Anesthesia and Pain Medicine Evidence-Based Guidelines (Fourth Edition). Reg Anesth Pain Med. 2018 Apr;43(3):263–309.
46 Wagner J, Lock JF, Kastner C, Klein I, Krajinovic K, Löb S, Germer CT and Wiegering A. Perioperative Management of Anticoagulant Therapy. Innov Surg Sci. 2019;4(4):144–151. Published 2019 Jul 18. doi: 10.1515/iss-2019-0004.
47 Wagner J, Lock JF, Kastner C, Klein I, Krajinovic K, Löb S, Germer CT and Wiegering A. Perioperative Management of Anticoagulant Therapy. Innov Surg Sci. 2019;4(4):144–151. Published 2019 Jul 18. doi: 10.1515/iss-2019-0004.
48 Leitch J and van Vlymen J. Managing the Perioperative Patient on Direct Oral Anticoagulants. Can J Anaesth. 2017 Jun;64(6):656–672. English. doi: 10.1007/s12630-017-0868-2. Epub 2017 Apr 20. PMID: 28429198.
49 Wagner J, Lock JF, Kastner C, Klein I, Krajinovic K, Löb S, Germer CT and Wiegering A. Perioperative Management of Anticoagulant Therapy. Innov Surg Sci. 2019;4(4):144–151. Published 2019 Jul 18. doi: 10.1515/iss-2019-0004.
50 Leitch J and van Vlymen J. Managing the Perioperative Patient on Direct Oral Anticoagulants. Can J Anaesth. 2017 Jun;64(6):656–672. English. doi: 10.1007/s12630-017-0868-2. Epub 2017 Apr 20. PMID: 28429198.
51 Ward C, Conner G, Donnan G, Gallus A and McRae S. Practical Management of Patients on Apixaban: A Consensus Guide. Thrombosis J. 2013;11:27. doi: 10.1186/1477-9560-11-27.

52 Patel G. Personal Communication, May 18, 2022.
53 Douketis JD, Spyropoulos AC, Duncan J, Carrier M, Le Gal G, Tafur AJ, Vanassche T, Verhamme P, Shivakumar S, Gross PL, Lee AYY, Yeo E, Solymoss S, Kassis J, Le Templier G, Kowalski S, Blostein M, Shah V, MacKay E, Wu C, Clark NP, Bates SM, Spencer FA, Arnaoutoglou E, Coppens M, Arnold DM, Caprini JA, Li N, Moffat KA, Syed S, and Schulman S. Perioperative Management of Patients With Atrial Fibrillation Receiving a Direct Oral Anticoagulant. JAMA Intern Med. 2019 Nov 1;179(11):1469–1478. doi: 10.1001/jamainternmed.2019.2431. PMID: 31380891; PMCID: PMC6686768.
54 Douketis JD and Lip G. Perioperative Management of Patients Receiving Anticoagulants. Updated January 2022. Accessed 6 February 2022. https://www.uptodate.com/contents/perioperative-management-of-patients-receiving-anticoagulants.
55 Horlocker TT, Vandermeuelen E, Kopp SL, Gogarten W, Leffert LR, and Benzon HT. Regional Anesthesia in the Patient Receiving Antithrombotic or Thrombolytic Therapy: American Society of Regional Anesthesia and Pain Medicine Evidence-Based Guidelines (Fourth Edition). Reg Anesth Pain Med. 2018 Apr;43(3):263–309.
56 Gotoh S, Yasaka M, Nakamura A, Kuwashiro T, and Okada Y. Management of Antithrombotic Agents During Surgery or Other Kinds of Medical Procedures With Bleeding: The MARK Study. J Am Heart Assoc. 2020 Mar 3;9(5):e012774.
57 Gotoh S, Yasaka M, Nakamura A, Kuwashiro T, and Okada Y. Management of Antithrombotic Agents During Surgery or Other Kinds of Medical Procedures With Bleeding: The MARK Study. J Am Heart Assoc. 2020 Mar 3;9(5):e012774.
58 Omran H, Bauersachs R, Rübenacker S, Goss F, and Hammerstingl C. The HAS-BLED Score Predicts Bleedings During Bridging of Chronic Oral Anticoagulation: Results From the National Multicentre BNK Online bRiDging REgistRy (BORDER). Thromb Haemost. 2012 Jul;108(1):65–73. doi: 10.1160/TH11-12-0827. Epub 2012 Apr 26. PMID: 22534746.
59 Polania Gutierrez JJ and Rocuts KR. Perioperative Anticoagulation Management. [Updated 2021 Aug 11]. In: StatPearls [Internet]. Treasure Island (FL): StatPearls Publishing; 2022 January. Available from: https://www.ncbi.nlm.nih.gov/books/NBK557590/.
60 Eliquis Product Insert.
61 Available from: https://www.drugs.com/newdrugs/fda-approves-eliquis-reduce-risk-stroke-blood-clots-patients-non-valvular-atrial-fibrillation-3618.html.
62 Clodiprogrel Monograph. Drug Information 2006. American Hospital Formulary Service. ASHP, Bethesday, 2006.
63 Deposition testimony of plaintiff's cardiologist expert, 4/17/20.
64 Price MJ, Coleman JL, Steinhubl SR, Wong GB, Cannon CP, and Teirstein PS. Onset and Offset of Platelet Inhibition After High-Dose Clopidogrel Loading and Standard Daily Therapy Measured by a Point of Care Assay I Healthy Volunteers. Am J Cardiol. 2006;98:681–684.
65 Plavix Package Inset. Sanofi, 2017.
66 Available from: https://www.accessdata.fda.gov/drugsatfda_docs/label/2009/020839s044lbl.pdf.

Part III

Pharmacists, Pharmacy, and Pharmacy Practice

26 Pharmacy Practice, Managed Care, and Manufacturers

F. Randy Vogenberg and Rita Marcoux

Editorial Assistance by Christopher Hartley

SYNOPSIS

26.1 INTRODUCTION TO PHARMACY AND THE RELATED MANAGED HEALTHCARE ENVIRONMENT

Managed healthcare and federal reimbursement policy shifts have affected pharmacy policy and practice to different degrees over the past 15 years. This chapter will focus on how specific changes at the federal level have reverberated through pharmacies in all settings including hospitals, long-term care facilities, and retail. Since 2013, institutional revenue streams were realized from successful, short hospital stays and single day surgical procedures. The number of admissions across all types of hospitals fell as did patient days into 2018. Yet, the number of hospital days per 1,000 *non*-Medicare HMO members continued to grow somewhat, while Medicare HMO patients rose at a higher rate of growth in general [1]. From 2016 to 2017, the average length of stay (ALOS) per Medicare length of stay increased, with the largest year to year increase and the longest recorded ALOS in 2017. Increase in length of stay with chronic disease states such as acute coronary syndrome, asthma, diabetes mellitus, hypertension, prostate cancer, rheumatoid arthritis, and stoke could point toward an increase in the number of patients who require these services or could mean that they are staying longer to prevent readmission at discharge. Another CMS initiative (Never Event Policy) was to hold hospitals accountable for outcomes of care post-discharge typically in a 30-day window. Managed care totals of Medicare spending decreased between 2017 and 2018, representing the first reduction

DOI: 10.1201/9781003615323-29

in share since 2006. This dip occurred while Medicare Advantage (MA) enrollment grew at a faster rate in 2018 that continued into 2021. What the effect of the pandemic which started in 2020–2023 will have on Medicare remains to be seen [2].

The impact of COVID-19 has been far-reaching for all healthcare delivery or medical office entities. COVID care dominated the inpatient setting, pushing off elective and increasingly more emergency care that can be managed at home or alternate care sites. Similarly, COVID-19 dampened the rising rate of outpatient or day surgeries being performed in the United States, while COVID testing has dominated Urgent Care sites affiliated or not affiliated with hospitals/health systems.

Commercially insured lives can dominate healthcare utilization and out-of-hospital care—which is where managed care has incented plan members to get care. Drugs used in both scenarios of care setting must be efficacious, possessing few side effects or other interactions that could interfere with these goals. Pharmacists must be more attuned to patient outcomes being achieved quickly and safely, including the avoidance of troublesome returns to the hospital after discharge especially in light of Center for Medicare and Medicaid Services (CMS) never-event policies.

A widely cited report on medication errors and their associated mortality, morbidity, and financial cost in the United States has been produced by the Institute of Medicine (IoM—renamed from the National Academy of Medicine until July 2016). In the continuing response to the IoM—National Academy of Medicine's report and numerous articles highlighting the impact on quality of life and economic waste, The Joint Commission (TJC) has committed to assisting organizations in medication error prevention. The National Patient Safety Goal (NPSG) 03.06.01, focusing on medication reconciliation, has been part of its accreditation criteria for hospitals since 2005. Many hospitals have placed pharmacists in the emergency room to manage medication order verification and for ordering in their attempt to meet NPSG 03.06.01 requirements. In addition, many hospitals have increased their management of education regarding discharge from a hospital or outpatient encounter. Pharmacist-driven "Meds to beds" programs have continually popped up, as well as discharge counseling provided at bedside prior to discharge. However, organizations continue to struggle with the implementation and maintenance of effective processes in support of this NPSG. The Joint Commission understands the limitations on accurately documenting patient medication histories and seeks a good faith effort in meeting the goal in assessing performance. The Joint Commission's focus is on positively impacting the risk points on medication reconciliation for patients [3].

At the same time that hospital costs and quality are being monitored, patient satisfaction continues to grow in importance for determining who gets the inpatient care business from payers. This is known as integrating reasonable costs with highest possible quality, which some analysts try to calculate through a cost/quality ratio. Patient surveys to determine the degree of satisfaction with services provided often include questions about drugs and/or pharmacist services, if applicable.

How these many managed care changes are impacting the three major types of pharmacy settings can be described as follows. Systems of care for a geographic region have emerged through strategic alliances and organizational mergers. Each has reduced redundant services, including general pharmacies, and increased alternatives to hospital and physician care, including specialized pharmacies. This strategy optimizes drug use outcomes, while maintaining economic efficiency.

In July 1998, a new reimbursement program was implemented for Medicare's Part A services in long-term care, sub-acute care, and home care domains. This program is known as the Prospective Payment System (PPS) and operates similar to the way that Diagnosis-Related Groupings (DRGs) functioned in hospitals. Rather than being reimbursed on a fee-for-service basis, nursing homes and others must now categorize patients and their needs according to specific assessments required by the Centers for CMS. The PPS system's daily rates are adjusted for geographic differences in labor costs and case mix. Case mix adjustments are done using a system known as Resource Utilization Groups (RUGs). The RUGs classification assigns patients to groups based on the patient characteristics and services expected to be required. The number of groups within the RUGs has increased from 44 to 66 in RUGs IV. CMS released a proposal that would include new quality reporting programs and staffing information beginning in 2016 as required by the Social Security Act. The result of these changes continues to require these organizations to re-evaluate the way in which they do business, including contracting for pharmaceuticals and pharmacy consultative services. Pharmacists who provide drugs or monthly patient chart reviews will be challenged to maintain high quality in a lowered cost reimbursement environment. As seen in hospitals, larger organizations that can spread the financial risk over a greater number of patients or services will likely do better than independent operators.

All types of ambulatory and community-based care are growing in this environment. Outpatient visits for day surgery, disease monitoring, and preventive care have continuously grown over the past five years, to the point where most hospitals' occupancy rates can fall below 50%. In turn, however, intensive care units' (ICUs') occupancy remains strong and is growing, as people are sicker by the time they reach the hospital. As a result, changes have become necessary, as far as the number of staff and the personnel matrix required running a more acute care (compared to maintenance level) hospital service. Long-term care facilities now offer a wider range of services—including intravenous drug administration—that generate different staffing and pharmacy needs. Similarly, community-based (retail) pharmacists are supplying drugs and information to patients who otherwise would have been hospitalized in the 1990s to early 2000s. Increasing fiscal pressure combined with advances in care technology outside acute hospital care settings has furthered the movement of patients to receive care outside the traditional hospital institution. Furthermore, pharmacists are changing their roles to become more like drug information consultants, immunizers for vaccinations, and care or drug use documentation advisors (both for patients and prescribers).

From another perspective, in multihospital systems of care (compared to independent organizations) until the 2019 pandemic:

- Outpatient surgeries per day continued to increase overall
- Outpatient visits overall per day increased
- Emergency department visits per day increased slightly
- Average length of stay (ALOS) fell for all facilities slightly
- Total costs per admission increased due to care acuity and patient mix
- Acute care hospitals were staffed with more physician assistants and advanced practice nurses, along with utilizing hospitalists

These trends and figures overall speak to the efficiencies that may be gained from the new order of where healthcare delivery is provided, as well as the changes required by hospitals, long-term care facilities, and retail pharmacies [4–6]. The post-pandemic staffing and care levels for patients outside the hospital remain to seen. It is clear for now that telehealth and remote patient monitoring in the home had been used heavily during the pandemic are likely to continue forward, albeit at some reduced level.

Managed care has also played a role in various aspects of hospital but especially community based care. A significant portion of pharmacy benefit managers' (PBM) revenues are derived from retaining a percentage of the drug price or rebates obtained through negotiation. Therefore, a PBM's profit may be less with a lower-cost drug compared with a higher-priced medication. Employers still believe that their PBM is managing all the costs in the value chain; yet, there are significant issues with the current economic model, which result in higher costs, without equivalent value for employers. PBMs began as the broker and claims payer in the middle, negotiating the best price and service on the employer's behalf. Many became out-patient pharmacies by offering mail-order services, and some developed relationships with retail pharmacy chains. This created a channel conflict, with some PBMs pushing patients to preferred networks, formularies, and their own mandatory mail-order programs, which drove their profit [7].

All businesses are now facing new privacy obligations due to a 2020 California ballot measure known as proposition 24—the California Privacy Rights Act of 2020 (CPRA) [8]. Currently, the California Consumer Privacy Act of 2018 (CCPA) applies to any such business that meets any one of three main criteria [9]. In addition, now, despite CPRA being California legislation, any employer or business, regardless of where located, who has a California employee, accepts applications from California residents for positions anywhere in the nation, has customers in California who are natural persons, or otherwise does business in California (including internet) may be subject to the CPRA and CCPA. A big area of focus for these efforts is around data, and healthcare is reliant on an ever-expanding collection or use of data so this becomes relevant for the stakeholders mentioned in this chapter. Some exemptions are available, and implementation is planned for January 1, 2023.

26.2 PHARMACISTS AS HEALTHCARE PROFESSIONALS: TRAINING, SUPPORT STAFF, AND LIFE-LONG LEARNING

26.2.1 Registration, Certifications, Credentialing, Colleges of Pharmacy, and Accreditation Matters for Pharmacy Professional Staff

Like physicians and other licensed professionals, pharmacists are compelled to redefine their roles in the delivery system in the face of dominant market penetration by managed care pharmacy programs. Threatened by new technology-driven distribution channels for prescription drugs, pharmacists are increasingly searching for expanded areas to optimize their clinical expertise. The need for additional primary providers and the focus on improving the medication outcomes offer pharmacists an opportunity to expand their role in the system and maximize their significant advantage—frequent interaction with the patient. Pharmacists' direct patient contact has placed them in a unique position to play a vital role in Medication Therapy Management (MTM) and limited primary care services. In effect, pharmacists are positioned to be the driving force in delivering "hands-on" service to patients in dispensing drugs and monitoring their treatment, healthcare education, specific disease management, and other related services critical to patient treatment and positive medical outcomes.

The Pharm.D. (Doctor of Pharmacy) is the sole educational degree for pharmacists in the United States as of June 2005. The Pharm.D. curriculum emphasis is on advanced biopharmaceutical sciences, pharmacotherapy, and clinical rotations. Disease management in various patient-care settings is a critical component of the programs. This degree may require six to eight years of academic education. Nontraditional learning programs have emerged in pharmacy, enabling expanded numbers of pharmacists with baccalaureate degrees to learn via remote, collaborative, or online courses. These programs lead to the Pharm.D. degree for B.Sc. pharmacists seeking an advanced clinical focus. Some institutional programs allow entrance from high school. In contrast, other institutions require two years of pre-pharmacy courses and the PCAT exam passage before students may apply to their program.

According to the American Association of Colleges of Pharmacy (AACP), there were 142 U.S.-based schools and colleges of pharmacy with accreditation status as of December, 2023.[1] This number has increased from about 80 programs in 2002 [10]. Class sizes range from 34 to over 300 students as enrollment at institutions grew, along with the number of colleges and schools. The student demographics have shifted over the last 25 years. Today, students comprise over 60% women and 17% underrepresented minorities [11]. Institutions reported 50,842 applications for the 2020–21 academic year, significantly reduced from the peak of 109,150 applicants in 2009 [12]. The number of students completing the Pharm.D. degree in May 2019 was 14,8000. Accreditation Council for Pharmacy Education (ACPE) released new standards for colleges' accreditation in January 2016. The new standards incorporated feedback from stakeholders and emphasized developing a curriculum that offers students the opportunities to develop the competencies and confidence needed to be part of a multidisciplinary healthcare team, emphasizing practice and communication skills. ACPE standards' objectives ensure that students are practice-ready upon completion of their terminal degree. The curriculum's goals are to develop professionals and lifelong learners. The 2016 standards increased the number of experiential hours required for the completion of the program [13]. Pharm.D graduates are required to pass a national licensure exam for state licensure. The National Association of Board of Pharmacy (NABP) coordinates the North American Pharmacy Licensing Examination (NAPLEX). This comprehensive exam evaluates the general practice knowledge of graduates. NABP limits a candidate to five-lifetime attempts at passage. Candidates apply for licensure for specific states at the time of examination. However, NABP allows NAPLEX scores to be transferred to additional states to meet the state's licensure requirements. In addition to the NAPLEX exam, most Boards of Pharmacy administer a Multistate Pharmacy Jurisprudence Exam (MPJE) to graduates seeking licensure within their state. Graduates must demonstrate the knowledge of federal and state-specific laws and regulations applicable to pharmacy practice across all practice settings. Idaho has recently removed the MPJE requirement for licensure. Idaho's applicants for licensure must attest to the knowledge of state and federal laws and regulations in place of taking an exam. Other states Boards of Pharmacy are discussing the merits of the MPJE versus an attestation of regulatory knowledge.

While in the final year of their Pharm.D. program, many students opt to continue their educational experiences through one- or two-year residency or fellowship programs. Most students apply for residencies through the American Society of Hospital Pharmacy (ASHP). ASHP has 5,327 accredited residency positions, including Post Graduate Year 1 (PGY1) and Post Graduate Year 2 (PGY2) sites [14]. There are also nonaccredited programs that attract graduating students. Under the guidance of a preceptor, the PGY1 resident receives applied training in various patient care settings. Residents are required to be licensed pharmacists while completing their PGY1 residency. Many PGY1 residents continue their education in a PGY2 program. PGY2 residency prepares the pharmacist in a specialized area of practice. Upon completing a PGY2 residency, pharmacists are ready to participate as medication experts in specialized areas such as transplants, critical care, pediatrics, oncology, and cardiac care. While students pursuing a residency are generally interested in clinical care, those seeking fellowships are interested in indirect patient care. Fellowships are typically based in corporate environments. Students develop skills in research, presentations, and critical thinking. These programs offer experience in regulatory affairs, clinical research and development, medical affairs, and the industry's commercial aspects. The fellowships may be one- or two-year programs. For example, Rutgers Institute for Pharmaceutical Industry Fellowships is a partnership with 17 companies, which offers over 250 fellowships for Pharm.D. and MDs [15].

To ensure licensed pharmacists' continued competency, all 50 state Pharmacy Practice Acts require pharmacists to acquire a minimum number of continuing professional education (CPE) hours for re-licensure. Most states require pharmacists to complete a minimum of 15 contact hours of CPE yearly. States vary on the specifics included within these 15 hours. The most common requirement is specified live or web-based activity hours. Some states require a limited number of hours dedicated to selected topics—such as regulatory, medication errors, or treatment for specific diseases such as substance abuse disorders. With the expanding scope of practice, Boards of Pharmacy have identified job-specific CPE, such as compounding and nuclear pharmacy. Pharmacists who wish to maintain active registration as an immunizing pharmacist or board-certified pharmacist or practice under a collaborative practice agreement must meet the area-specific CPE requirements. These CPE specific hours vary by state. In many states, pharmacists who fail to meet the CPE requirements are subject to immediate license revocation upon a pharmacy audit board. NABP has facilitated the record-keeping and monitoring of CPE through their online CPE Monitor. Pharmacists and Boards of Pharmacy can quickly query the system to monitor annual credit hours acquired and topic areas. Boards of Pharmacy use this system to verify the licensed pharmacist's attestation that the licensure requirements for CPE credits have been met.

While it is essential that pharmacists meet the state requirement for licensure, specific documentation around certifying the medical staff members is a required activity of hospitals and other entities. The inclusion of primary source verification in the credentialing process is an important development for current credentialing practices. Traditionally, hospitals and plans relied upon copies of documentation and other information supplied by the physician. However, the marketplace's demands for quality assurance and pressure from government regulators for greater accountability have forced the industry to focus its attention on increasing the performance standards in this area. This stringent requirement is reflected in the most recent standards adopted by industry accreditation bodies, including the National Committee for Quality Assurance (NCQA), American Accreditation Program, Inc. (AAPI), Utilization Review Accreditation Commission (URAC), and The Joint Commission. Many of these regulatory boards require re-certification or licensure approximately every three years. The federal government recognizes these boards that are typically nonprofit organizations to avoid potential claims of economic biases related to speed and standards or accreditation. Some of these organizations, particularly the NCQA, release publicly available report cards on the facilities that it certifies yearly, giving its accreditation slightly more weight than organizations that review facilities every few years.

In managed care, NCQA involves a process of certifying members of the medical staff and other primary care providers who come in contact with patients. Articles in insurance and professional journals underscore the practice changes for pharmacists and other allied health provider credentialing. Quality management in managed care covers a broad range of activities, which managed care plans must undertake to meet their industry's accreditation standards. Among these activities, credentialing of participating health professionals plays a critical role. As a management process, credentialing has evolved over the years and has been adapted to meet the managed care environment's unique needs. It is, in effect, an objective assessment process intended to both validate each provider's training and experience and serve as the vehicle to evaluate performance. In managed care credentialing, the emphasis is on individual performance. The need for managed care plans to credential network providers is now well-documented. Recent judicial decisions, imposing liability for physician malpractice on the plan, no longer permit plans to rely on a hospital's credentialing process [16]. Moreover, several empirical studies substantiate the need for greater accuracy in the credentialing process through the independent verification of credential's information from the primary (original) source of information [17].

In response to these changes, post-licensing education has expanded to allow pharmacists to specialize in specific areas. As early as 1976, the Board of Pharmaceutical Specialties, an autonomous division of the American Pharmacist Association, began offering certification in five specialties. Today, this organization has 50,000 pharmacists worldwide that are certified in 14 specialties [18]. The Council on Credentialing in Pharmacy (CCP) was founded in 1999. It is a coalition of 11 national organizations with a vested interest in the profession of pharmacy. These organizations focus on credentialing programs that impact or are relevant to pharmacy. Over the last 20 years, the organizations that form this coalition have developed standards for credentialing programs. Over 23 certification programs are currently available for pharmacists through one of these organizations [19]. Additionally, URAC has developed several accreditation programs focused on pharmacy services such as mail-order pharmacy, specialty pharmacy, PBM services, and drug therapy management. These accreditation programs are becoming a standard for entry into segments of the market. Board certification, continuing medical education, and other expert training and experience are becoming the entry-level expectation of practitioners. This emphasis on specialization is fueling the demand for residency programs across the country as newly graduating pharmacists are challenged to transition into these recently expanded practice models of care quickly.

With the expansion of pharmacists' services, the support personnel education and competencies have been at the state Boards of Pharmacy's focus. Many of the distribution functions performed by licensed pharmacists have been transferred to technicians and technology. Pharmacy technicians hold positions in a wide variety of healthcare settings, including community practice, military, long-term care, hospital, and managed care organizations, to name a few. The role of the technician has evolved to handle many of the technical aspects of dispensing prescriptions. A pharmacy technician works under the supervision of a pharmacist, responsible for the care of the patients. They may handle routine prescription refilling and assist with new prescription processing. As the technician's scope of services has increased, so has the number of states developing regulations governing the pharmacy technician's education, training, and responsibilities. Currently, 45 states regulate technicians through some type of licensure, registration, or certification process. Of these 45 states, 29 have regulations specific to the mandatory training of technicians. In 22 states, the Board of Pharmacy requires technicians to pass a national examination [20]. NABP and Council on Credentialing in Pharmacy have released proposals to encourage states to require certification of all technicians. The Pharmacy Technician Certification Board's (PTCB) certification program includes enrolling in their Education/Training program or completing 500 hours of work experience. Upon the completion of training, the candidate must successfully pass the Pharmacy Technician Certificate Exam. Candidates require criminal disclosures [21]. Alternatively, candidates may use the National Healthcareer Association's program and ExCPT to acquire their Certified Pharmacy Technician Certificate [22]. Like pharmacists, states may require criminal background screenings and fingerprinting to check criminal records before licensure and certification. In many states, potential technicians must have a high school diploma or equivalent and maintain a criminal record devoid of felony convictions or pending charges for five years. They may not have any previous felony convictions involving controlled substances found or used within the pharmacy. Most states have continuing education requirements to maintain licensure. In many states, this requirement is annual, although some states have a review every two years. State boards of pharmacy usually require between 5 to 10 continuing education credits per year. However, some states require job-specific training or certification for technicians. PTCB has 11 Advanced Certification options, including sterile compounding, immunization, and controlled substance diversion prevention. As of December 2020, PTCB worked with approximately 280,000 certified technicians [23].

States' regulations allow certified technicians to call physicians, take refill orders, immunize patients, and check other technicians before refilling medications. These certified technicians' job function is at the supervising pharmacist's discretion to the extent allowed under current state regulations. Many states have ratios in place to limit the number of supportive personnel that a pharmacist may supervise at any one time. These ratios would include registered or certified technicians, in addition to a pharmacist intern (or extern, in some states). For example, a state may allow no more than three supportive personnel per pharmacist (a three-to-one ratio), provided that at least one of the three supportive personnel is a certified pharmacy technician or an intern. With the increasing level of education required by technicians, states are beginning to re-evaluate these ratios. As these support personnel take over many of the dispensing tasks, pharmacists can manage their patients' more complex medication problems and embrace the expanding regulations that allow the pharmacists to prescribe within newly passed regulations. Regardless of certification and regulations, the ultimate responsibility for the technician's work remains with the responsible pharmacist.

26.3 PRACTICE SITES: INPATIENT, AMBULATORY/COMMUNITY, SPECIALTY, LONG-TERM CARE, AND OTHER (COMPOUNDING, NUCLEAR)

26.3.1 Practice Settings, Practice Site Certification, Pharmacist Practice versus the Business of Pharmacy, Credentialing, and Accreditation Matters

Managed care plans have begun exercising greater selectivity in contracting with medical professionals in response to employer and government requirements for greater quality assurance and transparency. Quality and accountability are significant themes heard in today's healthcare marketplace—including managed care organizations, employers, and payers. Increasingly, both government and private sector purchasers of healthcare services are searching for ways to differentiate the many healthcare providers in this highly competitive market. While most of the attention is presently focused on the physicians' role, all healthcare professionals are being subjected to increasing scrutiny of their qualifications and performance.

Traditionally, pharmacists have worked within the walls of the pharmacy. However, the last two decades have seen an expansion of their practice sites in institution, ambulatory, and community settings. The advanced education and credentialing of these practitioners have expanded expectations to include a wide range of responsibilities outside the distribution of medications. This expansion has resulted from the profession pushing the boundaries of practice to utilize their training and a need for primary care providers to meet patient care demands. Specialized medicine and the aging baby boomer population continue to create the perfect environment for advanced practice pharmacists. Pharmacists are already servicing many of these patients as data from the National Health and Nutrition Examination Survey and the Canadian Health Measures Survey indicates that 69% of adults between 40 and 79 years of age took 1 drug in the last 30 days while 22.4% took 5 drugs. Many of these patients are taking medications to manage chronic diseases such as diabetes, cardiovascular, and depression [24]. Additionally, nearly nine in ten Americans live within five miles of a community pharmacy or have access through telepharmacy [25]. The pharmacist is the member of the healthcare team most easily accessible to patients.

Pharmacists continue to push for legislation that allows for providers' status and the ability to be reimbursed for clinical services provided. Currently, pharmacists have provider status in over 37 states and territories [26]. Although each state's Board of Pharmacy regulates pharmacy practice, CMS continues to innovate the Medicare and Medicaid programs with an emphasis and payment pressure for quality of care and cost-effective use of resources supporting the expanded practice for pharmacists. A significant component of the Medicare Part D program is the Medication Management Therapy (MTM) programs offered by plan sponsors. MTMs are Comprehensive Medication Review (CMR) and disease management programs. These programs monitor patients for medication appropriateness, adherence, and complications that may lead to adverse events. The sponsor plans must include patients with multiple chronic diseases taking multiple Part D drugs and are likely to reach a certain annually determined drug cost threshold. These programs are patient-centered and include high-touch interventions to engage patients in their care. CMS requires that these programs be developed in cooperation with licensed and practicing pharmacists and physicians. CMS has approved pharmacists as providers for services reimbursed under the MTM provision and made significant changes in plan sponsor requirements for MTM programs in 2010. They also increased the number of beneficiaries who qualify for this intervention with expanded criteria and elimination of the opt-in method of patient enrollment. At a minimum, the plan sponsor must offer an annual comprehensive medication review that is interactive, person to person, or using telehealth technology. The CMR should be by a pharmacist or qualified provider and includes OTC and herbal products to qualifying enrollees targeted at least quarterly for enrollment [27]. In 2017, CMS launched Part D Enhanced Medication Therapy Management Model with a five-year performance period ending December 2021. CMS selected six sponsor plans for the program and offered payment incentives and regulatory flexibility to participate. The goal was innovative strategies to optimize medication and improve therapeutic outcomes through appropriate changes to MTM services. The second annual independent evaluation reported changes to MTM service that broadened eligibility, enhanced analytics on measurements, and added new interventions. The report's review of programs did not find a significant impact on Medicare expenditures. While inpatient and skilled nursing services' cost declined, outpatient spending increased. The model found similar difficulties of the traditional model in getting prescribers to adopt and implement recommendations. Also, more significant prescriber–patient interaction could be leading to the increase in outpatient use and spending [28]. These findings do not detract from the improvement in patient care seen by the reduction in inpatient and skilled nursing service, 300,000 more services that were delivered, and a significantly larger percentage of enrollees eligible for 2 plus interventions in year 2 [29].

CMS routinely audits sponsors' MTM programs. Plan sponsors are responsible for measuring and reporting to CMS on the outcomes of their MTM programs. Increasingly, purchasers are limiting contracts to health plans and providers with demonstrated quality services. MTMs continue to offer pharmacists opportunities to market their clinical expertise as recognized providers under CMS. Many pharmacists work independently with enterprises such as OutcomesMTM, Cardinal Health, and Mirixa Corporation. In contrast, other pharmacists work with their employers to consult with patients and bill plan sponsors for MTM assessment and interventions. Colleges/schools of pharmacy have included MTM skills in their curriculum as required by ACPE Standards 2016 for accreditations. Their CPE offices offer the American Pharmacists Association certification program to ensure that licensed pharmacists employ best practice guidelines when offering MTM services [30].

Many pharmacists continue to develop their practices under Collaborative Practice Agreements (CPAs) with prescribers. CPAs create formal relationships between pharmacists and physicians or other providers, which allow for expanded services the pharmacist can provide to patients and the healthcare team. CPAs define the specific patient care functions that a pharmacist can autonomously provide under defined situations and conditions. Nationally recognized guidelines are essential components of these CPAs. Currently, 47 states allow pharmacists to participate in some form of CPAs. However, the requirements might include the pharmacist's board certification, limiting the functions to modify or adjust but not initiate therapy, including the administration of medications and therapeutic substitution [31].

Advanced practice competencies are essential in the Specialty Pharmacy sector. Specialty medications account for close to 50% of the U.S. drug spend [32]. Some of these medications are monitored through a Risk Evaluation and Mitigation Strategy (REMS) by the FDA. The REMS requirement may be simply the mandate for dispensing with a specific patient information leaflet. However, many require the tracking of adherence, limited distribution of the product, and patient registries. Increasingly, the pharmaceutical industry manages the REMS by limiting the distribution of their product to select pharmacies capable of interacting and overseeing the patients on the medication. Often, the specialty providers have pursued accreditation through URAC, The Joint Commission, or other organizations in this arena. Many of their clinical pharmacists are board-certified in specialty areas to manage patients with complex health issues and complex medications. The pharmacists may work under CPA with physicians to manage dosing and side effects and request the required prior authorization from insurers. Pharmacists are essential in helping physicians evaluate the newly released biosimilars available for treatment. Product selection that minimizes adverse drug events and reduces cost for patients enhances adherence. Adherence is critical to optimize health outcomes in these patients. Specialty pharmacies stress their ability to facilitate access to the correct specialty medication, ensuring cost-effective, therapeutic management of these high-cost patients.

Now consider the typical acute hospital patient today who is over age 65 with multisystem diseases. These patients are being admitted and managed at hospitals for one or more acute exacerbations of their underlying diseases. Upon arrival, pharmacy initiates a medication reconciliation to assure a safe entry into the system's care. Pharmacy personnel identify the most accurate list of medication that a patient is taking. The importance of initial drug assessment with medication reconciliation, aggressive polypharmacy intervention, and coordination in pharmaceutical care has been highlighted for older adult patients by healthcare professionals and payors such as CMS. Pharmacists are playing a pivotal role in assisting these institutions in meeting these quality measures. Their job goes beyond medication distribution to include direct patient care. As members of the medical team, pharmacists consult with prescribers on diagnosis, review charts, and recommend medication treatment for patients. They monitor patients for adverse drug events and adjust dosing. Pharmacists are visible in intensive care units, emergency rooms, surgical suites, and other medications intensive specialties such as transplants and oncology. The trend toward value-based payment models necessitates the clinical expertise of advanced practice pharmacists. The pharmacists' recommendations reduce readmission and prevent never-events such as deep venous thrombosis (DVT) and hospital-acquired infections. Pharmacists monitor patient medications and develop patient transition of care plans from hospital to home or rehabilitative facilities. These plans address the modification to previous medication therapy that routinely occurs for hospitalized patients. Pharmacists work with patients to facilitate medication availability upon discharge to help minimize adherence issues, resulting in non-billable readmission. CMS continues to push for quality improvement with its initiatives, such as identifying 11 hospital-acquired conditions resultant from noncompliance with best practice guidelines and its process of care measure data requirements that support initiatives such as the Hospital Care website. This CMS-sponsored website allows consumers to compare local hospitals based on patient surveys on quality of care as well as objective data on efficaciousness of treatment for key conditions such as heart attacks, pneumonia, and infection rates [33].

While many hospital pharmacists work on patient units, others are located in the various outpatient clinics within these health systems. These outpatient clinics offer patients the opportunity to manage their chronic diseases with system-based practitioners. The clinics have a range of specialties such as oncology, pulmonology, cardiology, behavioral health, and transplants. Advance practice pharmacists are critical members of the staff. They work with prescribers to manage the medication regimens, address adverse drug events, and minimize the organizations' cost. The extent of services provided by the pharmacists is governed by the system's policies and procedures and state regulations.

Consider the number of these patients who resided in the community and restricted adult communities, continuing care, or long-term care facilities. Changes in our healthcare delivery system, including healthcare reform efforts, have forced providers and consumers to become more astute in understanding the system. They must consider the quality and cost of use for all healthcare services and their choice of direct care clinical provider. Consumers (patients) are now in the challenging position of either developing a better understanding of their healthcare choices or aligning themselves with their family caregiver, primary care physician, or an independent patient advocate who may guide them through or refer them to a preferred plan. This new role is particularly difficult for older adults who may be at the highest medical risk and have the greatest need to access healthcare services without advocacy assistance. The pharmacist's role on a geriatric assessment team (GAT) has been shown to provide value to the older adult patient, hospital, and non-pharmacist team members. There are some examples of the value of the pharmacist's role, such as in the Programs for the All-inclusive Care of the Elderly (PACE), programs designed to assist the elderly in remaining in the community despite qualifying for nursing home care. Drug therapy is a key component of these programs, and pharmacists can be found as members of the patient's healthcare team. Medicare has launched a Facebook page and eMedicare site that offer beneficiaries a host of plan and coverage information [34].

Home-care services are becoming a greater part of healthcare as more and more states are looking to manage the care of chronically ill patients in their homes for as long as feasible. Home-care services allow patients to maintain their autonomy and the quality of life and permit states to reduce the overall cost of long-term care. Home-care services consist of a spectrum of healthcare services delivered in various settings. This is not unlike the change happening in hospitals transforming themselves into integrated or continuing care delivery systems (IDS, CCDS). Home-care services may be a part of an IDS or, more frequently, part of an affiliated, independent arm of the acute-care hospital.

Community pharmacists have seen the greatest expansion of their services in the last 10 years. In 2019, retail pharmacies filled over 3.7 billion prescriptions [34]. States have passed regulations allowing retail pharmacies to use central fill pharmacies and low-volume stores to assist in managing the workflow in high-traffic pharmacies. Central fill pharmacies are backend facilities that prepare the prescription and send it to the retail store to be dispensed to the patient. Drug utilization and data entry may be performed at slower retail pharmacies within the same chain. The scan prescriptions are reviewed and processed through to the dispensing retail outlet. Electronic prescriptions and technology-based dispensing units assist the pharmacists in managing the distribution function with the aid of certified technicians. In addition to their distribution responsibilities, states require pharmacists to counsel patients on new medications and any changes in therapy. Despite the lack of provider status and reimbursement avenues, pharmacists have experienced a significant increase in the expectation of their clinical services. Pharmacists have assumed a significant portion of the immunization for influenza, shingles, and pneumonia. The major retail pharmacies offer vaccinations without the need for appointments. This ease of access has made the pharmacy a significant advantage for patients. Some states have expanded the administration role of the pharmacists to include long-acting antipsychotics. States across the country have been increasing the prescriptive authority of pharmacists to meet the primary care needs of patients. Pharmacists are utilizing POC test to help monitor patients and prescribe acute therapy for urinary tract infections and Strep A. Pharmacists have been a critical player in the opioid epidemic through the distribution of naloxone under state-wide protocols. Many of these services continue to be tied to the reimbursement of the product [35].

Finally, the availability of on-site medical services in pharmacies or at employer clinics has created new potentially integrated mid-level care systems that feature pharmacist-provided care, including MTM. Examples of this include CVS/Caremark and Walgreens, where acquisitions by these corporations have created a combination of retail, PBM/mail order, and mid-level practitioner limited care sites in hundreds of locations across the United S. With the continued shortage of primary care physicians, states continue to expand the scope of practice for nurse practitioners and physician assistance to fill the void.

26.4 ISSUES FOR PHARMACY PRACTICE, INSURANCE, AND MANAGED CARE IN THE NEAR FUTURE

26.4.1 The Landscape of Practice Sites and Changing Business of Health Landscape

Third-party payment for pharmaceutical products is now the predominant form of payment in all types of pharmacy settings. The pharmacy benefit from healthcare insurers is widely prevalent across all types of managed care. The passage of the Medicare Modernization Act of 2003 expanded prescription coverage for those on Medicare with the addition of Part D. Part D prescription coverage went into effect in 2006 and is offered to 60 million elderly and disabled beneficiaries. Medication coverage is available through private plans that are either stand-alone prescription drug plans (PDPs) or Medicare Advantage prescription drug plans (MA-PD). A Medicare Advantage plan includes all Medicare benefits. In 2020, CMS reported that more than 46 million beneficiaries had enrolled in a Medicare Part D program [36].

Consolidation continues to occur within every segment of the healthcare industry. The pace of change continues to be rapid; however, both federal and state regulators have taken mostly conservative positions that have slowed mergers. Affected market segments employing pharmacists included pharmacy benefit management firms, healthcare insurers, physician practice management (PPM) companies, hospitals, pharmacy chains, and pharmacy wholesalers.

Consumer advocacy and patient protection continue as a priority, resulting in several pieces of legislation that impacted healthcare delivery decisions. Managed care organizations and other healthcare providers are working continuously to improve their data systems' security and managed access to protected health data. The federal and state courts are increasingly imposing sanctions against organizations for the violation of Health Information Portability and Accountability Act (HIPAA) provisions. An example of these sanctions includes a national pharmacy chain agreeing to a $2.25 million settlement for a HIPAA violation in which their pharmacies were inappropriately disposing of labeled medication vials [37]. The American Recovery and Reinvestment Act (ARRA) of 2009 has significantly increased the monetary penalties for HIPAA violations, further increasing the stress for secure systems and processes.

At the beginning of 2014, the Office of Civil Rights (OCR) announced that it would focus on auditing for compliance with the Health Information Technology for Economic and Clinical Health (HITECH) Act, enacted as part of the American Recovery and Reinvestment Act of 2009 and HIPAA. OCR has been diligent in auditing and assessing penalties for security breaches of patient data. In 2018, OCR announced a resolution agreement settlement totaling $16 million dollars from Anthem to resolve a potential HIPAA violation from a data breach in 2015 in which the records of 78.7 million of its members were stolen by cybercriminals. Anthem paid $39 million to 43 states and DC for the data breach and settled a class action suit for $115 million [38]. Another ARRA provision that OCR is focusing on extends the application of the main provisions of HIPAA to business associates of the covered entities and requires periodic compliance auditing of covered entities and their business associates. Covered entities must ensure that the organizations they are contracting with have policies and procedures that meet the HITECH and HIPAA standards of covered entities. In September 2020, CHSPSC LLC, a business associate service entity, agreed to a $2.3 million settlement with OCR to settle potential violations for a data breach impacting six million individuals in 2014. OCR has also been actively enforcing patients' right to their health data. Under HIPAA, entities are required to provide timely access to health records at a reasonable cost. In 2019, OCR announced its Right to Access Initiative. On December 22, 2020, OCR announced its 13th settlement with Dr. Peter Wrobel for $36,000 for potential violation of failure to provide records [38]. Lastly, individuals must be notified of a breach in their confidential information if the information was in an unsecured format. OCR must be informed immediately of all breaches of 500 or more patients. Pharmacy organizations must also be diligent in monitoring the activities of their employees. An Indiana Court of Appeals upheld a ruling in the lawsuit against Walgreens. In this suit, a pharmacist accessed prescription data for personal reasons and disclosed it in violation of HIPAA regulations [39]. Connecticut, Missouri, West Virginia, and North Carolina courts have allowed negligence cases in which individuals' privacy under HIPAA regulations was violated to move through the courts [40]. HIPAA regulations are defining patient's expectations for confidentiality from their healthcare providers.

Federal reimbursement changes continue to be phased in as a result of the Balanced Budget Act (BBA) of 1997 and CMS, which continues to encourage Medicare and Medicaid beneficiaries to move into managed care where available. The continuing economic burden of healthcare on state budgets has required significant changes to be made to most Medicaid programs. In 2002, Michigan and Vermont received approval from CMS to implement a preferred drug list for beneficiaries in fee-for-service Medicaid programs. Preferred drug lists (PDL) allowed states to contract with manufacturers for additional supplemental rebates for position on the preferred drug list. Currently, over 40 states have PDLs in place. In addition, states have implemented additional cost containment strategies such as co-pays for certain segments of their programs, limiting the number of monthly prescriptions and implementing quantity limits to manage increasingly tight budgets. States continue to lower reimbursement through the application of strategies such as maximum allowable cost reimbursement on generics, dispensing fee reductions, and the implementation of pricing algorithms working from a percentage off the acquisition cost of each branded medications. All of these changes to the healthcare marketplace have significantly affected the role of a pharmacist in delivering patient-care services. Pharmacists today, in all settings, face continued pressure to maintain low-cost, high-quality pharmacy services with fewer personnel. Much of the cost pressure will continue to increase due to the demographics of our aging society along with the physician's reliance on medications as a primary form of treatment for most diseases. Given the number of new drugs, including novel or therapeutically important agents, pharmacists today face an economic and drug knowledge challenge unlike that of previous generations.

26.5 CURRENT AND NEAR FUTURE ISSUES FOR PHARMACISTS

26.5.1 Landscape of Pharmacy Practice, the Changing Professional Marketplace

As clinical expectations for pharmacists have grown over the last decade, so has the passage of state regulations that oversee the practice. Pharmacists are currently allowed to immunize patients in 50 states, although the patient's age and type vary by state. In 2016, California and Oregon passed legislation that allowed a pharmacist to dispense contraceptives without a prescription to women. In 2020, 14 U.S. jurisdictions had statutes or regulations that allowed pharmacists to prescribe contraceptives without a collaborative practice agreement: California, Colorado, District of Columbia, Hawaii, Idaho, Maryland, Minnesota, New Hampshire, New Mexico, Oregon, Utah, Vermont, Virginia, and West Virginia [41]. Medical marijuana is legal in 21 states, and 11 states allow recreational and medical marijuana within state limits. Seven states, Arkansas, Connecticut, Louisiana, Minnesota, New York, Pennsylvania, and Utah, mandate pharmacists' involvement. Connecticut's medicinal marijuana regulations mandate that only a licensed pharmacist who has received a dispensary license from the Department of Consumer Protection can dispense medical marijuana. Louisiana requires patients to obtain their marijuana from one of the nine state-licensed pharmacies. Some states require pharmacists as a consultant to dispensaries or patients [42]. States have also turned to pharmacists to help address the opioid crisis. Emergency regulations were passed in states allowing pharmacists to dispense naloxone to patients without a prescription. Emergency regulations allowed pharmacists to dispense this legend medication under a CPA with a prescriber or in some states under a state-authorized protocol. States modified their regulations to allow the dispensing of prescription medications to individuals who were not the patients. Also, some states have passed laws that allow pharmacists to prescribe autonomously under state protocols or independently, with the regulations deferring to national guidelines as guidance. States have focused on therapeutic areas which entail more short-term medication utilization or disease prevention. Many of these areas have well-established national guidelines or Point of Care (POC) tests performed in a pharmacy. POC testing involves performing a diagnostic test outside of a laboratory. These tests produce a rapid and reliable result, helping the pharmacist identifying or managing chronic diseases and acute infections such as Strep A, influenza, and Hep C. These tests are waived under the Clinical Laboratory Improvement Amendments (CLIA) of 1988. Pharmacists prescribe medication for smoking cessation, travel medication, epinephrine injections, and fluoride. Under protocol and using the POC test, pharmacists prescribe medications for uncomplicated Strep A and influenza [43].

TABLE 26.1
Degree of Integration Matched to the Stage of Managed Care.

Number of Components, Number of Delivery Components, and Number of System-Wide Contracts
(Stage 2)
Including lab and diagnostic imaging only; few if any system-wide contracts
(Stage 3)
Only hospital and physician care contracts; limited but growing system-wide contracts
(Stage 4)
Nearly-all to all components of diagnostic and care delivery across the continuum of patient-care settings via system-wide contracts

Changes continue to impact the current and foreseeable future of pharmacy practice. Movement from stage two to stage three status in managed care takes less time today than it did three years ago. Even within a six-month period, subtle shifts that impact pharmacists or pharmacy services for prescription drugs can be seen in most markets. Multiple pressures on the pharmacy as a result of this dynamic marketplace put cascading pressure on the pharmacist in the dispensing of drugs and drug information to patients and other providers. This can result in the potential for more medication-related errors by all providers—including the pharmacist. Concern around medication errors has been the subject of several journal articles and reports by the National Academy of Medicine, focusing on both the system cost of these various errors and the opportunities for system improvement to eliminate potential errors through changes in practice patterns. These changes toward quality improvement include the use of automation, new generations of computer software to check for drug-related prescribing errors, and requirements for better training of healthcare professionals, which are documented to verify improvement in personal professional practice. While technology such as bar coding continues to be stressed as a key to achieving significant impact on the estimated $21 billion dollars in wasteful spending attributable to errors, Boards of Pharmacy are taking a role in educating and engaging their pharmacists on medication errors and safety. Over 20 states require pharmacies to have quality programs within their retail settings and 7 states have continuing education requirements on medication errors [44]. A few states' Boards of Pharmacy are mandating pharmacies use investigative techniques such as root cause analysis to understand, document, and redefine workflow issues to prevent the reoccurrence of medication errors.

This is significant in relations to the U.S. Food and Drug Administration (FDA trend toward a less paternalistic approach to medication oversight). Over the last 20 years, there has been a consistent movement of legend (prescription) medication to OTC status. This movement has been seen in a number of categories including sinus, inflammation, and gastric acid products. In addition, individual states have passed regulations on medicinal marijuana, immunizations, naloxone initiatives to prevent overdose and pharmacist dispensing of oral contraceptives. These regulations have an impact on the pharmacist's ability to manage patient care in a comprehensive manner as the availability of complete medical and prescriptive data including OTC products does not exist within the current practice setting. As the scope of their practice continues to expand, pharmacists have lobbied for their right to not dispense a medication for ethical and moral reasons. These conscience clause issues have involved such products as emergency contraceptives, naloxone, and the right to die drugs. Boards of Pharmacy and states have enacted laws addressing the right of pharmacists to refuse to fill a valid prescription based on personal rather than clinical considerations. Pharmacists' rights vary by states, but in all states, the pharmacist or pharmacy is required to assist the patient in finding alternative venues for the medication to ensure that their care will not be affected.

TABLE 26.2
Continuum of Acute-To-Chronic Patient-Care Settings. Intensity of care related to need for hands-on nursing care and/or 24-hour professional-services support.

Highest-Care Intensity
Acute care
Subacute/transitional care
Rehabilitation
Nursing home/long-term care
Hospice
Assisted living
Freestanding medical infusion
Urgent care
Specialty office-based care delivery
Primary care
Home
Lower-care intensity

Note: The complexity of drug treatment can remain constant across the continuum.

In addition to patient care, pharmacists have always been considered the gatekeepers who manage access to legally approved and prescribed controlled substances. This role has expanded with the introduction of Prescription Drug Monitoring Programs (PDMPs) by the states. In an effort to monitor the volume of controlled substances being prescribed and dispensed, 49 states and the District of Columbia require the prescription data for controlled substances be submitted to the state agency at regular intervals. Physicians and pharmacists are able to access the state database to view patient prescription history for the duplication of therapy as well as physician and pharmacy shopping, The National Association of Boards of Pharmacy (NABP) has developed a system, NABP PMP Interconnect, to assist states in allowing their practitioners to view data across state lines. Regulations vary by state on whether a prescriber or pharmacist must review this data before prescribing or dispensing a controlled substance. Recently, West Virginia's Supreme Court ruled that pharmacists and physicians who negligently prescribe and dispense addictive medications can be sued for enabling patient's addiction [45]. In 2020, the DEA announced a settlement with Purdue Pharma. The manufacturer agreed to pay over $5 billion in criminal fines and forfeiture. Purdue also agreed to pay $2.8 billion to resolve civil liability under the False Claims Act. The Sackler family agreed to pay $225 million in damages to resolve a civil False Claim Act [46]. Other manufacturers, Mallinckrodt, Endo, Teva, and Insys, are also part of the sweeping opioid investigations. Wholesalers such as McKesson, Cardinal Health, and AmerisourceBergen (ASB) are part of the multistate lawsuit for their lack of oversight on the distribution of opioids to pharmacies. The DEA continues to investigate prescribers for their role in the opioid crisis. Many prescribers have paid settlements, lost their license, and are serving sentences for the inappropriate prescribing of opioids. The DEA audits pharmacies to ensure that pharmacists are meeting their corresponding responsibility in the dispensing of controlled substances. Pharmacists must ensure that the prescription has been written for a valid medical reason. This mandate often places the pharmacists in a difficult position as they do have access to patient medical records. DEA expects pharmacists to play a significant role in preventing the diversion of controlled substances and a limited number of noncontrolled substances.

The Drug Enforcement Agency's (DEA's) war on illicit drugs continues to include monitoring by the pharmacies of a very common cold preparation, pseudoephedrine, which is used in the manufacturing of methamphetamine. The product remains available to consumers but is managed by store personnel as this product is used to manufacture methamphetamine. Many retail stores have moved this product to the pharmacies to be managed by pharmacy personnel to ensure appropriate and controlled use. DEA-approved stores require a photo ID before the product is sold to a consumer, and logs of the purchase are recorded as consumers are limited to a 3.6 gm daily per purchaser and 9 gm

TABLE 26.3
Spectrum of Out-of-Hospital to Home-Care Settings in Which Pharmacy and/or Pharmacist Services May Be Provided.

Adult day care*
Ambulatory/Out-patient clinic*
Assisted living*
Community/public health programs*
Congregate living*
Continuing-care community (life care
Home healthcare) **
Hospice**
Palliative care*
Rehabilitation facilities**
Respite care*

Note: **Services provided in ambulatory/home or at a facility/building outside of hospital setting.**Both in-patient hospital and ambulatory/home-based services.*

a month. Retail pharmacies may use the National Precursor Log Exchange (NPLEx), a real-time electronic compliance system, to track pseudoephedrine purchases. NPLEx is utilized in 33 states to comply with the DEA regulations of this chemical [47].

However, the function as gatekeeper of controlled substances must not become viewed as the sole mission of pharmacists in the community setting. With FDA approval of Suboxone®, community pharmacists play an increased role in the management of patient addiction. Traditionally, patients seeking addiction treatment were managed by opioid treatment programs, and the availability of Suboxone® has moved treatment to mainstream healthcare settings. This transition has allowed patients to maintain their treatment in a less conspicuous environment. While the community setting has been evolving as an addiction treatment model, drug abuse and opioid overdose deaths have also been increasing. Many states have responded by passing legislation allowing the distribution of naloxone kits to prevent overdoses. State emergency response teams have been educated on the use of this product. Individuals addicted to opioid agents as well as their families and friends are being trained on how to administer naloxone. Naloxone kits are being made available in pharmacies by statewide collaborative agreements with practitioners or states' departments of health.

The pharmacist's role has traditionally been one of distribution, not administration. States vary on the number of medications that pharmacists are allowed to administer. Long-acting antipsychotic medications and vaccines are the most commonly allowed. This expansion of practice has been particularly needed in many rural areas lacking the necessary health personnel to manage the immunization process. Pharmacists have been identified as a potential key to improve immunization rates in all areas, but especially rural areas, because of their easy accessibility. Immunization at pharmacies continues to grow as state regulations expand the types of vaccines allowed and allow pharmacists to vaccinate children. To help address the increase in volume of work the pharmacist managed, states passed regulations allowing certified technicians to administer the vaccines once a patient has been assessed by the pharmacist. This expanded scope has been instrumental in helping states meet the volume of vaccinations required due to COVID-19.

Another area of change has been with the dispensing of medication as written by the physicians. Traditionally, pharmacists filled prescriptions as written by the physician. However, most states enacted generic substitution laws that required pharmacists to dispense generic equivalents unless specified by the physician that a brand medication was necessary. This mandate to fill generically has saved managed care and federal and state governments billions of dollars while having a minimal effect on patient care as the two products are chemically equivalent. This practice is generally acceptable to physicians and has becoming increasingly requested by most patients as the burden of medication cost is shifting to them through deductibles and co-pays. However, some states have started allowing therapeutic substitution of medications in which a product from the same therapeutic class is selected over the prescribed choice of the physician. The COVID-19 pandemic and drug shortages have strengthened this initiative. The selection would be based on formulary criteria and patient history. Physicians and advocacy groups oppose this practice. Pharmacists working in collaboration with physicians may have individual practitioners' approval to intervene, and hospital pharmacists often make therapeutic substitutions within the hospital's formulary. However, pharmacists in these practices have the information necessary to make informed decisions. Until the information exchange between practitioners is developed, pharmacists in the community would find it challenging to gather the information necessary to make informed decisions [48].

As states' regulations expand and redefine the role of the pharmacists in the healthcare delivery team, there has been a corresponding increase in the expectation of these practitioners. Traditionally, physicians have been held responsible for warning patients about the side effects and adverse outcome of the medications being prescribed. Pharmacists have used the Learned-Intermediary-Doctrine to shield them from civil negligence suits due to adverse drug events. Traditionally, courts have agreed to the premise that pharmacist might erode the physician–patient relationship if they were allowed to question physician prescribing. However, courts have begun to allow civil cases to move forward under specific situations. The courts have begun to hold the pharmacist accountable in duty to warn cases where the pharmacist has had specific knowledge of a drug interaction, side effect, or known allergies but did not warn the patient and or physician that a problem might exist. In *Happel v Walmart Stores, Inc.*, 766N.E.2d 1118 (Ill. 2002), the pharmacist had knowledge of the patient's allergy but dispensed a drug without warning the patient or calling the physician about the contraindication. In *Riff v. Morgan Pharmacy,* 508 A.2d 1247 (Pa. Super. Ct. 1986), the pharmacist typed the directions as written. Unfortunately, the directions were inadequate to prevent harm to the patient. The court ruled that the pharmacist had a duty to notify the physician of the inadequate directions that created substantial risk to the patient. These cases illustrate the court's recognition of the relationship between the pharmacist and the patient. Given specific knowledge, the pharmacist is expected to inform the prescriber or patient when there is an issue or concern in medication treatment. Pharmacists are being recognized as medication experts by the courts, and they have a role in managing a patient's medication.

As their clinical role has expanded, the financial business of the pharmacy has changed. Reimbursement shifts have driven profits out of drug distribution. Managed care and public sector payers have extracted discounts from retail selling prices to the point where reimbursement formulas are now indexed on near acquisition prices to retail (plus a fixed fee for dispensing). Conflict between employer and employee escalated as pharmacists with exempt status argued for overtime compensation. The court rulings largely depended on state laws. For example, California requires overtime for individuals who work more than seven days in a row to be paid overtime for the seventh day. Pharmacists are specifically identified in the law. A retailer was denied using a Sunday to Saturday work week to circumvent the law [49]. The pressure to fill these openings is waning as the newly established academic programs completed their first cycle of pharmacy candidates. Currently, most market indices reflect an appropriate supply for the national demand. The next decade may see this shift to an oversupply as the new colleges begin to graduate a full cadre of students. Graduates have begun to see a downward trend in salaries and offers upon graduation.

The personnel issue continues to exert pressure on the industry as it strives to meet increasing managed care, consumers, and regulatory demands. In response to these pressures, retailers have increased the rate of implementation of technological advances in automation and computer software. Rural areas and small community hospitals are using telepharmacy to service their patients. A pharmacy technician fills the prescription using scanning technology that enables the pharmacist to see the prescription and medication dispensed. A computer system enabled with audio-visual capability allows the pharmacist in an off-site location, sometimes hundreds of miles away, to verify and approve prescriptions filled by technicians and counsel patients who would otherwise lack access to prescription services. Hospitals have utilized telepharmacy to cover their 11 p.m. to 7 a.m. shift, which traditionally has been difficult and costly to staff. Using this technology, one hospital pharmacist may verify prescriptions at a number of off-site hospitals and approve the dispensing of medications through automated dispensing machines. These automated systems allow nurses to access medications from patient-profile-based automated dispensing machines. In addition, the availability of computer physician order entry that directly routes orders to robotic dispensing systems allows pharmacists the opportunity to spend more time on patient floors and in consultation with physicians. Hospital pharmacists are now located on patient floors and in specific clinics monitoring patients, including anticoagulant, asthma, and diabetes clinics.

These robotic dispensing systems also assist in processing the ever-increasing volumes at the retail stores. The systems are integrated with interactive voice response systems to decrease the volume of calls handled by store personnel and to facilitate customer service. Many larger chain retailers are developing central prescription processing sites to handle refills and nonemergency prescriptions for a large geographic area of retail stores. These central fill locations are mail-order type facilities able to handle large volumes of prescriptions using the latest prescription-processing technology and automated systems. In addition, many of these retail chains have launched call centers consolidating functions and optimizing the workload of store personnel. The call center's staff assists in third-party processing issues, physician calls, and patient inquiries. The call center allows store personnel to assist in-store customers and be available to offer patient MTM type services. Another advanced technique for managing excess volume in stores has been the triaging of calls between high-volume and lower-volume stores. Pharmacies with excess pharmacists' capacity are reviewing and managing the prescription processing steps up through the actual dispensing of medication in their stores via the chain computer system. State boards of pharmacy have worked collaboratively with community chains to modify or rewrite regulations so that the practice of pharmacy maximizes the clinical role of pharmacists in the healthcare delivery team while utilizing the available resources for the dispensing function of pharmacy.

Lower margins resulting from this reimbursement have caused retail pharmacies to move faster into automated dispensing techniques and to seek to use non-pharmacist personnel to increase the productivity of pharmacists. Other pharmacies have gone into compounding and other specialties in pharmacy that do not have the strict reimbursement provisions seen in the mainstream pharmacy business. By contrast, the pharmacist who is not involved in the distribution of drugs is focused either on direct patient-care monitoring and education or is working as a member of the healthcare team (whose job includes advising others about the appropriate use of medications for individual patients). The role of the individual pharmacist in our emerging healthcare delivery system will continue to be debated and redefined. New national and local programs targeted toward pharmacists have begun to capitalize on their strengths and to position pharmacists as quality managers who can contribute to better medical outcomes for patients. Pharmacist academicians and many associations have adopted this patient-care focus as the future value of pharmacists in the community or institutional delivery settings.

Barriers to expanding the pharmacists' capabilities in this new integrated, patient-oriented environment include database information, consensus on the pharmacist's role, and training opportunities reflective of the changing role of the pharmacist. To assist in achieving a standardized approach and maintaining appropriate levels of quality, long-term care (LTC) and home care have followed other levels of care in moving toward patient-care guidelines and focusing on consistent, cost-effective care. This has led rehabilitation facilities and nursing homes to incorporate best practices into their daily routines, including improved communication of patient data [50, 51].

The need for information and assessment is being pushed in efforts to decrease medication errors in order to improve the quality of care and reduce excess cost in the present system. Organizations continue to assist in monitoring healthcare delivery. The FDA has used the MedWatch form as a mechanism to track adverse drug events. The industry continues to look out for organizations with missions to address medications' safety. For example, the Institute for Safe Medication Practice, formed in 1975, assists healthcare providers with medication error prevention and safe medication use. The organization tracks medication errors and develops strategies and educational programs to help address these potentially life-threatening events. The Patient Safety and Quality Improvement Act of 2005 also addresses the healthcare system's need to improve its recording and analysis of medication errors. This act establishes a voluntary reporting of errors and provides federal privilege and confidentiality protection for patient safety work product and information gathered during analysis and data gathering for error analysis. Patient Safety Organizations (PSO) collect, analyze, and assist organizations in using the information to make changes to prevent future errors.

While the states push practitioners to analyze their workflows and errors, a significant event such as the fungal meningitis outbreak of 2014 brings radical change quickly. In October 2014, the New England Compounding Center (NECC) was implicated in the fungal meningitis deaths occurring in multiples states. The fungal infections were linked to steroid injections that had been compounded by NECC. To date, there have been 64 deaths linked to the products compounded by NECC. Pharmacists have traditionally been allowed to compound prescriptions for individual patients, but NECC was allegedly compounding products for fabricated patients and shipping large quantities to facilities in multiple states. NECC did not adhere to the good manufacturing practices (CGMP) imposed upon pharmaceutical manufacturers as it was licensed and operated as a pharmacy. The FDA and state Boards of Pharmacy have sought to enact regulations defining traditional compounding versus manufacturing. The Drug Quality and Safety Act (DQSA) of 2013 addressed many of the violations found within the NECC facility as well as other pharmacies licensed as pharmacies but operating as large-scale compounding facilities. The DQSA clearly defines compounding allowed within a pharmacy under section 503A of the Food Drug and Cosmetic Act (FDCA). The DQSA created a new section of the FDCA, Section 503B, which allows a compounder to qualify as an outsourcing facility, exempt from the product approval process and from the labeling requirements of direction for use. Outsourcing facilities under Section 503B must comply with CGMP requirements, be subject to FDA inspections, and have specific reporting requirements to the FDA.

Information management is an essential component of the integration within healthcare- delivery systems. Some of the obstacles to merging the various databases in healthcare, particularly for pharmacists, have been reported in the medical and information management literature over many years. Important barriers for the hospital–LTC interface include patients who are members of a health plan but who do not universally have pharmacy benefits. They also include patients with plan limits (which would mean that some prescription services would not be captured in the claims system). Also, current data captured may not be sufficient for meaningful outcomes analysis, and the reporting of utilized services is usually incomplete when those services are reimbursed by prospective payment schemes such as capitation. This has been a historical challenge as providers submit data for the purpose of payment and not utilization review or research, thus the information analyzed may not be robust or precise enough to allow for clinical evaluation. The challenges encountered using payment data for utilization analysis and quality review may be addressed with CMS' latest initiative on ICD-9-DM. In January 2009, CMS released a final rule that requires the use of ICD-10-CM diagnostic codes beginning in October 2013. A few of the enhancements with ICD-10-DM include greater specificity in diagnosis codes, expanded injury codes, and diagnosis/symptom code combination that will decrease codes submitted. The replacement of ICD-9-CM with the greatly expanded ICD-10-CM code set will help support quality reporting, pay-for-performance, bio-surveillance, and other activities critical to the management of patient claims [52].

The information barriers are important to the hospital pharmacist, who is being asked to become more involved (through integrated delivery systems)—both in preventing LTC readmissions and in expediting discharges, as these relate to individual patient drug therapy issues. Without adequate information from inside the hospital or the outside older adult sources, it can be difficult to make those decisions on recommendations for patient drug therapy interventions. A significant investment has been made in Electronic Health Record (EHR) systems which are becoming mature in the healthcare market and are including pharmacy interfaces with other care provider organizations such as hospitals and medical groups. Physicians and healthcare organizations are subject to meaningful use requirements, set by U.S. Department of Health and Human Services (USDHHS), but retail pharmacies are not which may have initially limited the interest in connectivity with community pharmacy practitioners.

This continuous striving to better manage patient care increased in momentum with two CMS initiatives. These initiatives linking quality of care to reimbursement are Hospital Acquired Conditions (HAC) and Hospital Quality Measure Reporting. Increased morbidity and the cost of patient care due to hospital-acquired conditions (HAC) have been documented in a number of studies and cited in the National Academy of Medicine reports. The National Academy of Medicine's report "To Err is Human: Building a Safer Health Systems" estimates that the total national costs of these errors, due to lost productivity, disability, and healthcare costs, could be between $17 and $29 billion [53]. Under HAC, CMS will no longer pay hospitals at higher rates for the increased cost of care for patients harmed by one of several conditions that they did not have upon hospitalization or for conditions that could have been reasonably prevented. The hospital will be reimbursed as if these conditions did not exist for discharges occurring on or after October 1, 2008. The HAC conditions are commonly referred to as never-events and will continually be updated by CMS. Two new conditions are deep venous thrombosis (DVT) and pulmonary embolism (PE) occurring after knee and hip surgery. Medication therapy will be a consideration in managing many of these conditions and patients, further emphasizing the need for pharmacists to be part of the team working to prevent HAC events. Furthermore, CMS has issued a Medicaid Directors guidance letter on the coordination of Medicaid payment policies in consideration of the newly enacted Medicare HAC policies. Many states and insurers have followed CMS' lead and developed a list of events that will not be reimbursed [54].

The second initiative is the Hospital Quality Measure Reporting, which is used to develop payment algorithms for hospitals. The program requires most hospitals to submit data for specific quality measures for health conditions common among people with Medicare and that would typically result in hospitalization. The information gathered is intended for use by consumers in making healthcare decisions, while also encouraging hospitals and providers to continually improve the quality of inpatient care provided to all patients. The information is available to the public at www.hospitalcompare.hhs.gov.

In the near future, patients stand to gain the most from these and other changes in the increasingly better managed healthcare marketplace. Managed care has injected price competition into all sectors of healthcare delivery. It has also changed provider behaviors, created novel opportunities within the business of healthcare, and moved healthcare toward a defined and measurable standard of quality [55].

Pharmacists need to be aware of the differing perspectives and common goals in this marketplace as integrated systems evolve. The hospital integrated care systems will demand that pharmacists perform certain tasks as part of various performance improvement initiatives. Pharmacists, whether in a retail, hospital, or LTC setting, must be knowledgeable of the healthcare system environment and understand what the desired goal is for the patient, hospital, and payer. Ultimately, all pharmacist providers must communicate and work together in order for these novel older adult-care systems to truly provide effective patient care (including pharmaceutical care).

Increasingly, capitated or prepayment-reimbursement methods are creating incentives for both providers and payors to promote wellness. This can lead to incomplete data, unusual referral patterns for care, and unreported services (due to billing methods used in prepayment). In contrast to those information problems, some of the outcome goals include increased patient satisfaction, cost-per-case-day reduction, and decreased admission–readmission rates—all of which are more difficult to determine in many current prepayment schemes. For LTC facilities and hospitals, an interface that uses fewer, or avoids, inpatient days stands out as an important element to the success of a continuum of care (or IDS). In some LTC settings, additional value may be created when service and equipment redundancy can be eliminated, which can have the additional benefit of avoiding an emergency room visit or hospital admission.

There are providers, including pharmacists, who are now being asked to deliver patient- oriented care for older adult patients—regardless of the tradition or existing bureaucracy barrier that has flourished to date. This has required an adjustment in the job function as well as perspective among the hospital pharmacist, retail pharmacist, or home-care services consultant pharmacist as their traditionally disparate workplaces now reflect the implementation of medication reconciliation, transition of care, and medication therapy management programs by health plans and CMS. Today's marketplace has become team-based wellness management, performance assessment, and integration of services along the healthcare continuum.

26.6 PHARMACEUTICAL MANUFACTURER THROUGH WHOLESALER AND DISTRIBUTION SUPPLY CHAIN

Pharmaceutical industry marketplace historically started at the manufacturer and product was distributed through a supply chain led by a wholesaler (pharmacies) or distributor (medical offices), and then was available for dispensing to an individual patient. Efficiencies of scale and delivery distribution drove relationships and product supply from manufacturer to consumers or patients until disruption started in the late 20th century. Such disruption or innovation as some would call it continues today in the early 21st century.

Functioning as an intermediary between prescription drug manufacturers and consumers is a lot more complicated than it used to be. Until the 1980s, the only place to have a doctor's prescription filled was a local pharmacy. The drug supply chain moved in a relatively straight line, from the manufacturer to the wholesaler to the pharmacy and, finally, to the consumer. Now, there are a variety of alternate distribution channels or oversight entities in place, including preferred or high-performing pharmacy providers, mail-order services, in-house pharmacies, specialty pharmacies, and internet pharmacies—all part of efforts designed to capture prescription business, increase efficiency, and attempt to contain rising drug claim costs. The distribution supply chain for high-cost specialty drugs varies from that for traditional prescription drugs or nonbiologic products. Unlike the very large number of retail pharmacies, there is a smaller but growing number of specialty pharmacies, around 700 today, including several large publicly traded or owned by a drug wholesaler (McKesson, ASB) or health system. Few retail pharmacies today are in this highly controlled supply chain due to many differences from the larger population dispensing of lower cost product seen with traditional prescription drugs versus specialty drugs. Many of the specialty drugs are administered by or under the supervision of a physician, so there also is direct distribution to medical offices in addition to hospitals [56].

Changes in the healthcare system have led drug wholesalers to broaden the services they offer to pharmacies, physicians, and hospitals or health systems. This expansion has enabled pharmacists to extend the services they offer to patients in a variety of settings. Traditionally, wholesalers served as the middleman—a distribution hub between the pharmaceutical manufacturer and the pharmacy. This industry has undergone merger-and-acquisition (M&A) activity, leaving a few national leaders and a handful of local or regional firms. Leaders in this industry are the publicly traded corporations McKesson, Cardinal Health, and ASB, which collectively control 92% of all drug wholesaling as of 2017 [57].

The trade association for this segment of the pharmacy industry is the National Wholesale Druggists Association (NWDA). Wholesalers are expanding current services or developing new services that manage assets and support the needs of manufacturers and pharmacies. The offerings by wholesalers include decision support software for clinicians, barcode scanning technology, and healthcare information technology software and computer hardware to support the required infrastructure for secure electronic transactions across healthcare delivery settings. As a result, pharmacists are able to offer more patient care-oriented services in their practice settings. Back in 1999, chain pharmacies were the dominant wholesaler customer base (30.5%), and independent pharmacies were second (18.3%) [58]. More recently, that base shifted although chain pharmacies were still dominant (27%), followed by hospitals, clinics, or other service providers (26%), then chain warehouses (18%), independent pharmacies (16%), and then mail-order pharmacies (13%) [58]. While pharmacy chain retailers remained dominant, independent pharmacies have enjoyed a resurgence in numbers in the past few years with a strong support from wholesalers such as ASB's Good Neighbor Pharmacy program.

Requirements from federal and state agencies related to the distribution of products (supply chain), product safety for patient use, and product efficacy have pushed the drug industry to develop a complex network of middlemen, which delivers supply chain or product access solutions interdependent on one another, resulting in a longer and more complex system. Depending on the condition, there can be multiple entities involved in drug supply from the manufacturer to patient. Similarly, managing access to drugs along with implementing plan designs involves multiple entities.

Since 1987, wholesalers are key players in the new prescription drug pedigree regulations known as the Prescription Drug Marketing Act of 1987 [59]. More information on this can be found in Section 48.14. The wholesalers will be responsible for verifying the pedigree of products sold to customers and ensuring the pedigree of products purchased from secondary markets. If the federal government's implementation precedes the States', a national standard may ease the burden being placed on wholesalers as the gatekeepers against counterfeit products. However, state-specific requirements varying from a national standard may prevent the distribution of products on a timely basis and impact the availability of products to consumers.

Pedigree implications going forward in 2021 to 2023 include the following:

- PDMA granted FDA authority to require non-manufacturers to provide prior sales, purchase, or trade records of all drugs that are used in prescription drugs or repackaged.
- The FDA recommends that standardized numerical identifiers (SNIs) for prescription drugs be used.
- By November 2018, manufacturers and repackagers must affix a unique product identifier (UPI) to their package and homogenous case.
- By 2019, wholesalers must follow above UPI rule.
- By November 2023, the DSCSA requires a full system electronic, interoperable product track and trace system be implemented for prescription drugs for human use
  - Exceptions
  - Homeopathic drugs, compounded drugs, and radioactive drugs— transactions for first responders

The FDA has designated 503A compounding pharmacies as those that compound according to prescriptions specific to particular patients and are required by state boards of pharmacy to comply with USP and other guidelines. These facilities (state licensed pharmacies) are limited to dispensing only for home use and are not allowed to compound large batches, an ability that can lead to lower product costs.

Compounding in large batch quantities for healthcare office use is now governed by FDA section 503b regulation. So-called 503B suppliers are outsourcing facilities that may manufacture large batches with or without prescriptions to be sold to healthcare facilities for office use only. They require full compliance of current good manufacturing practices (CGMP).

- Comply with USP <795> and <797>, state Board of pharmacy, and 21 CFR Part 210 and 211 (cGMP)
- Need environmental monitoring program
- Need their own independent entity of operation and sales: Complete autonomy for investigations and releasing products
- Required to register with each board of pharmacy, DEA, and FDA and report their product list to the FDA biannually [60].

At $4.6+ billion, the overall U.S. compounding pharmacies market size is set to exceed $6.8 billion by 2026 according to the Global Market Insights March 2020 research report. As a special pharmacy group, the sales leaders held around 54% of U.S. compounding pharmacy market share in 2019. Major players in this market segment include B. Braun, Baxter, Dougherty's pharmacy, Fagron, Fresenius Kabi, ImprimisRx, Institutional Pharmacy Solutions, McGuff Company, Pencol Compounding Pharmacy, Rx3 Compounding Pharmacy, Triangle Compounding Pharmacies, and Wedgewood Village Pharmacy [61].

In March of 2020, Congress made long-awaited reforms in healthcare product approvals through the Food & Drug Administration (FDA). Specifically, reforms to over-the-counter (OTC) drug monograph change were included in the Coronavirus Aid, Relief, and Economic Security Act (CARES ACT of 2020) intended to allow more nimble OTC oversight and potentially new safety and innovation via an OTC monograph. Appropriate new product aspects and recipe for formulating a product generally recognized as safe and effective (GRASE) can eliminate premarket requirement for review and approval by FDA [62].

Another area impacting wholesalers and distributors is physicians dispensing of drug products, especially controlled substances. Owing to the opioid epidemic and prescribing reduction efforts over the past several years, there remains a huge cost of physicians dispensing through a major safety and financial risk [63, 64]. Such dispensing includes worker compensation services, clinics, and traditional medical offices or clinics that offer some form of prescription drug dispensing. As part of the crackdown on opioid prescribing and use through licensed physicians, drug dispensing is another area of legal exposure for all those involved in the drug distribution supply chain.

26.7 MANUFACTURERS: TRADITIONAL AND INNOVATIVE SEGMENTS

The dominance of managed care along with the implementation of the ACA (Affordable Care Act) has had a significant impact on the financing and delivery of healthcare services. The faster paced, dynamic changes taking place today have forced everyone in the healthcare industry to adopt new strategies or tactics in the marketplace. Nowhere are those changes more pronounced today than in the pharmacy industry. As a result of recent M&A activity and rapid growth in biotech-based products, the largest firms today include Allergan (formerly Actavis), BristolMyersSquibb, Celgene, Amgen, AbbVie, Novartis, Merck, AstraZeneca, Biogen, Johnson & Johnson, Roche, Glaxo-Smith Kline, Sanofi, and Pfizer [65].

While the introduction of third-party prescription drug programs by the insurance industry in the early 1980s foretold the intrusion of third-party payers into the traditional healthcare distribution channels, now hospitals are accelerating more change. Group purchasers (GPOs and health systems) and their managed care advisors have now usurped the exclusive "directing" role previously enjoyed by physicians in the healthcare delivery decision-making process, including the prescribing of prescription drugs.

Pharmacy benefit management, plan design, and cost issues have been increasing in importance to pharmaceutical companies over the past five years. The 2020 Employer Health Benefits Survey from Kaiser Family Foundation provides a comprehensive overview of the current state of prescription drug coverage costs and plan designs. Some of the key findings from the report are included next [66]:

- Employers established drug plan designs to share some portion of drug costs with members.
- Seventeen percent of employers provide financial incentive for workers to use a retail health clinic, such as a minute clinic, instead of visiting a traditional physician's office.
- Three or more tier plan designs are used by 89% of employers. The most commonly used cost sharing approach is a three-tier copayment design (generics, preferred brand, and non-preferred brand).
- Companies with a fourth tier included things such as lifestyle drugs as well as biologics.
- Deductible spending has increased from $917 in 2010 to $1,644 in 2020.
- Generic drug use continues to rise. Employers are using incentives for generic dispensing in retail and mail service.
- Employees who work at large firms with a least one separate tier for specialty drugs have a 45% copayment for specialty drugs, and 53% have coinsurance.

26.7.1 Non-Biologic Medications

The realization that the patient's immune system was responsible for reacting to infections and potentially ridding the body of pathogens took several hundred years. The ability of a doctor to cure or ameliorate disease only began to increase substantially during the 1930s. Chemical or natural products expanded rapidly in the 20th century including the manufacturer-patented or brand drugs that yielded many financially blockbuster products. Generic or patent-expired drugs that are chemically similar and interchangeable followed with robust growth in the late 20th century. More recently from 2020 till date, innovative new drug delivery formulations of established drugs emerged that typically improved distribution in the body; reached targeted parts of the body; combined multiple ingredients into one tablet or capsule; or allowed for easier medication absorption, administration, or use by the patient versus older formulations. All of these new formulations came at a much higher cost than the original brand or generic products. Since 2000, the number of new drugs that are biologic-based products has rapidly increased, again at much greater cost than non-biologic drugs. Along with rising healthcare costs in general, managed care increasingly focused on managing pharmacy insurance benefits and drug formularies outside of the hospital setting.

After the implementation of ACA in 2012, plan designs changed somewhat in compliance with new provisions for coverage in ACA but were fundamentally similar for pharmacy benefits. Change begun in 2012 and has accelerated since 2014 around the use of high deductible health plans (HDHPs). HDHPs have had indirect and some direct impacts on members. Adults aged 18–64 with employment-based coverage had an increase in enrollment with an HDHP with an HSA from 4.2% in 2007 to 18.9% in 2017 [67].

According to several industry reports which track drug-related benefit trends (i.e., The Express Scripts Drug Trend Report, CVS Caremark Drug Trends, EMD Serono Specialty Digest, Magellan Rx Management, Access Market Intelligence Trend Reports, and IMS Health), the top priorities in managing benefits include implementing site-of-care infusion management, incentivizing telemedicine and retail health-clinics, providing payment reforms, and integrating specialty management across benefits [68]. Third-party payer strategies continue to include prior approval, use of limited distribution networks, multiple coverage tiers, co-payment for specialty, and site-of-service/care incentives. A majority of both HDHP and traditional benefit plans feature a specialty cost-share tier into 2015.

During this same period of time from early 2000 through 2020, spending on specialty pharmaceuticals was on the rise. Specialty drugs require complex biological manufacturing, and the drugs themselves are frequently administered by medical professionals, often at higher-cost treatment sites such as hospitals. The Pharmaceutical Care Management Association (PCMA, the PBM trade group) estimates that spending in this category can reach $1.7 trillion in 2030. This reflects an increase from 24% of total drug spend to an estimated 44% of a health plan's total drug expenditure in 2030 [69]. That figure does not include the associated laboratory and clinical support services that are required for patients who use these drugs.

The trend forecast for the top five specialty therapy classes, such as inflammatory conditions, multiple sclerosis, oncology, hepatitis C, and HIV/AIDS, shows double-digit growth from 2015 through 2017 [70]. Inflammatory conditions demonstrated a spending increase of 17.1%, Oncology 7.2% higher unit cost, Diabetes 5.2% increase in spending, HIV 8.1% spending increase [70].

This significant trend has changed the approach taken by plan sponsors, administrators, and providers to more aggressively control the rapid dollar expenditure while providing quality care that can deliver good outcomes of care for commercial plan members.

Given the variety of options along with changes in practice settings where pharmaceutical care and prescription drugs are purchased, stored, and delivered to patients, the industry supplying these medications has had to change. One change is the consolidation occurring among manufacturers, as they seek to gain research benefits to fuel future offerings in generic and brand-marketed drugs (biologic and specialty drugs) and increase their clout in the marketing of drugs in a fiercely competitive U.S. marketplace. Additionally, the world marketplace has further intensified the competition among manufacturers for long-term survival.

The pharmaceutical drug manufacturers aggressively contract with pharmacy purchasers in the United States, who themselves are under increasing fiscal pressure to reduce costs. Group purchasing in all pharmacy settings continues to be the norm today. These groups are much larger than they were just several years ago and offer a more concentrated purchasing power to manufacturers. The need to drive better contracts has forced purchasers to buy bigger volumes of product and drive real, versus promised, purchasing from manufacturers. Manufacturers have become strict about their contracting terms and require performance in order for the organization to gain contractual discounts or purchased product rebates. Competition among manufacturers and the plethora of drug options have caused manufacturers to use multiple strategies to maintain market share and to be able to research new pipeline drugs for the future [71].

An increasingly important market force on manufacturers has been legislation at the state and federal levels to introduce pedigree requirements for pharmaceutical products. Pedigree is a record, either paper or electronic, that documents the transaction of the product throughout the course of its manufacturer and sale. The Prescription Drug Marketing Act (PDMA) of 1987 had language to address many of the issues of counterfeit, misbranded, and adulterated drugs. The subsequent amendments to the PDMA added and clarified language on pedigree and extended implementation until January 2010. With the continued extension of the PDMA implementation, individual states began to address the pedigree issue. California's requirement was an electronic pedigree and was scheduled to be implemented on January 1, 2009, but had been delayed until 2011 and further delayed as a phased approach through 2020. By November 2023, the DSCSA requires a full system electronic, interoperable product track and trace system be implemented for prescription drugs for human use. Exceptions include homeopathic drugs, compounded drugs, and radioactive drugs—transactions for first responders.

The Drug Supply Chain Security Act (DSCSA) of 2013 mandates the eventual use of unique codes (serial numeric identifiers or SNIs) on each container of drug products moving from manufacturers to pharmacies and retailers—item level serialization. Similarly, Unique Device Identification (UDI) is the system mandated by the FDA Amendments Act of 2007 and made final by rulemaking in 2013 [72]. The impetus for these efforts and this legislation is to combat counterfeit drugs that have entered the market and to be able to trace products for recall. The negative impacts from counterfeiting and piracy are projected to drain $4.2 trillion from the global economy and put 5.4 million legitimate jobs at risk by 2022 [73]. With the outsourcing of manufacturing to other countries and with many manufacturers based in other countries, the opportunity for counterfeit products of FDA-approved products continues to increase [73]. The previous manufacturing issues with heparin from China and the continuing proliferation of counterfeit sales of high-visibility products such as Viagra® have the FDA and manufacturers aligned to implement a system that meets the goal of a safe distribution system. The most promising technology to date for pedigree has been Radio Frequency Identification (RFID), but other electronic and paper systems could be possible as interim steps in the process of a standard national system. Two major hurdles have been the cost of these systems as well as the time to implement a tracing system from the initial ingredient to sale to consumers.

With the continued emphasis on disease outcomes from commercial plans and ACA legislation, manufacturers are also aligning themselves with a variety of patient-centered disease prevention and treatment programs, where their drug would or could be part of a program that links providers and patients in driving better outcomes of care. Known historically as "disease management," these programs are developed and implemented by healthcare organizations in order to achieve better patient outcomes, which bolsters their presence in the marketplace. The synergy for manufacturers and healthcare providers is to use drug products appropriately and achieve a cost-effective, positive outcome for the patient.

Manufacturers continue to have several different types of field-based representatives calling on customers today. They also have staff members who collaborate with or help coordinate their resources on behalf of the customer to achieve sales and product movement. They include the following examples:

- National Account Managers (NAMs) are responsible for purchasing groups (such as Premier, Novation, and several others), large health systems (such as InterMountain Health, Kaiser, Catholic Health Initiatives), or national companies (such as Walgreens Boots Alliance, CVS/Health, Wal-Mart).
- Key Account Managers (KAMs) are responsible for key accounts or influential systems at the local and regional levels.
- Managed Care Managers (MCMs) are responsible for working with managed care organizations at the local, regional, or national level (such as Blue Cross, Aetna, United Health, and others).
- Sales representatives are responsible for calling on local physicians, their office or clinic personnel, and local pharmacists in pharmacies.
- Hospital representatives are responsible for calling on the local hospitals, including teaching institutions. They also work on establishing product in-roads with thought leaders in the medical community.
- Specialty representatives are responsible for product niche areas and the respective physicians or pharmacists who would use or purchase such a product. An example would be drugs for transplant patients or a drug for a rare medical condition.

26.7.2 Research-Intensive, Biologics, Gene, and Generic Segments

26.7.2.1 Biologic Medications

Biologic drugs are structurally mimic compounds found in the body. They include a wide array of products like vaccines, blood, blood components, allergenics, gene therapy, tissues, and therapeutic proteins created by biological processes in contrast to traditional proteins created by biological processes as opposed to chemistry [74].

In 2020, the FDA approved 53 novel drugs under new drug applications (NDAs) and therapeutic biologics under biologics license applications (BLAs) [75]. The number of 2020 approvals was significantly higher than the 48 drugs approved in 2019. Orphan (58%) and specialty drugs continue to dominate the new drug approvals. As of August 2016 till date, there are around 3,000 potential drugs in the pipeline. According to the PhRMA, more than 20% of these drugs are biotechnology products [76].

There are over 9,500 projects in clinical development: 731 gene therapy or cell therapy, 173 DNA or RNA therapeutics, and 188 conjugated monoclonal antibodies—all working toward gaining FDA approval. Typically, 40 out of 53 (75%) novel drugs were approved in the United States before any other country. Of those same 53 products, 21 (40%) were first-in-class medication products approved by the U.S. FDA [75].

Today, many firms are licensing from or purchasing new products from small upstart biotech-based companies rather than investing in early-stage research. As a result, many top-tier firms focus on late-stage research and FDA approval for new drugs as well as additional indications once marketed in the United States or around the world. Branded manufacturers saw therapeutic classes converted mostly to generic products as managed care organizations used their tools to shift market share quickly to newly released generic alternatives [77].

As these new drug entities became available, multiple generic manufacturers competed for the market, helping to quickly reduce the cost of these agents. In addition, patent expirations over the past five years rapidly diminished branded drug use in favor of generics. The top generic companies include Apothecon, Mylan, Teva, AbbVie (formerly Abbott), Watson, Schein, Geneva, Par, Pfizer (Greenstone and Hospira), Ranbaxy, Dr. Reddys', Sun, and Roxane. Interestingly, many of these firms are wholly owned subsidiaries of research-intensive manufacturers based in the United States, Europe, or other countries.

For biotechnology and molecular medicine (biopharmaceutical) manufacturers, efforts have resulted in Congress to allow follow-on biologics or biosimilar medications to be approved by the FDA. A biosimilar is a product that attempts to replicate a biologic product, which is a complex product manufactured through living organisms. These biologic products are difficult to replicate, and therefore biosimilar products would not be identical to the original as is the case with current generic products. As part of the Affordable Care Act, Congress enacted the Biological Price Competition and Innovation Act (BPCI) of 2009 which amends the Public Health Act and other statutes to create an abbreviated licensure pathway for biological products shown to be biosimilar to, or interchangeable with, an FDA-licensed biological reference product. The BCPI allows biopharmaceutical manufacturers at least 12 years' exclusivity from first licensure of the reference product. Most biological products are produced from living organisms, which makes the replication process exceedingly complex and challenging. The biosimilar agent must be highly similar to the reference product and show no clinically meaningful differences in terms of safety [78]. Due to the complexity and challenges faced by manufacturers in producing a biosimilar product, the European market, where several biosimilars have been available, has seen only a 20 to 30% savings from the original product. Although significantly less of a discount than what is seen from traditional generic products, the cost of these biosimilar products results in significant savings even at these reduced discounts.

A continuing challenge for manufacturers has been reimportation practices in the United States. Individuals struggling to pay for the cost of their medications have looked up to Canada and Mexico for brand name medications at reduced prices. This practice has been supported by legislation in a few states. The passage of the MMA 2003 and the patent expiration on a number of blockbuster medications have diminished the strong push for the importation of foreign products. The Medicare Part D programs offer prescription coverage to the largest group of Americans who had no prescription coverage, reducing the need to seek alternative sources of medications. In addition, an FDA study in 2003 found that a majority of U.S. citizens would spend less buying generic versions in the United States than branded products in Canada [79]. COVID vaccinations in 2020 were designed by the Federal government to be of no cost for patients, regardless of coverage or health plan type or none [80].

Under the 1997 Act, companies were permitted to distribute off-label usage information and health economic data to professionals. The FDA also relaxed its restrictions regarding direct-to-consumer (DTC) advertising of prescription medications [81]. In October 2002, President Bush signed the Prescription Drug User Fee Act (PDUFA III) that continues funding to the FDA to review activities that might help speed up new drug product approvals. Additionally, President Bush signed an Executive Order in October 2002 to speed the entry of generic drugs into the marketplace and limit branded product litigation against generic drug market entry to a single 30-month period. The Prescription Drug User Fee Amendment of 2007 (PDUFA IV) will enable the FDA to significantly expand its post-marketing surveillance of approved drugs and enhance its IT infrastructure to monitor and track adverse drug events.

Biologics, gene therapy, and digital health are more specific topics relative to reimbursement issues due to their very high costs (biologics and gene therapies) versus low-cost digital health solutions that now include therapeutic indications beyond just information capture or tracking. Donut hole coverage in 2021 Medicare prescription drug plans has now been fixed for Medicare part D members [82].

The development of biologic drugs is only possible through advances in basic science or genetic research and technologies that can now offer important treatment options where none were available nor successful before. Specialty drugs are being used to treat many types of difficult-to-manage conditions such as cancer, multiple sclerosis, rheumatoid arthritis, hepatitis C, diabetes, hemophilia, cystic fibrosis, among others. In addition, specialty drugs are also being used to treat infertility, neurological disorders, defective genes, and even high cholesterol levels.

What is the main difference between nonspecialty and biologic (specialty) drugs? Conventional nonspecialty drugs are chemical-based medicines, considered small molecules, and relatively easy and inexpensive to produce. In the majority of cases, their patents have expired, allowing for multiple sources of product. Even so, some small-molecule oral and infusible drugs cross the price threshold and could be considered specialty agents, but for the purposes of this discussion, specialty drugs will be limited to biologics only.

1. Biologics are made from living organisms (therefore a "biologic"), are usually very large molecules with complex structures, and are much more difficult and costly to make than a small-molecule drug. According to the FDA, biologics represent

> [A] wide range of products such as vaccines, blood and blood components, allergenics, somatic cells, gene therapy, tissues, and recombinant therapeutic proteins. Biologics can be composed of sugars, proteins, or nucleic acids or complex combinations of these substances, or may be

> living entities such as cells and tissues. Biologics are isolated from a variety of natural sources—human, animal, or microorganism.
>
> [83]

Biologics produce responses that may vary from patient to patient, including positive effects and adverse reactions. This is the result of their basic genetic or cellular biologic effects. Therefore, biologics may be very effective in patients with a specific identified genetic mutation or biomarker—providing the ability for what we refer to as personalized medicine.

The FDA has been working to review and respond to many of the changes that occurred with the provisions of the PDUFA. The FDA is responsible for overseeing the advertising of drugs and sending regulatory letters to manufacturers to halt the dissemination of materials that are in violation of DTC advertising regulations. The Government Accountability Office's (GAO) 2008 report on *Trends in FDA is Oversight of Direct-to-Consumer Advertising* highlights the difficulty the FDA has had in oversight of this area. The GAO reports that DTC reviews and advisory letters often arrive after the manufacturer has ceased the dissemination of the information [84]. The additional number of staff hired, through budget expansion in PDUFA IV, should help address this area.

Significant challenges continue to plague the FDA. The past decade has seen the agency deal with drug recalls such as Vioxx and the questions on the safety of the food supply with the widespread recall of tainted peanut products. Margaret Hamburg, M.D., who just stepped down as Commissioner in early 2015, was selected by President Obama as the individual capable of reshaping and redirecting this $2 billion agency. Dr. Hamburg had a history in public health as well as in bioterrorism and disease control. To date, her message has emphasized safety as well as efficacy, with the underlying message that the FDA is crucial to ensuring the welfare of U.S. citizens through oversight and accountability.

Additionally, in June 2009, President Obama signed landmark legislation that gave the FDA increasing authority over the tobacco industry. The new legislation will allow the FDA to ban misleading health claims, restrict marketing campaigns, and increase the health warnings associated with smoking all types of cigarettes as well as monitor the sales of tobacco products. Critics have voiced concerns that the FDA is currently overburdened with responsibilities and that the added burden of overseeing tobacco will further dilute the FDA's ability to oversee the activities within the pharmaceutical arena regulations.

Consumers continue to switch or be switched from brand to generic drugs as they increasingly become available. Generic substitution rates of over 90% are commonly seen in many health plans into 2020; yet, brand products account for 70% of managed care claims [81]. Generic manufacturers capitalized on a significant number of blockbuster branded medications losing patent protection over the last five to seven years. For the generic drug manufacturing industry, one big event in 1997 was Congress' passage of the Food and Drug Administration Modernization Act (FDAMA).

FDAMA included some benefits to generic drug manufacturers, as follows:

- Once the FDA and an applicant company agree on what bioavailability or bioequivalence studies are needed for the approval of an Abbreviated New Drug Application (ANDA), the FDA cannot change the rules (without a compelling reason).
- The unavailability of data from the FDA field office cannot be used to delay generic drug approvals.

FDAMA also gives certain innovator drugs that treat severe or life-threatening illnesses an extra six months of marketing exclusivity in exchange for manufacturers conducting pediatric clinical studies of the drug. Congress continues to tinker with FDA legislation and regulation that balance the marketing rights among traditional research-oriented and generic drug firms. Other regulation and legislation that are still debated but not fully resolved include (1) FDA-proposed guidelines to hold drug manufacturers or any other PBM owner responsible for false or misleading prescription marketing or promotion; (2) a CMS proposal to require hospitals to demonstrate a medication error rate lower than or equal to 2%, in order to receive Medicare funding; and (3) a congressional equal access bill to prohibit health plans from favoring one type of pharmacy provider (e.g., mail order over local retail pharmacy) by inclusive contract or by financial incentives such as co-pay differentials.

FDAMAs' success was expanded further through The Food and Drug Administration Safety and Innovation Act of 2012 (FDASIA), which is a piece of American regulatory legislation signed into law on July 9, 2012. It gives the United States Food and Drug Administration (FDA) the authority to collect user fees from the medical industry to fund reviews of innovator drugs, medical devices, generic drugs, and biosimilar biologics [85]. The latest law through Congress was the 21st Century Cures Act 2016: Streamline drugs intended to treat certain serious or life-threatening diseases [86].

26.7.2.1.1 Marketing Settlements

A number of class action lawsuits have resulted in billions of dollars in settlements. At the core of many of these suits has been the role of the manufacturer in convincing physicians to prescribe these medications for patients with conditions outside FDA indications. Physicians have always had the authority to prescribe drugs for off-label use, but manufacturers are limited to discussing labeled indications. One manufacturer settled a lawsuit alleging that their antipsychotic product was promoted the FDA approved label (i.e., off-label) and that the manufacturer minimized the risk of diabetes. The manufacturer set aside $1.42 billion for a potential settlement that subsequently resulted in another manufacturer settlement described next. In another case, the government has assessed a manufacturer $2.3 billion in criminal and civil penalties for violating drug marketing rules.

Perdue and Sackler Family reached a government settlement in 2020 of more than $8 billion and dissolution of company and its assets entirely for the public's benefit. Included was:

- One count dual-object conspiracy to defraud the United States and violate Food, Drug, and Cosmetic Act, and two counts of conspiracy to violate the federal Anti-Kickback Statute.
- Criminal fine of $3.544 billion and additional $2 billion in criminal forfeiture. Civil settlement of $2.8 billion to resolve civil liability under False Claims Act. Separately, Sackler family will pay $225 million in damages to resolve civil False Claims Act liability [87].

Another issue facing drug manufacturers is the number of products that have had black box warnings added to their drug labeling. A black box warning is the strongest safety warning the FDA requires and usually gives details as to the risk. Manufacturers are required to change their package insert to include the black box warning, and notification is sent out to prescribers. The anti-smoking drug Chantix® and the newer, second-generation antidepressants as well as some older medications such as propoxyphene and metoclopramide recently received black box warnings for significant adverse drug events.

Patent expiration of some blockbuster drugs valued around $20 billion has occurred over the last decade. Legal maneuvering usually delays the actual marketing of generic products, and research-intensive manufacturers also will license early marketing for as long as possible to a subsidiary or marketing partner to better manage the profitability of their products [77].

As the manufacturers of traditional medications strive to develop new products to replace these blockbuster drugs, patent protection has allowed the products of biotechnology companies in the United States to remain unchallenged.

26.7.2.2 Digital Health and Medication Therapy Management (MTM)

Digital health has emerged since 2020 as a full continuum of technology solutions, which includes mobile health, health info technology, wearable devices, telehealth and telemedicine, and personalized medicine [88, 89]. The promise and purpose for digital health for healthcare use include addressing

- Improved access
- Reduced costs
- Increased quality
- Help to make medicine more personalized
- Increase in easy access of patients. to medical information technology like "MyChart" as electronic medical records. One benefit example is to be able to look into specific patient care information such as receiving a COVID vaccination injection.
- Increase in popularity of apple watches/fit bits. Being able to use ECG and oxygenation saturation to track and detect AFib/COVID. Being able to detect falls with the fall alert on apple watches.
- Pharmacists are integral parts of the care team. For example, pharmacists can receive fees for managing medications for patients with multiple chronic diseases under Medicare Part D by the Centers for Medicare/Medicaid Services (CMS) 42 C.F.R. 423.153(d)
  - Required for costs covered in Part D drugs greater than or equal to $3,000 increase by annual percentage (2.85%). In 2020, the cost was $4,255, and in 2021, it was $4,376.
  - Aimed at reducing costs

As with changes in presidential administration (Obama, Trump, and Biden), President Joseph Biden entered in a state of flux from the election to the start of his term. As a result of political differences, over 40 executive orders were once again changing the regulatory landscape outside of the normal legislative process through Congress passing laws.

26.8 PHARMACEUTICAL MANUFACTURER CUSTOMERS

26.8.1 Organization and Operations

Pharmaceutical companies in the United States have traditionally been organized into three operational areas to fulfill their mission: (1) Research and development (R&D), (2) sales and marketing, and (3) manufacturing and distribution.

R&D operations are primarily focused on the discovery of new compounds that will be safe and effective in treating targeted disease states. In the past, R&D was accomplished within the organization. Pharmacists are employed in various aspects of R&D, including drug formulation, clinical research, and medical communications about drug information. Companies estimate that spending on research exceeds $2 billion and approximately 10 years to successfully obtain FDA approval to market a drug in the United States, including discovery, drug development, and clinical testing [90]. Today, most companies also license new drugs or technology created by start-up firms who are more willing to assume risk (in order to capture investor funding). In fact, biotechnology today remains one of the hottest areas for investment by Wall Street and Venture Capital investors. Various biotechnology and pharmaceutical formulation firms have marketing agreements with traditional manufacturers who offer sales and marketing expertise, as well as the recognition in the complex and fast changing U.S. healthcare marketplace.

Sales and marketing is the other main engine driving pharmaceutical companies. Some players believe that if a company discovers a drug for which there is no other marketplace competition, doctors will prescribe it, and patients will purchase it. More commonly, however, marketing and sales expertise is necessary to achieve success in the face of obstacles such as being a non-breakthrough drug, pricing problems, or fierce competition. Typical sales personnel are recruited from colleges with a degree in a health-related area such as pharmacy, nursing, or medicine. All manufacturers require continuing education in salesmanship and conduct rigorous sales training.

At some point in their career, nearly all marketing personnel have spent time in the field. Marketing, although uniquely different from sales in many other industries, has remained intertwined with sales in the pharmaceutical industry. This is probably due, in part, to the regulation, the nature of the product being sold, and the way in which the product is ordered through the prescriber. Pharmacists do hold sales and marketing positions in most pharmaceutical companies.

Rising in prominence today has been the role of drug pricing by manufacturers, which is the domain of marketing personnel. Oncologists have been the most active on this issue in 2015, but other professional groups as well as Congress have begun to enter the fray on pricing owing to the price tag for hepatitis C products marketed by Gilead Sciences in California. Pushback from insurers and PBMs has caused manufacturers to evaluate their pricing strategies for drugs currently on the market as well as those that have yet to receive FDA marketing approval. In addition, as the competition in most classes of new drugs allows formulary decision makers to exclude one of the new drugs from its formulary or make its formulary decision based on the company providing the best price, if clinically equivalent in terms of efficacy and safety.

Contract models for drugs that are clinically similar can include some of the following types.

1. Financial risk-based contracts: Evaluating drugs based on data on evidence from the real world, not just from clinical trials
2. Health-outcomes based contracts: Full or partial reimbursements if the patient does not respond to therapy or does not reach a targeted outcome.
3. Mortgage model: Spreading the cost of an expensive drug out over time, instead of paying it all up front
4. Subscription/Netflix model: "All you can treat" arrangement. Novel concept from Australia for HCV drugs [91].

Manufacturing and distribution of pharmaceutical products occur among all types of pharmaceutical manufacturers. Employment of pharmacists in this capacity is common (and, currently, there is a high demand for pharmacists to fill this role). Personnel in this area prepare the oral, liquid, and topical drug products that ultimately are sold by the manufacturer to a pharmacy. Actual distribution of the product may go through the drug wholesaler or directly from the manufacturer to a pharmacy or other licensed customer. Strict regulations surrounding the compounding, manufacture, and distribution of prescription pharmaceutical products demand a wide area of knowledge (of which the pharmacist has a solid, basic understanding).

26.8.2 Other Targeted Customer and Class of Trade Segments

Other customer segments, sectors, or trade categories include PBMs, specialty pharmacies, repackagers (typically hospitals or retail chain subsidiaries), federal (Medicare) or state government (Medicaid, Ryan White) programs, military, and the Veterans Administration. Manufacturers and wholesalers typically have separate account management and support for conducting business with these categories of pharmaceutical trade.

Unlike the private sector, public sector and military trade categories operate under different procurement rules and requirements, as well as have compliance with legislative or regulatory pricing guidelines. For example, the Federal Supply Schedule (FSS) is a key determinant for authorized purchases of all categories of products, including pharmaceuticals. This includes the VA and the military as well as some federally funded and qualified health centers (FQHCs) or federally qualified programs through legislative mandates.

From a medical and pharmacy practice perspective, professionals follow common standards of patient care as appropriate for their settings of care. In fact, cross innovation between private and public sector professionals has led to increased roles for pharmacists as active members of the patient care team. For example, pharmacists who can practice under a physician collaborative agreement evolved largely from VA hospital and clinic practices as well as select academic hospitals around the country.

26.8.3 Contracting and Change in the Pharmaceutical Industry

Just as pharmacists in pharmacies have changed in response to marketplace pressures, the manufacturers have adjusted personnel and resources to better compete in the future. One strategy is to focus on new drug entities that have no competitors and that offer a clear advancement in the diagnosis or treatment of a disease. Another strategy is to focus on select categories, as opposed to a broad-based range of conditions that may dilute the marketing capabilities of the organization across too many prescriber types. Some manufacturers are renting sales-force personnel through co-promotional alliances, where they do not have to compete in order to achieve faster market share accumulation.

Other manufacturers are more aggressively forming strategic marketing alliances and research partnerships to augment their own capabilities, in order to help them speed toward market approval and generate sales dollars. For manufacturers that do not focus on new drug marketing, competition has remained strong. Most recently, profits had lagged under the weight of purchaser consolidation, driving deeper discounts on multi-source (generic) drug products. This trend is leveling off, while many new drugs are coming off of patent protection and into generic firms, leading to a renewed profit opportunity for these marketers [81]. Deflation on all generics decreased by 11% but tends to hold at 15% year-over-years in the not-for-profit 46 Brooklyn December 2020 reports [81].

Manufacturers, pharmacies, and MCOs usually market the drug price savings associated with generic drug products to consumers. Now, even single-source brand name products may be marketed to consumers in an effort to capture market share by influencing the prescribers of prescription drug products.

Finally, all manufacturers continue to face scrutiny in their marketing practices due to various federal and state laws or regulation of pharmaceutical products. These include, but are not limited to, the distribution of drug samples, drug advertising (21 C.F.R. 202.1, 201.2), reminder advertising (21 C.F.R. 200.200), direct-to-consumer advertising (21 C.F.R. part 202), and the use of approved drugs for unapproved conditions.

Reimbursement regulations—such as those emanating from the Omnibus Budget Reconciliation Act of 1990 (OBRA), which mandated drug use rebates to Medicaid—can also affect manufacturers' pricing and marketing position. Managed care organizations, as well as federal and state programs, have traditionally provided reimbursement to pharmacies and clients as a percentage of the average wholesale price (AWP). The MMA 2003 and the Deficit Reduction Act have language requiring reimbursement be based on alternatives to AWP. The Deficit Reduction Act requires pricing using Average Manufacturer Price (AMP), which has traditionally been a confidential price used to calculate federal rebates for the Medicaid Programs. National Pharmacy Organizations have been challenging the use of AMP as a reduction in reimbursement to pharmacy providers. The MMA requires that Medicare reimbursement be based on Average Sale Price, a number submitted by manufacturers quarterly to CMS. In addition, First Data Bank, a national publisher of AWP, has agreed to cease publishing AWP as a part of its settlement in a lawsuit that accused First Data Bank of artificially inflating prices with the wholesaler McKesson [92].

The lawsuit alleges that the actions of FDB and McKesson cost Medicaid agencies, health plans, and private payers in excess of $7 billion. Given the marketplace changes, even regulations may have to be amended or repealed—or new regulations may have to be promulgated—to keep pace with the changing pricing algorithms used to determine fair and reasonable reimbursement.

Fraud and abuse within the healthcare system are another area that has gained local and national attention. HIPAA allowed for the creation of the National Health Care Fraud and Abuse Control Program (HCFAC). Responsibility for the security rules and administrative simplification standards of HIPAA was a CMS responsibility until Health and Human Services (HHS) Secretary Kathleen Sebelius granted the authority for administration and enforcement of HIPAA's privacy and security rules to the Office of Civil Rights. CMS retained its authority over the administrative simplification standards of HIPAA. On March 19, 2015, HHS issued a press release announcing that the Department of Justice and HHS had recovered $27.8 billion in returns in their joint efforts to combat healthcare fraud [93]. CMS expects the new ICD-10-CM codes (70,000) to improve the fraud and abuse initiatives that have been in place since the enactment of HIPAA in 1996 [94]. Federal fiscal year 2019 fraud and abuse issues continue to be an area of focus for the Department of Justice and Health and Human Services [95, 96]. Data security has rapidly emerged as an important area as healthcare increasingly uses and relies upon its IT infrastructure to manage population health. With an increased desire for interoperability comes an increased need for security. Recent health plan breaches or hacks have compromised a huge amount of clinical as well as reimbursement information of patients and providers that can be sold on the black internet market. HIPAA alone is not going to keep patient-level data safe. Allocating sufficient funds and resources to data security has become a necessity for healthcare entities throughout the drug distribution and clinical services delivery streams.

26.9 HEALTHCARE INDUSTRY CHANGES IN THE NEAR FUTURE

Among other changes or shifts in healthcare, there has been a changing number of community or retail-based pharmacies. For example, independent pharmacies in 2010–2019 had a relative increase of 12%, whereas chain pharmacies had a relative decrease of 0.2% [97].

- Pharmacists have been shifting to helping more in practice/ambulatory care, whereas people who are in community continue to shift toward machines [98].

A long-awaited Supreme Court of the United States (SCOTUS) decision came down in December 2020 ruling in favor of the states' interests of patients and community pharmacies in regulating PBMs. This SCOTUS case 592 U.S. 18. 504 (2020) was from the Arkansas Attorney General Leslie Rutledge versus the Pharmaceutical Care Management Association (PCMA) [99–101]. In essence, the State of Arkansas was ruled correct in promulgating legislation regulating PBMs to protect their businesses (pharmacies) and plan patients from overreach in pharmacy benefit plan management. Questions raised in this case supported by 16 additional states included that shall PBMs pay pharmacies at or above what the pharmacy paid the wholesaler? Are clawbacks on pharmacies by PBMs allowed? Are gag clauses enforceable in contracts?, and are requirements for use of mail order in place of community-based pharmacy dispensing allowed? This ruling focused on the ERISA Pre-emption rule only so additional related lawsuits are still pending, including a North Dakota case ruling that was sent back to the Federal Appeals Court by SCOTUS for review in light of the Rutledge decision.

Medical benefit drug products refer to the type of coverage for the cost of the drug or medication being used to manage a clinical condition. Rules for reimbursement are different and generally more lenient in medical benefits for drugs versus pharmacy benefits managed by PBMs. Lack of transparency in costs through the supply chain remains an issue here as in pharmacy benefits. Drugs covered in the medical plan typically require clinician administration (IV, IM) or observation period required by the FDA in their product labeling. An example of the difference in drug coverage by insurance benefit coverage type, medical versus pharmacy, is shown in Table 26.4 for different drug classes used in a chronic condition.

For commercial insurance coverages, there has been a growing argument for comprehensive benefit solutions in-line with consumerism and patient-centered care. Due to the numerous benefit design options offered (insurer/employer) and manufacturer support programs versus third-party (insurer or PBM) implications from their management, there are significant inconsistencies in the out-of-pocket impact on consumers and their prescription drugs.

How will healthcare or insurance reform as well as managed care affect hospitals and other care settings? It is useful to review some of the principles in the evolving marketplace influenced by managed care. There are several stages of managed care presence used by experts to determine the degree of saturation by managed care organizations (MCOs). One simple model to follow, developed between 2000 and 2010, has four stages:

TABLE 26.4
Drug Coverage by Insurance Benefit Coverage Type, Medical Versus Pharmacy.

Therapy/Benefit Design Example	Drug Type
Jardiance® oral diabetes therapy, with tier 2 co-pay	Pharmacy benefit
Remicade® infusion for rheumatoid arthritis, with flat co-pay, max out of pocket	Medical benefit
Remicade® infusion for rheumatoid arthritis; high-deductible health plan ($6,000), co-insurance, max out of pocket	Medical benefit

- Stage one represents an unstructured market with virtually no elements of managed healthcare. This is, essentially, the traditional fee-for-service market (which is now starting to enter into the sphere of MCOs). Stage one is common in rural areas and suburban pockets around the United States.
- Stage two represents more elements of managed healthcare—such as system evolution and contracting. Examples of cities/MSAs that were fully into stage two included: Atlanta, Georgia; Charlotte, North Carolina; Dallas, Texas; Philadelphia, Pennsylvania; and St. Louis, Missouri. In 2019, many of these cities/MSAs were in Stage 3.
- Stage three shows provider and institutional consolidation. Healthcare systems evolve from those changes. Examples of cities/MSAs that were among the many at this stage included Boston, Houston, Salt Lake City, and Phoenix. In 2019, many of these cities are moved to Stage four.
- Stage four is distinguished by clear coalitions of caregiver organizations and integrated systems of patient care across the continuum-of-care settings. Of the few cities/MSAs where this has occurred, Hershey, PA; Minneapolis, MN; Los Angeles, CA; and Worcester, MA are prime examples.

When examining a region's managed care evolution pre-pandemic, a determining factor has been the degree of vertical integration throughout the care system. Key aspects to evaluate include the number of components of care, components in the delivery of care, and the number of system-wide contracts. While there has been more merger and acquisition activity in healthcare before and during the pandemic, the basic staging or assessment has remained. National corporate entity vertical alignments play out more at the state level commercially due to law and regulatory structures in place for healthcare.

Future shifts based on pre-pandemic experience in providing care include moving from a system focused on short-term care to a system focused on a chronic or long-term continuum of care. Aging in the U.S. population continues to place an enormous strain on the resources of the U.S. healthcare delivery system, including access to drugs and pharmacists. Reimbursement changes such as prospective payment systems, shared risk contracting, and alternative quality contracts are aligning incentives among care providers to utilize the lowest level of care necessary for adequate patient-care outcomes. An increasingly important part of that outcome is related to drug therapy—a paradox for pharmacists and payors, as drug treatment can further increase the ambulatory cost of care. However, if a drug is not available due to access barriers such as cost sharing or if patients do not use it regularly, they will have adverse outcomes and will have to utilize more expensive levels of care such as the emergency room or hospital.

Integrated information systems (Electronic Health Record, Electronic Medical Record) are required to aid in refining the treatment process and obtaining patient outcome information. The ACA included incentives for physicians and other provider entities to implement integrated information systems and meet so-called meaningful use guidelines as criteria to receive the monetary incentives or avoid penalties by 2016. While pharmacies have long been fully computerized, they are not yet fully linked to other segments of the care delivery system. This lack of connection, even in stage four cities, remains a major barrier to fully achieving the promises of appropriate drug utilization and receiving any positive impact from pharmacists' patient care. Most MCOs have been spending increasing amounts of money on information systems, especially in those stage four markets, to remain competitive and achieve the benefits that shared information can bring to geographically separated members of the healthcare system. The focus of various electronic platform initiatives does include pharmacy but, primarily, medical care providers or facilities where most healthcare spending occurs in the United States. For example, prescriptions today are already primarily sent electronically by prescribers (physicians, nurse practitioners, physician assistants, and in some states pharmacists) in place of hand-written prescription paper given to the patient to take to the pharmacy.

In 2018, Congress passed Substance Use-Disorder Prevention that Promotes Opioid Recovery and Treatment (SUPPORT) for Patients and Communities Act. SUPPORT mandates that all Medicare Part D Providers electronically prescribe controlled substances (EPCS) by 2021.

- In 2017, 32% of office-based physicians prescribed controlled substances electronically; however, around 90% of all noncontrolled substances were sent electronically [102, 104].

Group purchasing of drugs by healthcare delivery systems as a single class of trade had emerged since 1998 as a major shift in purchasing policy and continues today by a wider variety of purchasing decision entities. Aside from a licensed retail pharmacy, all other care settings can purchase jointly and maximize their purchasing power, while still achieving a measure of cost containment. Formulary management has led to managed care entities operating in a group purchasing mode since they had demonstrated their impact on product market share by optimizing generic or select brand utilization over other options. Employer coalitions and other payors have similarly leveraged group purchasing as part of strategies to optimize drug product and pharmacist services efficiency.

Legislation impacting formularies has remained a problem with MCOs, as part of the historical consumer backlash over reduced access to care, which has once again surfaced in the healthcare reform debate. Mandated opening of drug benefits and access to prescription drugs (in general or in niche categories) have become a new problem for managed care to handle, especially in light of the continually rising costs of healthcare. Traditionally, closed formularies and narrow drug benefit policies had been used to create a consistent level of quality in drug utilization and to try to contain costs. Today, cost sharing has supplanted open formularies and easier prior approval processes that are more the norm. More drug choices along with new biotechnology and molecular medicine therapies in the pharmacies have contributed to almost double-digit increases in MCOs' pharmacy segment costs. As a result of that and ACA implementation, many plans have changed their budgeting to global costs-of-care assessments and increasing a shared financial risk model with physicians for drug utilization expenditures.

26.10 SUMMARY AND CONCLUSIONS

As with most areas of business, the business of healthcare has continued to evolve and change along with technological innovations in all aspects of healthcare. Consolidation of entities, streamlined work processes, increased FDA, new drug approvals, and the more rapid entry of IT solutions have all combined to drive change into traditional pharmacy, managed care, and manufacturer activities pre-pandemic 2020. What has been seen during the pandemic have been nothing short of remarkable in the breadth and depth of practice changes by all those professional constituencies in addressing a rapid response to the COVID-19 pandemic.

Looking at pharmacy alone, there remain high-risk areas including practice scope itself for pharmacists, technician supervision across an expanding area of support services and number of support personnel, and downstream impacts of the drug pedigree, and counterfeit drug supply chain participation as the final dispenser of prescription drug products to a patient at the point of service.

Other areas still being determined in the healthcare marketplace include pharmacy availability in local communities versus some form of package delivery, pharmacies being allowed or financially able to operate 24 hours 365 days a year, pharmacy and pharmaceutical care access by geographic MSA—especially in rural areas of the United States, and professional practice scope for pharmacists along with benefit design criteria providing reimbursement to the licensed pharmacies.

Managed care over the past decade had been increasingly scrutinized because its drug reimbursement management overreach, tactics, and role within the healthcare system are becoming outsized as middlemen are not clearly contributing a value proposition, beneficial to the end user. Most recently, Amazon has begun expansion into various aspects of healthcare that included prescription drug delivery with the acquisition of PillPack and grocery store chain Whole Foods Market that operated in-store pharmacies. As boundaries are changing along with the players, managed care will be challenged in ways, new and different from its historic beginnings in adjudication of Medicaid claims for a state agency. The relationship between managed care and manufacturers has also become strained as business models have changed among those two market stakeholders too.

Manufacturers of prescription drug, device, or diagnostic products have felt a similar scrutiny over the changes in products today versus less than 10 years ago, which were available for treating an ever-increasing number of medical conditions but at an unsustainable price pointing to the health plan or consumer. The trend of shifting from non-biological small molecule products rapidly into biologic large molecule or gene-based products has escalated drug price concerns even more than in the past. How these new drug products are covered in plans, managed by third parties, and utilized by consumers have grown increasingly complex in both the clinical journey as well as in the flow of funds among the parties.

There are numerous implications now at play in a rapidly transitioning healthcare marketplace that includes heavily regulated professions for plaintiff and defense attorneys and other judicial officials. The clash between economic costs and the value of clinical outcomes has never been more intensified, somewhat reflective of the political landscape resulting from the 2020 Presidential election. Where those attitudes and beliefs lead us through judicial actions will likely set even newer directions for healthcare delivery for decades.

Gray areas remain or emerge in healthcare despite efforts to close questions or gaps in law and regulation. Some of those areas still being determined include medical or pharmacy benefit insurance coverages in both full- and self-funded benefit programs; PBM and manufacturer relationships around product pricing or reimbursement practices; consumerism and fiduciary responsibility of plans that protect the interests or needs of the patient as a consumer; how to review and approve digital health products now currently managed by the FDA; and medical or general marijuana legalization along with its impact on workforce and workplace safety.

Few can accurately predict the future impact of the latest healthcare reform efforts underway in the United States on the pharmacist, pharmacy, and pharmaceutical industry, let alone supply chain or managed care. Even with health reform passed in some form, it would require significant time to effectively deal with the precision necessary at the federal level and for implementation in all state jurisdictions. Given the turmoil and rapid changes in the care delivery system in just the past 18 months into 2021, it is clear that all pharmacy-related stakeholders will feel some effect of planned system changes on their individual role within the healthcare system. However, some trends have emerged, and experts are attempting to focus a more lasting, thoughtful change in healthcare, including changes in pharmacy along with its supply chain, third-party reimbursement, manufacturer of product, and the pharmacist's role.

Recent and emerging changes in providing pharmacy services include

- integrated healthcare (merged, alliance) systems with fewer independent and rural pharmacies;
- a renewed emphasis on drug therapy management techniques with use controls to achieve documented, optimal patient outcomes;
- the decrease in privatization of public sector and not-for-profit institutions or organizations;
- the expanded use of alternative group purchasing organizations (GPOs) for optimizing care delivery performance or alternative risk arrangements and employer purchasing coalitions for value-based contracting;
- the changing role of the pharmacy wholesaler in the distribution system, going beyond being just a purveyor of products to becoming an integral, diversified partner in drug distribution with the manufacturer and pharmacy;
- general management and legal or regulatory issues particular to pharmacy professional services as part of a team-based care delivery system of regulated (licensed) professionals.

The use of non-dispensing pharmacist services, such as medication therapy monitoring (MTM) and immunizations administered by pharmacists, has been shown to have a significant positive impact on the quality and cost of patient care by optimizing drug therapy or access to vaccines, which, in turn, results in positive patient-care outcomes. To enable the pharmacist to engage in these non-dispensing activities, pharmacy services will necessarily require adequate compensation as well as to continue the process of automating the preparation and dispensing of drugs. The roles and responsibilities of pharmacy technicians and other non-pharmacist personnel will grow commensurate with changes in pharmacists' direct patient-care responsibilities. In the hospital, clinic, and home-care settings, pharmacists moving to decentralized patient-care areas will require an increased use of supportive personnel in nonjudgmental tasks of pharmacy operations. These changes will require or have already resulted in regulatory and personnel development changes in the field of pharmacy. Similarly, the increased use of automation in nonhospital settings will require or have already resulted in regulatory approval and retraining of personnel in pharmacy.

As the traditional dispensers of medication, pharmacies and pharmacists will be playing a greater role in drug identification, safety, and monitoring for optimal use of medication therapy. As a result, future pharmacy operations will continue to become more patient centered, regardless of the healthcare delivery setting. Performance will be measured by the actual data of patient outcomes, collected by the healthcare organization having primary responsibility for providing total healthcare, and reimbursement will be linked to those measures of outcome performance.

Total cost of care and various prepayment or reimbursement methods will continue but will increasingly allow for the compensation of pharmacists separate from product dispensing. This becomes necessary in order to achieve successful financial and patient-care outcomes for total healthcare value that can appeal to both sides (dispensing and clinical) within the current pharmacy profession along with those purchasing or paying for care. In addition, pharmacists are now permitted to administer vaccinations in most states, such as the flu vaccine, and play an emerging public health role in pandemic or emergency management planning. This was on clear display during the COVID-19 pandemic in 2020 to 2021.

This chapter provided an overview of pharmacy, pharmacists, managed care, and manufacturers as they relate to drug-use issues in various healthcare delivery settings, reimbursed through managed care. These health professional settings included the retail or community pharmacy and acute care hospital, as well as the subacute, outpatient, long-term, home, and physician office care settings. Healthcare professionals in all settings, including pharmacists, need to be aware of the differing perspectives and common goals for providing pharmacy services in the U.S. marketplace as integrated systems evolve. The integrated care system, in which they are a participant through a hospital or health plan, will expect pharmacists to perform tasks as part of various performance improvement initiatives, leading toward improved patient care outcomes.

Pharmacists, regardless of the healthcare settings in which they practice, must be knowledgeable of the U.S. healthcare system environment and understand the goals of the patient, hospital, and managed care payer. Ultimately, all pharmacists, as healthcare service providers, must communicate and work together with the entire healthcare ecosystem or integrated organization and their respective patient-oriented care delivery team in order for the new coordinated care systems to truly provide documented care. Optimal patient care outcomes today have clearly established the need for timely, clinically safe, and cost-effective drug treatment within a more integrated, electronically interconnected care program managed by healthcare professionals.

NOTE

1 https://www.aacp.org/article/academic-pharmacys-vital-statistics, Accessed 4/8/2025.

REFERENCES

1. *Managed Care Digest Series: Hospitals/Systems Digest.* Vol. 3. Bridgewater, NJ: Sanofi Aventis; 2014.
2. *Managed Care Digest Series: Public Payer Digest.* Bridgewater, NJ: Sanofi; 2019. https://www.managedcaredigest.com/ereader/2019PublicPayerDigest/37/index.html#zoom=z.
3. "Hospital: 2021 National Patient Safety Goals." The Joint Commission, Joint Commission Resources, 29 October 2020. www.jointcommission.org/standards/national-patient-safety-goals/hospital-national-patient-safety-goals/.
4. *Novartis Pharmacy Benefit Report.* 1998 ed. Totowa, NJ: Emron; 1998.
5. *Managed Care Digest Series: Institutional Digest.* 1998 ed. Kansas City, MO: Hoechst Marion Roussel; 2001.
6. *Managed Care Digest: Integrated Health Systems Digest.* Kansas City, MO: Hoechst Marion Roussel; 2001.
7. Drawing a Line in the Sand: Employers Must Rethink Pharmacy Benefit Strategies. Midwest Business Group on Health, September 12, 2017.
8. "California Privacy Rights Act: An Overview." Privacy Rights Clearinghouse. privacyrights.org/resources/california-privacy-rights-act-overview#:~:text=The%20California%20Privacy%20Rights%20Act%20clarifies%20that%20people%20can%20opt,personal%20information%20to%20third%20parties.&text=The%20California%20Privacy%20Rights%20Act%20expands%20this%20to%20cover%20data,includes%20a%20username%20and%20password.
9. Assembly Bill No. 375 Chapter 55: AB 375, Chau. Privacy: Personal Information: Businesses. https://leginfo.legislature.ca.gov/faces/billTextClient.xhtml?bill_id=201720180AB375.
10. Brown, DL. "Years of rampant expansion have imposed Darwinian survival-of-the-fittest conditions on US pharmacy schools." American Journal of Pharmaceutical Education, vol. 84, no. 10, 2020, p. ajpe8136.
11. Maine, Lucinda L. "It Really Isn't That Simple." American Journal of Pharmaceutical Education, vol. 83, no. 4, 2019, p. 7593. doi:10.5688/ajpe7593.
12. The Pharmacy Student Population: Applications Received 2018–19, Degrees Conferred 2018–19, Fall 2019 Enrollments Jamie N. Taylor, Nancy T. Nguyen, and Estela J. Lopez. American Journal of Pharmaceutical Education July, vol. 84, no. 7, 2020, p. ajpe8207. doi:10.5688/ajpe8207.
13. "Academic Pharmacy's Vital Statistics." AACP. www.aacp.org/article/academic-pharmacys-vital-statistics; https://www.aacp.org/article/academic-pharmacys-vital-statistics.
14. ACPE Standard Revision 2016. Web. 31 July 2015. https://www.acpeaccredit.org/deans/StandardsRevision.asp.
15. "ASHP 2020 Residency Match Phase I Signals Steady Growth in Positions." ASHP. www.ashp.org/News/2020/03/13/ASHP-2020-Residency-Match-Phase-I-Signals-Steady-Growth-in-Positions.
16. Rutgers Institute for Pharmaceutical Industry Fellowships. "FAQs." Rutgers Institute for Pharmaceutical Industry Fellowships, 28 August 2020. pharmafellows.rutgers.edu/FAQs.
17. Wickline v. State of California, 239 Cal. Rptr. 810 (Ct. App. 1986).
18. Porcaro ET. Final Report of Phase I SBIR Grant #97-P-08080/3-011994.
19. "History." Board of Pharmacy Specialties. www.bpsweb.org/about-bps/history/.
20. The Council on Credentialing in Pharmacy. *Scope of Contemporary Pharmacy Practice: Roles, Responsibilities, and Functions of Pharmacists and Pharmacy Technicians.* Washington, DC: Council on Credentialing in Pharmacy; 2009.
21. *Survey of Pharmacy Law.* National Association of Boards of Pharmacy; 2021, pp. 1–185.
22. "Choose PTCB. Choose Excellence." PTCB. www.ptcb.org/resources/state-regulations-and-map.
23. "Pharmacy Technician Certification (KPHT): NHA Certifications." Pharmacy Technician Certification (CPhT)|NHA Certifications. www.nhanow.com/certifications/pharmacy-technician.

24. "Choose PTCB. Choose Excellence." PTCB. www.ptcb.org/resources/state-regulations-and-map.
25. "Products—Data Briefs—Number 347—August 2019." Centers for Disease Control and Prevention, Centers for Disease Control and Prevention, 14 August 2019. www.cdc.gov/nchs/products/databriefs/db347.htm.
26. "Get to Know Your Pharmacist." Centers for Disease Control and Prevention, 4 January 2021. www.cdc.gov/heartdisease/pharmacist.htm.
27. Weitzman, Debbie. "Provider Status for Pharmacists: It's About Time." *Pharmacy Times*, 7 October 2020. www.pharmacytimes.com/news/provider-status-for-pharmacists-its-about-time.
28. Center for Medicare and Medicaid Services. Medicare Part D Medication Therapy Management (MTM) Programs, 2019. www.cms.gov/Medicare/Prescription-Drug-Coverage/PrescriptionDrugCovContra/Downloads/CY2019-MTM-Fact-Sheet.pdf.
29. "CMS Perspective: Enhanced Medication Therapy Management . . ." Center for Medicare and Medicaid Innovation, U.S. Department of Health and Human Services, October 2020. innovation.cms.gov/data-and-reports/2020/mtm-secondevalrpt-perspective.
30. "Part D Enhanced Medication Therapy Management Model (MTM . . ." Evaluation of the Enhanced Medication Therapy Management (MTM) Model: At a Glance, U.S. Department of Health and Human Services. innovation.cms.gov/data-and-reports/2020/mtm-secondevalrpt-fg.
31. "PharmD Program Accreditation." Accreditation Council for Pharmacy Education, 23 February 2021. www.acpe-accredit.org/pharmd-program-accreditation/.
32. *Survey of Pharmacy Law.* National Association of Boards of Pharmacy, 2021, pp. 1–185.
33. Biosimilars in the United States 2020–2024. IQVIA Institute for Human Data Science, October 2020. www.bigmoleculewatch.com/wp-content/uploads/sites/2/2020/10/iqvia-institute-biosimilars-in-the-united-states.pdf.
34. Department of Health and Human Services. *HIPAA Administration Simplification: Modifications to Medical Data Code Set Standards to Adopt ICD-10-CM and ICD-10-PCS.* Washington, DC: Department of Health and Human Services; 2009: 3328–3329.
35. Find a Medicare Plan. https://www.medicare.gov/plan-compare/#/?year=2022&lang=en.
36. Adams, Alex, and Krystalyn Weaver. "Pharmacists' Patient Care Process: A State 'Scope of Practice' Perspective." Innovations in Pharmacy, vol. 10, no. 2, 2019, p. 7. Crossref, doi:10.24926/iip.v10i2.1389.
37. "An Overview of the Medicare Part D Prescription Drug Benefit." *KFF*, 14 October 2020. www.kff.org/medicare/fact-sheet/an-overview-of-the-medicare-part-d-prescription-drug-benefit/.
38. Federal Trade Commission. *CVS Caremark Settles FTC Charges: Failed to Protect Medical and Financial Privacy of Customers and Employees; CVS Pharmacy Also Pays $2.25 Million to Settles Allegations of HIPAA Violations.* Washington, DC: Federal Trade Commission; 2009.
39. Greiter, Elizabeth, and Alissa Smith. "2020's a Bust, but HIPAA Enforcement Is on a Roll!" *Health Law*, 20 March 2018. dorseyhealthlaw.com/2020s-a-bust-but-hipaa-enforcement-is-on-a-roll/.
40. Foster Freedmen, Linn. "Walgreen Case Opens Door For State Law HIPAA Claims." LAW 360. Nixon Peabody LLP, 25 November 2014. Web. 25 August 2015. http://www.law360.com/articles/598691/walgreen-case-opens-door-for-state-law-hipaa-claims.
41. Gerdes Long, Laura. "Another State Rules That Patients Can Sue For Negligence for Violating HIPAA Regulations." Beyond The Fine Print RSS. Danna McKitrick, P.C. Attorneys at Law, 11 November 2014. Web. 25 August 2015. http://www.dannamckitrick.com/beyond-the-fine-print/2014/11/another-state-rules-that-patients-can-sue-for-negligence-for-violating-hipaa-regulations/.
42. "Pharmacist Prescribing: Statewide Protocols and More." National Alliances of State Pharmacy Associations, November 2018. naspa.us/resource/swp/.
43. Schmitz, Natalie, and Lucas Richert. "Pharmacists and the Future of Cannabis Medicine." Journal of the American Pharmacists Association, vol. 60, no. 1, 2020, pp. 207–211. Crossref, doi:10.1016/j.japh.2019.11.007.
44. Adams, Alex, and Krystalyn Weaver. "Pharmacists' Patient Care Process: A State 'Scope of Practice' Perspective." Innovations in Pharmacy, vol. 10, no. 2, 2019, p. 7. Crossref, doi:10.24926/iip.v10i2.1389.
45. *Survey of Pharmacy Law.* National Association of Boards of Pharmacy; 2021: 1–185.
46. "West Virginia Supreme Court Rules Addicts Can Sue Pharmacies, Doctors." American Pharmacist Association. Web. 25 August 2015. http://www.medpagetoday.com/Blogs/EPMonthly/53199.
47. "Justice Department Announces Global Resolution of Criminal and Civil Investigations with Opioid Manufacturer Purdue Pharma and Civil Settlement with Members of the Sackler Family." The United States Department of Justice, 28 January 2021. www.justice.gov/opa/pr/justice-department-announces-global-resolution-criminal-and-civil-investigations-opioid.
48. "NPLEx." Appriss Health, 24 August 2020. apprisshealth.com/solutions/nplex/.
49. "COVID-19: Therapeutic Interchange." *NASPA*, 3 December 2020. naspa.us/resource/covid-19-therapeutic-interchange/.
50. Lowery, Mark, ed. "CVS Settles Three Pharmacist-overtime Lawsuits." *Drug Topics*, 28 July 2015. http://drugtopics.modernmedicine.com/drug-topics/news/cvs-settles-three-pharmacist-overtime-lawsuits?page=full.
51. Cassidy J. Targeting Treatment in Rehabilitation. Subacute Care, vol. 10, no. 4, 1995, pp. 31–32.
52. Wagner L. Guidelines Leading the Way to Best Practices in Long-Term Care. Provider, vol. 21, no. 12, 1995, pp. 43–48.
53. Department of Health and Human Services. *HIPAA Administration Simplification: Modifications to Medical Data Code Set Standards to Adopt ICD-10-CM and ICD-10-PCS.* Washington, DC: Department of Health and Human Services; 2009: 3328–3329.
54. Institute of Medicine. *To Err is Human: Building a Safer Health System*; 1999.
55. "ICD-10 HAC List." *CMS.* www.cms.gov/Medicare/Medicare-Fee-for-Service-Payment/HospitalAcqCond/icd10_hacs.
56. Navarro RP. Measuring the Effect of Change. Medical Interface, vol. 8, no. 9, 1995, p. 13.
57. Pharmacy Benefits for Nonspecialty Drugs: Access and Management by F. R. Vogenberg, PhD, FASHP AMI Publications, Trumbull, CT. Copyright© 2018 F. R. Vogenberg ISBN 978-1-729-00088-5.

58. "Publications." The Role of Distributors in the US Health Care Industry, 2019. www.hda.org/resources/the-role-of-distributors-in-the-us-health-care-industry.
59. Yadav, Prashant. "When Fewer Is Better: Pharmaceutical Wholesaling and Distribution in Low- and Middle-Income Countries." *Center for Global Development*, 24 January 2020. www.cgdev.org/blog/when-fewer-better-pharmaceutical-wholesaling-and-distribution-low-and-middle-income-countries.
60. Dingell, John D. "Text—H.R.1207–100th Congress (1987–1988): Prescription Drug Marketing Act of 1987." *Congress.gov*, 22 April 1988. www.congress.gov/bill/100th-congress/house-bill/1207/text.
61. "503A Vs. 503B: A Quick-Guide to Compounding Pharmacy Designations & Regulations." *The FDA Group*. www.thefdagroup.com/blog/503a-vs-503b-compounding-pharmacies.
62. Ugalmugle, Sumant, and Rupali Swain. "U.S. Compounding Pharmacies Market Trends: Statistics Report 2027." *Global Market Insights, Inc.*, February 2021. www.gminsights.com/industry-analysis/us-compounding-pharmacies-market.
63. Courtney, Joe. "Text—H.R.748–116th Congress (2019–2020): CARES Act." *Congress.gov*, 27 March 2020. www.congress.gov/bill/116th-congress/house-bill/748/text.
64. Kuehner-Hebert, Katie. "Addressing the Physician Dispensing Challenge." *Risk & Insurance*, 24 August 2017. riskandinsurance.com/addressing-physician-dispensing-challenge/.
65. "Opioids Archives." *Risk & Insurance*. riskandinsurance.com/category/risksrm/opioids/.
66. Ipharmaservices. "Top 20 Pharmaceutical Companies by Revenues in 2020: Top 10 Pharma Companies by Revenues in 2020." *Ipharmacenter*, 2 March 2021. www.ipharmacenter.com/post/top-10-pharmaceutical-companies-by-revenues-in-2020.
67. "2020 Employer Health Benefits Survey—Section 9: Prescription Drug Benefits." *KFF*, 20 October 2020. www.kff.org/report-section/ehbs-2020-section-9-prescription-drug-benefits/.
68. Cohen, Robin A., and Emily P. Zammitti. "Products—Data Briefs—Number 317—August 2018." *Centers for Disease Control and Prevention*, 9 August 2018. www.cdc.gov/nchs/products/databriefs/db317.htm.
69. "2020 Employer Health Benefits Survey—Section 9: Prescription Drug Benefits." *Kaiser Family Foundation*, 20 October 2020. www.kff.org/report-section/ehbs-2020-section-9-prescription-drug-benefits/.
70. "Overview of a Specialty Drug Trend: Succeeding in the Rapidly Changing U.S. Specialty Market." *IMShealth*, 2015. Web 25 August 2015. https://www.imshealth.com/deployed-files/imshealth/Global/North%20America/United%20States/Managed%20Markets/5-29-14%20Specialty_Drug_Trend_Whitepaper_Hi-Res.pdf.
71. "2019 Drug Trend Report." *Express Scripts*, 2020. www.express-scripts.com/corporate/drug-trend-report#2019-by-the-numbers.
72. New Drug Therapy Approvals 2020. https://www.fda.gov/drugs/new-drugs-fda-cders-new-molecular-entities-and-new-therapeutic-biological-products/new-drug-therapy-approvals-2020.
73. Celeste, R. Does Healthcare Benefit From a Unified Approach to Item-Level Serialization and UDI? *Pharmaceutical Commerce*, July/August 2015, p. 6.
74. Hardy, Jeff. "Estimating the Global Economic and Social Impacts of Counterfeiting and Piracy." *World Trademark Review*, 18 May 2017. www.worldtrademarkreview.com/anti-counterfeiting/estimating-global-economic-and-social-impacts-counterfeiting-and-piracy.
75. Vogenberg, FR. *Glossary of Common Drug-Related Benefit Terms & Acronyms*. Trumbull, CT: Access Market Intelligence; 2018.
76. US Food and Drug Administration. "Advancing Health Through Innovation: New Drug Therapy Approvals 2020." Web. 21 January 2021. https://www.fda.gov/media/144982/download.
77. The biopharmaceutical pipeline: Innovative therapies in clinical development (Analysis Group) PhRMA, 2017.
78. Marsh, Tori. "43 Drugs Going Generic in the Next 5 Years (2018–2022)—GoodRx." *The GoodRx Prescription Savings Blog*, 26 July 2018. www.goodrx.com/blog/drugs-going-generic-2018-2019-2020-2021-2022/.
79. US Food Drug Administration. "Biosimilars: Questions and Answers Regarding Implementation of the Biologics Price Competition and Innovation Act of 2009 Guidance for Industry." April 2015. http://www.fda.gov/downloads/Drugs/GuidanceComplianceRegulatoryInformation/Guidances/UCM444661.pdf.
80. Bernstein IBG, Shuren J. The Food and Drug Administration's Counterfeit Drug Initiative. Journal of Pharmacy Practice, vol. 19, no. 4, 2006, pp. 250–254.
81. "Press Release Trump Administration Acts to Ensure Coverage of Life-Saving COVID-19 Vaccines & Therapeutics." *Center for Medicare & Medicaid Services*, 28 October 2020. www.cms.gov/newsroom/press-releases/trump-administration-acts-ensure-coverage-life-saving-covid-19-vaccines-therapeutics.
82. "May Your Holidays Be Filled with Generic Drug Deflation!" *46brooklyn Research*, 29 December 2020.
83. Cubanski, Juliette, and Anthony Damico. "Medicare Part D: A First Look at Medicare Prescription Drug Plans in 2021." *Kaiser Family Foundation*, 29 October 2020. www.kff.org/medicare/issue-brief/medicare-part-d-a-first-look-at-medicare-prescription-drug-plans-in-2021/.
84. Center for Biologics Evaluation and Research. "What Are 'Biologics' Questions and Answers." *U.S. Food and Drug Administration, FDA*, 6 February 2018. www.fda.gov/about-fda/center-biologics-evaluation-and-research-cber/what-are-biologics-questions-and-answers.
85. "Generics: Making a Comeback." Drug Topics Supplement, vol. 142, no. 15, 1998.
86. "Food and Drug Administration Safety and Innovation Act (FDASIA)." *U.S. Food and Drug Administration, FDA*, 28 March 2018. www.fda.gov/regulatory-information/selected-amendments-fdc-act/food-and-drug-administration-safety-and-innovation-act-fdasia.
87. "21st Century Cures Act." *U.S. Food and Drug Administration, FDA*, 1 March 2020. www.fda.gov/regulatory-information/selected-amendments-fdc-act/21st-century-cures-act.
88. "Justice Department Announces Global Resolution of Criminal and Civil Investigations with Opioid Manufacturer Purdue Pharma and Civil Settlement with Members of the Sackler Family." *The United States Department of Justice*, 21 October 2020. www.justice.gov/opa/pr/justice-department-announces-global-resolution-criminal-and-civil-investigations-opioid.
89. "What Is Digital Health?" *U.S. Food and Drug Administration, FDA*, 22 September 2020. www.fda.gov/medical-devices/digital-health-center-excellence/what-digital-health.

90. "Healthcare—Apple Watch." *Apple.* www.apple.com/healthcare/apple-watch/.
91. "Biopharmaceutical R&D the Process Behind New Medicines." *Pharmaceutical Research and Manufacturers of America*, 20 August 2015. www.phrma.org/Report/Biopharmaceutical-R-and-D-The-Process-Behind-New-Medicines.
92. Comer, Ben. "Six Drug Pricing Models Have Emerged to Improve Product Access and Affordability." *PricewaterhouseCoopers*, 23 September 2019. www.pwc.com/us/en/industries/health-industries/library/6-drug-pricing-models.html.
93. 244 F.R.D. 79 (D. Mass 2007) New Eng. Carpenters Health v. First Databank in violation of 18 U.S.C. (double s symbol) 1964. https://casetext.com/case/new-england-carpenters-health-v-first-databank-3.
94. "Departments of Justice and Health and Human Services Announce Over $27.8 Billion in Returns From Joint Efforts to Combat Health Care Fraud." *U.S. Department of Health & Human Services, HHS.gov*, 19 March 2015. wayback.archive-it.org/3926/20170127185611/www.hhs.gov/about/news/2015/03/19/departments-of-justice-and-health-and-human-services-announce-over-27-point-8-billion-in-returns-from-joint-efforts-to-combat-health-care-fraud.html.
95. "White Paper: The Impact of ICD-10 on Fraud, Waste, and Abuse Detection." *General Dynamics Information Technology*, 2012. https://www.govexec.com/media/gbc/docs/gdit_-_6973_healthit-wp1_-_3.19.pdf.
96. "Health Care Fraud and Abuse Control Program Report Fiscal Year 2019." *Health Care Fraud and Abuse Control Program Report Office of Inspector General, U.S. Department of Health and Human Services*, June 2020. oig.hhs.gov/reports-and-publications/hcfac/index.asp.
97. "CMS Fraud Prevention Initiative: New Tools to Fight Fraud and Protect Taxpayers Dollars." *Center for Medicaid and Medicare Services*, July 2011. https://www.cms.gov/Outreach-and-Education/Outreach/Partnerships/Downloads/BackgrounderFraudPreventionInitiative.pdf.
98. Hatemi, Pete, and Christopher Zorn. "Independent Pharmacies in the U.S. Are More on the Rise Than on the Decline: Analysis." *Pharmaceutical Care Management Association*, 5 March 2020. www.pcmanet.org/independent-pharmacies-in-the-u-s-are-more-on-the-rise-than-on-the-decline/.
99. John, Christopher. "The Changing Role of the Pharmacist in the 21st Century." *The Pharmaceutical Journal*, 8 January 2018. pharmaceutical-journal.com/article/opinion/the-changing-role-of-the-pharmacist-in-the-21st-century.
100. "Rutledge v. Pharmaceutical Care Management Association." *SCOTUSblog*, 2021. www.scotusblog.com/case-files/cases/rutledge-v-pharmaceutical-care-management-association/.
101. Bianchi, Alden J., and Tara E. Swenson Dwyer. "Supreme Court Holds That ERISA Does Not Preempt Arkansas PBM Law: The Impact on Employer Sponsored Group Health Plans." *The National Law Review*, 31 December 2020. www.natlawreview.com/article/supreme-court-holds-erisa-does-not-preempt-arkansas-pbm-law-impact-employer.
102. "Rutledge V. Pharmaceutical Care Management ASSN." *Cornell Law School: Legal Information Institute.* www.law.cornell.edu/supremecourt/text/18-540.
103. Getting, Andrew, and Thomas A. Mason. "The ONC Doctors' Perspective: Electronic Prescribing of Controlled Substances (EPCS) Is on the Rise, and We Must Work Together to Address Barriers to Use." *Health IT Buzz*, 3 October 2019. www.healthit.gov/buzz-blog/health-it/the-onc-doctors-perspective-electronic-prescribing-of-controlled-substances-epcs-is-on-the-rise-and-we-must-work-together-to-address-barriers-to-use.
104. "E-Prescribing." *U.S. Centers for Medicare & Medicaid Services*, 5 August 2020. www.cms.gov/Medicare/E-Health/Eprescribing.

27 The Pharmacist's Utilization of the National Patient Safety Goals to Contribute to Safe and Effective Medication Use[1]

Jennifer Splawski and Heather Minger

SYNOPSIS

27.1 INTRODUCTION

This chapter will explore how hospital pharmacists can improve the safety and efficacy of medications by satisfying The Joint Commission (TJC) National Patient Safety Goals (NPSGs) related to anticoagulation therapy and medication information. TJC established NPSGs in 2002 to help accredited organizations address specific concerns of patient safety. These goals discussed in this chapter are specific to the Hospital National Patient Safety Goals effective from January 1, 2020.[1]

27.1.1 Overview of "the Goals"

In 2002, a panel of patient safety experts was developed by the TJC to construct a patient safety newsletter called the Sentinel Event Alert.[2] Over time, this panel has morphed into what is now known as The Patient Safety Advisory Group. This group advises TJC on creating and updating the NPSGs and comprises safety experts to include physicians, nurses, pharmacists, risk managers, clinical engineers, and other experts on safety. The panel of experts meets annually to recommend which NPSGs TJC should

[1] The views expressed in this chapter are those of the author's and do not necessarily represent the views of The Joint Commission.

DOI: 10.1201/9781003615323-30

adopt, and then TJC determines the highest priority safety issues and addresses the goals accordingly.

The purpose of the NPSGs is to provide a system-wide approach to improve specific areas of patient safety. TJC provides evidence and expert-based methods to achieve the goals. The partnership between TJC and healthcare systems promotes changes in daily work with the ultimate goal to reduce patient harm.

The pharmacist can make the most impact within Goal 3. Goal 3 pertains to improving the safe use of medications relating to anticoagulation and communication about medications.

27.2 GOAL 3 AND THE PHARMACIST'S ROLE

27.2.1 NPSG.03.05.01 Relating to Anticoagulation

27.2.1.1 Introduction

Goal 3 is focused on improving the safe use of medications. NPSG 03.05.01 specifically discusses reducing the chance of patient harm associated with the use of anticoagulant therapy. This goal applies to hospitals providing prophylactic or long-term anticoagulation where the associated laboratory values for monitoring will remain elevated and outside the values of the standard reference range. The reason for this goal is that anticoagulant medications have a possibility to cause harm if not properly monitored due to complex dosing and pharmacodynamic interactions.

Pharmacists are an ideal healthcare resource to play a role in anticoagulation. There are several options for pharmacists to become experts in anticoagulation management. Anticoagulation is taught extensively in pharmacy schools, and during experiential rotations, students have the option of rotating through pharmacist-run anticoagulation clinics. Upon graduation from pharmacy school, graduates have the opportunity to complete a pharmacy practice residency and further gain experience by completing a second-year pharmacy specialty residencies (PGY2). Many post-graduate year 1 (PGY1) residencies have the option to rotate through a specific rotation geared to increasing experience with anticoagulant medications. For example, in the PGY1 program at the University of California at San Francisco, residents have the opportunity to spend one to three days a week for three months in a pharmacist-run anticoagulation clinic at San Francisco General Hospital.[3] There are currently no specialty residencies dedicated solely to anticoagulation; however, specialty residencies focused on cardiology, ambulatory care, and internal medicine allow residents to gain additional anticoagulation experience. Table 27.1 identifies certifications in anticoagulation available for pharmacists to pursue.

TABLE 27.1
Available Anticoagulation Certifications for Pharmacists.

Certification	Provider
Certified Anticoagulation Provider (CACP)	National Certification Board for Anticoagulation Providers
Anticoagulation Management Certificate Program	University of Southern Indiana
Anticoagulant Therapy Certificate Program	University of Florida
Board Certification in Ambulatory Care Pharmacy	Board of Pharmacy Specialties
Anticoagulation Traineeship	University of Connecticut Health Center, Farmington, Connecticut
Anticoagulation Certificate Program	Arizona Pharmacy Association
Anticoagulation Certificate Training Program	California Pharmacists Association

27.2.1.2 Warfarin Overview

One of the most common anticoagulants used is warfarin. Warfarin is a vitamin K antagonist (VKA) approved for the prevention and treatment of thrombosis and embolism.[4] Dosing for warfarin is individualized, and the pharmacodynamic response to warfarin therapy is often hard to predict. A trained healthcare provider must be able to consider the patient in their entirety to be able to dose warfarin appropriately. One must consider the following factors: Age, nutritional status, cardiac function, concurrent medication therapy, risk of bleeding, hepatic function, and, if possible, genetic factors. The pharmacodynamic response to warfarin is measured by an international normalized ratio (INR). Due to the long half-lives of vitamin K-dependent clotting factors (VII, IX, X, II), patients may not have stable INRs until five to six days after the initiation of therapy. Pharmacists can impress upon the patients through counseling the importance of follow-up laboratory testing of the INR and adherence to a specified dosing regimen based on the INR testing.

27.2.1.3 Patient monitoring

Several studies review the efficacy and safety of anticoagulation management when pharmacists are involved compared to physician-managed care. In 1995, Dager et al. compared a historical cohort of 60 consecutive pharmacist-managed warfarin patients randomly matched with 60 physician-managed patients in 1992.[5] An anticoagulation pharmacist was assigned to review the patients' medical record and provide a written consult each day with dosing recommendations. The pharmacist used their clinical experience in addition to assessing the patient's INR trends, hemoglobin, hematocrit, liver function tests, platelets, albumin, concurrent medications and medical problems, and previous warfarin dosing to assist with the dosing recommendations.

Pharmacist management of warfarin therapy resulted in a significant decrease on patient length of stay compared to physician management from 9.5 + 5.6 days to 6.8 + 4.4 days ($p = 0.009$). Pharmacists significantly reduced supratherapeutic INR values (> 3.5 and > 6). Bleeding complications were less in the pharmacist group; however, this was not statistically significant. Lastly, only 6 patients in the pharmacist group received a drug with a major drug–drug interaction with warfarin, whereas 13 patients from the physician-managed group received a major interacting medication ($p = 0.02$). The benefits of pharmacist consultation in this case achieved treatment goals while reducing the length of stay.[6–9]

These results can be replicated in different facilities and patient populations. Other studies demonstrating increased time inside the INR range and decreased length of stay have been summarized in Table 27.2.

27.2.1.4 Patient Education

TJC states "to achieve better patient outcomes, education through face-to-face interaction with a trained professional who works closely with anticoagulation therapy and patients" is a vital component. This trained professional should be able to discuss the risks and benefits of anticoagulation therapy.

Pharmacists have the ability to educate patients on anticoagulants. Content that should be covered in a patient-friendly language includes providing the indication for warfarin, meaning of the INR, when to seek medical care, drug–drug and drug–food interactions. These education points should also be provided in a written format in the patient-specific language.

27.2.1.5 Direct Oral Anticoagulant

In 2010, dabigatran (Pradaxa) became the first of four direct oral anticoagulants (DOACs) to be approved for the prevention of stroke and embolism in patients with non-valvular atrial fibrillation.[10] In 2014, the indication was expanded to include the treatment of deep vein thrombosis

TABLE 27.2
Literature Demonstrating Increased Time inside the INR Range and Decreased Length of Stay when a Pharmacist is a Member of the Healthcare Team.

Ref no.	Design	Patient Population	Outcome	Results
6	Retrospective, observational cohort study with a combined historical and parallel control group comparing a pharmacist-run anticoagulation service versus usual care at Kaiser Permanente of Colorado	Intervention group: 3,323 patients Control Group: 3,322 patients	Primary: Occurrence of anticoagulation therapy-related complications. Secondary: Proportion of time spent in target INR range	Primary outcome: Patients in the pharmacist-run group were 39% less likely to experience a complication (HR 0.61; 95% CI [0.42–0.88]). NNT to prevent a complication was 52. Secondary: Pharmacist group spent 63.5% of study days in target INR range compared to 55.2% in control group ($p < 0.001$)
7	Retrospective cohort study to compare pharmacist managed anticoagulation compared to physician management in a community hospital	Intervention group: 179 patients Control group: 179 patients	Mean time to therapeutic INR, mean time within goal, frequency of supratherapeutic INRs, bleeding, thrombotic rates, and mean INR on discharge	The pharmacist-managed group had a lower incidence of supratherapeutic INRs (29 versus 43). Significantly more time within INR goal ($p = 0.017$, 95% CI 0.12–1.17) No statistically significant difference in the mean time to therapeutic INR
8	Prospective nonrandomized trial comparing whether a detailed warfarin-dosing protocol administered by pharmacists significantly reduced the proportion of hospitalized patients with a supratherapeutic INR at the Mayo Clinic community teaching hospital.	Intervention group: 217 patients Control group: 293 patients	Using a dosing protocol managed by pharmacists could reduce the number of patients with an INR > 5	Pharmacist group had less INRs > 5 than control group. (7.85% versus 1.85% $p = 004$)
9	Single-center cohort study in a 1,200-bed teaching hospital in Singapore comparing a pharmacist-run anticoagulation service to physician care	Intervention group: 144 patients Control group: 26 patients	Percentage of INR achieving therapeutic range within 5 days. INRs > 4 during titration. Subtherapeutic INRs on discharge	Percentage of INR achieving therapeutic range within 5 days was higher in the pharmacist group 88% vs 38% ($p < 0.001$) Pharmacist had a reduction in INRs > 4 during titration. 27% vs 2% ($p < 0.001$) Subtherapeutic INRs on discharge were less in pharmacist-managed group 15% vs 0% ($p < 0.001$)

and pulmonary embolism. Dabigatran is a direct thrombin inhibitor that works by inhibiting coagulation by preventing thrombin-mediated effects. Advantages compared to warfarin are the removal of routine laboratory monitoring because there is no need to monitor lab values such as an INR, no food–drug interactions, and less drug–drug interactions. One of the disadvantages is that the medication needs to be adjusted renally, and there is a significantly higher risk of gastrointestinal bleeding compared to warfarin.[11,12] As of October 2015, idarucizumab (Praxbind) was FDA approved as a reversal agent for dabigatran.

Other DOACs currently available are apixaban (Eliquis), edoxaban (Savaysa), and rivaroxaban (Xarelto), which are oral, factor Xa inhibitors that exert their actions through selective and reversible inhibitor of factor Xa in both the extrinsic and intrinsic coagulation pathways. These medications are also irreversible, require renal adjustment, and in the case of apixaban also require dose adjustments based on age and weight. As of May 2018, andexanet alfa (Andexxa) was approved for the reversal of rivaroxaban and apixaban.

Even though extensive INR monitoring is not needed for these agents, a pharmacist can still be made available to provide renal dose adjustments and provide guidance to practitioners regarding the need to stop the DOAC for an invasive procedure. Pharmacists are also excellent resources regarding drug–drug interactions and when transitioning between one anticoagulant to another.

St John Medical Center in Detroit, Michigan, is a 772-bed hospital that evaluated the role of pharmacist management of dabigatran between May 2011 and August 2012.[13] A retrospective review was done of 176 patients. During hospital admission, 46% of patients required intervention, and 1.7% of patients needed permanent discontinuation of dabigatran due to a bleeding complication. This study demonstrated that pharmacists contributed to the safe and appropriate use of dabigatran. Types of interventions are described in Table 27.3.

TABLE 27.3
Pharmacist Intervention of Dabigatran Usage.

Intervention	Percentage of Patients Requiring Intervention
Admitted on inappropriate home dose	18.6%
Transition between dabigatran and other anticoagulants	74.2%
Renal dose adjustment or discontinuation	6.3%
Procedural anticoagulation	6.8%

The University of Michigan evaluated the outcomes of a pharmacist-led outpatient DOAC service. They found that when a patient was seen by a pharmacist, more patients were prescribed the appropriate DOAC and dosage at baseline compared with the usual care group (93% versus 79.1%; adjusted odds ratio [OR], 3.0; $p = 0.009$), and they also had higher levels of adherence.[14] Pharmacists were able to use motivational interviewing and patient counseling to increase the understanding of DOAC therapy, ensure awareness of adverse effects, and to emphasize the importance of medication adherence. The pharmacists were also able to assist with finding financial medication assistance programs for patients to potentially improve adherence.

A retrospective review of the electronic medical records of 585 patients on DOACs was done by Pearlman et al. Clinical pharmacists were able to make 258 consultations for 210 patients regarding their anticoagulation management.[15] Consultations included alerts regarding potentially inappropriate DOAC doses and recommendations to increase (29%) or decrease (5%) the dose, potentially inappropriate concomitant antiplatelet agents (20%), need for DOAC level monitoring (23%), and alerts regarding other drug-related problems (23%). More than 70% of recommendations were accepted by the attending physician.

Due to the novelty and complexity of DOAC management, the potential of drug-related problems is common.[38] Pharmacist involvement can mitigate these errors and promote strategies to reduce risk with these medications.

27.2.1.6 Anticoagulation Reversal Overview

Multiple reversal agents for anticoagulants have arrived on the market in recent years. DOACs have several advantages over warfarin including less frequent monitoring, no dietary restrictions, more predictability, less liable anticoagulant effect, less drug–drug interactions, and less cumbersome to bridge for procedures. In regard to major bleeding events, apixaban and edoxaban were superior to warfarin in reducing major bleeding episodes, while rivaroxaban and dabigatran are similar to warfarin.[16] Recently, several reversal agents have been approved by the FDA; here, we will discuss the agents currently available.

Four-Factor Prothrombin Complex (Kcentra) (4-Factor PCC) contains human coagulation factors II, VII, IX, and X, along with the antithrombotic protein C and protein S. 4-Factor PCC was approved in 2013 for the indication of urgent reversal of acquired coagulation factor deficiency induced by VKA therapy in patients with acute major bleeding.[10] 4-Factor PCC was found to be an effective resource to rapidly control hemorrhage in the setting of emergency anticoagulation reversal.[17]

Idarucizumab (Praxbind) is a monocolonal antibody approved in 2015 to reverse the anticoagulant effects of dabigatran.[10] Idarucizumab is known to completely reverse the anticoagulant effect of dabigatran within minutes of administration.[18]

Andexanet alfa (Andexxa) is a recombinant modified human Factor Xa protein approved in 2018, indicated for patients treated with apixaban or rivaroxaban in which anticoagulant reversal is needed due to uncontrolled or life-threatening bleeding.[10] Andexanet alfa provides markedly reduced anti-factor Xa activity in patients with acute major bleeding.[19]

27.2.1.7 Anticoagulation Reversal Programs

From warfarin to DOACs strategies for reducing harm associated with anticoagulation therapy are important goals for hospitals to improve patient safety, and pharmacists are one of the resources which can potentially increase safety and efficacy of these high-risk medications.

In patients with intracranial hemorrhage who are on VKA antagonists, prompt reversal is key, and the use of 4-Factor PCC has been shown to reverse the INR faster than fresh frozen plasma (FFP).[20] In a study completed by Corio and colleagues, a pharmacist-driven protocol was created for the ordering, preparation, and delivery of 4-factor PCC compared to usual care which was completed by the blood bank at the study's institution. When the pharmacist-driven protocol was reviewed, the time for the medication to reach bedside was 35 minutes (interquartile range [IQR] [25–62]; range, 11–133) compared to the blood bank, which was 70 minutes (IQR [34–89]; range, 14–244) in the pre-protocol group ($p = 0.034$). In this study, the pharmacist was available at bedside for questions regarding dosing and monitoring of the patient. The drug was also more accessible to the staff.

In another institution, a study was completed to determine if a pharmacist at bedside impacted the time to administration of 4-factor PCC.[21] The median time to 4-factor PCC administration was significantly shorter in the PharmD group (66.5 versus 206.5 min, $p < 0.001$). The pharmacist at bedside was the only factor independently associated with reduction in time to 4F-PCC. In this study, the pharmacist completed a thorough medication history to determine anticoagulant use and time of last dose, assess accurate weight, and recommend necessary laboratory parameters. In addition, pharmacists recommend concomitant vitamin K administration for warfarin-associated bleeds and against concomitant FFP due to the increased thromboembolic risk. Lastly, the pharmacist played a key role in communicating with the intravenous preparatory area of the pharmacy to make sure the medications are expedited and compounded with priority. In addition to time to delivery of the drug, this study showed that in the PharmD group, patients had a shorter length of stay in the intensive care unit and hospital.

27.2.1.8 Patient Education

TJC states that to achieve better patient outcomes, education through face-to-face interaction with a trained professional who works closely with anticoagulation therapy and patients is a vital component. This trained professional should be able to discuss the risks and benefits of anticoagulation therapy.

Pharmacists have the ability to educate patients on anticoagulants. What should be covered in a patient-friendly language includes providing the indication for warfarin, meaning of the INR, when to seek medical care, and drug–drug and drug–food interactions. These education points should also be provided in a written format in the patient-specific language.

A critical issue regarding counseling on DOACs is medication adherence, given their short half-lives.[22] The potential consequence of missed doses could be a venous thromboembolism or stroke. Due to the lack of routine monitoring with DOACs, there is also less routine monitoring for adherence. Pharmacists are one of the most accessible healthcare providers and can provide this counseling at the community setting when assessing for refills. During this valuable interaction time with the patient, pharmacists should also assess for bleeding risk as well as any drug interactions.

27.2.2 NPSG.03.06.01 Relating to Reconciling Medication Information

27.2.2.1 Introduction

The Institute of Medicine estimates that adverse drug events account for an estimated 1 in 3 of all hospital adverse events and can prolong hospitalization by 1.7 to 4.6 days.[23] Patients who take multiple medications and have complex medication regimens make medication reconciliation an important safety concern. The process of medication reconciliation involves a 'qualified individual', identified by the hospital, comparing the medications a patient should be ordered to take to the new medications that are currently ordered and resolving any differences. TJC includes errors of omission, contraindications, and duplication as well as errors involving drug–drug and drug–disease interactions.[1].NPSG.03.06.01 is to "record and pass along correct information about a patient's medicines" and review safe practices for medication reconciliation. TJC understands that there are challenges with medication reconciliation due to the difficulty in obtaining an accurate list from every patient at every encounter; therefore, a good faith effort will satisfy this NPSG. In addition to reconciliation, patients should be educated on safe medication use and how to communicate this information to their providers.

27.2.2.2 The Process of Medication Reconciliation

The American Society of Health Systems Pharmacists (ASHP) created a position statement on the pharmacist role in medication reconciliation. ASHP believes that pharmacists should maintain key roles in the medication reconciliation process.[24] The responsibilities that ASHP describes are as follows:

- Providing leadership in designing and managing patient-centered medication reconciliation systems
- Educating patients and healthcare professionals about the benefits and limitations of the medication reconciliation process
- Serving as patient advocates throughout transitions of care.

The pharmacist should provide leadership in developing medication reconciliation policies and procedures; implement and process improvement medication reconciliation activities; train to make the staff competent to be involved in medication reconciliation; develop information systems for data extraction of medication reconciliation activities; and advocate services to providers, nurses, and the community.

27.2.2.3 Improved Accuracy

Fewer errors are found when a pharmacist completes a patient's medication reconciliation versus physicians. The next couple of paragraphs describe specific instances when a pharmacist's intervention on medication reconciliation showed improved accuracy versus other healthcare professionals.

A total of 55 patients were included in an evaluation comparing physician-obtained medication histories with pharmacist-obtained medication histories. Pharmacists in this study not only identified a larger number of medications a patient was taking compared to the physicians, 614 versus 556 identified by the physicians ($p <= 0.001$), but also the pharmacists identified 353 discrepancies, 58 of which were not previously found by the physicians.[25]

Another study focused its attention on the emergency department, measuring if a pharmacist-obtained medication history reduced the number of medication discrepancies. The pharmacist intervention in the emergency department reduced overall discrepancies by 33% ($p < 0.0001$), with omission being the most common cause of the discrepancy.[26]

Other studies have looked at pharmacist-obtained medications histories versus nurse-obtained medication histories. Compared to the nurses, pharmacists identified a significantly higher number of medications taken per patient, also including over the counter (OTC) drugs and herbal supplements ($p < 0.001$). Pharmacists also contacted patients' community pharmacies significantly more often than nurses ($p < 0.001$). In addition, this study concluded that the amount of time spent by pharmacists completing medication histories was efficient and worthwhile to the patient's care.[27]

27.2.2.4 Decreased Mortality

In 2007, Bond and Raehl investigated which hospital-based clinical pharmacy services were associated with mortality rates.[28] Fourteen clinical pharmacy services were assessed from the National Clinical Pharmacy Services database, which is the largest in the United States. When pharmacists provide admission drug histories versus hospitals without this service, 3,988 deaths were avoided. This is further elucidated in Table 27.4. The study cited above demonstrates article a prime example of why pharmacists can play a vital role in contributing to a hospitalized patient's healthcare.

27.2.2.5 Allergy Identification

A complete medication history also includes the identification of any allergies a patient may have and discerning between true allergies versus an intolerance. A pharmacist is uniquely suited to interview patients regarding allergies due to their familiarity with drug information such as brand and generic names, dosing regimens, and possible side effects of certain medications. In one study, not only was the time to recording of allergy information decreased when a pharmacist conducted the history versus a nurse ($p =< 0.005$), but this act also decreased delays in drug dispensing due to waiting on allergy clarification.[27]

27.2.2.6 Discharge Medication Reconciliation

Another aspect of medication reconciliation occurs when patients are discharged. Medication discrepancies that occur at transitions of care can negatively impact patient care. Farley and colleagues compared usual care versus pharmacy case manager (PCM) involvement.[29] The study compared a control group (nurse or physician-managed medication reconciliation) versus the minimal involvement of a PCM (medication counseling and detailed medication reconciliation) and enhanced intervention with a PCM (everything which was done in the minimal intervention group and faxing the plan to their community physician and pharmacy). In the enhanced intervention group, it was shown that medication discrepancies of high significance in physician records were lower in the enhanced intervention group after 30 days ($p = 0.013$). This study demonstrates the significant impact pharmacists can have regarding medication-specific outcomes after discharge.

A study was conducted out of Northwestern Hospital in 2012 where in the intervention group, pharmacists conducted medication reconciliation at admission and discharge, including discharge counseling, and assessed their interventions on 30-day readmission rates.[30] All medication discrepancies were assessed before discharge.

TABLE 27.4
A Pharmacist's Contribution to Decreased Mortality When Completing Medication Admission Histories.

	No. Admissions/ Hospital/Year with This Service (Mean + SD)	No. of Deaths/ Hospital/Year with This Service (Mean + SD)	No. of Deaths/ Hospital/Year without This Service (Mean + SD)	No. of Reduced Deaths	No. of Reduced Deaths/Hospital (Mean + SD (%))
Admission Drug Histories	11,239 + 4,462	38.29 +19.67	47.88 + 40.18	3,988	107.78+87.6 (20.15)

Medication follow-up calls were completed at days 3, 14, and 30. Authors reported 380 discrepancies in the intervention group (46.2%) compared to 205 (19.9%) in the usual care group ($p < 0.0001$). In terms of hospital readmission, the intervention group had 24.8% compared to 39% readmission in 30 days ($p = 0.001$). This study showed that pharmacists were key in rectifying discharge medication reconciliation and can continue to help patients post-discharge with their medication regimens.

27.2.2.7 Utilization of the Pharmacist Extenders in Medication Reconciliation

With proper training, pharmacy technicians may take on expanded roles to participate in the medication reconciliation process. Throughout their training, pharmacy technicians get familiar with dosage forms, strengths, and usual dosing schedules for a wide variety of medications.[31] In addition, they are familiar with over-the-counter medications and are trained to ask about them when interviewing a patient. Through the medication reconciliation process, pharmacy technicians can document pre-admission medication histories from patients, from outpatient pharmacies, and other healthcare providers. Technicians can also help resolve discrepancies in medication lists and allow pharmacists to clinically intervene with the healthcare team improving patient care. By using technicians to complete the task of obtaining a medication history, the pharmacist can then use their expertise to assess the appropriateness of therapy.

Pharmacy technicians can fulfill the requirements to be a certified Pharmacy Technician (CPhT). Currently, 21 states require pharmacy technicians to have a CPhT certification, and the Pharmacy Technician Certification Board (PTCB) has granted over 700,000 CPhT Certifications, with 117,950 CPhT renewals issued in 2019.[32] To be eligible to earn the PTCB CPhT certification, the technician must have completed a PTCB-recognized training program or have equivalent work experience of 500 work hours and attest to fulfilling specific knowledge requirements, disclose criminal background, comply with PTCB certification policies, and pass the Pharmacy Technician Certification Exam. A list of PTCB-Recognized programs can be found at https://www.ptcb.org/educators/ptcb-recognized-education-training-program-directory.

The Pharmacy Technician Accreditation Commission (PTAC) is a collaboration between ASHP and the Accreditation Council for Pharmacy Education (ACPE) boards.[33] This collaboration was established to provide an accrediting review committee to specify the accreditation standards of quality pharmacy technician education and training programs in the United States. A list of accredited pharmacy technician education and training programs as well as information on preparing for an accreditation survey can be found on the ASHP website www.accreditation.ashp.org.

ASHP has provided a model curriculum for pharmacy technician education and training programs. Included in this curriculum are instructional objectives and teaching strategies which could be used to meet the goals set forth in the ASHP Accreditation Standard for Pharmacy Technician Education and Training Programs. The purpose of the model curriculum is to provide criteria for new programs in establishing a technician training program and assist current programs in preparation for an accreditation survey.[24] The model curriculum has dedicated an entire goal objective to assist pharmacists in medication reconciliation.

A PTCB Medication History Certificate is available for pharmacy technicians who show competency in gathering accurate medication histories, identifying potential errors and resolving with necessary clarifications, and completing medication reconciliation administrative functions. To be eligible, the technician must have a current PTCB CPhT certification and either must have completed a PTCB-recognized Medication History education and training program with at least six months' experience completing medication history tasks or must have at least one year of experience conducting medication histories without completing a program.

Pharmacy technicians are a safe alternative to complete medication histories when compared to other healthcare professionals. A program using pharmacy technicians to obtain medication histories at Fairview Health Center in Minnesota found that potential errors were reduced by 82% when trained pharmacy technicians obtained medication histories.[34] The errors included incomplete or incorrect information, illegible orders, and serious drug interactions. Additional studies have demonstrated that pharmacy technicians are able to complete a medication history with a 95% accuracy rate, and their involvement decreased time spent by physicians, nurses, and pharmacists at the time of admission.[31] In a study done by Markovic et al. at an academic medical center, when pharmacy technicians completing medication histories were compared to nursing staff, the pharmacy technician error rate was 5.6% compared to an error rate of 86% for the nursing staff.[35] Another study at a regional medical center showed that when medication histories are taken by technicians in an emergency department, the error rate was 15%, compared to a 65% error rate for nurses and other non-pharmacy personnel.[36]

Utilizing pharmacy technicians to complete medication histories is not only efficient as discussed earlier but also cost effective. A study done out of MultiCare Health System in Tacoma, Washington, showed that personnel cost for 3.5 FTE pharmacy technicians was $141,000, and the return on investment was $2.3 million dollars.[37]

Pharmacy technicians have a greater understanding of medication lists and medication-taking behaviors than non-pharmacy personnel. Through advanced training, technicians can be trained to perform this task with greater accuracy than nurses and other hospital staff. Utilizing pharmacy technicians will allow pharmacists more time to effectively prevent, identify, and resolve drug therapy problems.

27.3 SUMMARY AND CONCLUSIONS

Certainly, the pharmacist plays a clear role in improving the safe use of medications in the hospital setting while ensuring that those medications are effective. Hospitals should include pharmacists as members of the multidisciplinary team to assist the organization in the development and sustainability of processes to ensure the Hospital National Patient Safety Goals are utilized in the organization to provide the utmost environment of patient safety.

REFERENCES

1 National Patient Safety Goals, 2020. Retrieved April 19, 2020, from https://www.jointcommission.org/-/media/tjc/documents/standards/national-patient-safety-goals/2020/simplified_2020-hap-npsgs-eff-july-final.pdf.

2 Facts About the Patient Safety Advisory Group. Retrieved August 24, 2015, from http://www.jointcommission.org/facts_about_the_patient_safety_advisory_group/.

3 PGY1 Residency: Pharmacy Practice, n.d. Retrieved November 16, 2020, from https://pharm.ucsf.edu/residencies/pgy1-pharmacy.

4 Coumadin™ (Warfarin) Package Insert. Research. Princeton, NJ: Bristol Myers-Squibb, 2011.

5 Dager WE, Branch JM, King JH, et al. Optimization of inpatient warfarin therapy: Impact of daily consultation by a pharmacist-managed anticoagulation service. Ann Pharmacother. 2000 May;34(5):567–572.

6 Witt DM, Sadler MS, Shanahan RL, et al. Effect of centralization clinical pharmacy anticoagulation service on the outcomes of anticoagulation therapy. Chest. 2005 May;127(5):1515–1522.

7 Chilipko AA, Norwood DK. Evaluating warfarin management in a community teaching hospital. Consult Pharm. 2014 Feb;29(2):95–103.

8 Dawson NL, Porter IE, Klipa D, et al. Inpatient warfarin management: Pharmacist management using a detailed dosing protocol. J Thromb Thrombolysis. 2012;33:178–184. DOI: 10.1007/s11239-011-0655-9.

9 Wong YM, Quek YN, Tay JC. Efficacy and safety of a pharmacist-managed inpatient anticoagulation service for warfarin initiation and titration. J Clin Pharm Therapeut. 2011;36:585–591.

10 Lexi-Comp, Inc. Lexi-Drugs. Lexi-Comp, Inc., November 20, 2020.

11 Bloom BJ, Filion KB, Atallah R, et al. Meta-analysis of randomized controlled trials on the risk of bleeding with dabigatran. Am J Cardiol. 2014;113:1066–1074.

12 Connolly SJ, Ezekowitz MD, Yusuf S, et al. Dabigatran versus warfarin in patients with atrial fibrillation. N Engl J Med. 2009;361:1139–1151.

13 Tedders KM, Lucey MF, Edwin SB. Evaluation of pharmacist-managed dabigatran in an inpatient setting. Ann Pharmacother. 2013 Dec;47(12):1649–1653.

14 Ashjian E, Kurtz B, Renner E, et al. Evaluation of a pharmacist-led outpatient direct oral anticoagulant service. Am J Health Syst Pharm. 2017;74(7):483–489. DOI: 10.2146/ajhp151026.

15 Perlman A, Horwitz E, Hirsh-Raccah B, et al. Clinical pharmacist led hospital-wide direct oral anticoagulant stewardship program. Isr J Health Policy Res. 2019;8(1):19. Published 2019 Feb 1. DOI: 10.1186/s13584-019-0285-9.

16 Hellenbart EL, Faulkenberg KD, Finks SW. Evaluation of bleeding in patients receiving direct oral anticoagulants. Vasc Health Risk Manag. 2017;13:325–342. DOI: 10.2147/VHRM.S121661.

17 Pabinger I, Brenner B, Kalina U, et al. Prothrombin complex concentrate (Kcentra) for emergency anticoagulation reversal: A prospective multinational clinical trial. J Thromb Haemost. 2008;6:622–631.

18 Pollack CV Jr, Reilly PA, van Ryn J, et al. Idarucizumab for dabigatran reversal: Full cohort analysis. N Engl J Med. 2017 Aug 3;377(5):431–441. DOI: 10.1056/NEJMoa1707278. Epub 2017 July 11. PMID: 28693366.

19 Connolly SJ, Crowther M, Eikelboom JW, et al. Full study report of andexanet alfa for bleeding associated with factor Xa inhibitors. N Engl J Med. 2019 Apr 4;380(14):1326–1335. DOI: 10.1056/NEJMoa1814051. Epub 2019 Feb 7. PMID: 30730782; PMCID: PMC6699827.

20 Corio JL, Sin JH, Hayes BD, et al. Impact of a pharmacist-driven prothrombin complex concentrate protocol on time to administration in patients with warfarin-associated intracranial hemorrhage. West J Emerg Med. 2018;19(5):849–854. DOI: 10.5811/westjem.2018.6.37932.

21 Masic D, Hidalgo DC, Kuhrau S, et al. Pharmacist presence decreases time to prothrombin complex concentrate in emergency department patients with life-threatening bleeding and urgent procedures. J Emerg Med. 2019 Nov;57(5):620–628. DOI: 10.1016/j.jemermed.2019.06.027.

22 Leblanc K, Semchuk WM, Papastergiou J, et al. A pharmacist checklist for direct oral anticoagulant management: Raising the bar. Can Pharm J (Ott). 2018;151(2):102–106. Published 2018 Feb 9. DOI: 10.1177/1715163518756926.

23 Adverse Drug Events, 2020, FebruaryFebruary 5. Retrieved May 18, 2020, from https://health.gov/our-work/health-care-quality/adverse-drug-events.

24 American Society of Health-System Pharmacists. ASHP statement on the pharmacist's role in medication reconciliation. AM J Health-Syst Pharm. 2013;70:453–456.

25 Reeder T, Mutnick A. Pharmacist-versus physician-obtained medication histories. Am J Health-Syst Pharm. 2008;65:857–860.

26 Becerra-Camargo J, Martinez-Martinez F, Garcia-Jimenez E. A multicentre, double-blind, randomised, controlled, parallel-group study of the effectiveness of a pharmacist-acquired medication history in an emergency department. BMC Health Serv Res. 2013;13:337.

27 Nester T, Hale L. Effectiveness of a pharmacist-acquired medication history in promoting patient safety. Am J Health-Syst Pharm. 2002;59:2221–2225.

28 Bond CA, Raehl CL. Clinical pharmacy services, pharmacy staffing, and hospital mortality rates. Pharmacotherapy. 2007;27(4):481–493.

29 Farley TM, Shelsky C, Powell S, et al. Effect of clinical pharmacist intervention on medication discrepancies following hospital discharge. Int J Clin Pharm. 2014;36:430–437.

30 Phatak A, Prusi R, Ward B, et al. Impact of pharmacist involvement in the transitional care of high-risk patients through medication reconciliation, medication education, and postdischarge call-backs (IPITCH study). J Hosp Med. 2016;11(1):39–44. DOI: 10.1002/jhm.2493.

31 Remtulla S, Brown G, Frighetto L. Best possible medication history by a pharmacy technician at a tertiary care hospital. Can J Hosp Pharm. 2009;62(5):402–405. DOI: 10.4212/cjhp.v62i5.828.

32 PTCB Certification Eligibility Requirements to Change in 2020, 2019, February 2. Retrieved April 22, 2020, from https://www.ptcb.org/news/ptcb-certification-eligibility-requirements-to-change-in-2020.
33 Pharmacy Technician Education Accreditation Collaboration, 2017, September 8. Retrieved April 22, 2020, from https://www.acpe-accredit.org/pharmacy-technician-education-accreditation-collaboration/.
34 Michels R, Meisel S. Program using pharmacy technicians to obtain medication histories. Am J Health-Syst Pharm. 2003;60:1982–1986.
35 Markovic M, Mathis AS, Ghin HL, et al. A comparison of medication histories obtained by a pharmacy technician versus nurses in the emergency department. PT. 2017;42(1):41–46.
36 Rubin EC, Pisupati R, Nerenberg SF. Utilization of pharmacy technicians to increase the accuracy of patient medication histories obtained in the emergency department. Hosp Pharm. 2016;51(5):396–404. DOI: 10.1310/hpj5105-396.
37 Medication Reconciliation Technician, n.d. Retrieved May 18, 2020, from https://www.ashp.org/Pharmacy-Technician/About-Pharmacy-Technicians/Advanced-Pharmacy-Technician-Roles/Medication-Reconciliation-Technician?loginreturnUrl=SSOCheckOnly.
38 Julia S, James U. Direct oral anticoagulants: A quick guide. Eur Cardiol. 2017;12(1):40–45. DOI: 10.15420/ecr.2017:11:2.

28 Pharmacist Malpractice and Liability

James T. O'Donnell and James J. O'Donnell III

SYNOPSIS

DOI: 10.1201/9781003615323-31

28.1 INTRODUCTION

As every healthcare worker (and attorney) knows, drug mishaps are nothing new. In fact, studies dating back several years[1] show that about 2% of hospital patients experience preventable adverse drug events, although the majority of these are not fatal. Medication error has been cited as the cause of death for 1 out of 131 outpatient deaths and 1 out of 854 in-patient deaths. It is estimated that 6.7% of hospitalizations result in an adverse drug reaction, and in 0.32% of these cases, fatality occurs. This extrapolates to about 2,216,000 cases annually in hospitalized patients and 106,000 deaths.[2] Of course, it does not take a lawyer to figure out that this adds up to an excessive number of potential lawsuits against medical personnel.

Originally, these lawsuits were almost always aimed at physicians and nurses, but pharmacists are now increasingly becoming the target of malpractice litigation. This phenomenon, predictably, has resulted in the development of strategies to help reduce the risks of medication errors and to manage pharmacist liability. Jill F. Bechtold and Alison A. Hofhematologister, civil defense lawyers in Jacksonville, Florida at the Marks Gray Firm, published an article examining the increased liability of pharmacists in the *National Trial Lawyer*. They report that Florida courts have traditionally held that pharmacists merely have a duty to exercise "due and proper care in filling [a] prescription" and that "Courts are beginning to hold pharmacists liable in negligence and wrongful death actions involving overdoses or adverse reactions to lawful prescriptions filled as written by the prescribing physicians."

The Florida Fifth District Court of Appeals' recent decision in *Oleckna v. Daytona Discount Pharmacy* highlighted a changing area of Florida law, which has been seen nationwide. For the last decade, Florida courts have appeared to expand the traditional liability for a pharmacist, seemingly bringing the common law a step closer to the duties outlined by the statutory and administrative laws.

28.2 THE SCIENCE OF RISK MANAGEMENT

The risk management of pharmacist malpractice includes identifying theories of liability through the examination of case law and civil litigation. Pharmacists are to protect their patients from harm and must collaborate with physicians and healthcare team members in an efficient way so that medical mistakes are avoided or corrected to avoid serious injury.

Another method of analysis and perhaps prevention of errors is to analyze claims against insured pharmacists. Two claims studies are reported in this chapter. Not surprisingly, the tables, incidences and types of errors, drugs involved, and report discussions and conclusions are strikingly similar.

28.3 CLAIMS STUDIES

28.3.1 The Pharmacists Mutual Claims Study

The first is the Pharmacists Mutual Claims study. This study was first published in the early 1990s and has been

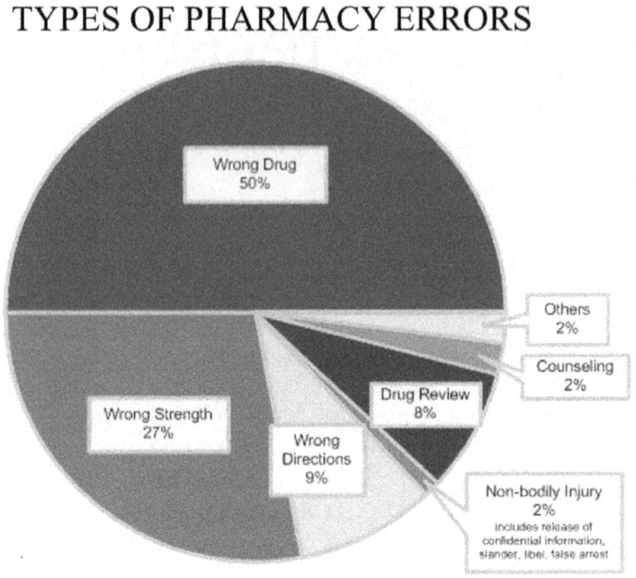

FIGURE 28.1 Categories of Medication Errors.

continuously updated on the company website.[3] It has frequently been discussed in the pharmacy and risk management literature. This study has identified the most common categories of errors and omissions that are most responsible for claims made against pharmacists for malpractice. Figure 28.1 depicts, in order of frequency, the categories of pharmacy errors that are given as follows:

- Wrong drug
- Wrong strength of drug
- Wrong directions
- Lack of drug review (which can result in allergies or contraindicated combinations of drugs being administered)
- Failure to properly counsel patients on medication usage
- Non-bodily injury
- Other (miscellaneous)

The Pharmacists Mutual Claims Study was updated in 2020.[4] This study highlights drugs that are commonly involved in claims. The claims result from dispensing the wrong drug and the wrong strength or dispensing a prescription with incorrect directions. Many of the drugs commonly involved in these claims are not surprising. Both hydrocodone and oxycodone are on the list at numbers 8 and 11, respectively. What is revealing is the reason that drugs are on the list beyond the fact that they are widely dispensed. Hydrocodone and oxycodone are available in a number of different strengths and combinations. This presents challenges in the dispensing process to make sure that the correct product is dispensed.

The number one drug involved in claims is warfarin. A closer look at warfarin errors reveals that incorrect directions are seldom the error involved. Almost two-thirds of the time, it is dispensing the wrong strength. Levothyroxine, at number two, is similar with strength errors accounting for over two-thirds of its claims. Considering the number of strengths of these two products available, these results are not surprising.

Toprol® comes in at number five in the study. It is commonly dispensed in place of Topamax® (and vice versa). Here, about two-thirds of the errors are dispensing the wrong drug. It is easy to see how that could happen. Claims involving oral hypoglycemic drugs, primarily glyburide, are in third place on the list. These claims also involve the patient receiving the wrong drug. But here, it is a whopping 90% of the errors!

Our last example is prednisone, which comes in at number nine. Prednisone claims are spread almost equally among wrong drug, wrong strength, and wrong direction categories. Again, this is not surprising, given the variability of dose and duration for different patients and conditions.

The key to a successful risk management program is data. Knowing where dispensing errors occur is helpful. Knowing why they occur is much more useful. Performing a root cause analysis allows you to better understand not only the how and where but also the why. Knowing the why allows you to implement a risk management program that is both efficient and targeted. Increased accuracy should follow as the data shows you where changes are needed.

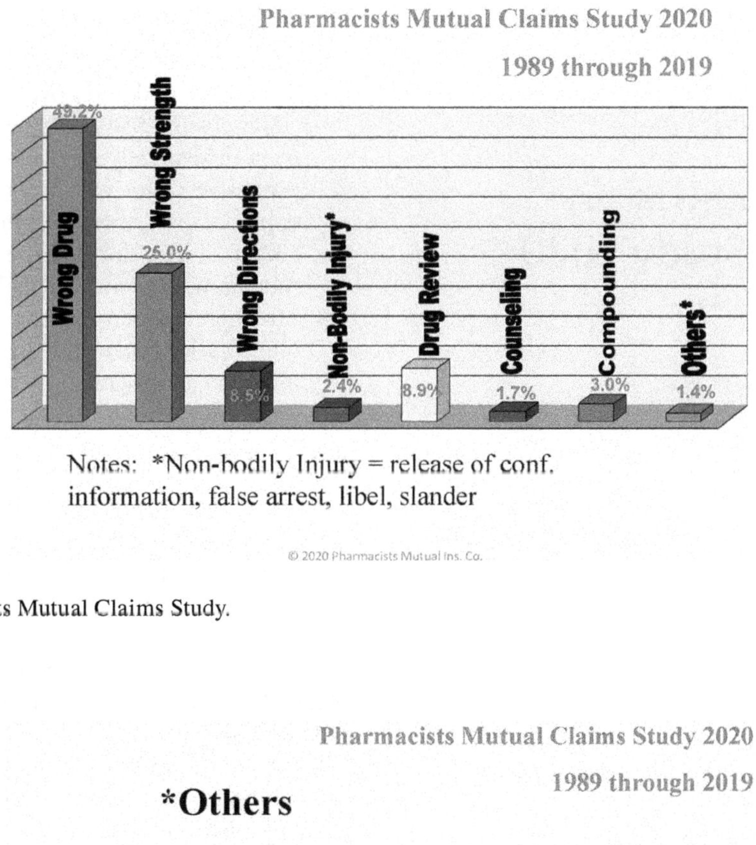

FIGURE 28.2 Pharmacists Mutual Claims Study.

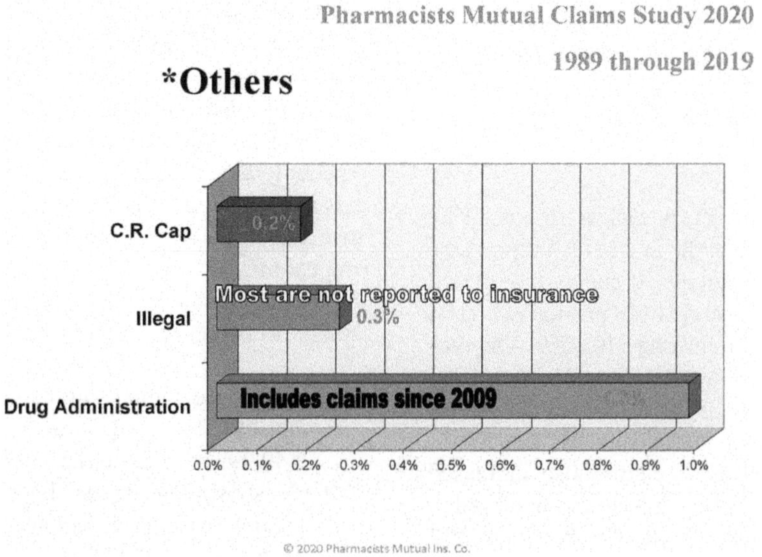

FIGURE 28.3 Pharmacists Mutual Claims Study: Others.

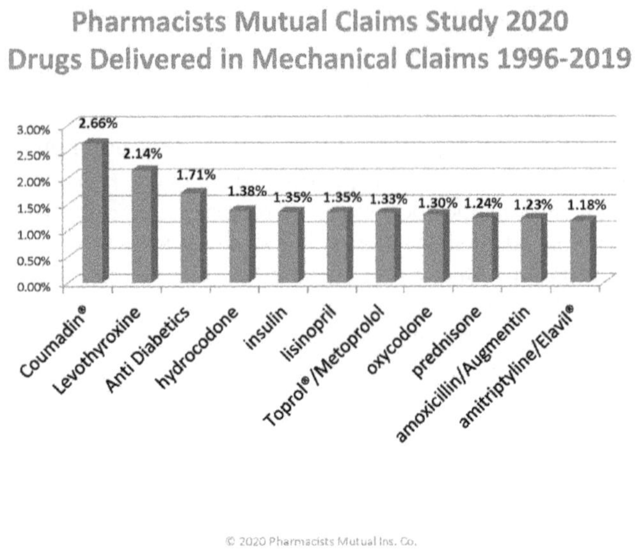

FIGURE 28.4 Pharmacists Mutual Claims Study: Drugs Delivered in Mechanical Claims.

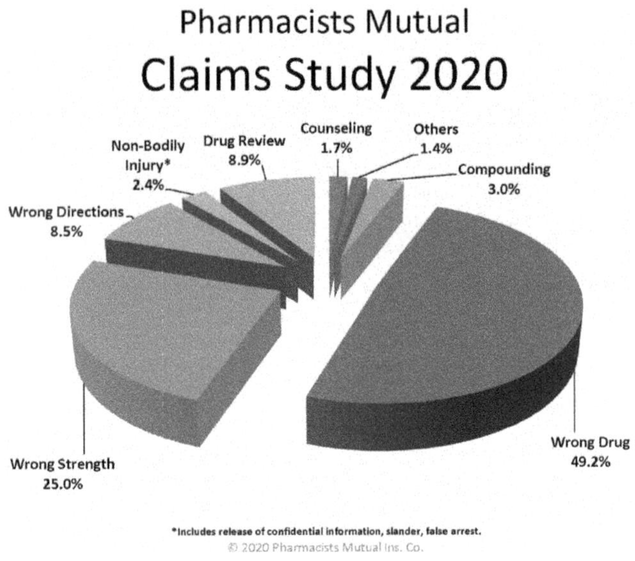

FIGURE 28.5 Pharmacists Mutual Claims by Type.

Eight key points from the Pharmacists Mutual Claims study are:

1. The total cost of pharmacy claims increased by 22.8% since 2013, when the first edition report was released. That report analyzed claims from 2002 to 2011 and showed a total of $18 million in claims with an average claim costing $101,269. The second edition report showed $25 million in total claims with an average claim costing $124,407, though the study time was only half as long.
2. The number of pharmacy claims also increased from the first report, when only 162 were closed in a 10-year period, versus 184 closed between 2012 and 2016.
3. Most of the claims filed between 2012 and 2016 were against pharmacists (96.2%), rather than pharmacy technicians (3.8%).
4. The majority of claims were filed against independent or individually owned pharmacies (55.4%). The next most common targets were compounding.
5. The most common claims were for dispensing the wrong drug (36.8%) and dispensing the wrong dosage (15.3%).
6. The most expensive claims were filed against hospital pharmacies, with an average claim costing $273,338—more than twice the overall average—and compounding specialty pharmacies, with an average claim costing $256,381. The least expensive claims were against pharmacists in homecare environments, with an average claim costing $5,063.
7. The most expensive type of claim reported was for failure to identify overdosing, with an average claim costing $544,600. However, it was also the most infrequently reported claim. The next most expensive claim was a compounding calculation or preparation error, with an average claim costing $324,819. The third-costliest claim was for libel/slander, with an average claim costing $300,000.
8. The most frequent types of closed claims involving injuries were for gastrointestinal distress, infection, and death.

28.3.2 CNA Claims Study (CNA/HPSO)

CNA Insurance, a second major insurer of pharmacists and pharmacies, reported pharmacists' claims experiences in the CNA/HPSO Claims Study 2019.[5] Through their partner Healthcare Providers Service Organization (HPSO), CNA Insurance released a significant closed claims analysis for insured pharmacists covering 10 years of experience from 2002 to 2012 on professional liability of pharmacy practice in the United States.[6]

There is little difference in types of errors and claims reported and analyzed by this claims study and the Pharmacist Mutual Study. Subsequent discussion will analyze and provide commentary on the CNA/HPSO study. The real value of such a study is to examine history so that it is not repeated—that is, to recognize trends and promulgate the study so that pharmacists learn from it and not "repeat history."

A comparison of total Claim (average) incurred (2013 and 2018) is presented here:

- Of closed claims with total incurred cost of at least $1, 67.6% of claims resolved between $1 and $49,999, similar to the 2013 dataset.
- As shown later in the chapter, there are 10% fewer claims closing with an average total incurred cost in the $1 to $9,999 range in 2018 compared with 2013.

- In 2018, there has been a shift to more claims closing in the $50,000 to $499,999 range when compared to 2013.
- There was a small but significant increase in claims that closed with a total incurred amount of $1 million. This increase is largely due to the rise of claims against a pharmacist, which involved multiple patients. One example involves a pharmacist's failure to follow established procedures when compounding, which led to the contamination of medications or parenteral nutrition (PN) to multiple patients.

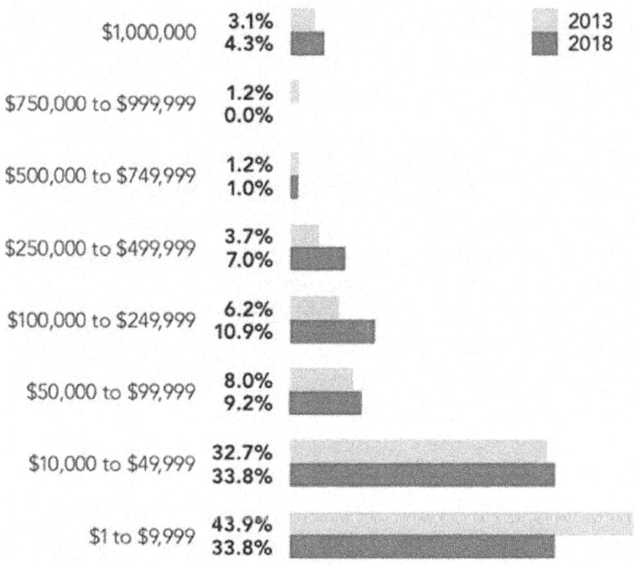

FIGURE 28.6 Comparison of Average Total Incurred Cost: 2013 and 2018.

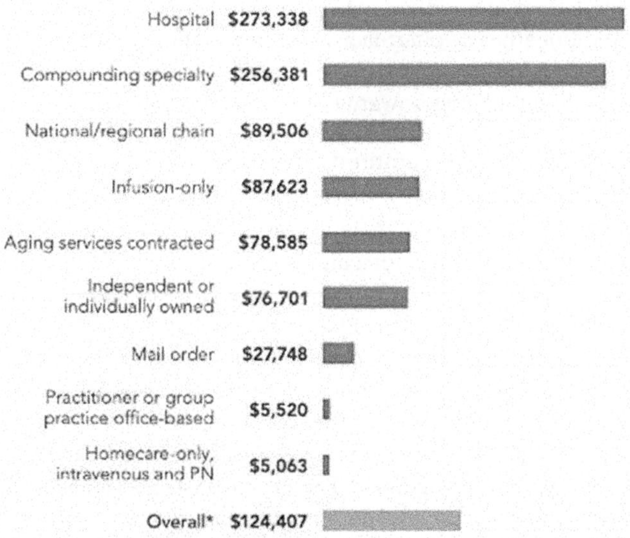

FIGURE 28.7 Severity by Pharmacy Type.

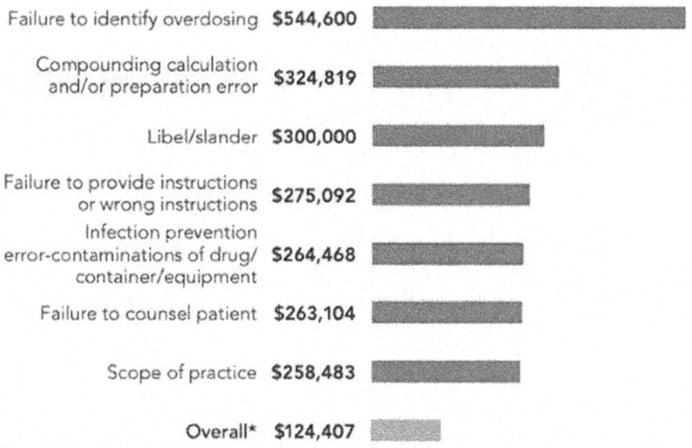

FIGURE 28.8 The Severity of Allegations.

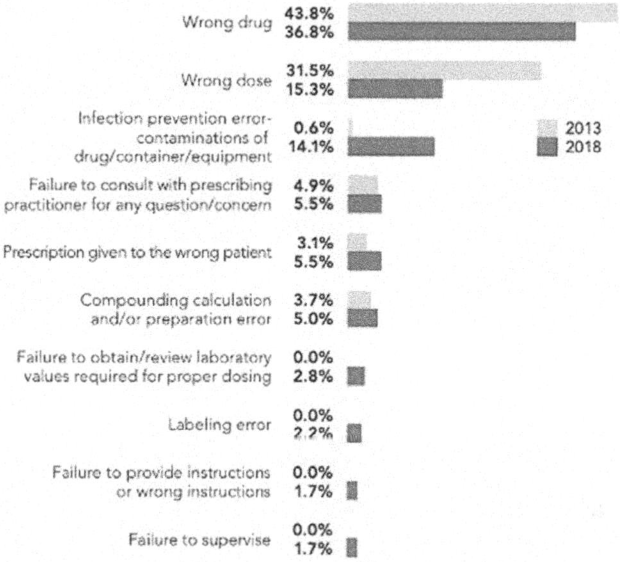

FIGURE 28.9 Distribution by Allegation Errors.

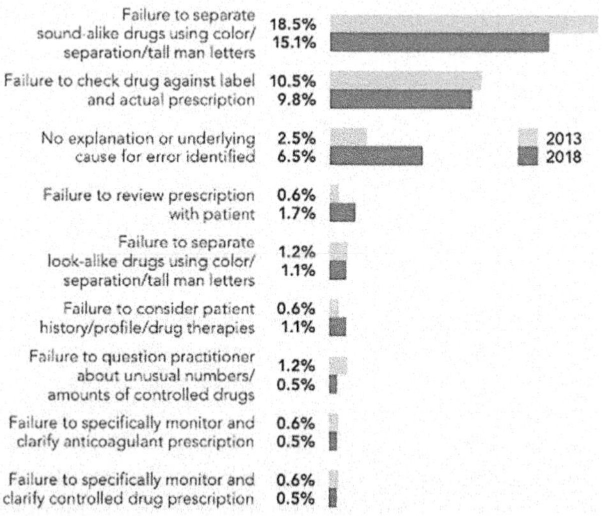

FIGURE 28.10 Distribution of Wrong Drug Closed Claims by Factors Impacting Wrong Drug-Dispensing Errors.

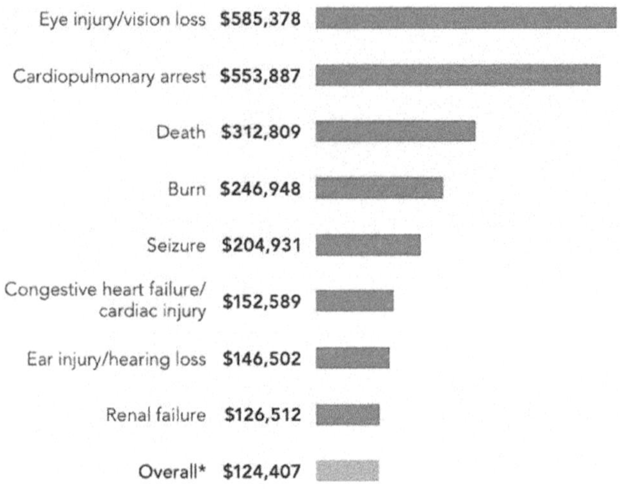

FIGURE 28.11 Severity of Injury/Illness/Adverse Outcome by Injury/Adverse Outcome.

Injury	Distribution of Closed Claims
Gastrointestinal distress	11.9%
Infection/abscess	11.9%
Death	10.3%
Emotional/psychological harm/distress	8.2%
Syncope/fainting	6.0%
Vertigo/dizziness/light-headedness	5.0%
Neurological deficit/damage	5.0%
Congestive heart failure/cardiac injury	4.3%
Eye injury/vision loss	4.3%
Seizure	3.8%
Total of the highest distribution of closed claims by injury/illness/adverse outcome	70.7%

FIGURE 28.12 Distribution of Closed Claims by Injury/Illness/Adverse Outcome.

Medication errors expand beyond the borders of a pharmacist's role in the health-care system. Learning from mistakes allows for the improvement of practices, reduces the risk of making errors, and prevents history from repeating itself. An insurance company (Company) does the same, yet on a larger scale. Unlike an individual practitioner or practice site, the Company collects large numbers of claims. The Company analyzes the circumstances leading to the claims. In addition, it examines the financial outcomes resulting in claims that are settled (dollars paid for the claim) or results of jury verdicts if there is an adverse finding in a case that goes to trial. To minimize the number of costly claims, the Company must undertake such a project and inform their insureds. The Company must also consider the financial incentive involved. In doing this, there may be less claims, less exposure, and less money paid out, and therefore, greater profits will be earned by the Company. The alternative is to raise the premiums for the insureds.

TABLE 28.1
Reasons Given by Pharmacists for the Errors—Pharmacists Mutual Claims Study.

SALAD (Sound-Alike Look-Alike Drug)
Ambiguity
CS dosing (now PMP responsibility) (opiates)
Unusual Rx
Wrong instructions/directions
Failure to check history (allergy-interactions)
High workload/lack of attention/interruptions – quotas – workplace conditions – breaks
Reliance on technology – continuous computer system changes

28.3.2.1 CNA Database and Methodology

The database includes closed claims which resulted in money payments, as described before. HPSO insures approximately 70,000 pharmacists, representing a variety of pharmacy practice sites, including community, hospital, infusion centers, long-term care, and compounding pharmacies. From 2002 to 2012, liability patterns and trends were highlighted in the study, and the circumstance which created adverse experiences were examined. Over the 10-year period, there were 1,409 reported medication-related incidents; adverse patient outcomes; and actual claims against pharmacists, pharmacy technicians, other pharmacy personnel, and pharmacy entities insured through the CNA/HPSO program. The study also included the costs incurred to defend of pharmacists before Boards of Pharmacy. The CNA/HPSO report contains several detailed case studies and high-level risk management recommendations, which, if implemented, can enhance medication safety and minimize the likelihood of patient injuries and pharmacist liability exposures. Additionally, a pharmacist self-assessment checklist is included in the study report intended to aid pharmacists in enhancing their risk awareness and safety practices.

28.3.2.2 Most Common Categories of Errors

The 2013 CNA/HSPO Pharmacist Claims Report has identified the most common categories of errors and omissions that are responsible for claims made against pharmacists for malpractice. Wrong drug (47%) and wrong dose (34%) represent 77% of all the closed claims reported. Note that the majority of errors/claims are mechanical (wrong drug/wrong dose); the contribution of wrong dose has increased, thus lowering the contribution of wrong drug, compared to the Pharmacists Mutual Claims Study reported earlier in this chapter (See Section "The Pharmacists Mutual Claims Study" and see the preceding figures).

Three National Coordinating Counsel for Medication Error Reporting and Prevention (NCC MERP) disability categories had a higher average paid indemnity compared to the overall average paid indemnity. This accounted for 32.7% of all the closed claims in the analysis. Examples of each type of error are shown next.

1. 11.7% of the errors resulted in patients suffering permanent brain damage:
   a. An infant underwent a premature birth due to the dispensing of a wrong drug (use of Prostin instead of progesterone).
   b. A child received improperly compounded total parenteral nutrition.
   c. An adult received simultaneous overdoses of Phenergan and fentanyl.
2. 11.7% of errors resulted in patient deaths:
   a. A child died from a clonidine-compounding error
   b. A child died from a dispensing error of the wrong drug.
   c. An adult died from intrathecal morphine.
3. 9.3% of errors required an intervention to sustain the patient's life:
   a. The first claim involved a fentanyl wrong dose resulting in respiratory arrest, resuscitation, and permanent brain damage.
   b. The second claim involved a wrong dose of tacrolimus which led to the failure of the patient's transplanted liver and led to a second liver transplant operation.

28.3.2.3 Claim Analysis by Insurance Source and Licensure Type: Pharmacists versus Technicians

The vast majority, 93.8%, of the claims analyzed in the CNA/HPSO involved CNA-insured pharmacists with individual professional liability policies, while 5.6% of the claims involved pharmacists employed by a CNA-insured corporate entity. Only one closed claim, constituting 0.6% of the total claims analyzed, involved a lawsuit against a pharmacy technician. That technician was employed by a CNA-insured corporate entity.

28.3.2.4 Factors Impacting Wrong Drug-Dispensing Errors

Some elements have emerged that appear to have contributed to the percentage and/or severity of such errors. The most common causes of wrong drug-dispensing errors included pharmacist failures in differentiating among Sound-Alike Look-Alike Drugs (SALAD) and checking the drug against the label and the actual prescription. Three factors were identified for wrong drug closed claims that experienced a higher paid indemnity than the overall average paid indemnity:

1. Failure to question the prescribing practitioner about any unusual prescription accounted for 1.9% of wrong drug closed claims.
2. Failure to question the practitioner about unusual numbers/amounts of controlled drugs accounted for 1.2% of wrong drug closed claims.
3. Failure to obtain the patient history/profile/drug therapies accounted for 0.6% of wrong drug closed claims.

Distractions in the pharmacy are another common and unavoidable part of every workday. Label switches can result due to a pharmacist's "multitasking" or filling multiple prescriptions for a single patient. A patient may have a prescription for Coumadin once a day and Lasix twice a day, for example. If the labels are switched, and the patient ends up taking Coumadin twice a day, he may suffer a serious hemorrhage.

28.3.2.5 Drugs Involved in Claims

The drugs commonly reported in the Claims Study, in order of frequency, include the following: Warfarin (Coumadin®), levothyroxine, amoxicillin/Augmentin®, amitriptyline, prednisone, Lipitor®, hypoglycemic drugs/sulfonylureas, beta blockers, ACE inhibitors, and opioids. These are depicted in Figure 28.13. Note that the order and frequency of the drugs reported in the CNA Claims study are very similar to those reported in the cumulative Pharmacists Mutual Study, discussed earlier in this chapter. Table 28.2 describes the "Usual Suspects" in pharmacy drug errors.

28.3.2.6 Most Common Error: Wrong Drug

Since 1990, the number of "wrong drugs" administered has remained relatively consistent (49.2%), although the reasons for these errors appear to be varied. In one case, the pharmacist took a prescription over the phone from a doctor's office for digoxin. The pharmacist prepared the label, counted the correct drug into the tray, and then poured it into the bottle. As he placed the bottle next to the completed label, the phone rang again, with a request for warfarin. The pharmacist filled the prescription for warfarin in the same manner, but, somehow, the two labels were mixed up. The warfarin bottle received the digoxin label and was given to the wrong patient.

In another case, a technician simply took the wrong bottle from the shelf and counted out the wrong drug. If a busy

TABLE 28.2
Usual Suspects in Pharmacy Drug Errors.

Warfarins, direct thrombin inhibitors, heparins
Hypoglycemics, insulin
Synthroids
Penicillin—cross allergy
Opiates—fentanyl patches, high doses to naïve patients
Beta blockers—Lisinopril
Amitriptyline
Prednisone
Lipitor/statins

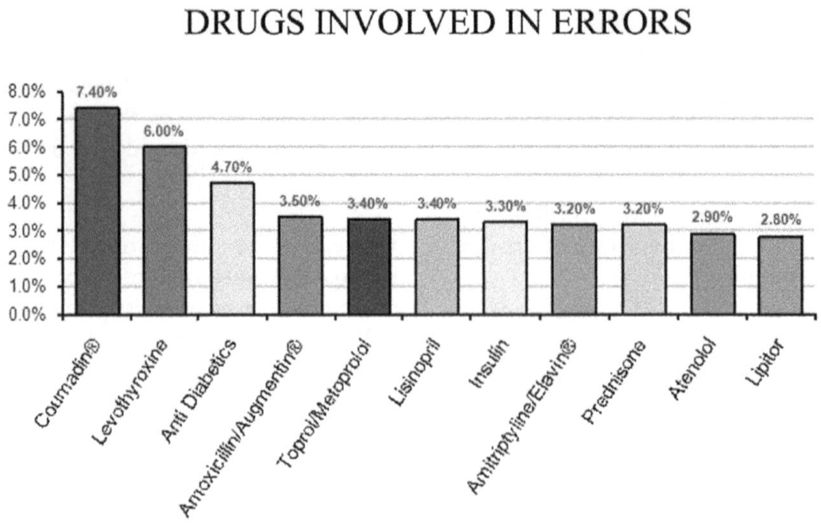

FIGURE 28.13 Drugs Involved in Errors.

pharmacist does not catch the error when he performs his check, or does not check the technician's work, the results can be serious.

A more thorough reliance on NDC# checks, notations by technician/verification by the pharmacist, can help eliminate this type of error. An enhanced technology, bar code scanning, is even more helpful in preventing wrong drug errors. When the drug product is selected in the computer system, a bar code is printed on the "fill sheet" and printed prescription label. When the technician (or pharmacist) takes the bulk drug product off the shelf, the bar code is scanned, and it must match the (bar code) identification linked to the selected drug. Bar coding or at least NDC# checking is almost universal in pharmacies. The bar code is unique for a drug, dosage form, strength, and manufacturer/distributor.

28.3.2.6.1 The Sound-Alike Look-Alike Drug (SALAD) Problem

Sometimes drug names look alike. For example, prescriptions for Navane can be mistaken for Norvasc, Prilosec for Prozac, and Lasix for Losec. Interestingly, the Lasix/Losec error precipitated a name change by the Losec manufacturer (it was renamed Prilosec). After that, Prilosec and Prozac began to be mistakenly dispensed in place of one another. This problem occurs so frequently that a special committee of the United States Pharmacopeia (USP) has been formed to look at the selection of new drug names. There is an evolving science in understanding and preventing this error of fine distinction. An update to the *Confused Names* list in 2019 may be found on the ISMP.ORG website.

28.3.2.6.2 Physician's Handwriting

Physicians' handwriting is another cause of pharmacist error. Often the subject of jokes, the typical physician's scrawl presents the most dangerous type of pharmacist error. There is an increased interest in electronic prescribing, which would help obviate such interpretative errors between the physician and pharmacist. It has been estimated that 50% of prescribing is now "e-prescribing," and many hospital systems and clinics prohibit the use of handwritten prescriptions. Washington state requires typed or block letter printing on prescriptions, no cursive, as an effort to avoid handwriting misinterpretations and errors.

E-Prescribing allows for the prescriber to electronically send accurate, error-free, and easy-to-understand prescriptions directly to a pharmacy from their point-of-care. This is a significant step in advancing the quality of patient care. The inclusion of electronic prescribing in the Medicare Modernization Act (MMA) of 2003 gave momentum to the movement, and the July 2006 Institute of Medicine report on the role of e-prescribing in reducing medication errors received widespread publicity, helping to build awareness of the role of e-prescribing in enhancing patient safety. Adopting the standards to facilitate e-prescribing is one of the key action items in the government's plan to expedite the adoption of electronic medical records and build a national electronic health information infrastructure in the United States.[7]

The SUPPORT for Patients and Communities Act, signed into federal law in October of 2018, includes an electronic prescribing requirement for all controlled substance prescriptions under Medicare part D drugs. The deadline to comply with the bill, implemented to address the opioid abuse epidemic, was January 1, 2021.

Through EPCS, providers can easily prescribe Schedule II–V controlled substances and noncontrolled prescriptions. This simplified workflow will ultimately lead to improved patient safety and reduce opioid prescription abuse and misuse. Following the federal mandate, many states have put forth legislations with similar laws. New York, for example, was the first state to mandate EPCS back in 2016. Today,

21 states have an EPCS mandate in place. An additional 17 states have future effective dates, and 5 have proposed EPCS legislations.[8]

28.3.2.6.3 E-Prescribing Information. 856 IAC 1–40: Electronic Prescribing. What Is an Electronic Prescription?

The only difference between a regular prescription and an electronic prescription is that an electronic prescription contains the electronic signature of the practitioner and is transmitted in accordance with relevant law.[9] E-scribing (electronic prescribing), with the prescriber selecting a drug and instructions in the patient's record, is automatically and digitally forwarded to a selected pharmacy. This is touted as an error reduction strategy. It has been evaluated in the past few years, and some findings have been published in several publications from several countries.

28.3.2.7 Wrong Drug Strength

The second largest category of claims (25%) shown in the Pharmacists Mutual Study is "wrong strength." A common example would be receiving a prescription for digoxin 0.125 mg, and filling it in error with digoxin 0.25 mg. In fact, misplacement of a decimal point is a very common way these errors occur. Another error is picking up the wrong bottle when filling the prescription. Perhaps the drug is correct, but the dosage is wrong. Depending upon the drug prescribed, the results of selecting the wrong strength can be dangerous, even fatal. Another common outcome is a lack of efficacy. For example, if too low a dose of an anticoagulant (such as Coumadin) is administered, it could fail to prevent a fatal clot.

Even old, familiar drugs are subject to this kind of error. The drugs that are filled most frequently are going to be involved in more errors, simply as a matter of statistics. For example, Haldol is used for senile dementia. It would be unusual for Haldol 5 mg to be prescribed for an ambulatory elderly patient. A more common dosage is 0.5 mg. The drugs with the greatest numbers of available dosage forms offer the greatest probability for a dosage error.

The drugs that can cause the most toxicity are also those that will result in claims. If the patient suffers some type of damage or adverse effect—even if the patient only has to present to an emergency room because of the error—this can result in a cause of action against the pharmacist and the pharmacy.

CASE REPORT

FACTS OF THE CASE

Hailey, a three-year-old toddler girl of 14.6 kg weight, was inadvertently prescribed oxycodone concentrate, 20 mg/1 ml, 0.5 ml, every 4 hours as needed (for pain). The child's mother took the prescription to a (national chain) pharmacy near her workplace. The prescription was filled and verified and dispensed by a pharmacist on July 17, 2016. Mom gave the child one dose (0.5 ml /10 mg) on the evening of 9/18/16 (or early morning/1 AM 9/19/16). The next morning, 9/19/16, the child was unresponsive and stiff. CPR was administered. 911 was called. EMS came and continued CPR and took Hailey to a local hospital where continued CPR was unsuccessful. An autopsy and toxicology testing were performed. The Medical Examiner ruled the cause of death: Oxycodone overdose. The Medical Examiner ordered separate toxicology testing of the prescription bottle dispensed to the child.

OPINIONS

My opinions are expressed with reasonable pharmaceutical certainty.

1. The pharmacist should **not** have filled the prescription.
2. The pharmacist **overrode** a "HARD STOP" HIGH DOSE alert. He
   a. Did not consult with the prescriber
   b. Did not consult the patient
   c. Did not document the reason for override
   d. Did not check any literature resources and document same
3. The pharmacist did not adequately perform a Drug Utilization Review (DUR). DUR requires a safe dose check, which was obviously ignored, and, in fact, a HARD STOP alert was overridden (see #2 cited above). This is a Plaintiff Pharmacist Expert on of the Pharmacy Company Policy & Procedures, as well as OAC 4279-5-20 (5).
4. The product packaging states **(IN BOLD)**: **ONLY FOR USE IN PATIENTS WHO ARE OPIOID TOLERANT**
   a. The pharmacist ignored the warning—he should have heeded the warning and stopped the process.
   b. The pharmacy computer alert did not contain this warning—it should have!

   c. The pharmacy company "How To Use this Information" (Patient Prescription Information—PPI) did not contain the **bolded ONLY FOR USE IN PATIENTS WHO ARE OPIOD TOLERANT**it should have.
5. Prescription mentioning the use of syringe required demonstration to the patient. Based upon the mother's testimony, no special counseling or syringe demonstration was provided to her.
6. It is not certain that the manufacturer's provided syringe was not given to the mother.
   a. Mother's deposition only described volume measures, not dosage increments, which are on the manufacturer's syringe.
7. The pharmacist verified and dispensed a dosage dose that delivered (10 mg = 0.5 ml of 20 mg/ml) 400% to 1300% of the recommended dose for pediatrics (0.05–0.15 mg/kg;15 kg of child).[10]
8. The pharmacist departed from the standard of care,[11] the Ohio Pharmacy Practice Act, and pharmacy company's own Policy and Procedure in multiple ways, as described before.
9. There were multiple omissions by the pharmacist: Deliberately ignoring a HARD STOP High Dose Alert, failure to consult with the prescriber (opiate tolerant; toxic dose), failure to consult with the mother ("this contains a toxic dose—I can't provide it to you").
10. The pharmacy company was negligent in failure to include the bolded **ONLY FOR USE IN PATIENTS WHO ARE OPIOID TOLERANT** in the alert software as well as in the Patient Prescription Information.
11. The gross negligence of the pharmacist as well as the omissions of the pharmacy company significantly contributed to the child's death from oxycodone overdose.
12. A reasonable physician, when contacted by a pharmacist with a toxic dose warning, as well as the alert **ONLY FOR USE IN PATIENTS WHO ARE OPIOID TOLERANT**, would have canceled the prescription thus, in this case, avoiding the tragic death of this three-year-old child.

28.3.2.8 Wrong Directions

At 7.8% of all claims, "wrong directions" represents a significant number of the claims reported in the Pharmacists Mutual Study. These cases involve incorrectly entering the directions into the computer. For example, in one case, a pharmacist entered a new prescription for birth-control tablets into the computer and inadvertently typed: "Take two tablets daily." For nine months, this patient refilled her birth-control prescription every 15 days, while following the erroneous label directions, apparently without anyone at the pharmacy noticing the discrepancy. The most dangerous "wrong-directions" claims are for children's prescriptions (and especially prescriptions for children under the age of six years).

As a consultant, I (JTOD) always recommend that pharmacists check the label directions against the "hard-copy" prescription. Another good idea is for the pharmacist to follow a standard procedure of removing the prescription from the bag as he counsels each patient. The pharmacist should read the written directions to the patient and ask, "How did your doctor explain you were to take this medication?" The pharmacist can use similar words to determine whether the patient understands what the directions mean. This serves two additional purposes: It allows the pharmacist to double check the label directions, and, by removing the prescription from the bag, it creates the appearance of a professional service rather than merely sales of a "commodity" in a sack.

28.3.2.9 Wrong Route of Administration

CASE REPORT

NON-STERILE TOPICAL LOTION DISPENSED IN PLACE OF R_X FOR STERILE EYE DROPS

OPINIONS

The pharmacist testified that she made an error in filling the prescription. Actually, she made multiple serious errors and violations of the Pharmacy Law, Pharmacy Company Policies, and the Standards of Practice of the Profession of Pharmacy, as follows:

1. Filled the prescription with the wrong product
2. Filled the prescription with a 4 oz bottle; 15 ml was prescribed

3. Filled the prescription with a shake-well auxiliary label—a solution was prescribed
4. Filled the prescription with a topical lotion labeled for external use to treat acne—an ophthalmic solution was prescribed
5. Filled the prescription with a non-sterile topical suspension; a sterile solution was prescri
6. Dispensed a misbranded and adulterated prescription
7. Filled a prescription labeled for use in the eye that was/is predictably toxic and injurious to the eye. Indeed, the prescription she dispensed caused a chemical burn and continues to cause LM disabling pain and suffering as well as impaired vision. The chemical burning, hyper-irritability, inflammation, and pain are caused by the chemical environment of the NON ophthalmic. Ophthalmic products, by necessity and definition, must be isotonic, of reasonable viscosity, with minimal (or no particulates), sterile, and pyrogen free.[12] The best-described toxic mechanism to any product introduced to the physiological cells is that of tonicity—the solute load. Physiologic cell environment is "isotonic." The acne lotion sulfacetamide is HYPER-TONIC, as well as containing many additional ingredients with known toxicity and irritability to the eye (MSDS—Material Safety Data Sheets). Hypertonic exposure to any cell in the body can lead to cell death (permanent injury to the function of the organ) if not rapidly corrected. This phenomenon is well described and not just limited to ophthalmic cells.
8. Failed to counsel LM on the appropriate use of the "eye drop" prescription. Had she done so, it is likely that she would have realized her mistake.[13] The Pharmacy Company Policy requires counselling all patients on new prescriptions.
9. Failed to consider the safety and utility of dispensing a topical non-sterile lotion for use in the eye (part of the mandated DUR (Drug Utilization Review)).
10. The Pharmacy Company contributed to this unsafe behavior by not enforcing its policy to Counsel and not disciplining this pharmacist when the serious error was reported.

This is not just a "mistake" or "error." This is gross negligence! The pharmacist's behavior was dangerous, irresponsible, and multifactorial and demonstrated a conscious disregard for patient safety. She did not recognize a need to counsel LM on the appropriate method to administer a sterile eye drop. Industry standards and pharmacy company Policy required the patient be counseled with new prescriptions, and this is especially important given that this was an eye drop. The pharmacist had no memory of any response to the offer to counsel. The standard of practice for the profession of pharmacy is to COUNSEL a patient on all new prescriptions, especially ophthalmic prescriptions, as the patients cannot be expected to know how to safely and effectively use the eye drops.[14]

28.3.2.9 Lack of Drug Review

OBRA-90 (Omnibus Budget Reconciliation Act) requires pharmacists to review all prescriptions prior to filling them—checking for interactions, allergies, and a list of other potential problems. Especially because pharmacy technicians are increasingly being used to reduce the pharmacist's workload, this area of claims—previously almost unheard of—now represents over 9% of all claims.

Drug review was first described in "The Standard of Practice of the Profession of Pharmacy."[15] The American Pharmacists Association (APhA), in concert with the American Association of Colleges of Pharmacy (AACP), has defined standards of practice for the profession of pharmacy. Many or all of the requirements that were eventually legislated and mandated by the OBRA were already components of the standards of practice, even before this legislation. OBRA requires medication profiles, as well as review for therapeutic duplication, allergy, cross-sensitivity, drug-induced disease, and contraindications. A failure to provide meaningful patient drug review has resulted in claims and lawsuits that plead the error of omission.

One way that a pharmacist can easily ensure that each prescription has been reviewed is to personally hand it to the patient, while counseling on its use. The pharmacist can take the prescription out of the bag and examine it while explaining to the patient how the drug should be used, the goal of therapy, contraindications, and so on. By the time the pharmacist then hands the drug to his patient face-to-face, 90% of the errors that occur in the filling process will have been detected.

A recent article by Appold[16] in *Drug Topics* echoes the importance of counseling and references a 1997 survey that reported that an approximate 83% of errors are discovered during counseling and corrected prior to a patient leaving the pharmacy.[17] It is therefore critical to routinely offer counsel for every patient. During each visit, the actual medication should be presented to the patient, rather than handing it to a patient in a sealed bag. Completion of this process provides an important opportunity for the patient to confirm the medication is consistent with what they are used to taking.

The Supreme Court of Illinois reviewed and issued an opinion on a case involving Walmart Pharmacy, where the patient told all of her physicians that she was allergic to aspirin. After a medical procedure, the patient was given a prescription for Toradol, a drug contraindicated for patients allergic to aspirin. She took the prescription to the Walmart Pharmacy, which (appropriately) asked her if she had any drug allergies. As always, the patient responded that she was allergic to aspirin. The Walmart Pharmacy filled the Toradol prescription anyway. The patient developed a life-threatening anaphylactic shock after taking the drug (although she recovered after an emergency treatment). Of course, she later sued the pharmacy.

Precedent cases involving the same theory have accumulated, eliminating any doubt that the pharmacist has a duty to screen for cross-allergenicity. The standard of care requires that the pharmacist should have called the physician and informed him that his patient was allergic to aspirin. Because there is cross-sensitivity for Toradol in patients allergic to aspirin, giving Toradol was contraindicated. The pharmacist should have suggested an analgesic with no cross-allergenicity to aspirin. In any case, he should have refused to dispense this drug to a patient at risk.

28.3.2.10 Counseling: A Powerful Weapon against Liability

Progressive pharmacy companies make it a standard business practice to actually counsel each patient on every new prescription, instead of merely offering a perfunctory option to the patient of obtaining counseling if they have any questions for the pharmacist. (Rather than actually requiring counseling, OBRA requires that the pharmacist only *offer* to counsel the patient.) With critical-care drugs, failure to counsel leads to predictable and serious problems. Inadequate or incomplete counseling and lack of documentation or proof of counseling are omissions that can indicate that the pharmacist is providing a lower-than-standard level of care. The patient cannot be expected to understand everything in the patient package insert without professional advice and guidance from the pharmacist.

Counseling is also a growing area of claims (compared to just a few years ago). Most of these claims are for "failure to counsel," but a few involve allegations of "inadequate" or "incorrect" counseling. Patients often report that the pharmacist failed to counsel, when, in reality, they did receive counseling (but there is no record of this having taken place). This is also a growing increasingly frequent reason for boards of pharmacy to administer disciplinary actions.

28.3.2.10.1 California Lawsuits against CVS and Walgreens

Mark Lowery, Content Editor for *Drug Topics*, reports in the August 19, 2015 edition of two lawsuits against large pharmacy companies (Walgreens and CVS) by the State of California for failure to counsel pharmacy patients. Walgreens has agreed to pay $502,200 to settle charges that some of its pharmacists in California failed to provide patient consultations as required by law. "Pharmacist consultations prevent drug errors and ensure that patients have the right prescription for their condition," San Diego County District Attorney Bonnie Dumanis said. "Without these checks and balances, dire consequences could result."

28.3.2.10.2 Rite Aid Settles Patient Consultation Lawsuit

Pharmacists are required to provide patient consultations when customers receive new prescriptions or new dosages of existing prescriptions. Walgreens did not admit any liability. The agreement stipulates that Walgreens will be subject to an injunction requiring full compliance with California's standards for proper patient consultations and that the retail chain must implement an internal compliance program. Previously, both CVS and Rite Aid have also faced charges alleging their pharmacists at some California locations failed to provide required patient consultations. In 2013, a $658,500 judgment was issued against CVS; and in June 2014, a $498,250 judgment was issued against Rite Aid. Several district attorneys' offices in California worked with the California State Board of Pharmacy (CSBP) to conduct undercover investigations of the major pharmacy chains in the state.

28.3.2.10.3 Drug Interaction Case Report—Affidavit of James T. O'Donnell

At the trial of this matter, the plaintiff intends to call James T. O'Donnell.

Dr. O'Donnell will explain the process by which medications, in general, including Diflucan and Zofran, are approved by the FDA. On average, it takes 12 years and over $350 million to get a new drug from the laboratory through the approval process. Once the drug is developed, it undergoes approximately 3 ½ years of testing before an application is made to the FDA to begin testing the drug in humans. Less than one out of ten of 1% of the medications that are laboratory tested ever make it to human testing. If the FDA allows human testing, the "investigative" drug enters a three-phase clinical trial. The first phase uses 20–80 healthy volunteers to establish a drug's safety and profile. Phase 1 takes approximately one year. Phase 2 involves 100 to 300 patient volunteers to assess the drug's effectiveness. Phase 2 takes approximately two years. In phase 3, 1,000 to 3,000 patients in clinics and hospitals are monitored carefully to determine the effectiveness and identify adverse reactions. Phase 3 is approximately a three-year process. Following the clinical trials, the developing company submits an application to the FDA for approval. If the medication is approved, it becomes available for prescription and sale. This process has been used for drug approval for decades. Both Diflucan and Zofran were subjected to this process.

Despite the rigorous steps in the process of drug development, the true picture of the product safety actually evolves over the months and years that make up the product's lifetime in the marketplace. FDA programs allow for the reporting of problems and safety issues with medications after approval. These programs allow information regarding medications to be constantly assessed and updated. The information obtained from the approval process and post-marketing drug safety monitoring is used by entities that publish and market drug to drug interaction computer programs. The program utilized by Thrifty White in 2014 was based on FDA information. The FDA post-marketing surveillance programs are codified in 21 CFR 310.305, 21 CFR 312.32, and 21 CFR 314.80.

The aforementioned process leads to the development of prescribing information for each medication approved. Attached hereto as is the prescribing information for fluconazole/Diflucan and the prescribing information for ondansetron/Zofran. The prescribing information for Diflucan provides, in pertinent part, that "some azoles, including fluconazole, have been associated with prolongation of the QT interval on the electrocardiogram." "Fluconazole is a potent CYP2C9 inhibitor and a moderate CYP3A4 inhibitor." " There is a potential risk for increased plasma concentration for other compounds metabolized by the enzymes CYP2C9 and CYP3A4 co-administered with fluconazole. Caution should therefore be exercised when patients are administered these drug combinations." The product information for Diflucan, including the post-marketing experience includes "QT prolongation and torsades de pointes." Finally, the product information states "coadministration of other drugs known to prolong the QT interval and which are metabolized via the enzyme CYP3A4 such as cisapride, astemazole, pimozide, and quinidine are contraindicated in patients receiving fluconazole." Ondansetron is known to prolong the QT interval and is metabolized via the enzyme CYP3A4. The product information for Zofran provides "ECG changes including QT interval prolongation has been seen in patients receiving ondansetron." "Avoid Zofran in patients . . . taking other medicinal products that lead to QT prolongation." Diflucan is a product that leads to QT prolongation.

The interaction involved in this case is a drug-to-drug interaction between the prescription of 100 mg of fluconazole with that of 8 mg of Zofran every 8 hours as needed. The prescriptions from the pharmacy identify the route, dosage, and frequency with which the medications were to be taken. The plaintiff testified that his wife was taking the medications as ordered. A drug-to-drug interaction warning was triggered at the pharmacy for the prescriptions of fluconazole and Zofran to his wife. The warning was triggered on the basis of the route, dosage, and frequency prescribed by her doctors. The patient warning identified the interaction as severe and stated "do not take these drugs together. Discuss possible alternative treatment options with your prescriber." The pharmacy warning states "concomitant administration of fluconazole and drugs that both prolong the QT interval and the CYP3A4 substrate is contraindicated according to the FDA approved product labeling."

The science leading to the warnings in this case is neither "novel" nor considered "junk science." The FDA approval process has been the sole method of approving medications such as Diflucan and Zofran in the United States for decades. The FDA is the highest authority in the United States on drug safety. All pharmacists and prescribing physicians rely on the information generated through the approval process and post-marketing investigation. That information is generally accepted in the pharmaceutical and medical community. The scientific methods and principles used to develop the drug-to-drug interaction information in this case are evidence-based and are further based on epidemiological evidence. Accordingly, defendant's assertion that "[p]laintiff's have failed to present any evidence, opinion, or authority to support a contention that these medications in these doses are known to prolong the QT interval" (Def. Motion, page 15) is patently false and ignores the warnings in this case that are based on the best available evidence on drug safety.

Dr. O'Donnell has reviewed the articles cited by the defense experts. None of the articles address the interaction between fluconazole and ondansetron. None of the articles were designed to challenge the product information developed by the FDA for fluconazole and ondansetron. None of the articles, or the principles discussed therein, have led to a withdrawal of the warnings for oral Zofran. None of the articles stand for the proposition that patients concomitantly taking fluconazole 100 mg and Zofran 8 mg three times daily as needed do not experience clinically significant QT prolongation or are not at risk for sudden death due to cardiac arrythmia. In fact, the FDA Drug Safety Communications from 2011 and 2012 all reiterate that patients taking Zofran, alone, have demonstrated QT prolongation and torsade de pointes. Patients taking Zofran and other medications that prolong the QT interval are at "particular risk" for QT prolongation. The literature cited does not "establish" that low oral doses of fluconazole and ondansetron do not cause QT interval prolongation.

The FDA does not issue warnings based on "novel" science. In order for a warning to be issued, the approval process and/or post-marketing surveillance have established "sufficient risk" for the warning. The manufacturer's duty to warn arises when a reasonable association exists between the medication and the danger. Both clearly exist here.

The opinions Dr. O'Donnell holds and to which he will testify at the trial of this matter are all held to a reasonable degree of probability in his field of expertise. His opinions are based on his education, training, and pharmacological and pharmaceutical experience and on his knowledge of the accepted standards of practice that apply to healthcare providers caring for patients like the decedent. Dr. O'Donnell's opinions are formed through the application of well-known and generally accepted principles of pharmacy and science related to the management of patients who present to pharmacies where severe drug-to-drug interactions are identified. In forming his opinions, Dr. O'Donnell has relied on his education; training; experience and expertise as well as his knowledge of the medical literature; his care of patients such as the decedent and his review of her medical records, pharmacy records, autopsy report, documents produced through discovery; and the depositions in this case including exhibits.

The court rejected the defense motion and ruled that Dr. O'Donnell would be allowed to testify. The defendants settled the case with the plaintiff.

28.3.2.11 Non-Bodily Injury

"Personal injury" is an insurance term. These types of claims are also referred to as "non-bodily injury" claims. These claims involve libel, slander, false arrest, and/or unauthorized release of confidential records. Unauthorized release of confidential records accounts for approximately one-half of these types of claims. This is another fast-growing area of professional liability claims against pharmacists. These claims usually involve the pharmacist or technician, but it also may involve any employee in the pharmacy or hospital.

The risk of being sued increases when there are confidentiality or breaches related to mental health issues, sexually transmitted diseases, use of birth control, or the release of prescription records to a relative. For example, one technician filled a prescription for an AIDS drug and recognized that the man was receiving treatment for HIV. The patient's son was acquainted with the technician's own children, and the technician told her children not to associate with their friend anymore. When the patient discovered that the pharmacy had disclosed information about his HIV treatment, he brought a suit against the pharmacy.

28.3.2.11.1 Judge Rules Pharmacists' Comments to a Patient are Privileged and Therefore a Defense for a Slander Suit

A recent case analysis by the pharmacist attorney David Brushwood (*Pharmacy Today*, March 15, 2015) involves a physician suing a pharmacy for slander, claiming that pharmacists had made defamatory statements to patients about the physician's "qualifications as a medical doctor." The pharmacy filed a motion to dismiss the case, claiming a qualified privilege. The court noted that malice is an essential element of slander. False statements that suggest someone has committed a dishonest or illegal act are defamatory and clothed in a "presumption of malice."

However, the presumption ceases to exist if the defendant has a qualified privilege to make the statements. The court explained that a statement is privileged if it is (1) made in good faith, (2) with an interest to be upheld, (3) made on a proper occasion, and (4) made in a proper manner.

The court reasoned that the statements at issue in this case were made by pharmacists to patients at the time patients attempted to have medication dispensed, pursuant to prescriptions, and that the apparent purpose of the statements was to inform the patients about the physician who had issued the prescriptions.

The court noted that the "pharmacists acted in good faith and were upholding a legitimate interest since the statements were made while the pharmacists were filling prescriptions and giving general advice as they have a duty to do."

The court noted its ruling from a prior case, concluding that pharmacists have a duty to provide competent advice to patients and that this duty is not satisfied by "a robotic compliance with the instructions of the prescribing physician." Applying this standard to the allegations in the present case, the court said the pharmacists "exercised their due diligence."

28.3.2.12 Miscellaneous Errors

At the end of the list of medication errors reported by Pharmacists Mutual Claims Study is a category for "other." This category may include several types of miscellaneous errors' responsibility for a significant number of claims.

One relatively new area of claims involves using proper safety caps on prescription bottles. Safety-cap claims either involve the pharmacist not following federal law or the pharmacist being unable to prove it was the patient who requested "no safety cap." From Pharmacists Mutual claims experience, the pharmacist cannot rely on a notation in the computer nor on the testimony, "I always use safety caps, unless the patient requests otherwise." For the pharmacist's protection, the patient or caregiver should be required to sign a written request for each new prescription ordered without a safety cap. A once-a-year blanket release is inadequate.

Another area of miscellaneous claims involves the use of generic drugs. In these claims, the pharmacist usually believes that a generic product is equivalent to the brand-name drug but is mistaken. Inadequate generic substitution may result in therapeutic inefficacy, adverse reactions, or allergies.

28.3.2.12.1 Compounding Errors

Hospital and home-care pharmacy therapy involving the preparation of intravenous (IV) solutions for treating acutely ill patients is another area where critical mistakes occur. These solutions are usually mixed in the pharmacy (called "compounding"). Close coordination between the medical staff and the compounding pharmacist is of vital necessity here. There is a greater risk for errors with this activity, and when errors occur, they tend to result in more serious outcomes, such as, for example, from life-threatening infections. Examples include the substitution of insulin for heparin, overdoses of sodium, excessive or no glucose, and alterations and errors in almost any ingredient. Many deaths and permanent injuries have been reported as a result of compounding errors in hospital and home-care pharmacies.

One home-care pharmacist was reported to have dispensed syringes filled with potassium chloride, instead of sodium chloride, which resulted in an infant patient's sudden cardiac arrest. Profound brain damage was the result.

An investigation revealed that technicians had mislabeled the refrigerator storage bags. The case was eventually settled out of court.

In other case, in Springfield, Missouri, a hospital inaccurately compounded a cardioplegia solution, with fatal results. The hospital was sued and was subjected to a punitive-damage award.[18]

When it comes to compounding, pediatric patients are at the greatest risk. In one case, a child in Boston was given a 125 times overdose of a drug, causing prolonged low blood pressure and serious brain damage. The family was awarded a multi-million-dollar judgment. Another child in a Wisconsin hospital received a 10-fold overdose of digoxin due to a dosage miscalculation by a hospital pharmacist. The nurses did not detect the error. The child died. The hospital was sued and subsequently settled the case. The State Pharmacy Board of Wisconsin learned of the lawsuit and settlement and charged the pharmacist and the hospital pharmacy director with failure to report the error (a little-known regulation in Wisconsin—one that exists in only a few states).

28.3.2.12.2 Home Healthcare Pharmacist Monitoring

Some classes of drugs seem to lend themselves to medication errors and adverse events. For example, the aminoglycosides, such as gentamicin, have a well-known ability to cause damage to the kidneys, as well as to both the auditory and vestibular portions of the inner ear. This toxicity is both dosage- and time-dependent, requiring careful monitoring of serum drug concentrations. Lack of monitoring can cause catastrophic kidney and ear damage to patients and liability for the pharmacist and physician. The vestibular damage can result in terrible balance problems for the affected patients. In fact, there are so many patients who have suffered vestibular damage from gentamicin that they have created their own website.[19]

28.3.2.12.3 NECC Pharmacy Compounding Explodes into the News

The abstract for the June 27, 2013 *New England Journal of Medicine* describes an outbreak of fatal fungal meningitis infections, which was first reported in the Fall of 2012 and identifies a single compounding pharmacy (New England Compounding Center) as the source of adulterated and contaminated "sterile" methylprednisolone acetate injections intended for epidural use. Since the outbreak, the company has gone bankrupt, $100,000,000 in insurance claims has been paid and coverage exhausted, the pharmacists have surrendered their pharmacist licenses, and at least one pharmacist has been charged with murder! Portions of the abstract are presented as follows:[8]

At the outset of the outbreak, the persistence and progression of neutrophilic meningitis of unknown cause were the triggers for obtaining the history of a recent epidural injection of methylprednisolone. Once this association was highlighted, other physicians realized that they too had struggled to find a cause for similar cases. Of interest, the mold causing meningitis was reported to be Aspergillus fumigatus, an organism that has not been detected in any of the subsequent 700-plus cases. It has since been determined that the major culprit is Exserohilum rostratum, a plant pathogen that rarely causes human disease. This mold has been cultured or identified by means of a polymerase-chain-reaction (PCR) assay from cerebrospinal fluid or tissues in 152 patients and has been detected in unopened vials from two of the three implicated lots of methylprednisolone.

Shortly after the Tennessee Department of Health was notified on September 18, 2012, the implicated lots were quickly identified, all centers that had received the implicated lots were alerted, and patients who had received injections from these lots were notified of the potential for fungal infection. More than 13,400 patients could have been exposed to contaminated methylprednisolone from one of the three implicated lots. The compounding pharmacy producing the drug, New England Compounding Center (NECC), was closed, and all products (not just the implicated lots) were recalled. The Centers for Disease Control and Prevention (CDC) provided timely information regarding appropriate diagnostic testing and treatment on its website (www.cdc.gov).

After years of criminal investigations, the case was tried in Federal Court in Boston. Penalties and prison sentences were given for pharmacist owner, pharmacist in charge, and pharmacists and a technician for their dangerous pharmacy compounding practices that caused dozens of deaths and debilitating meningitis due to contaminated "sterile" products compounded at their pharmacy.

28.3.2.13 Wrong Directions

In a recent Colorado case, a sloppy auxiliary label occluded the 1 in the 12 on the label, changing the instructions for taking 1 tablet every 12 hours, to taking 1 tablet every 2 hours, with resultant gastrointestinal toxicity that led to severe illness and loss of wages.

28.3.2.14 Lack of Drug Review

OBRA-90 (Omnibus Budget Reconciliation Act) requires pharmacists to conduct a DUR on all prescriptions prior to filling them—checking for interactions, allergies, and a list of other potential problems. Because pharmacy technicians are increasingly being used to reduce the pharmacist's workload, this category of error, previously almost unheard of, now represents about 8% of all claims. Reports from the field indicate that technicians frequently override DUR alerts and do not involve the pharmacist, leading to errors and injuries.

OBRA requires medication profiles, as well as reviews for therapeutic duplication, allergy, cross-sensitivity, drug-induced disease, and contraindications. Failure to provide a meaningful patient drug review has resulted in claims and lawsuits that plead error of omission.

An application example could be a pain medication (Toradol®) where the patient has a documented aspirin allergy. The standard of care requires that the pharmacist call the physician and inform him of the patient's aspirin allergy. Because there is cross-sensitivity for Toradol® in patient's allergy to aspirin, it means that product is contraindicated. The pharmacist should have suggested an analgesic with no cross-allergenicity to aspirin. In any case, the pharmacist should have refused to dispense a drug to a patient who is at risk.

28.3.2.15 Avoiding Errors and Malpractice

Based upon the claims made, both the Pharmacists Mutual and the CNA/HPSO Claims Studies also provide risk management recommendations to avoid errors and thus injuries and claims. HPSO states: "Dispensing of any medication involves potential risk, and every possible safeguard must be undertaken to prevent errors." Some of the strategies are as follows:

1. Do not dispense any unfamiliar drug without performing appropriate research regarding its uses, contraindications, and hazards.
2. Ensure that each pharmacy computer is programmed to offer comprehensive current drug research, which is automatically updated.
3. Consider any override of a computerized warning to be an incident and regularly review all system errors, incomplete formulary, inadequate or inaccurate Sig codes, practitioner ordering issues, or pharmacist or technician competency issues.
4. Never assume that similar sounding names (SALAD) are equivalents. Sound-alike names are one of the major factors in pharmacy errors. Effective measures should be taken to separate and clearly identify sound-alike drugs, including the use of conspicuous warning labels.
5. Contact the prescriber regarding any questions related to the prescribed drug, including contraindications and potential interactions, and consult with the supervising pharmacist or pharmacy director as needed.
6. Ensure that all prescriptions are checked prior to dispensing, preferably by a second pharmacist. In a single pharmacist setting, the pharmacist must check each prescription against the original order; verify that the proper drug, dosage, and quantity are dispensed; and confirm that the label, patient instructions, and any warnings are correct.
7. Maintain and consistently adhere to appropriate policies, protocols, and systems to identify problems caused by new drugs, including possible interactions between a newly prescribed drug and other prescribed drugs, OTC medications, and dietary supplements used by the patient.
8. Maintain a current patient history and drug information, updating the information at each encounter.
9. Provide written patient instructions and counsel the patient regarding medication regimens.
10. Offer each patient the opportunity to ask questions during and after medication counseling and document the patient's response to this offer.

William Kelly (PharmD, FASHP), an esteemed pharmacist and professor, offered "Top Ten" recommendations for avoiding pharmacist malpractice:

1. Think, rather than just do. Question everything. Ask "why?"
2. Counsel every patient.
3. When in doubt, ask another pharmacist or call the prescriber.
4. Be leery when you have to open many vials or dispense large quantities.
5. Do not let technicians bypass ANY safety alerts. Never give the technician your bypass code. This is the Pharmacist's responsibility!
6. Read and know and follow your employer's pharmacy policies and procedures.
7. Document ALL errors.
8. Have someone else (even a technician) check your calculations.
9. Always review the patient medication history before dispensing a medication.
10. Always list the patient's drug allergies and document what happens when they take the drug they are allergic to.

28.3.2.16 Alert Fatigue

28.3.2.16.1 Risk Management Recommendations

The following risk control strategies are designed to serve as a starting point for pharmacists seeking to assess and enhance risk control practices. They complement the recommendations that follow the detailed closed claim analysis. Other valuable resources and tools can be utilized and may be accessed at HPSO, the Agency for Healthcare Research and Quality (AHRQ), and ISMP.

According to the Agency for Healthcare Research and Quality (AHRQ), the term "alert fatigue" describes how busy healthcare providers become desensitized to safety alerts and, as a result, may bypass, override, ignore, or otherwise fail to respond appropriately to warnings, potentially leading to patient harm. Alert fatigue is caused by an excess of alerts and/or warnings in the clinical environment, most but not all of which are less than urgent. This unintended consequence of the computerization of healthcare has become a significant hazard in many healthcare settings.

The AHRQ Patient Safety Network online resource Alert Fatigue discusses this phenomenon in detail. The following steps, adapted from the AHRQ resource, can help pharmacists avoid medication errors, as well as foster a working environment that regards patient safety a top priority.

1. Reduce or eliminate clinically inconsequential alerts.

2. Removing/deleting insignificant alarms should be performed using a structured review process, and an individual pharmacist should not be allowed to make these changes without organizational review/approval.
3. Tailor alerts to patient characteristics and critical integrated clusters of physiologic indicators. For example, incorporate renal function laboratory results into the alert system so that alerts for nephrotoxic medications are triggered only for patients at high risk.
4. Tier alerts according to severity. Warnings may be presented in different forms, in an effort order to focus clinicians to alerts that are more clinically consequential.
5. Apply human factors principles when designing alerts, carefully choosing the format, content, legibility, and color of alerts.
6. Periodically, evaluate the pharmacy computer system for clinically insignificant and false positive alerts and take action to minimize alert fatigue (Medication Errors Involving Overrides of Healthcare Technology).
7. Review all system reports on alerts to determine which alerts are overridden and the reasons for the overrides.
8. Require that pharmacists document rationale when overriding a serious alert, such as exceeding a maximum dose or a serious drug interaction (Medication Safety Self Assessment® for Community/Ambulatory Pharmacy).

28.4 SPECIFIC PHARMACIST MALPRACTICE CASE REPORTS/TOPICS

Pharmacists discuss their worst mistakes in a new Column in *Drug Topics,* August 19, 2015. Dennis Miller, a retired pharmacist and the author of *Pharmacy Exposed*, states:

> Sometimes errors occur inexplicably, for none of the above reasons. Miller writes, "discussing real world errors among pharmacists can be educational, and it surely makes pharmacists more careful."

Some of the "The nightmare cases" described by Miller in his book include:

- $30.6 million award in California: Pharmacist dispensed 100 mg of phenobarbital to Bryn Cabanillas instead of 15 mg prescribed, resulting in brain damage
- $31.3 million award in Illinois: Pharmacist dispensed diabetes drug glipizide to Leonard Kulisek instead of gout drug allopurinol, leading to renal failure, stroke, and death
- $25.8 million award in Florida: Pharmacist dispensed blood thinner warfarin in 10 times the dose prescribed to Beth Hippely, causing cerebral hemorrhage; it was a teenage pharmacy technician's error
- $21 million judgment in Illinois: Pharmacist dispensed adult diabetes drug glipizide to infant girl Alexandra Gehrke instead of anti-seizure drug phenobarbital
- $18.5 million jury award in New Jersey: Pharmacist prepared contaminated chemotherapy, which was injected into the spine of Anton Weck, causing paralysis
- $16 million award: Pharmacist dispensed adult diabetes drug Glynase to a young girl instead of Ritalin, resulting in brain damage

28.4.1 Duty to Warn?

In a case discussed in *Pharma-Law e-News* in August 2008, the court dismissed the plaintiffs' claims for failure to provide expert testimony on a claimed duty of Walgreens' pharmacists to refrain from filling prescriptions for Vytorin and/or gemfibrozil when the patient was also taking cyclosporine. The patient developed rhabdomyolysis. Plaintiffs moved for reconsideration, arguing that the parties had agreed not to engage in discovery and the hiring of experts until the court decided the legal question of whether the defendants owed a duty to the plaintiff to refrain from filling the prescriptions in question. Walgreens disputes that such an agreement existed and that the alleged agreement was not before the court at the time its ruling was made.

On reconsideration, the court noted that—as conceded by plaintiffs—Indiana does not recognize a duty to warn on the part of a pharmacist, unless the prescriber directs the pharmacist to do so. However, pharmacists have a duty to cease filling a prescription under certain circumstances. In *Hooks SuperX*, the patient was consuming the medication more frequently than ordered by the physician.[20] The Indiana Supreme Court held that 1) pharmacists possess expertise regarding the dispensing of prescription drugs; 2) the relationship between pharmacist and patient is sufficiently close to justify a duty; and 3) it is foreseeable that one who consumes excessive quantities of habit-forming drugs may become addicted to them, and "such an addiction carries with it certain reasonably foreseeable consequences." Finally, the Court concluded that public policy favors preventing intentional and unintentional drug abuse. Having found a duty, the *Hooks SuperX* court found that the pharmacist must exercise the same degree of care that an ordinarily prudent pharmacist would under the same or similar circumstances.

The district court then examined whether, applying similar tests, the Indiana Supreme Court would "find that pharmacists have a duty to refrain from filling a prescription that is incompatible with medication previously dispensed to the customer at a different store location." It began by noting that such a duty is not well settled; however, the relationship test is met such that the Walgreens pharmacists do owe the plaintiff a duty. The Court held that

> [T]he issue is whether it is reasonably foreseeable to a pharmacist filling a valid prescription that a customer will suffer harm from an adverse drug interaction with other medications. In the absence of special circumstances placing the pharmacist on notice that the customer is taking other adverse medications, the resulting harm isn't foreseeable.

According to the facts of the case, a cyclosporine prescription was filled by Walgreens in May of 2004, but all additional supplies of cyclosporine were provided to the plaintiff by the University of Nebraska Medical Center. The Court ruled that "nothing in the record could establish that Walgreens knew or should have known that Ms. Bobay was taking Cyclosporine in April/May 2005. . . . The foreseeability factor weighs against imposing a duty in this case."

Finally, in the absence of special circumstances, the Court held that the public policy stance in *Ingram* remains in force; the interest in patient safety permits, but does not require, a pharmacist to act to refrain from filling a lawful prescription, and thus, "relying on the reasoning [in *Ingram*], this court finds that the public-policy concern of customer safety in this instance isn't paramount to the policy concern of avoiding interference with the physician-patient relationship." The Court granted anew Walgreens' motion for summary judgment, albeit on new grounds.

The risk management of drug malpractice includes identifying theories of liability through the examination of case law and civil litigation. Pharmacists have an independent duty to protect their patients from harm and must consult with prescribing physicians in a positive way so that mistakes and misunderstandings can be avoided or corrected. The volume of daily work that each pharmacist must perform has created a role for pharmacy technicians to perform many of the steps in filling a prescription. Each and every prescription must still be checked and approved by a licensed pharmacist. This is mandated both by law and by professional obligation. All of these obligations are in force for all prescription drug products—but even greater scrutiny is required for investigational drugs, because of the greater risk of toxicity and because of the possibility of adverse effects that may not yet be well understood or reported.

28.4.2 Wrong Drug

A recent case in the Midwest deserves discussion. A middle-aged man was required by his prescription drug insurance plan to obtain his chronic medications from a Mail Service Pharmacy. He did this for several years without any incident. However, after receiving his 'Xanax" prescription, he suffered a series of inexplicable serious and life-threatening hypoglycemic reactions—inexplicable until the pills in his "Xanax" bottle were identified as Glimepiride (Amaryl), an oral sulfonylurea hypoglycemic agent. This was identified as a prescription mis-fill (error) by physicians at Mayo Clinic as well as by the patient's primary care physician. At the Mayo Clinic, the patient was evaluated by a psychiatrist and found not to be exhibiting factitious behavior —that is, fabricating the error—and that he was not nor had he been suicidal (taking a lethal dose of drugs FOUR times). The patient injured his left leg during his first hypoglycemic coma event where his leg was trapped under his body for several hours, and he continues to suffer pain and neurological deficit from this insult such as sciatica, neuropathy, regional pain syndrome—LLE. He tried but was unable to work after the series of hospitalizations, and he has had IME and FCE and Neurology rulings of disability. His ability to work is limited to sedentary activities, which is incompatible with his work as a mortician.

Three Mail Service Pharmacy employees testified. At least one employee of the three admitted that errors in filling prescriptions have occurred. However, all three pharmacy employees testified that the "system" "cannot make mistakes" and checking computer records "proves" that alprazolam—not glimepiride—was in the patient's Xanax prescription bottle in August 2010 and therefore disproves any mistake by the Mail Service Pharmacy.

28.4.2.1 Opinions

1. More likely than not, glimepiride, not alprazolam, was in the bottle delivered to in August 2010, and thus, the Mail Service Pharmacy and its pharmacists provided the wrong drug, the bottle was mislabeled and contained the wrong fill date, and, in doing so, the pharmacists were negligent and departed from the standard of care of reasonable and prudent pharmacists.
2. All pharmacies, unfortunately, commit errors, even with good systems. The most frequent pharmacy error is dispensation of the wrong drug.
3. If glimepiride, not alprazolam, was in the bottle delivered in August 2010, then the pharmacy and its pharmacists provided the wrong drug, mislabeled it, and provided the wrong fill date; in doing so, they were negligent and departed from the standard of care of reasonable and prudent pharmacists.
4. Glimepiride, a second-generation oral sulfonylurea agent, given to an euglycemic patient, will lower blood sugar and, if the blood sugar is lowered too much, may lead to dangerously low blood sugar levels, with resultant metabolic and encephalopathy and other neurological sequalae.
5. The pharmacy error is the proximate cause of several life-threatening experiences, a permanent disability to the patient's (left leg), and cognitive deficits.

28.4.2.2 Basis for Opinions

Pharmacists have a duty to dispense the correct drug, label the prescription container, identify the prescriber and the patient, and note the date that the prescription is filled on the prescription label and receipt. These are universal requirements throughout the United States. To provide the wrong drug, wrong instructions, wrong fill date, wrong name, etc., is a departure of pharmacy practice act and is negligence. When an incorrectly dispensed drug is taken by a patient and the patient is injured, the pharmacist's error/negligence is proximately related to the injury.

The patient's hypoglycemia is documented in several hospitalizations as caused by his unintentional and accidental consumption of glimepiride. His chronic sciatic neuropathy is traced to an injury to his leg when he nearly died following the first hypoglycemic injury. Other experts have evaluated and found him disabled, having limited work capacity, and cognitively impaired, all related to his initial hypoglycemic reactions.

28.4.3 Quotas and Metrics: Contributing to the Problem?

Debates about quotas or metrics for production in clinical operations or services have emerged as well. Metrics have increasingly become part of the business landscape to optimize efficiency and cost effectiveness for activities needed to deliver cost-efficient care and "value-based purchasing," a term used by the Centers for Medicare & Medicaid Services (CMS).

Additionally, efforts to cut costs and increase the volume of prescriptions filled seem to contribute to the problem of pharmacy errors. Jim Aichelman, a California pharmacist, reported to *Drug Topics* in July of 2009 that most community/retail pharmacists fill about 250 prescriptions a day and up to 1,300 per week. Of course, such volume increases the opportunity for errors to occur. There is also a necessity for more pharmacy technicians to assist, which require more management on the part of the pharmacist. The result is less counseling, less attention to detail, and fewer breaks—tired minds make mistakes. Aichelman's team also found that pharmacists who must skip breaks to keep up with an ever-increasing workload were less likely to counsel or "go out of their way" to help patients. This, too, may contribute to increased error rates.

There have been many lawsuits over metrics and quotas in pharmacy. It is troubling when there is an outcry of complaints about lack of counseling, while at the same time termination of employment is based solely on "metrics." To be sure, this metric measure, or quota, is not unique to pharmacy practice. Physicians air the same complaints that they are measured solely on the number of complaints and not on the quality of the care they provide. One problem is that metrics can be used as an age discrimination vector; they can also be used to penalize pharmacists and other health workers for taking extra necessary time to solve a patient's problem.

There are also reports about quotas and metrics in community and hospital pharmacists. A recent survey on the topic conducted and reported by Ukens in *Drug Topics* comments on the adoption of quotas by pharmacies. Some drugstore chain executives and independent owners have established daily prescription quotas that their pharmacists are expected to fill. Such quotas are a fairly recent phenomenon, but they have already become a highly emotional issue with some pharmacists.

Proponents tout quotas as a management tool ensuring productivity, fair workload distribution, and efficient staffing levels. Critics counter that quotas add up to trouble—more medication errors, more pharmacist stress, and less patient counseling. Drugstore owners/managers who use quotas are sometimes vilified as bean counters obsessed with black ink and the patient be damned.

Ukens conducted a nationwide survey of pharmacists. Fourteen percent of the 1,259 respondents have quotas imposed, and 90% of those pharmacists report that the quota is merely a guideline, not a must. Quotas are most prevalent in chain drugstores, where 12% reported working under quota system.

"Machines, we're not"—quotas are unpopular with pharmacists:

The quota system may not have taken pharmacy by storm yet, but the majority of the pharmacies *Drug Topics* surveyed hope it never does. Quotas got a thumbs down from 66% of all the respondents, who also believe they should be eliminated.

An overwhelming majority, 84%, of all the pharmacists surveyed would not apply for a job that included a quota. "Stop and take a gut check to see if this is what you went to school for," urged an Ohio independent. "Those who work for pharmacies with quotas perpetuate the problem and lower the professional level of all pharmacists—and eventually patient care," said a chain pharmacist in Virginia.

'Not unreasonable' —opinions of pharmacists who work under quotas:

Familiarity does not seem to breed contempt in the case of quotas. Pharmacists who actually work with quotas were more upbeat than pharmacists in general. Two-thirds of quota pharmacists would sign on for a similar position. Some 33% said quotas greatly contribute to stress, 23% reported they greatly increase medication errors, and 24% said they greatly curtail patient counseling. Those figures were nearly balanced by quota pharmacists with opinions at the other end of the 10-point scale; 29% said a quota has no effect on error rates, and 22% said it does not restrict patient counseling. In terms of stress, however, only 12% see no increase. "Normally, quotas are not set at unreasonable rates," said a pharmacist in a Pennsylvania hospital and ambulatory clinic. "If the staffers of the facility work together, (quotas) do not present as great an obstacle as they are made out to be."

When pharmacists who actually work under quotas are looked at separately, 70% find the system has good and bad points, but only 20% would eliminate them altogether. Another 4% think that quotas are good for pharmacy and should be encouraged. Not so, counter quota opponents, who worry about Rx foul-ups, pressure, and neglected patients. Of all the pharmacists surveyed, 69% believe that quotas contribute to errors, 57% see the stress level rising as a result of quotas, and 56% think there is less time to counsel when quotas are in effect.

ISMP's Cohen and Smelter discuss the matter of quotas in their book, *Preventing Dispensing errors:*

> Explicit or tacit quotas for dispensing put pharmacists under stress and increase the risk of error. Demands to dispense a certain number of prescriptions per shift are put in place by misguided supervisors or companies that value productivity over accuracy. One state pharmacy association has served notice that pharmacists shall not dispense and permit holders shall not allow a pharmacist to dispense prescription drugs at such a rate per hour or day as to pose a danger to public health or safety; the statement mentions a threshold of 150 prescriptions per pharmacist per day. Clearly, pushing people past their limits for safe professional practice can lead to errors.

Ken Baker, a noted pharmacist attorney, in a published article on Ethical Decisions in *Drug Topics,* writes:

> "I told them if they didn't get me more help, we would kill someone." This sentence was part of a three-page handwritten letter sent to a board of pharmacy investigating a prescription error that led to the death of an elderly woman patient of a chain pharmacy. The pharmacist who wrote the letter had filled the woman's prescription for a diuretic with digoxin instead. While there was a medical question of whether that mistake had caused the death, it probably was a factor. A reading of the pharmacist's entire letter left little doubt as to its meaning: "It wasn't my fault, it was the boss's fault." The patient's family later introduced this letter into the civil trial against the pharmacy chain.

28.4.4 Systems Failure of Medication Reconciliation Results in Brain Damaged Patient and $20.5 Million Verdict

A middle-aged woman was screened and pre-admitted for thyroidectomy surgery. As part of the pre-admission orders, methylene blue dye was ordered, which is commonly used to help the surgeon visualize the thyroid and parathyroid gland structures.[21] A home medication history included venlafaxine (Effexor—Pfizer). The hospital pharmacy prepared an IV methylene blue (500 mg) in 500 ml NS infusion, which was administered 1 hour before surgery. Following surgery, the patient did not wake up and experienced blood pressure swings and tonic-clonic seizures. She was admitted to the ICU. A diagnosis of serotonin syndrome (SS) was identified, most likely caused by the interaction of methylene blue (MB) and venlafaxine. Coma was induced and maintained for three weeks. The comatose patient was transferred to a University Hospital where she did recover but with significant neurological deficits (brain damage). She did return to work three months later but at a much lower function and retired early due to cognitive problems.

The injured patient sued the surgeon and the hospital for administering the dangerous combination of MB and venlafaxine. Medication reconciliation was performed on admission. The pharmacist testified that they did not usually consider home medications, nor did the hospital and pharmacy software screen home meds against new medication orders, and so it was not automatically done. The pharmacist testified that they received the MB orders a few times a year, although a pre-printed order set was used. The pharmacist also testified that because she was not familiar with MB, she checked the package insert and found no warnings about interactions between venlafaxine and MB. She did not, however, check the venlafaxine package insert, which contraindicates the MB combination, or any external drug interaction software such as Drugs.com.[22] The website www.drugs.com identifies the combination interaction risk as follows:

> *Major methylene blue venlafaxine*
> *Applies to: methylene blue, venlafaxine*
> **CONTRAINDICATED**: Co-administration of methylene blue with serotonergic agents may potentiate the risk of serotonin syndrome, which is a rare but serious and potentially fatal condition thought to result from hyperstimulation of brainstem 5-HT1A and 5-HT2A receptors.

A search and analyses of the United States Food and Drug Administration MedWatch database were conducted for methylene blue and interaction medications and adverse events.[23] Serotonin syndrome is the most commonly reported adverse reaction when methylene blue is reported as a suspect or interacting medication in an adverse event case. Specifically, 43.7% of cases that report methylene blue also report serotonin syndrome (199 out of 455 cases). One of the authors (JTOD) provided an affidavit in the case, critical of the pharmacist and the hospital for the following:

1. Failure to detect and warn about the interaction between venlafaxine and methylene blue.
2. Failing to have a computer system or other reliable and functioning system in place which screened the September 10, 2013 order for methylene blue for the patient against her known home medications, including venlafaxine, for potential harmful interactions.
3. Failure to have in place policies and procedures directing the pharmacists and assistants to confirm that the order for methylene blue was screened against her known home medications, including venlafaxine, for potential harmful interactions.

Both the surgeon and the anesthesiologist testified that they relied on the pharmacist to screen for drug interactions. Hospital policy and procedure described a screening duty, as do ASHP Practice Guidelines. Interestingly, the pharmacist also agreed with the duty to screen for drug interactions—but blamed the oversight and thus life-threatening interaction on the absence of the warning in the MB package insert. After learning this testimony, attorneys for the injured patient sued Akorn, the manufacturer of methylene blue injection that was used in the case. Akorn admitted knowledge of the interaction. However, Akorn claimed that since MB was a grandfathered drug, not the subject of an NDA, they were not able to include the interaction warning about serotonin syndrome with SSRIs. A different manufacturer of MB, American Regent, provided the warning in their package insert for the product, even before they were awarded an NDA for MB.

The hospital (pharmacy/ist) and the surgeon were dismissed from the case before the trial. A trial was conducted with Akorn as the only defendant. Akorn maintained its position that they could not warn and blamed the pharmacist for not warning the surgeon and avoiding the drug interaction injury. An FDA labeling expert testified that Akorn had a duty to include the warning and could have done so. The Jury found Akorn liable, negligent, considered their behavior egregious for not providing a warning of the drug interaction risk, and awarded compensatory and punitive damages to the injured patient, totaling $20.5 million dollars. After the trial, the jury was polled—they attributed no fault to the pharmacist or the surgeon.

Incidentally, after the incident, the pharmacy learned that their software had a feature to screen home medications with active orders—they just had not activated it. After the injury, home medication screening was included in software-driven drug interaction screening.

28.4.5 Failure To Follow Rules and Regulations/Use of Regulations and Standards of Practice to Prosecute or Defend Cases Against Pharmacists

CASE REPORT

Allegation of miscommunication and failure to have adequate drugs on hand for the treatment of patient.

ASSIGNMENT

Review the records and testimony and reports and provide opinion(s) on whether or not the defendant hospital pharmacy/pharmacists complied with the standard of care of reasonable and prudent hospital pharmacists.

FACTS OF THE CASE

The plaintiff, a hemophiliac who underwent planned outpatient hemorrhoid surgery, developed post-operative bleeding and required re-hospitalization and rehab care.

Allegations of Deviations from Pharmacy Standards of Care

1. Failure to stock adequate supplies of Factor VIII
2. Failure to communicate with prescribers and follow up and execute orders
3. Failure to document all patient interactions in the hospital record ("chart")

OPINIONS

All my opinions are expressed with reasonable pharmaceutical certainty.

1. Defendant hospital pharmacy/pharmacists complied with standards of care of reasonable and prudent hospital pharmacists.
2. Defendant hospital pharmacy/pharmacists complied with the Positions and Guidance Documents in *ASHP Best Practices*.
3. Nothing defendant hospital pharmacy/pharmacists did or did not do contributed to or caused Mr. Plaintiff's post-operative bleeding.

Rebuttal of Plaintiff's Pharmacy Expert

The plaintiff's pharmacist expert submitted a 28-page report, summarizing testimony, reciting facts and data, and expressing opinions on departures from the standard of care (SOC) and recklessness by pharmacists at the defendant hospital, specifically the Director of Pharmacy.

In my rebuttal report, I will excerpt and *emphasize* opinion statements (including some bases for opinions) and then agree, rebut, comment, and affirmatively state my opinion(s) and bases for rebuttal opinions.

Plaintiff Pharmacist Expert Opinion on Documentation in Chart

"As a pharmacist this is also very concerning that care, treatment, and interactions with patients such as Mr. Plaintiff are happening that are not being documented in the chart. This is concerning because when others would review Mr. Plaintiff's chart at a later point this interaction with Mr. Plaintiff would not be documented and would not know what was done or not with Mr. Plaintiff. Based on my experience, I would consider this an immense deviation from the acceptable standard as a Pharmacist as well as reckless to not have documented this/these interaction(s)."

Rebuttal: The Director of Pharmacy's (DOP) testimony describes her inquiry, follow-up, and reasons why the interaction with Mr. Plaintiff, and similar *supply* interactions, were not and are not documented in the patient's chart. The defendant hospital pharmacy P&P, DOP's testimony, and actions comply with the *ASHP Best Practices* (2012–13). No chart documentation was necessary; the circumstances and actions (or lack thereof) by the DOP do not violate any SOC and are certainly not reckless. No harm did, could, or would come to the Plaintiff by not documenting an interaction identifying that an order was entered for the Plaintiff to use his own Advate. The attending physician, residents, nurses all knew that that was the case, as the hematologist's order was documented on the chart. Further, at no time did the Plaintiff miss any dose of or treatment with Factor VIII; Factor VIII was always administered as ordered, either from the hospital's supply (morning of June 9) or with the patient's Advate (other administrations noted in the records).

Effective Communication/Coordination of Care; Need for Factor VIII

"For certain, there is a lack of effective communication/coordination of care between the hematologist, Hematology and Oncology and Associates, and the hospital. This lack of effective communication/coordination of care directly led to the lack of Factor available for the Plaintiff when he presented to the Hospital and the transfer of the Plaintiff to another Medical Center was a severe deviation from the acceptable practice, and clearly is reckless."

Rebuttal: There was no "lack of Factor available for the Plaintiff." There is no evidence of any notification of the defendant hospital pharmacy; in fact, the Director of Pharmacy, in addition to denying such notification, had it been received, has testified that adequate supplies of additional Factor could have been obtained through overnight ordering or borrowing from local hospitals. The defendant hospital pharmacy P&Ps describe this routine supply/inventory process, which also complies with the *ASHP Best Practices*. Factor VIII was available, either by using the Plaintiff's Advate, or using the hospital's equivalent source of Factor VIII. No doses of Factor VIII were missed; Factor VIII was always available.

Plaintiff Pharmacist Expert Opinion: Failure to Transfer

"Regardless, there is a lack of effective communication/coordination of care between the Hematologist, Hematology and Oncology and Associates, and defendant hospital and the Pharmacy. This led to the lack of Factor available for the Plaintiff when her **[sic]** presented to defendant hospital bleeding, the transfer of the Plaintiff to another Medical Center etc. All these actions and inactions by the Pharmacy and its staff were a severe deviation from the acceptable practice, and reckless."

Rebuttal: There was no "lack of Factor available for the Plaintiff." There is no evidence that the defendant hospital pharmacy was notified in advance of Mr. Plaintiff's planned surgery. The Plaintiff signed himself out of the ER against medical advice on June 8, 2013, stating that he preferred to be treated at Transfer. Mr. Plaintiff told a resident in the ER that the defendant hospital pharmacy did not have (*his*) Factor VIII. In actuality, defendant hospital did not have Advate, Plaintiff's favored brand of Factor; however, defendant hospital did indeed have an appropriate substitute Factor VIII, which was administered on the morning of June 9, 2013, prior to his transfer to another facility. The resident has testified that he called the pharmacy and claims that he was told there was no Factor. Inventory records document the presence of Factor. If a call had been received, action would have been taken to initiate purchase or borrowing of the product by a supervisor or Director of Pharmacy. Both Nurses testified that they would have contacted the pharmacy if a resident had claimed none was available, as residents who are new to the system do not always know the procedures and processes in place. It is clear that the pharmacy had Factor VIII, as it was administered to the patient prior to his transfer to Transfer. The transfer was made to Transfer because the Plaintiff expressed his desire to continue his care there and was not impacted by anything the pharmacy did or did not do. There is no "severe deviation from the acceptable practice, and reckless."

The lack of Factor for Mr. Plaintiff led to a transfer to Transfer via life-flight

"IF defendant hospital Pharmacy was notified of the need for adequate amounts of Factor for Mr. Plaintiff, and failed to order such, I would consider this a severe deviation form [sic] the acceptable practice and reckless. **If** the Pharmacy director was not notified by Hematologist (Hem/Onc), I would defer to a Hematologist regarding this as outlined more fully in in their opinions" (**emphasis added**).

Rebuttal: Plaintiff Pharmacist Expert's opinion is speculative, stated conditionally ("**if**"... "then") and based upon unsupported conjecture. The hematologist did not send a letter to the defendant hospital pharmacy. No one called the defendant hospital pharmacy. No other experts expressed opinions that the defendant hospital pharmacy failed to act on any (undocumented) notice to the defendant hospital pharmacy. Nevertheless, the defendant hospital pharmacy had Factor on hand (some was administered to the Plaintiff). If notified, they would (as they did) advise that Advate was not their contract Factor VIII, supplies would have been ordered (as they were), and if commercial/distributor sources were not timely, borrowing Factor from another hospital would all comply with the SOC. There is certainly no negligent, let alone reckless practice exhibited.

Factor VIII ordering and inventory management at defendant hospital pharmacy

"All of the above are very concerning for several reasons. It seems defendant hospital through its Corporate Designee has answers that change depending on what is most beneficial to escape from any liability from this incident. From the testimony of Director of Pharmacy, it is not clear by even the hospital's own staff of any policies and procedures regarding this. Second, specific to the Plaintiff, it is further unclear **if** the hospital was notified of the Plaintiff's need for Factor prior to his surgery by the hematologist and Hematology and Oncology Associates, or **if** the hospital was notified, it appears that the hospital did not attempt to keep any Factor separate for the Plaintiff despite prior notice. As a pharmacist, I would consider all of this a severe deviation from the acceptable standard and reckless." (**emphasis** added)

Rebuttal: A series of speculative and unsupported suppositions (**If**s) do not form the bases for a deviation from a pharmacist's standard of care. There is no evidence that the defendant hospital pharmacy was notified in advance of the June 6 surgery. There was no departure from the standard of care.

Record Keeping

"The level of difficulty the hospital has in simply answering whether the Pharmacy had Factor when the plaintiff presented is concerning. A simple review of the records if kept in order would answer this question. This a severe deviation from the acceptable practice to not have this information accurately documented, or kept on record, and reckless. "

Rebuttal: Record keeping is a business practice, not a standard of care. The inquiry, as Plaintiff Pharmacist Expert points out, was held six years after an incident, and, on further investigation, the Director of Pharmacy demonstrated both that Factor was on hand (and it was given to the Plaintiff on June 9) and that, when ordered, it was replaced. Clearly, pharmacists have a basic responsibility to control medications in a hospital. The defendant hospital pharmacists did so; their P&Ps demonstrated how, and their execution of this basic inventory management task comports with the *ASHP Best Practices*.

Further opinion on lack of documentation

"I would again reiterate my prior opinions regarding the lack of documentation within the plaintiff's records by the Pharmacy as should have been done, and lack of communication even within the Hospital by the pharmacy and physician, both of which as a Pharmacist I consider a severe deviation from the acceptable practice and reckless."

Rebuttal: The Director of Pharmacy's testimony describes her inquiry, follow-up, and reasons why the interaction with the plaintiff and similar supply interaction were not and are not documented in the patient's chart. The defendant hospital Pharmacy P&P, Director of Pharmacy's testimony, and actions comply with the *ASHP Best Practices* (2012–13). No chart documentation was necessary; the circumstances and actions (or lack thereof) by the Director of Pharmacy do not violate any standard of care and are certainly not reckless. No harm did, could, or would come to Mr. Plaintiff by the pharmacy for not documenting an interaction identifying that an order was entered for the plaintiff to use his own Advate. The attending physician, residents, and nurses all knew that that was the case as the hematologist's order was documented in the chart. Further, at no time did the plaintiff miss any dose of or treatment with Factor VIII; Factor VIII was always administered as ordered, either from the hospital's supply (morning of June 9) or with the patient's Advate (other administrations noted in the records).

Difficulty to Confirm Inventory level

"It is concerning how difficult it is for the Hospital to confirm whether or not it had adequate Factor, or even how much Factor, the Hospital had on the date(s) the Plaintiff presented. To not be able to properly document how much Factor was available when Mr. Plaintiff presented is a severe deviation from the acceptable standard as it led to much of the confusion discussed within this report by the hospital pharmacy, including confusion with medical professionals at the hospital attempting to treat the Plaintiff when he presented in the ER/ICU. This lack of effective communication/coordination led to the plaintiff bleeding, being transported and cared for at another hospital. The delay in such, and is shown through the records, when even the Director of Pharmacy cannot give a simple answer **if** there was enough Factor available for the Plaintiff when he presented. I would consider all of this a severe deviation from the acceptable standard and beyond reckless."

Rebuttal: This opinion is a re-hash of previous opinions regarding failure to document how much inventory was on hand and alleged confusion with (various) medical professionals. Previous rebuttal opinions have addressed this communication issue. However, in this opinion, Plaintiff Pharmacist Expert states (for the first and only time): "This lack of effective communication/coordination led to Mr. Plaintiff bleeding."

This is an opinion that has no basis and is simply wrong. Plaintiff Pharmacist Expert is not qualified to express a medical opinion as to the cause of bleeding. The Plaintiff had a congenital blood clotting disorder and had recently had a surgery. Indeed, no physician expert has testified that Plaintiff ever missed any doses of Factor, his own or the hospital's Factor, or that any missed doses caused his bleeding. The medical record establishes that the Plaintiff received all recommended dosages prescribed by the hematologist. The Plaintiff was bleeding on presentation to the ER, not as a result of a lack of Factor in the ER. Earlier rebuttal and the medical record provide evidence that Factor was available and administered.

Proper drug inventory in the hospital

"**If** the Hospital did have notice that Mr. Plaintiff would be needing Factor pre and post-surgery, then this "loan" process described is a severe deviation from the acceptable standard, as, but not limited to, doing this when Mr. Plaintiff was in need of factor would already be too late, cause delays in his ability to obtain Factor, and reckless in light of prior notice of needing Factor." (**emphasis** added)

Rebuttal: Director of Pharmacy had Factor in inventory. Diligent and cost-conscious inventory control is essential, especially with high cost and short shelf-life biologics like Factor. Plaintiff Pharmacist Expert's opinion is speculative and predicated on an unsubstantiated supposition. There is no evidence that the HOSPITAL or its pharmacy had been provided notice, and even without notice, with a basic minimum inventory (which they had), as well as the routine practice of borrowing and 24-hour ordering, the Plaintiff's needs were met.

(IF) Failure to follow orders

"**If**-Hospital or its Pharmacy or staff disregarded and/or did not follow the orders the Hematologist and Hematology and Oncology Associates of NEPA, this action and inaction would be a severe deviation from the acceptable standard of care, and reckless in light of the prior notice by the hematologist at Transfer."

Rebuttal: This is another speculative opinion predicated upon unsubstantiated supposition. The Hematologist placed an order in the chart which was followed. There is no testimony by the Hematologist or any other physician that an order was ignored by the pharmacy.

Case Conclusion

All of the opinions expressed by Plaintiff Pharmacist Expert which start with the word "**If**" are speculative, conditional, and based upon unsupported conjecture. Director of Pharmacy's testimony and exhibits produced support hospital pharmacy compliance with standard of care. At all times, the pharmacy had an appropriate Factor product and at all times Mr. Plaintiff received Factor in accordance with the orders of the hematologist. If the ER resident misunderstood and transferred the patient, that is not a deviation by the pharmacist. If a call was made by an ER physician to a pharmacist on duty, that pharmacist, even if Advate was requested, would have no reason to deny availability, as everyone in this case, including Plaintiff Pharmacist Expert, agrees that the generic Factor VIII (recombinant) is therapeutically equivalent to Advate. Any pharmacist practicing at the hospital would know the Policy on contract brands/generic-therapeutic equivalence, would have advised the resident of that policy, and dispensed the (proven available) Factor to the ER. The medical record clearly shows that the hospital pharmacy dispensed Factor VIII which was administered to Mr. Plaintiff prior to his transfer to the Medical Center.

Finally, Plaintiff Pharmacist Expert cites no authorities, references, Pharmacy Practice Acts, Societies, etc., supporting his opinions on documentation, communication, inventory control, and pharmacy order execution. He opines that hospital pharmacy violated standards of care and was reckless. Had he compared the Hospital P&Ps with the *ASHP Best Practices*, as well as the Director of Pharmacy's testimony, he would see that the hospital pharmacists complied with the *ASHP Best Practices*.

The hospital pharmacy, its Director of Pharmacy, pharmacists, and support staff complied with the standard of care of reasonable and prudent hospital pharmacists. Nothing they did or did not do increased the Plaintiff's risk of post-operative bleeding or the actual bleeding itself.

CASE RESOLUTION

The case was tried to a jury in May 2021, resulting in a not-guilty verdict in favor of the hospital and the defendant hematologist.

28.4.6 Controlled Substances Violations by Pharmacists

28.4.6.1 Criminal and Civil Charges against Pharmacies

A press release by the United States Attorney in Florida (Contact: Public Information Officer May 13, 2015, Number: 954-660-4602) reported that the "United States Reached $22 Million Settlement Agreement with CVS for Unlawful Distribution of Controlled Substances." CVS Health agreed to pay $22 million to resolve allegations that two of its retail stores located in Sanford, Florida, distributed controlled substances based on prescriptions that had not been issued for legitimate medical purposes by a healthcare provider acting in the usual course of professional practice. CVS acknowledged that its retail pharmacies had a responsibility to dispense only those prescriptions that were issued on the basis of legitimate medical need. CVS further acknowledged that certain of its retail stores dispensed certain controlled substances in a manner not fully consistent with their compliance obligations under the Controlled Substances Act (CSA) and the related regulations.

The CSA authorizes the United States to seek civil penalties for a pharmacy's failure to fulfill its corresponding responsibility to dispense only those prescriptions that have been issued for a legitimate medical purpose by a healthcare provider acting in the usual course of professional practice. Knowingly filling an illegitimate prescription subjects a pharmacy to civil penalties under the CSA. This settlement caps an investigation that began as part of DEA's crackdown on pill mills in Florida. Prescription drug addicts were travelling to Florida, known as the nation's epicenter for the illegal distribution of prescription drugs, for access to physicians who were prescribing pain medication without regard to medical need and to pharmacies that were filling the prescriptions despite red flags that they were illegitimate. The investigation led to DEA's execution of administrative inspection warrants at two CVS stores in Sanford. As a result, the DEA registrations of both stores were revoked in June 2012.

Frequent litigation results from drug abusers seeking illegal prescriptions. In these circumstances, when pharmacists violate the Good Faith requirement of the CSA and provide the prescription drugs without a legitimate medical purpose, it can be quite challenging to defend that pharmacist in a malpractice claim against another pharmacist who alleges the defendant pharmacist departed from the standard of care, and that deviation harmed or killed the patient.

CASE REPORT

PHARMACIST VIOLATION OF CONTROLLED SUBSTANCES ACT

A patient of a national pharmacy company, as a motorist, was involved in two collisions on the same day; the second resulted in another motorist's death. After the collision, the negligent driver's blood was tested and found positive for alprazolam, morphine, meprobamate, trazodone, carisoprodol, doxylamine, and other substances. The alprazolam was at a very high level (120 ng/ml). He was prosecuted for DUI Homicide and convicted and is imprisoned at a Florida prison.

Prior to the accident, the motorist and his mother had numerous prescriptions filled at a pharmacy in Indiana. Both were prescribed alprazolam by a Florida physician while they were living in Indiana. The mother was also seeing Indiana doctors who prescribed alprazolam and other medicines for her. Examination of defendant pharmacy's prescription records and pharmacy patient's Bank of America (BofA) records shows that the motorist wrote a check for both his and his mother's alprazolam, which he paid for with a single check. He twice stated falsely that it was for a "co-pay." (His portion was not.) An examination of BofA records indicate that the motorist picked up all of these prescriptions—nine (9) in all.

The defendant pharmacy expert opined that:

1. The pharmacists complied with the standard of care "through the correct process of transferring and filling of prescriptions from the state of Florida to the state of Indiana", "when evaluating the transfer of controlled substances from . . . Florida to . . . Indiana . . . by utilizing professional judgment of the pharmacist for the purpose of eliminating abuse, misuse and diversion."
2. The pharmacists "utilizing(ed) professional judgment of the purpose of eliminating, abuse, misuse and diversion, met the corresponding responsibility of a pharmacist."
3. The pharmacy and associated staff met the standard of care, by not discriminating the filling of prescriptions based on appearance, communications, or means of payment. Further, the pharmacy and associated staff met the standard of care by not creating any HIPAA violations.
4. Responsibilities of pharmacist(s) to help curve (sic) the opioid crises within the United States has developed over a long period of time. The tools, rules, and laws from 2011 to 2018 are vastly different. The interpretation of such information must consider exclusively the time of the incident (2011) not of present day, and any application otherwise is negligent.

OPINIONS

My opinions are expressed with reasonable pharmaceutical certainty.

1. There is no evidence or identified materials reviewed by the defense pharmacy expert to conclude that the pharmacist "utilizing(ed) professional judgment of the purpose of eliminating, abuse, misuse and diversion, met the corresponding responsibility of a pharmacist." No depositions of the pharmacists have been taken, nor has the expert spoken with any Kroger pharmacist.
2. Indiana was identified as a State with a high substance abuse/diversion problem and implemented a prescription drug monitoring program as early as 2003.[24] While the opioid crisis worsened after 2012, it was an acute problem in 2010, and pharmacists' diligence and standard of care for identifying and preventing substance and diversion were substantially the same in 2011 as in 2018.
3. DEA "Red Flags" for identifying substance abuse existed prior to 2010 and in fact is mirrored in the pharmacy SOPs provided as Answers to Discovery.[25]
4. Based on the DEA and discovery records, several "red flags" were present to alert pharmacists to problems of controlled substance abuse with the motorist's alprazolam prescriptions, including the following:
   a. Distance to prescribing doctor (Indiana to Florida)
   b. Multiple family members receiving same controlled substance
   c. Multiple doctors writing prescriptions for patients, including Controlled Substances
   d. Motorist picking up the same prescription drug for himself and his elderly mother
   e. Odd writing on checks
   f. Each had their own insurer
5. Pharmacy Discovery is devoid of any warnings or alerts from the motorist and his mother's pharmacy (internal) records. "Screen shots" documenting interactions and warnings created by combinations of

the Florida doctor's prescriptions used with Indiana doctors' prescriptions contemporaneous use of these medications. Such interaction warnings should have occurred, and documentation of the warning and any pharmacist(s)' override would be documented in the record.

6. Pharmacy Discovery and Answers deny any high-dose alert warnings were part of the pharmacy software system. "High dose" alerts are common for the industry, and it is quite surprising that this pharmacy, a company with thousands of pharmacies, has no such alert/safety built into their screening software. Assuming that no such alert exists, notwithstanding, the pharmacists must have recognized that the daily dose of alprazolam prescribed for the motorist exceeded the maximum.

Anxiety Disorders and Transient Symptoms of Anxiety

Treatment for patients with anxiety should be initiated with an alprazolam dose of 0.25 to 0.5 mg given three times daily. The dose may be increased to achieve a maximum therapeutic effect, at intervals of three to four days, to a maximum daily dose of four mg, given in divided doses. The lowest possible effective dose should be employed, and the need for continued treatment reassessed frequently. The risk of dependence may increase with dose and duration of treatment.

Pharmacists are concerned and predictably warn patients about driving while initiating benzodiazepine drugs, when using at a new dose, or when using with another CNS depressant (i.e., opioid). Indeed, two of the most common warning labels (and verbal cautions) by pharmacists to patients are "may cause drowsiness: use caution when driving" or "do not drive or use alcohol when using this medication." Pharmacists know the significant risk of patients using CNS depressants and driving.

The alprazolam present in the motorist's blood after the accident was consistent with the excess amounts that bank and pharmacy records show he obtained and were sufficient to cause significant impairment.

Summary and Conclusion

I agree with the defense pharmacy expert's simplistic opinion that the Controlled Substance transfer process was according to regulations but strongly disagree that the pharmacists did not violate the standard of care. In my opinion, the pharmacists failed to exercise diligence and their "corresponding responsibility" with the Xanax (and other) prescriptions for the motorist and his mother.

CASE REPORT

EXCESSIVE DISPENSING OF CONTROLLED SUBSTANCES; DEATH OF PATIENT

The prescribing physician in this case was a notorious over-prescriber of controlled substances without legitimate medical need. The U.S. Department of Justice, Drug Enforcement Administration investigated the physician's irregular, excessive, and suspicious prescriptions for non-legitimate medical purposes of Schedule II and Schedule III medications that were being filled at the defendant Pharmacy Company by various individuals, including the Patient.

From my review of these materials, I have concluded on the basis of my education, training, and experience that there is a reasonable and meritorious cause for filing this action against the defendant, Pharmacy Co., concerning its pharmacy practice in filling and dispensing medications, namely schedule II narcotics, from putative prescriptions from Prescribing Physician, for reasons more fully set forth in this report.

By way of an abbreviated synopsis, the materials show a pattern and practice by the Prescribing physician for a period of years of writing prescriptions for schedule II and schedule III medications that were irregular and suspicious and should have been known by Pharmacy Co. to have been for non-legitimate medical purposes, including those specifically to the patient. The pharmacy would have known that prescribing physician was being investigated by the U.S. Department of Justice, Drug Enforcement Agency for his irregular, excessive, and non-legitimate schedule II and III prescriptions. A pharmacist employed by the pharmacy gave a statement to investigators documenting the prescribing physician's suspicious and unusual prescriptions of these addictive/habit-forming narcotics and indicated that the Prescribing Physician was likely part of a drug ring.

The materials further disclose that the prescribing physician wrote an unusual frequent amount of schedule II and schedule III prescriptions to an individual named patient, which were in high combined dosages/quantities beyond those normally prescribed. The Pharmacy Company would have had this data known to its pharmacists through its computer Prescription Profile for the patient.

The highly addictive medications were prescribed in such amounts and circumstances that pharmacy company knew or at least reasonably should have known were being used for non-legitimate medical purposes, including the illicit drug trade. Indeed, the DEA investigation file noted that several pharmacies other than Pharmacy in the local areas correctly refused to fill and dispense Schedule II and Schedule III controlled substances, pursuant to prescriptions from the prescribing physician, due to the illegitimacy and irregularities of those prescriptions, including potential criminal conduct involving drug trade and abuse.

The records provided indicated that the patient, on numerous occasions, had sold her prescriptions to others, including to a "Divertor." The records indicated that Divertor would then take the prescription(s) to the defendant pharmacy to have it filled, dispensed, and take possession of the medication even though the prescription was not written for him. The records indicated that the patient was on public assistance; yet the Divertor would pay cash for the prescription. This is another indicator to Pharmacy that the prescription was not for legitimate medical purposes and used for invalid/illegal purposes.

The records indicate that Divertor paid the patient for her prescription from the prescribing physician for yet additional prescriptions for Schedule II narcotics—Oxycontin and Duragesic. The Divertor then took that prescription to the defendant pharmacy and had that prescription filled by its pharmacists. The pharmacy improperly gave Mr. Divertor these medications for a cash payment. The divertor then took these medications to his home where he provided and shared some of the Oxycontin with another man—the decedent. The decedent then suffered a cardiac arrest as result of the acute toxicity of the Oxycontin.

It is my opinion, to a reasonable degree of pharmacy certainty, that it was contrary to accepted pharmacy customs; practices; and the Illinois Controlled Substance Act, Codes and Federal Regulations for the pharmacy through its pharmacists to have filled and dispensed the prescribing physician's prescriptions to another person for 90 tablets of 40 mg Oxycontin and 10 Duragesic (Fentanyl) 100 mcg/hour patches to a divertor for a cash payment. I have formulated opinions that pharmacy company deviated from the standard of care in this matter.

CASE REPORT

PHARMACIST DUTY/CONTROLLED SUBSTANCES

This is a recent New Mexico Appellate Court opinion that affirms the pharmacists' duties with respect to Controlled Substances' dispensing, Good Faith, and Standard of Care. Relevant sections are excerpted and included here for the reader's edification.

OAKEY ESTATE OF LUCERO v. MAY MAPLE PHARMACY INC
Court of Appeals of New Mexico.
Kathleen M. OAKEY, Personal Representative of the ESTATE OF Tawana LUCERO, deceased, Plaintiff-Appellant, v. MAY MAPLE PHARMACY, INC., Defendant-Appellee.
NO. 34,914
Decided: April 13, 2017

This appeal rises from a lawsuit brought by the personal representative of the estate of Tawana Lucero, who died at the age of 19 from an overdose of physician-prescribed medications, including opioids classified under federal and state law as Schedule II controlled substances because of their high potential for abuse and addiction. As relevant here, the personal representative (Plaintiff) asserts claims of negligence and negligence per se against May Maple Pharmacy, Inc. (the pharmacy). The pharmacy moved for summary judgment, contending that it was entitled to judgment as a matter of law because "a pharmacist's standard of care is to dispense appropriately prescribed medications to a patient in accordance with a proper medical doctor's prescription[,]" and the pharmacy met that standard in filling the prescriptions at issue. The district court entered an order granting the motion, dismissing all claims against the Pharmacy with prejudice, and awarding costs to the pharmacy. We reverse.

Dr. John Tyson of Doctor On Call, LLC, a medical clinic focusing on pain management, wrote prescriptions for Oxycodone, Oxycontin, and Alprazolam to treat Lucero's pain and anxiety, which the Pharmacy dispensed to

Lucero from May 28, 2009 through November 16, 2009. Oxycodone was prescribed in 5 mg dosages, and Oxycontin was prescribed in dosages between 20 mg and 80 mg. The Pharmacy sometimes dispensed medication to Lucero "early," i.e., prior to the time the previously prescribed amount should have lasted if taken as directed.

The Pharmacy does not dispute Plaintiff's interpretation of the record as showing that the Pharmacy filled Oxycontin prescriptions for Lucero between 2 and 23 days "early" on at least 7 occasions between May 28, 2009 and September 21, 2009. At least some of these prescriptions contained the words "OK to fill early" or a similar indication that the prescription could be filled "early." On a few occasions, Lucero paid a substantial amount of cash to purchase Oxycontin from the Pharmacy and at least once paid $1,107 for 90 Oxycontin 80 mg pills in September 2009. An October 2009 "addendum" note by Doctor on Call's Dr. Maron with the subject "Rx FRAUD?" indicates receipt of a call from an unidentified pharmacist reporting that Lucero had "presented to pharmacy for early refill" and had offered to pay over $1,000 cash, despite that she would have received the medication free via Medicaid three days later.

Plaintiff initially sued Dr. Tyson and Doctor On Call, asserting claims for malpractice, negligence, and wrongful death (among others), based on allegations that Dr. Tyson had prescribed excessive amounts of dangerous medications to Lucero. A subsequent amended complaint also asserted claims against the Pharmacy, as follows: (1) negligence, based on allegations that the Pharmacy breached its "duty of care to apply the knowledge ordinarily used by reasonably well-qualified pharmacists" by dispensing "excessive quantities of Schedule II or other dangerous drugs" to Lucero; and (2) negligence per se, based on allegations that the Pharmacy, by dispensing "excessive quantities of medications" to Lucero, "departed from the standard of care, knowledge, and skill of a reasonably trained pharmacist" and breached regulatory duties to "properly and reasonably dispense controlled medications" mandated by 16.19.20.41(A) NMAC and 16.19.4.16 NMAC.

The Pharmacy moved for summary judgment, dismissal with prejudice, and costs, based on the argument that

> [A] pharmacist who accurately fills prescription medication as prescribed by the doctor has no liability exposure to one who is injured by the drugs on claims the amounts were excessive, unless the pharmacist has some reason to know the specific customer will be harmed [,]

and that the Pharmacy "accurately dispensed what Lucero's doctors prescribed and otherwise met all applicable standards of care." The Pharmacy's motion discussed no standard other than its proffered clerical accuracy standard, for which it relied on case law from other jurisdictions. The motion made no mention of any statutes or regulations applicable to pharmacy practice or controlled substances and no argument concerning Plaintiff's claim of negligence per se, nor did the Pharmacy's reply brief,[3] although Plaintiff addressed these points in opposing the motion. The Plaintiff argued that genuine issues of material fact precluded summary judgment because the parties' experts gave contrary opinions concerning the conduct required of a retail pharmacist in these circumstances, pursuant to statutes, regulations, and public policy, and whether the Pharmacy's conduct deviated from the standard of care.

The parties' expert affidavits reflect differing opinions concerning the standard of care for retail pharmacists dispensing Schedule II drugs and whether the Pharmacy's conduct met that standard. The Pharmacy's expert, Dr. Matthew C. Lee, stated that "[t]he appropriate standard of care for a retail pharmacist is that he or she has a duty to dispense appropriately prescribed medications to a patient" and that if the pharmacist "does not dispense medication in accordance with the medical doctor's prescription, that pharmacist risks interfering with the doctor/patient relationship and may be inappropriately practicing medicine without a license." According to Dr. Lee, there were instances in this case "where the customer presented with an early refill," but Dr. Tyson had approved "those early refills for reasons medically indicated by the doctor [,]" and physician-approved "early refills" are valid and should be filled by the pharmacist.

Dr. Lee stated that

> [I]f the retail pharmacist does find discrepancies in either the prescriptions ordered or in fact has evidence of drug abuse, the pharmacist should call the prescribing physician to ensure that the prescriptions presented are in fact what the physician intended to order [,]

noting but not identifying "certain indications in the record" that the Pharmacy "did consult with personnel at Doctor[]on[]Call[.]" Dr. Lee added,

> [T]here is nothing unusual or inappropriate about either the level or amount of narcotic medication prescribed which should have led any retail pharmacist to question or refuse to dispense the prescription. Although the dosages are considered high, specifically for Oxycontin, there is nothing unusual in this dosage level as prescribed for patients with chronic pain. In other words, all prescriptions of Dr. Tyson and filled at the May Maple Pharmacy are valid and legitimate."

Dr. Lee's affidavit did not explain the basis for his opinions or identify any source materials supporting them, other than his background in pharmacy and his review of certain case documents, including prescriptions, medical records, and deposition transcripts of the medical examiner and a state police officer. Although he cited no authorities—legal or professional—Dr. Lee said he "found no violation of any federal or New Mexico statutory or regulatory requirements dealing with the practice of pharmacy [,]" and concluded without further explanation that the Pharmacy "accurately filled all prescriptions according to the terms and instructions written by Dr. Tyson" and "met all applicable standards of care which apply to the practice of retail pharmacy."

Plaintiff's expert, Dr. James T. O'Donnell, relied not only on his background in pharmacy and review of record materials but also on his review of other materials, including the Standards of Practice for the Profession of Pharmacy, the New Mexico Pharmacy Practice Act, provisions of the federal Controlled Substances Act, and materials addressing the responsibilities of pharmacists under the Controlled Substances Act. Dr. O'Donnell disagreed with Dr. Lee's opinions that the prescriptions at issue were facially valid and that the standard of care for retail pharmacists required nothing more of the Pharmacy in these circumstances than that it accurately filled facially valid prescriptions. He said that prescriptions indicating "OK to fill early" were illegal and could not be filled "no matter what the prescriber has written on the prescription" because they were for Schedule II controlled substances, which cannot be "refilled"[5] or authorized as "OK to fill early." According to Dr. O'Donnell, a pharmacist faced with an "early" request to fill a prescription for a Schedule II controlled substance "has a duty to inquire [of] the patient why, and then speak to the physician and get authorization from the physician."

Dr. O'Donnell said that such "early" requests are "evidence of excessive use of the [c]ontrolled [s]ubstance, in excess of the prescribed dose." Excess use "places the patient at risk ([of] death or serious injury), increases abuse, dependence, and addiction, and may be evidence of diversion." A pattern of such "early" requests "is highly suspicious of abuse and[/]or diversion, and would preclude the pharmacist" from filling the prescriptions; to do otherwise would violate requirements of "[g]ood [f]aith, [r]easonable [j]udgment, and [c]orresponding [r]esponsibility" imposed by federal and state law. According to Dr. O'Donnell, provisions of the federal Controlled Substances Act, the New Mexico Pharmacy Act, and their respective implementing regulations "require the pharmacist to consider issues beyond the face legality of the prescription" such as abuse, diversion, and whether the prescription is for a legitimate medical need. He concluded that the Pharmacy breached the "[s]tandard of [c]are of the [p]rofession of [p]harmacy" and violated the New Mexico Pharmacy Practice Act, NMSA 1978, § 61-11-1 (1997); 16.19.20.41 NMAC; and the federal and state Controlled Substances Acts, 21 U.S.C. § 829 (2016); 21 C.F.R. § 1306.04(a) (2017); and NMSA 1978, § 30-31-1 (2005).

The district court's order granting summary judgment contains no analysis but necessarily reflects the court's conclusion that Dr. Lee's affidavit sufficed to satisfy the Pharmacy's burden to establish a prima facie case of entitlement to judgment as a matter of law as to the applicable standard of care, the Pharmacy's compliance with the standard, and the court's rejection of Plaintiff's argument that the differing opinions of the parties' experts demonstrated the existence of a genuine dispute of material fact on those issues. In addition, the district court's dismissal of the Pharmacy "from this suit [] with prejudice" necessarily reflects the dismissal of all claims against the Pharmacy—the negligence claim and the separate claim for negligence per se.

We reverse, based on our conclusions that (1) the Pharmacy's motion did not establish a prima facie case of entitlement to judgment as a matter of law as to the standard of care or the Pharmacy's compliance with the standard; (2) even if the Pharmacy had met that burden, Plaintiff's expert affidavit sufficed to establish a genuine dispute of material fact concerning these material issues; and (3) dismissal of the Pharmacy from the case was improper because the motion did not demonstrate the Pharmacy's entitlement to summary judgment on the separate claim of negligence per se, and there is no indication that the district court even considered that issue.[26]

This case involves a question of first impression in New Mexico: The conduct required of retail pharmacists in filling prescriptions for controlled substances with a significant potential for abuse and addiction, such as Oxycodone and Oxycontin. The few New Mexico negligence cases involving the conduct of pharmacists provide no guidance. See, e.g., Johnson v. Primm, 1964-NMSC-217, ¶¶ 6, 15–16, 74 N.M. 597, 396 P.2d 426 (reversing summary judgment in favor of the pharmacy in a case alleging that the pharmacy failed to exercise due care in selling the plaintiff a drug in excess of the prescribed amount based on consideration of contributory negligence and proximate cause without addressing the standard of care); Wilcox v. Butt's Drug Stores, Inc., 1934-NMSC-060, ¶ 12, 38 N.M. 502, 35 P.2d 978 (affirming judgment against a pharmacy in a case in which the plaintiff sought damages for the death of her dog from a dangerous drug, applying the "controlling" principle that

> [A] druggist who negligently delivers a deleterious drug when a harmless one is called for is responsible to the customer for the consequences, as being guilty of a breach of the duty which the law imposes on him to avoid acts in their nature dangerous to the lives of others (internal quotation marks and citation omitted);

Thompson, 2012-NMCA-014, ¶¶ 19–23 (declining to reach question of a consulting pharmacist's duty to patients of nursing facility).

We recognize the importance of this question, especially in light of the nation's ongoing "opioid crisis," the subject of news reports and commentary almost daily. But the factual record and the law potentially relevant to this determination were not adequately developed below, nor did the district court actually rule on the issue,[7] leaving us with an insufficient basis for appellate review. Accordingly, we reverse and remand for these reasons as well. See Garcia-Montoya, 2001-NMSC-003, ¶ 48 (remanding for district court to consider an issue in the first instance and, if necessary, to develop additional facts); Brown, 1995-NMSC-050, ¶ 15 (stating that summary judgment is inappropriate "when the facts before the court are insufficiently developed or where further factual resolution is essential for determination of the central legal issues involved" (internal quotation marks and citation omitted)); Horner v. Spalitto, 1 S.W.3d 519, 524 (Mo. Ct. App. 1999) (reversing summary judgment where the appellate court did not have "in the record presented sufficient detail to determine whether [the defendant] fulfilled his duty as a pharmacist").

The pharmacy's expert advocates what amounts to a clerical-accuracy standard, requiring only that a retail pharmacist fill a prescription accurately, unless the prescription is facially invalid or the pharmacist has personal knowledge that filling the prescription would harm a specific customer, and contends that the pharmacy met that standard. Plaintiff's expert contends that the pharmacy's proffered standard is insufficient to fulfill the pharmacist's duty of care in the context of prescriptions for Schedule II controlled substances, relying on statutes and regulations as well as facts indicating potential abuse or diversion.

The motion concluded that Plaintiffs did not allege a failure to warn or that the Pharmacy filled prescriptions inaccurately but that "the doctor improperly determined the appropriate drug, quantity, and dosage for Lucero, an error not discovered by [the pharmacy]." Dr. Lee's affidavit "squarely rejected" this allegation, the Pharmacy contended, by opining that the prescriptions were valid and legal and that

> [T]here was nothing on the face of the prescriptions, including the amounts, dosage levels, or quantity dispensed which would indicate to a prudent pharmacist that the customer was being improperly medicated or over prescribed for the condition of chronic pain.

Although Dr. Lee said that he "found no violation of any federal or New Mexico statutory or regulatory requirements dealing with the practice of pharmacy[,]" and that the Pharmacy "met all applicable standards of care which apply to the practice of retail pharmacy[,]" his affidavit cited no statutes, regulations, or other authorities supporting that conclusion or his proffered clerical-accuracy standard.

Among the specific responsibilities of pharmacists imposed by the New Mexico Administrative Code is the mandatory responsibility ("shall") to review the patient's profile and, "[p]rior to dispensing any prescription," to identify issues including "clinical abuse/misuse" and "incorrect drug dosage." 16.19.4.16(D)(1)(a), (e) NMAC.

> Upon recognizing any of the above, a pharmacist, using professional judgment, shall take appropriate steps to avoid or resolve the potential problem[, which] may include requesting and reviewing a controlled substance prescription monitoring [program] report [(PMP)], consulting with the prescriber and counseling the patient.
>
> **16.19.4.16(D)(2) NMAC**

The New Mexico Administrative Code provides additional guidelines and responsibilities applicable to opioid prescriptions, including that "[a] pharmacist shall use professional judgment based on prevailing standards of practice in determining whether to obtain and review a PMP report before dispensing an opioid prescription to that patient," 16.19.4.16(E) NMAC; and, further, "shall request and review a PMP report covering at least a one[-]year time period" if the pharmacist, for example,

> [B]ecomes aware of a person currently exhibiting potential abuse or misuse of opioids (i.e. over-utilization, early refills, multiple prescribers, appears overly sedated or intoxicated upon presenting a prescription for an opioid, or paying cash when the patient has prescription insurance),
>
> **16.19.4.16(E)(1)(a) NMAC**

or the "pharmacist receives an initial prescription for any long-acting opioid formulations," 16.19.4.16(E)(1)(d) NMAC; or the "pharmacist becomes aware of a patient receiving an opioid concurrently with a benzodiazepine [,]" 16.19.4.16(E)(1)(e) NMAC. "Upon recognizing any" of these conditions, "a pharmacist, using professional judgment, shall take appropriate steps to avoid or resolve the potential problem[,]" which "may include consulting with the prescriber and counseling the patient." 16.19.4.16(E)(3) NMAC. In addition,

> [A] pharmacist shall use professional judgment base[d] on prevailing standards of practice, in deciding the frequency of requesting and reviewing further [PMP] reports [e]xcept that PMP reports shall be reviewed a minimum of once every three months during the continuous use of opioids for each established patient.
>
> **16.19.4.16(E)(4) NMAC**

As noted, neither the motion nor Dr. Lee's affidavit mentions any statutes, although Plaintiff's complaint does, in its allegations supporting the claim for negligence per se. It is not for this court to determine a professional standard of conduct for pharmacists in these circumstances. Nevertheless, we conclude that a party cannot establish a professional standard of care as a matter of law with an expert affidavit that fails to account for law applicable to the professional and/or to the particular circumstances in which the professional has acted or failed to act. Spencer, 2013-NMSC-010, ¶¶ 14–19 (holding that the New Mexico Rules of Professional Conduct are relevant to establish the appropriate standard of conduct for attorneys and that the determination of whether or not the defendant attorney conformed to the standard of conduct required by those rules "will depend on the evidence introduced at trial" and concluding that genuine issues of material fact existed concerning whether the defendant attorney failed to exercise reasonable skill and care in his representation of client).

In sum, Dr. Lee's affidavit, which does not address any regulatory requirements applicable to the practice of pharmacy, or to prescriptions for Schedule II drugs, or to prescriptions for opioid medications, is insufficient to satisfy the pharmacy's burden to demonstrate a prima facie case of entitlement to judgment as a matter of law. See Brown, 1995-NMSC-050, ¶¶ 15–16 (reversing the summary judgment because the moving party failed to develop sufficient facts to satisfy "the burden of showing the absence of any genuine issue of material fact, and also that the undisputed facts supported judgment in its favor as a matter of law"). If, on remand, the pharmacy wishes to renew its motion for summary judgment based on the argument that it fulfilled its duty to Lucero because it conformed its conduct to the standard of care required in the circumstances presented here, it must adduce competent evidence that accounts for statutes and regulations relevant to the professional responsibilities of pharmacists filling prescriptions for the controlled substances at issue.

We disagree with the district court's view that Dr. O'Donnell's affidavit failed to show the existence of a genuine dispute of material fact because it did not "take on Dr. Lee." The affidavit leaves much to be desired, but so does Dr. Lee's affidavit. Nevertheless, Dr. O'Donnell's affidavit suffices to establish a genuine dispute about the material issues of the applicable standard of care and the pharmacy's compliance with that standard. See Trujillo, 1984-NMCA-050, ¶ 27 ("Expert testimony from a qualified doctor in the same field, familiar with the circumstances of [the] defendant's practice, the standard of care of physicians, and the testimony of [the] plaintiff, is generally sufficient to raise questions of material fact."); Garcia-Montoya, 2001-NMSC-003, ¶ 7 ("If there is the slightest doubt as to the existence of material factual issues, summary judgment should be denied." (internal quotation marks and citation omitted)); Lasley, 880 P.2d at 1134 (concluding that "[o]n this record, we cannot say as a matter of law that [the pharmacy] did not breach the standard of care for the duty it owed to [the customer]" in light of expert affidavit concerning pharmacist's standard of care); Hooks, 642 N.E.2d at 519 (affirming denial of summary judgment in pharmacy case after recognizing that "[w]hat constitutes due care in a particular case will depend upon the circumstances of that case, and will usually be a question of fact [,]" including such issues as

> [T]he frequency with which the pharmacist filled prescriptions for the customer, any representations made by the customer, the pharmacist's access to historical data about the customer, the manner in which the prescription was tendered to the pharmacists, and the like);
>
> **Dooley, 805 S.W.2d at 386**

(The fact that the pharmacy owes its customer a duty in dispensing prescription drugs is without question. [The defendant] simply argues that the duty to warn of potential drug interactions is not a part of its duty. The plaintiffs here have introduced expert proof disputing this assertion. Therefore, whether the duty to warn of potential drug interaction is included within the pharmacist's duty to his customer is a disputed issue of fact preventing the granting of summary judgment).

We hold that the dismissal of the Pharmacy from the case was improper because the motion did not demonstrate the Pharmacy's entitlement to summary judgment on the separate and distinct claim of negligence per se, and the district court did not decide the issue.

CONCLUSION

For the reasons set forth herein, we reverse and remand for proceedings consistent with this opinion.

IT IS SO ORDERED.

CASE REPORT

Pharmacist overrides high dose alert; pharmacist ignores manufacturer's (OXYCODONE CONCENTRATE) warning FOR USE IN OPIOID TOLERANT PATIENTS.

FACTS OF THE CASE

A three-year-old boy was inadvertently prescribed oxycodone concentrate, 20 mg/1 ml; 0.5 ml every 4 hours as needed (for pain). His mother took the prescription to a pharmacy near her workplace. The prescription was filled, verified, and dispensed by a pharmacist on July 17, 2016. His mother gave the child one dose (0.5 ml /10 mg) on the evening of 9/18/16 (or early morning/1:00 am 9/9/16). The next morning, 9/19/16, Hailey was unresponsive and stiff. CPR was administered, and 911 was called. EMS came and continued CPR. EMS took the child to a local hospital where continued CPR was unsuccessful. An autopsy and toxicology testing were performed. The Medical Examiner ruled the cause of death: Oxycodone overdose. The Medical Examiner ordered separate toxicology testing of the prescription bottle dispensed to the mother Checking and will delete if repeated.

OPINIONS

My opinions are expressed with reasonable pharmaceutical certainty.

1. Pharmacist should not have filled the prescription
2. Pharmacist overrode a "HARD STOP" HIGH DOSE alert
3. Did not consult with the prescriber
4. Did not consult the patient
5. Did not document the reason for override
6. Did not check any literature resources and document same
7. Pharmacist did not adequately perform a Drug Utilization Review (DUR). DUR requires a safe dose check, which was obviously ignored, and, in fact, a HARD STOP alert was overridden (see #2 above). This is a violation of the pharmacy's Policy & Procedures, as well as OAC 4279-5-20 (5).
8. The product packaging states: ONLY FOR USE IN PATIENTS WHO ARE OPIOID TOLERANT
9. The Pharmacist ignored the warning—he should have heeded the warning and stopped the process.
10. The pharmacy computer alert did not contain this warning—it should have!
11. "How To Use this information" (Patient Prescription Information—PPI) did not contain the bolded ONLY FOR USE IN PATIENTS WHO ARE OPIOD TOLERANT—it should have.
12. Prescription requiring the use of syringe required demonstration to patient. Based upon the mother's testimony, no special Counseling or syringe demonstration was provided to her.
13. Manufacturer's provided syringe not given to the mother.
14. The mother's deposition only described volume measures, not dosage increments, which are on the manufacturer's syringe.
15. The pharmacist verified and dispensed a dosage dose that delivered (10 mg = 0.5 ml of 20 mg/ml) 400% to 1300% of recommended dose for pediatrics (0.05–0.15 mg/kg;15 kg per child)[27]
16. The pharmacist departed from the standard of care, the Ohio Pharmacy Practice Act, and pharmacy's own Policy & Procedure in multiple ways, as described before.
17. There were multiple omissions by the pharmacist, deliberate ignoring a HARD STOP High Dose Alert, failure to consult with the prescriber (opiate tolerant; toxic dose), and failure to consult with the mother ("this contains a toxic dose—I can't provide it to you").
18. The pharmacy was negligent in showing failure to include the bolded ONLY FOR USE IN PATIENTS WHO ARE OPIOID TOLERANT in the alert software as well as in the Patient prescription information.
19. The gross negligence of the pharmacist as well as the omissions the pharmacy significantly contributed to the child's death from oxycodone overdose.
20. A reasonable physician, when contacted by a pharmacist with a toxic dose warning, as well as ONLY FOR USE IN PATIENTS WHO ARE OPIOID TOLERANT, would have canceled the prescription; thus, in this case, avoiding the tragic death of this three-year-old child.

28.4.6.2 Wrong Dose: 50 mcg for 5 mcg Liothyronine

CASE REPORT

FACTS OF THE CASE

The patient was being treated by his PCP with a combination of levothyroxine (T4) and liothyronine (T3). He had been on a 5 mcg dose of liothyronine in 2016. In early 2017, he requested a refill of the T3 and was told he had no more refills. He contacted his doctor, who emailed (eScript) for liothyronine 0.005 mg (5 mcg) to the pharmacy. The pharmacist filled the prescription with 50 mcg liothyronine, a 10-fold overdose. They provided 3 refills with the 10-fold overdose. The patient experienced heart, anxiety, fatigue, and other symptoms of iatrogenic hyperthyroidism. He underwent an invasive coronary procedure to control his atrial fibrillation.

One of the pharmacists and the Board of Pharmacy (BOP) auditor discussed the DUR (drug utilization review), the error he made, and that he entered the medication and verified it. The pharmacist admitted the data entry was incorrect. He reviewed the DUR with the Board of Pharmacy investigator and admitted he overrode the DUR. The pharmacist downloaded the ADR form and gave it to the BOP representative, and it stated that incidents are supposed to be reported within 15 days. The pharmacist forgot about the 15 days' requirement. One section of the form states, "please describe the significant adverse event," and the pharmacist put in atrial fibrillation, resolved. The attorney asks why resolved and the pharmacist responds, that's my guess because he stopped taking those medications that he claims were causing the issue. The attorney asks how he knows that, and he responds that he looked at the refill history.

1/14/2017 @ 3:37: Patient prescriber was reviewed
Scanned by eRX @15:26 (124)
Patient prescriber review @15:37 (124)
Unsure who entered it on 1/14, does not say (124)

The patient discovered the error while he was in the heart institute; he was not concerned about what pills were in the bottle; he was more concerned about "not stroking out." He did not notice while taking the February Rx that they were 50 mcg tabs instead of 5 mcg tabs.

OPINIONS

My opinions are expressed with reasonable pharmaceutical certainty.

1. These pharmacists committed multiple errors when incorrectly filling liothyronine 5 mcg prescription with 50 mcg. These include the wrong drug, incorrect verification, failure to counsel, failure to note the prior dose in DUR/automatic DUR override, failure to inspect original eScript on first prescription, ignoring the obvious 10-fold overdose created by providing 50 mcg for a 5 mcg prescription. These actions of pharmacists are not "mistakes." They show careless, reckless disregard for the safety of the patient. As they noted in the incident report, workload and leading zeros may be a contributing factor to the error. Two ways are there to correct this situation: Slow down, perform all duties diligently, or demand more staffing from the corporate. They did neither.
2. The manager of the Pharmacy did not submit the error report until visited by an inspector. He was told to delay "by higher ups." He is licensed by the State and not by the company. He, as well as company "higher ups," violated this regulation.
3. These pharmacists argued that a dosage increase from 5 to 50 mcg is not a concern and not necessary to contact the prescribing physician. In my opinion, they never performed the DUR, for, if they had, a reasonable pharmacist would have noted the 10-fold dosage increase and taken action to contact the prescriber.
4. In addition to the verification step, the DUR provided an opportunity to correct the mistake in selecting a 10-fold overdose (50 for 5). Additionally, on the first refill, the DUR also provided a complete list of 5 mcg refills, providing an additional opportunity for correction of the error.
5. No counselling is noted on the incident report. The company Policy requires counselling on new prescriptions. Had these pharmacists performed a DUR and noted the 10-fold dose increase, they would HAVE to

ask the patient about it. Asking the patient "do you have any questions for the pharmacist" is not counselling. In this case, with a requisite DUR review, and an automatic override without consideration, these shortcuts caused Dr. Patient serious health injuries and risks. Repeating, this is more than a "single mistake." It is a combination of an understaffed pharmacy staffed with pharmacists who take dangerous shortcuts to keep up with the workflow at the risk and expense of patients.

6. The dosage of 0.005 mg could not be clearer. Any reasonable pharmacist who viewed this prescription should select a 5 mcg dose.
7. Pharmacy Management failure to counsel or discipline the pharmacists demonstrates the company's attitude toward and acceptance of their grossly negligent practices.
8. Verifications, DUR, a second look on first refills, and mandatory counselling are all standards of practice and are also now the pharmacy company Policy. These responsibilities and policies do not protect patients if they are not followed. Lack of compliance is caused by the inability to perform the work, not enough staff, or lack of enforcement by the management.

28.4.7 Methotrexate (MTX) Errors

Methotrexate (MTX) is an antimetabolite that has been used in treating leukemias and other blood cancers for more than 50 years. Approximately 30 years ago, rheumatologists found that MTX, in substantially lower doses and dosed ONCE weekly, was effective in treating rheumatoid arthritis. In this use, it is classed as a disease-modifying antirheumatic drug (DMARD). Unfortunately, physicians, nurses, and pharmacists contribute to errors and serious injuries by ordering, filling, and/or administering the MTX DAILY instead of WEEKLY, oftentimes with fatal consequences. Despite the frequent news reports of MTX errors, the Joint Commission Sentinel status, and a High Alert drug status by ISMP, these errors continue to occur.

Cases of fatal reactions to low-dose oral methotrexate due to interactions and dosing errors highlight the need to improve safety measures. ISMP (Institute for Safe Medication Practices) published "tips" for hospital and community pharmacists and nurses to avoid methotrexate errors:

1. Create a forcing function to ensure that every oral MTX prescription is reviewed with the patient or family member.
2. If folate has not been prescribed, check with the prescriber to suggest initiation of this supplement (it limits the toxicity of the MTX).
3. Ensure that any drug interaction alerts generated during order entry and verification are communicated to and resolved with the prescriber and/or the patient.
4. When possible, dispense only a four-week supply of methotrexate at a time (community only).
5. When possible, dispense low-dose methotrexate for non-oncologic indications as a dose pack (e.g., Rheumatrex), which helps guide patients to take the proper dose weekly.
6. Ensure that every patient receives education or counseling when prescribed oral methotrexate or when filling a prescription for oral methotrexate.
7. Double check all printed medication lists and instructions to ensure that they indicate the correct dosage regimen for oral methotrexate prior to providing them to the patient.
8. Ensure that the process for providing education or counseling for oral methotrexate includes clear verbal and written instructions. Ideally, EHRs and pharmacy computer systems should automatically generate this written information for patients receiving oral methotrexate.
9. Specifically review the dosing schedule with patients.
10. Ask the patient or caregivers about the use of specific prescription and OTC medications that may interact with MTX.

CASE REPORT

A few years ago, a pharmacy malpractice case went to trial in the Southwest against a hospital and its contract pharmacy. A woman was sent to a rehabilitation hospital. She was being treated with weekly methotrexate for her rheumatoid arthritis. The order was correctly written. The order was correctly interpreted and entered by the hospital pharmacist, creating a correct MAR. Inexplicably, nurses administered daily doses of methotrexate, and six doses were given over six days, instead of one dose WEEKLY. The error was compounded and actually facilitated by pharmacy technicians who dispensed TWO doses of methotrexate into an automatic dispensing cabinet (ADC) and refilled the ADC when the arbitrary PAR level alerted the refill (less than two doses). Consequently, the ADC drawer was filled three times, when only a single dose should have been available to the nurses caring for the patient. The hospital pharmacist approved the ADC refills but did not question the refilling of several doses of methotrexate. She missed the opportunity to stop the dispensing. Clearly, the nurses were negligent—they admitted negligence—but the pharmacist, in obfuscating control of the methotrexate to the technicians, facilitated the error. Had the pharmacist not dispensed the extra drug, the nurses could not have administered the overdose. In this case, the pharmacists claimed they did nothing wrong, denied any knowledge of the High Alert status of methotrexate, and did not provide extra alerts in their pharmacy computer or in the packaging of the drug. The Jury in the case found the pharmacist negligent who contributed to the error and serious injury to the patient—who fortunately survived.

28.5 PHARMACISTS NEED TO DO THE RIGHT THING

The following essay was published on the Medical Accountability Network website in 2006. The website is no longer active, but the message remains relevant.[28]

Pharmacists have a duty to patients. Pharmacists need to do the right thing. I'm concerned, based on some recent personal observations, that pharmacists are not doing the right thing. Pharmacists are not exercising their duties to patients. Pharmacists are abdicating their duties to corporate employers or allowing assistants/technicians to overextend their technical duties into the professional pharmacist arena, resulting in substandard care, potential and actual harm to patients, and a clear violation of professional duties.

I've had a varied 37-year practice, 20 years in hospital, working in drug stores, consulting to pharmaceutical companies, editor of the *Journal of Pharmacy Practice*, editor of 4 books, 3 of which focus on drug injury and pharmacists duties. I am currently an Associate Professor of Pharmacology at Rush University where I teach a clinical pharmacology course, and a member of the faculty at the University of Illinois College of Medicine where I serve on committees and participate in special educational programs. I also have an extensive litigation consulting practice, and in consultations, I frequently examine pharmacy malpractice cases. In addition, I spend about one day a month as a pharmacist, usually in a 'chain' drug store. In the past year, I've been assigned to multiple stores in 4 or 5 different chains.

I'd like to share some of my experiences of 'floating' from store to store and chain to chain, from the perspective of a 'working' pharmacist. I look at this from my consultative perspective by analyzing a set of circumstances surrounding an alleged prescription error or deviation from the standard of care for pharmacists.

There are two primary observations that concern me and are the bases of my statement above, that pharmacists are not doing the right thing. First, pharmacists should be counseling patients by explaining the use of new medications but that is not happening. Second, technicians are performing professional tasks which by regulation and standards should be reserved for the pharmacist. Both of these issues have great potential to place patients at harm. "Do you have any questions about your prescription?" asks the technician/cashier who was scanning the bar code on the prescription as she directed the patient to sign the screen indicating she was receiving the prescription. What the patients usually don't know is that when they sign the screen, or the paper log, they are waiving counseling by the pharmacist. "No" is the usual response by the patient. Incredibly, this question is sometimes asked by the technician who receives the prescription from the patient on intake. However, unless the patient is counseled, told/confirmed what the medication is for, how to take it, how to store it and any special precautions, how can the patient have any questions? Indeed, the 'offer to counsel' is an OBRA 90 (Omnibus Budget Reconciliation Amendment) requirement that beneficiaries of federally funded programs be provided a Drug Utilization Review (DUR) and Counseling. Last minute negotiations and compromises resulted in the counseling requirement being reduced to an 'offer to counsel'. While the offer to counsel may be made by a pharmacist or designee, the actual counseling may only be provided by a pharmacist or student pharmacist under direct supervision of a pharmacist.

One of my introductory statements I make as I walk into a new pharmacy is "I counsel every patient on every new prescription." As I check the prescription, I make a notation on the bag or receipt that 'counseling' is indicated. To my dismay I've seen and discovered that technicians, under my temporary supervision, ignore my direction. Instead, they ask the simple question, "Do you have any questions?", or proceed to provide the patient counseling themselves! Why am I concerned? It has been written and demonstrated that the last act, of picking up the prescription bottle, describing the drug and the label to the patient, asking some clarifying questions and generating questions by the patient can detect 90 to 95% of prescription errors. It has also been written and demonstrated that educated patients are compliant patients. Therefore, the act of counseling, wherein the pharmacist talks with the patient about his drug therapy, is valuable. Effective counseling is not supplanted by a patient package insert. Indeed, some companies have adopted a business policy of counseling all patients with new prescriptions. These companies recognize that this is a good practice, and it is good business. A few states have pharmacy regulations requiring counseling by the pharmacist on new prescriptions. I've asked technicians in these various stores, "Do your pharmacists counsel patients, or do they wait for the patients to ask questions?" It almost unanimous to the latter! What a tremendous lost opportunity. An additional grave concern is that technicians are overstepping the functions that they are allowed to do in a pharmacy. In many cases technicians are performing tasks that should be reserved for a pharmacist.

For those readers who are not pharmacists, let me briefly describe the prescription filling process. A prescription comes in on paper, fax or as a telephone call (email will happen too). It is "interpreted," and the data/prescription information is entered into a computer. Computer software screens the new drug order for high/low doses, drug interactions, allergies and in some programs, drug/disease interactions. If the program detects one of these an alert is flashed on the screen. The alert requires review followed by an override by a pharmacist in order for the prescription order to proceed. I instructed all of my technicians that I was to be notified of and would determine if the alerts could be overridden. Almost universally this instruction was new to them, as it was routine for the alerts to be overridden by technicians. My concern here is that the technicians in these stores were routinely allowed to do the alert overrides in the first place! This is not, however, an isolated experience. There have been surveys and studies in the pharmacy literature that report alert overrides are commonplace, both by pharmacists and inappropriately by technicians. Sometimes this has severe consequences in a patient such as drug interactions, severe allergic reactions and overdoses. There can even be a failure to recognize that therapeutic duplication has occurred—that is, a copycat drug is being given.

An actual example is a pending case where a patient that was known to be allergic to sulfa was prescribed the sulfa drug Bactrim (sulfamethoxazole/trimethoprim—Roche, Nutley, NJ). The patient took one tablet and had a severe allergic reaction which provoked his body to attack some of his own blood elements (acute hemolytic thrombocytopenia) and caused his kidneys to fail. The patient has recovered somewhat but he is not the same robust man he was before his nearly fatal event. The pharmacy computer had information that the patient was allergic to sulfa. The pharmacy computer records also indicated that someone in the pharmacy called the doctor who approved the prescription. The pharmacy computer also indicated that a mandatory counseling needed to take place based on 'serious allergic risk'. Someone overrode the alert. Was it a technician? I don't know. The prescribing doctor denies he was called. The doctor stated he would have cancelled the prescription—of course! Why didn't the counseling take place? There was supposed to be a bright colored sticker on the bag indicating counseling and advising the cashier to contact the pharmacist. The patient's neighbor swore there was no bright sticker, and that no one talked to her about her neighbor's prescription that she was picking up. The patient and his wife also denied being contacted by the pharmacist about the allergy risk. Technicians are not trained in the sciences. They cannot know the significance of rotely 'clicking through' the alerts, sometimes with tragic results. An additional inappropriate action is technicians taking prescriptions from doctors or doctors' offices, either on the phone or from messaging systems. I discovered this as I was checking a telephoned prescription, one that I did not take or write. When I inquired the technician stated, "The pharmacists trust us to do this." Professional pharmacy practice cannot be based on 'trust' of technicians, whose duties are strictly circumscribed by the law! There are nuances in voice, considerations of dose range and questions that are raised when the prescription is being given. The background and training of the pharmacist bears on this interaction, but all of that is lost when this basic duty is delegated to a technician. It is downright dangerous. It is a violation of every pharmacy board regulation that I have read.

The patient's current medication regimen ('profile') is not routinely reviewed in most stores. In one store there is a review policy for the pharmacist to perform a Drug Utilization Review (DUR), in which he is assisted by a computer printout of the profile. In the absence of a pharmacist DUR everyone is relying on the computer software, which does not and should not replace the pharmacist's judgment. In addition, they are relying on the technician to NOT override alerts generated by the computer DUR. In most cases professional Drug Utilization Review is simply not happening. One of my last prescriptions filled was for a young child who was prescribed a liquid codeine/acetaminophen '1 to 2 milliliters every 4 to 6 hours for dental pain.' I took the prescription from the Dentist on the phone. The prescription was entered into the computer by a technician. The computer printed a label. I poured the codeine syrup into a prescription bottle. As I was checking the label, I read '1 to 2 teaspoonful every 4 to 6 hours'. I couldn't believe my eyes. I re-read the prescription. It was an obvious input error. I pointed this out to the order entry technician, explaining the significance of a 500% dosage error of codeine in a child. It occurred to me later that the technician must have overridden the 'high dose alert' which would have been generated by the computer based on the child's young age. The consequences are obvious! The child could have died! These are my recent 'hands on' experiences. Such practices have been apparent in many litigation cases that I have examined. By the time the cases get to me, as a consultant in litigation and expert witness, patients have been harmed. Each error could be a fatal error. The sum total of the lack of counseling, technicians performing pharmacist's functions, and a lack of performance of DUR is an ethical and professional violation. Such sloppy business practices rob patients of basic protections. I like to use the term 'safety net'; the pharmacist, as a professional with an independent duty to a patient, provides a 'safety net' to add to the safe and effective use of medication. If pharmacists abdicate these duties to non-professionals, patients will suffer. Please don't take this essay as an attack on technicians. Throughout my career I have championed the use of technicians, supportive personnel, to free up pharmacists for professional duties. Pharmacists need to do the right thing.

Our patients' lives depend on it.

28.6 STEPS TOWARD A BETTER OUTCOME

Errors contributing to the death of a patient or causing serious harm are every pharmacist's worst nightmare. Regardless of the setting—be it a hospital, a chain pharmacy, or a community pharmacy all run this same risk. And the results can be disastrous, from the pharmacist losing his/her license to huge monetary awards in court. Several studies show that the chances of such mistakes are about 1 in 30 in a retail pharmacy and about 1 out of 1,000 in a hospital pharmacy. According to a study conducted by Betsy Flynn (RPh, PhD) and colleagues at the Center for Pharmacy Design at Auburn University in Alabama, dispensing errors at retail pharmacies across the nation have actually gone up (from 22 to 24%) between 1995 and 2009. The rate of critical injury fell by 1% in the same time period. Even counseling rates have decreased—from 43% in 1995 to 27% in 2009, despite legislation mandates. Things are getting worse, not better, despite evidence that counseling is an effective means of decreasing error.

28.7 SUMMARY AND CONCLUSIONS

As a pharmacy-liability consultant, I (JTOD) am often asked, "How can we avoid malpractice?" My response has always been "to practice at a high level." When pharmacists do their jobs well, drugs will be used more efficaciously and safely, and patients will suffer fewer drug injuries. I tell pharmacies to slow down and hire more staff—not to attempt to take on more work than can be safely done in a specified period of time. I tell them to make counseling their standard practice, supervise support staff, and to employ quality-assurance techniques. I tell pharmacists to stay up to date with the pharmacy literature and to read and circulate the Institute for Medication Safety Practices' newsletter.[29]

I tell pharmacists to speak up—to communicate with physicians on a regular basis. Pharmacists cannot read physicians' minds (even if they are used to reading their handwriting!). Pharmacists must have the determination to actually call and ask for help in interpreting a confusing prescription. When the pharmacist observes what appears to be an error in the physician's prescription, it is negligence to avoid calling the physician to diplomatically address the problem and offer an alternative.

Although pharmacy errors (and, thus, pharmacy malpractice) will never be completely eliminated, the entire profession must continue our efforts to minimize our mistakes and protect the lives of our patients. This has to be addressed as a team, with each member of the team, especially the pharmacist, providing a safety net to identify and stop mistakes before the drug gets to the patient and has the potential to cause harm.

The following discussion references the Institute for Safe Medication Practices discussion, and Figure 28.14 depicts the safety net (Swiss Cheese Model).[30] According to a report from the Institute for Safe Medication Practices (ISMP) in Horsham, Pennsylvania, "the first step in setting up an error reduction program is to establish a multidisciplinary team to improve medication use." This team, the Institute explained, must collaborate to assess medication safety and innovative foolproof systems of checks and balances to prevent errors from occurring.

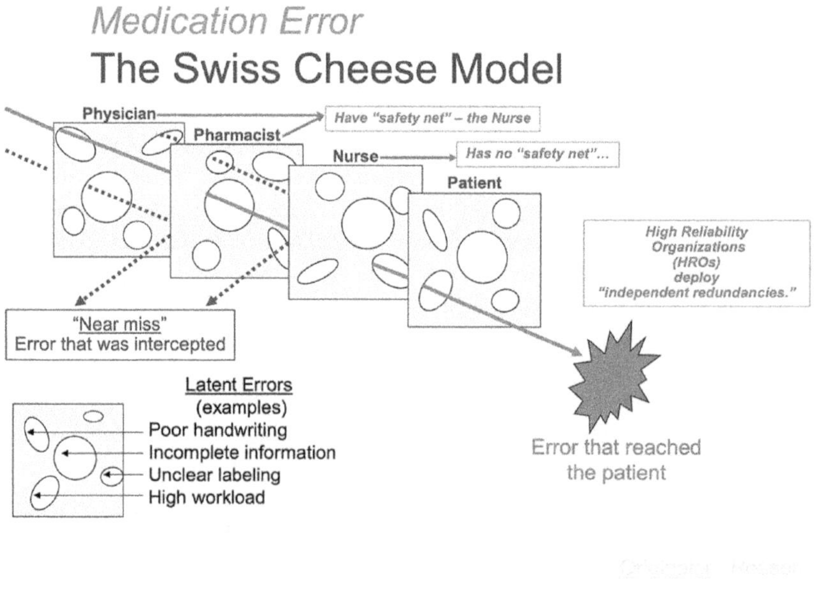

FIGURE 28.14 Medication Error: The Swiss Cheese Model.

Such checks should include a system for reporting errors, understanding the root causes of medication errors, and educating practitioners thoroughly about the systems in place for preventing errors. The report recommended Computerized Prescriber Order Entry (CPOE), bar-coding systems, infusion pumps with pre-programmed dose limits, automated dispensing cabinets, and an integrated pharmacy order-entry system that can communicate with other computerized systems in the hospital.

Teamwork can result in error reduction, patient harm and injury, and eventually costs associated with litigation.

Pharmacists are taught to be a "safety net" for every patient who is given a prescription. (see Figure 28.14). But even the best-laid plans for drug development, research, and physician diagnosis can go awry if pharmacists give the patient the wrong drug, the wrong strength, or the wrong instructions. Even when dealing with conscientious professionals, Murphy's Law still applies—and what can go wrong sometimes does go wrong. Errors and negligence can harm or even cause death.

NOTES

1 Institute of Medicine (IOM). *To Err Is Human: Building a Safer Health System.* National Academy Press, Washington DC, 2000.
2 Lazarou J, Pomeranz BH, Corey PN. Incidence of adverse drug reactions in hospitalized patients: A meta-analysis of prospective studies. *JAMA.* 1998 Apr 15;279(15):1200–1205.
3 http://www.phmic.com. Accessed September 25, 2021.
4 Reiner G, Pierce SL, Flynn J. Wrong drug and wrong dose dispensing errors identified in pharmacist professional liability claims. *J Am Pharm Assoc 2003.* 2020 Sep–Oct;60(5):e50–e56. doi: 10.1016/j.japh.2020.02.027. Epub 2020 Mar 23. PMID: 32217085.
5 Gross A. HPSO report examines pharmacist liability. In *Pharmacy Today November (CNA and HPSO Pharmacist Liability Claim Report*, 2nd ed, 2019. www.cna.com, www.hpso.com.
6 https://www.hpso.com/risk-education/individuals/Pharmacist-Claim-Reports. Accessed September 25, 2021.
7 https://www.cms.gov/Medicare/E-Health/Eprescribing.
8 https://hellohealth.com/blog/epcs-regulations-mandatory-states/.
9 https://www.in.gov/pla/2987.htm.
10 Taketomo CK, Hodding JH, Kraus DM, Eds. *Pediatric Dosage Handbook*, 13th ed. Lexi-Comp/American Pharmacists Association, 2006–2007, 1063–1066.
11 Kalman SH, Schlegel JF. Standards of practice for the profession of pharmacy. *Am Pharm.* 1979 Mar;NS19(3).
12 Ophthalmic drug chapter. In *Remington's Pharmaceutical Sciences*, 14th ed. Mack Publishing, Philadelphia, 1988.
13 Cohen M. Counselling discovers 95% of prescription errors. Institute for Safe Medication Practices, Personal Communication.
14 Kalman SH, Schlegel JH. APHA standards of practice for the profession of pharmacy. *Am Pharm.* 1979 Mar; NS19(3).
15 Kalman SH, Schlegel JF. Standards of practice for the profession of pharmacy. *Am Pharm.* 1979 Mar;19(3).
16 Appold K. How to prevent 7 common prescription mistakes. *Drug Topics.* https://www.drugtopics.com/view/how-to-prevent-7-common-prescription-mistakes?utm_source=sfmc&utm_medium=email&utm_campaign=10132020_ELS-20-DRD0163_DRTP_eNL_US_Only&eKey=amltQHBoYXJtYWNvbnN1bHRhbnRpbmMuY29t
17 Ukens C. Deadly dispensing: An exclusive survey of Rx errors by pharmacists. *Drug Topics.* 1997;100–111. https://www.questia.com/magazine/1P3-11192915/deadly-dispensing.
18 Lester B. *Cobb Memorial Hospital*, Springfield, MO vs. Baxter Laboratories, 1989.
19 http://www.wobblers.com.
20 Hooks SuperX v. McLaughlin, 642 N.E.2d 514 (Ind. Supr. Ct. 1994).
21 Kuriloff DB, Sanborn KV. Rapid intraoperative localization of parathyroid glands utilizing methylene blue infusion. *Otolaryngol Head Neck Surg.* 2004 Nov;131(5):616–622.
22 https://www.drugs.com/interactions-check.php?drug_list=1604-0,2296-&types[]=major&types[]=minor&types[]=moderate&types[]=food&types[]=therapeutic_duplication&professional=1.
23 Danese P. *FDAble LLC*, Glaston, CT, November 22, 2016. FDAble.com.
24 https://obamawhitehouse.archives.gov/sites/default/files/docs/state_profile-indiana.pdf.
25 Carter RA. DEA. Combating Pharmaceutical Diversion, March 2013.
26 Robert L. Cottam vs. CVS Pharmacy, SJC 08497, Lexis 146 (Supreme Judicial Court of Mass. 2002).
27 Taketomo CK, Hodding JH, Kraus DM, Eds. *Pediatric Dosage Handbook*, 13th ed. Lexi-Comp/American Pharmacists Association, 2006–2007, 1063–1066.
28 Previously available from: http://www.medicalaccountability.net/Articles_jodonnell.html, July 2006.
29 www.ismp.org.
30 www.ismp.org.

29 Regulation of Pharmacy Practice

Ned Milenkovich

SYNOPSIS

29.1 INTRODUCTION

Unlike professional groups such as retail merchants, who are typically regulated by outside entities, pharmacists made a conscious decision to become a self-governing body of healthcare professionals. This decision was made in the post-Civil War era in the United States, when pharmacy distinguished itself from the rest of the retailing world as a purveyor of medicaments, a crucial ingredient in the country's nascent, yet developing, health care system.

Shortly thereafter, regulations arose that governed public commercial transactions of toxic substances, along with criteria for the effective labeling and accurate recordkeeping of sales of such products. Nineteenth-century lawsuits conducted against pharmacists also established precedents for pharmacist liability, in disputes ranging from negligence cases (where patients were dispensed incorrect or improper medications) to the sale of debased products (essentially, products that were purported to be legitimate but in fact were knock-offs of one sort or another).

29.2 LICENSURE OF PROFESSIONAL ACTIVITIES

Licensure requirements for health care providers are self-evident. Patients (or consumers) of medication, who

DOI: 10.1201/9781003615323-32

are not healthcare professionals, are understood as being unable to differentiate between a qualified and an unqualified provider. From the patient's perspective, licensure helps safeguard individuals from seeking health care from unqualified providers.

As far as pharmacists are concerned, licensure has three goals or objectives:

1. To improve the nature of health care services being provided
2. To cut health care costs
3. To prevent illegal drug diversion and use

The licensure of pharmacists is intended to improve health care services by (1) ensuring that patients receive the right medication and (2) having an accredited individual supervise their drug therapy. Licensure also controls the cost of health care, because pharmacists can help ensure that patients do not receive unnecessary medications and are provided with the lowest-cost medication selected from a range of suitable alternatives available in the marketplace. The permanent objective of preventing illegal abuse is achieved by creating a self-contained distribution system for drugs that are likely to be abused, and by restricting the right to dispense such drugs, a privilege available only to licensed health care personnel.

State laws that govern the pharmacy profession, often referred to as pharmacy practice acts (PPAs), normally regulate the pharmacy profession, pharmacies, and ancillary personnel (e.g., pharmacy technicians) within each state. Furthermore, PPA provisions typically vest a state's board of pharmacy with the power to issue regulations in accordance with the PPA and to enforce such provisions that regulate the practice of pharmacy. Some states treat the governing board of pharmacy as the supreme authority overseeing the profession of pharmacy, while other states have diminished the role of the pharmacy board to that of an advisory body serving a more centralized state government entity.

In contrast with their 19th-century intentions, the modern pharmaceutical profession and licensed pharmacists are regulated by state-level governmental bodies that have been vested with the authority to protect public health, welfare, and safety. These governmental bodies (1) conduct public meetings to discuss a variety of issues related to the profession as well as the public good, (2) conduct disciplinary proceedings to compel adherence to statutes and regulations, (3) submit cases to adjudication when suitable, and (4) issue new and rescind obsolete regulations that no longer serve a beneficial function.

29.2.1 Boards of Pharmacy—A Closer Look

State PPAs provide a framework that permits the creation of an administrative agency, otherwise known as the "state board of pharmacy." The board is mandated to protect public health, safety, and welfare. Some pharmacists may erroneously suppose that a board of pharmacy makes decisions that are not in the best interests of the pharmacy profession; however, they must bear in mind that the board of pharmacy exists to protect the public and not necessarily look out for the monetary interests of the pharmacy profession.

Generally speaking, the board of pharmacy is composed of practicing pharmacists. However, it may also include members of the public, consumers, and/or representatives of related health care professions among its number. Typically, a state's governor directly appoints members to the board of pharmacy.

Many state boards of pharmacy endeavor to include a chain pharmacist and a hospital pharmacist among their members in an attempt to faithfully reflect the entire range of pharmacy practice. Some PPAs, state laws, and pharmacy regulations stipulate that pharmacists from different fields of practice and major branches of the profession be appointed to the board. For instance, representatives from retail pharmacy, hospital pharmacy, long-term care pharmacy, and so on may each have provision for their inclusion. In general, the largest group represented on a pharmacy board comprises licensed pharmacists, who are sometimes joined by a few public members who are not pharmacists.

Some PPAs require feedback from special interest groups, such as state pharmacy associations, while they oversee the profession. Even though some PPAs require that each branch of the pharmacy profession be represented on the board, many states lack such a requirement. Naturally, some pharmacy professionals from practice areas that are not represented on a state board of pharmacy may judge this to be unfair. They maintain that ignorance of the fine points of a certain practice area may result in the promulgation of laws and regulations that do not serve the needs of the practice area in question and do not necessarily benefit the general public.

Each state PPA may determine the number of members on its state pharmacy board, the length of the members' terms, the manner of nomination and appointment, as well as eligibility requirements. The PPA may be amended at the discretion of the state legislature, provided, however, that the governor signs the PPA into law. Provisions may only be changed in this manner.

In many states, a board member is directly answerable to the governor, who is vested with the authority to appoint board members. A few states require board member campaigns and elections, but it is much more common for a board member to obtain a seat on the board by gubernatorial appointment.

Membership on a state board of pharmacy offers an opportunity to participate in the regulation of the pharmacy profession. Normally, periodic public meetings are conducted during which matters pertaining to the general public are examined. A host of topics may be discussed at such meetings, ranging from local matters that involve an individual pharmaceutical entity to sweeping issues that affect the entire profession of pharmacy, if not society as a whole. Stakeholders in the practice of pharmacy frequently attend these meetings to voice their insights. More specifically, representatives from state pharmacy associations almost always attend these meetings and are typically joined by major stakeholders from a cross section of pharmacies, all of whom wish to keep abreast of regulatory changes and developments.

The state pharmacy board must often handle disciplinary action when a pharmacy, pharmacist, or pharmacy technician is alleged to have broken state laws or regulations. Disciplinary hearings before a pharmacy board typically deal with licensure matters, as well as drug theft, diversion and abuse, and a broad spectrum of other transgressions of the PPA and its promulgated rules. Off-the-record hearings are often conducted by pharmacy board members, in conjunction with state prosecutors, in which settlements are proposed before the case is submitted to adjudication before a hearing officer or the court system.

29.2.2 National Association of Boards of Pharmacy

The National Association of Boards of Pharmacy (NABP) (http://www.nabp.net) serves as an independent non-governmental organization that unites individual state boards of pharmacy. The NABP supervises the standardized examination process that states rely on to determine the qualifications of applicants for pharmacy licensure and acts as an arena for the discussion and development of pharmacy policies and standards. The NABP also drafts models of proposed legislation and regulations that it makes available to member boards, oversees licensure transfer between states, and enables communication and cooperation between states when disciplinary action is initiated against a pharmacist.

29.3 PRACTICE STANDARDS

Each state may determine (1) the qualifications of individuals necessary for the practice of pharmacy, (2) the requirements for the physical premises in which pharmacy may be practiced, and (3) the orderly manner in which the profession of pharmacy is practiced. Pharmacists adhere to these fundamental standards—for example, dispensation in approved containers that bear printed labels—because they have been memorialized in the law. Additional practice standards found in many states include the requirement that a pharmacist be present in a pharmacy when the pharmacy department opens for business; otherwise, there is a risk that unqualified individuals would have access to drugs liable to abuse, as well as the risk that patients might be precluded from asking the pharmacist questions about treatment when they receive medications.

Since pharmacy is a self-governing profession, laws and regulations often codify already long-established standards of practice. For instance, verifying the prescriptions that have been filled by a technician is required by the law, but most pharmacists would likely verify the work of non-pharmacist support staff even if there were no such laws because verifying prescriptions is crucial to the successful treatment of a patient. A standard operating procedure that becomes codified in a law or regulation facilitates the enforcement of these standards if anyone departs from them. Even so, laws and regulations cannot encompass all the aspects of typical operating procedures that support the highest standards of practice.

Despite the fact that states directly oversee the professional pharmacy practice, the federal government may indirectly impose regulations on the pharmacy practice. The federal government controls the drug product and it likewise provides accompanying requirements for the product that a pharmacist must fulfill by acting in a certain manner. Also, the federal government may create requirements for participation in programs that it funds (or partially funds) by stipulating that states must adhere to such conditions to qualify for federal funds. For example, OBRA ’90 created such conditions for participation in the Medicaid pharmaceutical program.

29.3.1 Legally Circumscribing Pharmacy Practice

The manner in which a state circumscribes the practice of pharmacy is crucial. At first, states’ definitions of the practice of pharmacy were restricted to regulations relating to the dispensation of medicine. Nowadays, many states have definitions that cast a much wider scope for the practice of pharmacy, and they incorporate the clinical responsibilities that pharmacists assume. These responsibilities include, in part, drug utilization review (DUR), participation in clinical consultations with other healthcare professionals and patients, and making immunization services available to the public.

The broader the scope of the definition, the greater the interpretive powers available to the state board to regulate the growing pharmacy practice and its servicing of new markets. In many cases, state board regulations are preferable to the demands of passing new legislation. A broad definition of the practice of pharmacy also creates professional identity, which is instrumental in advising courts and other administrative bodies as to when they must judge issues set before them about the pharmacy practice. To foster such dialogue, many states have legally defined pharmacy as a learned profession, to differentiate pharmacy practice from ordinary retailing.

The manner in which the practice of pharmacy is legally defined is crucial for a host of other reasons. It distinguishes between pharmacists and physicians, since a pharmacist, without such definition, could stand accused of posing as a physician. The law protects a health care provider whose practice overlaps with that of another profession because it does not treat such a provider as having practiced medicine illegally, even though the function such an individual is performing may be interpreted as the practice of medicine. Therefore, a pharmacist overseeing drug therapy, which is circumscribed by the definition of pharmacy practice, may not be considered as having practiced medicine without a license, but an unlicensed individual who supervises drug therapy would, of course, be considered as practicing medicine without a license.

The manner in which pharmacy practice is defined by the law also helps differentiate those tasks only a licensed pharmacist may execute from pharmacy-related tasks that may be performed by an unlicensed technician or other ancillary staff member. Technicians shall be precluded from executing tasks that fall within the legal confines of pharmacy practice, except, of course, if the law contains provisions allowing technicians to perform them. Similarly, just as pharmacists may now be permitted to perform some tasks that had been heretofore assigned only to physicians, so too pharmacy technicians may now execute certain tasks that only pharmacists have performed in the past. The mutual growth and penetration of the pharmacist practice into medicine, as well as that of the pharmacy technician into the practice of pharmacy, is, nevertheless, strictly defined by the law.

Additional questions that should be addressed by the state include the following: Is an individual, who selects the medications to be used for a managed care organization's official list of medicines that may be prescribed, practicing pharmacy? Is an individual who reviews drug utilization, and then decides if a patient may receive a certain medication, practicing pharmacy? May pharmacy be practiced outside the premises licensed as a pharmacy? Determining exactly which functions properly belong to the practice of pharmacy, and where such functions may be performed, can have an important impact on the quality of care a patient receives; however, many states have not yet addressed these issues.

29.4 LICENSURE PROCESS TO PRACTICE PHARMACY

29.4.1 Licensing

The fundamental responsibility of the State Board of Pharmacy is to license pharmacists and pharmacies. Thus, the state board of pharmacy guarantees that pharmacists, the premises in which they work, and the business organization they elect to form have met requisite professional criteria.

29.4.2 Licensing of Pharmacists

States may have somewhat different criteria for the licensure of pharmacists, but most stipulate that candidates who wish to practice pharmacy must meet five requirements:

1. A diploma from an accredited school of pharmacy
2. Fulfillment of requisite internships
3. Fulfillment of a minimum age requirement
4. A passing grade on the state's licensure examination
5. Possession of good moral character

Typically, a pharmacist candidate must have received a diploma from an accredited school or college of pharmacy or the equivalent. The American Council on Pharmaceutical Education (ACPE) confers accreditation to schools of pharmacy in the United States. For candidates who have studied pharmacy abroad, the NABP administers the Foreign Pharmacy Graduate Equivalency Examination, which gives state boards of pharmacy the opportunity to determine whether the education the graduate of a foreign pharmacy school has received is equivalent to that of a U.S. graduate. A state board, judging the candidate's scores on this examination, may allow the candidate to take the state board licensure examination or it may request further education before allowing the candidate to sit for the examination.

The student must complete the standard curriculum from the accredited educational institution, and many states also stipulate that the student pharmacist, often in their first year of pharmacy school, must serve as a licensed or registered intern for a minimum number of work hours to have on-site experience and before taking any licensure examination. The state must approve the pharmacy training site, and the student pharmacist must submit proper documentation in support of the hours worked at the site.

The training hours worked at the pharmacy must be certified by a supervising pharmacy preceptor, who is responsible for the student pharmacist's progress. Interns are permitted to perform any task that a pharmacist does, provided, however, that the intern is under a pharmacist's direct supervision. Some states establish pharmacist/intern ratio requirements; others do not.

All states require the North American Pharmacy Licensure Examination (NAPLEX) to be the written test administered for licensure. The NAPLEX examination, a national standardized test, evaluates the candidate pharmacist's knowledge in broad areas of pharmacy practice.

Furthermore, before a candidate is allowed to practice pharmacy, states require the successful completion of an examination on state and federal laws, whether the state's own examination or the Multistate Pharmacy Jurisprudence Exam (MPJE), which is given under the aegis of the NABP. Although they vary by state, requirements that must be fulfilled before taking the examination on state and federal laws typically include clearance of a criminal background check, attainment of a specified number of hours of classroom work, and a minimum, fixed grade point average. Some states additionally require a practical demonstration of ability, an oral patient consultation examination, or an interview.

The MPJE examination evaluates the candidate pharmacist's understanding of laws and regulations that govern the pharmacy profession. Laws governing the practice of pharmacy are relatively consistent from state to state, but important variations do exist. Thus, the MPJE is tailored to each state's legal construct of the pharmacy practice. Pharmacy candidates who successfully complete these exams are granted state licensure and registration to practice pharmacy, and they are deemed competent to serve the general public.

It may not be necessary for licensed pharmacists from one state to take the state board of pharmacy examination in another state to receive licensure in that second state.

State boards of pharmacy may permit a transfer of licensure. The credentials of a candidate under consideration for licensure transfer are reviewed by the NABP, so a license may be awarded in a state other than the original licensing state in which the qualification for licensure was determined by examination.

29.5 THE DIFFERENT TYPES OF PHARMACY LICENSES

The PPA, pharmacy regulations, and pharmacy boards normally govern licensure for several categories of licensed pharmacy practice (e.g., registered pharmacist, clinic permit, wholesaler, sterile compounding). Some states have stipulated that pharmacy technicians must be subject to certification, and they have also extended the continuing education (CE) requirement to include pharmacy technicians. Pharmacy technicians may also be required to accumulate pharmacy technician education credits that parallel those for pharmacists.

Pharmacy licenses may be further sub-categorized. For instance, there are states that have created specific licenses for retail pharmacy, institutional pharmacy, nuclear pharmacy (pharmacists who compound and dispense radioactive drugs for diagnosis or treatment), or specialty pharmacy. Furthermore, some states may stipulate additional state licensure for controlled substances, which is separate from federally mandated requirements of the Drug Enforcement Administration (DEA). Even though such licenses are normally not bound by any DEA registration requirements, the issuing state would retain jurisdiction over the pharmacy in addition to any federal laws that must be followed by the pharmacy.

29.5.1 Disciplinary Actions

State boards of pharmacy avail themselves of wide-ranging discretionary powers in taking disciplinary actions against pharmacists and pharmacies. Many states have provisions that enable the temporary suspension of licenses or, in extreme cases, permanent revocation. However, there are a range of penalties between these two extremes that include monetary penalties, public reprimands, and probation. Each state pharmacy board provides guidelines for various categories of disciplinary action to be taken against a pharmacist, a technician, or a pharmacy premises. Before penalties are meted out to violators, the state pharmacy board typically must adhere to administrative procedures and take into consideration a variety of factors, including, for example, potential or actual harm to the public, aggravating evidence, and prior warnings, as well as any mitigating factors.

29.5.2 Causes of Disciplinary Action

State PPAs typically define a wide range of causes for disciplinary action against a pharmacist or pharmacy. Punishable offenses may be classified in ascending tiers of severity. Punishable offenses may be self-evident, such as providing false information in a license application, alcoholism, or the dispensation of an incorrect drug, or they may be less evident, such as a conviction for failure to meet child-support obligations or drug trafficking, which may be construed as an immoral act in many states.

Some state boards may revoke a pharmacist's license for committing an act that results in criminal prosecution, despite the fact that the pharmacist may be absolved of such charges later in a court of law. This is attributable to the mechanism of administrative procedure, which stands apart from procedures in criminal prosecution. Prosecutors in administrative procedures are not required to meet the high burden of proof that is required in criminal procedures. The rules of evidence in administrative procedures may also allow the decision maker(s) to permit the admission of testimony and documents into evidence that would otherwise be barred in a criminal case.

PPAs tend to avail themselves of ambiguous, broadly interpretable phrasing that casts a wide net and may trap pharmacists who adhere to the letter, but not to the intent, of the law. A vague category such as "unprofessional conduct" is intended to include actions for which there is no specific legal prohibition. Such phrasings and categories may provide grounds for a disciplinary proceeding, even though the hypothetical pharmacist in question has violated no specific statute or regulations. While there have been cases that challenged these categories as being unconstitutionally vague, many courts have upheld the discretionary use of such broad phrasing to justify disciplinary action by state boards of pharmacy.

29.5.3 Practice Focus on Licensure

In the spirit of American entrepreneurship, some pharmacies take the initiative with new business opportunities that transcend the traditional dispensation of drugs. Keeping pace with technological innovation, pharmacy is expanding into realms of patient treatment that involve complex compounding methods, specialty pharmaceutical drugs, and related supply-chain issues.

Varying legal concerns arise for any dispensing pharmacy whose business transcends the confines of its licensure. The case of a pharmacy that enters wholesale distribution is relatively straightforward: it would require a separate wholesaling license. The case of a hypothetical Internet-based drug distribution business that crosses state lines is, however, complex. In evaluating licensure requirements for a business crossing state lines, a complete review of the laws and regulations of each state in question should be undertaken to guarantee that full legal compliance is being met, since drug supply-chain dispensing/distribution activities are normally governed by the laws of each state. Federal law may also need to be examined.

A state board of pharmacy (or other enforcement entity) may undertake an enforcement action in the case of the unauthorized pharmacy practice or wholesale distributor of drugs if it is determined that full licensure is lacking. Disciplinary action may result in monetary penalties, suspension, or revocation of existing licenses; such actions are contingent, of course, on the gravity of the unauthorized activity. A pharmacy practice or wholesaler/distributor may expect, at the very least, that as-yet unauthorized business activity would be suspended until such necessary licensure is granted or until such a time as the pharmacy practice or wholesaler/distributor mounts a successful challenge to the charges.

29.5.4 Ongoing Professional Education

After having been licensed as a registered pharmacist, the PPA, as well as concomitant state regulations, requires the pharmacist licensee to fulfill CE requirements to successfully renew the license and to continue to practice in the profession. CE programs in pharmacy practice are ubiquitous and often take the form of written preparatory materials for examination, as well as webinars, webcasts, and live conferences.

A failure to comply with the minimum required CE requirements will initially trigger a suspension; a subsequent failure to remedy the lack of CE credit hours could in turn trigger a revocation of a pharmacist's license to practice pharmacy. All pharmacists are required to produce—upon the request of the licensing board of pharmacy—a certificate attesting to the fulfillment of the requisite CE hours.

The pharmacy profession has acknowledged the significance of CE or continuing pharmacy education (CPE) for many years, but CE did not become a legal requirement for re-licensure until the 1970s. It is now mandated by each state, which typically demands 15 hours or 1.5 continuing education units (CEU) per year, or 30 hours (3 CEUs) biennially. However, that is where many CE-related similarities end.

Some states stipulate that a fixed number of CE hours or units must be devoted to a specific subject, while other states stipulate that a fixed number of those hours be devoted to live programs. Some states require that CE hours or units must be approved by the ACPE; in other states, the pharmacy board is permitted to approve CE hours. Still, other states accept qualification by either body. Generally speaking, many states grant pharmacists extensions for demonstrable cases of hardship. If a pharmacist elects inactive licensure status, the CE requirement is waived in most states.

The NABP, ACPE, and ACPE providers, in a joint effort called CPE Monitor, have united to enable pharmacists and technicians to register on an Internet-based system to simplify the monitoring of completed CPE credits. License holders can register and receive an e-profile ID number at http://www.nabp.net/programs/cpe-monitor/cpe-monitor-service. ACPE providers must have this ID number to receive CPE credit. State boards of pharmacy may conduct periodic audits to determine compliance with CPE requirements.

29.5.5 Support Personnel

The practice of pharmacy has recently begun to redefine its goals by moving away from strictly dispensing functions to providing professional patient care services. Support staff, who may execute routine dispensing tasks that do not require a decision to be made by the pharmacist, will thus be able to make the pharmacist's time available to provide cognitive professional services to patients.

A pharmacy technician may legally perform certain functions, which are generally uniform from state to state, in a community pharmacy setting; however, the qualifications, licensure requirements, degree of supervision, and pharmacist/technician ratio are treated differently by states. In some states, no qualifications are required to be a pharmacy technician, yet, in others, pharmacy technicians must complete a board-approved program. Still, other states require national certification. States in this latter group require that a pharmacy technician pass a nationally administered standardized examination to obtain certification.

Some states have created two categories of technicians, certified and noncertified; however, the NABP amended its model act to ensure that all technicians be certified by 2015. Although many states do not specify that technicians be licensed or registered with the state board, there is a rising national trend to license or register technicians.

29.6 FEDERAL DRUG LAWS

Pharmacists and pharmacies must also comply with federal regulations as well as those of state PPA and Board of Pharmacy regulations. The Federal Food and Drug Administration (FDA) generally does not regulate pharmacy practice matters directly, but when it construes certain activities to be consistent with drug manufacturing and safeguarding the drug supply chain, the FDA may invoke its authority.

29.6.1 OBRA '90

The Food, Drug, and Cosmetic Act (FDCA) and the Controlled Substances Act (CSA), both federal laws, imposed on pharmacists new guidelines concerning the verifiability and transparency of drug distribution to patients. These laws do not directly govern those who handle medications; instead, the new regulations were applied to the drug product. Even so, federal law did not directly regulate practice standards for pharmacists until 1990. The Omnibus Budget Reconciliation Act of 1990 (P.L. 101–508, commonly referred to as OBRA '90) took a quantum leap beyond the regulations governing drug products set forth in the FDCA and the CSA. OBRA '90 profoundly altered the manner in which pharmacy is actually practiced. OBRA '90 acknowledged a public expectation of pharmacists that transcends the mere supervision of drug distribution by requiring the detection and resolution of problems with drug therapy.

Previously, state legislators, administrative agencies, and courts of law had instituted numerous laws, regulations, and decisions that regulated the practice of pharmacy. Even so, none of these pre-OBRA '90 requirements were as all encompassing as this federal legislation. None of the ideas in OBRA '90 are innovative; however, their uniform imposition in all states signaled thoroughgoing augmentation of pharmacy practice standards. In this fashion, OBRA '90 is probably the most significant pharmacy-related law that history has ever witnessed, so it deserves undivided attention.

OBRA '90 is chiefly concerned with issues related to government funding. There are only a few sections of OBRA '90 that are concerned with pharmacy practice; however, these sections have exercised an unprecedented effect. The creation of a federal policy that mandated DUR to guarantee that drug therapy is as safe and effective as possible represented a quantum leap that imposed new levels of responsibility for pharmacists. OBRA '90 placed public trust in the pharmacist's competence to make decisions to improve the quality of drug therapy and increase the chances of satisfactory results.

The chief objective of OBRA '90 is to cut costs. The U.S. Congress, the most significant financial supporter of health care reimbursement in the United States, acknowledged that it bears the burden of guaranteeing that taxpayer dollars are spent prudently. Congress, obviously driven by the belief that improvements in the quality of drug therapy would cut health care costs, decided to guarantee that patients in need of medications would get them, that patients who were not in need of medications would not get them and, finally, that patients use medications in the safest and most effective manner possible. Raising quality and cutting costs cannot be viewed as self-contradicting objectives in federal legislation.

29.6.2 Medicare

Congress created Medicare in 1965 to provide health care for those over the age of 65, regardless of income or medical history. Medicare is title XVIII of the Social Security Act of 1935 (42 U.S.C. §§ 1395 and 1396; 42 C.F.R. § 405.1 et seq.). It also provides federal health insurance for those who suffer a permanent disability, for those who have end-stage renal disease, and for those who have been exposed to environmental toxins. The Centers for Medicare & Medicaid Services (CMS), a component part of the Department of Health and Human Services, administers Medicare and Medicaid.

Medicare is divided into four parts. Part A covers hospitalization insurance for which eligible beneficiaries, such as workers and their dependents who receive Social Security checks or railroad retirement checks, are not required to pay a monthly premium. Part B covers beneficiaries for outpatient medical services. Part C, at a minimum, combines the benefits offered under original Medicare (Parts A and B). Part C is called Medicare Advantage, and it gives beneficiaries the option to choose a managed care plan. Part D is the prescription drug benefit added in 2003 and fully implemented in 2006; it is discussed in the following section.

Most beneficiaries pay a monthly premium for Part B or C and Part D and may choose to drop this coverage. Part A not only covers hospitalization costs, including medicines administered by the hospital, but it also ensures time spent in certain skilled nursing facilities, visits made to the patient's home by healthcare professionals, and hospice care. Part B ensures a percentage of outpatient diagnostic services, including X-rays and laboratory tests; outpatient hospital, physical, and speech therapy; some colostomy supplies; rental and purchase of medical appliances and equipment; and certain ambulance services. Part B also treats prescription medicines that the patient may not administer to himself/herself, which are provided by a physician or hospital outpatient department in the course of the physician's professional service and are not charged separately. Durable medical equipment, certain vaccines, and diabetic supplies are also insured.

29.6.3 Medicare Part D

In 2003, the Medicare Prescription Drug, Improvement, and Modernization Act of 2003, known as Medicare Part D, was signed into law. It was the most significant and controversial modification to the program since its founding in 1965. Soon afterward, CMS published regulations that clarified aspects of the law (70 Fed. Reg. 13397 (March 21, 2005)).

29.6.4 Medicaid

Salient Medicaid requirements that impinge on pharmacy practice may be found in the OBRA '90 provisions. Additional Medicaid provisions are also applicable to pharmacy practice because they concern reimbursements for drugs pharmacists provide to patients. Title XIX of the Social Security Act of 1934, Medicaid (42 U.S.C. § 1396 et seq.), covers health care costs of certain categories of indigents, including:

- The blind
- The disabled
- The aged
- Members of families with dependent children

Income and assets define an individual's eligibility. Dual eligibility is possible for some patients who are eligible for both Medicare and Medicaid. Medicare Part D rather than Medicaid provides for prescription drug benefits for dual-eligible patients.

29.6.5 Prescription Drug Coverage

Medicaid treats prescription medicine coverage as an elective service. A state has the option of providing such insurance; all states now elect to cover it.

Forty years ago, the federal government determined that reimbursements to pharmacies by many state Medicaid agencies were too costly and responded accordingly. By relying on recommendations for the use of generic drugs and the creation of a more standardized drug benefit program in each state, the government determined the maximum allowable cost for drugs program in 1975 (42 C.F.R. part 19) in an attempt to remedy such high reimbursements and lower costs. This program was amended in 1987 (42 C.F.R. parts 430 and 447). According to the 1987 law, reimbursement to a pharmacist is contingent upon whether the medication is a multiple-source drug for which CMS has created a specific upper limit (called the federal upper limit) or another drug. Multiple-source drugs are medications that are produced and marketed by at least two manufacturers.

29.6.6 Fraud, Waste, and Abuse

Pharmacists must take heed of the Medicare and Medicaid fraud, waste, and abuse statute (42 U.S.C. § 1320a-7b), particularly because the Part D program demands that pharmacies employ a comprehensive program to prevent and correct fraud, waste, and abuse during the dispensation of products and services to Medicare and Medicaid patients. This statute criminalizes the conscious falsification of a material fact in any application for a benefit or payment. Some examples include billing for non-existent prescriptions (filled but never picked up), splitting prescriptions to receive additional dispensing fees, and inappropriate use of DAW codes.

The law also takes action against kickbacks. The anti-kickback provision prohibits anyone from knowingly and willfully soliciting, receiving, offering, or paying any remuneration in exchange for inducing referrals or furnishing any goods or services paid for by Medicare or Medicaid. Violation of the fraud and abuse statute will constitute a felony punishable by a maximum fine of $25,000 per violation, five years imprisonment, or both. Each prescription claim for reimbursement that is illegally submitted to Medicare or Medicaid would be considered a separate false claim. Violators also will likely be expelled from the Medicare and Medicaid programs as well as face civil penalties from Department of Health and Human Services (HHS). The agency within HHS charged with enforcing this aspect of the fraud and abuse statute is the Office of the Inspector General.

29.6.7 340B Drugs

In 1992, section 602 of the Veterans Health Care Act (P.L. 102–585) enacted section 340B of the Public Health Service Act, and it stipulates that drug manufacturers make outpatient drugs available at discounted prices to select covered entities that cater to neglected and uninsured populations. This became known as the 340B program. The 340B program limits participation to certain federally qualified health centers (such as Critical Access Hospitals—Disproportionate Share Hospital, Migrant Health Centers, Health Care for the Homeless, Office of Tribal Programs, or urban Indian organizations); family planning projects; state-operated AIDS Drug Assistance programs and similar types of clinics, facilities, and hospitals; and, most recently, children's hospitals (74 Fed. Reg. 45206, September 1, 2009). A covered entity may contract directly with a manufacturer or wholesaler and receive 340B prices.

Covered entities that do not want the responsibility of providing drugs may contract with a pharmacy to inventory and dispense the drugs. Such a contract provides that the covered entity owns the inventory but that the drugs are delivered directly to the pharmacy. Following a prescription, the pharmacy dispenses the medications to beneficiaries of the covered entity, while in return it receives a dispensing fee. Pharmacies are not required to keep a separate physical inventory of the 340B drugs, if inventories are accounted for by means of an electronic or virtual database. Federal law prohibits the covered entity or pharmacy from dispensing or selling a 340B drug to anyone other than a 340B beneficiary or "patient," the definition of which has recently undergone scrutiny. Some states classify such acts as unprofessional conduct.

29.6.8 Pharmacy Compounding

The FDA governs the manufacture of drugs; state laws regulate pharmacy compounding. Even so, legal ambiguities arise if the FDA determines that pharmacy compounding is tantamount to manufacturing.

In 2013, President Obama signed the Drug Quality and Security Act (DQSA), legislation that contains important provisions relating to federal oversight of the compounding of human drugs.

Section 503A of the DQSA describes the conditions under which certain compounded human drug products are entitled to exemptions from three sections of the federal FDCA requiring (a) compliance with current good manufacturing practices (CGMP); (b) labeling with adequate directions for use; and (c) FDA approval prior to marketing.

The DQSA also creates a new section 503B in the FDCA. Under section 503B, a compounder can become an "outsourcing facility." An outsourcing facility will be able to qualify for exemptions from the FDA approval requirements and the requirement to label products with adequate directions for use but not the exemption from CGMP requirements. Outsourcing facilities (a) must comply with CGMP requirements; (b) will be inspected by the FDA according to a risk-based schedule, and (c) must meet certain other conditions, such as reporting adverse events and providing the FDA with certain information about the products they compound. If compounders register with the FDA as outsourcing facilities, hospitals, and other health care providers can provide their patients with drugs that were compounded in outsourcing facilities that are subject to CGMP requirements and federal oversight.

If a compounder chooses not to register as an outsourcing facility and qualifies for the exemptions under section 503B, the compounder could still qualify for the exemptions under section 503A of the FDCA. Otherwise, it would be subject to all of the requirements in the FDCA applicable to conventional manufacturers. The FDA and state pharmacy boards are intended to work together on the issues of pharmacy activities that rise to the level of manufacturing as well as the continuing traditional compounding aspects of pharmacy practice.

29.6.9 FDA REMS

Risk Evaluation and Mitigation Strategies (REMS) originated in 2007, as a result of federal legislation. It grants the FDA the power to require REMS for certain drugs and biological products to guarantee that the benefits of such products outweigh the risks.

Briefly stated, REMS is an FDA risk-management plan that is concerned with prescription drugs and biologicals, and it necessitates the use of assessment tools that transcend the routine labeling and dispensing of prescriptions. The FDA determines what kind of REMS assessment is necessary on a drug-specific basis and whether the particular drug requires pre-approval or post-approval treatment.

REMS may, in the end, influence the manner in which pharmacies dispense drugs, despite the fact that the FDA's regulatory authority is confined to manufacturers in this regard. But should a manufacturer be found to be out of compliance with REMS requirements, the FDA may (1) ban the drug from the market, (2) determine the drug to be misbranded, and (3) impose civil penalties on manufacturers. Therefore, REMS, which are intended to regulate drug manufacturing, may ultimately influence prescribers and pharmacists at the level of professional practice.

29.6.10 DEA

The DEA is the principal federal enforcement agency that regulates controlled substances. A pharmacy, besides being regulated by any PPA and state board of pharmacy requirements, may not dispense controlled substances unless it is registered with the DEA and is in good standing. The CSA of 1970 is a federal law that provides the underlying framework for the DEA's operations. The DEA has also issued a wide variety of regulations that further clarify the CSA and provide additional mandates in connection with the purchase, control, storage, security, dispensing, and disposal of controlled substances.

29.7 PHARMACY PRACTICE: PUTTING IT TOGETHER

The state PPAs, as well as additional board regulations, control the ordinary practice of pharmacy. Throughout these laws and regulations, a common thread is woven into the fabric of regulatory thinking. For instance, prescriptions dispensed for outpatients and in-patients must be prescribed for legitimate medical reasons by an authorized individual in the normal course of professional practice.

Furthermore, prescription medications must be prepared and dispensed by pharmacy personnel according to relevant federal and state statutes and regulations governing the practice of pharmacy. Pharmacy staff must also confirm that all requisite information—which may include but is not limited to patient name, address, date of birth, sex, weight, allergies/idiosyncrasies, drug name and strength, directions for use, quantity, refills, and proper prescriber identifiers—is gathered prior to updating the patient's medical profile with a prescription for a drug.

The law may further require that drug orders be recorded either manually or electronically into a patient's medical record or chart in a clinical setting by an authorized prescriber or their agent, according to either a manual process or an automated process commonly known as a Computerized Prescriber Order Entry.

State laws will routinely require that prescriptions be accepted by a pharmacy by either a physical handwritten prescription or by a prescriber (or designated agent thereof) via telephone, facsimile, or electronic means via a secure computer-to-computer transmission. After the patient profile or chart has been updated with the pertinent data, most states demand that a pharmacist perform DUR before dispensing any new prescriptions or drug orders. The DUR process confirms that a vaccine, device, biological, or drug is suitable for the patient's age, weight, and disease state and is intended to confirm that the medication does not interact negatively with the patient's other medications or diet.

After having filled and labeled a prescription order, state laws normally require that the pharmacist verify the product visually to further guarantee that the correct medication is being dispensed. Most states require that the initials or unique identifiers of the pharmacist and/or technician who executed each component function of the prescription or medication order process be entered into the patient profile and that such data be readily available. This is known as an audit trail. Pharmacy workflows and practice settings may vary; however, component functions of these processes typically include data entry, data verification, DUR, product fulfillment, final product validation, and consultation. Each element of the process may be executed by one or more pharmacists and/or technicians, which is contingent on how the workflow has been designed and what the law permits.

Once a drug order has been verified and dispensed, the law usually mandates that, in an institutional environment, it be administered to the inpatient by another healthcare professional. On the other hand, in a retail environment, most states stipulate that a consultation or offer to counsel be recorded before prescriptions are dispensed to patients or their representatives. In the mail-order environment, most states mandate that printed hardcopy instructions be included, as well as a toll-free telephone number so that the patient may speak to a pharmacist in case there are questions about the medication or treatment.

29.7.1 Pharmacy Practice: An Ongoing Progression

In addition to support staff, pharmacists may rely on automation for assistance. Automated dispensing systems and robots have enabled pharmacists to dispense drugs faster, more efficiently, and with fewer errors. As a result, the question arises as to whether a pharmacist may be required to verify a prescription dispensed by automation. A state board may not have legal grounds to charge a pharmacist for a violation if a prescription has not been verified, yet the pharmacist may remain legally liable for any error in dispensation, either as the result of a state board action or as the result of a negligence lawsuit, or both. Therefore, it is easy to postulate that a pharmacist must verify automatically dispensed prescriptions as standard operating procedure.

As the number of prescriptions grows and profit margins decline, executive management in all areas of pharmacy practice increasingly relies on computerization and automation to meet growing patient needs. States have acknowledged advances in technology and many are supporting new workflow management methods by making reasonable amendments to the law. However, technology develops faster than state laws can adapt, and corresponding amendments in the laws and regulations have thus become a matter of concern.

Despite as-yet unaddressed concerns, approved technological advances that have been put in place via legal amendments include prescription image routing, remote data entry, automated dispensing systems, bar code scanning devices, central fill facilities, common electronic files, and automated prescription drug pick-up kiosks. Each of these technological advances has permitted pharmacists and pharmacies to handle data entry, fulfill products, complete product validation, and document distribution components of the filling process much faster and with fewer mistakes.

29.7.2 Collaborative Practice Agreements

Pharmacy has long entertained the idea of broadening the scope of practice to the point where a pharmacist, by relying on the diagnosis of another healthcare professional, may prescribe, regulate, and supervise a patient's drug therapy regimen. This idea has become a reality in more than 40 states through new laws sanctioning collaborative practice agreements. The requirements differ from state to state, but, broadly speaking, many states do presently allow a pharmacist to develop or adjust a patient's drug therapy regimen in accordance with a written agreement executed between a prescriber and a pharmacist. Such an agreement would enumerate the policies and procedures to which the pharmacist must abide, and the agreement would provide an official list of medicines that may be prescribed, known as a forwarding of therapeutically interchangeable charges. The prescriber and pharmacist would determine the range of discretion granted to the pharmacist under the agreement typically pursuant to some form of peer-reviewed process.

29.7.3 Drug Utilization Review

OBRA '90 mandated that pharmacies make prospective DUR a component part of the dispensing process. State regulations that stipulate screening, counseling, and the maintenance of patient medication documentation have broadened the range as well as the criteria of practice. Many states have incorporated the language of OBRA '90 into their DUR regulations. But a small number of states still mandate that the pharmacist must counsel the patient instead of simply allowing the pharmacy to propose a consultation, as permitted by OBRA '90. Very few states restrict their DUR requirements exclusively to Medicaid patients.

29.7.4 Other Mandates Impacting Pharmacy Practice Quality Assurance Regulations

States also affect the practice of pharmacy through quality assurance regulations, but these regulations are not uniform from state to state. Some states mandate a comprehensive peer review program, continuous quality improvement initiatives, and/or compulsory drug error reporting, while other states simply require that an audit trail be maintained for each prescription. The variations are so pervasive that one state may demand remediation through additional coursework in the form of CE, while another state may impose a civil fine on a pharmacist or even suspend or revoke the pharmacist's license either temporarily or indefinitely.

Pharmacies in every state must rely on a coordinated and extensive set of tools designed to prevent drug prescription errors, but, when required by state laws or regulations, most pharmacies will only institute a process-driven, system-based approach to monitoring quality assurance.

29.7.5 Health Insurance Portability and Accountability Act of 1996, as Amended

The enactment by Congress of the Health Insurance Portability and Accountability Act of 1996 (HIPAA) was intended, among other goals, to protect the health care system's electronic medium through privacy and scrutiny safeguards. HIPAA inaugurated sweeping changes in pharmacy practice as well as throughout the health care system (P.L. No. 104–191, 110 Stat. 1936 (1996)). HIPAA is a broad, complex law whose overriding goal is to raise the level of the functional utility of the health care system. The law seeks, on the one hand, to make improvements to the portability and continuity of health insurance coverage, while on the other hand outlawing discrimination in health coverage. HIPAA also governs the privacy and security of health care information, and it invests the HHS with the power to establish pertinent regulations in response to public concerns over the use, efficiency, security, and abuse of electronic records.

HIPAA focuses on four components of health information, for which HHS has subsequently developed regulations: (1) privacy, including the use and disclosure of protected health information (PHI), (2) security of electronically protected health information (EPHI), (3) transaction and code sets that standardize reporting, and (4) national provider identifiers (NPIs) to identify covered health care providers.

In February 2003, HHS instituted the complete regulations dealing with electronic data transactions and code sets (68 Fed. Reg. 3434), which came into force on May 23, 2005. On this date, health care providers could start the application process for an NPI number. HIPAA-covered health care entities were obliged to obtain and start using the NPI by the compliance deadline of May 23, 2007. Prior to the enactment of the NPI, a provider typically had a unique identification number for each of its different plans. By limiting each provider to a unique NPI, HIPAA achieved uniformity, administrative simplicity, and cost savings.

The Final Rule on Security Standards, which took effect in February 2003, complimented the privacy rule and sought to protect electronic PHI (68 Fed. Reg. 8334). It established administrative, physical, and technical safeguards that covered entities (i.e., health plans, health care clearinghouses such as billing services and community health information systems, and health care providers) were obliged to implement to shield EPHI from unauthorized access, alteration, deletion, and transmission. Participating entities may design their own security policies, provided, however, that they meet the criteria established in the regulations.

State laws may further define federal requirements, thus imposing privacy responsibilities on the pharmacy as well as the pharmacist. Some of the added obligations imposed on the pharmacist professional include the implementation of full policy and procedures to protect all electronic information and contracts executed with pharmacy business partners.

30 Emergency Department Pharmacist

Victor Cohen, Samantha P. Jellinek-Cohen, and Megan Musselman

SYNOPSIS

30.1 INTRODUCTION

In June 2015, the Board of Directors of the American College of Emergency Physicians (ACEP) authored a policy statement confirming the role of clinical pharmacy services in the emergency department (ED).[1] In addition, in 2017, the American College of Medical Toxicology (ACMT) released a position statement endorsing clinical pharmacists as integral to the safety and care of all patients in the ED.[2]

One important aspect is having awareness that the ED is a complex environment presenting unique challenges for medication selection, dosing, administration, monitoring, and caring for high-risk populations such as the critically ill, geriatric patients, pediatric patients, those with limited healthcare access, and those with multiple comorbidities that often requires the use of high-risk medications and the need for time-sensitive medication decisions; both ACEP and ACMT believe that pharmacists serve a critical role in ensuring efficient, safe, and effective medication use in the ED and advocates for health systems to support dedicated roles for pharmacists within the ED.

Both organizations state that the emergency medicine pharmacist (EMP) should serve as a well-integrated member of the ED multidisciplinary team who actively participates in patient care decisions including resuscitations, transitions of care (TOC), and medication reconciliation to optimize pharmacotherapy for ED patients. The exact delivery method for these services can vary among institutions depending on size, financial resources, presence of academic programs, and other factors. Additionally, ACEP encourages emergency medicine rotations for pharmacy residents and clinical research regarding pharmacist access in the ED. Furthermore, in February 2020, the Board of Pharmacy Specialties (BPS) formally recognized emergency medicine pharmacy as a specialty practice area. This was based on a petition created jointly by the American College of Clinical Pharmacists and the American Society of Health-System Pharmacists with multiple supporting

DOI: 10.1201/9781003615323-33

letters from the medical community. The acknowledgment of emergency medicine pharmacy as a specialty solidified the role of EMPs as specialized in the delivery of direct patient care at the bedside and care for patients across diverse populations and acuity levels. It further defines EMPs as critical members of the interprofessional emergency medicine team, able to anticipate pharmacotherapy needs in the fast-paced environment of the ED, and have expertise in the management of time-dependent emergencies, pre-hospital medicine, emergency preparedness, public health, and toxicology.[3]

The recognition of emergency medicine pharmacy as a specialty by BPS and the ACEP policy statement affirms the advanced practice role of the pharmacist as a necessity and not a luxury and yet many institutions continue not to employ a dedicated ED pharmacist or clinical pharmacy services for the ED. As seen in a survey by Pedersen et al., 6.8 percent of hospitals had a pharmacist practicing in the ED.[4] Pharmacists prospectively reviewed a limited percentage of ED medication orders prior to first dose delivery, and only 40.7 percent of hospitals retrospectively reviewed ED medication orders for prescribing errors.[4] In 2015 in a similar survey by Pedersen et al. on dispensing and administration, pharmacy directors were asked about situations in which nurses or other non-pharmacy personnel compound medications in their hospital.[5] Most frequent times occurred in emergency situations (81.4 percent) and in the ED (27.0 percent). On the positive side, however, since 2002 the percent of all hospitals where pharmacists are required to review and approve medications before dispensed in the ED has risen from 4 percent in 2002 to 5 percent in 2005, 9.3 percent in 2008, 9.1 percent in 2011, and 20.2 percent in 2014 (average sample size surveyed was 503 hospitals). Interestingly, almost half (40 percent) of hospitals surveyed with > 600 beds or more did require a pharmacist to review and approve medication orders before drug administration, whereas smaller hospitals ranged from 9.4 percent in hospitals with 50–99 beds, 14.3 percent if < 50 beds, 20.8 percent in hospitals with 100–199 beds, 31.9 percent in hospitals with 200–299 beds; and 29.3 percent in hospitals with 300–439 beds; 32.3 percent in hospitals with 400–499 beds; suggesting a trend such the larger the hospital, the more likely that pharmacists are required to review and approve medication orders in the ED. Sin et al. published the results of a retrospective cohort study evaluating the feasibility and impact of prospective medication review.[6] They concluded that prospective medication review does not adversely affect patient care by creating delays to medication therapy as evidenced by a median order verification time of three minutes (interquartile range = one to seven minutes).

Despite these advances being made and the support of the highest authority in emergency medicine for the deployment of pharmacists in the ED, hospitals continue to operate at risk by not deploying a team of well-trained clinical pharmacists within the ED. The question remains: Can facilities continue to endure the liability of operating under less than the highest standard of care and best practice? Even more important is the risk to patient care, the patient experience, and the quality of care. As satisfaction surveys could be enhanced by deploying pharmacists in the ED, can institutions endure the cost of poor performance on satisfaction surveys?

The risk is bidirectional—as EMPs are considered advanced practitioners with significant training in responding to medical emergencies—deploying a less than optimally certified and qualified pharmacist can pose risk. In fact, the courts have held that pharmacists owe purchasers of prescription medication

> the highest practicable degree of prudence, thoughtfulness and vigilance and the most exact and reliable safeguards consistent with the reasonable conduct of the business in order that human life may not constantly be exposed to the danger flowing from the substitution of deadly poisons for harmless medicines.[7]

For example, it is stated that a pharmacist who inaccurately fills a prescription is therefore liable to the customer for resulting harm. A pharmacist is bound to safely fill a medication. A pharmacist may be held liable for adverse outcomes, particularly if a medication is knowingly dispensed in a way that the pharmacist judges to be harmful.

An example of this was found in *Brooks v Wal-Mart Stores*, where a patient was prescribed prednisone 80 mg QID (four times a day), an excessive dose.[7] The pharmacist called the physician to confirm the dose and filled the prescription as written. The medication error was recognized 10 days later; however, the patient developed Nocardia pneumonia and cerebral aspergillosis. He underwent numerous hospitalizations and surgeries and suffered renal failure. The court ruled, "A pharmacist must exercise his own judgment as to whether any dosage prescribed, even if confirmed by the prescriber, would be harmful to the patient. If he determines the dosage would be harmful, he has an obligation not to fill it." The patient was awarded $2.5 million.

Further liability may be bidirectional when the clinical pharmacist performs consulting duties. Although there are no cases of liability against pharmacists in the ED as of yet—the physician collaborating on team care with the pharmacist must be aware of prior decisions of courts that have deemed the physician ultimately responsible.

Burnout can lead to poor quality work, job turnover, and personal or familial struggles and presents as emotional exhaustion, depersonalization, and a decreased sense of personal accomplishment. Rozycki et al. identified the prevalence of burnout among EM pharmacists during three separate four-week time periods.[8] Burnout was identified in 69.8, 67.1, and 68.5 percent of respondents. Younger age, more ED visits per year, level 1 trauma center designation, and a lower percentage of direct patient care time were associated with increased odds of burnout.

This chapter is designed to illustrate the inherent risks associated with the use of medications in the Department of Emergency Medicine and to demonstrate the impact of clinical pharmacy services in detecting, mitigating, and preventing drug injury. The objectives of this chapter are (1) to introduce the reader to drug injury occurring in the ED, (2) to describe the role of a specialized, trained clinical pharmacist in mitigating the risk or improving the quality, (3) to discuss the methods used for preventing drug injury, and (4) the potential liability of not practicing at the highest standard or best practice that warrants the ED pharmacist.

30.2 EPIDEMIOLOGY OF DRUG INJURY AND CONTRIBUTING RISK FACTORS

Multiple small-scale epidemiological studies have been published that provide a glimpse into the incidence and prevalence of drug injury in patients visiting the ED. For example, Zed et al. conducted a prospective study to evaluate the frequency, severity, and preventability of drug-related visits to the ED over a 12-week period.[9] Of the 1,017 patients included in the study, 122 patients were identified as having drug-related visits, while 83 of these visits were deemed to be preventable. For the 122 cases detected, severity was classified as mild in 16 percent, moderate in 75 percent, and severe in 10 percent. The most common drug-related visits were due to adverse drug reactions (43 percent), non-adherence (28 percent), and the utilization of the wrong drug (12 percent). Rates of hospital admission and length of stay were increased in patients presenting to the ED with a drug-related event. These preventable adverse events that occur outside the hospital contribute to the large number of patients that EDs must manage.

A plethora of data has emerged attempting to identify the incidence or prevalence of drug injury associated with the treatment by clinicians providing emergency care. Schenkel reported that an estimated 108,000 people die each year from potentially preventable iatrogenic injury and one in 50 hospitalized patients experience a preventable adverse event.[10] Up to 3 percent of these injuries and events take place in EDs. Chin et al. found that 3.6 percent of older persons were prescribed an inappropriate medication in the ED and 5.6 percent upon discharge from the ED.[11] Caterino et al. conducted a retrospective analysis of ED visits in the 1992–2000 National Hospital Ambulatory Medical Care Survey and found that an estimated 16 million, or 12.6 percent, of elderly ED patients received inappropriate medications in the ED.[12] The medication error incidence has been reported to be 43 percent in a study reviewing the medical records of critically ill children in four northern California EDs.[13]

Pham et al. conducted a cross-sectional study of all ED errors reported to the MEDMARX system between 2000 and 2004.[14] Their findings included an error rate of 78 reports/100,000 visits. Most errors occurred during the administration phase of the medication administration process and during times of peak ED crowding (Mondays and during the evening shift). Improper dose or quantity, unauthorized drugs, and omissions accounted for the top three error types.

Hafner et al. reported 321 suspected adverse drug events (ADEs) identified from 13,004 ED charts.[15] Thirteen ADEs were caused by the ED therapeutic intervention, representing 6 percent of total ADEs. Herr et al. evaluated the incidence of potential adverse drug interactions (ADIs) with any new medication given in the ED.[16] They discovered that, out of 199 visits, 26 percent of ED patients had been exposed to a potential ADI, and 3 percent had experienced clinically significant reactions, as determined by a three-member physician-review panel. Using a retrospective design, Beers et al. revealed a 10 percent rate of exposure to potential ADIs among ED patients who received at least one prescription.[17] In addition, charts failed to indicate that the prescribing clinician was aware of such a potential interaction (thus classifying the event as an error).

30.2.1 Contributing Risk Factors

The ED's fast pace and unpredictability, in general, make it a high-risk area for medication errors.[18] However, there are other unique systems challenges that place patients at risk.[19] For example, ED physicians do not know the patients they treat. Unlike their primary care physicians, ED physicians, oftentimes, are treating their patients for the first time; are unfamiliar with their pertinent medical information such as their comorbidities, concurrent medications, and allergy histories; and have limited, if any, access to their medical records. Not only do ED physicians have limited knowledge of their patients' histories, but they also have limited knowledge of medications that patients have taken prior to coming to the ED. This is becoming more prevalent as the number of medications available on the market continues to increase. EDs never close. Therefore, there are times when an ED must dispense medication directly to the patient because the patient must begin taking the medication immediately and all local pharmacies are closed. This places the patient at risk since the crucial safety checks by the pharmacist are not taking place. Crucial safety checks are also eliminated when medications are administered in the ED during an emergency. Verbal orders which may be misinterpreted or ambiguous and administration of medications via high-risk routes (e.g., central lines) also increase the risk of medication errors.

Research has also suggested that overcrowding, availability of providers, poor teamwork, availability of inpatient beds, and availability of alternative sources of medical care may be further contributing to medical errors in EDs.[20] Pham et al., in their cross-sectional study of all ED errors reported to the MEDMARX system, identified that the three most common factors contributing to medication errors were distractions, emergency situations, and workload increases.[14] Scott et al. reported that medication errors related to patient identification, allergy status, and medication omissions occur more frequently in the ED when the ED is overwhelmed, the ED has patients with more severe presentations, and the staffing is not at appropriate staffing levels.[21]

Goldberg et al. reviewed ED records from two different hospital settings, examining a specific population of patients previously shown to be at high risk for ADIs.[21] Inclusion criteria specified patients on three or more medications, who were 50 years or older and who were taking at least two medications. Drug regimens were analyzed for potential ADIs using the Drug Master computer-software program. Drug interactions that were moderate to high were included in the analysis. Eighty-nine out of 191 patients (49 percent) had a total of 226 potential ADIs—50 percent of which were related to ED treatment. As expected, the potential for ADIs rose dramatically with the number of medications administered. For example, 13 percent of patients taking two medications were at risk of ADE versus 38 percent for patients taking five medications and 82 percent for patients taking seven or more medications. Of the 226 potential drug interactions, 11 drugs accounted for 223 of them (98 percent). The significance of risk was achieved with digoxin, furosemide, theophylline, nifedipine, enalapril, ranitidine, and glyburide; but not with prednisone, prochlorperazine, phenytoin, or aspirin. Goldberg et al. also reported that 44 of 205 patients (21.5 percent) had a total of 94 potential drug–disease interactions. Thirty-two (34 percent) were related to ED treatment. The leading drug–disease interactions included patients with congestive heart failure, renal disease, hypertension, and diabetes. Based on this data and the high-risk population, the authors suggested that this population is at substantial risk of drug–drug and drug–disease interactions. The authors also suggest that half of the drug–drug or drug–disease interactions are attributable to medications administered or prescribed in the ED. ADIs increase with the number of medications administered, from 13 to 82 percent, as the number of medications increased from two to seven. Others have found that 90 percent of potential ADIs are related to ten specific drugs: aspirin, digoxin, steroids, propranolol, phenytoin, aminophylline, prochlorperazine, quinidine, penicillin, and carbamazepine.[21]

Although this data has significant legal implications, there is little information confirming the clinical significance of these interactions. Estimates of the rate of clinical significance of these interactions range from 1 to 23 percent.

In summary, ADEs are not uncommon in the ED and may represent substantial annual costs. ADEs in the ED are significant. They represent the chief complaint of the patient, are more common in the elderly and in those taking multiple drugs, and are associated with treatment initiated in the ED. Therefore, they warrant scrutiny and vigilance when managing patients in the ED. An ED pharmacist can aid in the prevention of potentially harmful medication errors reaching the patient.[22,23]

30.3 ETIOLOGY AND SOURCES OF DRUG INJURY IN THE ED

The fast pace of the ED does not permit for an accurate, detailed medication history. This situation often results in time wasted and medication errors. Rusnak et al. reported that most medication errors occurred at the interface of care—for example, at admission, transfer, or discharge.[24] The ED encompasses all three interfaces, thereby constituting a great risk for medication error.

The etiology of these events is multifactorial based on the nature of the ED. Oftentimes, medications are dispensed, prepared, and administered without pharmacist double check, overcrowding and boarding of patients with limited adequate staffing capabilities, undifferentiated and unfamiliar patients with lack of data, and, most importantly, the emergent nature of the care provided.[25] Other challenges to safe medication use in the ED include point-of-care orders, verbal orders, incomplete medical records, multitasking with frequent interruptions and distractions, and the high prevalence of information gaps for patients.[26]

A survey of ED nurses identified the most common perceived barriers that hinder the ability to provide safe medication practices. Barriers identified included the absence of standard handoff communications between physicians and other nursing personnel, lack of independent double checks of nurse-prepared intravenous medications, and failure to consistently use read-backs for verbal orders.[27] Moreover, some clinicians have the impression that a "stat dose," given only once, cannot cause drug injury. The "barroom" culture of the ED—where visitors are permitted, and clinicians are frequently interrupted—is potentially the cause of a medical error. Patients may harbor a drug interaction during acute stabilization, but because there is a lack of accurate, essential, and believable information, a general approach to stabilization is instituted, as opposed to a more informative approach. These interventions, which are often instituted without complete information, may worsen the situation or prolong hospitalization.

Another source of drug injury in the ED is discharge prescriptions. Wingert et al. found that 33 percent of 2,213 prescriptions written by house staff in a California pediatric ED contained a dosing error, and 95 percent were incomplete, considering broader specifications, including that all prescriptions contain the medication quantity, dosage interval between doses or hours to be given, as well as any appropriate instructions.[28] Community pharmacists corrected these errors less than 10 percent of the time, and most errors made it to the patients' medicine cabinets. Johnson et al. conducted a follow-up study on written original prescriptions and discharge instructions, comparing them to instructions written on the labels of the bottles provided by the pharmacist.[29] They found discrepancies in 12 percent of 192 pediatric patients. Half of the errors were related to the original prescription, while 3 percent were transcription errors. It was also noted that the packaging was distinctly different than what the discharge instructions assumed, increasing the risk of error and confusion. In summary, all components of the medication process—prescribing, transcribing, dispensing, procuring, administering, and monitoring—are at risk for error, due to the nature of emergency care.

30.4 CLINICAL PHARMACY IN THE ED: A HISTORICAL PERSPECTIVE

Historical accounts of clinical pharmacy services provided to the ED date back to the early 1970s. In 1971, accounts of clinical pharmacy faculty from the University of Florida at Shands Teaching Hospital establishing a consultant toxicology service where they asked to be notified when poisoning cases were admitted to the ED were described.[30] Pharmacists' participation in "code 500's," also known as cardiac or respiratory arrest at the University Hospital in Lexington, Kentucky, as part of their health care resuscitation team and documentation of their associated outcomes dates back to 1972. The pharmacist's role included (1) serving as a source of drug information to the physician regarding the choice of drug, dose, and possible incompatibilities; (2) coordinating and directing the flow of drugs and supplies to the physician; (3) providing advice about equipment for special procedures; (4) setting up and operating many pieces of special emergency equipment; and (5) recording all actions.[31,32] In 1977, R. M. Elenbaas stated that the major goal of clinical pharmacy services in the ED was to promote and assure rational pharmacotherapeutics for all aspects of healthcare offered by departments of emergency medicine.[33] The general activities of the pharmacist include practice, education, and research. Elenbaas' initial description of the key clinical activities included:

1. Bedside consultation with physicians and nurses to design, implement, and monitor patient-specific therapeutic plans using the most cost-effective and least toxic therapies.
2. Patient education directed toward increased understanding of medication use and maximizing chances of therapeutic success.
3. Assistance in maintaining ED compliance with pharmacy procedures and developing an appropriate ED medication formulary.

Further illustration of the pharmacist's clinical role was described by Lada et al.[34] The types of services provided by the pharmacist in the ED include drug information consultations, pharmacokinetic consultations, anticoagulation services, emergency resuscitation team participation, antimicrobial surveillance, patient recruitment for ongoing research, order entry and dispensing of medications, formulary interchange, and sample medication provision to indigent care patients.

In 2011, ASHP released guidelines on EMP services describing best practices. In 2021, a revision of the previously published guidelines was released. The guidelines not only defined the scope of pharmacists in the realm of safety and optimization of patient care in the ED but also promoted hospital leadership to continue to further develop the expansion of ED pharmacy services.[35]

Despite the well-defined historical role of the pharmacist in the ED, the presence of pharmacists in the ED is still slow growing. In 2016, Thomas et al. conducted a survey to describe pharmacy practice in the ED. A total of 187 survey responses were received. The majority of respondents were from community hospitals (59.6 percent) or academic medical centers (36.1 percent). A pharmacist's presence in the ED of more than eight hours per day on weekdays and weekends was commonly reported (68.7 percent of respondents); 49.4 percent of institutions provided more than eight hours of coverage daily. However, nearly one in three institutions (34.8 percent) provided no weekend ED pharmacy staffing.[36]

30.5 THE ED PHARMACIST PLAYS A DUAL ROLE AT MAIMONIDES MEDICAL CENTER

The following is a description of clinical pharmacy services provided at the Department of Emergency Medicine with case-based illustrations. These progressive services were developed by the author (V. Cohen) while practicing at the Maimonides Medical Center (MMC).

The Department of Emergency Medicine at MMC is a primary teaching facility for the medical school of the State University of New York, also serving the Boro Park community of Brooklyn, New York. The department sees 130,000 patients annually, with an admission rate of 25 percent. The acute adult facility is divided into three main areas, consisting of four critical-care beds, 23 general beds (with two quiet rooms), one obstetrics-and-gynecology room, an isolation room, and an asthma-treatment area—all staffed with board-certified emergency medicine physicians and nurses. Nurse practitioners and physician assistants staff a "fast-track" area. Board-certified pediatric emergency medicine physicians staff the pediatric ED.

Clinical pharmacy services were offered to the department by the pharmaceutical department at MMC through an affiliation with the Arnold and Marie Schwartz College of Pharmacy and Health Sciences at Long Island University in July 1998. Since the Department of Emergency Medicine has a medical residency program and a training program for the Fiorello H. Laguardia Community College paramedic program, a clinical pharmacist specializing in emergency medicine seemed mutually beneficial. The ED would be used as a pharmacy practice-training site for entry-level Pharm.D. students, with the goal of the specialized clinical pharmacist to establish a practice.

The pharmaceutical department provided a centralized, 24-hour distribution support service to the Department of Emergency Medicine. A medication room located in the ED stores most of the necessary medications. The room can fit five persons for the procurement of medications. The central pharmacy refills the floor stock daily and sends medications that are not floor stock through the translogic CTF 30 pneumatic-tube system. Drug and poison information is provided as needed. Emergency medicine pharmacy research protocols are developed, designed, and implemented. The Department of Emergency Medicine at Maimonides is busiest during the hours of 9 am and 2 am. The ED pharmacist provides a dual role that includes a traditional and contemporary practice of pharmaceutical care. The ED pharmacist specializes in acute stabilization of the critically ill patient, while also providing a traditional pharmacy role to provide optimal pharmaceutical care.

The Department of Emergency Medicine at MMC initiated a Division of Pharmacovigilance. Pharmacovigilance is traditionally defined as the post-marketing surveillance for adverse drug reactions, to minimize their occurrence. MMC has applied this definition to the ED. The Division of Pharmacovigilance conducts post-prescribing surveillance for medication errors, potential ADEs, and drug misadventures within the department. The goal is to minimize their occurrence.

Using the ED Information System (EDIS), MMC has created safeguards at the point of prescribing. First, they created a restricted emergency medicine-specific drug formulary, based on the most common medications charged for and then added this list as floor stock. Chemotherapeutic agents were omitted, because of their rarity for use in an ED setting (they placed a safeguard that includes a prior approval from an oncologist before using any of these agents).

Through the ED's computerized physician order entry (CPOE) system, they created a clinical alert system that warns the clinician that the use of the medication being prescribed has been designated a high-risk medication, as described by the Institute of Safe Medication Practices. For example, a double asterisk is used to trigger clinicians to double-verify the medication order for appropriateness. Some high alerts include medications requiring dose adjustment, such as enoxaparin, as well as antibiotics and medications that should be dose-adjusted for the elderly (such as ketorolac and opiates). Alerts to the use of potassium supplements and insulin have also been developed.

The ED pharmacist is involved in constant surveillance of real-time medication orders while in the ED (or while in the office, via a unique tracking board available through the hospital-wide intranet). An electronic pill-bottle icon has been added to the tracking board screen to permit the pharmacist to quickly verify medications for appropriateness. When placing the computer cursor over the pill bottle, the medication orders appear. The pharmacist uses a paper ED screening form to document a therapeutic assessment of the prescribed order and verifies the order for appropriateness. A verification pill bottle (in yellow) on the screen notifies the physician and nurse of a modification made to an incompletely transcribed order, or simply an inappropriate order. The nurse and physician are verbally notified before the change, to ensure that they agree with it. Qualitative examples of the effectiveness of this surveillance system are illustrated in the following cases.

Case #1: A physician assistant completed orders during the shift change (at 7:30 A.M.). Upon review of the orders, the ED pharmacist noticed two discrepancies: a digoxin order was written for 1.25 mg by mouth daily, and an order for Diovan was written for 800 mg by mouth daily. The ED pharmacist noticed this discrepancy and notified the nurse to hold the order. The ED pharmacist conducted a medication history and corrected the orders.

Case #2: The ED pharmacist identified an order written for aminophylline 75 ml, to be administered over a period of 30 minutes. A concentrated dose of 75 ml would have resulted in a serious and life-threatening overdose—especially if given over a half-hour period. The prescribing physician was educated on how to properly order an aminophylline infusion. A drug misadventure was avoided.

Case #3: A patient was started on an incorrect infusion rate of tirofiban (an antithrombotic). Usually, an initial bolus dose must be administered, followed by a maintenance infusion. The nurse, who was unfamiliar with procurement, started the patient on a maintenance infusion dose, but without the bolus dose that had been ordered by the cardiology fellow. Upon survey, the ED pharmacist detected this discrepancy and adjusted the rate. He also educated the nurse.

Case #4: An oncology patient on chronic opioid therapy consisting of morphine 30 mg PO three times a day was brought to the ED with altered mental status. Upon arrival to the ED, the patient was subsequently intubated. An ED medical resident converting the patient's home oral medications to intravenous (IV) regimens ordered a 1:1 conversion of oral morphine (30 mg PO three times a day) to IV morphine (30 mg IV three times a day). The ED pharmacist reviewed the patient's medication history prior to verifying the IV morphine and noticed the three-fold error. The order was changed to morphine 10 mg IV three times daily and education was provided to the medical resident regarding conversion of morphine between oral and IV formulations.

In summary, various safeguards have been put into place at the prescribing interface to pre-empt any medication-related events.

30.6 THE ED PHARMACIST: A SUB-SPECIALIST IN EMERGENCY MEDICINE

30.6.1 Training and Education

As stated earlier, the ACEP (the nation's largest professional organization of emergency medicine physicians) Board of Directors released a statement on clinical pharmacist services in the ED.[1] The statement advocates for health systems to support dedicated roles for pharmacists within the ED. It specifically states that "the EMP should serve as a well-integrated member of the ED multidisciplinary team who actively participates in patient care decisions including resuscitations, TOC, and medication reconciliation to optimize pharmacotherapy for ED patients." While the number of EDs with dedicated clinical pharmacy services continues to increase, it is still not optimal, and those pharmacists employed do not all possess the ideal credentials. Ideally, an ED pharmacist is one who has earned a Doctor of Pharmacy (PharmD) degree from an accredited College of Pharmacy. They have also completed two residencies, a Post Graduate Year One (PGY-1) pharmacy residency and a Post Graduate Year Two (PGY-2) specialized residency in emergency medicine. Vollman et al. conducted a survey to determine the prevalence and nature of EM pharmacy training available to pharmacy students and residents.[37] Colleges or schools of pharmacy reported EM Introductory Pharmacy Practice Experiences and Advanced Pharmacy Practice Experiences at 12/57 (21.1 percent) and 44/53 (83 percent), respectively. There are currently only 77 PGY-2 EM pharmacy residency programs in the United States.[38] While this number has doubled since the last edition of this text was published in 2015, it pales in comparison to the other specialties, such as critical care where 166 different programs are offered.[39] Since there are such few pharmacists with ED specialty training, we often see pharmacists with years of experience in other venues or those who are trained in critical care assuming the role of the ED pharmacist. While this may fill the position and offer some services to a unit which was never previously serviced by a pharmacy, this practice lends itself to error. The ED pharmacist possesses experience and skills which a pharmacist without this specialized training does not have. For example, the ED pharmacist has likely been cross-trained to do procedures such as phlebotomy, attaining an ECG, placing a patient on a cardiac monitor, and assisting with intubation. These procedures are all important for the team approach to acute stabilization of the patient.

30.6.2 Certification

In 2019, ASHP launched an Emergency Medicine Certificate Program aimed at providing pharmacists with the foundational knowledge and skills needed to provide optimal patient care in the ED.[40] The course focuses on evidence-based pharmacologic and non-pharmacological treatments for conditions commonly encountered. An EM specialist should be well-versed in medication management and pharmacology in areas such as airway management, rapid sequence intubation, and post-rapid sequence intubation sedation; ambulatory care; cardiology; critical care; general medicine; infectious diseases; pediatrics; procedural sedation; psychiatry; and toxicology, drugs of abuse; and overdose. As stated previously, in February 2020, EM Pharmacy was officially recognized as a new specialty, the 14th pharmacy specialty recognized by the BPS.[3] The first examination is anticipated to be administered during the fourth quarter of 2022. As such, until board certification in EM is made available, ED pharmacists should possess board certification in pharmacotherapy, also known as BCPS. The ED pharmacist should also be certified in American Heart Association (AHA) Basic Life Support, AHA Advanced Cardiac Life Support (ACLS), AHA Pediatric Advanced Life Support, American Academy of Clinical Toxicology Advanced Hazardous Materials (also called "HazMat") Life Support, American College of Surgeons Advanced Trauma Life Support and Emergency Neurological Life Support. Certifications for specializing in poison information; the American Stroke Association National Institutes of Health Stroke Scale; and toxicology (Diplomate of the American Board of Applied Toxicology, DABAT) also exist.[41] The ED pharmacist may also be a Certified Medical Investigator—important for detecting drug injury and providing expert testimony. These credentials are all essential to providing the immediate life-saving emergency care described by Schwerman and Schwartau in the 1970s.[42] These authors suggested that the involvement of a pharmacist during cardiac arrest allows for the physician to focus on the diagnosis and immediate treatments needed, while the pharmacist focuses on the preparation, dosage, and appropriateness of necessary therapy—thus making this a collaborative, team-oriented activity resulting in a high rate of success. The ED pharmacist provides a rapid approach upon anticipation at the bedside pharmacotherapy consultation to support the medical staff's procedures during the stabilization of the patient. The ED pharmacist monitors for life-threatening dysrhythmias and recommends immediate action and intervention. The ED pharmacist also documents medications administered during a cardiac arrest. Research has demonstrated hospital mortality rates are improved as well as compliance with ACLS treatment guidelines when pharmacists participate on the resuscitation team.[43] In addition, the ED pharmacist—depending on the personnel available—may support the clinicians with intubations, chest compressions, phlebotomy, and other nontraditional roles (such as manually ventilating patients until the patient is placed on a respirator by the respiratory therapists).

However, the ED pharmacist's role is not limited to acute stabilization. The ED pharmacist also has a role in providing general pharmaceutical care for patients admitted or discharged from the ED. The generalist role of the ED pharmacist includes (1) ensuring an optimal continuum of care; (2) detecting, preventing, and managing drug injury; and (3) building a defense system against the risk of medication misadventures.

30.7 THE ED PHARMACIST AS A GENERALIST

According to the American Society of Health Systems Pharmacists' EMP services guidelines, the goal of the pharmacist is to provide safe, optimized medication therapy-related patient care. This is accomplished by serving as a well-integrated member of the multidisciplinary team involved in direct patient care activities including completion of bedside patient care evaluations, medication selection, medication therapy monitoring, participation in procedures that require high-risk medications (i.e., procedural sedation, rapid sequence intubation), medication procurement and preparation, documentation of associated interventions, and the prescribing process.[35] The pharmacist is also a provider of medication information, involved in resuscitative efforts, facilitates the delivery of patient care involving high-alert medications or procedures, medication procurement, medication order review, medication therapy monitoring, patient and caregiver education, care of boarded patients, medication reconciliation, and TOC services. Administrative roles include identification and leading of quality improvement initiatives, ensuring medication safety, providing interdisciplinary education, and preparing for and responding to emergencies. Romano et al. describe in their systematic review, three key emerging areas of practice for the EM pharmacist that are associated with positive patient outcomes including management of critically ill patients, antimicrobial stewardship roles, and ordering of home medications for administration in the ED.[44] Vest and Musch describe the role of the EM pharmacist as one who brings medication therapy and pharmacy services to the bedside and is charged with designing collaborative, best practice programs that integrate pharmacy operations into direct, patient-centered care. Using this approach which ensures that all aspects of the medication use system are utilized, the pharmacist can manage patients with an array of different clinical conditions and needs ensuring that the pharmaceutical care they receive is comprehensive and individualized.[45] Advances in technology, specifically the use of clinical decision support surveillance systems have become increasingly popular as a means to improve cost containment, patient safety and TOC.[46] Carter et al. describe how the generalist role of the ED pharmacist can be applied with a pharmaceutical care approach.[47] The ED pharmacist conducts a drug therapy assessment in order to identify any problems with medication orders. The assessment includes the following nine pharmaceutical care questions concerning the drug therapy prescribed in the ED: (1) Is there an immediate indication? (2) Are there any absolute or relative contraindications that are clinically relevant that prohibit the use of this medication? (3) Is this drug the safest and most cost-effective therapy available to facilitate the attainment of positive outcomes, or at least improve the patient's immediate quality of life? (4) Are there any untreated illnesses that require immediate therapy? (5) Is the dosing regimen correct (dose, route, and rate)? (6) Are there any immediate adverse drug reactions that would worsen the critical condition of this patient (precluding the use of this agent)? (7) Are there any drug interactions that have an immediate onset, an unpredictable duration, or major severity, which I must prevent from occurring? (8) Is this the most cost-effective drug? (9) What monitoring parameters must be assessed before and after therapy and how frequently should the patient be monitored while in the ED? It is not always feasible to provide answers to all of these questions—due to lack of information, higher-priority activities, and immediate transfer. However, the goal is not the quantity—but the improved quality—of care provided to the patient. This systematic approach allows the ED pharmacist to be efficient and ensure a continuum of care from the ED to the inpatient setting.

30.8 THE ED PHARMACIST ENSURING OPTIMAL CONTINUUM OF CARE

30.8.1 The ED Pharmacist and Infectious Diseases

In 1998 the ED pharmacist was immediately engaged in activities related to antimicrobial stewardship in the ED. He/she was charged with solving problems, such as delays in treatment of serious infections or overutilization of antimicrobials throughout the ED and IV to PO conversions.

> **Quality of Care Improvement Case Study #1:** Through collaboration between pharmacy, infectious disease (ID), and emergency medicine, a clinical infectious disease "pathway" was developed. This pathway was initiated in the ED and implemented in October 1999. Information cards containing the clinical pathway were disseminated to the medical staff. A restricted antimicrobial empiric-therapy card was developed to allow ED clinicians to request the antibiotics indicated from the central pharmacy. The ED pharmacist was responsible for the maintenance of this clinical service. After three months of service, 231 restricted antimicrobial cards had been sent to the pharmacy by the ED clinicians, with a 95 percent rate of compliance with the clinical ID pathway recommended by the Antibiotic Surveillance Committee. The incidence of inappropriate selection was 10 percent, which was deemed an "acceptable" level (due to confounding clinical presentation). "Door-to-needle" times for treatment of serious infectious diseases improved dramatically—to less than one hour from the time of the order written by the physician. The ED pharmacist has intervened and consistently streamlined and de-escalated therapy, assuring optimal cost-effective antibiotic therapy.

As part of continuous quality improvement, the Medical Director for the Department of Emergency Medicine is notified in cases of inappropriate selection (and education is provided to the prescribing physicians when necessary). For continuity, this antimicrobial guideline is used across the medical center and has gained wide acceptance.

Because of the initial success of the empiric antibiotic-approval program in the ED, target quality-assurance programs were developed to optimize the treatment of the most common infectious diseases, such as community-acquired pneumonia (CAP). Pre-printed antimicrobial guides with the recommended indications were provided to the ED, via the same antimicrobial approval card. The antimicrobial approval card tagged the patient for follow-up by the ED pharmacotherapy team. ED approval was granted for 24 hours, after which the physician (in the inpatient setting) would either discontinue therapy, switch to alternative therapy, or—if a diagnosis of CAP was confirmed—order gatifloxacin, the preferred CAP therapy, through a novel CPOE CAP pathway. The CPOE CAP pathway required the physician to consider renal adjustments, to plan for streamlining therapy, or to make an automatic switch from IV-PO therapy (minimum time permitted was within 48 to 72 hours), and to screen for allergies or co-morbid conditions that would make gatifloxacin alone an inappropriate selection for that patient. Two years after the implementation of the integrated ED-ID approval system and the CPOE CAP pathway, the quality of patient care has improved, as demonstrated by a reduction in the average length of stay from 4.3 to 3.34 days. This program has improved the medication use process, enhanced the quality of patient care by reducing the average length of stay in the hospital, and enhanced the safety and effectiveness of the use of antimicrobial agents in the institution.

ANTIBIOTIC STEWARDSHIP: Qualitative Case Study of Direct Patient Care: An example demonstrates the role of the pharmacotherapist as an essential team member in providing an important continuum of care in patients with infectious diseases. A patient with a brain abscess on a CT scan was initially managed with ceftriaxone 2 g IV. The ED pharmacist's surveillance suggested that this patient was at risk of drug-resistant streptococcal pneumonia and anaerobic organisms. The ED pharmacist recommended metronidazole and vancomycin to assure broad-spectrum coverage. The recommendations were well accepted. Initial empiric therapy was enhanced.

Other ED pharmacists have also engaged in antimicrobial stewardship activities by assuring the appropriate selection of therapy for treated and released patients who are prescribed an antibiotic. The ED pharmacists are involved in reviewing culture reports and modifying antimicrobial therapy based on the results. For example, in 2009, Randolph describes the ED pharmacist's involvement in the management of patients who have a culture obtained in their ED.[48] If the patient is not receiving appropriate therapy, a new prescription is called in to the patient's outpatient pharmacy. Patients are also contacted by the ED pharmacist regarding their culture results and to receive counseling for the new antimicrobial regimen.

Acquisto and Baker in 2011 published their observations of antimicrobial stewardship implemented in the ED.[49] Their paper summarizes the experiences of developing an ED pharmacist-managed antimicrobial stewardship and culture follow-up program from two separate institutions. Specifically, they focus on a description of the steps for establishing an ED pharmacist-managed antimicrobial stewardship program, a description of the culture follow-up process, managing the culture data and cultures that require emergent notification and review, medical/legal concerns, and barriers to implementation. Outcomes data available from institutions with similar ED-based antimicrobial stewardship programs are also reviewed.

The medical-legal issues stem from communicating follow-up information and therefore the Health Insurance Portability and Accountability Act plays an important role in communicating follow-up information with patients discharged from the hospital or the ED. The authors suggest that the ED pharmacist must be cautious and use appropriate language and content when leaving messages on answering machines, when talking to family members of the patient, and when sending health information via mail or electronically.

The outcomes of ED-managed outpatient antimicrobial stewardship activity were also described. At the Carolinas Medical Center—NorthEast, a non-for-profit hospital with a 47-bed ED and 85,000 ED patient visits per year, conducted a retrospective review of physician-managed cultures (June 2007—June 2008, n = 2278) was compared to pharmacist-managed cultures (July 2008—July 2009, n = 2361).[50] The total number of cultures that required adjustment was similar between groups [275 (12 percent) versus 355 (15 percent)]. However, in evaluating readmission rates within 96 hours for the same chief complaint, a greater proportion of patients presented to the ED in the physician-managed group than in the pharmacist-managed group [432 (19 percent) versus 165 (7 percent), $p < 0.001$]. Reasons for readmission included treatment failure, noncompliance with medication regimen due to cost or otherwise, and allergic reactions to the antimicrobial prescribed. Not only did the Emergency Pharmacist (EPh)-managed program result in the optimization of the antimicrobial regimen, but the workload of the EM physicians was reported to be reduced as well. The time required for review and antimicrobial adjustment as well as time required for communication and documentation surrounding the process was estimated to be approximately 15 minutes for each positive culture result. Based on the time savings shown to the EM physicians in this study, it may be possible to justify to ED and institutional leadership supplemental salary support or cost transfer salary support for the EPh.

In another a retrospective case-control study of all patients discharged from the ED with subsequent positive cultures was performed at URMC.[51] Two congruent time periods were included to compare the antimicrobial stewardship process before and after the implementation of an EPh-managed antimicrobial stewardship program; 212 positive cultures were identified, 132 in the pre-implementation group (November 2007—January 2008) and 80 in the post-implementation group

(November 2008—January 2009). Of those, 104 in the pre-implementation group and 73 in the post-implementation group required follow-up. The authors found that the median time to positive culture review and follow-up [2 days (range: 0–4) versus 3 days (range: 1–15), $p < 0.0001$] and median time to the patient or primary care provider notification [2 days (range: 0–4) versus 3 days (range: 1–9), $p<0.01$] were shorter in the post-implementation group compared to the pre-implementation group. These data show that the EPh was able to perform culture reviews in a timelier fashion than the previous MLP-managed program. This is expected given the perhaps heavier patient load of a traditional role of an MLP in the ED.

In summary, despite the retrospective nature of these studies, the data supports a trend toward outcome benefits and the impact of an ED pharmacist in antimicrobial stewardship activities. However, this does bring up the issue of the potential liability of a delay in culture follow-up, and as such institutions could be held liable if they fail to have a robust culture follow-up process. Additionally, due to the TOC nature of this role, erroneous or improper recommendations may occur, resulting in the risk of drug injury and liability. Pharmacists must be assured of standard operating procedures to ensure no criminal or civil action can be taken against them as a result of providing care within this novel scope of practice.

30.8.2 The ED Pharmacist and the Ambulatory Care Interphase

The discharge-prescription program (DPP): the ED pharmacist initiated the DPP in the ED. For this service, the ED pharmacist provides the discharge prescription, counsels the patient on use, and verifies that the patient comprehends the instructions for the use of the medication prescribed before her discharge from the ED. The ED pharmacist surveys for discharge prescriptions in the ED fast track, pediatric, and acute-care areas. The ED pharmacist processes the prescriptions and conducts a therapeutic assessment (as described above), while the outpatient pharmacy procures the medication. The patient is provided with the medication at the bedside and with demonstrations on how to use the medication (during a formal counseling session). The ED pharmacist documents the counseling sessions in the patient's medical chart.

Since the inception of the program, the ED pharmacist has referred 700 prescriptions to the outpatient pharmacy. Future goals of this program include assessing the impact of counseling on compliance and outcomes and attaining reimbursement for counseling and follow-up (for patients who return to the same pharmacy and visit the ED pharmacist for medication management). This program is likely to prevent unwarranted visits to the ED. Examples of the DPP's impact on reducing drug injury are illustrated here:

Case #1: A 51-year-old white female was given a prescription for two weeks' worth of ketorolac 30 mg PO every six hours. The ED pharmacist providing the discharge prescription reviewed the prescription, conducted a therapeutic assessment, and deemed that—among other things—the dose was actually an intravenous dose, the duration of therapy was too long, and the patient had a prior history of peptic ulcer disease and hypertension. The ED pharmacist intervened, recommended alternative therapy, and avoided the potential overdose and drug misadventure.

Case #2: A pediatric resident wrote a prescription for oral amoxicillin, to be administered to a child. An ED pharmacist student was called to provide the discharge prescription at the bedside. Upon review, the pharmacy student noted that the dosage on the prescription was double the recommended maximum dose. The student notified the ED pharmacist, and the dosing was corrected. The patient was discharged with a positive outcome.

Case #3: A 71-year-old male was prescribed enoxaparin 100 mg SC every 12 hours for a total of five days and warfarin 5 mg PO daily for an acute deep-vein thrombosis. The ED pharmacist was paged to provide discharge counseling for the patient and his wife regarding the administration technique of enoxaparin and his new medications. Enoxaparin is a weight-adjusted and renal-adjusted medication, considered a high-risk, high-alert drug by the Joint Commission, and requires a safety check. Upon review of the patient's electronic medical record (EMR) by the ED pharmacist, it was discovered that the most recent set of laboratory values assessing renal function for this patient was completed two years prior; understating the variation of this set of tests, the ED pharmacist wanted to assure that the current levels were not abnormal (as this would require a dose adjustment). The ED pharmacist notified the attending physician and a new set of values was ordered and completed. The new tests revealed some degree of renal impairment that subsequently required a dose adjustment for the enoxaparin, from the initially prescribed twice-a-day dosing to once-daily dosing. The prescription was clarified and re-written and the potential harm of hemorrhage and readmission was avoided.

30.8.3 The ED Pharmacist and TOC

To date, there are no studies regarding emergency department pharmacists (EDP) as a TOC therapy provider in the observation unit, despite the pharmacist's extensive role in comprehensive medication management in other settings. Kaiser Permanente was able to reduce all-cause mortality by 76 percent with a clinical pharmacy cardiac risk service.[52] Beyond medication management, EDP has proven to be effective in reducing medication reconciliation discrepancies in home-to-hospital TOC by over 30 percent compared to physicians.[53] Okere et al. found that pharmacy student medication history collection in the ED led to increased patient satisfaction, gave patients greater confidence in taking their medications, and decreased 60-day readmission rates.[54]

The ACEP has deemed that observation of appropriate ED patients in a dedicated area is a "best practice" that requires the commitment of clinical staff and hospital resources.[55] The care provided to patients in the observation unit is understandably focused on a specific acute diagnosis, rather than chronic conditions not requiring acute management. In 2005, to prevent these TOC issues, the Joint Commission published National Patient Safety Goal #8 to "accurately and completely reconcile medications across the continuum of care" including emergency and urgent care.[56] We attempted to elucidate where the pharmacist can fit into the observation unit model as a TOC provider. The primary objective is to implement a process that would allow pharmacists to safely continue chronic therapy in these patients that is adaptable for other EDs, feasible, and efficient.

The EDP, when present, supervised a pharmacy-led TOC program in the observation unit in the MMC ED, in which each patient is initially interviewed by pharmacy students or residents to obtain a medication history. Due to the diverse patient population, translated questionnaires were available in Creole, Korean, Mandarin, Russian, Spanish, and Yiddish using Google Translate©. If the patient was unable to provide a medication history, alternative sources of information such as pill bottles, personal medication lists, or discussions with the patient's caregiver were utilized. This list was then confirmed via the hospital discharge medication list or by contacting the patient's outpatient pharmacy. If the medication was confirmed by both sources, the ED pharmacist (EDP) determined if it was contraindicated based on the treatment plan or admitting diagnosis. Some common examples where medications were held were beta-blockers and stress testing or antiplatelets and hemorrhage. Next, they assessed compliance within the past 24 hours and performed therapeutic interchange per hospital protocol or calculated dosage conversion (i.e., insulin.) Orders were then discussed with the physician and transcribed in the EMR. Medications were then dispensed from the satellite to the nurse for the time remaining in the observation unit, which routinely is no greater than 24–48 hours. If the medication could not be confirmed with a pharmacy profile or discharge orders from previous admissions, then the pharmacist assesses the patient for signs or symptoms of the condition, or the primary care provider is contacted if available to ascertain the need for therapy. The EDP then determines if treatment is indicated by reviewing laboratory data, vital signs, expected treatment plan, half-life of the drug, and the last administration time. The physician then signed off on all medication orders in the EMR. All medication histories acquired were transcribed into the patient's EMR to ensure proper TOC from ED to inpatient with a complete and accurate medication history in the event the patient was admitted. The ED pharmacist continually assessed the patient for the efficacy and safety of the medications that were continued.

The pharmacy team assessed 290 patients, of whom 51 percent were male with a median age of 65 ± 18 years. There were 1,533 chronic medications collected during the medication history interview. The ED Pharmacist continued 987 medication orders in the observation unit, in addition to 184 therapeutic interchanges. The top five medication classes continued by the EDP were antihypertensive (n = 281, 28 percent), antiplatelet (n = 126, 13 percent), hypercholesterolemia (n= 100, 10 percent), anti-hyperglycemics (n = 79, 8 percent), and gastrointestinal drugs (n = 79, 8 percent). The interviewers spent a median of 28 minutes gathering patient information prior to the interview, 22 minutes interviewing the patient for medication history, and 23 minutes with ED Pharmacist transcribing the orders and preparing medication to be dispensed. The total time to complete medication management from interview to completion of history has the potential to save providers 51 minutes/patient/visit (MPPV). Patients > 55 years old were more likely to require continuation of chronic therapy than those 181–54 years old (17.5 percent vs 82.4 percent, p = 0.0001; OR = 4.71).

The expanding role of the pharmacist is undeniable, and HR 592 has recently been introduced to the U.S. Senate to recognize pharmacists as providers under the Centers for Medicare & Medicaid Services.[57] Exploring safe and feasible processes that allow EDPs to be providers of TOC therapy in an observation unit could provide more pharmacists with direct patient care opportunities. Potentially revenue-generating services could serve to justify additional positions while concurrently decreasing medication reconciliation errors, with less financial impact on departmental budgets. ED Pharmacists performing continuation of chronic therapy management during the transition from ED to observation unit to either admission or discharge is a valuable service, not only associated with saving provider MPPV but also in the prevention of potential chronic disease state exacerbations that may be of considerable value to the hospital.

30.8.3.1 Medication Admission Notes in the ED

Unintentional medication discrepancies on hospital admission are common, occurring in up to 67 percent of inpatients. Such discrepancies include interruption of regularly used medications, inconsistent dosing or frequency of home medications, and provision of incorrect medications that differ from those normally prescribed.[58] Up to 27 percent of all hospital prescribing errors have been attributed to incomplete medication histories at the time of admission.[59] Research has shown that at least 1 medication is omitted in more than 57 percent of patients admitted to an ED. Traditionally, medications are identified in the histories taken by physicians or nurses. However, when a pharmacist is involved in obtaining a medication history, there is a 43–84 percent relative risk reduction.[53] It is essential to attain a verified, reliable, and accurate medication history upon ED admission to ensure an optimal continuum of care.

Having access to a complete and accurate medication history is important since it may unveil reasons for the patients' illnesses, such as noncompliance or adverse drug reactions, and patients' at-home medication regimens are often continued during and after hospitalization. However, obtaining a medication history is a cumbersome, time-consuming (17 minutes on average) and challenging process. Assuming the patient is awake and alert, the clinician begins by asking the patient what prescription and non-prescription medications they take. The information may be retrieved from a list, the medication bottles, or the patient's memory. The information retrieved from the patient's memory may vary from a complete list (the patient accurately recalls each medication name, the dose, and how frequently they take it) to describing the characteristics or color of individual medications to not being able to recall any information about the medications they are taking at home. The patient's inability to recall medications can sometimes be a limitation or a source of error. The clinician may attempt to obtain the medication history information from the medical chart of previous ED or clinic visits or hospital stays. Alternatively, the clinician may attempt to contact the patient's outpatient pharmacy or primary medical doctor assuming the patient is able to provide this information and that they are open.

The Joint Commission's National Patient Safety Goal (NPSG) on medication reconciliation requires providers at accredited organizations to find out what medications patients are taking when they arrive at the facility and compare that information with any new medications ordered and provide patients with written information about their medications when they leave the hospital.[60] To achieve the medication reconciliation NPSG, the ACEP has described a three-tiered approach to medication reconciliation that is used in the ED, which is simpler and minimizes the documentation requirements.[61] The first tier is called screening reconciliation, and in this approach the triage nurse asks the ED patient about current medications. The second tier is called focused reconciliation, in which the emergency physician could obtain additional information such as the exact dosage and route of the medications from the patient's pharmacy and primary care physician and family. If a patient is admitted to the hospital, the third tier, full medication reconciliation should be completed by the inpatient unit and pharmacist. Various other tools have been published which attempt to improve the accuracy and completeness of documented information and minimize the time to acquire accurate medication histories.[62,63]

Recent clinical data supports the notion of pharmacists obtaining medication histories in the ED and has shown that pharmacists obtain more accurate medication-related information from patients than either nurses or physicians. Carter et al. affirmed that clinical pharmacists obtain more complete medication histories for patients upon admission.[64] Pharmacists identified 1,096 home medications compared to 817 that were identified by ED physicians, medical students, or nurses. The most common discrepancy was the omission of the dosing information (78 percent) or the omission of a home medication (25 percent). Bond et al. report an annual cost savings of $7 million per hospital, as well as a reduced annual rate of deaths, for a group of 128 hospitals with pharmacists taking medication histories, compared with a control group of hospitals that did not have pharmacists on staff to take histories.[65] Currently, only 3 percent of hospitals employ pharmacists in this role, and even fewer EDs are equipped with this resource. Nester et al. demonstrated that pharmacist-conducted medication histories improved rates of clinical interventions, as compared to nursing-acquired medication histories (34 percent versus 16 percent, $p < 0.001$).[66] The authors also suggested that, perhaps, a pharmacist could work in areas such as the emergency room or admission areas during certain hours to conduct medication histories as patients are admitted to the hospital. Nester et al. suggested targeting certain populations, such as those at high risk, the elderly, and those admitted due to drug-related morbidity. Interestingly, however, the authors reported that this clinical pharmacy service was curtailed at their institution, due to major personnel and budgetary changes—even though this service was found to reduce cost and mortality. Lastly, Hayes et al. examined the effect of pharmacist-conducted medication reconciliation in the ED on compliance with the NPSG.[67] The medication reconciliations not conducted by pharmacists were designated as the control group, and the pharmacist-conducted medication reconciliations were designated as the study group. In the eight-week study period, a total of 117 errors were identified on the medication histories conducted by the control group compared to only two errors for the study group ($p = 0.001$). Also, allergy documentation was recorded for only 62 patients in the control group (79 percent) versus all 60 patients in the study group (100 percent) ($p = 0.001$).

The ED pharmacist conducts a comprehensive medication history as an initial triage of patients entering the ED. The data collected includes:

1. Medications prior to admit
2. Medications taken right before the event
3. Over-the-counter medications used regularly
4. Herbal products taken regularly
5. Illicit drug substances used
6. Social history
7. Allergies and reactions
8. Immunization history
9. Initial vital signs and quick assessment
10. Compliance history
11. Medications needed immediately to prevent withdrawal reactions
12. Identification of foreign medications
13. Identification of medication taken in overdose
14. Adverse drug reactions

The ED pharmacist will immediately alert the ED clinicians to the potential risks involved with mixing ED-initiated therapy with current therapies or if the pattern of care indicates a potential drug-related admission. This information may assist with the disposition and optimal management of the patient.

An example of the impact of attaining comprehensive medication histories is seen in the following cases:

Case #1: A 54-year-old Russian female presented in a catatonic state. After the ED pharmacist conducted an extensive medication history, it was revealed that the patient was self-administering Kavololum—a Russian tonic for anxiety—that had phenobarbital as its main ingredient. This explained the patient's initial presentation.

Case #2: A 31-year-old female taking carbamazepine for a seizure disorder was recently started on treatment for Helicobacter pylori. The private physician started the patient on a combination regimen containing clarithromycin and lansoprazole. The patient presented to the ED with a clinical presentation of dizziness, nystagmus, and ataxia, as well as an elevated level of carbamazepine. The ED pharmacist identified the drug interaction between the carbamazepine and clarithromycin and treated accordingly, by reducing the dose of carbamazepine. The patient was subsequently discharged within six hours. Data has also been published demonstrating the ability of trained pharmacy technicians in obtaining medication histories in the ED. Hart et al. evaluated medication history errors before and after implementation of a pharmacy-technician-based medication reconciliation program in the ED.[68] The primary objective was to determine any differences in the percentage of patients with accurate medication histories prepared by nurses compared with pharmacy technicians. Medication histories conducted by pharmacy technicians were accurate 88 percent of the time compared with 57% of those conducted by nurses ($p < 0.0001$). Johnston et al conducted a study to determine whether pharmacy technicians could obtain the best possible medication history in the ED with accuracy and completeness similar to that of pharmacists.[69] They found no significant difference between pharmacists and technicians in terms of discrepancies involving prescription drugs or over-the-counter medications. Hiring a pharmacy technician to perform medication reconciliation in the ED rather than a pharmacist would result in a significant cost saving to the department and institution and could free up the pharmacist to assess and resolve clinical medication-related problems.

30.8.4 The ED Pharmacist as a Clinical Toxicology Consultant

As described in 1979 by Czajka et al., the pharmacist has three main functions in clinical toxicology consultations.[70] The first is assisting in obtaining the patient history and conducting a patient assessment of the toxicological problem. He next recommends a plan for management and, thirdly, counsels the patient and caregiver on poison prevention to prevent reoccurrences. The ED pharmacist at MMC is consulted for these services. This pharmacist conducts a comprehensive investigation of the patient medication history, counts pills, assesses other medication the patient may have had access to, and identifies foreign medications. He also recommends a management plan. In addition—and most importantly—the pharmacist provides bedside care during the initial supportive care of the toxicological emergency in the form of assisting with gastric decontamination, administering activated charcoal, or gastric lavage. The ED pharmacist recommends and procures antidotes too—especially those that are not commonly used, such as the cyanide antidote kit, dantrolene, flumazenil, methylene blue, sodium bicarbonate, glucagon, and ethanol infusion drip. The ED pharmacist evaluates drug levels, arterial blood gas, toxicodynamics, and toxicokinetics, to assist with the disposition of the patient. In addition, ED pharmacists can also become board-certified toxicologists with the American Academy of Clinical Toxicology, providing them with knowledge, experience, and competence to provide toxicological expertise in emergent and non-emergent situations. The impact of the ED pharmacist is demonstrated in the following cases:

Case #1: A 24-year-old Asian male presented with an acute altered mental status. The physician requested a consult from the ED pharmacist and requested that Ceftriaxone IV be administered for suspected bacterial meningitis. The ED pharmacist questioned the patient, and through patient assessment, noticed widely dilated pupils and a moderately confused sensorium, like what is seen in anticholinergic toxicity. Although the patient had difficulty remembering, the ED pharmacist was able to obtain evidence that the patient attempted suicide. The patient's family corroborated this. After further investigation, the patient admitted to taking 30 Unisom tablets Unisom is a well-known over-the-counter sleep aid that contains diphenhydramine 50 mg. The patient was given activated charcoal and supportive care. Antimicrobial therapy was discontinued.

Case #2: A seven-year-old child treated with risperidone for aggressive behavior had a dystonic reaction in school, according to the guidance counselor. After further evaluation, the physician determined that this was an expected event. The ED pharmacist conducted a further investigation and discovered that the instruction on the medication bottle was incorrect, and that a pipette dispensing tool used to deliver the medication orally had been used inappropriately, resulting in the mother administering at least ten times the recommended dose. Hence, this reaction was a drug misadventure due to the overdose—not necessarily an expected untoward effect of the drug. A rechallenge at normal doses was negative, permitting the reinstitution of risperidone therapy, which led to a positive outcome. The ED pharmacist was trained in detecting drug errors. Without his investigation, another accidental overdose might have occurred, or the physician might have unnecessarily discontinued risperidone in a patient who had been effectively managed on this therapy.

Case #3: A 28-year-old male was brought into the ED for a suspected overdose of his sister's naproxen prescription. He presented with the bottle and his sister who identified the medication to be her naproxen prescription. Upon arrival at the ED, the patient was admitted to medicine for psychiatry clearance. The clinical ED pharmacist reviewing the case prior to transfer to the floor opened the vial and noted the presence of acetaminophen 500 mg tablets rather than naproxen tablets. An acetaminophen concentration was ordered, and an occult acetaminophen overdose was identified.

Case #4: A 49-year-old male patient, a frequent flier to the ED, presented with suspected alcohol-related seizures for the seventh time over the previous four months. Upon presentation, the patient had altered mental status and was unable to give an adequate medical history. Based on his admission laboratory results, it was noted the patient had an anion gap acidosis. The medical team attributed these laboratory findings to be due to a suspected seizure that occurred prior to presentation to the ED. A pharmacist reviewing the patient's progress six hours after initial presentation noticed an anion gap acidosis still present and suggested toxic alcohol levels be sent to the laboratory for testing. Based on these results, an ethylene glycol ingestion was discovered, and the patient was initiated on antidotal therapy.

30.8.5 The ED Pharmacist and the Cardiology Interface

Prior to clinical pharmacy service, the "door-to-needle" time for initiating fibrinolytic therapy for acute myocardial infarction was estimated at three hours. A primary goal of the medical director was to reduce this time to the standard of less than one hour. To this end, the emergency nurse specialist, medical director, and the ED pharmacist at MMC developed and implemented the first chest-pain order form. The chest-pain order form was created to ensure that initial standard medications were considered and immediately requested by the treating clinician, barring any contraindications that might be listed on the form. The chest-pain order form served as a reminder of the medications recommended by the ACC/AHA guidelines for use during an acute coronary syndrome. As a result of the chest-pain order form, the "door-to-needle" time improved from three hours to less than one hour—within just three months of implementation. Interestingly, when the ED pharmacist was present, there were case reports of administration of fibrinolytic therapy within 15 minutes. This rapid approach to instituting life-saving medications improves the goal of salvaging myocardium, while assuring safe and appropriate use of the fibrinolysis. The importance of assuring appropriate procurement and administration of fibrinolysis cannot be overstated, as reported by Cannon et al., who demonstrated that mistakes with the administration of fibrinolysis result in outcomes worse than in those who never received fibrinolysis.[71] To provide greater safety, fibrinolytic kits are now available in the MMC's ED, with instructions and guidelines for dosing, administration, procurement, and monitoring. A medication use evaluation card is attached to the kits for future pharmacovigilance studies. The goal of the card is for real-time data collection on the use of fibrinolytics. The hope is that a review of the annual medical charts will indicate which strategies have been most successful in acute myocardial infarction, and provide information on the preferred fibrinolytic, and any adverse outcomes that may have resulted.

The ED pharmacist uses epidemiological tools, such as the thrombolysis in myocardial infarction (TIMI) risk score, to estimate the risk of morbidity and mortality for patients presenting with symptoms of acute coronary syndromes. The TIMI risk score will compare the risk of death if the patient is left untreated with the risks incurred by treatment with antithrombotics. The ED pharmacist intervenes when the risk of antithrombotic therapy outweighs its benefits or to avoid potentially harmful dosing regimens with anticoagulants (e.g., heparin, enoxaparin, and abciximab). The ED pharmacist also ensures appropriate and immediate preparation and administration by conducting direct observation of therapy at the bedside.

At MMC the ED pharmacist is providing even more intense direct patient care through the management of physician-approved protocols. In 2009 the ED pharmacist has been managing the rate control of atrial fibrillation/flutter patients to ensure the achievement of endpoints and sustained rate control. To date, 48 patients have been managed by the pharmacist. The program has been shown to be safe and effective and has resulted in increased patient satisfaction with intense monitoring and ED physician approval, allowing the ED physician to manage the surge and enhance the throughput.

Other institutions have also demonstrated the impact of the ED pharmacist in cardiovascular emergencies. For example, as current guidelines recommend door-to-balloon times of 90 min or less for patients presenting to the ED with ST-segment elevation myocardial infarction (STEMI), it is essential to have an efficient process. Acquisto et al. conducted a retrospective observational cohort study of ED patients with STEMI requiring urgent cardiac catheterization.[72] A multivariate analysis conducted in 120 patients determined that the ED pharmacist presence is associated with a mean 13.1-min and 11.5-min decrease indoor/diagnosis-to-CCL and door-to-balloon times, respectively. Patients were more likely to achieve a door/diagnosis-to-CCL time ≤ 30 min and≤ 45 min and a door-to-balloon time ≤ 90 min more likely when the EDP was present. The authors concluded that the EDP presence during STEMI presentation to the ED is independently associated with a decrease indoor/diagnosis-to-CCL and door-to-balloon times.

30.8.6 The ED Pharmacist and Neurological Emergencies

The ED pharmacist observes at the bedside during neurological emergencies. The pharmacist provides immediate recommendations and procurement of neurological emergency pharmacotherapy and makes a bedside assessment of contraindications, to avoid any medication-related problems with the use of t-PA for stroke.

30.8.7 The ED Pharmacist and Pulmonary Emergencies

The ED pharmacist is involved in acute status asthmaticus, in the procurement of medications at the bedside as requested by the physician, and consultation, as illustrated by the following case presentation. A patient (who happened to be a cardiologist) presented at the ED for acute status asthmaticus unrelieved by aggressive bronchodilator therapy. The ED physician was ready to intubate the patient, as recommended by the pulmonologist. The ED pharmacist suggested aminophylline. The pulmonologists consulting on the case disagreed and stated that aminophylline no longer had a role in status asthmaticus. However, to avoid intubation, the ED physician agreed with the pharmacist. The aminophylline infusion provided instant alertness and appeared to improve extra-pulmonary ventilation, allowing the patient to express himself (which, minutes before, he had been unable to do). Intubation was avoided and the patient was discharged a day later. The cardiologist suggested publishing this case supporting the use of aminophylline in acute status asthmaticus. This intervention prevented substantial morbidity and a prolonged length of stay in the intensive-care unit.

30.8.8 The ED Pharmacist and Public Health Services in the ED

Several public health programs have been developed and initiated within the ED. The ED pharmacist has engaged in screening and brief intervention for smoking cessation and for preventing exposure of children to second-hand smoke from their family members. One hundred thirty-four patients have been screened and counseled on methods for preventing second-hand smoke exposure to their children.

Between 2008 and 2010, the ED pharmacist trained hundreds of community and hospital pharmacists in administering vaccinations and has been granted approval by the institution to administer influenza and pneumococcal vaccines to treated and released patients. Over 70,000 patients who visit the ED are treated and released. Many of these patients do not get vaccinated appropriately, so this newly granted access may improve the vaccination rates of the community. The ED pharmacist has collaborated with the Department of Health to provide vaccinations during the H1N1 pandemic at health fairs, resulting in the vaccination of hundreds of people. In 2010, the ED pharmacist screened patients for the need for vaccinations from the ED.

Additionally, the ED pharmacist conducts emergency preparedness and training of all staff for disasters and has educated the media and the population about risk and mitigating strategies in the event of a terrorist attack.

30.9 BUILDING LAYERS OF DEFENSE AGAINST DRUG INJURY

30.9.1 Detecting and Preventing Drug Injury in the ED

The ED pharmacist has many responsibilities—for example, drug-related injury (detection/prevention), reviewing discharge prescriptions, trauma services, and code participation.[73] Furthermore, the ED has been recognized high-risk area for patients (60 percent) to be subjected to medication-related errors.[74–76] Most medication errors occur during the prescribing and administration phases of the drug delivery process. Boarded patient status, increasing number of medication orders, increasing number of medications administered, and part-time nursing status are associated with an increased risk of medication error.[77] Gregory et al. reviewed discharge prescriptions over a three-year period and identified a 16.5 percent error rate.[78] Rothschild et al. reported a medication error recovery rate (7.8 and 2.9 percent, respectively, for patients and medications) following a pharmacist review of medications—47.8 percent of mitigated errors were considered to be serious.[23] Stasiak et al. reported a pharmacist-identified prescription error rate of 3.2 percent—with respect to the prescriptions reviewed during a 25-day study period.[79] Prescription errors, as defined by Stasiak et al., are wrong dosing (28.3 percent), incomplete prescription (27.3), "other" medication errors (17.2), wrong frequency (15.2 percent), wrong medications (11.1), and wrong route (1 percent). Risk factors identified as contributing to prescription errors included age greater than 65, multiple prescriptions written for patients, and resident-written prescriptions.[79] In another study, Cesarz et al. reported an ED pharmacist intervention rate of 10.1 percent for discharge prescriptions—53.4 percent of ED discharge medications were prescribed during the operational hours of the ED pharmacy.[80] However, following the differentiation of pharmacist interventions for prescription-related errors, between adult and pediatric populations, a disparity is presented (8.5 and 23.6 percent, respectively). The types of interventions pharmacists made were similar between correcting medication errors versus optimizing medication therapy. Pharmacist discharge interventions (83.8 percent required ≤ 5 minutes) neither deterred from other pharmacist-related discharge activities, decreased the ED patient discharge efficiency, nor disrupted standard ED operations.[80] A refreshing observation from the study is that, counter to previously held opinions, decreased ED efficiency should not be attributed to pharmacists.[81] With up to 66 percent of adverse events related to medication error, occurring post-discharge from the hospital, pharmacist review of discharge medications lowers the rate of outpatient drug-related injury.[82]

Patanwala et al. compared pharmacist activities resulting in medication error interception. During the duration of their study, 2.2 percent of ED prescriptions resulted in medication errors. ED pharmacist consultation resulted in the greatest medication error interception (51.4 percent) compared to medication review of orders (34.9 percent). The majority of these errors occurred during the prescribing phase (82.4 percent), with only 9.3 percent of errors being minor.[83] Similar to previous studies, medication dosing was the cause of the majority of errors.[14] Pharmacist consultation can positively impact medication order clarification, the acquisition of accurate medication histories, and drug therapy recommendations.[83]

Greenwalt et al. implemented a series of interventions aimed at reducing weight-based dosing medication errors due to inaccurate estimated weights on patients presenting to the ED.[84] At baseline, 13.8 percent of patients had an estimated weight documented that varied more than 10 percent from later measured admission weights. After the implementation of the interventions, which included the removal of barriers to weighing patients, storytelling to engage staff and change culture, and removal of the estimated weight documentation field in the EMR, the number of errors decreased to zero.

Perez-Moreno et al. evaluated the clinical relevance of pharmacist interventions on patient care in a prospective observational study;[85] 991 interventions were recorded in 557 patients. Medications were considered severe in 57.2 percent of cases and 64.9 percent were considered relevant (based on a modified assessment scale of Overhage and Lukes). The severity of the medication error and the clinical significance were correlated.

Narcotic-opioid use is another area where ED pharmacists can assist with drug-related injury (prevention/detection). Opioid analgesic abuse is increasing in the United States, and the number of unintentional prescription overdose deaths has almost quadrupled since 1999.[86] Opioid prescriptions have increased from ~76 million (1991) to a peak of 219 million prescriptions (2011).[86] Patient mortality resulting from opioid overdose escalated to 16,651 and ED opioid prescriptions increased by 49 percent in 2010.[87,88] The increase in opioid prescriptions does not match the slight increase (8 percent) of patient admission to the ED. Hoppe et al. reported that the majority of ED opioid prescriptions (primarily immediate-release formulations) were small volume and were primarily written for immediate-release formulations.[89] Pharmacist intervention can result in a decrease in opiate-related patient mortality via the use of state-specific controlled substance monitoring databases and selecting alternative pain-relief medications. In light of the growing epidemic of narcotic abuse,[90] ED pharmacists, along with ED physicians, can not only assist opioid-dependent patients by decreasing both drug abuse and opioid-related injury but ultimately with opioid cessation. D'Onofrio et al. studied the effect of ED-initiated buprenorphine/naloxone administered to randomized ED patients and reported that, when coupled with a referral to a primary addiction service, ED patients were more likely to be both engaged with their addiction treatment and had greatly reduced the weekly frequency of illicit opioid use.[91]

A separate chapter on Dangers of Opiates is found in this book.

30.9.2 The ED Pharmacist and Community Surveillance for Adverse Drug Reactions

An adverse drug event or reaction (ADER) results in increased ED patient admissions; as high as 21 percent for adult patients and 0.5–3.3 percent for pediatric patients.[92,93] Hohl et al. reported a low rate (6.8 percent) of reported ADER resulting from outpatient medications compared to all possible identified ADER (28.1 percent).[94] As part of pharmacovigilance, MMC actively surveys and reports ED visits due to adverse drug reactions. Before July 1998, MMC's ADER reporting was accomplished by using an ADR "stat" line. The healthcare professional would leave a voice recording of the name and medical record number of the patient who had experienced the ADER. Although this system is convenient for pharmacies, it has little utility in a busy ED. The presence of the ED pharmacist and students surveying the computerized tracking board and assessing for ADERs to report (but also to confirm and assist in management) is convenient. The ED pharmacist's presence is beneficial, because it allows the pharmacist to track medication-related visits and medication-related problems that occur in the community and to visit the ED. Through this surveillance, the community clinicians are notified and educated about the event.

The ED pharmacist surveys for ADER and then records and files the reaction. An evaluation of the ADER is made using the Naranjo Algorithm. A report to MedWatch-FDA is filed, based on the severity of the reaction. The ADER is filed for in-hospital review and TJC requirements. The Naranjo Algorithm is detailed fully in the Evaluation of Medical Causation chapter by Marks elsewhere in this book.

Feedback on the ADER that occurred in the ED and methods of prevention are provided to the medical director and clinical staff. The following case illustrates the importance of ED pharmacist surveillance for potential ADERs.

A patient presented with shortness of breath and a headache. In the past, the patient was treated with subcutaneous sumatriptan for relief of migraine headaches. Prior to laboratory evaluation, the patient was given a subcutaneous dose of 6 mg of sumatriptan. The patient immediately developed chest pain and back pain. At the time there was no cardiac monitoring. It was concluded that this adverse event, because of its temporal relation, was sumatriptan-induced. The ED pharmacist requested an electrocardiogram (ECG) to ensure that there was no further ischemia. No changes were detected on the ECG. As the patient's clinical manifestations ran their course, it was clear that the initial headache was due, in part, to a urinary tract infection—not the migraine headache. The physician was educated on the fact that sumatriptan must be used with caution and with appropriate monitoring. Acetaminophen alone might have relieved the headache associated with this patient's infection. The patient was discharged and released from the ED with antibiotics. To further educate the clinicians, case reports of sumatriptan-induced vasospasm were provided, with certain predictive risk factors that would help them be alert to the risk factors for such an event.

30.10 PHARMACY PRACTICE IN THE ED: PHARMACOTHERAPY SPECIALTY

A clinical pharmacist may prevent drug injury through the use of consultation services. As discussed previously, pharmacy consultation is the leading contributor to the detection and prevention of drug-related injury via drug therapy recommendations—most frequently, recommendations are with respect to antimicrobial agents.[73] Berry et al. reported that a clinical pharmacist consultation service yielded consultation in 3 percent of all ED cases. The service was most highly used in July for new house staff.[95] Powell et al. described a 24-hour satellite pharmacy in a 75-bed ED.[96] From the satellite, the pharmacist mixed and distributed drugs, tracked inventory, took part in work rounds, instructed residents and students, and concurrently reviewed all medication orders. The authors describe the substantial benefits to patient care as a result of the pharmacist's clinical, distributive, and educational services. Aldridge et al. established a 24-hour clinical ED pharmacy program within the Veterans Affairs San Diego Healthcare System.[97] During the six-month implementation period, 9,568 interventions were recorded that were deemed to have a high probability of preventing serious harm to the patient. After the initial implementation period, providers and nurses were asked to identify the most important and beneficial duties provided by the ED pharmacist. The three most important roles identified were consultations with the clinical staff (27 percent), patient education (26 percent), and prospective medication order review (13 percent).[97] A survey conducted by Coralic et al., evaluating ED staff perception of the ED pharmacist, reported that a majority of ED staff strongly supported the presence of an ED pharmacist and agreed that they were more likely to consult [antimicrobial selection (89 percent) and non-anti-biotic medications (94 percent)] a pharmacist when they were on-site.[98] Inquiries relating to drug interactions were posed during all pharmacist consultations. A majority of the ED staff also agreed that pharmacists must/should be consulted for all high-risk medications or high-error potential medications.[98] In the survey of ED staff, Cesarz et al. almost all ED staff agreed that the pharmacist service improved patient safety. Similar to data reported in previous surveys, a majority of ED staff consulted/contacted the ED pharmacist at least once during their previous five shifts.[80] Treu et al. evaluated nursing satisfaction prior to the initiation of an EM pharmacist and one year after implementation.[99] All general pharmacy questions were improved at one year with timely resolution of pharmacy-related issues, medication procurement, and satisfaction with pharmacy services achieving statistical significance. The impact of the ED pharmacist on providing specialist consultation in the ED is demonstrated in the following case examples:

Case #1: A patient who ingested a quart of "OOPs" latex remover presented to the ED. The patient was stable at the time. The ED pharmacist was consulted for this toxicological emergency. The ED pharmacist investigated the case and provided recommendations that ensured that the standard of care was maintained. "OOPs" is considered a hydrocarbon; therefore, supportive management was recommended. However, the ED pharmacist recognized that the patient may have been a chronic alcoholic, and raised concerns about possible alcohol withdrawal. The "OOPs" contained ethyl alcohol. After further investigation, the son stated that his mother was a chronic alcoholic. The ED pharmacist estimated the alcohol level and recommended that alcohol-withdrawal management be initiated as soon as possible, to avoid delirium tremens. The patient was admitted to the medical intensive-care unit without going into alcohol withdrawal. She recovered and was subsequently discharged from the hospital. Thus, acute suffering due to delirium tremens was prevented.

Case #2: A stray cat bit a 61-year-old Caucasian female. The ED pharmacist was consulted to determine whether the patient, who was on warfarin, should receive intramuscular injections of rabies vaccination. After a review of the CDC guidelines, and of the patient's history and the circumstances of the bite, he concluded that the recommendation for the rabies vaccination was justified. The patient was counseled and the pharmacist verified her understanding of the risk for rabies. The patient agreed to have the rabies vaccine. Because of the empathic counseling and assurances provided by the ED pharmacist, the patient sent a letter to the chairman of the department, describing the excellent care she received in the ED. In summary, the generalist role of the ED pharmacist requires a diverse knowledge of pharmacotherapy.

Another commonly encountered ED problem, which could be positively impacted via pharmacy consultation, concerns the growing number of patients seeking primary care from the ED. Based on the results reported by the National Hospital Ambulatory Medical Care Survey, approximately 8 percent of ED visits were categorized as non-urgent.[12] Rising et al. reported access to timely follow-up appointments, increased convenience, and timely results are among the factors contributing to nine-day ED patient re-visit.[100] Baise et al. reported that telephone follow-up for patients (≥ 65 years old) were more likely to result in patient follow-up visits to their primary care provider—no change in the rate of prescription medication acquisition was observed and instances of pharmacist-initiated patient medication education were not evaluated.[101] Previous studies have shown that up to one-third of ED patients do not have their prescription(s) filled, even when the medication(s) are classified as priority medication(s) for the treatment of an acute condition.[102] Pharmacy intervention can lead to medication optimization and increased compliance.

30.11 SUMMARY AND CONCLUSIONS

Drug injury in the ED is not uncommon and represents a potential source of liability. Clinical pharmacists specially trained in acute stabilization—while providing general pharmaceutical care—may reduce this liability and help reduce risk by detecting, mitigating, preventing, and treating drug injury. Presently the role of the ED pharmacist is growing and becoming well accepted and desired by emergency healthcare teams. Outcome-based studies are emerging to demonstrate the operational and quality improvement associated with pharmacists practicing in the ED. Institutions not including pharmacists in the ED may be held liable if not including a pharmacist in the ED. Additionally, the risk is bidirectional—the ED pharmacist may have their scope of practice extended toward a provider role that makes their practice potentially risky if an adverse event occurs related to their expanded roles and functions.

REFERENCES

1. American College of Emergency Physicians. Clinical Pharmacist Services in the Emergency Department. https://www.acep.org/Clinical---Practice-Management/Clinical-Pharmacist-Services-in-the-Emergency-Department/. Accessed November 24, 2015.
2. American College of Medical Toxicology. ACMT Position Statement: The Role of Clinical Pharmacists in the Emergency Department, August 4, 2017. https://www.acmt.net/_Library/Po sitions/ACMT_Position_Pharmacist s.pdf. Accessed February 20, 2021.
3. Board of Pharmacy Specialties. Emergency Medicine Pharmacy Recognized as New Specialty. https://www.bpsweb.org/2020/02/21/emergency-medicine-pharmacy-recognized-as-new-specialty/. Accessed February 22, 2021.
4. Pedersen CA, Schneider PJ, Scheckelhoff DJ. ASHP national survey of pharmacy practice in hospital settings: Dispensing and administration—2008. Am J Health Syst Pharm. 2009;66(10):926–946.
5. Pedersen CA, Schneider PJ, Scheckelhoff DJ. ASHP national survey of pharmacy practice in hospital settings: Dispensing and administration—2014. Am J Health Syst Pharm. 2015;72(13):1119–1137.
6. Sin B, Lau K, Tong R, et al. The feasibility and impact of prospective medication review in the emergency department. J Pharm Pract. 2018 Feb;31(1):22–28.
7. Moore JJ, Matlock AG. Shared liability? Consultants, pharmacists, and the emergency physician: Legal cases and caveats. J Emerg Med. 2014;46(5):612–616.
8. Rozycki E, Bilhimer M, Bridgeman P, et al. Evaluation of burnout among emergency medicine pharmacists. J Am Coll Clin Pharm. 2020;3:1423–1433.
9. Zed PJ, Abu-Laban RB, Balen RM, et al. Incidence, severity and preventability of medication-related visits to the emergency department: A prospective study. CMAJ. 2008;178(12):1563–9.
10. Schenkel S. Promoting patient safety and preventing medical error in emergency departments. Acad Emerg Med. 2000;7(11):1204–1222.
11. Chin MH, Wang LC, Jin L. Appropriateness of medication selection for older persons in an urban academic emergency department. Acad Emerg Med. 1999;6(12):1232–1242.
12. Caterino JM, Emond JA, Camargo CA Jr. Inappropriate medication administration to the acutely ill elderly: A nationwide emergency department study, 1992–2000. J Am Geriatr Soc. 2004;52(11):1847–1855.
13. Marcin JP, Dharmar M, Cho M, et al. Medication errors among acutely ill and injured children treated in rural emergency departments. Ann Emerg Med. 2007;50(4):361–367, 367.e1–367.e2.
14. Pham JC, Story JL, Hicks RW, et al. National study on the frequency, types, causes and consequences of voluntarily reported emergency department medication errors. J Emerg Med. 2011;40(5):485–492.
15. Hafner JW Jr, Belknap SM, Squilante MD, et al. Adverse drug events in emergency department patients. Ann Emerg Med. 2002;43(3):258–267.
16. Herr RD, Caravati EM, Tyler LS, et al. Prospective evaluation of adverse drug interactions in the emergency department. Ann Emerg Med. 1992;21(11):1331–1336.
17. Beers MH, Storrie M, Lee G. Potential adverse drug interactions in the emergency room: An issue in the quality of care. Ann Intern Med. 1990;112(1):61–64.
18. Dabaghzadeh F, Rashidian A, Torkamandi H, et al. Medication errors in an emergency department in a large teaching hospital in Tehran. Iran J Pharm Res. 2013;12(4):937–942.
19. Peth HA Jr. Medication errors in the emergency department: A systems approach to minimizing risk. Emerg Med Clin North Am. 2003;21(1):141–158.
20. Burroughs TE, Waterman AD, Gallagher TH. Patient concerns about medical errors in emergency departments. Acad Emerg Med. 2005;12(1):57–64.
21. Scott BM, Considine J, Botti M. Medication errors in ED: Do patient characteristics and the environment influence the nature and frequency of medication errors? Australas Emerg Nurs J. 2014;17(4):167–175.

22. Goldberg RM, Mabee J, Chan L, et al. Drug-drug and drug-disease interactions in the ED: Analysis of a high-risk population. Am J Emerg Med. 1996;14(5):447–450.
23. Rothschild JM, Churchill W, Erickson A, et al. Medication errors recovered by emergency department pharmacists. Ann Emerg Med. 2010;55(6):513–521.
24. Rusnak RA, Stair TO, Hansen K, et al. Litigation against the emergency physician: Common features in cases of missed myocardial infarction. Ann Emerg Med. 1989;18:1029–1034.
25. Weant K, Bailey A, Baker S. Strategies for reducing medication errors in the emergency department. Emerg Med. 2014;4:45–55.
26. Stiell A, Forster AJ, Stiell IG, et al. Prevalence of information gaps in the emergency department and the effect on patient outcomes. CMAJ. 2003;169(10):1023–1028.
27. Juarez A, Gacki-Smith J, Bauer MR, et al. Barriers to emergency departments' adherence to four medication safety-related Joint Commission national patient safety goals. Jt Comm J Qual Patient Saf. 2009;35:49–59.
28. Wingert WA, Chan LS, Steward K, et al. A study of quality prescriptions issued in a busy pediatric emergency room. Public Health Rep. 1975;90:402–408.
29. Johnson KB, Butta JK, Donohue PK, et al. Discharging patients with prescriptions instead of medications: Sequelae in a teaching hospital. Pediatrics. 1996;97(4):481–485.
30. Roberts RW, Russell WL. A pharmacist-based toxicology service. Drug Intell Clin Pharm. 1978;12(11):665–670.
31. Rapp RP, Piecoro JJ, Swintosky JV. The value of emergency care situations in the clinical education of a pharmacist. Ann Pharmacother. 2006;40(4):742–746.
32. Edwards GA, Samuels TM. The role of the hospital pharmacist in emergency situations. Am J Hosp Pharm. 1968;25(3):128–133.
33. Elenbass RM, Waeckerle JF, McNabey WK. The clinical pharmacist in emergency medicine. Am J Hosp Pharm. 1977;34:843–846.
34. Lada P, Delgado G Jr. Documentation of pharmacists' interventions in an emergency department and associated cost avoidance. Am J Health Syst Pharm. 2007;64(1):63–68.
35. Ortmann MJ, Johnson EG, Jarrell DH, et al. ASHP guidelines on emergency medicine pharmacist services. Am J Health Syst Pharm. 2021;78:21–275.
36. Thomas MC, Acquisto NM, Shirk MB, et al. A national survey of emergency pharmacy practice in the United States. Am J Health Syst Pharm. 2016;73:386–394.
37. Vollman KE, Adams CB, Shah MN, et al. Survey of emergency medicine pharmacy education opportunities for students and residents. Hosp Pharm. 2015;50:690–699.
38. ASHP. Online Residency Directory. Emergency medicine pharmacy. https://accreditation.ashp.org/directory/#/program/residency. Accessed March 2, 2021.
39. ASHP. Online Residency Directory. Critical care pharmacy. https://accreditation.ashp.org/directory/#/program/residency. Accessed March 2, 2021.
40. ASHP Launches Emergency Medicine Certificate [Press Release]. Bethesda, MD, June 6, 2019. https://www.ashp.org/news/2019/06/06/emergency-medicine-certificate?loginreturnUrl=SSOCheckOnly. Accessed March 2, 2021.
41. Fairbanks RJ, Rueckmann EA, Kolstee KE, et al. Clinical pharmacists in emergency medicine. In *Advances in Patient Safety: New Directions and Alternative Approaches (Vol. 4: Technology and Medication Safety)*. Rockville, MD: Agency for Healthcare Research and Quality (US), 2008 August. http://www.ncbi.nlm.nih.gov/books/NBK43767/pdf/Bookshelf_NBK43767.pdf. Accessed November 24, 2015.
42. Schwerman E, Schwartau N, Thompson CO, et al. The Pharmacist as a member of the cardiopulmonary resuscitation team. Drug Intell Clin Pharm. 1973;7:299–308.
43. Draper HM, Eppert JA. Association of pharmacist presence on compliance with advanced cardiac life support guidelines during in-hospital cardiac arrest. Ann Pharmacother. 2008;42:469–474.
44. Roman C, Edwards G, Dooley M, et al. Roles of the emergency medicine pharmacist: A systematic review. Am J Health-Syst Pharm. 2018;75:796–806.
45. Vest TA, Musch KLE. Expanding pharmacy services in the ED. *Pharmacy Purchasing & Products*, May 2019. Accessed March 2, 2021.
46. McCoy S. *Optimizing Pharmacists' Role in the Emergency Department.* Wolters Kluwer. Accessed March 2, 2021.
47. Carter B. How many of us provide pharmaceutical care. Pharmacotherapy. 1997;17(4):845–846.
48. Randolph TC. Expansion of pharmacists responsibilities in an emergency department. Am J Health-Syst Pharm. 2009;66:1484–1487.
49. Acquisto NM, Baker SN. Antimicrobial stewardship in the emergency department. J Pharm Pract. 2011;24(2):196–202.
50. Randolph TC, Parker A, Meyer L, et al. Effect of a pharmacist-managed culture review process on antimicrobial therapy in an emergency department. Am J Health Syst Pharm. 2011 May 15;68(10):916–919.
51. Baker SN, Acquisto NM, Ashley ED, et al. Pharmacist-managed antimicrobial stewardship program for patients discharged from the emergency department. J Pharm Pract. 2012 Apr;25(2):190–194.
52. Sandhoff BG, Kuca S, Rasmussen J, et al. Collaborative cardiac care service: A multidisciplinary approach to caring for patients with coronary artery disease. Perm J. 2008 Summer;12(3):4–11.
53. Becerra-Camargo J, Martinez-Martinez F, Garcia-Jimenez E. A multicentre, double-blind, randomised, controlled, parallel-group study of the effectiveness of a pharmacist-acquired medication history in an emergency department. BMC Health Serv Res. 2013;13:337.
54. Okere NA, Gessert C, Renier C, et al. Effects of medication reconciliation service provided by student pharmacists. Pharm Pract. 2013;4(2):1–9.
55. American College of Emergency Physicians. *State of the Art: Observation Units in the Emergency Department.* Policy Resource and Education Paper. http://www.acep.org/workarea/DownloadAsset.aspx?id=82436. Accessed December 29, 2015.
56. The Joint Commission. Using medication reconciliation to prevent errors. http://www.jointcommission.org/assets/1/18/SEA_35.pdf. Accessed December 29, 2015.
57. Yap D. *Federal Bill for Provider Status Recognition Reintroduced.* American Pharmacists Association, January 28, 2015. Web. May 26, 2015.
58. Cater SW, Luzum M, Serra AE, et al. A prospective cohort study of medication reconciliation using pharmacy technicians in the emergency department to reduce medication errors among admitted patients. J Emerg Med. 2015;48(2):230–238.
59. Tam VA, Knowles SR, Cornish PL, et al. Frequency, type and clinical importance of medication history errors at admission to hospital: A systematic review. CMAJ. 2005;173(5):510–515.

60. The Joint Commission. *National Patient Safety Goals Effective January 1, 2015*. Hospital Accreditation Program. http://www.jointcommission.org/assets/1/6/2015_NPSG_HAP.pdf. Accessed November 24, 2015.
61. Schneider ME. Reconciliation standards debut July 1. *ACEP News*. http://www.acep.org/Content.aspx?id=80781. Accessed November 24, 2015.
62. De Winter S, Vanbrabant P, Spriet I, et al. A simple tool to improve medication reconciliation at the emergency department. Eur J Intern Med. 2011;22(4):382–385.
63. Australian Commission on Safety and Quality in Health Care. *National Medication Management Plan User Guide*. ACSQHC, Sydney, 2009. http://www.safetyandquality.gov.au/wp-content/uploads/2010/01/Medication-Management-Plan-User-Guide.pdf. Accessed November 24, 2015.
64. Carter MK, Allin DM, Scott LA, et al. Pharmacist-acquired medication histories in a university hospital emergency department. Am J Health Syst Pharm. 2006;63(24):2500–2503.
65. Bond CA, Raehl CL, Franke T. Clinical pharmacy services and hospital mortality rates. Pharmacotherapy. 1999;19(5):556–564.
66. Nester TM, Ladonna HS. Effectiveness of a pharmacist-acquired medication history in promoting patient safety. Am J Health Syst Pharm. 2002;59(22):2221–2225.
67. Hayes BD, Donovan JL, Smith BS, et al. Pharmacist-conducted medication reconciliation in an emergency department. Am J Health Syst Pharm. 2007;64(16):1720–1723.
68. Hart C, Price C, Graziose G, et al. A program using pharmacy technicians to collect medication histories in the emergency department. *Pharm Therapeut*. 2015;40(1):56–61.
69. Johnston R, Saulnier L, Gould O. Best possible medication history in the emergency department: Comparing pharmacy technicians and pharmacists. Can J Hosp Pharm. 2010;63(5):359–365.
70. Czajka PA, Skoutakis VA, Wood GC. Clinical toxicology consultation by pharmacists. Am J Hosp Pharm. 1979;36:1087–1089.
71. Cannon CP. Thrombolysis medication errors: Benefits of bolus thrombolytic agents. Am J Card. 2000;85(8A):17C–22C.
72. Acquisto NM, Hays DP, Fairbanks RJ, et al. The outcomes of emergency pharmacist participation during acute myocardial infarction. J Emerg Med. 2012;42(4):371–378.
73. Cohen V, Jellinek SP, Hatch A, et al. Effect of clinical pharmacists on care in the emergency department: A systematic review. Am J Health-Syst Pharm. 2009;66:1353–1361.
74. Kohn LT, Corrigan J, Donaldson MS, eds. *To Err is Human: Building a Safer Health System*. Washington, DC: National Academy Press, 2000.
75. Kulstad EB, Sikka R, Sweis RT, et al. ED overcrowding is associated with an increased frequency of medication errors. Am J Emerg Med. 2010;28:304–309.
76. Patanwala AE, Warholak TL, Sanderset AB, et al. A prospective observational study of medication errors in a tertiary care emergency department. Ann Emerg Med. 2010;55:522–526.
77. Shahis S, Shafqat S. Emergency pharmacist: A safety valve in hospital emergency. Bangladesh J Med Sci. 2013;12(1):10–16.
78. Gregory H, Cantley M, Calhoun C, et al. Incidence of prescription errors in patients discharged from the emergency department. Am J Emerg Med. 2020 Jul 25;46:266–270.
79. Stasiak P, Afilalo M, Castelino T, et al. Detection and correction of prescription errors by an emergency department pharmacy service. CJEM. 2014;16(3):193–206.
80. Cesarz JL, Steffenhagen AL, Svenson J, et al. Emergency department discharge prescription interventions by emergency medicine pharmacists. Ann Emerg Med. 2013;61(2):209–214.
81. Sorelle R. EM groups persuade Joint Commission to temper pharmacy review policy. Emerg Med News. 2007;29:1–4. Editorial.
82. Forster AJ, Murff HJ, Peterson JF, et al. The incidence and severity of adverse events affecting patients after discharge from the hospital. Ann Intern Med. 2003;138(3):161–167.
83. Patanwala AE, Sanders AB, Thomas MC, et al. A prospective, multicenter study of pharmacist activities resulting in medication error interception in the emergency department. Ann Emerg Med. 2012;59(5):369–373.
84. Greenwalt M, Griffen D, Wilkerson J. Elimination of emergency department medication errors due to estimated weights. BMJ Qual Improve Rep. 2017;6:u214416.w5476.
85. Perez-Moreno MA, Rodriguez-Camacho JM, Calderon-Hernanz B, et al. Clinical relevance of pharmacist intervention in an emergency department. Emerg Med J. 2017;34:495–501.
86. Owens P, Mutter R, Stocks C. Substance Abuse and Mental Health Services Administration. *Drug Abuse Warning Network, 2007: National Estimates of Drug-Related Emergency Department Visits*. National Library of Medicine.
87. Mack KA. Drug-induced deaths: United States, 1999–2010. MMWR Surveill Summ. 2013 Nov 22;62(Suppl 3):161–163.
88. Amirshahi M, Mullins P, Rasooly L, et al. Rising opioid prescribing in adult U.S. Emergency Department visits: 2001–2010. Acad Emerg Med. 2014;21(3):236–243.
89. Hoppe JA, Kim H, Heard K. Association of emergency department opioid initiation with recurrent opioid use. Ann Emerg Med. 2015;65(5):493–499.
90. Centers for Disease Control and Prevention (CDC). National hospital ambulatory medical care survey: 2011 emergency department summary tables. http://www.cdc.gov/nchs/data/ahcd/nhamcs_emergency/2011_ed_web_tables.pdf. Accessed December 29, 2015.
91. D'Onofrio G, O'Connor PG, Pantalon MV, et al. Emergency department–initiated buprenorphine/naloxone treatment for opioid dependence: A randomized clinical trial. JAMA. 2015;313(16):1636–1644.
92. Queneau P, Bannwarth B, Carpentier F, et al. Emergency department visits caused by adverse drug events: Results of a French survey. Drug Saf. 2007;30(1):81–88.
93. Zed PJ, Haughn C, Black KJ. Medication-related emergency department visits and hospital admissions in pediatric patients: A qualitative systematic review. J Pediatr. 2013;163(2):477–483.
94. Hohl CM, Kuramoto L, Yu E, et al. Evaluating adverse drug event reporting in administrative data from emergency departments: A validation study. BMC Health Serv Res. 2013;13:473.
95. Berry NS, Folstad JE, Bauman JL, et al. Follow-up observations on 24-hour pharmacotherapy services in the emergency department. Ann Pharmacother. 1992;26:476–480.
96. Powell MF, Solomon DK, McEachen RA. Twenty-four hour emergency pharmaceutical services. Am J Hosp Pharm. 1985;42:831–835.

97. Aldridge VE, Park HK, Bounthavong M, et al. Implementing a comprehensive, 24-hour emergency department program. Am J Health-Syst Pharm. 2009;66:1943–1947.
98. Coralic Z, Kanzaria HK, Bero L, et al. Staff perceptions of an on-site clinical pharmacist program in an academic emergency department after one year. West J Emerg Med. 2014;15(2):205–210.
99. Treu CN, Llamzon JL, Acquisto NM, et al. The impact of an emergency medicine clinical pharmacist on nursing satisfaction. Int J Clin Pharm. 2019 Dec;41(6):1618–1624.
100. Rising K, Padrez K, O'Brien M, et al. Return visits to the emergency department: The patient perspective. Ann Emerg Med. 2015;65(4):377–386.
101. Biese K, Lamantia M, Shofer F, et al. A randomized trial exploring the effect of a telephone call follow-up on care plan compliance among older adults discharged home from the emergency department. Acad Emerg Med. 2014;21(2):188–195.
102. Kajioka EH, Itoman EM, Li ML, et al. Pediatric prescription pick-up rates after ED visits. Am J Emerg Med. 2005;23(4):454–458.

31 Pharmacy Case Law Review

Roger N. Morris and William J. Stilling

SYNOPSIS

DOI: 10.1201/9781003615323-34

31.1 ADMINISTRATIVE LAW

31.1.1 Due Process—Pharmacist Licensure

31.1.1.1 *Berjikian, et al. v. Franchise Tax Board et al.*, No. CV 13—06301 DDP, 2015 WL 1185472 (C.D. Cal. March 12, 2015)

RELIEF SOUGHT: Plaintiffs, "tax delinquents," filed a motion for summary judgment after suing the California Tax Board, DMV, and Board of pharmacy, alleging violation of their due process rights under the Fourteenth Amendment.

ISSUE: Did state agencies deprive plaintiffs of due process under the Fourteenth Amendment by not providing a hearing before depriving them of driver's licenses and pharmacy licenses?

FACTS AND PROCEDURAL HISTORY: A pharmacist, Berjikian, was listed on California's Franchise Tax Board's "top 500 tax delinquents." The pharmacist did not deny she owed approximately $450,000 in state income taxes. Pursuant to California law, the Board of Pharmacy suspended her pharmacy license because of the tax delinquencies. The plaintiff filed a summary judgment motion stating that she was not provided the opportunity to challenge the tax liability or the resulting license suspension.

REASONING: California law did not afford the pharmacist a meaningful opportunity to be heard at a meaningful time regarding the suspension of her license, and operated retroactively to penalize her for past conduct. "Courts have long recognized that licenses which enable one to pursue a profession or earn a livelihood are protected property interests for purposes of a Fourteenth Amendment analysis." At the time, the state notified the pharmacist that she would lose her license, and her right to a hearing regarding the tax debts had expired.

The Board of Pharmacy did not provide an opportunity to challenge the license revocations. The court also found that the pharmacist's license was subject to protected property interests under the Fourteenth Amendment and could only be removed subject to procedural due process.

HOLDING: The court granted the pharmacist's motion for summary judgment because California deprived her of due process by not affording her a meaningful opportunity to be heard.

31.2 ANTITRUST

31.2.1 State Regulatory Boards Immunity

31.2.1.1 *North Carolina Bd. of Dental Examiners. v. Federal Trade Commission,* 135 S. Ct. 1101 (Feb. 25, 2015)

RELIEF SOUGHT: FTC sought injunctive relief against the North Carolina Board of Dental Examiners to stop the Board from: (i) prohibiting non-dentists from providing teeth whitening services or products, (ii) discouraging the provision of such goods or services, and (iii) communicating to third parties that such provision violated state law.

ISSUES:

1. Were the Board's actions anti-competitive?
2. Were the Board's actions protected by state-action immunity?

FACTS AND PROCEDURAL HISTORY: The North Carolina Dental Practice Act stated that the Board was "the agency of the state for the regulation of the practice of dentistry," and that the Board may file suit to enjoin any person from unlawfully practicing dentistry. The statute required an eight-member board: (i) six members to be licensed dentists; (ii) one to be a dental hygienist; and (iii) one to be a "consumer" appointed by the Governor.

The Board began to receive dentist complaints about non-dentists conducting teeth whitening services. Few of the complaints warned of potential harm to clients, but most focused on low prices charged by non-dentists. These individuals competed directly with teeth-whitening services from dentists. The Board opened an investigation in response to complaints. The dentist member led the inquiry while the hygienist and consumer members did not participate.

The Board sent multiple "cease and desist" letters on Board letterhead to the unlicensed individuals seeking to impose fines or other liability for unlicensed practice of dentistry, a violation of the Dental Practice Act. The Board also convinced the "North Carolina Board of Cosmetic Art Examiners to warn cosmetologists against providing teeth whitening services."

The letters were effective. Non-dentists stopped offering teeth whitening in NC. No Board rule or regulation was developed, even though the Act did not specify that teeth whitening be considered dental practice. FTC challenged the Board's actions, claiming actions to be anti-competitive and an unfair method of competition. The Board argued it was operating under its state regulatory powers to protect the health and safety of North Carolina citizens ("State Action Doctrine"). The Board sought immunity under the doctrine.

An ALJ denied the Board's motion to dismiss and concluded the Board's actions were anti-competitive, unreasonably restrained trade, and violated federal law. The Fourth Circuit affirmed.

REASONING: The U.S. Supreme Court explained that anti-trust laws are a "central safeguard" for a free market. However, states often pass laws and regulate economic activities that would normally run afoul of antitrust laws as restrictions on occupations or other restrictions on competition to further other public objectives. Therefore, states acting within their sovereign powers are not subject to antitrust laws. This is known as *Parker* immunity after the *Parker v. Brown*, 317 U.S. 341, 63 S.Ct. 307 (1943), the case that established state immunity from antitrust laws.

The N.C. Board argued the state gave its members the power of the state to regulate dentistry and the *Parker* immunity protected them from antitrust claims. The court rejected this argument because:

> A nonsovereign actor controlled by active market participants—such as the Board—enjoys *Parker* immunity only if it satisfies two requirements: "first that 'the challenged restraint . . . be one clearly articulated and affirmatively expressed as state policy,' and second that 'the policy . . . be actively supervised by the State.'"

The court and the parties assumed the first requirement for a clearly articulated and affirmatively expressed state policy had been met. The law prohibits the unlicensed practice of dentistry. However, the law does not address teeth whitening. However, the Board did not receive active supervision from the state when it interpreted the law to prohibit teeth whitening by non-dentists and issued cease-and-desist letters to non-dentists. Here, the dentist Board members were market participants who could gain financially from limiting competition by non-dentists, which the court noted is the "very risk of self-dealing" that the active supervision requirement was created to address.

The question that must be answered in evaluating sufficient state supervision "is whether the State's review mechanisms provide 'realistic assurance' that a nonsovereign actor's anticompetitive conduct 'promotes state policy, rather than merely the party's individual interests.'" The court noted a few constant requirements of active supervision: [i] The supervisor must review the substance of the anticompetitive decision, not merely the procedures followed to produce it; [ii] the supervisor must have the power to veto or modify particular decisions to ensure they accord with state policy; and [iii] the "mere potential for state supervision is not an adequate substitute for a decision by the State[; and iv] . . .the state supervisor may not itself be an active market participant. In general, however, the adequacy of supervision otherwise will depend on all the circumstances of a case" (citations omitted).

HOLDINGS: The Supreme Court affirmed the Fourth Circuit's decision, finding:

1. The Board's actions were anti-competitive.
2. The Board's actions were not protected by state-action immunity.

NOTE: After the Supreme Court's decision in *North Carolina Bd. of Dental Examiners*, the FTC issued *FTC Staff Guidance on Active Supervision of State Regulatory Boards Controlled by Market Participants* to help states evaluate whether their regulatory boards will receive *Parker* immunity. This guidance can be found at: https://www.ftc.gov/system/files/attachments/competition-policy-guidance/active_supervision_of_state_boards.pdf

31.3 CIVIL PROCEDURE

31.3.1 Spoliation of Evidence—Pharmacy's Duty to Maintain Evidence of Misfill

31.3.1.1 *Burton v. Walgreens Co.*, 2015 WL 4228854 (D. Nev. July 10, 2015)

RELIEF SOUGHT: Patient sought sanctions against pharmacy for willful spoliation of evidence after Walgreens destroyed the bottle and the pills returned after a misfill.

ISSUES:

1. Did Walgreens have a duty to preserve evidence (bottle/pills)?
2. Was Walgreens on notice of potential litigation due to misfill?

FACTS AND PROCEDURAL HISTORY: Walgreens' patient received a prescription for an antihypertensive prescription (Diovan). The prescription instructed the patient to take one tablet of Diovan by mouth daily. A Walgreens pharmacist misfiled a patient's prescription with a mix of Diovan and Lithium pills (same color, but differently shaped pills). The patient took it as instructed. The wife noticed two differently shaped pills, reported it to Walgreens, and returned the pills/bottle to the pharmacy. The patient experienced numbness and weakness in his left hand and was later hospitalized. Hospital records showed patient took approximately one 300 mg lithium pill per day for 5 days. The patient claimed the hospital learned of lithium intake from communication with Walgreens pharmacists.

As the patient's symptoms worsened over time, he was diagnosed with carpal tunnel syndrome and polyneuropathy as a result of improper ingestion of lithium. The patient underwent surgery on the hand/arm but suffered residual pain and stiffness. The patient sued Walgreens alleging various claims of negligence. During the initial discovery, the patient asked for Walgreens policies for dealing with misfills and for the returned medications and original bottles so the suspect pills could be tested to determine if they were actually lithium. Walgreens informed the patient that the bottle and pills were destroyed in accordance with store policy.

The plaintiff filed a motion for spoliation sanctions and asked the court to strike the defendant's answer and affirmative defenses on liability and causation. The plaintiff also sought a bench trial to determine the sole remaining issue of the plaintiff's damages. As an alternative, the plaintiff requested an adverse inference jury instruction, which would have allowed the jury to presume the missing evidence would have supported the plaintiff's negligence claim. The plaintiff further asked the court to exclude any evidence that would controvert the adverse inference. Finally, the plaintiff sought attorneys' fees and costs expended to prepare the motion for sanctions.

REASONING: "Spoliation is the destruction or significant alteration of evidence or the failure to preserve property for another's use as evidence pending or reasonably foreseeable litigation." The court reasoned, "When a defendant destroys evidence according to its internal policies or the normal course of business, that defendant has not engaged in the spoliation of evidence if the defendant had no notice of the evidence's potential relevance in future litigation." No evidence showed Walgreens' pharmacist purposefully and willfully destroyed evidence. Medication was destroyed as directed by store policy.

Further, Walgreens was on notice of potential litigation due to its error. Return of incorrectly filled medication by the patient, triggered the duty to preserve evidence. Walgreens had a duty to preserve, but the plaintiff faced no prejudice from spoliation because Walgreens admitted the misfill. The plaintiff had ample evidence to show lithium caused harm.

HOLDING: The court denied the plaintiff's motion because Walgreens admitted the error and there was no prejudice from the destruction of the prescription.

1. Walgreens did not have a duty to preserve evidence because the evidence was destroyed in accordance with its internal policies. The evidence was not destroyed purposefully or willfully.
2. Walgreens was on notice of potential litigation.

31.4 CONSCIENTIOUS OBJECTION

31.4.1 Emergency Contraception

31.4.1.1 *Stormans, Inc. v. Wiesman*, 794 F.3d 1064 (9th Cir. 2015)

RELIEF SOUGHT: Pharmacy and pharmacists with religious objections to dispensing emergency contraceptives, brought action against the Washington Pharmacy Quality Assurance Commission challenging the rules requiring a pharmacy to deliver or dispense drugs.

ISSUE: Are Washington's pharmacy regulations, requiring pharmacies and pharmacists to deliver and dispense drugs, unconstitutional?

FACTS AND PROCEDURAL HISTORY: Stormans Inc., which owns Ralph's Pharmacy, declined to stock the pharmacy with emergency contraceptive drugs, like Plan B or Ella "because the pharmacy owners have religious objections to their use." The pharmacists were also unwilling to dispense the emergency contraceptives for religious reasons. If a patient requested these drugs, the pharmacists would refer the patient to another pharmacy. Washington's pharmacy rules permit a "religiously objecting individual pharmacist to deny delivery, so long as another pharmacist working for the pharmacy provides timely delivery. But, unless an enumerated exemption applies, the rules require a pharmacy to deliver all prescription medications, even if the owner of the pharmacy has a religious objection." Stormans challenged the rules on Free Exercise, Equal Protection, and other constitutional grounds. In 2007, the district court granted a preliminary injunction prohibiting enforcement of the delivery rule. In 2009, the Ninth Circuit reversed the decision, finding the regulations (requiring pharmacists to stock emergency contraceptives) did not target religious conduct. In 2012, the district court found the regulations unconstitutional. Defendants appealed.

REASONING: "The right to own, operate, or work at a licensed professional business free from regulations requiring the business to engage in activities that one sincerely believes lead to the taking of a human life," is not a fundamental liberty interest. Under the Free Exercise Clause, "Congress shall make no law prohibiting the free exercise of religion." The right to free exercise of religion "does not relieve an individual of the obligation to comply with a valid and neutral law of general applicability on the ground that the law prescribes conduct that his religion prescribes."

The pharmacy rules apply to "all objections to delivery that do not fall within an exemption, regardless of the motivation behind those objections." Any refusal to dispense a medication violates the rules, regardless of whether the refusal is motivated by religion, morals, ethics, etc. "The delivery requirement also applies to all prescription products—not just Plan B or ella." The rule's effect would "extend beyond Plan B, for example, by guaranteeing access to medications for HIV patients." A law is not generally applicable if it "in a selective manner, imposes, burdens only on conduct motivated by religious belief." Further, as held in the earlier opinion, "the enumerated exemptions are 'necessary reasons for failing to fill a prescription' in that they allow pharmacies to operate in the normal course of business." The exemptions "increase access to medications by making it possible for pharmacies to comply with the rules, further patient safety, and maintain their business." Because the pharmacy rules are neutral and generally applicable, the Court reviewed the rules using a rational basis standard. Under rational basis review, the Court must uphold the rules if they are rationally related to a legitimate governmental purpose.

HOLDING: The delivery rules are constitutional. They are "rationally related to Washington's legitimate interest in ensuring that its citizens have safe and timely access to their lawful and lawfully prescribed medications."

SUBSEQUENT ACTIVITY: A petition for a writ of certiorari is pending before the U.S. Supreme Court. A response to the petition is due on March 7, 2016.

31.5 CONTROLLED SUBSTANCES

31.5.1 Duty to Verify DEA Registration

31.5.1.1 *Farmacia, Yani*, 80 Fed. Reg. 29,053 (May 20, 2015)

31.5.1.2 *JM Pharmacy Group Inc., d/b/a/ Farmacia Nueva and Best Pharma Corp.*, 80 Fed. Reg. 28,667 (May 19, 2015)

RELIEF SOUGHT: In two separate DEA actions against pharmacies, each pharmacy appealed the decision of an administrative law judge ("ALJ") to deny applications for DEA registration.

ISSUE: Does a pharmacy have a duty to verify the DEA registration of prescribers under the DEA's corresponding liability regulation?

FACTS AND PROCEDURAL HISTORY: In *JM Pharmacy*, the DEA claimed two pharmacies filled more than 170 prescriptions for a physician whose DEA registration had been revoked. *Farmacia Yani* involved allegations that the pharmacy filled more than 200 prescriptions for controlled substances for a physician whose DEA registration had been revoked. Both cases involved additional, detailed facts that the ALJ used as bases for denying the registrations. The most important basis for denial for purposes of this summary is ALJ's finding that the pharmacies could have checked the prescribers' registration on the DEA diversion website, contacted the local DEA office, or contracted with a private service to obtain DEA verifications.

REASONING: The DEA Administrator (Administrator) reviewed the ALJ's decision and analyzed the corresponding liability section of the DEA regulations and other applicable laws and regulations.

§ 1306.04 Purpose of issue of prescription.

(a) A prescription for a controlled substance to be effective must be issued for a legitimate medical purpose by an individual practitioner acting in the usual course of his professional practice. The responsibility for the proper prescribing and dispensing of controlled substances is upon the prescribing practitioner, but a corresponding responsibility rests with the pharmacist who fills the prescription. An order purporting to be a prescription issued not in the usual course of professional treatment or in legitimate and authorized research is not a prescription within the meaning and intent of section 309 of the Act (*21 U.S.C. § 829*) and the person knowingly filling such a purported prescription, as well as the person issuing it, shall be subject to the penalties provided for violations of the provisions of law relating to controlled substances.

The Administrator noted that under this section, the pharmacist must act knowingly or intentionally. Moreover, there is no requirement in the Controlled Substances Act or DEA regulations that require a pharmacist to verify a prescriber's DEA registration before dispensing a controlled substance prescription. To meet this requirement, a pharmacist must have knowledge or reason to know a prescription is not valid. The Administrator explained the pharmacists violated a duty to periodically check whether a prescriber had retained authority to practice medicine and dispense controlled substances. The Administrator further noted that the DEA must provide some guidance on the scope of this duty before the DEA will do anything more than give "nominal weight" to such a duty. The Administrator concluded that a pharmacist must have knowledge that a prescription is not valid but also mentioned an amorphous duty to verify DEA registration. In *JM Pharmacy,* the Administrator denied the registration case because the pharmacy had falsified its application for registration.

HOLDING: In the *Farmacia Yani* case, the Administrator afforded minimal weight to the failure to verify DEA registrations and held the DEA application in abeyance for six months until the pharmacy personnel completed a course on controlled substances dispensing and corresponding liability. In *JM Pharmacy Group*, the Administrator likewise gave nominal weight to the pharmacists not ensuring the DEA numbers were current but denied the registration because the pharmacy falsified its renewal application.

31.5.2 Constitutionality

31.5.2.1 *McFadden v. United States,* 135 S. Ct. 2298 (June 18, 2015)

RELIEF SOUGHT: Defendant appealed jury's conviction for distribution of controlled substance analogues because the jury instructions failed to include the applicable mental state required for the crime.

ISSUE: Did the district court's jury instructions fail to convey the correct mental state as required by the Analogue Act?

FACTS AND PROCEDURAL HISTORY: In 2011, Police were investigating the use and distribution of bath salts. Using informants and investigators, police received information that bath salts were being sold by McFadden. McFadden was indicted on eight counts of distribution of controlled substance analogues. The government sought a jury instruction requiring only that the defendant knowingly and intentionally distribute a mixture or substance that was a controlled substance analogue with the intent that it be consumed by humans. McFadden sought a more demanding instruction requiring that the defendant knew that the substances he was distributing possessed the characteristics of controlled substance analogues.

The district court compromised and instructed the jury that the statute required that the defendant knowingly and intentionally distribute a mixture or substance that has substantially similar effects on the nervous system as a controlled substance and that the defendant intended for the mixture or substance to be consumed by humans. At trial, McFadden argued that he did not know the substances were regulated as controlled substances under the Analogue Act. McFadden was convicted on all nine counts. On appeal, McFadden insisted that the district court erred in refusing to instruct the jury that the government was required to prove that he knew that the substance had characteristics of controlled substance analogues.

Court of Appeals rejected McFadden's argument and affirmed, stating that the intent element "requires [only] that the government prove that the defendant meant for the substance at issue to be consumed by humans." McFadden appealed.

REASONING: "The Analogue Act requires a controlled substance analogue, if intended for human consumption, to be treated 'as a controlled substance in schedule I.'" The Controlled Substance Act makes it "unlawful for any person knowingly . . . to distribute . . . a controlled substance" § 841(a)(1). "The word 'knowingly' applies not just to the statute's verbs but also to the object of those verbs—'a controlled substance.'" Thus, §841(a)(1) requires a defendant to only know that the substance he is dealing with is some unspecified substance listed on the federal drug schedules. For example, this requirement "may be met by showing the defendant knew he possessed a substance listed on the schedules, even if he did not know which substance it was"; or, by showing that the defendant knew the identity of the substance he possessed.

How does the knowledge requirement apply to controlled substance *analogues*? Because the requirement of §841(a)(1) carries over to controlled substance analogues, the government must prove the defendant knew the substance was a controlled substance. This requirement can be established and satisfied in two ways. The government can provide evidence that a defendant knew: (i) the substance is some controlled substance, regardless of whether he knew the particular identify; or (ii) the specific analogue he was dealing with, even if he did not know its legal status as an analogue.

The court determined that the court of appeals did not adhere to this standard and did not apply the correct mental state requirement. "Instead, it concluded that the only mental state requirement for prosecutions involving controlled substance analogues" is the "intended for human consumption" requirement. This is inconsistent with the statutes. The district court's instructions to the jury did not fully convey the mental state required by the Analogue Act. Although the government contended that, any error in the jury instructions was harmless because no rational jury could have concluded that McFadden was unaware that bath salts were controlled, SCOTUS recognized that even the omission of an element from a jury charge is subject to the harmless error analysis.

HOLDING: The court vacated the judgment because jury instructions failed to convey the correct mental state as required by the Analogue Act and remanded the case to the Fourth Circuit.

31.6 CRIMINAL

31.6.1 Violations of Pharmacy Law Applied to Non-Pharmacists

31.6.1.1 *Moore v. State of Florida*, No. 1D14-3527, 2015 WL 4464689 (Fla. Dist. Ct. App. July 21, 2015), Reh'g Denied (Sept. 1, 2015)

RELIEF SOUGHT: Defendant sought reversal of judgment and sentence after he was found guilty of violation of the Florida Controlled Substance Act and Pharmacy Act.

ISSUE: Can Florida criminally charge a non-pharmacist for violation of its pharmacy practice act (Fla. Stat. Ann. § 465.015) for dispensing a prescription drug without a prescription?

FACTS AND PROCEDURAL HISTORY: The defendant faced drug charges for: (Count I) possession of oxycodone with intent to sell, in violation of § 893.13(1)(a) of Florida's Controlled Substance Act and (ii) (Count II) selling or dispensing a prescription drug without first being furnished a prescription, in violation of § 465.015(2)(c) of Florida's Pharmacy Law.

The state presented evidence the defendant sold or delivered an oxycodone tablet to a confidential informant in a cigarette box. The informant exchanged the tablet for a $20 bill and returned the box to the defendant. At the close of the state's case, the defendant moved for acquittal, arguing §465 did not apply to him because he was not a pharmacist.

The defendant argued that the part of § 465.015(2)(c) that prohibited dispensing a drug without a prescription was not applicable to him because he was not a pharmacist. The trial court rejected his argument and the jury returned a guilty verdict on both counts. Defendant appealed.

REASONING: The court noted there are two prohibited acts in § 465.015(2)(c). The first is selling a prescription drug. Selling is not defined in chapter 465, but the court in *Block v. State*, 437 So.2d 792 (Fla. 2d DCA 1983) instructed the jury that "sell means to transfer or deliver something to another person in exchange for money or something of value, or a promise of money or something of value." The court agreed with *Block* that § 465.015(2)(c) applies to a non-pharmacist for selling a prescription drug.

However, the court based its decision on the second legal action prohibited by § 465.015(2)(c)—"dispensing a prescription drug without a prescription." Dispensing only applies to pharmacists. The definition of "dispense" excludes "the actual sales transaction and delivery of such drug" and includes actions carried out by a licensed pharmacist. The court found that § 465.015(2)(c) is not available to the State to prosecute the dispensing of a drug without a prescription by a person who is not a pharmacist.

HOLDING: The state may not prosecute a non-pharmacist for dispensing a prescription drug without being furnished a prescription under §465.015(2)(c). The court reversed the guilty verdict for Count II and affirmed the guilty verdict for Count.

31.6.2 PMP Records

31.6.2.1 *Lundy v. State,* 26 N.E.3d 656 (Ind. Ct. App. Feb. 20, 2015)

RELIEF SOUGHT: Criminal defendant appealed the court's decision to grant the Indiana Board of Pharmacy's refusal to provider her prescription records pursuant to INSPECT—Indiana's electronic prescription monitoring program.

ISSUE: Did the court err by ruling Lundy's INSPECT records were not discoverable because Lundy knew where she could possibly obtain records of her prescription?

FACTS AND PROCEDURAL HISTORY: Lundy was arrested for possession of hydrocodone pills. Indiana charged Lundy with Class D felony possession of a controlled substance without a valid prescription. Lundy claimed she had a valid prescription.

Lundy served a subpoena on the Indiana Board of Pharmacy requesting a copy of her INSPECT report. At the time of the request, Lundy "knew where she could possibly obtain records of her prescription." INSPECT information is confidential and may be disclosed only to certain individuals, but not patients. Indiana Board filed a motion to quash the subpoena on the grounds that the records were confidential.

The trial court granted the motion to quash because (i) Lundy must "make a threshold showing that she could not get her prescription records elsewhere"; and (ii) Lundy did not present any such evidence.

REASONING: On appeal, Lundy contended the court erred by ruling that she had to "make a threshold showing that she could not get her prescription records elsewhere."

The court applied the Indiana Supreme Court's three-part test for discoverability of records by a criminal defendant:

(1) there must be sufficient designation of the items sought to be discovered (particularity); (2) the requested items must be material to the defense (relevance or materiality); and (3) if the first two requirements are met, the trial court must grant the request unless there is a showing of a "paramount interest" in nondisclosure.

The court determined "particularity" requires a showing that the information was not "readily available" elsewhere. "The particularity requirement is not to be construed strictly against the defendant but should be administered so as to maximize pretrial discovery." Just because Lundy knew where she could *possibly* obtain her prescription records, did not mean they were readily available.

HOLDING: The court reversed and remanded. Lundy was entitled to her INSPECT report from the Board.

31.6.3 Second Degree Murder

31.6.3.1 *U.S. v. Barry J. Cadden, et al.,* 2014 WL 7151586 (D. Mass. Dec. 16, 2014)

INDICTMENT OF NECC, EXECUTIVES, AND EMPLOYEES: Federal prosecutors filed charges, including second-degree murder, racketeering, conspiracy, and mail fraud against defendants involved in the New England Compounding Center ("NECC").

FACTS AND PROCEDURAL HISTORY: In 2012, NECC was at the center of a deadly meningitis outbreak caused by tainted epidural steroid injections. NECC sent injections to clinics in 23 states. 751 people were diagnosed with a fungal infection and 64 people died. An investigation uncovered unlawful conduct, such as grossly unsanitary production practices and fake descriptions used to mislead regulators.

CHARGES: December 2014: Federal prosecutors charged NECC President and head pharmacist (Cadden) and pharmacist (Chin) with second-degree murder under the RICO Act for acting in wanton and willful disregard of the likelihood that the natural tendency of their actions would cause death or great bodily harm.

- There were 131 counts in the indictment and roughly, 14 people (managers and pharmacists) were charged.
- Alleged Cadden and Chin and other employees consistently failed to ensure that the drugs were sterile and failed to properly test them for sterility.
- Alleged Cadden instructed a sales company to falsely represent to customers that NECC was complying with USP, though the drugs fell well short of USP standards.
- Alleged Chin instructed pharmacy technicians to falsify cleaning records.
- Alleged Chin and other senior pharmacists had knowledge the drugs they were making were made in a thoroughly contaminated lab and they failed to comply with basic health standards.
- Alleged Cadden and Chin conspired to profit from selling the sterile injections, knowing that they had not been properly sterilized or tested.

STATUS: At this point, the federal government has seized more than $18 million from three shareholders of NECC, which is now bankrupt.

31.7 DEFAMATION

31.7.1 Physician Against Pharmacist

31.7.1.1 *LeFrock v. Walgreens Co.,* 77 F. Supp.3d 1199 (M.D. Fla. Jan. 16, 2015)

RELIEF SOUGHT: Physician sued Walgreens for alleged defamatory statements made by Walgreens pharmacists.

ISSUES:

1. Did pharmacists commit slander against physicians during consultation with patients?
2. Were comments made during the consultation privileged?

FACTS AND PROCEDURAL HISTORY: The physician brought a defamation claim against the pharmacy. The physician claimed pharmacists at Walgreens made defamatory statements to patients regarding his medical reputation and ethics when they attempted to fill prescriptions. "The apparent purpose of the statement was to inform customers about the physician who wrote the prescription."

The plaintiff claimed Walgreens' employees committed slander per se when they "conveyed defamatory statements" regarding his qualifications as a medical doctor. Walgreens moved for summary judgment.

REASONING: To prevail in a claim for slander under Florida law, a plaintiff must prove: (i) a false and defamatory statement; (ii) an unprivileged publication to a third party; (iii) fault amounting to at least negligence by the publisher; (iv) either an actionable statement irrespective of harm or the existence of special harm caused by the publication. Malice is an essential element of slander. Malice is presumed when a false statement states or suggests a person committed a dishonest or illegal act. When a statement is privileged, the presumption of malice does not apply.

Statements are privileged if: "(1) made in good faith, (2) with an interest to be upheld, (3) made on a proper occasion, and (4) made in a proper manner."

Pharmacists acted in good faith and upheld a legitimate interest because statements were made while filling scripts and giving advice required by law. Pharmacists have a duty to provide competent advice to customers "beyond merely following the doctor's instructions robotically."

Pharmacists exercised due diligence by informing customers of relevant information regarding the prescribing physician. Statements were made in the proper location and manner. Statements were limited in scope to the specific prescriptions and were not mere generalizations. Therefore, pharmacists' statements were protected by privilege; the plaintiff cannot overcome qualified privilege because he failed to present evidence that statements were made with express malice.

HOLDINGS:

1. Pharmacists did not commit slander against physicians during consultation with patients.
2. Comments made during the consultation were privileged.

31.7.2 Duty to Fill

31.7.2.1 *Kadambi v. Express Scripts,* 2015 WL 475373 (N.D. Ind. February 5, 2015)

RELIEF SOUGHT: Physician and eight patients sued mail-order pharmacies for breach of duty to honor prescriptions and to fill as written. The physician sued for defamation.

ISSUES:

1. Does Indiana pharmacy law, purportedly requiring pharmacists to honor all prescriptions from a physician, create a private cause of action?
2. Does the Indiana anti-SLAP (strategic lawsuit against public participation) statute bar the plaintiff's defamation claim?
3. Are pharmacist statements to patients regarding the reason for refusal to dispense protected by qualified privilege?

FACTS AND PROCEDURAL HISTORY: Dr. Kadambi, an endocrinologist, prescribed HGH for patients claiming HGH was medically necessary and approved by insurance companies. Defendant pharmacies refused to fill HGH prescriptions from Dr. Kadambi. Pharmacies claimed refusal was based on concern of violating 21 U.S.C. § 333(e). Section 333(e) makes distributing HGH for off-label use a felony. Pharmacists claimed they learned Dr. Kadambi prescribed HGH for off-label use or he was associated with organizations advocating for off-label use. Pharmacies explained to patients their refusal was based on suspect prescribing. The plaintiffs first alleged pharmacy violated Indiana Code § 25-26-13-16 requiring pharmacists to "exercise his professional judgment in the best interest of the patient's health" and that "a pharmacist has a duty to honor all prescriptions from a practitioner." Pharmacists must take "reasonable steps" to determine whether a prescription has complied with applicable law.

Patients sued pharmacies alleging (i) violation of Indiana pharmacy law/breach of duty to honor prescription and (ii) defamation.

Indiana Code § 25-26-13-16 granted immunity for criminal and civil liability for refusing to honor a prescription if (i) it would be contrary to law, (ii) be in the best interest of the patient, (iii) aid or abet an addiction or habit, or (iv) is contrary to health and safety of the patient. Plaintiffs argued that because the code provided civil immunity for failure to honor prescriptions, the logical implication is that immunity would not be necessary if there was no private right of action.

Defendants moved to dismiss under state anti-SLAP law (designed to reduce lawsuits brought to chill freedom of speech—used as a defense against a plaintiff's defamation claim). Pharmacies argued that statements made to patients regarding refusal to honor HGH prescriptions were in furtherance of free speech on a public issue. Defendants argued statements were too narrow and patient-specific for anti-SLAP protection and statements were not made in public interest. Defendants also argued defamation claim was barred by qualified privilege. Under Indiana law, a statement is privileged if: (i) made in good faith; (ii) with an interest to be upheld (iii) made on a proper occasion; and (iv) made in a proper manner.

Defendants claimed Dr. Kadambi: (i) wrote prescriptions for cosmetic reasons; (ii) is a plastic surgeon; (iii) is on a list of physicians involved with sports medicine and anti-aging medicine; and (iv) issued fraudulent and illegal prescriptions.

Dr. Kadambi's alleged statements were not made in good faith because they turned a blind eye to key information that the defendant had discovered about Dr. Kadambi in a previous suit. Pharmacies argued statements were made in good faith after investigations regarding HGH prescriptions by Dr. Kadambi.

REASONING: The court reasoned Indiana Code § 25-26-13-16 did not provide a private right of action. The law benefits the public at large, not any specific individual.

The court also held the anti-SLAP law did not protect pharmacies. There was no public interest in statements made to patients regarding Dr. Kadambi's prescribing of HGH. Statements were not in furtherance of free speech but were communicated to patients about reasons for not dispensing and to protect the pharmacy from liability under federal law. A genuine issue of material fact existed as to whether the defendant's statements were made in good faith.

HOLDINGS:

1. As to claim under Indiana pharmacy law, the court granted the pharmacies' motion to dismiss the pleadings.
2. The court denied the motion to dismiss under the anti-SLAP law because the law did not afford protection to pharmacies.
3. The court denied the defendant's motion for summary judgment on qualified privilege because a fact question existed about whether statements to patients were made in good faith.

31.8 EMPLOYMENT

31.8.1 Discrimination (Pregnancy)

31.8.1.1 *Torres-Skair v. Medco Health Solutions, Inc.*, 595 F.App'x 847 (11th Cir. Dec., 4, 2014)

RELIEF SOUGHT: Plaintiff sued former employer for pregnancy discrimination.

ISSUE: Did Medco discriminate on the basis of pregnancy and retaliate against a former employee in violation of Title VII and the Florida Civil Rights Act?

FACTS AND PROCEDURAL HISTORY: Medco is "a third-party manager of prescription benefits for health insurers that provides prescription drugs by mail and prescription claims-processing services for insured persons." The plaintiff worked for Medco as a clinical care pharmacist, primarily working over the phone. In 2010, she started working from home but experienced, and complained of, equipment trouble that persisted throughout her tenure. In 2010, Medco instituted production quotas that included (i) weekly goals for prescriptions converted from retail to mail order and (ii) goals relating to the number of calls made and the percentage of idle time.

Medco found out about the plaintiff's pregnancy in October 2010. Before this, there was concern about the plaintiff's production. The plaintiff's manager (without knowledge of pregnancy) told her that her job performance was deficient with respect to her numbers. The plaintiff informed the manager that she was pregnant shortly after review.

In January 2011, Medco increased its performance goals again. During this time, the plaintiff informed Medco that she had been placed on medical restrictions by the physician due to her pregnancy. The supervisor made comments to the plaintiff such as (i) she was "moody" and "her pregnancy was affecting her effectiveness" and (ii) "that doctor's notes that she was giving were reducing her production" because she was not on the phone as often. In her March 2011 evaluation, the plaintiff was consistently below goals, her performance declined, and she received no bonus or stock options.

The plaintiff filed an anonymous complaint with the Medco hotline and then claimed retaliation for expressing concerns about the job. The complaint was investigated with no action taken. The plaintiff notified Medco of FMLA leave in anticipation of maternity leave. Two days later, the plaintiff was put on administrative leave pending an investigation regarding additional performance issues. The plaintiff was terminated 11 days later. The investigation found she hung up on the customer (a terminable offense) and continued poor performance.

The plaintiff filed an EEOC charge of discrimination. The district court granted Medco's motion for summary judgment, concluding plaintiff failed to establish a prima facie claim of pregnancy discrimination. The court also concluded that the plaintiff could not establish a prima facie claim that Medco's adverse actions were pretextual or that she faced retaliation.

REASONING: The Eleventh Circuit affirmed the district court, dismissing the plaintiff's case. Title VII and the Florida Civil Rights Act prohibit discrimination based on sex, including on the basis of pregnancy, childbirth, or related medical conditions. When the court evaluated the conditions that existed for the plaintiff, it explained, "Only the most blatant remarks whose intent could be nothing other than to discriminate on the basis of some impermissible factor constitute direct evidence of discrimination." The plaintiff presented no evidence to meet this standard. Comments that the plaintiff was moody and hormonal did not show direct evidence of discrimination.

Because there was no evidence of discrimination on the basis of pregnancy on the record, the court applied the "burden-shifting framework of the McDonnell Douglass Test, which was first applied in *McDonnell Douglas Corp. v. Green*, 411 U.S. 792, 93 S. Ct. 1817 (1973). This test requires a plaintiff to show that she was "(1) pregnant; (2) qualified to do the job; (3) subjected to an adverse employment action; and (4) treated differently than similarly situated non-pregnant employees, in that employment or disciplinary policies were differently applied to her." The court determined that the plaintiff did show that she was (1) pregnant, (2) qualified for the job, and (3) subject to adverse action, but **did not** show she was (4) treated differently than other employees. The court found plaintiff's pregnancy was not a motivating factor for the adverse action. Poor performance reviews came before knowledge of pregnancy and continued after management became aware of her pregnancy. Medco provided multiple non-discriminatory reasons for placing the plaintiff on administrative leave and terminating her. The plaintiff's hanging up on customers was particularly important, as it was an automatic terminable offense.

HOLDING: The plaintiff's retaliation claim was without merit. The plaintiff complained that she was retaliated against after making complaints regarding comments about her pregnancy. The plaintiff failed to show that the adverse action would not have occurred but for the protected activity. Further, any causal connection between her protected conduct and the adverse action was far too indirect and attenuated to be actionable.

31.8.2 Employment at Will

31.8.2.1 *Hoven v. Walgreens Co.*, 751 F.3d 778 (6th Cir. June 2, 2014)

RELIEF SOUGHT: Employee sued his former employer for wrongful termination.

ISSUES:

1. Was Walgreens' termination of the employee in violation of public policy?
2. Was the employee wrongfully terminated for exercising his rights of self-defense, defense of others, and to carry a concealed weapon?

FACTS AND PROCEDURAL HISTORY: Hoven has been a Michigan-licensed pharmacist for Walgreens Co. since 2006. In 2007, he was held up at gunpoint in the pharmacy. After the incident, Hoven asked Walgreens to install extra security precautions, such as a panic button, but Walgreens refused to implement the requested installments. In 2008, Hoven obtained a state-issued permit and gun for protection. He began carrying his gun to work. In 2011, two men held up the pharmacy and held two employees hostage at gunpoint. Seeing Hoven, the robbers attempted to shoot him several times but failed. Hoven returned fire. The robbers fled the scene. No one was hurt during the attempted robbery.

Five days later, Hoven was informed that he had violated the store's non-escalation policy and a policy against carrying firearms in the workplace. Hoven refused to resign and was terminated. Hoven sued alleging wrongful termination because he was fired in violation of a public policy grounded in state law that permits individuals to defend themselves and others from the imminent threat of violence. The trial court dismissed the case because Hoven could not identify the source of any public policy to support his claim. Hoven appealed.

REASONING: The Sixth Circuit Court of Appeals affirmed the trial court's dismissal for two reasons: (i) Hoven was an at-will employee, and (ii) Hoven failed to identify a public policy source that supported his claim. At-will employees can be terminated at any time for any reason, or no reason. However, Michigan recognizes a limit on the general rule of at-will employment: The Doctrine of Termination in Violation of Public Policy.

This doctrine recognizes that some reasons for terminating an employee are simply "so contrary to public policy as to be actionable." A termination violates public policy when an employee is discharged: (i) in violation of an explicit legislative statement prohibiting the discharge of employees who act in accordance with a statutory right or duty; (ii) for the failure or refusal to violate the law in the course of employment; or (iii) or exercising a right conferred by a well-established legislative enactment.

Hoven argued that the third exception applied due to the Second Amendment (right to bear arms). Under Michigan law, constitutional provisions may not be the source of a claim for termination in violation of public policy against a *private* employer.

HOLDINGS: The Court affirmed dismissal because:

1. Walgreens' termination of employee did not violate public policy.
2. The pharmacist was not terminated for exercising his rights of self-defense, defense of others, or to carry a concealed weapon.

31.8.3 Americans With Disability Act

31.8.3.1 *Stevens v. Rite Aid Corp., et al.*, 6:13-cv-00783 (N.D.N.Y., September 23, 2015)

RELIEF SOUGHT: Pharmacist sued former employer for violation of the Americans with Disabilities Act (ADA) and the New York State Human Rights Law (NYSHRL).

ISSUES:

1. Did the employer violate the ADA and the NYSHRL after terminating a pharmacist who refused to provide vaccinations because of trypanophobia (needle phobia)?
2. Is trypanophobia a recognized disability?
3. Did Rite Aid fail to provide reasonable accommodations to the employee?
4. Were awarded damages excessive?

FACTS AND PROCEDURAL HISTORY: Pharmacist Christopher Stevens was a pharmacist at Eckerd Pharmacy in upstate New York. Rite Aid purchased the pharmacy in 2007. Rite Aid required all pharmacists to undergo mandatory immunization training. Stevens had never undergone such training. Stevens provided HR and district managers with letters from the physician stating he has trypanophobia—needle phobia. Stevens contended that it would be unsafe for him to provide immunizations to patients.

Rite Aid warned Stevens he would be terminated if he did not undergo immunization training. Stevens refused and was fired days later. Stevens filed a complaint with the EEOC. During the investigation, Rite Aid admitted Stevens was fired because he refused to administer flu shots.

Rite Aid argued that trypanophobia was not a disability defined by the ADA and that firing was on a "legitimate, nondiscriminatory" basis. A jury found:

(1) [Stevens] was discharged because of a disability in violation of the ADA; (2) Rite Aid failed to provide a reasonable accommodation in violation of the ADA; (3) [Stevens] was retaliated against in violation of the ADA; (4) [Stevens] was discharged because of a disability in violation of the NYSHRL; (5) Rite Aid failed to provide a reasonable accommodation in violation of the NYSHRL; and (6) [Stevens] was retaliated against in violation of the NYSHRL. The Jury awarded Plaintiff $485,633.00 in back-pay damages; $1,227,188.00 in front-pay damages (encompassing 4.75 years from the date of the verdict, i.e., January 22, 2015); and $900,000.00 in non-pecuniary damages.

Pharmacy filed motions for judgment as a matter of law seeking to overturn the jury verdict, or, in the alternative, seeking a new trial.

REASONING: The court first addressed whether the pharmacist had a *physiological or psychological disability*. The EEOC defines physical or mental impairment to mean:

Any physiological disorder or condition, cosmetic disfigurement, or anatomical loss affecting one or more body systems, such as neurological, musculoskeletal, special sense organs, respiratory (including speech organs), cardiovascular, reproductive, digestive, genitourinary, Immune, circulatory, hemic, lymphatic, skin, and endocrine.

A physician testified the pharmacist exhibited an "unprepared, spontaneous reaction . . . that could not be rehearsed" that included turning white, looking annoyed, and almost fainting when the physician pierced his own skin with an insulin syringe and drew blood.

The court concluded there was sufficient evidence that the *impairment was a "substantial limitation,"* which means the impairment substantially limits the ability of an individual to perform a major life activity as compare to "most people." However, an impairment "need not prevent, or significantly or severely restrict, the individual from performing a major life activity in order to be considered substantially limiting." A physician testified that the trypanophobia significantly restricted the pharmacist from performing any job involving the administration of injections.

The court also found sufficient evidence that *trypanophobia is a neurological impairment* based on expert testimony that the impairment impacted the pharmacist's neurological function through the "sympathetic branch of the nervous system," which caused anxiety, which in turn caused the pharmacist to avoid the thing he was phobic about.

The court then evaluated whether giving immunizations was an *essential job function*. If an employee cannot perform an essential job function with or without reasonable accommodation, the employer is not required to eliminate the function. Rite Aid District Manager did not include immunizations in his description of the plaintiff's duties. None of the 16 "essential duties and responsibilities" in the job description included immunization. Thus, there was sufficient evidence that immunization was not an essential job function. However, the court found that the pharmacist did not present sufficient evidence that Rite Aid failed to reasonably accommodate his disability by providing desensitization therapy, hiring a nurse, giving him a technician position, or assigning him to a dual-pharmacist store.

The court turned to damages and sustained all damages except for the $900,000 of compensatory damages based largely on emotional distress because such damages would shock the judicial conscience.

HOLDINGS:

1. The court held there was sufficient evidence to support each of the jury's findings except for the finding that Rite Aid failed to provide reasonable accommodation by not allowing time off for "desensitization."
2. The jury's damages award was proper except for the non-pecuniary award of $900,000, which the court reduced to $125,000, or the plaintiff could try the case again.

31.8.4 Overtime Class Action

31.8.4.1 *Baugh v. CVS Health, et al.*, 2:15-cv-00014 (E.D. Penn., July 27, 2015)

RELIEF SOUGHT: CVS sought summary judgment against pharmacist who filed a putative class action complaint alleging CVS denied overtime to floater pharmacists in violation of the Fair Labor Standards Act (FLSA) and Pennsylvania Wage Payment and Collection Law ("WPCL").

ISSUE: Was Baugh entitled to the longer three-year statute of limitation ("SOL") rather than the standard two-year SOL under FSLA?

FACTS AND PROCEDURAL HISTORY: Baugh worked as a floater for CVS from October 2011 through his termination in October 2012. He filed suit on January 5, 2015. Baugh alleged that CVS violated the FSLA and WPCL because it failed to pay floating pharmacists who fill in for absent pharmacists time-and-a-half for all hours worked over 40. The plaintiff claimed that paychecks and the internal CVS payroll system demonstrate that pharmacists work 50-hour work weeks or more. However, CVS only paid straight-time rates. Baugh asked to certify a class of subordinate and floater Pennsylvania pharmacists who have worked at one of CVS's 400+ Pennsylvania locations.

CVS filed a motion for summary judgment seeking to dismiss the lawsuit because: (i) Baugh was an exempt employee under the FSLA and (ii) filed his claim past the two-year SOL and failed to show evidence that CVS acted willfully, which would have extended the SOL to three years.

RULING: An FSLA plaintiff must institute a claim for wages due within two years of the date of the last paycheck for the pay period upon which the claim is based, unless the violation was willful. If willfulness is shown, the SOL is three years. The plaintiff failed to show CVS's failure to pay overtime wages was willful.

> Following the review of the record evidence and the oral argument, Baugh adduces no evidence leading this court to find CVS knew or showed reckless disregard for whether its conduct toward him violated the FLSA during the relevant period sufficient to create a genuine issue of material fact.

In fact, CVS relied on an opinion of a federal court, *Anani v. CVS Rx Services, Inc.*, 788 F.Supp.2d 55 (E.D.N.Y. 2011), that held CVS's pay arrangements for pharmacists did not violate the FSLA. Therefore, there was no justification to expand SOL from two to three years.

California case similar to Baugh dismissed. California CVS pharmacists tried to certify as a class but failed. Plaintiffs argued that CVS's internal personnel login and prescription software demonstrated pharmacists worked in stores more than 40 hours per week. District court judge disagreed, noting that employees often used each other's login IDs and expert software analysis resulted in multiple false positives.

HOLDING: The court dismissed Buagh's Complaint because he filed too late (past the two-year SOL) for claimed wages under FLSA. However, his claims under WPCL survived and Baugh will have to pursue them in state court.

31.8.5 Medical Marijuana

31.8.5.1 *Coats v. Dish Network*, 350 P. 3d, 849 (Colo. June 15, 2015)

RELIEF SOUGHT: The terminated employee appealed the dismissal of his suit against his employer, alleging that his termination was based on his "lawful" state-licensed use of medical marijuana.

ISSUE: Was the plaintiff's use of medical marijuana under Colorado's Medical Marijuana Amendment lawful under Colorado's law that prohibits employment discrimination for "lawful" activities (Colo. Rev. Stat. §24-34-402.5)?

FACTS AND PROCEDURAL HISTORY: Coats claimed Dish Network violated Colorado's "lawful activity" law (§24-34-402.5) by discharging him for his state-licensed use of medical marijuana at home during non-working hours. Under §24-34-402.5, firing an employee for lawful activities outside of work is an unfair and discriminatory labor practice. The trial court dismissed Coat's complaint for failure to state a claim after finding that medical marijuana was not lawful under §24-34-402.5.

REASONING: The court reasoned that marijuana use is illegal under federal law and nothing in §24-34-402.5 limited the term "lawful" to state law. The term was used in its general unrestricted sense, indicating that a "lawful" activity is one that complies with all state and federal laws.

HOLDING: The Colorado Supreme Court affirmed because the employer did not terminate the plaintiff for a "lawful activity" (see §24-34-402.5).

31.9 FRAUD AND ABUSE

31.9.1 False Claims

31.9.1.1 *United States v. Express Scripts, Inc.*, 602 F. App'x 880 (3rd. Cir. Feb. 20, 2015)

RELIEF SOUGHT: *Qui tam* relator appealed the district court's dismissal of his False Claims Act ("FCA") claims.

ISSUE: Were the relator's FCA claims precluded by the public disclosure rule?

FACTS AND PROCEDURAL HISTORY: Morgan, a pharmacist, claimed he discovered widespread price inflation of brand-name drugs "through his diligence." This amounted to eyeball comparisons of two publicly available price listings. Morgan says he became aware of communications between First Databank and price listing publisher AmerisourceBergen, after noticing price discrepancies and while conducting an audit. This communication indicated First Databank knew of price differentials.

The district court dismissed Morgan's FCA claims for lack of subject matter jurisdiction. The district court concluded relator's claims were based on publically disclosed allegations whose "original source" was not Morgan. Morgan's original claim alleged that various defendants, including Express Scripts, CVS Caremark, Medco, First Databank, etc. profited from artificially inflated AWP prices for brand-name drugs.

The district court found that Morgan's third amended complaint "does not demonstrate that Morgan had any direct knowledge of any alleged wrongdoing" as to the myriad of defendants. District Court dismissed claims due to lack of subject matter jurisdiction.

REASONING: Morgan's allegations that the PBMs profited from inflated AWPs and secret spread pricing had been disclosed via multiple sources. Morgan's allegations that PBMs knew First Databank fraudulently inflated profits echoed allegations from previously filed lawsuits, including one where Morgan served as an expert. "Knowledge of a scheme is not direct when it is gained by reviewing files." This was the full extent of Morgan's diligence.

Morgan's knowledge of the pharmaceutical industry did not make him an original source. Morgan was not a party to the allegedly conspiratorial communications. The fact that Morgan quantified the AWP differential does not remove his allegations from the public disclosure realm. Morgan's 4.16% differential indicates an AWP based on a 25% markup over wholesale acquisition cost, a markup disclosed in a congressional report predating Morgan's complaint.

The congressional report provided Morgan with the essential elements needed to arrive at the 4.16% price differential. Consequently, Morgan was not the original source of the allegations contained in his complaint. The public disclosure bar precluded FCA claims.

HOLDING: The third Circuit affirmed the district court decision because the relator was not the original source of information that served as the basis for the FCA claims.

31.9.2 False Claims—Generic Substitutions

31.9.2.1 *Doe v. Houchens Indus., Inc.*, No. 1:13-CV-00196-RLY, 2015 WL 133706 (S.D. Ind. Jan. 9, 2015)

RELIEF SOUGHT: Relator brought *qui tam* claims under the federal FCA and the Indiana False Claims Act alleging defendant misrepresented drug prices.

ISSUE: Did the relator sufficiently allege a FCA claim by claiming the pharmacy's reward program allowed patients to purchase prescriptions at a lower price than the pharmacy used for usual and customary price calculations?

FACTS AND PROCEDURAL HISTORY: Defendant developed a pharmacy rewards program permitting cash-paying customers to pay a small fee to participate in the program, which offered flat discounted fees for hundreds of generic medications.

The relator (a former employee) was instructed to "collect a small fee from the enrollees and give them a gift card in the same amount to offset the fee." The defendant also instructed the relator "when billing Medicare Part D and other third parties for a generic drug on the program list," *not* to "change the price to the discounted price unless the co-pay exceeded $3.99." Relator claimed the defendant overcharged the government by seeking reimbursement for the generic drug in an amount in excess of the "usual and customary" price it typically charged cash-paying customers. Relator alleged that this violated the FCA and the Indiana FCA. The defendant moved to dismiss.

REASONING: The FCA imposes liability on anyone who "knowingly presents, or causes to be presented, a false or fraudulent claim for payment or approval," or who "knowingly makes, uses, or causes to be made or used, a false record or statement material to a false or fraudulent claim." Pharmacies that "contract with Medicare Part D plan sponsors are required to price prescriptions *at the contracted rate or U & C rate, whichever is lower.*" U&C price is the amount a provider would charge cash customers for a prescription, exclusive of sales tax.

Defendant argued that the special pricing it offered members who enrolled in the Rewards program was not the U & C price because that price was not offered to the general public, but only to those who enrolled. However, this argument was rejected in *United States ex rel. Garbe v. Kmart Corp.*, 968 F.Supp.2d 978, 982–83 (S.D. Ill. 2013).

In *Garbe*, the court found that members of Kmart's generic discount program were considered a part of the general public because anyone could join. Here, the enrollment process was simple and open to anyone who filled prescriptions at the pharmacy.

HOLDING: The court denied a motion to dismiss because the relator stated plausible claims under the FCA.

31.9.3 False Claims & Anti-Kickback Statute

31.9.3.1 *U.S. Ex Rel. Kester v. Novartis Pharm. Corp.*, No. 11 CIV. 8196 CM, 2015WL 1650767 (S.D.N.Y. Apr. 10, 2015)

RELIEF SOUGHT: Relator brought *qui tam* action against pharmacy defendants alleging violation of the False Claims Act (FCA) and the Anti-Kickback Statute (AKS).

ISSUE: Should the State of Washington's motion for leave to file an amended complaint-in-intervention be granted?

FACTS AND PROCEDURAL HISTORY: Novartis develops, manufactures, and markets prescription drugs, and then sells them through various specialty pharmacies. Novartis used Accredo Health Group (specialty pharmacy and subsidiary of Express Scripts, Inc.) to sell Exjade, an iron-reducing drug given to patients who receive blood transfusions. Former Novartis employee alleged that Accredo received additional patient referrals and other benefits from Novartis in exchange for bolstering refills of Exjade.

Due to the decreasing sales of Exjade, Novartis would refer more patients with Exjade prescriptions to "participating specialty pharmacies" in exchange for the pharmacies assigning employees to call Exjade patients to encourage them to adhere to their regime and refill their prescriptions. Novartis also gave the pharmacy volume-based rebates, as well as performance-based rebates. The program was not designed for patients' benefit. Instead, pharmacy employees would secure additional refills by providing patients with incomplete information by downplaying Exjade's serious and potentially life-threatening side effects.

At no point did Novartis disclose to health plans, patients, or physicians that it paid specialty pharmacies financial incentives based on their performance in driving up sales of Exjade. Nor did Accredo disclose to patients that Novartis paid it based on its success in increasing the quantity of Exjade dispensed.

The relator brought *qui tam* action against Novartis alleging violation of the FCA and the AKS. Several states subsequently intervened as co-plaintiffs against Novartis. "Before the court is the State of Washington's motion to file an amended complaint under Rule 15(a). Washington seeks to (1) add Accredo as a defendant; and (2) recover from Novartis for damages arising out of its relationship with Accredo."

ANALYSIS: Under Fed.R.Civ.P. 15(a)(2), "a party may amend its pleading only with the opposing party's written consent or the court's leave. The court should freely give leave when justice so requires." The Supreme Court has explained that the standard embodied in Rule 15 is a liberal one:

> If the underlying facts or circumstances relied upon by a plaintiff may be a proper subject of relief, he ought to be afforded an opportunity to test his claim on the merits. In the absence of any apparent or declared reason such as undue delay, bad faith, or dilatory motive on the part of the movant, repeated failure to cure deficiencies by amendments previously allowed,

undue prejudice to the opposing party by virtue of allowance of the amendment, futility of amendment, etc. the leave sought should, as the rules require, be "freely given."

The court denied Washington's motion for leave to file an amended complaint because Washington delayed moving for leave to amend for over a year without an adequate explanation. Further, the motion was denied because allowing the amendment would prejudice Accredo by prolonging the disposition of the case and requiring additional discovery.

HOLDING: Washington's motion was denied because it delayed moving for leave to amend and granting the motion would be prejudicial to Accredo.

SUBSEQUENT HISTORY—SETTLEMENT: In May 2015, Accredo Health Group agreed to pay $45 million to federal authorities to settle claims that it had participated in patient referral kickback schemes. Novartis continues to dispute the allegations. In November 2015, Novartis agreed to pay $390 million to the U.S., New York, and other states.

31.9.4 Consumer Fraud

31.9.4.1 *City of Chicago v. Purdue Pharma L.P.*, 2015 WL 2208423 (N.D. Ill. May 8, 2015)

RELIEF SOUGHT: Defendants moved to dismiss the City's complaint alleging multiple violations of the Chicago Municipal Code and state law in connection with pharmaceutical manufacturers' marketing of certain drugs.

ISSUE: Were the City's allegations sufficient to state a claim that pharmaceutical manufacturers' marketing practices violated the Chicago Municipal Code?

FACTS AND PROCEDURAL HISTORY: The City sued several drug manufacturers (e.g., Purdue Pharma, Teva Pharmaceuticals USA, Johnson & Johnson, Endo Pharmaceuticals) to recover payments made to drug manufacturers for opioid drugs prescribed to City employees HMO, PPO, and worker's compensation plans. City specifically alleged defendants misrepresented that opioids were effective for more than short-term treatment of cancer pain.

The City alleged that the defendants launched a coordinated effort to promote long-term opioid therapy through (i) medical journal articles on the therapy, (ii) misuse of continuing medical education programs (CME) programs to market the therapy, and (iii) use of professional and patient advocacy groups as marketing tools. Additionally, the City alleged defendants overstated the effectiveness of opioids and downplayed the effectiveness of alternatives and understated or hid addiction risks.

The City alleged violations of Chicago Municipal Code §2-25-090 for consumer fraud or deceptive practices. Defendants moved to dismiss.

REASONING: Elements of an Illinois Consumer Fraud and Deceptive Business Practices Act (which the Municipal Code section cites as an interpretative guide) claim include (i) a deceptive act or practice by the defendant; (ii) the defendant's intent that the plaintiff relies on the deception; and (iii) occurrence of the deception during a course of conduct involving trade or commerce.

Defendants denied violating §2-25-090 arguing only advertisements are actionable under §2-25-090. The City claimed the defendant's unbranded materials (i.e., materials that identify a drug but not a specific company's drug) were indirect attempts to persuade doctors to prescribe, and consumers to purchase, opioid products and that the defendants acted or used deception, fraud, false pretenses, or concealment with the intent that others rely on such concealment in connection with the sale of any merchandise.

The district court dismissed most of the City's claims because the City did not show defendants had editorial control over materials that they allegedly sponsored or funded and the City did not show where or when defendants made alleged misrepresentations to doctors or consumers.

The court explained:

> The City does not explain what editorial control, if any, the Endo entities had over materials they allegedly sponsored or funded. Further, it does not allege that the Endo entities distributed the educational materials or advertisements to Chicago doctors or consumers, that Chicago doctors attended the continuing medical education programs, that Chicago doctors or consumers visited the websites or otherwise indicate when, how, and to whom the alleged misrepresentations were made. Without such allegations, the City has not stated viable §§ 2–25–90 and 4–276–470 claims against the Endo entities.

As to Purdue, the court further explained:

> Though most of these allegations suffer from the same flaws as those leveled against the other entities, the allegations that, starting in 2005 and continuing to the present, the Purdue entities made misstatements about opioids on their own websites with the intention that Chicago doctors and consumers rely on those misrepresentations are sufficient to state claims against the Purdue entities for violations of Code §§ 2–25–90 and 4–276470.

In July 2015, the court denied Purdue's motion to reconsider its refusal to dismiss the case.

HOLDING: The court dismissed claims as a matter of law against all defendants except Purdue because the City failed to allege facts sufficient to meet all the elements of the applicable code section. The Court dismissed claims against Purdue except for two claims that survived because Purdue made statements about opioids on its website that could have been seen by area physicians and patients.

31.10 NEGLIGENCE

31.10.1 Duty to Provide Medication

31.10.1.1 *Davies v. Virginia CVS Pharmacy, LLC, et al.,* 7:14-CV-00175, 2014 WL 6460787 (W.D. Va. Nov. 17, 2014)

RELIEF SOUGHT: Pharmacy moved to dismiss claims by the estate of a deceased patient that sued pharmacy claiming the pharmacy's delay in providing anticoagulation medications caused the patient's death.

ISSUE: Does a pharmacy have a duty to dispense drugs without payment after telling a patient the pharmacy has the drugs in stock?

FACTS AND PROCEDURAL HISTORY: The decedent was involved in a car accident and was treated for a broken leg at the hospital. The hospital pharmacy could not provide two needed prescriptions (anticoagulants). The decedent was discharged from the hospital on the condition that he obtains and takes anticoagulants. A CVS employee told the plaintiff (representative of the decedent's estate) that the medicine was available and that it would be provided to the plaintiff for the decedent's use. When the patient went to the pharmacy to fill the prescription, pharmacy employees told the patient there was a problem with the medications being approved for payment, that they could not fill them at that time, but they could fill them after payment was approved. The decedent never received or consumed the anticoagulants and died several days later as a result of not taking the medications. The plaintiff sued CVS and the decedent's insurer, alleging, in CVS's case, negligence for failure to provide medication. CVS moved for summary judgment for failure to state a claim, arguing that it had no duty to dispense prescriptions without payment.

REASONING: The complaint does not allege CVS told the plaintiff or anyone that it would provide the medication free, and it was under no legal obligation to do so. The plaintiff argued CVS had assumed a voluntary duty to act when its employee told her or the decedent that CVS would provide the anticoagulation medicine. There is no legal precedent suggesting that by telling a potential customer it would provide medication to the customer, a pharmacy assumes a legal duty to provide that medication for free. Instead, a retail pharmacy like CVS understandably requires payment for medications it dispenses.

HOLDING: The court ruled CVS had no duty to fill the prescriptions free and granted CVS's motion to dismiss.

31.10.2 Duty Not to Dispense

31.10.2.1 *Oleckna v. Daytona Disc. Pharmacy,* 162 So. 3d 178 (Fla. Dist. Ct. App. 2015)

RELIEF SOUGHT: Patient's widow appealed the dismissal of her claims against pharmacy and pharmacist for filling controlled substances too often, which she claimed resulted in her husband's death.

ISSUE: Did the pharmacy and its pharmacists have a duty to inquire into or refuse to fill prescriptions being prescribed too often?

FACTS AND PROCEDURAL HISTORY: The patient (decedent) was diagnosed with stress syndrome and the treating physician prescribed Xanax and hydrocodone or oxycodone. The complaint alleged that for two years the doctor repeatedly prescribed the drugs before the patient was due for a refill and the pharmacy filled at least 30 of these prescriptions even though the prescriptions were issued too frequently. The patient died due to combined drug intoxication of Xanax and hydrocodone. The plaintiff sued the pharmacy for negligence, alleging pharmacy owed several duties to the patient, including a duty not to dispense or fill prescriptions that were unreasonable on their face or in light of the circumstances. The trial court granted a motion to dismiss for the failure to allege facts to support the violation of the duty of care. Plaintiff appealed.

REASONING: A pharmacist's duty to use due and proper care in filling a prescription extends beyond simply following the prescribing physician's directions. The pharmacy unquestioningly filled numerous prescriptions that were so close together that the pharmacy should have been put on notice that the patient was getting too many pills within a short period. "The prescriptions here were alleged to be unreasonable on their face because they were written in a quantity, frequency, dosage, or combination that a reasonable pharmacist would either have checked with the prescribing doctor or warned the patient." Court refused to "interpret a pharmacist's duty to use 'due and proper care in filling the prescription' as being satisfied by 'robotic compliance'" with the prescribing physician's instructions.

HOLDING: The court reversed the dismissal because a fact question existed as to whether the pharmacy and its pharmacists breached their duty to inquire into or refuse to fill prescriptions being prescribed too often.

31.11 PRIVACY

31.11.1 Patient Privacy—Vicarious Liability

31.11.1.1 *Walgreens Co. v. Hinchy,* 25 N.E.3d 748 (Ind. Ct. App. Jn. 15, 2015) Reh'g of, 21 N.E.3d 99 (Ind. Ct. App. Nov. 14, 2014)

RELIEF SOUGHT: Patient sued pharmacy and its employees for negligence, professional malpractice, and invasion of privacy.

ISSUES:

1. Is a pharmacy employer liable under the theory of *respondeat superior* for a pharmacist employee's access and divulging of patient information?
2. Did Hinchy's original complaint allege a viable claim of negligence/professional malpractice against Walgreens?

FACTS AND PROCEDURAL HISTORY: Peterson (♂) and Hinchy (♀) had an on-and-off again sexual relationship. Withers (♀), a Walgreens pharmacist, began dating Peterson in 2009. Hinchy was a pharmacy patient. Withers was notified by Peterson, her then-boyfriend that she may have been exposed to an STD. Fearful, Withers viewed Hinchy's prescription profile to determine whether Hinchy had taken STD medication.

Withers revealed some of the information she discovered to Peterson. Peterson then sent Hinchy a series of text messages concerning her prescription records, accusing her of failing to refill her birth control and becoming pregnant. Excerpts from the text messages follow.

I'm not trying to start any crap but I have a print out showing that you didn't even refill ur birth control perscription for July or august. The last time you filled ur prescription was June. I know uve lied to ur mom and harmony and anybody willing to listen but the printout does not lie. I know you lied to me wth tears and curse words and misplaced righteousness. U really should think about what you did . . . on ur own. You really should think about that FACT before you call me another name. What kind of person does something like that? (internal spelling and grammatical errors original)

Hinchy sent the following text to Peterson in response:

Print out. It's illegal for u to obtain any kind of information like that regarding me. And if u knew anything about my medical history u would know that I was on multiple types of birth control since I was 15[.] (internal spelling and grammatical errors original)

This prompted a reply from Peterson:

Abby, you ddnt refill ANYTHING at all. No type of birth control medication at all. June you did. You did NOT in july and august. Jeez . . . . r you really still trying to claim? Again, I'm not trying to start shit. What's done is done, but what's happening was totally avoidable. You are NOT a victim. You did something wrong abby. Very wrong. Ps . . . . it is not illigall for ME to have it. Ime being very technical here but I ddnt break any laws myself. (internal spelling and grammatical errors original)

Hinchy filed a complaint against Withers for negligence and various theories of invasion of privacy, and against Walgreens under *respondeat superior.* The jury awarded $1.4 million—Peterson was 20% liable, and Withers and Walgreens were jointly responsible for 80% of the damages.

REASONING: Under *respondeat superior, the* employer is responsible for actions of an employee acting within the scope of employment. The act must be incidental to the conduct authorized by the employer or it must further the employer's business. Conduct is within this scope if it is of the **same general nature** as that authorized or **incidental** to such conduct. As long as **some** of the employee's actions were authorized, the question of whether the actions were within the scope of employment is determined by the jury. Withers' actions were of the same general nature as those authorized by Walgreens. Withers was authorized to use the computer system and printer, look up customer information, and review patient prescription histories.

Withers' actions were also incidental to authorized actions because she was on the job and using store equipment when the improper access occurred. The Court of Appeals affirmed a $1.4 million jury verdict, finding Walgreens vicariously liable for a pharmacist employee's illegal review of a patient's prescription profile and divulging such records to a third person. Walgreens filed a petition for rehearing challenging whether Hinchy had sufficiently raised a claim against it. The court reached the same conclusion.

HOLDING:

1. Walgreens was liable under the theory of *respondeat superior* for pharmacist employees accessing and divulging patient information.
2. The court determined that while Hinchy did not explicitly raise a precise negligence/professional malpractice claim, Hinchy stated a viable claim with supporting argument and evidence.

31.11.2 Text Messages

31.11.2.1 *Thompson v. CVS Pharmacy, Inc.*, 6:204-cv-02081 (M.D. Fla. Dec. 19, 2014)

RELIEF SOUGHT: Plaintiff sued pharmacy for alleged violations of the Telephone Consumer Protection Act.

ISSUE: Did the pharmacy violate the Telephone Consumer Protection Act ("TCPA") when it sent robo-texts to patients' cell phones regarding pharmacy services without patients' consent?

FACTS AND PROCEDURAL HISTORY: In 2012, CVS implemented an automated system that included text message alerts related to prescriptions. The text messages would remind patients to pick up and refill prescriptions. The messages also included marketing notifications about flu shots and in-house services. CVS failed to acquire the written consent of consumers. Consumers were automatically opted in and had to opt out to avoid the repeated messages. CVS also failed to ensure that the text messages were being sent to the correct individuals. The TCPA prohibits contacting cell phones via automated calls, including text messages, except with prior express consent of the party called (or for emergency purposes). The TCPA authorizes the FCC to assess fines of up to $16,000 per violation.

Thompson, a CVS customer, received frequent and unwanted text messages directed to another person. Thompson continued to receive text messages even after she requested the pharmacy stop sending them. Thompson filed a lawsuit alleging that CVS violated the TCPA by sending text messages to consumers about their prescriptions without their consent. The lawsuit asked the court to certify a nationwide class of individuals who received unsolicited text messages and a class for those who attempted to opt out of the text messages and continued to receive them. In 2014, there were several class actions alleging that pharmacy prescription reminders violated the TCPA by sending automated calls or text messages without the required consent.

Recent class actions have yielded multimillion-dollar settlements.

31.11.3 Robocalls

31.11.3.1 *Kolinek v. Walgreens Co.*, 2014 WL 3056813 (N.D. Ill. July 7, 2014)

RELIEF SOUGHT: Kolinek sued Walgreens for allegedly violating the Telephone Consumer Protection Act of 1991 ("TCPA").

ISSUE: Did Walgreens violate the TCPA by making unsolicited calls to the cell phones of former and current patients?

FACTS AND PROCEDURAL HISTORY: Kolinek had a prescription filled at Walgreens. The pharmacist asked the customer for his phone number for "verification purposes." From then on, the customer began receiving automated reminders "robocalls" from Walgreens to his cell phone. Kolinek claimed he and thousands of other Walgreens customers did not consent to receive the robocalls on their cell phones and that Walgreens violated the TCPA. Walgreens moved to dismiss arguing that Kolinek had given prior express consent and that the call fell within the TCPA emergency purposes exception. The court originally granted Walgreens' motion to dismiss because Kolinek had voluntarily given his number to Walgreens. However, the judge later reconsidered and reversed his decision—holding that Walgreens could not assert a consent defense in its motion to dismiss.

SETTLEMENT: Walgreens agreed to pay $11 million to end the suit. The amount will be paid into a settlement fund to be used to pay class members' claims and will fund notice and settlement administration expenses. Included in this class are all consumers who received pre-recorded calls from Walgreens to their cell phones. Walgreens will improve its procedures for confirming that customers have consented to the prescription calls and may opt out.

31.12 PRODUCT LIABILITY

31.12.1 Learned Intermediary Doctrine

31.12.1.1 *Watts v. Medicis Pharm. Corp.*, 342 P.3d 847 (Ct. App. 2015), Review Granted in Part (Sept. 22, 2015)

RELIEF SOUGHT: Plaintiff who suffered from drug-induced lupus sued the pharmaceutical company for product liability and consumer fraud action. Plaintiff appealed the trial court's dismissal of her complaint.

ISSUES:

1. Is the LID inconsistent with Arizona's comparative fault tort system?
2. Does the Arizona Consumer Fraud Act apply to consumer advertising by a drug manufacturer or seller?

FACTS AND PROCEDURAL HISTORY: The patient sought treatment for chronic acne and was prescribed Solodyn. Solodyn is a prescription oral antibiotic manufactured by Medicis (an Arizona corporation). Before using Solodyn, the patient received two publications providing details about the drug, but neither disclosed any link between Solodyn and the development of autoimmune diseases.

FDA-approved patient labeling provided to physicians warned that joint pain, lupus-like syndrome, and autoimmune hepatitis were possible side effects of Solodyn. After taking Solodyn, the patient was diagnosed with drug-induced lupus and drug-induced hepatitis. The patient sued Medicis for consumer fraud, product liability, and punitive damages. Medicis' motion to dismiss was granted based on the LID. The patient appealed the dismissal.

REASONING: Under the Learned Intermediary Doctrine, "a manufacturer is not liable for failing to warn consumers of a product's potential risks so long as it provides a proper warning to the specialized class of people who are authorized to sell, install, or provide the product."

The court reasoned that a physician is an intermediary necessary for the consumer to receive a drug. A physician's failure to warn the patient of drug risks constitutes a superseding force that breaks the causal chain between a manufacturer and the patient's harm. Thus, LID shields Medicis from liability for insufficient warning if it provides adequate warnings to the physician.

However, "protecting a prescription drug manufacturer from possible liability for its own actions in distributing a product, simply because another participant in the chain of distribution is also expected to act, is inconsistent with UCATA [Uniform Contribution Among Tortfeasors Act]." Manufacturers are increasing direct consumer advertising to promote their products. This causes consumers to "ask, encourage, and even pressure their medical providers to prescribe these brand-name medications." While it is true that prescribers are gatekeepers, physicians are no longer consumers' sole source of information about the effects and risks.

Under AZ's comparative fault system, when the manufacturer of a product provides false or misleading information to the consumer, it should not be shielded from liability simply because it provided adequate warnings to a third party.

Elimination of the learned intermediary doctrine in these circumstances allows a fair allocation of fault under UCATA, and a consumer who is harmed by false or misleading information from either a manufacturer or the prescribing physician may recover in accordance with each defendant's percentage of fault. In short, the learned intermediary doctrine cannot coexist with UCATA.

HOLDING: The Court of Appeals reversed the dismissal and remanded.

1. The LID is inconsistent with Arizona's comparative fault tort system.
2. The Arizona Consumer Fraud Act applies to consumer advertising by a drug manufacturer or seller.

31.12.2 Product Liability (Applicability to Pharmacists)

31.12.2.1 *Randol Mill Pharmacy v. Miller*, 465 S.W.3d 612 (Tex. 2015), Reh'g Denied (Sept. 11, 2015)

RELIEF SOUGHT: Pharmacy appealed a denial of its motion to dismiss for failure to comply with Texas's expert report requirement in a negligence case for compounding a drug that caused an adverse reaction.

ISSUES:

1. Were the pharmacy and its employees engaged in "the dispensing of prescription medicines" under the Texas Medical Liability Act (TMLA) when they compounded an injectable lipoic acid?
2. Are the plaintiff's claims "health care liability claims" subject to the requirements of the TMLA?

FACTS AND PROCEDURAL HISTORY: In 2011, the plaintiff was diagnosed with Hepatitis C. The doctor prescribed and began administering weekly IV injections of 200 mg/ml of lipoic acid. The plaintiff underwent nine weeks of treatment without incident. Sometime later, she had a severe adverse reaction while receiving a lipoic acid treatment. The plaintiff alleged she was hospitalized for several weeks, received multiple blood transfusions, and is now permanently blind in both eyes. Randol Mill Pharmacy compounded the particular vial to which Miller reacted. "It was prepared as part of an order Dr. Tan had placed with Randol Mill for twenty-three 30-ml vials of lipoic acid for office use, without reference to any particular patient." The plaintiff sued the doctor and the pharmacy. Court dismissed claims against the doctor.

Plaintiff's claims against the pharmacy and pharmacists included: (i) negligence in compounding, inadequate and inappropriate warnings, and instructions for use, which resulted in the compounded lipoic acid being defective, ineffective, and unreasonably dangerous; (ii) failure to confirm the identity, strength, and sterility of the drug prior to its release; (iii) failure to implement reasonably safe design; (iv) failure to manufacture the drug in a reasonably safe condition; and (v) failure to accompany the drug with proper warnings regarding possible adverse side effects with information to medical providers regarding proper use.

Defendants moved to dismiss claims for failure to serve an expert report within 120 days of filing. The trial court denied the motion. The Court of Appeals affirmed, holding that the defendants were not health care providers and that the claims were not health care liability claims.

REASONING: The TMLA requires that plaintiffs serve expert reports early in the litigation process "for each physician or health care provider against whom a [health care] liability claim is asserted." Failure to do so results in the dismissal of the claim with prejudice. The TMLA defines a health care liability claim as:

> A "cause of action against a **health care provider** or physician for treatment, lack of treatment, or other claimed departure from accepted standards of medical care, or health care, or safety or professional or administrative services directly related to health care, which proximately results in injury to or death of a claimant, whether the claimant's claim or cause of action sounds in tort or contract."

A health care provider is defined as "Any person, partnership, professional association, corporation, facility, or institution duly licensed, certified registered, or chartered by the State of Texas to provide health care including . . . **a pharmacist.**"

Licensed pharmacists are health care providers under the act with respect to "those activities limited to the **dispensing** of prescription medicines which result in health care liability claims." The court turned to the definition of "dispense" under the Pharmacy Act.

> "Dispense" means to prepare, package, **compound**, or label, in the course of professional practice, a prescription drug or device **for delivery to an ultimate user or the user's agent under a practitioner's lawful order.**"

The court determined a physician could be considered the patient's agent. Pharmacy regulations allow pharmacists to "dispense or deliver reasonably quantity of a compounded drug to a practitioner for office use."

"A pharmacist who compounds a drug for office use pursuant to a practitioner's lawful order, as authorized by the Pharmacy Act, is 'dispensing' the drug whether or not the order identifies the patients to whom the drug will be administered."

In compounding lipoic acid for office use, pharmacists defendants were engaged in "activities limited to dispensing of prescription medicines" under the Act. The plaintiff's claims call into question the pharmacy's compliance with professional standards of care applicable to pharmacies performing compounding services. Determining whether defendants complied with these standards inevitably requires expert testimony. The court "cannot allow plaintiff to recast her malpractice claim as a breach of warranty and products-liability claims to avoid the Act's strictures." Consequently, the Act applied to the plaintiff's claims against pharmacist defendants. The plaintiff's failure to file an expert report within 120 days of her suit required dismissal.

HOLDING: The Texas Supreme Court reversed and remanded because:

1. Pharmacists were engaged in "the dispensing of prescription medicines" under the TMLA when they compounded an injectable lipoic acid.
2. The plaintiff's claims were subject to the requirements of the TMLA. The plaintiff's failure to file an expert report required dismissal with prejudice.

32 Pharmacy Compounding—Patient Injury and Regulatory Compliance

Willis C. Triplett

SYNOPSIS

32.1 INTRODUCTION

Compounding is an integral part of pharmacy and medical practice and is essential to the provision of quality healthcare. Compounding is a broad topic and difficult to correctly define, but federal law states, "The term 'compounding' includes the combining, admixing, mixing, diluting, pooling, reconstituting, or otherwise altering of a drug or bulk drug substance to create a drug." The activities involved in compounding range from simple (e.g., the addition of a liquid to a manufactured drug powder) to extremely complex (e.g., the preparation of a sterile, multi-component parenteral-nutrition solution).

Pharmaceutical compounding has been a core component of pharmacy throughout the history of the profession. Prior to 1860, **all** medicines were compounded, but in that year, John and Frank Wyeth opened their drugstore and research laboratory in Philadelphia and began to mass-produce popular and commonly prescribed drug compounds. Henry Bowers, a Wyeth employee, constructed a world-changing rotary press machine that was able to generate large batches of tablets in a very consistent way and with minuscule variation. This was the birth of the pharmaceutical industry.

When machines and automation began to apply to drug production, the calculus of risk shifted markedly. An error while preparing a million doses could injure a great many patients, whereas an error made compounding an individual compound, although tragic, will affect only one patient. The Quality Assurance ("QA") approach is necessarily different, not just because of the scale of production, but the scale of **economic cost**. Therefore, it has been critical to define compounding—as it contrasts with manufacturing—for purposes of regulatory enforcement at all levels of government.

Every state is a de facto government unto itself. Most state professional boards (pharmacy, medicine, and nursing) are invested with plenary authority to regulate their respective professions. Most pharmacy boards agree that compounding differs from manufacturing in that compounding involves:

- a genuine practitioner/patient/pharmacist relationship ("the Triad Relationship");
- a relatively small quantity of medication prepared; and
- limited conditions of sale, usually including a requirement for a specific prescription order from an authorized prescriber for an individually identified patient.

32.2 COMPOUNDING TRENDS AND DRIVING FORCES

During the first two-thirds of the twentieth century, pharmaceutical manufacturers provided a wide variety of dosage forms for their commercial products to accommodate infants, children, adults, and the elderly. However, in recent years, under economic pressure to contain costs and optimize profits, pharmaceutical manufacturers have markedly and steadily reduced the variety of dosage forms available. The production of many drug products that serve an obvious patient need was discontinued because the small sales volume was inadequate to meet corporate overhead

DOI: 10.1201/9781003615323-35

requirements. The same economic pressures, as well as interruptions in the supply chain, have served to make shortages of pharmaceutical formulations commonplace.

Simultaneously, independent pharmacy owners faced ever-shrinking margins in reselling FDA-approved manufactured products. Because third-party payers resist paying for compounded prescriptions, such preparations are very often paid for in cash, which is an attractive alternative to pharmacy owners. A separate, but important factor is that compounding pharmacists are often much more intimately involved in the clinical care of their patients than retail pharmacists selling repackaging manufactured forms. Compounding pharmacists often feel more professional fulfillment than chain store pharmacists.

Over the past five decades, patients have increasingly become more assertive in managing their own health. Patient demand for drugs, nutrients, "nutraceuticals," exercise, fitness, and beauty aids have all grown steadily. These combined trends have all contributed to the re-emergence of pharmacy compounding.

The resurgence in pharmaceutical compounding began in the 1970s and continued into the 1980s. By the early and mid-1990s, it was evident that compounding was making a dramatic comeback in pharmacy practice. Several reasons have been put forth to explain the increase in preparing patient-specific medications, including, but not limited to the following:

- Many patients need drug dosages different from those that are commercially available.
- Many patients need specific dosage forms (such as suppositories, oral liquids, topicals, or injections) that are not commercially available.
- Many patients are allergic to, or have idiosyncratic intolerance of, excipients used in the manufacture of certain commercially available products.
- Pediatric medications need to be prepared with liquids and flavored to enhance adherence. Children also frequently prefer alternative dosage forms (such as lozenges, "gummy bears" and ice pops).
- Some medications are not chemically stable and require preparation and dispensing every few days; such formulations are not well suited to be manufactured products.
- Many drugs and drug-delivery systems are reported in the literature but have not yet been manufactured. Pharmacists can compound these for their patients' use, even before they are commercially available.
- Many physicians desire to try drug products in innovative ways, and pharmacists often work with them to meet the specific needs of individual patients.
- The preparation of veterinary drugs can be very complex (due to the variety and size of the patients involved and their place of domicile, including pastures and stables); consequently, most drug products are not available for animals and must be compounded.
- Home healthcare and the treatment of an increasing number of patients in the home environment have resulted in the need to compound sterile and non-sterile preparations for home use.

32.3 SEEKING THE OPTIMAL REGULATORY BALANCE BETWEEN "MANUFACTURING" VERSUS "COMPOUNDING"

Pharmaceutical compounding is necessary to ensure an uninterrupted flow of needed medications to patients. Individualizing patient care is at the heart of pharmaceutical compounding and is core to the professional practice of medicine and pharmacy.

The Quality Assurance approaches in manufacturing are necessarily more rigorous than those in healthcare compounding, but it is vital that the oversight of healthcare compounding quality from all sources is sufficient to protect public health. Governmental and non-governmental agencies, boards, and professional groups all play important roles in protecting public health in matters related to compounding.

- **Governmental Oversight** of Compounding (power to impose legal consequences)
    - **Federal** oversight of drug manufacturing falls to the U.S. Food and Drug Administration ("FDA") as it continuously evolves its interpretation of the Food, Drug, and Cosmetic Act of 1938 ("FDCA").
        - The FDA's scope is incomprehensively vast, but its sole instrument for measuring regulatory compliance of drug production is Current Good Manufacturing Practices ("cGMP"). Its definition of "current" is in constant evolution and can change as often as the companies the FDA inspects find innovative ways to improve their performance. When the FDA inspectors observe and report a great technical advance, it will soon become "current" in GMP. Because "current" is such a dynamic concept, the bar for federal compliance can become higher every day.
        - The statutory language of cGMP rarely changes, but what changes more rapidly is the FDA's enforcement policy based on its "current thinking." Unfortunately, there is no written record published in "real time" to inform us of the FDA's current thinking. The only pathways available for regulated entities to glean insights regarding how to comply is to read the FDA's enforcement

actions and/or the "Draft Guidance" or "Guidance" documents published on www.fda.gov.

- The FDA cannot represent itself in federal court. To impose legal consequences on regulated entities, it must enlist the collaboration of the U.S. Department of Justice. This serves as an important step in the federal "checks and balances."
- The FDA's power to levy sanctions is crushing, but the pace at which it applies its sanctions is glacial. The only time the FDA moves rapidly is on those occasions when public health emergencies threaten patient harm. It is not unusual for 18 months to elapse between the issuance of a dismal Form 483 and the issuance of a corresponding Warning Letter informing the pharmacy entity for the first time that its shortcomings were categorized by the FDA as "Official Action Indicated."

- **State** oversight of compounding differs sharply from the FDA approach and varies markedly from state to state but virtually always falls to a state-appointed board of professional authority. For compounding, this most often falls to the various "state pharmacy boards," but, depending on state-by-state approaches, it could also fall to state medical boards, state nursing boards, state consumer protection agencies, or state boards of health. Each state government has the "power to empower" its unique approach to compliance oversight.
  - Virtually every state has a statute governing pharmacy practice ("Statutory Law"), and virtually every state pharmacy board has promulgated a set of published rules to be followed by pharmacists and pharmacies ("Administrative Law").
  - Whereas the FDA's interpretation of federal statute is dynamic and evolving, state pharmacy board decisions are typically static and based on existing precedent. If a pharmacist avoids breaking a state's straightforward, literal rules, their compliance risk is relatively low. Pharmacy boards are loath to apply the state equivalent of what the FDA calls, "enforcement discretion" because at a state/regional/local level discretion could easily be perceived as favoritism or cronyism.
  - State pharmacy boards are constituted by elected legislators and/or executives to impanel the professional leaders within the state to apply their judgment to the actions of the pharmacists and pharmacies they regulate. Although appointments are often political, pharmacy boards typically have plenary powers and quasi-judicial authority to impose abrupt sanctions upon licensed persons and establishments, including fines, suspensions, cease-and-desist orders, and even revocation of the license to practice.
- **Non-governmental** oversight of compounding (powerless to impose legal consequences but able to set standards that attach to other vital consequences, including ineligibility to obtain reimbursement).
  - The National Association of Boards of Pharmacy ("NABP") is a private association of state pharmacy boards that came into existence primarily as a clearinghouse to facilitate the transfer or reciprocation of pharmacist's licenses between states. It has grown to become the primary forum by which state pharmacy board administrators and members can share information, conduct dialogue on important topics, and discuss enforcement approaches regarding issues of national scope.
  - The United States Pharmacopoeia (USP) Convention is a private, not-for-profit standard-setting organization which predates the FDA. USP was formed in Philadelphia in 1820 at a convention of prominent physicians representing most of the states and territories to establish a "national" consensus on the scientific validity of the most popular drug treatments of the time. USP scientific standards for therapeutic substances are recognized in the FDCA as the basis of quality, purity, and certain scientific attributes. Producing drugs that fail to meet USP standards can be construed by the FDA and DOJ to constitute adulteration and or misbranding and can result in criminal convictions and prison time.
  - The Joint Commission ("TJC") is a private not-for-profit organization that sets voluntary quality standards for its members, which include hospitals and other healthcare organizations. It routinely and regularly performs compliance "surveys" of its members and accredits those which achieve and maintain sufficient scores. These surveys have critical consequences because loss of accreditation is typically accompanied by loss of the ability to bill the Medicare and Medicaid Programs and many private health plans.

Because the federal government is deeply committed to the new drug approval process and because all compounded drugs are categorized by the FDA as "Unapproved New Drugs," there has been tension surrounding pharmacy compounding compliance for decades. This tug-of-war between healthcare providers on one side and the FDA on the other has been marked by legislation, lawsuits, and a public health calamity, all of which are interrelated. Chronologically, the key milestones in the FDA's role include:

- Although not called the "FDA" until 1930, the agency traces its modern regulatory functions to the passage of the **1906 Pure Food and Drugs Act**, which prohibited interstate commerce in adulterated and misbranded food and drugs.
- The Sulfanilamide Disaster of 1937 set the stage for the passage of the **Food Drug and Cosmetic Act of 1938** (FDCA), which required all marketed drugs to be **safe** when used as directed. This public health event occurred when a respected drug maker distributed an oral liquid formulation of this popular anti-infective drug as "Elixir Sulfanilamide" Unfortunately, rather than alcohol and water as the vehicle, the product was formulated with diethylene glycol ("antifreeze") and water. More than 100 people were killed, while others were rendered permanently blind.
- The **Kefauver Harris Amendment of 1962** amended the FDCA to require drug manufacturers to prove scientifically that a medication was not only safe but also **effective**. Because the legislative course of the Bill overlapped with the thalidomide-induced birth defects that ravaged Europe, public sentiment galvanized solidly behind this legislative expansion which had these important effects:
  - Required that manufacturers prove the effectiveness of drug products before they go on the market, and afterward report any serious side effects.
  - Required that evidence of effectiveness be based on adequate and well-controlled clinical studies conducted by qualified experts. Study subjects would be required to give their informed consent.
  - Gave the FDA 180 days to approve a new drug application and required FDA approval before the drug could be marketed in the United States.
  - Mandated that the FDA conduct a retrospective evaluation of the effectiveness of drugs that had been approved for safety—but not for effectiveness—between 1938 and 1962.
  - Allowed the FDA to set good manufacturing practices for industry and mandated regular inspections of production facilities.
  - Transferred to the FDA the oversight of prescription drug advertising, which was required to include accurate information about side effects.
  - Controlled the marketing of generic drugs to keep them from being sold as expensive medications under new trade names.
- The **FDA Modernization Act of 1997** made many changes in the FDCA, including the insertion of Section 503A. This was a two-edged sword. On the one hand, 503A provided specific exemptions from certain key provisions of FDCA for pharmacists who adhere to specific practice requirements. On the other hand, 503A was also intended to prevent compounders from masquerading as manufacturers by establishing fixed federal conditions **within which** the practice was deemed appropriate and lawful.
- *Western States Medical Center v. Shalala (filed November 1998)*—Section 503A took effect on November 21, 1998, one year after the date of the enactment of the Modernization Act. That same month, the solicitation and advertising provisions of section 503A were challenged by seven compounding pharmacies as an impermissible regulation of commercial speech. The U.S. District Court for the District of Nevada ruled in the plaintiffs' favor. The FDA appealed to the U.S. Court of Appeals for the Ninth Circuit. On February 6, 2001, the Court of Appeals declared section 503A invalid in its entirety (Western States Medical Center v. Shalala, 238 F.3rd 1090 (9th Cir. 2001)). The government petitioned for a writ of certiorari to the U.S. Supreme Court for review of the circuit court opinion. The Supreme Court granted the writ and issued its decision in the case on April 29, 2002.
- The Supreme Court affirmed the 9th Circuit Court of Appeals decision that found section 503A of the Act invalid in its entirety because it contained unconstitutional restrictions on commercial speech (i.e., prohibitions on soliciting prescriptions for and advertising specific compounded drugs). The Court did not rule on (and therefore left standing) the 9th Circuit's holding that the unconstitutional restrictions on commercial speech could not be severed from the rest of section 503A. Accordingly, the entirety of section 503A was invalid.
- After section 503A was struck down, the FDA's approach to compounding by state-licensed pharmacies became less assertive. The FDA undertook several pharmacy inspections in 2008, but there was considerable pushback, and inspection frequency dropped again.
- **The Serratia marcescens Outbreak of 2001**—In 2001, an outbreak of meningitis was traced to bacterial contamination in one lot of compounded betamethasone repository injection prepared by Doc's Pharmacy, a state-licensed pharmacy in Walnut Creek, CA. Eleven patients experienced infection after injection, including eight patients with culture-confirmed *Serratia marcescens* and three others with unattributed organisms. Of the

11, 5 had meningitis, three of whom died; 5 others had epidural abscesses; and 1 had an infected hip joint. In the Accusation of Gross Negligence by the California Board of Pharmacy against the Pharmacist-in-Charge at the time of the outbreak, key facts included (1) the pharmacy prepared 300 ml of the betamethasone compound, then subdivided that amount into three 100-ml vials; (2) per their routine, they took the 100 ml vials to the office of a physician office (next door neighbor of the pharmacy) for autoclaving; (3) the instruction manual for the physician's autoclave stated on the first page in bold type, "Not recommended for sterilization of liquids intended for direct patient contact"; (4) the physician's autoclave could not be set to match the settings for the validated protocol that was being used and the temperature, pressure; and time settings all varied from the protocol requirements; (5) no positive control was used to demonstrate the effectiveness of the sterilization; (6) after the betamethasone was autoclaved and cooled, each of the 100 ml amounts were subdivided into non-sterile 10 ml vials. These non-sterile 10 ml vials had been prepared by so-called "cold sterilization." "Cold sterilization" involved squirting isopropyl alcohol into the vials and onto the stoppers and closures four times and allowing them to dry.

- This accusation documented a tragic series of fundamental misconceptions and unacceptable practices, including "borrowing" from a neighbor the use of an inappropriate autoclave that was incapable of the required adjustments, followed by the absurd belief that isopropyl alcohol can be treated as a trusted sterilant.
- **The Fungal Meningitis Outbreak of 2012**—In 2012, an outbreak of meningitis was traced to fungal contamination in three lots of compounded methylprednisolone suspension prepared by New England Compounding Center (NECC), a state-licensed pharmacy in Framingham, MA. The most frequently isolated organism was *Exserohilum rostratum*, but *Aspergillus fumigatus* was also isolated. Doses from those three lots were administered to more than 14,000 patients in 20 states. The usual method of administration bypassed the protective immunity of the skin and blood because the drug was injected directly into the epidural space. The result was the single largest patient injury event ever associated with pharmacy compounding.
- The Centers for Disease Control and Prevention ("CDC") set up a webpage with a map of affected states and a grid to tabulate the human cost. CDC updates of case counts on the webpage ceased after October 30, 2015, when the count of total cases reached 753 and total deaths reached 64. Ironically, although 20 states had citizens infected, *not a single case* was recorded in the Commonwealth of Massachusetts. In other words, the NECC recall totaled about 17,000 multiple-dose vials, but not one case of infection was recorded in its domicile state.
- Michigan (264 cases, 19 deaths) and Tennessee (153 cases, 16 deaths) were the states hardest hit. Many victims who did not die from the infections were saddled with crippling permanent morbidity and a need for lifetime treatment with antifungal drugs.
- In the aftermath of the outbreak, there was public and media outrage. The House Energy & Commerce Committee held a hearing on November 14, 2012, and the Senate Health, Education, Labor, and Pensions ("HELP") Committee held one the next day. There were bipartisan recriminations and castigation of the FDA, but Commissioner Margaret Hamburg held fast to her position that the FDA was eager to inspect pharmacies but believed it was prohibited by the Western States Decision. She repeatedly told the legislators that the law needed to be revised to satisfy the constitutional flaw identified in the judicial review of Section 503A.
- **The Drug Quality and Security Act of 2013**—In the end, the Congress did give the FDA a new law. The Drug Quality and Security Act ("DQSA") was passed on November 21, 2013, and signed into law by President Obama on November 27, 2013. This legislation changed (almost) everything in the world of pharmacy compounding, but its full impact has not been fully measured and may not be for several more years.
- The DQSA is composed of two Titles. Title I is the "Quality Compounding Act" and addresses the quality assurance of large-scale pharmacy compounding. Title II is the "Drug Supply Chain Security Act" and is the culmination of the federal agenda for drug pedigree tracking. There is more overlap between the two topics than many perceive, but I will limit my scope to Title I, the very succinct Quality Compounding Act (a mere 4,713 words, including preamble and page numbers), which altered the Food Drug and Cosmetic Act in the following ways:
    - Section 503A was reinstated but revised to make no restrictions on Commercial Free Speech.
    - Section 503A provides healthcare compounders **exemption** from three important requirements of FDCA:
        - Section 505 (concerning the approval of drugs under new drug applications or abbreviated new drug applications);

  - Section 502(f)(1) (concerning the labeling of drugs with adequate directions for use); and
  - Section 501(a)(2)(B) (concerning current good manufacturing practice requirements).
- To maintain eligibility for these three exemptions, the 503A healthcare compounders were required to comply with each one of the following conditions:
  - The drug product is compounded for an identified individual patient based on the receipt of a valid prescription order, or a notation, approved by the prescribing practitioner, on the prescription order that a compounded product is necessary for the identified patient (section 503A(a) of the FD&C Act). (Note: a lack of notation by a prescriber that a compounded product is necessary is deemed sufficient to invalidate the compounder's FDCA exemptions.)
  - The compounding of the drug product is performed:
    - By a licensed pharmacist in a state-licensed pharmacy or a Federal facility, or by a licensed physician on the prescription order for an individual patient made by a licensed physician or other licensed practitioner authorized by state law to prescribe drugs; or
    - By a licensed pharmacist or licensed physician in limited quantities before the receipt of a valid prescription order for such individual patient, and
- Is based on a history of the licensed pharmacist or licensed physician receiving valid prescription orders for the compounding of the human drug product; and
- Those orders have been generated solely within an established relationship between the licensed pharmacist or licensed physician and either such patient for whom the prescription order will be provided or the physician or other licensed practitioner who will write such prescription order (sections 503A(a)(1) and (2) of the FD&C Act).
  - The drug product is compounded in compliance with the USP chapters on pharmacy compounding using bulk drug substances, as defined in 21 CFR 207.3(a)(4), that comply with the standards of an applicable USP or National Formulary (NF) monograph if one exists.
  - If such a monograph does not exist, the drug substance(s) must be a component of an FDA-approved human drug product. If a monograph does not exist and the drug substance is not a component of an FDA-approved human drug product, it must appear on a list of bulk drug substances for use in compounding developed by the FDA through regulation (section 503A(b)(1)(A)(i) of the FD&C Act).
- The drug product is compounded using bulk drug substances that are manufactured by an establishment that is registered under section 510 of the FD&C Act (including a foreign establishment that is registered under section 510(i) of the FD&C Act) (section 503A(b)(1)(A)(ii) of the FD&C Act).
- The drug product is compounded using bulk drug substances that are accompanied by valid certificates of analysis for each bulk drug substance (section 503A(b)(1)(A)(iii) of the FD&C Act).
- The drug product is compounded using ingredients (other than bulk drug substances) that comply with the standards of an applicable USP or NF monograph, if one exists, and the USP chapters on pharmacy compounding (section 503A(b)(1)(B) of the FD&C Act).
- The drug product does not appear on the list, published at 21 CFR 216.24, that includes drug products that have been withdrawn or removed from the market because such drug products or components of such drug products have been found to be unsafe or not effective (section 503A(b)(1)(C) of the FD&C Act).
- The licensed pharmacist or licensed physician does not compound regularly or in inordinate amounts any drug products that are essentially copies of commercially available drug products (section 503A(b)(1)(D) of the FD&C Act).
- The drug product is not a drug product identified by the FDA by regulation as a drug product that presents demonstrable difficulties for compounding that reasonably demonstrate an adverse effect on the safety or effectiveness of that drug product (section 503A(b)(3)(A) of the FD&C Act). See section III.B.3.
- The drug product is compounded in a state that has entered into a memorandum of understanding (MOU) with the FDA that addresses the distribution of inordinate amounts of compounded drug products interstate and provides for appropriate investigation by a state agency of complaints relating to compounded drug products distributed outside such state; or, in states that have not entered into such an MOU with the FDA, the licensed pharmacist, licensed

pharmacy, or licensed physician does not distribute, or cause to be distributed, compounded drug products out of the state in which they are compounded, more than 5% of the total prescription orders dispensed or distributed by such pharmacy or physician (sections 503A(b)(3)(B)(i) & (ii) of the FD&C Act).

- **Section 503B—Registered Outsourcing Facilities**—In addition to reinstating Section 503A for healthcare compounding entities, The Quality Compounding Act inserted a new Section 503 B, which created a *de novo* category of compounding establishments, called "Outsourcing Facilities."
- Section 503B states that three important requirements of FDCA:
    - Labeling with adequate directions for use (section 502(f)(1))
    - Premarket approval requirements (section 505)
    - Drug supply chain security requirements (section 582)
- "**shall not apply** to a drug compounded by or under the direct supervision of a licensed pharmacist in a facility that elects to register as an outsourcing facility," so long as specified conditions are met.

Registration of state-licensed pharmacies as outsourcing facilities was intended by Congress (and the FDA) to be the sole legitimate pathway for interstate shipment of large-batch compounded preparations without the "Triad Relationship" and without the requirement that "The drug product is compounded for an identified individual patient based on the receipt of a valid prescription order, or a notation, approved by the prescribing practitioner, on the prescription order that a compounded product is necessary for the identified patient." The main tradeoffs for this enormous power were that the Registered Outsourcing Facility must:

- register with (self-identify to) the FDA;
- pay registration fees;
- open itself to regular, recurring FDA inspections and agree to pay reinspection fees should the FDA determine that follow-up is needed before the next routine inspection; and
- agree to perform **all** compounding (including non-sterile formulations) under cGMP conditions.

DQSA made registration under 503B completely voluntary, the theory being that, after the lessons of NECC, hospitals and physician practices would surely stop buying sterile preparations from unregistered compounding pharmacies. Thus, Darwinian-like market pressures would ensure that interstate shipment of compounded preparations would eventually be limited to formulations compounded under cGMP conditions. Estimates were that within five years, hundreds of busy 503A compounders would register as outsourcing facilities under 503B.

PharMEDium Services LLC registered all four of its facilities (MS, NJ, TN, TX) on December 11, 2013. The PharMEDium registration was followed in rapid succession that month, by:

- SCA Pharmaceuticals (AR) on the 13th;
- KRS Global Biotechnology (FL) on the 15th;
- Cantrell Drug Company (AR) on the 16th;
- Medi-Fare Drug & Home Health Center (SC) on the 17th;
- US compounding (AR) on the 20th;
- Kings Park Slope, Inc (NY) on the 23rd;
- Region Care (NY) on the 24th;
- Banner Health (AZ) on the 26th; and
- Allergy Laboratories Inc. (OK) on December 30th.

This represented a very promising start because Region Care (A subsidiary of North Shore Long Island Jewish, now renamed "Northwell Health") and Banner Health were subsidiaries of prominent hospital systems and PharMEDium, SCA, KRS, Cantrell, Medi-Fare, and U.S. Compounding were already among the most successful providers in the large-batch compounding sector.

By September 9, 2014, the total number of Registered Outsourcing Facilities had grown to 55. Unfortunately, the rate of increase plummeted after FDA inspections started in earnest, because healthcare compounders had great difficulty comprehending and adapting to the quality assurance requirements for compliance with cGMP. Registrations continued at an acceptable pace until the COVID-19 pandemic, but de-registrations, bankruptcies, and legal pressures have been so frequent that the total numbers of Registered Outsourcing Facilities have simply remained balanced in a narrow range from the end of 2016 to December 2021 Here are the numbers, using the FDA's own webpage entitled Registered Outsourcing Facilities:

- On December 16, 2016, there were 65 companies listed.
- On December 6, 2017, there were 72.
- On October 22, 2018, there were 74.
- On December 4, 2019, there were 76.
- On December 30, 2020, there were 74.
- On December 20, 2021, there were 76.
- On March 14, 2022, there were still just 74 entities on the FDA webpage.

These 74 currently registered entities include several others that are operating under an unclosed Warning Letter or under Regulatory Meeting Status. Seventeen of the 74 are listed by the FDA as "Not Yet Inspected." One of those uninspected facilities (Strukmyer Medical of Mesquite, TX) registered on February 8, 2019. Notwithstanding the reason, this entity has been registered with the FDA and has been producing sterile preparations for human consumption for more than 1,000 days but still has never been inspected.

The primary reason for these long lag times has been the advent and the aftermath of the COVID-19 pandemic, which sharply curtailed air travel. Another factor might be that one or more may have never commenced compounding operations and the FDA can only perform operational inspections after production is underway. Nonetheless, if any Outsourcing Facility had been operational for more than two years without an inspection and suffered a headline-making quality failure, this would seem to be a blow to the FDA's oversight. There have been no patient harm incidents by a 503B facility since the pandemic, but the risk still exists.

When the FDA inspected large compounding pharmacies, several who have tried to "move up" to outsourcing from the 503A sector have suffered some epic failures as a result. These business reversals and liquidations are well known among pharmacy owners and have served as disincentives to those who are still compounding in large batches under 503A at community pharmacies and hospitals. Here are three "cautionary tales" that are legendary among owners of large compounding pharmacies:

- PharMEDium
  - When NECC made headlines, PharMEDium had already been one of the largest of the sterile compounders for several years. It had achieved much of its size in absorbing the Compass business from Baxter. It had been on the FDA's "radar screen" for years and had even obtained a letter from the FDA in 2005 stating that the agency was willing to apply its enforcement discretion to allow the company to link a product to patient post-shipment. On February 5, 2013, the FDA sent a second letter reversing that position and criticizing PharMEDium for laxity in the linking process.
  - Even before PharMEDium registered all four of its sites on December 11, 2013, as Outsourcing Facilities, each location was inspected by the FDA during February and March of 2013 and each suffered serious Form 483 Observations regarding simple and straightforward issues. Warning Letters addressing the FDA's concerns were issued to all four establishments and even to the PharMEDium corporate headquarters on July 18, 2014.
  - Pharmedium Issued a Nationwide Recall of a Norepinephrine admixture on December 31, 2015, and PharMEDium Headquarters issued another 483 on January 4, 2016. There was a Regulatory Meeting for all sites on May 5, 2016, and a recall of bupivacaine on that same day.
  - On October 6, 2016, despite the regulatory pressures, AmerisourceBergen announced it was buying PharMEDium for $2.58 Billion in cash.
  - There was a recall of specific lots of Potassium Phosphate and Succinylcholine Chloride on June 26, 2017.
  - On May 22, 2019, a Consent Decree was entered against PharMEDium and two of its senior executives Production was shut down from its Memphis site.
  - In February 2020, AmerisourceBergen announced it was shuttering all PharMEDium sites and ceasing operations.
- Pharmakon Pharmaceuticals
  - Initially registered on January 23, 2014.
  - Its first inspection ended on March 13, 2014, and its second inspection ended on April 8, 2014, and dismal 483s accompanied both. The second was in such rapid succession due to a clumsy recall of mislabeled midazolam.
  - The firm was issued a Warning Letter on May 21, 2015.
  - The FDA received reports on February 16, 2016, of serious adverse events in three infants associated with the use of the recalled super-potent morphine sulfate products from Pharmakon.
  - An FDA inspection that began February 18 ended with a 483 issued on March 16, 2016, with an Observation that the FDA laboratories found potencies from 0% in some cases to 207% in others.
  - In the case of the morphine lot that had caused the adverse reactions in the infants, the shoddy practices culminated in Pharmakon's distribution of 2,460% (i.e., 24.6 TIMES-labeled strength) super-potent morphine sulfate, an opiate pain medication, to hospitals in Indianapolis and Chicago. The miscalculated morphine was administered to infants in the pediatric unit and three infants suffered adverse effects from the narcotic overdose. One infant required naloxone reversal and was sent by helicopter to a nearby hospital with a neo-natal intensive care unit. The evidence at trial indicated that the owner and his Director of Compliance collaborated in trying to prevent the FDA from finding the laboratory evidence of the sub- and super-potency.
  - The Compliance Director entered a plea agreement, but the owner was indicted in June 2017, found guilty on April 11, 2019, after an eight-day trial and, on September 19, 2019, was sentenced to 33 months in federal prison.

- Cantrell Drug Company
  - Cantrell was a family-owned pharmacy that had been in business for decades before it grew huge in sterile compounding for hospitals and physician practices. Its Quality Assurance practices operated at the level of the USP compounding chapters. Pharmakon's various actions, inactions, and potency errors clearly seem to warrant the fate it suffered, but, by contrast, Cantrell produced tens of millions of doses during its existence without any instance of patient harm attributed to its products. Nonetheless, like Pharmakon, its existence ended with a federally imposed Consent Decree:
  - As with PharMEDium, the FDA inspected Cantrell before the DQSA became law. The timing was
    - Cantrell's first inspection ran from October 15 to November 4, 2013;
    - President Obama signed DQSA into law on November 27, 2013;
    - Cantrell registered with the FDA on December 16, 2013; and
  - Cantrell's first 483 was issued November 4, 2013, and it listed 12 observations of variance from the principles of GMP. If those shortfalls had been expertly addressed immediately, adequate progress might have been made before its next inspection.
  - The FDA's next action was a Warning Letter based on the findings of the first inspection issued 443 days later, on January 21, 2015. (For pharmacists unaccustomed to the FDA's pace, silent lag times greater than 14 months might be interpreted as tacit approval of the facility's plan of correction, but this would be a false assumption. Long periods of silence from the FDA are more the rule than the exception.)
  - Cantrell wrote a Warning Letter Response Letter on February 10, 2015. The company asserted that the company did not concur that its processes put patients at risk. It then detailed multiple observation-specific remedial actions, some of which were performed at great expense. (Note: This exemplifies an important part of the paradigm shift which pharmacists must adopt when dealing with the FDA, because the agency does not accept a serial remediation approach such as "Item 1 needs fixed—here is how we fixed Item 1." The FDA expects regulated entities to evaluate the underlying processes that allowed each Observation to occur and to identify and remediate the root cause. The FDA's expectation is "Fix the **process**, not the Observation.")
  - Cantrell's next FDA interaction was an inspection that included 16 days on site between September 14, 2016, and October 14, 2016. A 483, an Amended 483, and a Second Amended 483 were issued on October 14, 2016, which noted 12 Observations of potential GMP non-compliance, including three "Repeat Observations" from the first inspection. (FDA issues Form 483 documents to create evidence of their most important concerns. There is no requirement to respond to a 483 in writing, but failure to do so may be interpreted as indifference. Repeat Observations are taken as negligence of quality concerns, and frequently lead to the slippery slope of serious Official Action.)
  - Cantrell performed a Recall of Select Sterile Drug Products Due to Lack of Sterility Assurance on November 18, 2016.
  - A third 483 was issued on June 29, 2017, after six days on site.
  - Cantrell issued a Voluntary Nationwide Recall of All Sterile Drug Products Due to Lack of Sterility Assurance on July 25, 2017.
  - The FDA issued a Press Release on March 1, 2018, entitled, "FDA Alerts Healthcare Professionals and Patients not to Use Compounded Drugs from Cantrell Drug Company; Agency Seeks Action to Stop Production and Distribution."
  - A fourth 483 was issued on March 22, 2018, after six days on site.
  - A Federal Judge entered a Consent Decree against Cantrell on April 19, 2018.
  - A fifth and final 483 was issued on August 22, 2018, after seven days on site.

Cantrell's experience served as a case in point of what can happen when prominent "big-batch" 503A pharmacies register with the FDA. The vicious cycle can be as follows:

- The pharmacy registers and, at its initial FDA inspection, it receives multiple Observations citing cGMP shortcomings.
- Some elect to bring in a cGMP consultant, but many determine to address the Observations on their own. Even those who hire a consultant, usually hire a "pharmacy compounding expert" rather than a GMP expert validation firm.
- Typically, the FDA will not inspect again for many months, but, when they do, they often find many "Repeat Observations" and their concerns escalate. They stay longer and dig deeper.
- Eventually the entity may need to perform a Recall. The financial pain of a Recall may range widely from:
  - One lot number of a solitary product;
  - All lot numbers of a solitary product;

- All lot numbers of all products in a specific category; to
- All products within expiry and a cessation of production until the FDA agrees with the entity's correctional plan.

- Any recall can threaten the financial viability of small Registered Outsourcing Facilities for several reasons:
  - Performing a Recall correctly is tantamount to a second "full time job" for the leadership and the staff of the entity, requiring many hours of unbudgeted overtime and weekend work;
  - As personnel costs jump, ongoing revenue from the recalled product lines drops to zero;
  - If the organization pauses production, their personnel must be paid during the interim or laid off. In either case, trained, seasoned staff are likely to find other jobs;
  - Recalls are disruptive and disquieting to existing customers and tend to degrade success in acquiring new ones.
  - Last, but not least, the entity must pay the high costs of refunding, returning, and destroying the affected products.

Consent Decrees are devastating to the companies and owners that are subject to them. They are a form of a legal contract that typically obligates the pharmacist who signs them (no matter where they practice in the future) to, operate in compliance with cGMP for all future compounding activities, pay heavy fines (sometimes thousands of dollars per day) in the event of any future failure to comply with cGMP, and pay the cost of all future the FDA inspections. This includes:

- Airfare
- Meals
- Lodging
- Ground transportation
- The **combined** per diem salaries of the FDA personnel who appear on site

Persons who have signed a Consent Decree face great financial peril if they ever again work in any job the duties of which could be remotely construed by the FDA to constitute "compounding." Hospitals and chain drug stores might hesitate to hire them, knowing they are potential "lightning rods" for FDA inspections.

Here is a non-exhaustive list of Registered Outsourcing Facilities that have signed Consent decrees:

- Downing Laboratories on January 11, 2016
- Medistat Rx LLC on July 06, 2017
- Isomeric Pharmacy Solutions on August 04, 2017
- Cantrell Drug Company on April 19, 2018
- Delta Pharma on June 08, 2018
- PharmD Solutions, LLC, on May 22, 2019
- PharMEDium (four sites) on May 22, 2019

Here is a non-exhaustive list of Registered Outsourcing Facilities that have conducted recalls:

- Avella of Deer Valley, Inc. (dba Avella Specialty Pharmacy), Phoenix, AZ
- Avella Specialty Pharmacy, (formerly Advanced Pharma, Inc.), Houston, TX
- Bella Pharmaceuticals, Inc.
- Cantrell Drug Company, Little Rock, AR
- Coastal Meds LLC, Biloxi, MS
- Downing Labs, LLC, Dallas, TX
- Fusion IV Pharmaceuticals, Inc., dba Axia Pharmaceutical, Los Angeles, CA
- Isomeric Pharmacy Solutions, LLC, Salt Lake City, UT
- Medistat RX, LLC, Foley, AL
- Pharmakon Pharmaceuticals, Noblesville, IN
- PharMEDium Services, LLC, Cleveland, MS
- PharMEDium Services, LLC, Memphis, TN
- Qualgen LLC, formerly registered as Amerilab LLC, Edmond, OK
- SCA Pharmaceuticals, Windsor, CT
- US Compounding, Inc., Conway, AR
- Wells Pharmacy Network

Despite the difficulties that many large-batch compounding 503A pharmacies have encountered after registering as Outsourcing Facilities, the sector is still ripe with potential because the public demand is large and rapidly growing. Therefore, we should understand the complexities required of those entities that decide to register. The statute states that, to maintain the exemptions afforded to a Registered Outsourcing Facility.

- The drug must be compounded under the direct supervision of a licensed pharmacist.
- The facility must register with the Secretary of Health and Human Services (via the FDA) and adhere to all the various requirements of registration, including:
  - Register its name, place of business, unique facility identifier, and a point of contact e-mail address;
  - Produce at least one sterile drug for administration to humans;
  - An Outsourcer may license as a pharmacy with any state, but there is no federal requirement to do so.
    - An Outsourcer may obtain prescriptions from valid prescribers for individually identified patients, but there is no federal requirement to do so.
    - Indicate whether it intends to compound a drug that appears on this list in effect under section 506E (i.e., the FDA drug

shortage list) during the subsequent calendar year.

- Upon initially registering; once during the month of June of each year; and once during the month of December of each year—each outsourcing facility must submit a report identifying the drugs compounded by such outsourcing facility during the previous 6-month period and electronically provide the FDA:
  - the active ingredient;
  - the source of the active ingredient;
  - the National Drug Code number of the source drug or bulk active ingredient, if available;
  - the strength of the active ingredient per unit;
  - the dosage form and route of administration of the compounded preparation;
  - the package description;
  - the number of individual units produced, and
  - the National Drug Code number ("NDC") of the final product. (if assigned)
- Submit adverse event reports in accordance with the content and format requirements established through guidance or regulation under 21 CFR 310.305 or successor regulations (MedWatch).
- Comply with federal restrictions against producing drugs that are "essentially a copy of an approved drug."
- Recognize that paying the federal registration fee does not relieve an outsourcing facility of any state pharmacy licensing fees that pertain.
- Acknowledge that if the FDA determines that more than one inspection is indicated in any given fiscal year, a reinspection fee will be assessed for each reinspection.

32.4 INVESTIGATIONS, INDICTMENTS, CONVICTIONS, AND ACQUITTALS AFTER THE FUNGAL MENINGITIS OUTBREAK

Very soon after the Fungal Meningitis Outbreak was traced to the compounding practices at NECC, federal and state investigators swarmed over the facility to compile facts and collect evidence. A concentric circle of trucks and reporters from media outlets set up just the other side of the yellow tape to inform the public. There was an outcry to identify those responsible and see that justice was done.

As the facts were released, the sense steadily grew that the Outbreak should have been prevented. The Committee Staff Report for the U.S. Senate HELP Committee provided this chronology:

- NECC was granted a special pharmacy license by the Board in June 1998 and had seriously violated state rules by April 1999 but was let off with a warning and a private non-disciplinary advisory letter.
- In June 2001, the Idaho Board of Pharmacy complained to the Massachusetts Board that NECC was, providing unapproved prescription forms in its solicitations to Idaho prescribers, but no documentation of this event was found in the Board records during the post-Outbreak investigations.
- In March 2002, a prescribing doctor reported to the FDA that as many as five patients became ill following an epidural injection of NECC-produced betamethasone repository injection products. He reported the illnesses to the FDA, alerted NECC about the issue, and returned unused doses to NECC but did not take samples. The FDA arrived to inspect NECC on April 9, 2002, but there were no records regarding the drugs in question. The FDA's Form 483 issued at the inspection's close enumerated 13 observations of faulty practices.
- In August 2002, two more patients were hospitalized with meningitis and NECC's methylprednisolone acetate ("MPA") was implicated. The Massachusetts Board initiated an investigation and the FDA sporadically joined in between October 2002 and February 2003. The FDA collected vials of purportedly sterile injectable drugs from NECC's inventory and found that 5 of the 16 tested were contaminated with bacteria and that other products were sub-potent or superpotent. In the wake of these incidents, the FDA concluded that enforcement was the realm of the Massachusetts Board but wrote, "Recommend firm be prohibited from manufacturing until they can demonstrate ability to make product reproducibly and dependably."
- In February 2004, the MBPR staff performed an inspection and concluded that NECC had addressed its 2002–2003 shortcomings but recommended a public reprimand. In September 2004, the Board voted to seek a public censure and probation, but NECC did not agree to the proposed Consent Decree transmitted to it by the MBPR on October 4, 2004. NECC counter-proposed a non-public disciplinary action. MBPR (apparently) referred the matter to state prosecutors, but there was no record of a formal order or hearing.
- A modified consent agreement was approved by MBPR on January 10, 2006. This agreement called for NECC to submit to two inspections six

months apart by a third-party evaluation firm in exchange for a period of non-public probation.

- NECC chose Pharmacy Support, Inc. ("PSI") to perform the inspections. The first visit by PSI found 18 shortfalls of the most elementary and fundamental principles of healthcare sterile compounding, including:
  - "No requirements for donning proper attire or hand washing";
  - "Floors in the unclassified/hybrid buffer area have not been sanitized in 3 months of use";
  - "Lot numbers are not assigned appropriately."
- NECC replaced some deficient equipment, undertook some staff training, and wrote some new SOPs and on April 7, 2006, PSI submitted a final report that stated, "New England Compounding Center has made significant Improvements over the past several months. They have demonstrated the ability to be compliant with all state and federal regulations." It went on to say, "The Pharmacist-In-Charge has committed to these enhancements and has put an action plan in place to assure compliance. PSI is satisfied with the progress to date and is confident that the remaining issues will be resolved in a short period of time."
- On June 2, 2006, the Board Informed NECC that it had fulfilled the requirements of its Consent Decree and that it considered the matter closed.

After the investigations concluded and the violations of law were assessed, 14 people were indicted in connection with the NECC and the Nationwide Fungal Meningitis Outbreak. The two main focal points of responsibility were Barry J. Cadden, a pharmacist, the managing partner, and a 25% owner of NECC, and Glen Chin, the Pharmacist-in-Charge, who was directly professionally responsible for the compliance of the business entity with state laws and rules. Lesser charges were brought against 12 lower-ranking owners and employees, but it was these two decision makers who faced the most serious charges. The various charges included:

- Twenty-five counts apiece (Cadden and Chin only) of second-degree murder in Florida, Indiana, Maryland, Michigan, North Carolina, Tennessee, and Virginia. Second-degree murder is defined broadly as an intentional murder with malice aforethought but is not premeditated or planned in advance. However, the precise wording of the second-degree murder charges seemed to vary state-by-state in the indictment in accordance with the definition of that crime in each individual state statute.
- The other 12 included six other pharmacists, the director of operations, the national sales director, an unlicensed pharmacy technician, two of NECC's other owners, and one other individual were charged with additional crimes, including:
- Violations of the Food, Drug, and Cosmetic Act.
- Mail fraud: Contaminated and mislabeled vials sent by interstate courier.
- Criminal contempt: Defined as conduct that defies, disrespects, or insults the authority or dignity of a court. Often, contempt takes the form of actions that are seen as detrimental to the court's ability to administer justice. These charges stemmed from the fact that the owners of NECC transferred millions of dollars in assets after the court issued a restraining order prohibiting the transfer of assets.
- Structuring: The practice of executing financial transactions in a specific pattern calculated to avoid the creation of certain records and reports required by law. These charges relate to the withdrawal of cash from certain accounts in a manner designed to avoid legal reporting requirements.
- Racketeering: The federal crime of conspiring to organize to commit crimes, especially on an ongoing basis as part of an organized crime operation.
- Thirteen of the fourteen individuals indicted were convicted of at least one charge, but Joseph Evanosky, a staff pharmacist, was acquitted of all federal charges. Convictions included:
- On December 20, 2016, Robert A. Ronzio, NECC's National Director of Sales., pled guilty to one count of conspiring to defraud the FDA.
- On July 29, 2016, Carla Conigliaro, the majority owner of NECC, and her husband, Douglas Conigliaro, each pled guilty to withdrawing cash from their bank accounts in a manner intended to defeat financial reporting requirements.
- On March 22, 2017, Barry Cadden was convicted of racketeering, racketeering conspiracy, mail fraud, and introduction of misbranded drugs into interstate commerce with the intent to defraud and mislead but was acquitted of 25 counts of second-degree murder. He was sentenced to 108 months in prison and three years of supervised release, and forfeiture and restitution in an amount to be determined later.
- On October 25, 2017, Glen Chin was convicted of racketeering, racketeering conspiracy, mail fraud, and introduction of misbranded drugs into interstate commerce with the intent to defraud and mislead but was also acquitted of 25 counts of second-degree murder. He was sentenced to eight years in prison, two years

of supervised release, and forfeiture and restitution in an amount to be determined later.

- On. August 17, 2018, Scott M. Connolly, who was working for NECC as an unlicensed Pharmacy Technician, pled guilty to 10 counts of mail fraud;
- On December 13, 2018, verdicts came down in a trial of six other NECC personnel:
  - Gene Svirskiy, a former NECC clean room pharmacist was convicted of racketeering, racketeering conspiracy, 10 counts of mail fraud, and two counts of introduction of adulterated drugs into interstate commerce with intent to defraud or mislead.
  - Christopher Leary, a former NECC clean room pharmacist, was convicted of three counts of mail fraud, one count of introduction of adulterated drugs into interstate commerce with intent to defraud or mislead, and two counts of introduction of misbranded drugs into interstate commerce.
  - Alla Stepanets, one of NECC's verification pharmacists, was convicted of six counts of introduction of misbranded drugs into interstate commerce. Sentencing was scheduled for March 26, 2018.
  - Sharon Carter, NECC's former director of operations, was convicted of conspiracy to defraud the United States.
  - Greg Conigliaro, a former owner of NECC, was convicted of conspiracy to defraud the United States.
  - On May 3, 2019, Kathy Chin and Michelle Thomas were convicted of four and two counts, respectively, of dispensing drugs without valid prescriptions with the intent to defraud or mislead government regulators. Both had served at NECC as served as verification pharmacists, signing off on drug orders prior to shipment to customers.
- In December 2018, the Michigan Attorney General filed 11 state counts of second-degree murder against both Barry Cadden and Glen Chin. The victims include all eight Michigan citizens included in the federal case, plus three other victims who were not included in the federal racketeering prosecutions. I do not believe this would violate constitutional protections against "double jeopardy," but expect this may become a defense argument as the state prosecution takes shape.
- On June 7, 2019, 2 of the 13 defendants initially convicted had their conviction overturned on appeal because the presiding District Court Judge found that Sharon Carter and Greg Conigliaro could not have tricked the FDA as to whether NECC was a drug manufacturer or a compounding center because the law never made a distinction between the two. Judge Stearns determined that their conviction was technically a "legal impossibility."
- On July 7, 2021, after the First Federal Circuit Court referred Barry Cadden's sentencing back to Judge Richard Stearns suggesting some aggravating factors should apply, Cadden's sentence was increased to 14.5 years.
- On July 21, 2021, following the same logic, Judge Stearns extended Glenn Chin's sentence to 10.5 years.

32.5 MEMORANDUM OF UNDERSTANDING

Section 503A(b) (3) (B) established that to qualify for the exemptions in section 503A, the drug product must be compounded in accordance with either of the following:

1. It was compounded in a state that had entered an MOU with the FDA that addressed the interstate distribution of inordinate amounts of compounded drug products and provided for investigation by a state agency of complaints related to compounded drug products distributed outside such state.
2. It was compounded in a state that had not entered such an MOU, but the licensed pharmacist, pharmacy, or physician distributes (or causes to be distributed) compounded drug products outside of the state in which they were compounded—in quantities that did not exceed 5% of the total prescription orders dispensed or distributed by such pharmacy or physician.

The apparent purpose of this MOU was to shift much of the legal responsibility of tracking out-of-state shipments by 503A pharmacies from the FDA to the pharmacy boards of the domicile states.

Signing the MOU would obligate the state to inspect and monitor interstate shipments of compounded drugs prepared by resident pharmacies (or physicians) and maintain adequate surveillance of complaints and untoward outcomes. The reward for signing the MOU is that domicile pharmacies could maintain their 503A exemptions from FDCA, but this is an advantage only for those licensees, not for the state government. For the state, there would be massive increases in responsibility, risk of blame and liability, and demand for resources, while these factors would be counterbalanced by any offsetting rewards.

Not only are the incentives weak for states to sign the FDA's "one-size-fits-all" boilerplate MOU, but even if the states wanted to sign, there are countless constitutional, legal, and administrative hurdles to overcome. Some state constitutions can be interpreted as prohibitive and even if signing were constitutional, the MOU decision belongs to the elected state government, not to the pharmacy professional authority. Consensus by the Governor, the state legislature, and the state Attorney General's office would be necessary. Even were such a consensus reached, there would be a vulnerability to one or more lawsuits after which the judiciary process would take over.

It may not be surprising that this statutory requirement, put in place in November 2013, is still not in effect in 2022. The FDA has proposed multiple versions of a monolithic Compounding MOU in the Federal Register and the versions have tinkered with the percentage of compounded preparations permitted to enter interstate commerce by pharmacies domiciled in MOU-signing states. The latest version has increased the interstate fraction to 50%, but, according to FDA.gov, its most recent proposal just two states ratified it—New Hampshire and Colorado.

On September 21, 2021, litigation filed by Reed Smith on behalf of Wellness Pharmacy et al. won a favorable decision from Judge Chris Cooper of the United States District Court for the District of Columbia. On February 22, 2022, this ruling was followed up by a Status Report to Judge Cooper by HHS Secretary Becerra and FDA Commissioner Robert Califf stating that the government is preparing a Notice of Proposed Rulemaking that will settle the definitions of dispensing versus distribution.

I do not believe an MOU will ever go into effect until or unless there is a meeting of the minds between the FDA and the individual state governments. Because there are 50 states, a District, and multiple Territories, I expect that many MOUs must be painstakingly negotiated with individual states or groups of states if more than a few ever ratify the concept. In the absence of an MOU. DQSA is clear that a 503A entity cannot legally ship more than 5% of its total prescription orders across state borders but the government's Status Report makes clear that the FDA will continue to exercise "enforcement discretion" regarding the 5% limitation and that the government concedes the MOU published on October 27, 2020, is suspended.

32.6 USP, NABP, AND THE STATE PHARMACY REGULATORY AUTHORITIES

32.6.1 Defining "Safe Enough"

The Quality Assurance principles of the FDA contrast sharply with those of the state health professional authorities and their various affiliated extra-governmental quasi-regulators. The disharmony arises from the basic incompatibility between manufacturing principles versus the principles of patient care as practiced by health professionals.

The FDA's focus is on manufacturing. This focus on massive size and scope is inherent in the FDA's approach because its core mission is interstate commerce of huge quantities of precisely uniform drug products that must, by federal law, be both safe and efficacious.

Medicine, pharmacy, nursing, and other healing professions focus on each individual patient in their care. Addressing the unique need(s) of each patient is their core mission. This mission is always pragmatic in nature because the choice and characteristics of the final drug preparation are merely a means of addressing the patient's complaint(s). The professional listens to the patient, makes a recommendation based on judgment, and prescribes a therapy.

After a reasonable trial time—and regularly thereafter—the professional and the patient meet to assess whether the intervention improved the patient's condition. Each therapeutic intervention is a "clinical study" with a patient population of one.

At these two extremes, the contrast in defining "acceptable risk" from the product is clear, but the middle ground between millions of manufactured doses and the unique need(s) of one patient for a compounded drug is murky and controversial. The middle ground is pertinent whenever the healthcare practitioner recognizes a frequently encountered patient need:

- For which no FDA-approved product is available on the market—but which
- Can be met with a standardized compounded formulation of a single drug or combination of drugs.

Health professionals may elect to compound in this middle ground when the efficiency of large-scale compounding becomes commercially feasible and financially enticing. NECC confronted this middle ground when methylprednisolone became unavailable from the manufacturer, and they went for the money without an effective Quality Assurance Program.

Depending on where the level of acceptable product risk is set, the middle ground's quality assurance balance will be set over a broad range of rigor. The issue becomes how society will determine to define the lowest level of rigor that constitutes "acceptable risk."

Although there is a naive notion in the current culture that 100% safety is always the only answer, perfect safety is never achievable and ignores the laws of economics. NECC notwithstanding, it is vital to understand that imposing a manufacturing level of quality assurance on all compounded preparations would render patient care economically unfeasible.

Business schools teach that a customer wants a product with three desirable characteristics:

- They want it to be always available.
- They want it to be inexpensive.
- They want it to be of the highest quality.

The laws of economics dictate that the customer can almost always have two of the three but can almost never have all three at once. Society must balance its choices and determine how safe is "safe enough."

Traditionally state pharmacy boards are composed of prominent pharmacy leaders with a good general grasp of professional pharmacy practices. Their role is to judge controversial judgments made by other pharmacy practitioners. However, board members of today are often administrative leaders of large pharmacy corporations or hospitals who have little understanding of compounding practices. The pharmacy boards needed guidance from a higher level of expertise and the United States Pharmacopeial Convention ("USP") stepped forward to fill that gap by forming an expert committee on pharmaceutical compounding in the late 1990s.

The USP's pristine reputation as a global standard-setting organization rested on the honest interpretation of hard, measurable scientific data by its expert committees, Unfortunately, USP constructed the Compounding Expert Committee to function more like a state pharmacy board. Its compounding chapters are not based on measurable scientific facts but on the idiosyncratic experiences, opinions, and judgments of its various members. As an analogy, if the rest of USP is like a news publication, the writings of the Compounding Committee are more like an Opinion/Editorial Page.

There is a fundamental disconnect between the quality expectations of the States and those of the FDA. It is vital that the practice of the health professions continue to be regulated by the states rather than a federal agency. However, compounding quality assurance must be rigorous enough to protect the public health. The state professional authorities must become better informed and should adopt an FDA-style evidence-based paradigm for quality assurance.

USP 797 and 795 treat quality assurance like a static checklist. This is in keeping with the thinking and approach of most healthcare practitioners. Pharmacists and physicians are accustomed to clearly written, unequivocal rules. They want to know that they are free to care for patients in any way that does not specifically violate such rules.

In the clinical training of physicians, pharmacists, and nurses, the favored learning process is "Watch One-Do One-Teach One." This very pragmatic approach starts novices at a very superficial level, but their acumen grows steadily over many years of professional training. This thinking lends itself to unexamined processes, "tribal knowledge," and prohibitions that are insufficiently detailed in the early stages of training but which evolve to the highest degree of professional knowledge over time.

Conversely, in the CGMP paradigm, there are no arbitrary and opinion-based "best practices." Instead, under CGMP, the drug makers can be freely innovative and flexible in their approach to production provided they validate their processes scientifically and statistically. The CGMP approach essentially imposes a requirement to perform unceasing scientific research on one's own production processes.

32.7 PHYSICIAN AND MEDICAL OFFICE COMPOUNDING

It is important to note that the language of DQSA covers not just pharmacists and pharmacies but also physicians and medical practices. Under federal law, compounding by pharmacy and medical professionals is exempt from the same three requirements of the federal code, so long as they adhere to the same conditions. The ability to practice certain medical specialties is financially dependent upon purchasing storing, preparing, and administering drug products to their patients. Examples of **traditional** medical specialties with drug-dependent revenue streams include, but are not limited to:

- Oncology, which depends on revenue from the administration of oral and injectable chemotherapy drugs and will include cellular, gene, and tissue therapies as soon as the FDA approves them for marketing.
- Rheumatology and Gastroenterology, which depend on the administration of infused biological agents in the treatment of rheumatoid arthritis, psoriatic arthritis, and inflammatory bowel diseases.
- Allergy/Immunology, which depends on the administration of pooled gamma globulins and dispensing of desensitization preparations.
- Ophthalmology, which depends on the administration of bevacizumab injections for wet macular degeneration and for compounded eyedrops and topical preparations for corneal conditions and procedures.

An example of a less traditional, but burgeoning medical specialty is the "Health and Wellness" sector. "Health and Wellness" prescribing encompasses distinct, but overlapping subsectors including, but not limited to:

- Bio-identical hormone replacement
- Weight loss
- Anti-aging
- Vitamin therapy
- Erectile dysfunction
- Beauty/tanning
- Exercise/fitness/body building
- Nutraceuticals

"Health and Wellness" ("H&W") is not yet recognized as a medical specialty by the American Board of Medical Specialties, but its financial significance is growing rapidly. The aggregation of patients and complaints of its subsectors may be largely attributed to the desire of lay people to take charge of their own health, even when doing so runs the risk of seeking therapies that are neither evaluated by the FDA nor paid for by "health insurance."

Driven by the same cultural and market dynamics as compounding pharmacy, many H&W physicians eschew submitting bills to health plans or pharmacy benefit manages, preferring instead to bill the patient directly. Declaring independence from "third-party payers" relieves both patient and physician from such valueless considerations as formulary tiers, "off-label" use, prior authorizations, and shopping "co-pays." The various "middle-men" and their respective profit margins are eliminated from the equation.

Personalized compounded preparations fit very naturally with the H&W segment and subscribe to the traditional principles of the free market. Unfortunately, the compounding quality assurance practices of physicians lag far behind those of compounding pharmacies. Although the USP Chapters <795> and <797> are open to valid criticism for being unscientific and opinion-based, they are far better than no standards at all. Physician practice owners are often unaware that <797> exists, let alone what it purports to require.

Traditional medical specialties (e.g., Oncology, Rheumatology, Gastroenterology, et al) typically start with FDA-approved parenteral products that arrive from drug manufacturers in a sterile state. The physician's staff members typically reconstitute, measure, or transfer the prescribed dose to a syringe, transfer the measured dose to a diluent bag, and immediately administer the dose to the patient via a timed infusion.

The lack of patient infectious risk (and patient harm) associated with this process owes to the very short interval between the initial puncture and the completion of the injection or infusion. Even with poor hand hygiene, poor air quality, and poor aseptic technique, there are rarely sufficient "doubling times" for bacteria or fungi to reproduce to a sufficient "critical mass" to cause clinical infection. The risk of patient harm escalates as the storage time between the completion of compounding and the administration of the preparation is prolonged.

Although to date, the FDA has rarely performed inspections in medical practices, physician compounding is subject to the same three exemptions from federal approval as pharmacies and pharmacists, but medical practice compounding can also be found ineligible for those exemptions for the same reasons.

There have been at least three FDA inspections related to drug compounding in physician practice entities:

- William R. Grace M.D. P. C., New York, NY—July 2016
  - This company was inspected by the FDA from June 28, 2016, to July 8, 2016, in response to an outbreak of *Exophiala dermatitidis* bloodstream infections in patients who had received intravenous medication prepared and administered in Dr. Grace's office. A Form 483 was issued that cited four Observations:
    - The cleaning disinfecting and upkeep of the equipment used to produce sterile drug products were inadequate.
    - Inadequate aseptic techniques were demonstrated by the operators who prepare and handle sterile drug products.
    - The facility design was inadequate to prevent microbiological contamination of sterile drug products.
    - Drug products purporting to be sterile were not tested to determine conformance with such requirements.

No Warning Letter was subsequently posted to the usual FDA webpage, but a Referral Letter was. The posted Letter was sent to the Commissioner of the New York City Department of Health and Mental Hygiene (NYC DOHMH) on August 8, 2017. The letter explained that although the FDA staff were able only to observe simulations, some observations may have constituted violations of FDCA. The letter noted Dr. Grace had committed to "meet recognized State requirements and other standards applicable to [a] physician office" and the FDA did not intend to take further action at that time. The FDA believed that corrective actions could be appropriately overseen by NYC DOHMH.

- CDC presented a webinar on April 18, 2017, entitled, "Lessons from an Outbreak Investigation: Improving Medication Preparation, Use, and Other Infection Control Practices in Outpatient Oncology Clinics."
  - The webinar summarized the results of a thorough scientific investigation which concluded that 17 patients developed bloodstream infections after having their implanted venous access ports flushed with an extemporaneously prepared flushing solution contaminated with *Exophiala dermatitidis* and/or *Rhodotorula mucilaginosa* at a New York City oncology clinic. The clinic was referred to as "Clinic A."
  - The investigation began on May 24, 2016, when infectious disease physicians at a hospital ("Hospital A") reported two cases of *Exophiala dermatitidis*—one on May 14 and another on May 15. This had caused a retrospective review of laboratory work and two more cases were identified—one from April 8 and another from April 22. This pattern caused the physician in Clinic A to call patients back in for surveillance blood cultures though they were not ill. On May 27, one of the surveillance cultures was positive, the FDA was notified, and a CDC team was assembled which arrived on May 27.
  - Because *Exophiala* bloodstream infections are extremely rare, the investigation was broadened to include blood cultures of all patients who had received intravenous treatment at the clinic since January 1, 2016. The clinic had seen 153 patients in the timeframe, but only 38 had received IV medications. Six had died before the investigation and 3 declined to participate, which left a cohort of 29 patients who could be evaluated. Of these 29 patients, 17 had positive blood cultures and 12 did not. Chemotherapy drugs and supportive drugs were ruled out as a common thread, but all 29 patients were exposed to the compounded flushing solution. Twelve of 17 positive cases

had a median number of flushes of 12 contrasted to a median number of 4 flushes for the patients with negative blood cultures.
    - The flushing solutions consisted of a 1000 ml normal saline bag with the addition of small amounts of vancomycin, ceftazidime, and heparin. This saline bag was stored in a refrigerator between uses, but the bag was accessed multiple times each business day with 10 ml aliquots being drawn into syringes as needed to meet demand over a period of four to eight weeks. During the investigational timeframe, three bags had been in use, but the first two had been discarded when empty. All 17 of the positive cases received flushes from the second bag, which was statistically significant ($P < 0.001$).
- Advanced Nutriceuticals, LLC (dba The Guyer Institute of Molecular Medicine), Indianapolis, IN—October 2020
- [*Note—although Nutraceuticals is spelled with an "a" rather than an "i," it is cited exactly as it was spelled on the FDA document.]
    - This company was inspected by the FDA from October 13 to October 29, 2020, and the two investigators issued a Form 483 that cited five Observations:
        - Aseptic processing was performed outside of a certified ISO 5 area;
        - The ISO 5 classified aseptic processing area was located within a non-classified room. Staff said that an IV with a [redacted] additive was produced inside the ISO 5 hood and labeled not to be used after "03-Oct-2020," but was shipped to a patient located in California on September 30, 2020, and arrived on October 1, 2020.
        - Staff touched surfaces outside the ISO 5 area with gloved hands, then performed aseptic processing without changing or sanitizing gloves.
        - The aseptic operator made rapid movements near open sterile units or instruments.
        - The aseptic operator conducted aseptic manipulations in an area that was blocked from first-pass air.

The company subsequently received a Warning Letter on November 10, 2021. The Warning Letter asserted that the firm did not receive valid prescriptions for individually identified patients for all drug products produced and compounded drugs that are not subject to an applicable USP or NF monograph, are not components of FDA-approved human drugs, and do not appear on the 503A bulks list. It concluded that because no new drug application was on file, the drugs were adulterated and misbranded within the meaning of the FDCA. The FDA added that they reviewed the firm's response letter to Form 483, and, although the firm ceased production and performed a voluntary recall, some of the corrective actions were inadequate.

The Warning Letter also noted that the practice "may have produced biological products" and biological products are not eligible for the exemptions for compounded drugs under sections 503A and 503B of FDCA. It further noted that the firm "may be exporting products to other countries," and, if products do not meet FDCA's domestic marketing requirements and are intended for export, then such exportation must comply with FDCA Chapter VIII—Imports and Exports.

- Age Management Institute Santa Barbara, Santa Barbara, CA
    - In February 2021, the FDA became aware of a 50-year-old female patient who was hospitalized and treated for suspected septic shock with multi-organ failure after receiving an IV vitamin infusion in her home. The patient's blood cultures grew *Pseudomonas fluorescens*, a gram-negative bacterium. The IV vitamin infusion was compounded by Age Management Institute Santa Barbara. The FDA collaborated with multiple state regulators and inspected the firm:
    - This company was inspected by the FDA from October 13 to October 29, 2020, and the two investigators issued a Form 483 that cited five observations:
        - Lack of a certified ISO-5 classified area for sterile compounding.
        - Contamination in compounding areas including peeling paint, stained work surfaces, visibly dirty equipment, and air vents with dust and grime.
        - Difficult to clean equipment and surfaces such as carpeting in the IV storage and mixing room.
        - Standing water in a refrigerated storage area used to store sterile vials.
        - Use of expired active pharmaceutical ingredients to prepare drug products intended to be sterile.

As of March 2022, no Warning Letter to Age Management Institute has been posted to the usual FDA webpage, but the agency decided to issue a Compounding Risk Alert about physician office compounding which included the following admonitions:

- The FDA has become aware of sterile compounding activities, such as adding vitamins to IV infusion bags, being performed by business entities such as IV hydration clinics, medical spas, and mobile IV infusion companies. It is unknown if drug products are prepared, packed, or held under insanitary conditions by these entities and whether a licensed practitioner is on site to evaluate patients and write prescriptions for the drug products intended to be sterile being administered. It is also uncertain whether entities producing these sterile products are following state regulations. It is the FDA's understanding that entities such as these can be found nationwide; however, the number of these entities and the compounding practices occurring at these entities are not fully understood given that compounders seeking to compound drugs under section 503A generally do not register with the FDA.

- The extent to which compounding of drug products is occurring at medical offices and business entities such as IV hydration clinics is not fully known; however, compounding, packing, or holding drug products intended to be sterile under insanitary conditions at any facility significantly increases the risk of serious product quality concerns, such as product contamination. Compounding drug products intended to be sterile under insanitary conditions, including employing poor aseptic practices, using dirty equipment, or working in a facility not properly designed to maintain appropriate levels of cleanliness, as noted in the examples described above, increases the risk of product contamination. The use of contaminated drug products intended to be sterile has led to serious patient illnesses, hospitalization, and death.

32.8 COMPOUNDING "CENTER OF EXCELLENCE" ("COE") AND THE QUALITY ASSURANCE PARADIGM SHIFT

In 2018, the FDA submitted a budget justification to the House Appropriations Committee that included a request for $25 million to create a "Center of Excellence on Compounding for Outsourcing Facilities." In that request, the FDA stated the following goals for the COE:

- It will allow the FDA will expand engagement with outsourcing facilities and states to help the pharmacy outsourcing industry grow to meet its intended function and adhere to higher quality standards to protect patient health.
- It will identify and propose solutions to market barriers to lower the cost for pharmacies to become outsourcing facilities.
- It will provide much-needed education and training to improve product quality, safety, and purchaser confidence.
- It will help the FDA adjust its regulatory oversight to better match the scope of production of an individual compounding pharmacy.
- It will create a venue for the FDA to work with the industry to improve manufacturing practices, create new programs relating to requested review of method design and stability study protocols, and work with state partners to reduce challenges associated with state regulatory diversity and support state-based oversight of pharmacies.

The Appropriations Committee approved partial funding for the COE initiative and the program was announced on December 19, 2019. Deloitte won the contract to perform the market assessment of the sector and, as of March 2022, is still speaking with leading stakeholders from the compounding sector regarding strengths, weaknesses, barriers, and opportunities of compounding pharmacies in general and outsourcing facilities specifically.

Although in relaxed moments, the FDA leaders might refer to the initiative as the "**Compounding** Quality COE," strong preferences are given to the 503B Outsourcing sector relative to all training that is more sophisticated than self-learning. The training is not produced by the FDA, but instead is provided by the Parenteral Drug Association. (PDA). PDA is a not-for-profit voluntary organization led by professionals from the pharmaceutical industry who are seasoned in sterile production. PDA was an excellent choice for subject matter expertise for ensuring that drug products inside final containers and closures are truly sterile. The ideal result will be a rapid leap forward in the understanding and acumen of aseptic practices on the part of the leaders of compounding pharmacies and outsourcing facilities.

32.9 CONCLUSIONS AND FORECASTS REGARDING PATIENT INJURY FROM HEALTHCARE COMPOUNDING

Risk cannot be avoided, and perfect safety can never be achieved, but it is prudent to calculate and constantly recalculate relative risks to the best of our ability. Every risk has a cost, so the more time and money we spend to increase safety, the more we increase the cost of the product or service. Inevitably, if we spend too much in the pursuit of safety, the product or service will be rendered unaffordable to the buyer.

Patients with health conditions seek drugs that mitigate or cure those conditions. Patients who agree to be injected or infused with drugs **always** run the risk of being injured or killed if their dose is prepared using an inadequate aseptic technique. This risk must be balanced against the risk of receiving no drug at all. These pressures—perfect aseptic safety versus lack of access to needed drugs—must be kept in balance and the patient needs to be both (1) well informed of the risk and (2) free to make the final judgment in accordance with the level risk he or she deems "acceptable."

There are many examples of fundamental quality assurance failures in healthcare sterile compounding, and it is indisputable that our quality assurance performance should be improved. It is less certain how patients will fare if they cannot receive their compounded drug therapies, but it is unlikely that they would abide by lack of access in any case. The best course would be to improve quality assurance practices as fast and as completely as possible while not interrupting patient access to drug treatment.

Compounding by healthcare professionals is not going away and for several years has grown rapidly. The sector needs more technical resources and third-party oversight to ensure that they are applying the most cost-efficient level of quality assurance that keeps patients safe within its compounding model. PDA is a tremendous resource from which to draw, but aseptic experts need to become much more available and affordable to pharmacies and physicians.

32.10 RECOMMENDED READINGS

1. CDC Streaming Health, director. *Lessons From an Outbreak Investigation. YouTube*, 2 May 2017. https://www.youtube.com/watch?v=dtM11QYCdZ8&t=530s.
2. Center for Drug Evaluation and Research. Advanced Nutriceuticals, LLC DBA the Guyer Institute of Molecular Medicine—615908–11/10/2021. *FDA*, 10 November 2021. https://www.fda.gov/inspections-compliance-enforcement-and-criminal-investigations/warning-letters/advanced-nutriceuticals-llc-dba-guyer-institute-molecular-medicine-615908-11102021.
3. Center for Drug Evaluation and Research. *FDA Highlights Concerns With Compounding of Drug Products by Medical Offices and Clinics Under Insanitary Conditions. U.S. Food and Drug Administration*, FDA, 25 October 2021. https://www.fda.gov/drugs/human-drug-compounding/fda-highlights-concerns-compounding-drug-products-medical-offices-and-clinics-under-insanitary.
4. Center for Drug Evaluation and Research. *Registered Outsourcing Facilities. U.S. Food and Drug Administration*, FDA, 27 July 2022. https://www.fda.gov/drugs/human-drug-compounding/registered-outsourcing-facilities.
5. "FDA Referral Letter." Received by Kimberly A. Leonard, Executive Secretary, New York State Board of Pharmacy, 8 August 2017, New York.
6. "The Federal Register." *Memorandum of Understanding Addressing Certain Distributions of Compounded Human Drug Products Between the State Board of Pharmacy or Other Appropriate State Agency and the Food and Drug Administration; Availability. Federal Register*, 27 October 2020. https://www.federalregister.gov/documents/2020/10/27/2020-23687/memorandum-of-understanding-addressing-certain-distributions-of-compounded-human-drug-products.
7. Food and Drug Administration. Department of Health and Human Services—Food and Drug Administration. *Fiscal Year 2019 Food and Drug Administration Justification of Estimates for Appropriations Committees*, 2019. https://www.fda.gov/media/112611/download.
8. Office of the Commissioner. *FDA Takes Efforts to Improve Quality of Compounded Drugs From Outsourcing Facilities Through Collaboration and Education as Part of New Center of Excellence. U.S. Food and Drug Administration*, FDA, 19 December 2019. https://www.fda.gov/news-events/press-announcements/fda-takes-efforts-improve-quality-compounded-drugs-outsourcing-facilities-through-collaboration-and.
9. Ritter JM, Muehlenbachs A, Blau DM, Paddock CD, Shieh WJ, Drew CP, Batten BC, Bartlett JH, Metcalfe MG, Pham CD, Lockhart SR, Patel M, Liu L, Jones TL, Greer PW, Montague JL, White E, Rollin DC, Seales C, Stewart D, Deming MV, Brandt ME, Zaki SR; Exserohilum Infections Working Group. Exserohilum infections associated with contaminated steroid injections: A clinicopathologic review of 40 cases. *Am J Pathol*. 2013 Sep; 183(3): 881–892. doi: 10.1016/j.ajpath.2013.05.007. Epub 26 June 2013. PMID: 23809916; PMCID: PMC4401815.
10. Schnirring L. House Committee Grills FDA Over Fungal Meningitis Outbreak. *CIDRAP*, 14 November 2012. https://www.cidrap.umn.edu/news-perspective/2012/11/house-committee-grills-fda-over-fungal-meningitis-outbreak.
11. Schnirring L. Senate Committee Raises More Meningitis Outbreak Questions. *CIDRAP*, 15 November 2012. https://www.cidrap.umn.edu/news-perspective/2012/11/senate-committee-raises-more-meningitis-outbreak-questions.
12. United States District Court for the District of Columbia. *Wellness Pharmacy, Inc., et al., v. Xavier Becerra*, 2 February 2022.
13. United States District Court for the District of Columbia. *Wellness Pharmacy, Inc., et al., v. AZAR et al, No. 1:2020cv03082—Document 59 (D.D.C. 2021)*, 9 September 2021.
14. United States, Congress, Food and Drug Administration. *FDA Form 483 Issued to Advanced Nutriceuticals LLC*, 2020.
15. United States, Congress, Food and Drug Administration. *FDA Form 483 Issued to Age Management Institute*, 2021.
16. United States, Congress, Food and Drug Administration. *FDA Form 483 Issued to William R. Grace M.D. P.C.*, 2016.

33 Compounding Pharmacy Fraud and Unethical Practices

James T. O'Donnell

SYNOPSIS

33.1 INTRODUCTION

The American Society of Pharmacy Law newsletter sets the stage for this chapter on pharmacy fraud and excessive pricing. The article is written by Nicholas H. Meza JD MPH and Michael S. Elkins, Partner and Associate at Quarles and Brady Law Firm Health & Life Sciences Group.

> On December 2nd, 2021 Florida pharmacy owner Peter Bolos was convicted by a federal jury in Tennessee for his role in a $174 million telemedicine pharmacy fraud scheme finding bolos responsible for at least $89 million of fraudulently paid Billings, the jury convicted bolus of 22 counts of mail fraud, conspiracy to commit mail fraud, and introduction of misbranded drugs into Interstate commerce. According to court documents and evidence presented at the trial, Bolos and his co-conspirators deceived pharmacy benefit managers, such as Express Scripts and CVS Caremark, into authorizing fraudulent claims worth more than $174 million. Private insurers also paid these claims and per court records, Bolos and two other individuals owned and operated Synergy pharmacy in Palm Harbor, FL. Synergy agreed with Florida telemarketer Healthright to generate prescriptions for Synergy. The prescriptions were typically for pain creams, scar creams, and vitamins that were often drugs those patients neither requested nor wanted. The Healthright telemarketing platform was used as a telemedicine service to call consumers and deceive them into agreeing to accept the drugs and to provide the personal insurance information. Healthright then paid doctors to authorize the prescriptions through its telemedicine platform, even though the doctors relied solely on the

DOI: 10.1201/9781003615323-36

telemarketer screening process as the basis for their authorizations, and never communicated directly with the patients. The trial resulted from a multi-year investigation conducted by 6 government entities including the HHS, FDA, USPS, FBI, DHS, and the office of Inspector General.

33.2 CRIMINAL PROSECUTIONS OF PHARMACY COMPOUNDERS

This is part of a stage set by the Department of Justice described in a news release on June 22, 2016, announcing "National Health care fraud takedown results in charges against 301 individuals for approximately 900 million in false billing". Several of the cases are described as follows:

In Tampa, Orlando, and elsewhere in the middle district of Florida, 15 individuals were charged with participating in a variety of schemes including compounding pharmacy fraud and intravenous drug fraud. In one case, the owner of several infusion clinics allegedly defrauded the Medicare program of over 8,000,000 dollars through a scheme involving reimbursement claims for expensive intervention intravenous prescription drugs that were never purchased and never administered to patients.

In the Southern District of California, 8 individuals were charged with health care related cases. In one case, five individuals including a doctor and a pharmacist were charged in a scheme to pay bribes and kickbacks to doctors and in exchange for prescribing expensive durable medical equipment and compound pain creams that were not medically necessary. The indictment alleges that approximately 27 million in false and fraudulent claims were submitted to insurers.

Tricare, a benefits program for Department of Defense beneficiaries, may have been the worst hit by this scheme. For the first four months of 2015 Tricare spent more than $1 billion on compounded drugs. While compounded drugs accounted for only 0.5% of the volume of medications reimbursed, they totaled 20% of the total cost. In May 2015 Tricare changed its compounded drug reimbursement rules to cover only compounds with FDA approved ingredients. As a result, Tricare saw compounded drug claims dropped by 74%, and compounded drug prescriptions went from 100 and 5200 per month to approximately 41,800. This translated to a 10 million per month decrease in spending. (DeLancey M. Compounding Pharmacies Should Expect Greater Scrutiny as Government Healthcare Budgets get Squeezed. Blake Rome LLP Newsletter July 10, 2020.)

Additional cases against individual pharmacies described in the Blank Rome newsletter include the following:

July 2017, a Mississippi pharmacist pled guilty to participating in a scheme where patients were provided unnecessary compounded drugs. The scheme involves selecting compounded drugs based on profitability as opposed to what patients needed or what was the most effective. The scheme is alleged to have involved 192 million in fraudulent claims submitted to Tricare.

July 2017, a False Claims Act is pending against Florida pharmacy solutions, five other compounding pharmacy, and numerous marketing companies' physicians and nurses. The suit alleges that a nationwide scheme to defraud Tricare of hundreds of millions of dollars to submit fraudulent inflated reimbursement claims to the government by recruiting beneficiaries to sign up for compounded drugs that were loaded with expensive and medically unnecessary ingredients.

July 2017, federal government intervened in a False Claims Act against the Tampa FL compounding pharmacy alleging that the pharmacy charged government health care plans 2000 percent to 2100% more for compounded drugs than it charged cash customers.

June 2017, six individuals pled guilty to a health insurance scheme which paid illegal kickbacks to doctors for writing compounded drug prescriptions, supplied preprinted prescription pads to doctors, and used mass marketing techniques and call centers to solicit patients. The individuals were sentenced between two and five years in prison forfeited more than $30 million in assets and were ordered to pay more than $130 million in restitution

March 2017 eight individuals were charged in a 158 million health care fraud scheme involving submission of false fraudulent claims for compounded drugs the individuals obtained control of compounding pharmacy and submitted claims to the Department of Labor office of worker's compensation obtaining reimbursement rates up to $28,000 per container for compounded creams. These prosecutions cover a broad range of issues including overbilling, automatically refilling prescriptions, creating products with little unknown medical value, large scale production without individual patient prescriptions, using ingredients and compounds that have not been approved for use in the United States and, creating copies of FDA approved drugs.

33.3 OVERPRESCRIBING AND OVERCHARGING OF COMPOUNDED DRUGS

Additional reports of fraud follow this discussion and then a special discussion regarding the overprescribing and overcharging for compounded pain medications and pain patches sold to patients in automobile no-fault (NF) prescription plans.

33.3.1 Department of Justice News Releases

News release from the Department of Justice US attorney's office district of New Jersey Tuesday, October 14th 2014, reports a pharmacist with a compounding pharmacy in Lakewood NJ admitted today to paying 10s of thousands of dollars in cash bribes to physicians for referring pain prescriptions, defrauding health care benefits programs of hundreds of thousands of dollars. The president and pharmacist in charge of Rx R Us, Vladimir Kleman, pleaded guilty to an information charging him with conspiracy to pay kickbacks and to commit health care fraud. According to court documents, from January 2013 to January 2014, claim and provided another individual with tens of thousands of dollars in cash and checks to provide bribes to physicians for referring prescriptions for compounded pain cream prescriptions to Rx R Us. Compounding pharmacies prepared the medication, using different types and dosages of drugs, to provide more personalized medication for patients. The compounded pain cream provided by prescriptions to Rx R Us in this case contains several components, including ketamine (Schedule 3 controlled substance), lidocaine, and diclofenac. The pharmacist admitted he knew certain insurance carriers, including federal health care benefit programs, did not cover compounded pain creams, but he nevertheless dispensed pain cream to these patients and obtained payment from their insurance carriers by falsely representing the pain cream to be other covered items. The pharmacist also acknowledged he defrauded healthcare insurers by making false claims and misleading representations about the quantity of the pain cream that he dispensed and the frequency with which he dispensed it. As a result, private insurance payers paid the pharmacy hundreds of thousands of dollars. A U.S. Attorney's Office news release of November 4, 2015, announced: Pharmacist sentenced to 20 months in prison for paying kickbacks for referrals and healthcare fraud.

33.3.2 News Reports in Newspapers

According to a report in the *Biloxi Sun Herald* newspaper, a Biloxi Doctor charged in a pharmacy scheme to defraud Tricare was indicted. By Robyn Fitzgerald, October 18, 2017.

The doctor is accused of writing prescriptions without examining patients and having the prescriptions filled by a Hattiesburg-based compounding pharmacy, according to a Justice Department press release. The indictment alleges that Dr. Diaz submitted false patient records for an audit for Tricare and indicated he had examined his patients before prescribing them compounded medications. The indictment is also related to the prosecutions of James May, the pharmacist in charge of Advantage Pharmacy in Lamar County, Mississippi, and the prescription market marketer Gerald J. Schar. Tricare, a health care benefit program for military veterans and their family members reimbursed the pharmacy more than $2.3 million for medications at Doctor Diaz had prescribed.

The *Pensacola News Journal* July 19th, 2019, headline reads Pensacola pharmacy co-owner indicted in federal court on fraud charges. A federal grand jury indicted the president and part owner of a Pensacola pharmacy Thursday for allegedly failing prescriptions that he knew were not based on legitimate doctor–patient relationships according to the United States Attorney for the Northern District of Florida. Andrew Fisher of Gulf Breeze is the president and part owner of a physician specialty pharmacy. He has been charged with conspiracy to commit healthcare fraud, wire fraud, and conspiracy to commit money laundering. Fisher paid commissions to the marketing representatives who recruited individuals to receive the compounded drug prescriptions. While Fisher is not a licensed pharmacist, the indictment further alleges that he directed his employees to use ingredient formulations for the drugs that would maximize the amount his pharmacy could bill Tricare and other companies without regard to what was medically necessary. One of the co-conspirators was sentenced to 21 months in prison.

An article in the *Dallas Morning News* on July 10, 2020, reads "Dallas firm that marketed compounded pain creams busted in massive healthcare fraud, kicked back case." The owners of a Dallas firm that marketed pain and scar creams for North Texas drug compounding pharmacies were arrested in connection with a large health care kickback scheme that bilked taxpayers out of $65 million, according to federal authorities. A Dallas compounding pharmacy, Trilogy Pharmacy, is one of the three indictments taking part in the scheme. The indictment says the pharmacies, which have not been charged with anything, paid kickbacks to the marketers for patient referrals. The marketer is accused of paying kickbacks to physicians—$60 for each compounded pain or scar cream prescription they wrote and $30 for each compounded vitamin prescription. They also paid kickbacks to Tricare beneficiaries.

An article in the *Nashville Tennessean* on February 8, 2019, reads a Tennessee clinic swindled the military out of $65 million. The crux of the cream conspiracy was choice MD in a now-shuttered clinic in Cleveland, TN, a manufacturing town near the Georgia border. A nurse practitioner Candice Michelle Craven has admitted she conducted fake telemedicine evaluations with marines in California so that two choice MD doctors, Susan Vergot and Carl Lindblad, could write nearly 4500 prescriptions to marines they had never met or diagnosed. Each prescription costs about $14,500 American taxpayers covered the cost. Vergot and Lindblad pleaded guilty to conspiracy to commit healthcare fraud. Craven pled guilty in November.

The reports, investigations, indictments, and convictions go on and are numerous. The scheme is the same. Enticing patients and prescribers to use and prescribe outrageously expensive, unnecessary topical compounded pain creams and billing the government or private insurers.

33.4 NOT YET CRIMINAL? INSURANCE COMPANIES FIGHTING BACK

Outside the obvious criminal fraud schemes, prosecution indictments, and convictions, private insurers are concerned about the medical necessity and excessive charges associated with pain creams and products described and dispensed in worker's compensation (WC) and NF insurance plans. The *New York Times* in an article by Andrew Pollack, August 14th, 2014 stated:

> It may be the biggest thing in diaper rash treatment, a custom-made product so to soothe a baby's bottom at the eye-popping price of $1600. Besides the $1600 ointment to treat diaper rash there was an $8500 cream to reduce scarring and the $2300 salve to relieve pain, recently billed to Catamaran, a pharmacy benefits manager. Alarmed that its spending on compounded drugs has quintupled in just two years, Catamaran has begun to review such claims more carefully. Other benefit pharmacy benefit managers owned by United Health and Blue Cross Blue shield plans are also reining in spending on compounding drugs, as are insurers like Harvard Pilgrim and various state workers compensation plans." While stating "there are absolutely situations where compounded medications are appropriate," but other cases in which the products are "unsafe and overly expensive," Dr. Sumit Dutta, Chief Medical Officer at the Schaumburg, Il. based PBM "if you remove the profit motive what is the baseline appropriate use of these products?

33.4.1 NF Pain Compounded and Topical Pain Product

This author has consulted in several compounded pain and pain patch prescription claims submitted to private insurers. While there are no allegations of fraud, conspiracy, bribery, or kickbacks, these companies are questioning the billing charges, medical necessity, and efficacy of the pain products provided to their insureds. A sample, anonymized case of one such claim in a Midwestern City follows.

33.4.2 Report Challenging the Pricing and Efficacy of a Compounded Pain Cream Prescription

An insurer received a claim/bill of $2,500 for a 240 gm (8 oz) seven-ingredient compounded pain cream. This consultant was tasked to review the pain cream prescription medication dispensed to the insured for safety, efficacy, reasonable pricing, and appropriate use.

> EXECUTIVE SUMMARY: The insured had nine (9) (multiple) pain locations/sources, including large (or deep) joints). The Formula "Ointment 8-NC" prescription contains multiple chemical ingredients that have limited or no proven efficacy when applied topically to the skin for the insured's painful conditions. The diclofenac and lidocaine ingredients in the prescription do have some efficacy; however, both diclofenac and lidocaine are available from commercial sources at substantially less cost to the payer. Considering the estimated actual costs to the Compounding Pharmacy, the overall prescription charge of $2,500.00 for 240 gm of the cream is excessively overpriced. The actual charges to the payer are likely to be a markup of 10–50-fold the actual cost to the Livonia Pharmacy.

This report will address each of the ingredients in the ointment and provide scientific and clinical supporting authorities applicable to each "active" ingredient contained in the ointment. A separate section will address the charges associated with each ingredient, documenting the estimated actual cost to the pharmacy, percent (%) markup over actual cost, the cost to the payer for an alternative commercial product used for the same purpose, and sale prices, supporting my opinions on the excessive charges.

Materials reviewed

- Medical and Pharmacy records, billings and invoices, literature on efficacy and pharmacokinetics of ingredients for topical pain creams
- FDA-approved package inserts, literature review on the efficacy of topical compounded pain ingredients, including mechanisms of topical absorption of drugs, bioavailability, resulting kinetics, and toxicity of topically applied analgesics and other medicaments.
- Commercial sources for bulk compounding (*chemicals/drugs (pharmacompass.com/price/)*
- U.S. Food & Drug Administration National Drug Code (NDC) Directory (https://labels.fda.gov/packagecode.cfm)

33.4.3 Ingredients and Costs of Pain Cream

33.5 GENERAL DISCUSSION

Overwhelmingly, the compounded pain topical medications (CPTM)—creams, lotions, and ointments (formula)—contain drugs approved by the Food and Drug Administration (FDA) and used clinically systemically (usually orally) for pain (analgesia) control, muscle relaxation, anti-inflammatory, and so on. The insured's prescription 8-NC Ointment contains amitriptyline, cyclobenzaprine, and diclofenac, which are FDA approved only for oral systemic use, except for diclofenac, which now also has an indication (proven use) for topical application to "amenable" joints. Otherwise, no scientific or clinical evidence (or FDA approval)[1] exists for the use of systemic drugs applied topically. Indeed, the incorporation of systemic drugs in topical products is an innovative concept.[2] This is not science; this is not proof of efficacy—that it works.

33.5.1 Evidence of Efficacy?

A recent controlled study evaluated the efficacy of CPTMs. Pain creams compounded for neuropathic pain (i.e., ketamine, gabapentin, clonidine, and lidocaine), nociceptive pain (i.e., ketoprofen, baclofen, cyclobenzaprine, and lidocaine), or mixed pain (i.e., ketamine, gabapentin, diclofenac, baclofen, cyclobenzaprine, and lidocaine) were assessed against placebo. No change was found in the mean reduction in pain scores between treatment versus control groups for patients with neuropathic pain, nociceptive pain, or mixed pain or for all patients. After one month, 72 participants (36%) in the treatment groups and 54 (28%) in the control group had a positive outcome. The authors conclude that the compounded pain creams did not show any better effect than placebo creams, and their higher costs compared with approved compounds should curtail routine use.[3]

Only a few reports support the efficacy of topical pain compounded creams/ointments.[4] Safaeian et al. reported on the successful treatment of radicular pain with a topical agent. These authors highlighted the need for a randomized, prospective study of both single and compounded topical agents for the treatment of radicular pain.[5]

Additional ingredients in the insured 8-NC include menthol, dimethylsulfoxide (DMSO), and lidocaine. The utility and efficacy of these ingredients will be discussed later in this report.

TABLE 33.1
Compounded Pain Ointment 8-NC

Ingredient	Quantity (gm)	Sell Price	Source	Sell Price per gram	Published Cost
Diclofenac pow sodium	24	$709.36	Medisca	$30.00	$1.00/gm
DimethylSulfoxide (DMSO)	14.4	$51.96	Medisca	$3.6	$0.10/gm
Cyclobenzaprine	4.8	$440.44	Medisca	$97.75	$1.00/gm[1]
Menthol crystal	12	$80.27	UNKNOWN	$6.68	$0.09/gm
Amitriptyline Pow HCL	19.2	$847.61	Medisca	$44.15	$0.50/gm[2]
Lidocaine	9.6	$179.85	Medisca	$18.75	$0.40/gm[3]
Ointment base emulsify	156	$197.51	Medisca	$1.26	$0.12/gm[4]
$2,500 per 240 gm jar = $10.41/gm					

Source: Medisca https://www.medisca.com/ is identified through the NDC # code on the Pharmacy document. Diclofenac, cyclobenzaprine, and amitriptyline published cost is 10X the highest wholesale cost listed on the Pharmacompass.com price list. DMSO, menthol, lidocaine, and ointment base are listed as ~5X published costs. Bulk prices are sold in 100 kg lots from India. The estimated cost is 5X the bulk cost listed in 2016. https://www.pharmacompass.com/price/diclofenac-potassium.

[1]https://www.pharmacompass.com/price/cyclobenzaprine

[2]https://www.pharmacompass.com/active-pharmaceutical-ingredients/amitriptyline-hcl

[3]https://thesmartshoponline.com/product/lidocaine-hydrochloride-purity-99-9-100-grams/?gclid=Cj0KCQjw38-DBhDpARIsADJ3kjmLW-awZ7lWklFJHZ8WLahX2rfCinkmGD7jNXPhtI6dc40zEjuWx-waAjGhEALw_wcB.

[4]https://www.amazon.com/DERMABASE-EMOLLient-CREAM-BASE-1LB/dp/B001V9X7VI

33.5.2 Expensive Ingredients

Many of the compounded pain creams contain very expensive chemical ingredients, for which little or no scientific proof exists on the extent of topical absorption and clinical efficacy. The clinical utility and concentration used in topical pain creams are theoretical and speculative. The role of topical (pain) preparations, when compared to traditional routes, has not been fully explored and thus remains unclear. Compounding pharmacists and prescribers of compounded pain creams/ointments state that the product contains "FDA-approved therapies." They commented that the ingredients of pain creams were all "FDA approved." These ingredients, overwhelmingly with only a few exceptions, are not "FDA approved" for topical use for pain treatment.

Topical compounded pain creams are associated with local skin hypersensitivity and are not without systemic toxicity.[6]

These "expensive" ingredients are surreptitiously inflated in actual acquisition cost with highly inflated average wholesale price (AWP) invoicing. Actual costs to the compounding pharmacy are listed on "member-only" websites cost invoicing, usually protected as proprietary.

33.6 INGREDIENT REVIEW FOR EFFICACY AND MECHANISM OF ACTION

33.6.1 Diclofenac

Diclofenac is a nonsteroidal anti-inflammatory drug (NSAID). NSAIDs work by inhibiting cyclooxygenase-1 and cyclooxygenase-2, which are responsible for producing prostaglandins (PGs). PGs contribute to inflammation and pain signaling. NSAIDs are used as a first-line therapy for pain and inflammatory conditions. Diclofenac was first approved by the FDA in 1988 under the trade name Voltaren®. Diclofenac is available in oral immediate and delayed-release tablets, topical solutions, topical patches, and topical gel (1% for arthritis) and 3% for actinic keratosis (AK). The 1% topical gel is now available over the counter (OTC—no prescription required) and from several generic sources.[7]

Diclofenac is indicated for use in the treatment of pain and inflammation from varying etiologies, including inflammatory conditions such as osteoarthritis, rheumatoid arthritis, and ankylosing spondylitis, as well as injury-related inflammation due to surgery and physical trauma. "Topical" pain medications direct the pain-relieving actions to tissues and nerves beneath the skin to which they are applied unless they are designed and dosed for systemic absorption and effect—that is, transdermal fentanyl (Duragesic) for systemic relief.

The official FDA-approved package insert/Highlights of Prescribing Information for Voltaren (diclofenac) 1% states the following:

> —INDICATIONS AND USAGE—
>
> Voltaren® Gel is a nonsteroidal anti-inflammatory drug indicated for the relief of the pain of osteoarthritis of joints *amenable* to topical treatment, such as the knees, elbows, hands, and ankle/feet/ankles. (Emphasis added)
>
> Voltaren gel was not evaluated for use on joints of the spine, hip, or shoulder.

In general, the systemic oral anti-inflammatory should be used first. It will relieve pain and inflammation in multiple locations. If the systemic product does not work, then a topical product can be tried.

33.6.1.1 Efficacy of Diclofenac Gel

A 2016 *Cochrane Database of Systematic Reviews* on topical NSAIDs for *chronic* musculoskeletal pain in adults notes the following:[8]

> Topical NSAIDs for chronic musculoskeletal pain in adults
>
> Bottom line: Topical diclofenac and topical ketoprofen can provide good levels of pain relief in osteoarthritis, but only for about 10% more people than get this result with topical placebo. There is no evidence for other chronic painful conditions.
>
> Background
>
> Chronic musculoskeletal pain occurs in conditions like osteoarthritis. Pain is typically moderate or severe in intensity, lasting for three months or more. Topical NSAIDs are applied where it hurts to unbroken skin in the form of a gel, cream, spray, or plaster. Topical NSAIDs penetrate the skin, enter tissues or joints, and reduce processes that cause pain in the tissue. Drug levels in the blood with topical NSAIDs are very much lower than with the same drug taken by mouth. This minimizes the risk of harmful effects.
>
> Key results
>
> Diclofenac and ketoprofen were the only two NSAIDS with good quality and longer duration studies, mostly in people aged over 40 years with painful knee arthritis. The comparison was between topical diclofenac or ketoprofen in a solution or gel, and the solution or gel without any drug in it (topical placebo). For diclofenac and ketoprofen, about 6 people out of 10 with osteoarthritis had much reduced pain after 6 to 12 weeks, compared with 5 out of 10 with topical placebo (moderate quality evidence). Clinical success with carrier (placebo) occurred commonly—in approximately half the participants in studies lasting 6 to 12 weeks. Both direct and indirect comparison of clinical success with oral placebo indicates that response rates with carrier (topical placebo) are about twice those seen with oral placebo.

33.6.2 Menthol (Methyl Salicylate)

Menthol is considered a rubefacient. Menthol/rubefacients have no efficacy for radiculopathy (bulging or herniated discs) or deep joint (shoulder/knee) injuries. The insured has nine multiple pain (diagnosed) loci (locations on the body), and the individual ingredients, including menthol, may provide some perceived relief of pain in a specific location but certainly not multiple pain locations. For example, a patient with multiple spinal complaints as well as a shoulder and a knee complaint will not benefit from a menthol in one location or the application of a topical ointment at a single or perhaps two locations. "Topical" pain medications direct the pain-relieving actions to tissues and nerves beneath the skin to which they are applied. The same limitation to efficacy on "amenable joints" as discussed earlier in the diclofenac topical gel applies to the CPTM.

Menthol topical has no documented scientific or clinical efficacy. The scientific and clinical literature include Cochrane reviews on rubefacients for acute and chronic pain, originally published in 2004,[9] and a follow-up in 2009, which conclude:[10]

> A topical medication is a one that is applied to body surfaces such as the skin to treat ailments. Topical products might be creams, foams, gels, lotions, and ointments. Topical products can include a large range of medicines. Rubefacients are drugs that cause irritation and reddening of the skin due to increased blood flow. They are believed to relieve pain in various musculoskeletal conditions and are available on prescription and in over-the-counter remedies. Salicylate (menthol—methyl salicylate) is a commonly used rubefacient. This review looked for evidence about the usefulness of topical rubefacients containing salicylate from randomized and double-blind studies. These studies were conducted in people with acute painful conditions like strains and sprains, or chronic painful conditions like osteoarthritis. We wanted to know whether topical salicylate-containing rubefacients helped with the pain.
>
> Evidence for topical salicylate-containing rubefacients is limited by the quality, validity, and size of the available studies. For both acute and chronic painful conditions, any evidence of efficacy came from the older, smaller studies, while the larger, more recent studies showed no effect. There is no good evidence that topical salicylate-containing rubefacients give useful pain relief. The evidence does not support the use of topical rubefacients containing salicylates for acute injuries or chronic conditions. They seem to be relatively well tolerated in the short-term, based on limited data. The amount and quality of the available data mean that uncertainty remains about the effects of salicylate-containing rubefacients.

A 2014 Cochrane review[11] on topical rubefacients concludes:

> The evidence does not support the use of topical rubefacients containing salicylates for acute injuries or chronic conditions. They seem to be relatively well tolerated in the short-term, based on limited data. The amount and quality of the available data mean that uncertainty remains about the effects of salicylate-containing rubefacients.

33.6.3 Lidocaine

Topical lidocaine has some efficacy and indeed widespread use for the relief of local muscle strain/pain. Many products (patches, creams, and ointments) exist in the OTC market (no prescription required) at a substantially lower price than the lidocaine ingredient charge in the 8-NC (~$180.00).[12] The efficacy, however, is limited to topical muscle and other tissues. Thus, it will have no appreciable analgesia for deep joint pain, such as shoulders, spinal column bulging disc/pain, or knees.

Cardiotoxic and neurotoxic adverse events (AEs) have been reported with lidocaine. While generally considered safe, an overdose of numbing medicine can be lethal if too much of the medicine is absorbed through your skin.[13] "Do not use large amounts of lidocaine topical or cover treated skin areas with a bandage or plastic wrap without medical advice (*Drugs.com*)." A Mayo Clinic website (*mayoclinic.*

org/drugs-supplements/lidocaine-topical-application-route/side effects) lists heart, allergy, breathing, swallowing, blistering, nervousness and dizziness, and headache all associated with topical lidocaine use.

33.6.3.1 Lidocaine Topical Toxicity

Lidocaine toxicity is manifested by confusion, dizziness, apprehension, delirium, paresthesia (lack of sensitivity/numbness), hypotension, central nervous system depression, and convulsions. These toxicities have been reported with topical use. A maximum of three patches of Lidoderm can be worn at a time for 12 hours on, followed by 12 hours off. Longer application times or multiple patches can result in increased absorption of lidocaine and high blood concentrations, leading to serious side effects. Lidocaine toxicity occurs with blood concentrations above 5 mcg/mL.

33.6.4 Amitriptyline

Amitriptyline is a prescription-only tricyclic antidepressant that is FDA indicated/approved for depression and nocturnal enuresis and is sometimes used as a sleep aid. It is only approved for the oral route of administration. Amitriptyline has not been approved for topical use. One study is reported wherein topical amitriptyline is combined with ketamine for the treatment of peripheral neuropathy. The study report notes. "It is not yet known whether topical amitriptyline and ketamine cream is more effective than a placebo in treating peripheral neuropathy caused by chemotherapy."[14]

Although it is recommended as a topical ingredient for neuropathic pain, no significant proof of efficacy exists.[15]

33.6.5 Cyclobenzaprine

Cyclobenzaprine is compounded and topically applied for pain disorder treatment. The efficacy and transdermal penetration of cyclobenzaprine has not been studied. Bryson et al. studied the effect of transdermal penetration of cyclobenzaprine using porcine skin. Cyclobenzaprine was compounded into commercially available bases: Lipobase, Lipoderm, and a poloxamer lecithin organogel. Cyclobenzaprine 5% yielded significant transdermal penetration, and a modest level of cyclobenzaprine was retained in the skin tissue administered with all bases tested. Systemically administered cyclobenzaprine (10 mcg/kg), but not topically administered cyclobenzaprine (1% and 5%), reduced nociception in an animal pain model.[16]

33.6.6 Dimethylsulfoxide

DMSO is an FDA-approved prescription medication for treating symptoms of painful bladder syndrome. It's also used experimentally to treat several other conditions, including shingles, and is sometimes used to increase the body's absorption of other medications. While it has widespread consumer use as a "liniment," its use as a pharmaceutical adjuvant or solvent is not FDA approved. Nor has there been any published research on the compatibility of DMSO with emulsifying bases or any of the chemicals added to the 8-NC ointment. Pharmaceutical-grade DMSO is advertised on the internet for less than $20.0 for an 8 ounces (240 ml/240 gm bottle).[17] This cost is just under $0.10 (10 cents/gm). The compounding pharmacy charge to the Insurer is $3.60/gm, a markup of ~ 3,600%.

A thorough review of DMSO use, therapeutics, and efficacy was published by Brayton.[18]

> DMSO readily penetrates skin. Within five minutes of cutaneous application radiolabeled DMSO can be detected in the blood, and characteristic garlic halitosis due to the reduction metabolism, dimethyl sulfide (DMS), is evident. Within 20 minutes, DMSO can be found in all organs of the body. Within one-hour, radiolabeled DMSO is detected in bones and teeth. DMSO may or may not reduce inflammation and edema in experimental models. In clinical situations, anti-inflammatory benefit from DMSO therapy is reported with acute musculoskeletal injuries, with acute, traumatic, and inflammatory disorders of the central nervous system, postoperatively when severe pain or swelling is expected. In chronic inflammatory conditions, results are less consistently achieved. DMSO effects blood coagulation. Mild hypocoagulative effects are reported. Accelerated clotting times and hypercoagulability induced by DMSO are reported. DMSO causes histamine release by mast cells. This effect is probably responsible for the local vasodilatation and cutaneous sensitivity commonly observed after application of DMSO.
>
> DMSO is readily absorbed through skin and relieves musculoskeletal pain when applied topically to painful areas. We studied the effects of DMSO on C-type nerve fibers, which mediate pain sensation. DMSO was applied directly to exposed cat sural nerves. C fiber conduction velocity was slowed by DMSO, even in low concentrations (5–7% v/v). Higher concentrations completely blocked C fiber conduction, with a minimum blocking concentration of 9%. Onset of nerve block was almost immediate with 15% DMSO or higher concentrations. C fiber blockade may account for analgesia with DMSO.[19] (Note: 8-NC is at the lower end of concentration associated with efficacy for analgesia for painful peripheral neuropathy.)

33.7 GLOBAL OPINIONS FOR THE PRESCRIPTION CPTM FORMULA 8-NC CLAIM CHALLENGE

1. The insured had multiple pain (diagnosed) loci (locations on the body), both peripheral joints and central (deep) joints (shoulders, legs, spine, and knees); yet the diclofenac is only indicated and proven effective in "amenable" joints, that is, knee, ankle/feet, elbow, and hand—joints that are not covered by large muscle masses (shoulders/spine) or are considered deep. Other topical products have limited efficacy (lidocaine 5%) or no proven efficacy (compounded pain creams). Alternative commercial sources are available without the need for compounding at substantially lower prices to the payer.

2. Sourcing bulk chemical costs and then inflating them by a factor of 10–100X as an estimated acquisition cost to pharmacy) and then examining the pricing of the component ingredients in the compounded pain creams has indicated that the AWP—that is used as a basis for pricing prescriptions as listed by the chemical wholesaler/supplier—is not in fact the charge to the pharmacy. This AWP/cost basis was a fictitiously and excessively inflated cost to support a substantially higher charge by the pharmacy to the payee. In this investigation, online sources of bulk chemicals used in 8-NC pain ointment are documented to be available for pennies on the dollar those charges that compounding pharmacy charged the insurance company.

33.8 DISCUSSION AND FURTHER BASIS FOR OPINIONS

Used primarily for pain management, compounded medications contain either a single active drug in an inactive base or several active drugs. Compounded medications are prepared and dispensed by compounding pharmacies, which are licensed by the Board of Pharmacy in the State in which they are located, with limited FDA oversight. Compounded medications are not subject to the rigorous drug review process that all commercially available prescription drugs must undergo to demonstrate safety and effectiveness prior to FDA approval. Further, compounded medications generally do not have standardized dosages and duration for use, and the protocols for preparing each compound are not standardized. Indeed, the inclusion of ingredients in pain creams, including concentrations therein, is based on theory and speculation.[20] Only a few studies on individual and multiple ingredient agents have been conducted, with limited efficacy, and calls for more research.[21]

CPTM preparations are likely to have batch-to-batch variability, and their sterility and purity cannot be guaranteed. Yet because of the time, effort, and expertise necessary for pharmacists to create compounded products, their costs are often much higher than those of standard medications, even without excessive inflation of acquisition costs.

Most CPTMs have not been proven to be effective at all, and certainly not more effective than commercially available, manufactured drugs (with rare exceptions).[22] CPTM advocates argue less systemic toxicity; however, this claim cannot be made without scientific and clinical proof documenting bioavailability, systemic blood levels, and toxic effects. CPTMs have not been approved for safety and efficacy by the FDA. Indeed, only sketchy published literature is available. Most of the literature concludes that there is no benefit[23] and increased risk involved with CPTM. Efficacy is non-existent for the most of drug ingredients in this review. Compounds are often not medically necessary. CPTMs are always substantially more expensive, often greater than $1,000 to several thousand dollars, resulting in significant money being wasted on ineffective and unnecessary therapies.[24]

A search of the literature to document bioavailability, tissue penetration and topical absorption, and systemic blood levels is sketchy at best—very little information is available. A few examples are previously discussed earlier in this report. The topical administration of medicaments for local and or systemic effects is well developed; the science is available to capture this information. These topical drug absorption concepts and mechanisms are routinely taught in medical and pharmacy schools.[25]

33.9 OVERBILLING OF TOPICAL DICLOFENAC GELS, LIDOCAINE CREAMS, AND OINTMENTS AND PATCHES

In other consultations, additional aggressive overbilling of topical pain commercial products has replaced some of the CPTM. Besides identifying excessive charges, these cases were evaluated for efficacy and medical necessity. Frequent single-ingredient topical pain products include diclofenac 1% and 3% gels, and topical lidocaine creams, ointments, and patches (with and without menthol and capsaicin).

Recall earlier discussion of fraud claims of compounding pharmacy and Pain treatment conspiracies selecting expensive ingredients and unnecessary treatments to inflate billing to payers.

Departing from that practice which had started in CPTM, the practice switched to prescribing commercial products—not requiring any compounding and charging highly inflated prices to insureds for patients in guaranteed benefit plans (e.g., workers compensation NF insurance). In doing so, not only is the patient exposed to increased toxicity, but, in many cases, the prescriptions (diclofenac 3%) should not be prescribed for the patients at all.

33.9.1 Diclofenac 3% (Solaraze)

In other consultations most insured were prescribed and dispensed one or more diclofenac 3% gel (100 or 200 gm); 3% diclofenac gel is not indicated, approved, or useful in topical pain and inflammation treatment and is associated with a greater level of toxicity due to the triple (3% v 1%) concentration of diclofenac in the product. The sell price by the pharmacies ranged from $943.60/100 to $1,700/200 gm. At the time, generic sources of diclofenac 3% gel were available for $100–200 per tube. Diclofenac 1%, at the time of the dispensations (pre-May 2020), lists the liberal retail price of $66.00 for 100 gm diclofenac 1% as an alternative (albeit not efficacious for most claimed painful conditions).

The diclofenac 3% is used to treat actinic keratoses, a condition that includes a rough, scaly patch on the skin that develops from years of sun exposure. AK is the most common precancer that forms on skin damaged by chronic exposure to ultraviolet (UV) rays from the sun and/or indoor tanning.

The FDA-approved prescribing information (package insert) for diclofenac 3% gel states:

- It is indicated for the topical treatment of actinic keratoses
- In clinical studies, localized dermal side effects such as contact dermatitis, exfoliation, dry skin, and rash were found in patients treated with Solareze® at a higher incidence than in those with a placebo.
- Adverse reactions of the 423 patients evaluable for safety in adequate and well-controlled trials, 211 were treated with Solareze drug product and 212 were treated with a vehicle gel. Eighty-seven percent (87%) of the Solareze-treated patients (183 patients), and 84% of the vehicle-treated patients (178 patients) experienced one or more AEs during the studies. Most of these reactions were mild to moderate in severity and resolved upon discontinuation of therapy. Of the 211 patients treated with Solareze, 172 (82%) experienced AEs involving skin and the application site compared to 160 (75%) vehicle-treated patients. Application site reactions (ASRs) were the most frequent AEs in both Solareze- and vehicle-treated groups. Of note, four reactions—contact dermatitis, rash, dry skin, and exfoliation (scaling)—were significantly more prevalent in the Solareze group than in the vehicle-treated patients; 18 percent of Solareze-treated patients and 4% of vehicle-treated patients discontinued from the clinical trials due to AEs (whether considered related to treatment or not). These discontinuations were mainly due to skin irritation or related cutaneous adverse reactions.
- Skin and appendage AEs reported for Solaraze at less than 1% incidence in *the Phase 3 studies*: skin hypertrophy, paresthesia, seborrhea, urticaria, ASRs (skin carcinoma, hypertonia, skin hypertrophy lacrimation disorder, maculopapular rash, purpuric rash, vasodilation).
- Post-marketing reports: Skin and appendages: rash, pruritus alopecia, urticaria, eczema, dermatitis, bullous eruption, erythema multiforme major, angioedema, Stevens-Johnson syndrome, excess perspiration, exfoliative dermatitis.

Independent medical examinations (IMEs—Peer Review) were filed for several of the insured receiving diclofenac 3% gel. For all those that received IMEs, the reviewers found the diclofenac 3% "not medically necessary."

Diclofenac 1% is also a frequent prescription for these beneficiaries. Noting the available retail price of $66.00 per 100 gm tube, invoices charging insured $700/100 gm tube and $1,300/200 gm tube were not unusual. There seems to be no justification for the substantially inflated price; perhaps the compounding pharmacy assumed that the charges would not be questioned as the benefits were guaranteed.

33.9.2 Lidocaine Topical Commercial Products

Earlier discussion addressed the inclusion, limited efficacy, and inflated charges for lidocaine ingredients in CPTM. In several consultations, various lidocaine topical products have been prescribed and dispensed for this same group of WC and NF beneficiaries. Frequently, lidocaine was prescribed in addition to diclofenac gels, and sometimes diclofenac oral systemic was prescribed with topical diclofenac gel—against labeling instructions.

Two (2) topical lidocaine products

- Lidocaine ointment 5%
- Lidoderm patch 5%

Many products (patches, creams, and ointments) exist in the OTC market (no prescription required) at a substantially lower price than the Lidoderm (lidocaine) 5% patches or lidocaine 5% ointments. As stated earlier, the efficacy is limited to topical muscle and other tissues.

Lidoderm (lidocaine) 5% patches were dispensed to the insured at very high prices—~$7.00 each. Incidentally, Lidoderm patches are not a covered medication and require prior approval by Blue Cross Blue Shield Federal Employee Program prescription plans. Lidoderm 5% patch is a prescription-only product. Equally (questionably) effective, and substantially less expensive, OTC lidocaine 4% patches are available from several commercial sources, including the brand SalonPas, or several generic 4% lidocaine patches, which sell for $1—$2.00 per patch at multiple retail outlets.

Lidocaine 5% ointment is a prescription-only product (NDC 65162-918-53). This product is available from several suppliers (generic) at relatively low prices compared to the sell price for lidocaine ointment 5% to several insureds. For example, in a previous consultation, an invoice was produced which indicates the wholesale cost to the pharmacy for 50 gm of lidocaine 5% ointment is $7.00 = $28.00/200 gm. Notably, the sell price to the insurer was $609.00/100 gm and $1,219.04/200 gm, which is a 2,100% markup over the pharmacy's actual cost.

33.10 RECOMMENDATION

Certain pharmacy compounding companies[26,27] aggressively promote CPTM as effective with less risk.[28] Conventional and current clinical pain medicine, therapeutics, and science question and refute these claims of superiority, efficacy, and less toxicity, and peer-reviewed publications support the conventional views. I share these doubts and questions about the utility and value of CPTM. This insured is not unique; it should not be assumed that Formula Ointment 8-NC would be effective, based on an enormity of scientific evidence to the contrary.

I recommend that you conduct an audit of the shipping invoices and payments for the products and ingredients discussed in this report, which were prescribed and dispensed to the insured to determine the actual costs, proof of payment to the suppliers, charges, markup, profits, and fees charged by the Livonia Pharmacy.

33.11 SUMMARY AND CONCLUSIONS

As a pharmacist, I'm embarrassed by these criminal acts by pharmacists discussed earlier in the chapter. They tarnish the image and reputation of pharmacists. It is also embarrassing to me to learn of the aggressive and unnecessary dispensing of questionable CPTM and commercial topical pain products at extraordinary charges. A review of the science and available product sources easily demonstrates what I consider as the least ethical violations, and perhaps the insured considers contract violations. To that end, I have learned that insured challenges to these excessive charges have usually resulted in a substantial reduction in the charges to the insured.

NOTES

1 Dose Response Information to Support Drug Registration: Guidance for Industry. FDA, November 1994 (CDVS2.CDER.FDA.GOV).
2 Jones M. Pharmacological interventions in the new millennium: A theory of efficacy. *IJPC.* 2000; 4(6): 6–15.
3 Brutcher RE, Kurihara C, Bicket MC, Moussavian-Yousefi P, Reece DE, Solomon LM, Griffith SR, Jamison DE, Cohen SP. Compounded topical pain creams to treat localized chronic pain: A randomized controlled trial. *Ann Intern Med.* 2019 Mar 5; 170(5): 309–318. doi:10.7326/M18-2736. Epub 2019 Feb 5. PMID: 30716769.
4 Somberg JC, Molnar J. Retrospective evaluation on the analgesic activities of 2 compounded topical creams and voltaren gel in chronic noncancer pain. *Am J Ther.* 2015 Sep–Oct; 22(5): 342–349.
5 Safaeian P, Mattie R, Hahn M, Plastaras CT, McCormick ZL. Novel treatment of radicular pain with a multi-mechanistic combination topical agent: A case series and literature review. *Anesth Pain Med.* 2016; 6(2): e33322. Published 2016 Mar 1. doi:10.5812/aapm.33322.
6 Cline AE, Turrentine JE. Compounded topical analgesics for chronic pain. *Dermatitis.* Sep–Oct 2016; 275(5): 263–271.
7 https://pubchem.ncbi.nlm.nih.gov/compound/Diclofenac.
8 Derry S, Conaghan P, Da Silva JAP, Wiffen PJ, Moore RA. Topical NSAIDs for chronic musculoskeletal pain in adults. *Cochrane Database Syst Rev.* 2016; 4.
9 Moore RA, Edwards JE, McQuay HJ, Derry S, Wiffen PJ; Cochrane Pain and Palliative Care Group. Systematic review of efficacy of topical rubefacients containing salicylates for the treatment of acute and chronic pain. *BMJ.* 2004; 328: 995.
10 http://www.cochranelibrary.com/cochrane-database-of-systematic-reviews/index.html.
11 Derry S, Matthews PRL, Wiffen PJ, Moore RA. Salicylate-containing rubefacients for acute and chronic musculoskeletal pain in adults. *Cochrane Database Syst Rev.* 2014; 11: Art. No.: CD007403. doi: 10.1002/14651858.CD007403.pub3.
12 https://www.cvs.com/shop/content/lidocaine-patches.
13 Marra DE, Yip D, Fincher EF, Moy RL. Systemic toxicity from topically applied lidocaine in conjunction with fractional photothermolysis. *Arch Dermatol.* 2006 Aug; 142(8): 1024–1026. doi: 10.1001/archderm.142.8.1024. PMID: 16924052.
14 https://clinicaltrials.gov/ct2/show/NCT00471445.
15 Leppert W, Malec-Milewska M, Zajaczkowska R, Wordliczek J. Transdermal and topical drug administration in the treatment of pain. *Molecules.* 2018 Mar 17; 23(3): 681. www.mdpi.com/journal/molecules.
16 Bryson E, Hartman R, Arnold J, Gorman G, Sweitzer S, Asbill S. Skin permeation and antinociception of compounded topical cyclobenzaprine hydrochloride formulations. *Int J Pharm Compd.* 2015 Mar–Apr; 19(2): 161–166. PMID: 26685496.
17 https://www.amazon.com/DMSO-Bottle-99-995-Dimethyl-Sulfoxide/dp/B01BSYQ0XC.
18 Brayton CF. Dimethyl sulfoxide (DMSO): A review. *Cornell Vet.* 1986 Jan; 76(1): 61–90. PMID: 3510103.
19 Evans MS, Reid KH, Sharp JB Jr. Dimethylsulfoxide (DMSO) blocks conduction in peripheral nerve C fibers: A possible mechanism of analgesia. *Neurosci Lett.* 1993 Feb 19; 150(2): 145–148. doi: 10.1016/0304-3940(93)90522-m. PMID: 8469412.
20 Jones M. Pharmacological interventions in the new millennium: A theory of efficacy. *IJPC.* 2000; 4(6): 6–15.
21 Barton DL, Wos EJ, Qin R, Mattar BI, Green NJ, Lanier KS, Bearden DJ, Kugler JW, Hoff JL, Reddy PS, Rowland KM, Riepl M, Christensen B, Loprinzi CL. A double-blind, placebo-controlled trial of a topical treatment for chemotherapy induced peripheral neuropathy: NCCTG trial N06CA *Support Care Cancer.* 2011 Jun; 19(6): 833–841.
22 Tricare Pharmacy Compound Screening.pdf.
23 Jorge LL, Feres CC, Teles VEP. Topical preparations for pain relief: Efficacy and patient adherence. *J. Pain Res.* 2014; 4: 11–24.
24 Walls AP, Johnson S, Nguyen M, O'leric K, Pokorney T, Randolph S. 2013. *Workers Compensation Drug Trend Report.* Express Scripts Lab. www.comppharma.com.
25 O'Donnell JT. *Syllabus.* Rush Medical College 502, Block 6, Spring 2014.
26 https://21centurypharmacy.com/services/compounding/. Accessed July 28, 2016.
27 www.atlanticcompounding.com. Accessed July 26, 2016.
28 www.bbpharmacy.com. Accessed July 28, 2016.

Part IV

Forensic and Toxicology Issues

34 Alcohol

James T. O'Donnell and James J. O'Donnell III

SYNOPSIS

DOI: 10.1201/9781003615323-38

34.1 INTRODUCTION

Expectations of the expert in forensic litigation involving alcohol include the following:

- Interpretation of the alcohol test
- Consider the methodology and margin of error of different alcohol testing
- Extrapolate the blood/breath alcohol concentration (BAC) from the time of an event to the time of the test
- Calculate the amount of alcohol consumed using the BAC test reports
- Calculate the metabolic rate of alcohol in the subject if more than one BAC test is performed
- Educate the jury or the judge on the pharmacology and toxicology of alcohol
- Apply the principles of pharmacokinetics (ADME—absorption, distribution, metabolism, excretion/elimination) of alcohol to the individual case
- Evaluate tolerance, delayed absorption, and altered metabolism of alcohol in patient-specific circumstances
- Opine on the intoxication and impairment of alcohol as it applies to an individual case scenario, including the manifestations of impairment, both cognitive and physical.

34.2 ALCOHOL INJURY EPIDEMIOLOGY

Alcohol is a cross-cutting, harmful factor considered in the United Nations' Sustainable Development Goals (SDG) Agenda 2030, illustrating the issue that disease burden attributable to high consumption should be effectively addressed. SDG 3.5 aims to "strengthen prevention and treatment of substance abuse, including narcotic drug abuse and harmful use of alcohol."[1] Alcohol consumption has been linked with more than 200 types of injuries and diseases, including road traffic and domestic accidents, cancer, liver cirrhosis, stroke, alcoholic cardiomyopathy, and infectious diseases, and it has been estimated that around 6% of total deaths could be attributable to alcohol consumption worldwide. The Institute for Health Metrics and Evaluation estimated that in 2016 1.6% of total disability-adjusted life years (DALYs) globally among females and 6.0% among males correspond to alcohol-related diseases. A total of 174,000 deaths were attributable to alcohol use disorders (AUDs) in that year in the Global Burden of Disease project. About 12% of global DALYs are due to road injuries, and 14–18.5% of those due to self-harm and interpersonal violence are attributable to alcohol use. Alcohol is also the main risk factor for death and/or disability among people between 15 and 49 years of age in some regions of the world.

Alcohol use disorder is a diagnosis that combines criteria for alcohol abuse and alcohol dependence from the 4th edition of the *Diagnostic and Statistical Manual of Mental Disorders* into a single disorder in the 5th edition,[2] negatively influences health, and is the third-leading preventable cause of death in the United States. According to the 2015 National Survey on Drug Use and Health, the prevalence of binge drinking, which is the consumption of an excessive amount of alcohol in a short period of time, and of heavy alcohol use was similar in males and females.[3] Likewise, a recent meta-analysis confirmed a greater increase in alcohol use and binge drinking in women versus men over the past 16 years,[4] representing a narrowing of the historically higher AUD rate in males.[5]

Alcohol consumption also generates an important economic burden. Rehm and colleagues showed that its weighted average cost was 2.5% of GDP-purchasing power parity among high-income countries, such as Canada, France, Scotland, and the United States.[6] Approximately one in ten deaths among working-age adults results from excessive drinking.[7]

34.2.1 Drinking and Driving

Each year in the United States, 85,000 deaths,[8] along with substantial disability from medical and psychiatric consequences, injuries, and "secondhand" effects (e.g., motor vehicle crashes), are attributed to the use of alcohol. Indeed, 10,076 (31%) people were killed in alcohol-impaired driving crashes where at least one driver had a BAC of.08 g/dl or higher. A total of 28.7 million people admitted to driving under the influence in 2013.[9] Approximately 290,000 persons were injured in drunk driving crashes in 2013.[10] Aside from the human cost, financially the estimated annual costs that are attributable to alcohol use are $223.5 billion in societal costs in the United States.[11] Considering the number of deaths and injuries associated with alcohol, via motor vehicle crashes and other modes, it is no surprise that alcohol plays a central role in criminal and civil litigation.[12]

Key facts:[13]

- Worldwide, three million deaths every year result from the harmful use of alcohol, this represents 5.3% of all deaths.
- The harmful use of alcohol is a causal factor in more than 200 disease and injury conditions.
- Overall, 5.1% of the global burden of disease and injury is attributable to alcohol, as measured in DALYs.
- Alcohol consumption causes death and disability relatively early in life. In the age group 20–39 years, approximately 13.5% of the total deaths are alcohol-attributable.
- There is a causal relationship between the harmful use of alcohol and a range of mental and behavioral disorders, other noncommunicable conditions, as well as injuries.
- The latest causal relationships have been established between harmful drinking and the incidence of infectious diseases such as tuberculosis as well as the course of HIV/AIDS.
- Beyond health consequences, the harmful use of alcohol brings significant social and economic losses to individuals and society at large.

Alcohol consumption can have adverse social, legal, occupational, psychological, and medical consequences. The risk of harmful consequences and disability exists on a continuum. Almost 9% of U.S. adults (approximately 13% of those who drink) meet the criteria for an AUD; the prevalence of AUDs is higher in clinical settings. Risk drinking is defined as an average of 15 or more standard drinks per week or 5 or more on an occasion for men and 8 or more drinks weekly or 4 or more on an occasion for women and people older than 65 years of age. A standard drink (i.e., 12 oz of beer, 5 oz of wine, or 1.5 oz of 80-proof liquor) contains 14 g of ethanol. High average consumption or frequent heavy drinking can be clinically silent yet have adverse health and social consequences. The prevalence of unhealthy use is 7–20% or more among outpatients, 30–40% among patients in emergency departments, and 50% among patients with trauma. Dependence (alcoholism) is best understood as a chronic disease, with peak onset by the age of 18. Moderate (i.e., less than risky) use of alcohol may have health benefits, but what constitutes "moderate" depends on age, sex, genetic characteristics, coexisting illnesses, and other factors. Observational studies indicate that for men under the age of 34 years and women under the age of 45 years, those who report no alcohol intake have the lowest mortality. Above these age cutoffs, weekly intakes of no more than five drinks for men or two drinks for women are associated with the lowest mortality.

Alcohol increases the risk of trauma and injury. The association of alcohol with injuries has been known since some of the earliest recorded history. Alcohol intoxication increases the risk of all types of traumas. A high percentage of seriously injured trauma center patients are at risk of having current psychoactive substance use (including alcohol) disorders. Available evidence implicates alcohol consumption as a major risk factor for almost every type of injury. Consequently, substantial litigation follows alcohol use. This litigation is in personal injury, motor vehicle, premises liability, drama and entertainment, government/police, employment, and family law. Just about any province or sector of life may be affected by alcohol, and, thus, alcohol is frequently involved in civil litigation. This drives the need for a competent scientist or clinician to serve and assist the trier of fact to determine the role of science in these varied forensic settings.

A brief summary of the intoxicating and impairing effects of alcohol is provided in the following paragraphs. The reader is referred to Caplan and Goldberger, *Garriott's Medicolegal Aspects of Alcohol*, 6th Ed, L&J, Tucson, for an in-depth discussion of the scientific issues and the literature references supporting those discussions.[14]

In April 2000, the National Highway Traffic Safety Administration (NHTSA) released a large-scale review of the literature (112 articles—from 1981 to 1997) on the effects of alcohol on driving-related skills including divided attention, drowsiness, vigilance tasks, tracking, perception, visual functions, cognitive tasks, psychomotor skills, choice reaction time, simple reaction time, and critical flicker fusion. (DOT HS 809 028). An excerpt from the abstract follows:

> Alcohol impairs some driving skills beginning with any significant departure from zero BAC. By BACs of 0.05 g/dL, the majority of the experimental studies examined reported significant impairment. By 0.08 g/dL, more than 94% of the studies reviewed exhibited skills impairment. Specific performance skills are differentially affected by alcohol. Some skills are significantly impaired by BACs of 0.01 g/dl, while others do not show impairment until BACs of 0.06 g/dl. All drivers are expected to experience impairment in some driving-related skills by 0.08 g/dl or less. In addition to automobile operators, motorcyclists also face increased risk from alcohol consumption. An April 2007 NHTSA report states: In 2004, 4,008 motorcyclists were killed and an additional 76,000 were injured in traffic crashes. Motorcyclist fatalities have been steadily increasing since 1997, when 2,116 fatalities were recorded.[15]
>
> It is apparent that alcohol use continues to be a significant problem in motorcycle crashes. In fatal crashes in 2004, motorcycle operators had higher blood alcohol concentration (BAC) levels (.08 grams per deciliter [g/dL] or

higher) as compared to other types of motor vehicle operators. The percentages for vehicle operators involved in fatal crashes were 27 percent for motorcycles, 22 percent for passenger cars, 21 percent for light trucks, and 1 percent for large trucks. In 2004, there were 1,264 motorcycle operators killed who had been drinking (BAC.01+), of whom 1,025 (81%) were intoxicated (BAC.08+).

34.3 ALCOHOL INTOXICATION EFFECTS IN LITIGATION

Thus far, attention has been primarily focused on drunk driving, despite the fact that drunk walking, drunk arguing, or even drunk sleeping, given fire and smoke hazards, are also dangerous. Contrary to popular belief, most alcohol-related injuries are due to violence and other factors, not just driving.

Overall, alcohol is involved in 43% of all unintentional deaths from injury. On weekend evenings, close to 50% of emergency department patients admitted for injury have a measurable BAC. Of all non-fatal injuries occurring in the home, alcohol intoxication is responsible for 22–30%. It's further implicated in 21–48% of all lethal falls and 50% of all lethal burns. Finally, alcoholics face a 3–16x greater risk of accidental death than non-alcoholics.

Thus, even if the anti-alcohol-driving programs are successful in reducing driving while intoxicated without reducing general ethanol ingestion, there is no guarantee that the overall severe injury rate will be significantly reduced.

34.4 DIFFERENCES BETWEEN CIVIL LITIGATION INVOLVING ALCOHOL FROM CRIMINAL/DUI

Some claimed injury has occurred; one party is trying to prove or make the jury aware of the use and effects of alcohol on an opposing party. In employment or family law, the question of fitness for duty or fitness as a parent may pivot on alcohol use.

Operation of a vehicle over the legal limit is an important consideration in itself (and frequently heavily litigated to get in or keep out of evidence), but the violation of DUI laws may not have occurred or be an important issue in cases involving alcohol. Even though injured intoxicated persons in non-motor vehicle activities are not violating any laws, the jury needs to be aware of alcohol use and its potential effects on the person. This issue was recently addressed in the *Petraski* case in Illinois (discussed and cited later in this chapter).

Depositions pretrial are not the rule in criminal cases; they almost never occur in DUI cases (at least in Illinois). In the DUI case, the first time the opposing attorney sees the alcohol expert is in the courtroom.

Most alcohol-related injury cases settle before trial; most litigants do not want to put an intoxicated party (at the time of an event) on a witness stand. The remaining sections of the chapter present case discussions and reports of civil alcohol actions in which the authors have consulted and/or given deposition and/or court testimony. Some additional cases are discussed. A few criminal cases are presented, as well as Family Law and Probation violations. These cases demonstrate the application of the science of alcohol pharmacodynamics, pharmacokinetics, and toxicology in a variety of alcohol-related cases.

34.5 SETTINGS FOR ALCOHOL-RELATED CIVIL LITIGATION

34.5.1 Employment

CASE REPORT: INTOXICATED WHILE WORKING

A municipal employee arrived at work; his supervisor suspected he was intoxicated. Government rules and union rules prohibited working with an alcohol BAC > 0.04 g/dL. An alcohol expert evaluated the arrest reports for a DUI the prior evening and was asked to calculate the worker's BAC at the time of arrival at work. At an employment termination hearing, the village attorney proffered the alcohol expert in the field of toxicology and extrapolation.

The expert was asked to assume the following facts as true:

> The employee was approached in his vehicle by police at 9:44 p.m. and arrested at 11:35 p.m. He submitted to two breath tests conducted by the police. The first was a Portable Breath Test conducted at 11:01 p.m. which revealed a BAC of 0.189 g/dL and the second test was conducted after a 20-minute observation period in which the employee/arrestee did not eat, drink, smoke, or ingest anything. The second breath test, conducted at 11:24 p.m. revealed a BAC of 0.188 g/dL. The employee's height was 5′7″ and he weighed 170 pounds.

Q. Based on these facts, do you have an opinion within a reasonable degree of scientific certainty as to what the employee's blood-alcohol level was the next morning at 6:30 a.m.? (Seven hours) What is that opinion?
A. 0.062 gm/dL
Q. What is the basis of that opinion?
A. Seven hours elapsed. Subtract the alcohol eliminated in seven hours (7 ×.018 g/dL/hour = 7* (0.018 g/dL BAC/hr) = 0.126 g/dL. 0.188–0.126 = 0.062)
Q. What variables, if any, may exist in making a determination?

A. Assume the average rate of metabolism.
Q. How does a person's weight, if at all, impact the rate of alcohol metabolism?
A. Not at all.
Q. What significance does the fact that his blood-alcohol level only went down 0.001 g/dL in 20 minutes have on your determination?
A. The first test is a portable breath test. The PBT does not have the reliability and accuracy of the breathalyzer machine used in (and certified) the police station.
Q. And at 6:45 a.m., do you have an opinion as to whether the employee's BAC would have been under or over 0.04 g/dL?
A. Over.
Q. And is that opinion one you hold to a reasonable degree of scientific certainty?
A. Yes.
Q. And in your opinion, at what point would a person with an average rate of alcohol metabolism have had their BAC drop below 0.04 g/dL?
A. Sometime between 7:30 and 8:00 a.m.
Q. And is this opinion one you hold to a reasonable degree of scientific certainty?
A. Yes.

CASE REPORT: WORKER'S COMPENSATION, PREMISES LIABILITY; ADDITIONAL SCIENTIFIC ISSUE—EXTREME ALCOHOL LEVELS/TOLERANCE

The hospital's record note:

- Security guard fell from a height of four feet at work (unwitnessed)
- Loss of consciousness
- Fractured his orbit and suffered a frontal brain contusion
- Chronic (alcoholic) ischemic changes of the brain are noted on the Computed Tomography (CT)
- +ETOH, "smells of ETOH," fall under ETOH; Alcohol abuse (chronic alcoholism) history of falls secondary to alcohol, history of loss of consciousness apparently from alcohol intoxication, no memory of the incidence of the falls
- "Drunk again?" per family
- Alcohol test 349 mg/dL at 4:55 p.m. on 7/26/00
- 74.4 kg (163 lb)
- Past medical history significant for alcohol intoxication/dependence

OPINIONS

1. Since the first note at the hospital, and when the blood was tested at 4:55 p.m., an elapsed time of 120 minutes is assigned from the time of the unwitnessed fall to the time of the test. The hospital tests serum, not whole blood. A blood test of 349 mg/dL on serum must be lowered by 18% to accommodate between whole blood and serum. (*http://www.isp.state.il.us/docs/alcoholt.pdf*). This lowering results in a new test level of 296 mg/dL. Using an above-average metabolic rate of elimination of alcohol (higher in alcoholics) of 0.02 g/dL per hour, 120 minutes (2.00 hour) would indicate that 0.040 g/dL of alcohol would be eliminated between the time of the test and the accident. Extrapolation from the time of the test to the time of the fall (296 + 40) results in a BAC of 336 mg/dL at the time of the fall. This is a substantially high blood-alcohol content, more than four times the presumptive level of intoxication (80 mg/dL × 4 = 320 mg/dL), defined by the Illinois Motor Vehicle Code. Thus, for purposes of this report, a final BAC of 336 mg/dL is used.
2. In my opinion, the plaintiff/guard was intoxicated and impaired by alcohol at the time of the fall. Intoxication with blood levels of 336 mg/dL causes a loss of critical judgment, impairment in memory, release of inhibitions, increased risk-taking, impairment in vision (peripheral and depth), and severe motor impairments, including delayed reflexes and balance.[12] This is the "falling down drunk" region for BACs. Intoxicated pedestrians are at greater risk for serious injury and death from motor vehicle accidents than sober individuals.
3. The blood-alcohol level of 336 mg/dL would indicate the presence of the equivalent of 14 drinks (glasses of one or mixed drinks with one ounce of 100-proof whiskey) in the intoxicated plaintiff's blood at the time of the fall.

This amount is calculated using the following equation:

BAC = 150 / wt × conc alc / 50 × ounces of beverage × 0.025gm/dL

(# drinks solved from equation BAC = (150/wt)(conc. Alcohol in beverage/50)(0.025%)(ounces of beverage)

Drinking over an extended period, during work or before work would necessitate additional alcohol consumption to replace the amount of alcohol metabolized and excreted over the drinking period and/or time from drinking cessation to the time of the fall. To calculate the amount of alcohol consumed by the intoxicated plaintiff, I have considered the following criteria:

- Time of the fall (~ 3 p.m.)
- 163 lb weight
- Male sex
- Time of the blood test (4:55 p.m.)

The blood-alcohol test provides definitive proof of the level of alcohol present, which allows a reference to the alcohol literature, which describes the type and extent of intoxication at specific alcohol levels.

4. Given the facts of the accident, the plaintiff's alcohol intoxication must be considered as a significant contributing cause of the fall. Further, it is my opinion that the plaintiff would have been too intoxicated and impaired to perform his job as a security guard.
5. Alcohol tolerance is dispositional and functional. Dispositional tolerance is defined as a diminution of a drug's effect after a period of administration of that drug. The drug becomes less effective after chronic use because there is less of it at its site of action. The rate of metabolic inactivation of the drug is increased after chronic administration; thus, a particular dose produces lower and shorter-lasting blood levels. Functional tolerance or tissue tolerance denotes an actual change in the sensitivity of the brain to a given concentration of the drug. Included in this definition are some types of behaviorally augmented or conditioned tolerance. The various forms of tolerance have different mechanisms and presumably different sites, time course, and dose relationship, even though all have the same ultimate effect in that the subject appears less intoxicated after chronic alcohol administration. In experiments documenting tolerance, heavy drinkers were less affected than moderate drinkers, and abstainers were the most sensitive to the effects of alcohol at equivalent doses.[16]

CONCLUSION

The plaintiff was significantly intoxicated by alcohol and in a cognitive and motor function impaired state at the time of his accident. 336 mg/dL is a significantly high blood-alcohol level, even for a chronic alcohol (tolerant) abuser. This significantly high alcohol level is the most likely cause of his fall and subsequent head injury. This opinion is supported by his history of falls associated with alcohol intoxication.

34.6 POLICE ACTIVITIES

In these cases, the decedents' families brought civil lawsuits against a municipality and its police department and sometimes individual police officers, claiming that the city police violated "police pursuit" orders and that the pursuit caused the crash. Other cases arise out of claims of excessive force and/or shootings of intoxicated subjects by the police. The defendant municipality engaged the services of a pharmacologist/alcohol expert to evaluate the toxicology reports and relevant facts of the case to determine if the victim/plaintiff was intoxicated and impaired at the time.

34.6.1 Police Pursuit

A driver drove with two friends to a soccer game. The driver testified that he had been drinking beer before, during, and after the game. After the game, a police officer clocked the vehicle at 44 mph in a 30 mph zone. After stopping for the police, the driver pulled away and eventually crashed into another vehicle, killing the other driver. The time of the collision was 7:44 p.m. The family of the decedent sued the city.

The passengers in the fleeing car testified that the driver was drinking that afternoon and evening and that he was drunk. Indeed, they had offered to drive the car for him, because he had had too much to drink. The driver gave various statements and testimony indicating he had as many as six or seven 12 oz beers. Both passengers testified that they begged the driver to slow down and stop for the police.

At the hospital, police noted that the driver had bloodshot eyes and slurred speech. A blood sample drawn at 8:13 p.m. was analyzed for alcohol at the State Police Laboratories. The result was reported as 0.206 g/dL. His weight was noted to be 160 lb on his driver's license.

34.6.1.1 Opinions

1. The driver was intoxicated and impaired by alcohol at the time of the motor vehicle crash which occurred at 7:44 p.m.
2. His BAC was 0.206 g/dL, approximately 30 minutes after the crash. Extrapolating backward (retrograde), it would be expected that he would have a BAC of 0.215 g/dL. This represents the alcohol equivalent of nine beers in his blood at the time of the test.
3. Since he started drinking earlier in the day, additional beers had to have been consumed beyond the amount (nine beers) calculated to be in his body at the time of the toxicology test.
4. His alcohol intoxication and impairment must be considered a significant contributing cause of the motor vehicle collision. The driver was significantly intoxicated by alcohol, and in a cognitive and motor function impaired state at the time he crashed his vehicle into the other vehicle while speeding and running a red light. Alcohol intoxication and impairment are well known to impair judgment, exacerbate emotions, and increase risk-taking.

34.6.2 Excessive Police Force

The driver, a member of a street gang, drove an automobile with the decedent as a front seat passenger, and two back seat passengers, on a winter evening. The four young men had been at a party. The driver answered interrogatories indicating that each of the four men consumed "3 to 4" beers that evening. The driver testified that he never saw any police and that they were not fleeing from the police; he heard no sirens and saw no (police) lights. Beer bottles were found in the vehicle.

Two police officers viewed the driver's vehicle. One of the officers testified that he saw a gun being displayed. The police reversed the direction of their unmarked police vehicle and followed the vehicle. The fleeing vehicle struck another vehicle that was parked and left the scene, later stating that they feared for their safety from the pursuing gang car. During a high-speed turn, the driver lost control of his vehicle, crashing the vehicle into a barricade at 2:25 a.m., killing the front-seat passenger.

The decedent was taken to the medical examiner's office where an autopsy toxicology report revealed a blood-alcohol level of 0.152 g/dL. The driver was injured in the crash; he was taken to a local hospital, where his blood was drawn at 3:30 a.m. for a DUI kit. The blood was tested at the State Police Lab: a result of 0.106 g/dL was noted. The driver pled guilty to reckless homicide/voluntary manslaughter and possession of cannabis and was sentenced to the Illinois Department of Corrections.

The officers testified that at no time were they in "pursuit," nor was their vehicle close to the vehicle. They discovered the crashed vehicle and radioed for ambulances and additional police support. The decedent's weight is noted to be 340 lb. The driver's weight is noted to be 230 lb. Police records indicate a weight of 160 lb. for the driver.

34.6.2.1 Opinions

The driver was intoxicated and impaired by alcohol during the early morning hours and at the time he crashed his car, killing his front-seat passenger.

The driver's BAC was approximately 124 mg/dL (0.124 g/dL) at the time of the crash. This represents the equivalent of five beers in his blood at the time of the crash. Since he testified that drinking started several hours earlier in the evening, his total consumption of alcohol that evening before the crash was most likely in excess of nine to ten beers.

34.6.2.2 Summary

The driver was intoxicated (more than one and one-quarter times the presumptive level of intoxication (80 mg/dL × 1.5 = 120 mg/dL) by alcohol), and in a cognitive and motor function impaired state at the time he crashed his vehicle while speeding. Alcohol intoxication and impairment are well known to affect judgment and increase risk-taking. The city settled the case for a nominal amount, "cost of defense."

34.6.3 Alcohol Effects on Aggression and Judgment

CASE REPORT: DECEDENT GRABS FOR OFFICER'S WEAPON

The decedent's mother testified that on the night of his death, her son was out celebrating a friend's birthday. They would drink alcohol every other day. Everyone was drinking gin during this time, including the decedent. A police cruiser started following the van. When the van stopped, several of the occupants jumped out and started running. A police officer detained the decedent. The police officer testified that the decedent tackled him and tried to grab his weapon. The officer shot the decedent, killing him.

OPINIONS

The decedent consumed alcohol leading to his impairment before the shooting. Testimony of his companions stated that they were drinking from a large bottle of Tanqueray gin. He also smoked marijuana. The decedent was experiencing the intoxicating effects of alcohol and marijuana at the time he tackled and attempted to disarm the police officer. His blood-alcohol test of 0.054 g/dL, vitreous alcohol of 0.033 g/dL, and urine alcohol test of 0.091 g/dL—all represent completely absorbed and distributed alcohol. This distribution of compartment tests is consistent with a rising BAC curve.

Intoxication with blood-alcohol levels of 0.054 g/dL causes disinhibition, increased impulsivity, increased risk-taking, and poor judgment. Marijuana, an illegal controlled substance Schedule I drug, may produce a variety of pharmacological effects including sedation, euphoria, hallucinations, and temporal distortion. It is described as a psychoactive drug. Alcohol-related aggression and violence is well recognized in the literature.[17,18,19,20,21]

SUMMARY OF OPINIONS

The decedent was impaired by alcohol and marijuana, and in a cognitively impaired state at the time he aggressively attacked the police officer. This is a clear example of extremely poor judgment and highly risky behavior. Alcohol, a known disinhibitor, increases aggressive behavior.

34.6.4 Foot Chase/Police Shooting/Excessive Force

Police officers responded to a call of "shots fired" and "man with a gun." They observed a vehicle moving fast with its lights off. The officers were in plain clothes and driving an unmarked police car. They turned on the MARS lights to pull this car over. The driver exited the car and began to run. He then turned into a gangway. One officer ran in pursuit and yelled "Stop! Police!"

One Officer ran through the gangway and then saw the suspect trying to push open a gate. The suspect moved a few feet and turned back to face the officer. The officer heard a gunshot and saw a muzzle flash. The officer drew his weapon and yelled "Police!" and then fired two shots at the suspect. When the suspect pivoted a second time, the officer fired four or five times because he thought the suspect would shoot at him again. The suspect then turned, jumped over a fence, and ran, again with the officer in pursuit. The suspect was found dead at the scene. While searching in the vicinity, an officer found a semi-automatic weapon in a yard near the shooting location.

The medical examiner performed the autopsy on the decedent. The postmortem BAC was 0.123 g/dL in central blood. The medical examiner testified that this level of alcohol would have impaired the decedent's judgment and diminished his motor skills. The medical examiner's report indicates a weight of 270 lb and 6′2″ height. The decedent consumed alcohol on the evening before his death.

34.6.4.1 Opinions

The decedent was intoxicated and impaired by alcohol at the time of his death. He had consumed at least the equivalent of eight to ten alcoholic beverages ("drinks") before the shooting; this consumption led to his alcohol intoxication. Alcohol intoxication impairs an individual's judgment and increases impulsivity, causes labile emotions, and increases aggression and violent acts.

34.7 MOTOR VEHICLE COLLISIONS

34.7.1 Vehicle/Vehicle

CASE REPORT: DRINKING AFTER THE CRASH

Two vehicles were involved in a collision. One fled the scene; a witness followed the fleeing vehicle and advised the police of its location (a friend's home). The driver first denied driving, stating he had been drinking and did not want to drive. He later admitted to driving, stating he left the scene because he was scared. A police officer noted alcohol effects, and the driver was arrested and given a breathalyzer test, which indicated an alcohol level of 0.127 g/dL. His friend testified that he had been drinking (and did not see any whiskey bottles). An officer noted he had slurred speech, bloodshot eyes, and smelled of alcohol. The driver's weight (200 lb.) and height (6′) are noted in the police report.

The driver testified that before the collision he was "hanging out with a large group of people, my peers." He denied ingesting drugs but when asked if he had anything to drink he said "Maybe a beer or two." He later states that each beer was "12-ounce cans." He stated that he might have had a beer or two perhaps on three occasions during the previous month.

After the crash, before the police arrived, he stated that he consumed hard alcohol while at his friend's house, Why? A: "I don't know. I was scared." He stated that he had one or two drinks out of a bottle. He also does not know the brand or type of liquor or bottle size. The officer interviewed the driver and noted that the driver had an odor of alcohol on his breath and had bloodshot eyes. His speech was a little slurred which indicated he had been drinking.

OPINIONS

The driver consumed alcohol leading to his intoxication before the collision. His testimony that he drank whiskey at his friend's house is inconsistent with the findings of the officer and of the friend. He would not appear intoxicated ("had been drinking") with bloodshot eyes and slurred speech immediately after drinking an unknown amount of alcohol (a few sips).

The driver was intoxicated and impaired by alcohol at the time of the crash. His alcohol test of 0.127 g/dL was taken 2.5 hours after the collision. The BAC would decrease 0.018 g/dL every hour through metabolism in the time between the collision and the alcohol test (this is based upon an average hourly metabolic rate of 18 mg/dL/hr. 18 × 2.5 = 45). This eliminated alcohol is added to the 0.127 g/dL, resulting in an extrapolated blood-alcohol level of 127 + 45 = 0.172 g/dL. This alcohol level is more than twice the level of presumed intoxication, as defined by the Illinois Motor Vehicle Code (2 × 0. 80 = 160 g/dL).

Based on the driver's 200 lb weight, the blood-alcohol level of 0.172 g/dL indicates the presence of the alcohol equivalent of at least nine 12-ounce beers. (Of note: 150 lb. man consuming one 12-ounce beer (4% alcohol) will develop a BAC of 0.025%.) If his drinking before the accident occurred over four to five hours, then he would have had to have consumed the equivalent of twelve 12-ounce beers, or ~15 drinks. If, indeed, whiskey had been consumed after the collision, approximately 12 ounces of 80-proof whiskey (the most common strength sold) would be required by the subject to have a BAC of 0.127 g/dL at the time of the breathalyzer test at the police station.

To calculate the amount of alcohol consumed by the driver, I have considered the following criteria:

- Time of the accident (10:48 p.m.)
- 200 lb weight
- Time of the blood test (01:14 a.m.)

SUMMARY

The driver was intoxicated by alcohol and in a cognitive and motor function impaired state at the time of the collision. In my opinion, he would have been an unsafe driver as a result of his intoxication.

(*Petraski v. Thedos* (County of Cook, Il) (Jury Should Hear Alcohol Expert) published opinion)

The Petraski Case is an important legal precedent establishing the admissibility of an expert's opinion that a BAC is 0.08 g/dL or greater. This case was tried twice; in the first trial, the judge barred the testimony of the defendant's pharmacologist expert (JTOD); the jury did not hear that the plaintiff's BAC was above 0.08 g/dL. A $35 million dollar plaintiff's verdict was awarded by the jury. The defendant (County of Cook, IL) appealed, and the case was reversed by the Illinois Appellate Court. One of the bases of the reversal was the Trial Court's barring the defendant's alcohol expert (JTOD). The case was retried, and a different alcohol expert (Jerrold Leikin, MD) testified that the plaintiff's BAC was greater than 0.08 g/dL and that she was impaired. The jury returned a verdict in favor of the defendant. The plaintiffs appealed, and the appellate court upheld the BAC testimony (referring to the first trial, but found that the court erred in allowing the alcohol expert to give testimony that the plaintiff was impaired as a result of alcohol intoxication). The case later was resolved by the parties. Excerpts related to the alcohol testing and interpretation are produced below.

PETRASKI v. THEDOS[22]

Michael PETRASKI, Guardian of the Estate of Margaret Petraski, a Disabled Person, Plaintiff—Appellee, v. Deborah THEDOS, Individually and as Agent/Employee of the Sheriff of Cook County, and Michael Sheahan, Sheriff of Cook County, Defendants—Appellants.

No. 1–10–3218.

—December 16, 2011

OPINIONS

On May 28, 2001, Margaret Petraski (Margaret) and Officer Deborah Thedos, of the Cook County Sheriff's Police Department, were involved in a motor vehicle accident at the intersection of the Midlothian Turnpike and Central Avenue in unincorporated Cook County. Officer Thedos admitted that she drove through a red light with her MARS lights activated. She had also activated her siren as she approached the intersection. Margaret was seriously injured in the accident and became a quadriplegic as a result of her injuries. Michael Petraski, Margaret's son and legal guardian, brought a personal injury suit on her behalf against Officer Thedos and the officer's employer Michael Sheahan, sheriff of Cook County.

At the first trial, a jury found for the plaintiff. Defendants appealed, claiming that evidence of Margaret's blood-alcohol content (BAC) should have been admitted at trial. This court agreed and reversed the judgment and ordered a new trial. *Petraski v. Thedos*, 382 Ill. App.3d 22, 320 Ill.Dec. 244, 887 N.E.2d 24 (2008).

At the second trial, the jury found for the defendants. Plaintiff filed a post-trial motion for a new trial, which was granted by the trial court on October 4, 2010. On November 3, 2010, the defendants filed a petition for leave to appeal the interlocutory order pursuant to Illinois Supreme Court Rule 306(a)(1) (eff. Feb.19, 2010). On January 6, 2011, this court granted the defendants' petition for leave to appeal.

On this interlocutory appeal, the defendants claim that the trial court abused its discretion by granting a new trial. The trial court found that it had committed three errors, each of which would independently require a new trial. The three errors were (1) the trial court should have granted the plaintiff's motion to bar the defendants' toxicology expert, Dr. Jerrold Leikin, from testifying that Margaret was in fact impaired, solely on the basis of her blood-alcohol level; (2) evidence of Officer Thedos' mental health history was improperly excluded; and (3) defense counsel made improper closing remarks about the societal impact of drunk driving.

***Cuellar V. Hout* (Published Opinion)**

This is an important case in that the retrograde extrapolation used by a defense expert pharmacologist (JTOD) was challenged on appeal, and an Illinois Appellate Court affirmed the defense verdict. Excerpts of the case are presented as follows:

> CUELLAR v. HOUT
> 168 Ill. App.3d 416 (1988)
> 522 N.E.2d 322
> TOMAS A. CUELLAR, Plaintiff-Appellant, v. ROBERT W. HOUT, Defendant (Winfield Township et al., Defendants-Appellees).
> No. 2-87-0414.
> Judgment affirmed.

OPINIONS

PRESIDING JUSTICE LINDBERG delivered the opinion of the court:

> Plaintiff, Tomas A. Cuellar, brought an action in the circuit court of Du Page County seeking damages for personal injuries he alleged resulted from the negligence of Roger W. Hout (Hout), Winfield Township (the township), and Winfield Township Highway Commissioner Arthur J. Lootens (Lootens). Plaintiff was taken to Central Du Page Hospital. At some time between 8:55 p.m. and 9:17 p.m. a blood sample was drawn to perform a blood-alcohol test. The test indicated a blood-alcohol level of.064 g/dL.

Defendants presented the testimony of James O'Donnell (JTOD), who was a pharmacologist, pharmacist, and nutritionist, as to whether the plaintiff had been intoxicated at the time of the accident. JTOD testified that "retrograde extrapolation" is accepted in the pharmacological community. Alcohol is eliminated from the body at an average rate of.015 to .02 per hour. JTOD used the .02-per-hour elimination rate on the basis that it was more likely correct due to elevated levels of certain enzymes in the blood indicating how the plaintiff's liver was functioning. Assuming the .02-per-hour elimination rate, and assuming that during the entire period after the accident plaintiff was in the elimination and not the absorption phase for the alcohol he had consumed, retrograde extrapolation indicated that the plaintiff had a blood-alcohol level of.104 at the time of the accident. JTOD was of the opinion that the plaintiff had been intoxicated at the time of the accident.

Austin Gibbons, M.D., a pathologist (who was also an attorney), testified as an expert for the plaintiff. He testified that retrograde extrapolation of a blood-alcohol level from a single measurement could not be relied upon. From that number, it is impossible to determine whether the person is still in the absorption phase or, if in the elimination phase, when the level had peaked. Trauma, the type of beverage consumed, and the type of food consumed could affect the absorption rate and so the validity of an extrapolation. Gibbons also testified that the enzymes JTOD had found significantly high were not much above normal levels and would be expected to be at higher than average levels for a period following trauma.

Plaintiff raises the following issues:

1. Whether the trial court ruled correctly in allowing defendants to place evidence of the plaintiff's drinking before the jury.
2. Whether the trial court ruled correctly in allowing opinion evidence that the plaintiff was intoxicated by one who did not observe the plaintiff, but who based the opinion on mathematical extrapolations and a statutory presumption.
3. Whether the trial court ruled correctly in excluding evidence of defendants' admission [that the intersection should have signs].

We affirm.

Plaintiff's first two issues are related. We will, therefore, follow the lead of the parties and discuss them together.

Under the first two issues, plaintiff challenges the admissibility of essentially three types of testimony. The testimony challenged concerned: (1) plaintiff's drinking of beer prior to the accident; (2) results of the blood-alcohol test showing a.064 alcohol level in plaintiff's blood; and (3) retrograde extrapolation from the blood-alcohol test results leading O'Donnell to the opinions that (a) plaintiff's blood-alcohol level was.104 at the time of the accident and (b) plaintiff was intoxicated at the time of the accident. Plaintiff's challenges to the admissibility of the blood-alcohol test and O'Donnell's testimony on retrograde extrapolation,

The judgment of the circuit court of Du Page County is affirmed.

Affirmed. INGLIS and NASH, JJ., concur.

People v. Floyd (2014 IL App (2d) 120507—Illinois Courts)[23]

More than 25 years later, The Illinois Appellate Court further clarified the use of retrograde extrapolation in alcohol cases.

Excerpts of the Court Opinion follow:

> Following a jury trial, defendant, Chrystal L. Floyd, was convicted of aggravated driving under the influence (DUI) pursuant to section 11-501(a)(2) of the Illinois Vehicle Code (625ILCS 5/11-501(a)(2) (West 2010)) and resisting arrest (720 ILCS 5/31-1(a) (West 2010)).

During the trial, the State introduced expert witness testimony on a "retrograde extrapolation" calculation in an attempt to demonstrate that defendant's BAC was at or above 0.08 at the time of her arrest. Retrograde extrapolation is premised on the theory that a person's BAC, derived from a breath or blood test at a particular time, can be extrapolated back to an allegedly higher BAC that existed at the time of a prior incident. The State also introduced evidence of other crimes that occurred before the defendant allegedly committed the offense of aggravated DUI.

OPINIONS

On appeal, defendant contends that the trial court erred by (1) allowing the (state's)expert witness's testimony on retrograde extrapolation when the expert did not have information necessary to conduct a reliable calculation; (2) allowing the State to admit other crimes evidence that was highly prejudicial, but minimally relevant; (3) allowing testimony, which lacked foundation, that defendant failed a horizontal gaze nystagmus (HGN) test; and (4) failing to instruct the jury that it could not draw a negative inference from the State's video recording of defendant's field sobriety tests, which the State failed to produce. For the following reasons, we reverse the defendant's DUI conviction and remand for a new trial.

Law enforcement officers administered a breath test to the defendant at 10:30 p.m., which registered her BAC at 0.069. At trial, the State produced John Wetstein, a forensic toxicologist (employed by the State), as an expert witness. Wetstein testified that, after conducting a retrograde extrapolation calculation, he determined that the defendant's BAC at 9:10 p.m. was between 0.082 and 0.095.

Wetstein explained that conducting a retrograde extrapolation calculation is possible because a person eliminates alcohol at a fixed rate of between 0.01 and 0.02 grams per deciliter of blood per hour. Wetstein explained that two conditions must be met for the calculation to be valid. First, the person metabolizes alcohol at a normal rate. Second, the person is in the postabsorption phase—that is, the person is no longer absorbing alcohol and is in the elimination phase—when the breath test is administered. Wetstein explained that, because the body absorbs alcohol primarily through the small intestine, a person's absorption rate will vary depending on many factors. These factors include the type of food that the person has eaten, the type of alcohol consumed, and the length of time during which the drinking occurred. Wetstein testified that after a person's last drink, a person can take from 15 minutes to 90 minutes or more to enter the postabsorption phase.

On cross-examination, Wetstein acknowledged that he did not know what the defendant had eaten that night, how long she had been drinking, or what type of alcohol she consumed. Wetstein admitted that he did not attempt to determine when the defendant had entered the elimination phase but, rather, assumed that she was in the elimination phase at 9:10 p.m. Wetstein explained that, if a person had not consumed any alcohol since 7:30 p.m., he would be "quite confident" that the person was in the elimination phase by 9:10 p.m.

The jury found the defendant guilty of aggravated DUI and resisting arrest. Based on two prior burglary convictions, the trial court sentenced the defendant as a Class X offender to a minimum of six years' imprisonment. The defendant appeals her DUI conviction but not her resisting arrest conviction.

The defendant's first contention on appeal is that the trial court erred in admitting Wetstein's testimony regarding Wetstein's retrograde extrapolation calculation. Defendant argues that, because Wetstein did not have the information necessary to perform a retrograde extrapolation calculation with any degree of certainty, the prejudicial effect of his testimony outweighed its probative value. Specifically, the defendant argues that Wetstein did the "simple part" of the retrograde extrapolation calculation by adding between 0.01 and 0.02 per hour to the result of the defendant's breath test, but he "assumed away" that the defendant was in the postabsorption, elimination phase. Thus, the gravamen of the defendant's argument is that, because a subject being in the elimination phase is necessary for a retrograde extrapolation calculation to be accurate and valid, Wetstein's testimony had little probative value because he merely assumed that the defendant was in that phase. Further, Wetstein's testimony was prejudicial because, as a "court-pronounced expert regarding retrograde extrapolation," the jury would listen to him anyway.

Thus, the reviewing court determined that the trial court did not abuse its discretion in excluding the retrograde extrapolation evidence. *Id.*

With respect to the retrograde extrapolation's probative value, we recognize that Wetstein's calculation would be relevant to whether the defendant's BAC was at or above 0.08 g/dL. Nonetheless, the inherent unreliability of Wetstein's calculation is reflected in his own testimony. Specifically, Wetstein testified that determining whether a person was in the elimination phase was a "complicated question." Wetstein testified that different circumstances could affect whether someone was in the elimination phase, such as when the person started and stopped drinking; a person's eating and drinking habits; how much and what food had been consumed; and the type of alcohol consumed. Wetstein acknowledged that he did not recall when the defendant started and stopped drinking. He testified that, if other relevant information on whether the defendant was in the elimination phase were available, he would have factored it into his calculation. However, Wetstein's testimony is devoid of any indication that he considered any other information to determine whether the defendant was in the elimination phase. Instead, Wetstein admitted that his "big assumption" was that the defendant was eliminating alcohol when law enforcement officers administered the breath test, and he admitted that if his assumption were wrong "the extrapolation [would not] be valid." Thus, because Wetstein's calculation was premised on the assumption that the defendant was in the elimination phase, without consideration of other relevant factors and without additional breath tests, we find the probative value of his testimony to be significantly diminished.

CASE CONCLUSION

In sum, because the State's expert witness acknowledged that he was unaware of many of the factors necessary to determine whether the defendant was in the elimination phase, and because the police conducted only one BAC test, we find the extrapolation calculation to be inherently unreliable. In addition, because the extrapolation evidence invited the jury to convict the defendant on the basis of a supposedly high BAC, the potential for prejudice from admitting that evidence was high. Because the prejudicial effect of the extrapolation substantially outweighed the probative value, the trial court abused its discretion in admitting the evidence. See generally *McKown*, 236 Ill. 2d at 314 (noting that the admissibility of scientific evidence is subject to the balancing of probative value and the risk of unfair prejudice). Further, given the conflicting nature of the other testimony at trial, including that the defendant passed some field sobriety tests while failing others, the trial court's admission of the extrapolation evidence was not harmless. See *id.* at 311 (rejecting a harmless error argument).

Nonetheless, although we are reversing, we find that, after viewing the evidence in the light most favorable to the State, there was sufficient evidence from which the jury could have found the defendant guilty of aggravated DUI beyond a reasonable doubt. See *People v. Lopez*, 229 Ill. 2d 322, 366–67 (2008) (noting that the relevant inquiry into whether double jeopardy prohibits another trial is whether, after viewing the evidence in the light most favorable to the State, including suppressed evidence, any rational trier of fact could have found the essential elements of the crime beyond a reasonable doubt). The evidence in this case included the improperly admitted extrapolation evidence, the field sobriety tests, and Drew's opinion testimony.

34.7.2 Motorcycle Cases

Motorcycles are frequently involved in collisions and injuries, and the literature (cited herein) documents an increased incidence of alcohol intoxication in motorcycle injuries and deaths associated with collisions.

Motorcycle v. Semi Tractor Trailer

Alcohol kinetic concepts involved: Two Alcohol Tests One Serum, One State Police Lab, Conversion, Extrapolation, Calculation of Metabolic Rate.

- Time of the Crash—9:20 p.m.
- Hospital serum alcohol 187 (0.187) at 10:25 p.m.
- ISP DUI Sample 0.128 at 11:29 p.m.
- Urine positive for Marijuana
- weight 220 lb., height 5′8″
- Time of drinking, 6 p.m.–8 p.m.; 3–4 Budweiser 12-ounce cans
- Last meal, breakfast, ~ 12 hours before the crash
- Usual weekly alcohol consumption: 12–18 beers

34.7.2.1 Opinions

The motorcyclist was intoxicated and impaired by alcohol at the time of the Crash. His BAC was 0.160 g/dL at the time of the Crash. This represents the equivalent of nine "beers" in his blood at the time of the Crash. Considering the alcohol metabolized from the onset of drinking until the time of the crash, the alcohol equivalent of three 12-ounce beers brings the total consumption to 12 beers. It is scientifically impossible for him to have consumed only three to four beers as he claims in the evening before the crash. The motorcyclist's alcohol intoxication and impairment was a significant contributing cause of the motor vehicle collision.

Available evidence implicates alcohol consumption as a major risk factor for almost every type of injury. Alcohol's effects on balance and motor coordination would be expected to have greater consequences for motorcycle riders than for car/truck drivers. Driving while intoxicated/under the influence (DWI) reports for 1984 and 1985 from the San Antonio, TX, Police Department were reviewed to evaluate motorcycle DWIs and to compare them with car/truck DWIs. Initiation of the DWI investigation of motorcycle riders was more frequently due to excessive speed, and, less likely due to an accident, when compared to car/truck investigations. Breath alcohol testing demonstrated a significantly lower BAC in motorcycle riders, 0.14 ± 0.05 g/dL, than in car/truck drivers, 0.16 ± 0.05 g/dL ($p = 0.016$). The results of this study suggest that alcohol influences motorcycle riders to a greater extent than it does car/truck drivers.[24,25,26]

34.7.2.2 Conclusion

Alcohol intoxication and impairment significantly contributed to the motorcyclist's collision into the rear wheel of the semi-truck.

CASE REPORT: *MOTORCYCLIST V. MOTORIST*

The motorcyclist was taken by ambulance to hospital, arriving at 11:55 p.m. Blood was taken for a variety of clinical tests, including a sample for serum ethanol (ETOH), the collection occurring at 12:15 a.m.). The result of the serum alcohol test was 0.174 gm/dL. Retrograde extrapolation to the time of the accident raised the serum alcohol level to approximately 0.185 g/dL. Some of the witnesses to the motorcyclist's activities prior to the accident have stated that he had consumed alcohol. The motorcyclist testified that he consumed two beers shortly after 9:30 p.m. at a bar, and had no other alcohol that evening.

OPINIONS

In my opinion, the motorcyclist was intoxicated and impaired by alcohol at the time of the accident. Intoxication at a level of 0.185 g/dL causes impairment in judgment, release of inhibitions, increased risk-taking, impairment in vision (peripheral and depth), and motor impairments, including delayed reflexes and balance. The risk of an accident occurring increases 25-fold. The motorcyclist was 200 pounds and six feet tall at the time of the accident. An adult male of his weight would require consuming the equivalent of ten 12-ounce beers before the accident for a 0.174 g/dL to be measured at 12:15 a.m.

I reviewed hospital records which include treatment for traumatic orthopedic injury following an accident wherein the motorcyclist fell off his motorcycle. The motorcyclist testified that he is 5′11″, 180 pounds, and his alcohol consumption on the day of the accident started at 2:00 p.m. with one beer, and that he might have had four to five beers between 3:30 and 8:30 p.m. The motorcyclist denied being intoxicated. He was admitted to the hospital through the emergency department shortly before midnight. His blood was tested for alcohol and reported at 12:06 a.m. to be 222 mg/dL. The medical records note a strong odor of alcohol (ETOH) on his breath, and that "he does consume a fair amount of alcohol."

CONCLUSION

In my opinion, the motorcyclist was intoxicated and impaired by alcohol at the time of the accident (11:35 p.m.). Impairments at the level tested include cognitive and gross motor control.

34.7.3 Boating

34.7.3.1 Intoxicated Guest Falls From Upper Deck

A partygoer fell backward off the upper deck of a party yacht shortly before 6 p.m. (EMS dispatch 5:50 p.m.) He was taken emergently to hospital emergency/trauma service, where he was diagnosed with multiple vertebral fractures and spinal cord injury. A blood sample was drawn at 6:30 p.m. and tested for alcohol, resulting in a BAC of 0.233 g/dL. Clinical notes include "intoxicated" and "had been drinking." The man testified that he drank one beer in the Limo on the way to the boat, was on the boat since around 12:30 p.m., and consumed beer, 2–3 per hour, ~ 10–12 all afternoon, and some soft drinks and food. Food was consumed early in the afternoon—1 to 2 p.m. A few dozen friends, business associates, family members, and friends were also on the boat for the afternoon. None of those questioned observed him to be intoxicated; a few described him as "mellow." None described him as slurring his speech, staggering, or having difficulty in any way associated with intoxication. He sat down on a white leather-like folding "bench" after the band stopped playing and was sitting on the bench for a few minutes before he fell backward to the lower deck. The bench is described by multiple witnesses as being positioned at the edge of the back of the upper deck of the boat. There was no railing at this deck location. He heard someone call him from a lower deck behind him. He turned his head in the direction of the voice, leaned back on the bench, and fell backward over the side of the upper deck to the deck below.

A toxicologist for the defense testified that the injured man was intoxicated and impaired by alcohol; (vision, cognitive, balance, walking ability, reaction times, attention, muscular coordination, and judgment); despite this opinion, he was unable to attribute any specific impairment to the fall, just a general attribution of alcohol intoxication as a "primary cause" of the fall. It impaired his ability to properly and safely function in performing normal functions. He further testified that the hospital serum BAC of 233 mg/dL must be lowered to 191 mg/dL (whole blood) and that the 191 mg/dL extrapolates to 209 mg/dL (an addition of 18 mg/dL). The toxicologist further testified that the injured man consumed 13 beers over the course of the afternoon to achieve the measured BAC.

34.7.3.2 Opinions

A pharmacologist expert (JTOD) retained by the injured man/plaintiff provided the following opinions:

> I agree that the injured man was intoxicated and impaired by alcohol. However, the injured man was consuming beer throughout the afternoon. Therefore, the BAC would not have peaked and be on a downward path at the time of the fall, rendering the retrograde extrapolation invalid. None of the "functions"—movements, thoughts, actions, muscle coordination, judgment, vision, etc.—attendant to responding to his name by turning his head and shoulders would be functions that would be "impaired" by alcohol. The injured man's alcohol impairment is not a cause, primary or contributory, to his fall.

34.7.4 Vehicle/Pedestrian

34.7.4.1 St. Patrick's Day Celebration

Mr. Plaintiff and Mr. Taxi Driver, the driver of a taxicab, collided in the westbound lane of Addison Street at 5 pm on Saturday, March 16. Mr. Plaintiff had been drinking since 1045 that morning. He was taken by EMS to a local hospital and treated for trauma injuries. While at the hospital, his blood was tested at 1730 (5:30 p.m.) for alcohol, and a serum alcohol of 0.233 g/dL was noted. Clinical notes indicated a reported consumption of seven beers, alcohol intoxication, and alcohol history was "a few beers or a glass of wine 2 or 3 times a week, on weekends." The plaintiff's weight was recorded as 209 lbs.

The plaintiff testified that he and his wife were hosting a late morning St. Patrick's Day celebration at their home. Mr. Plaintiff testified: " he had been drinking continuously throughout the day until around 4:30 Just prior to the impact, Mr. Plaintiff felt that he was buzzed, where I knew that I had probably reached my limit for the day of drinking." He looked both ways and entered the crosswalk. The intersection was backed up with traffic. When he emerged from the eastbound lane into the westbound lane, he did not look to his right—he was distracted by a disturbance in front of the Tavern. He was about three-quarters of the way through the eastbound lane when he saw a taxicab just before it crashed into him.

34.7.4.2 Taxi Driver

The taxi driver worked as a cab driver in Chicago for five to six months before the accident. The taxi driver recalls he was going at his own pace westbound on Addison at 20–25 mph when "a guy just popped out of nowhere" and he could not stop or act in any manner. Traffic in the eastbound lane was almost stopped at this point. He states that there were no other pedestrians in the crosswalk besides the one he hit. It did not occur to him to slow down because there were no pedestrians in the street. The eastbound lanes of Addison were almost stopped, but the westbound lanes were moving freely. The driver states that he did not see the pedestrian running across the street. He considers himself a safe driver and would not consider putting someone in harm's way.

34.7.4.3 Eye Witness

The witness testified that a group of pedestrians was crossing the street in the crosswalk when he saw an individual (the plaintiff) separate from the group and walk a little bit ahead of the group. He noticed a flash of orange, a vehicle, and heard a yell, a collision of some sort. When he turned back, there was an individual lying in the middle of the street. The pedestrian who was struck was not running, he appeared to be walking. He (Mr. Plaintiff) was at the front of his group and he was pulling away while crossing the street. The witness did not see the pedestrian look both ways and did not witness him look to the right for any westbound traffic.

34.7.4.4 Another Cab Driver—Witness

Mr. Driver 2 was working for a different Cab Company on Mar 16, 2013, He was driving eastbound on Addison and traffic was slow at 5–10 mph. A pedestrian was moving pretty fast and a cab struck him in the westbound lane. The pedestrian went into the air and fell onto his cab and then fell back to the street. "It means he might be kind of running." The cab going west was going 25–30 mph. The pedestrian was in the crosswalk when he was struck. "Maybe he (the pedestrian) was not looking. That's why—or something like this."

34.7.4.5 Opinions

1. The plaintiff was intoxicated and impaired by alcohol at the time he collided with the Taxi.
2. The alcohol test reported a 0.233 g/dL (233 mg%) on serum. This converts to a 0.197 g/dL. 0.233g / dL/1.18 = 0.197g / dL

3. Since the test was drawn 30 minutes after the collision, the 0.197 must be extrapolated back to the time of the collision. Alcohol metabolizes at a mean rate of 18 mg% (0.018 g/dL)/hour. Thus, an additional 9 mg% alcohol is added to the 197, resulting in an extrapolated alcohol level of 206 mg% (0.206 g/dL) at the time of the collision.
   0.197g / dL + 0.009g/dL = 0.206g / dL
4. Since the collision occurred 30 minutes after the drinking stopped, the alcohol content of the last beer is removed from the calculation, since the last beer may not have been completely absorbed by the time of the collision, falsely elevating any alcohol test at 1730.

Alcohol content (BAC) in a 209 lb man from one 4.2% 12 oz. beer is calculated as follows:

BAC = 150 / wt × conc of alc / 50× # ounces × 0.025g / dl (bac achieved in 150 bl man consuming one ounce of a 50% alcohol beverage)

BAC = 150 / 209 × 4.2%/ 50% × 12oz. × 0.025 = 0.018g/dl

Thus, the alcohol contribution of one 12 oz. bottle of Leinenkugel beer in a 209 lb man is approximately 18 mg%. Therefore, 18 mg% is removed from the extrapolated amount of 206 mg% (206–18) = 188 mg%, thus resulting in an adjusted extrapolated amount of 188 mg% (0.188 g/dL). (This adjustment accommodates unabsorbed alcohol from the last drink consumed, thus following the requisite considerations of *Floyd* as described earlier in this chapter.)

34.7.4.6 Summary

The plaintiff was intoxicated by alcohol, and in a cognitive and motor function impaired state at the time he collided with the taxicab.

CASE REPORT: *PEDESTRIAN V. MOTOR VEHICLE WESTERN COOK COUNTY*

At 9:24 p.m., John Pedestrian, while walking across Ogden Avenue against the light, was struck by the driver's vehicle. The pedestrian was taken emergently to a local Hospital and treated. While at the Hospital, his blood was tested; the blood test result at 2205 was 105 mg%. On the day of the motor vehicle crash (MVC), the pedestrian recalls several beers (at least two or three) at lunch between 1:00 and 3:00 p.m. He also took one Vicodin tablet on December 16, 2012, the day before the MVC.

A police officer who came to the scene noted alcohol. The pedestrian said he needed an ambulance. The officer asked him if he had been drinking and "He said he was just drinking beer, and that was it." In his police report the officer marked "pedestrian crossing against signal." The auto driver told the officer that she was driving through the intersection with the green light at 30 mph. Just before she reached the crosswalk, she saw the pedestrian crossing with a hood over his head and looking down. She locked up the brakes and slid into him.

OPINIONS

1. The pedestrian was intoxicated and impaired by alcohol at the time of the accident.
2. The pedestrian's Blood-Alcohol Concentration (BAC) was reported at 2205 as 105 mg%. Since this is a serum test, the result must be lowered by 18% (105/1.18 = 89 mg%)
3. The 89 mg% at 2205 (40 minutes after the Crash) extrapolates to 100 mg% (89 × 40/60 + 11; 11 + 89 = 100 mg). 100 mg% represents the equivalent of five (5) "drinks" in the pedestrian's blood at the time of the accident. Since he testified that he drank beer between 1 and 3 pm, substantially more beer than the five beers must have been consumed.
4. The urine toxicology tests were positive for opiates, barbiturates, benzodiazepines, and cannabis. The pedestrian testified that he took Vicodin the day prior; if he used barbiturates, benzodiazepines, and/or cannabis (marijuana) on the day/evening of the accident, the impairment/intoxication he was experiencing from alcohol would have been enhanced.

SUMMARY

The pedestrian was intoxicated by alcohol, and in a cognitive and motor function impaired state at the time of the accident.

CASE REPORT: PEDESTRIAN ON A DARK ROAD

Christopher Pedestrian was struck by a Driver's automobile shortly after 11 pm (~2320) on the evening. He was in the roadway in the Driver's traffic lane when he was struck. The Driver testified that she did not see the pedestrian until there was no time to stop or avoid the collision. She testified that she was unable to see due to high-beam headlights activated by another automobile, which was attempting to alert the Driver of the Pedestrian's presence in the roadway. EMS was called to the scene (2323); fluids were started, and he was taken emergently to a local hospital, arriving at 2355. In the Emergency Department, Mr. Pedestrian was resuscitated, he was given a total of 5,000 ml of crystalloids (fluid resuscitation), and multiple transfusions of packed cells and platelets in an attempt to keep him alive. Mr. Pedestrian was pronounced dead at 0246 despite the resuscitation efforts.

The police report notes that an earlier 911 call reported a man sitting on a curb near the scene of the accident. The police also note interviewing a bartender who testified that he knew Pedestrian, that the decedent came in that night, perhaps around 10 pm, and was "drunk," intoxicated, excessive slurred speech (he did have a speech impediment), poor balance, and wanted to buy alcohol. The bartender refused to serve Pedestrian.

A blood (serum) sample was drawn at 0001 and tested at the hospital laboratory for alcohol content, resulting in a BAC of 0.231 g/dL. A second blood sample was drawn by the medical examiner and sent to AIT Laboratory for alcohol and drug testing. An alcohol test was reported as 0.12 g/dL (120 mg/dL).

OPINIONS

1. Since the alcohol test was performed on serum, the serum result must be adjusted (corrected) to whole blood by lowering the result by 18%, to adjust for the difference between serum and whole blood readings. Physicochemical differences (water content) result in a higher reading in serum. An 18% reduction of a 231 mg% will lower the serum alcohol to an equivalent whole blood reading of 195 mg%.
2. The AIT (toxicology lab) test was performed on whole blood, and therefore the result (0.12 gm/dl) does not need to be adjusted.
3. Comparing the time and results of both of the tests (195 at 0001 and 120 at 0246—the time of death), it is my opinion that the two tests are inconsistent. Calculation of the metabolic rate (2.75 hours), 83 mg% = 30 mg/hour—quite high; however, the inconsistency could be caused by dilution of blood by the voluminous fluids and blood products. This means that the second blood test would have been higher but for the dilution.
4. Mr. Pedestrian was intoxicated and impaired by alcohol when he was struck by Ms. Driver's vehicle when he was in the roadway.
5. Extrapolation of both alcohol tests to the time of the accident results in BAC of 210 mg% (195 + 15 = 210 and 120 + 70 = 190). Both of these levels are substantially higher than twice the legal limit for intoxication, as defined by the Illinois Motor Vehicle Code (2 x 80 = 160).
6. Based on his autopsy weight of 154 lbs, Mr. Pedestrian had the alcohol equivalent of eight 12-ounce domestic beers (4% w/v) in his blood at the time of the accident

SUMMARY

The Pedestrian was significantly intoxicated by alcohol, and in a cognitive and motor function impaired state at the time he was struck by the Driver's vehicle. His alcohol tests corroborate the bartender's assessment that he was "drunk" shortly before the accident. The Pedestrian's intoxication must be considered as a contributory cause of this fatal accident. (Incidentally, the case was tried by a Jury. The plaintiff successfully barred the alcohol expert. The Jury found the driver not guilty, despite the lack of testimony about the pedestrian's significant intoxication.)

34.8 ALCOHOL AND FALLS

(This topic is extensively discussed in detail in the Falls chapter (Chapter 11) of this book).

34.8.1 Stairs—No Alcohol Test—Fall Down Bar Stairs

A 30-year-old woman fell and fractured her ankle while descending the last few steps of a stairway to the lower level (basement) location of a popular bar at approximately 11:30 p.m. She had been out for the evening with some business associates, following a business dinner. After the fall and her injury, police and an ambulance were called. She was taken emergently by ambulance to a nearby hospital emergency department.

She testified that she had only consumed one beer prior to her arrival at the bar. She was wearing heels. She was in the middle of the staircase and not using handrails that were on either side of the staircase. She stated her weight and height were 154 lb. and 5′10″.

Relevant clinical notes (and testimony) by the Emergency Department resident physician included:

- Positive check mark for alcohol
- Conjunctiva injected, so bloodshot eyes
- Diagnosis; acute alcohol intoxication
- Crying, intoxicated (at the time)

- Acute alcohol intoxication . . . results in impairment of balance, perception, ability to ambulate . . . can lead to problems with balance and problems walking downstairs
- Drunk people are more likely to miss a step and fall down
- Agrees that the patient's acute alcohol intoxication is a competent contributing factor to having a fall-down injury from losing your balance
- No blood-alcohol test was ordered/performed . . . in her case it seems as though it was clinically apparent to us and we didn't need to know what the exact number was.

34.8.1.1 Opinions

A pharmacologist was retained by the defendant. He testified giving the following opinions:

The woman's BAC was probably above (80 mg/dL), the legal presumption level of intoxication according to the Illinois Motor Vehicle Code. The clinical description of the patient is consistent with blood-alcohol levels above 0.08 g/dL (80 mg/dL).

34.8.1.2 Summary

The woman was intoxicated and impaired by alcohol when she fell on the stairs. It is scientifically impossible for the woman to only have consumed one beer a short time before she fell on the stairs, and then appear to be acutely intoxicated by alcohol at the hospital 30 minutes later. If the total consumption was only one beer before the fall, the clinician at the hospital would not have diagnosed her as acutely intoxicated by alcohol. If she consumed four drinks (as noted in the hospital record), then her BAC could have reached or exceeded 0.100 g/dL (100 mg/dL) BAC.

34.8.2 Stairs—Residential Stairs Fall—Adjustment of Calculated BAC Due to Morbid Obesity

A 48-year-old woman fell in a stairwell at the residence of "Kim," whom she had escorted home after an evening out. She testified that she consumed four 12 oz Miller Lite beers at a local restaurant starting from 7–7:30 p.m. to 9:30–10 p.m. She further testified that she consumed one beer and six pieces of pizza at the second bar from 10 p.m. to 11:30 p.m. When asked in her deposition, she testified that she was "not intoxicated (by alcohol)," and was not "feeling the effects of alcohol" when she fell and injured her right ankle. She had forgotten that she had walked up three flights of stairs, and on the descent, seeing light through a window at the first-floor landing (one flight up from the ground), walked straight forward, not knowing that another flight of stairs remained to descend. Consequently, she stepped down, injured her heel, and subsequently was found by her son, who took her to the hospital.

The hospital record notes:

- Arrived at the Hospital Emergency Department at 12:30 a.m.
- Patient tripped and fell down stairs; "missed one flight of stairs"
- Drinks occasionally
- Admits to eight beers, patient states they had ~ eight beers since 7 p.m. and dinner at 10 p.m.
- 48-year-old female 111 kg (245 lb) 5′3″ 213% IBW (Ideal Body Weight). No alcohol tests were reported in the Hospital record.

34.8.2.1 Opinions

Consumption of eight 12-ounce beers over the period of 4.5 hours would result in a blood-alcohol level of 0.111 g/dL at the approximate time of the fall in the stairwell (12:00 midnight).

The woman, weighing 245 lb with a height of 5′3″ was morbidly obese, 213% IBW. This is important and must be factored in calculating the distribution of alcohol in her body. Scientifically accepted equations and calculations for determining BAC are used taking the amount and type of beverage consumed, the weight of the patient, and a determination can be made with these criteria for a BAC.

The equation is as follows:

$$\text{BAC} = 150 / \text{wt} \times \text{conc alc} / 50 \times \text{ounces of beverage} \times 0.025\text{gm/dL}$$
$$= 150/150 \times 4.19/50 \times 96 \text{ ounces} \times 0.025\text{gm/dL}$$
$$= 1\times 0.0838 \times 96 \times 0.025\text{gm/dL} = 0.201\text{g/dL}$$

Thus, 0.201 g/dL is the maximum achievable alcohol. Since five hours elapsed from the time of onset of drinking to the time of the accident, then the alcohol metabolized/eliminated in that five-hour period is subtracted from the 201 mg/dL figure. A metabolic rate of 18 mg/dL/hour is selected (mean alcohol elimination rate). 5 ×18 = 90 mg/dL.

Thus, 90 mg/dL is subtracted from the 201 mg/dL, leaving a calculated BAC of 111 mg/dL at the time of the accident. Again, this calculation is based on the statement of consumption of eight beers, as noted in the emergency department records.

Since the woman is 213% IBW, the "wt" used for calculating the BAC in the previous equation must be adjusted to accommodate for her calculated weight to be used for determining a BAC. With an IBW of 115 lb, in my opinion, a reasonable (and conservative) body weight figure to use for the woman is 150 lb. This adjustment is necessary since alcohol distributes to lean body mass, not adipose (fat) tissue. This means that the lean body weight is closer to the IBW than the actual body weight. There are several authoritative texts and literature sources which teach this concept of volume of distribution and distribution of alcohol, and these references are listed as endnotes, and relevant text excerpts are provided for the edification of the reader.[39]

Assuming the eight-beer statement given by the woman is accurate, then, in my opinion, she was intoxicated and impaired by alcohol at the time of her fall on the stairwell at Kim's residence.

34.8.2.2 Summary

Given the facts of the stairs fall, her alcohol intoxication must be considered as a contributing cause of the accident. The fact that she "forgot" she climbed three flights of stairs, and on the descent, "walked toward the light" is evidence of impairment to memory and judgment.

34.8.3 Tripped on Threshold—Sued Condominium Association

Threshold Faller (Threshold Faller) was fit and in good health. Threshold Faller and his roommate and friend went to a Festival. They arrived around 5:00 p.m. and stayed until around 8:30 and returned to their condo around 9:00 to 9:15 p.m. Threshold Faller states that he had about four beers and also ate a dinner. His friend did not drink; he drove home to their condominium. While walking from their parking spot to their residence in the condominiums, Threshold Faller stepped on a threshold and slipped. When he tried to catch himself by grabbing the handrail, the handrail collapsed and he fell to the next landing level and severely injured himself. Threshold Faller has testified that he was too impaired to drive but he was otherwise not too impaired to walk or use the stairs. "I was functioning within normal limits."

Threshold Faller denies being under the influence of any drugs at the time of his fall. He does not contest the ER blood-alcohol level of 0.229 g/dL, which was drawn about one hour after the fall.

34.8.3.1 Opinions

Threshold Faller was severely intoxicated and significantly impaired by alcohol at the time of the trip and fall. Intoxication with blood levels of 212 mg% is the beginning of the "falling down drunk" region for BACs. This is a substantially high BAC, almost three times the presumptive level of intoxication (80 mg%) defined by the Illinois Motor Vehicle Code. The blood-alcohol level of 212 mg% would indicate consumption of ten 12-ounce beers (domestic 4% alcohol).

The notations by the ambulance personnel (admits to drinking, speech slurred/aphasic, confusion), and the hospital notations of intoxication, are corroborative of alcohol intoxication. The blood-alcohol test provides definitive proof of the level of alcohol present, which allows a reference to the alcohol literature, which describes the type and extent of intoxication at specific alcohol levels.

34.9 DRAM SHOP (BAR LIABILITY FOR SERVING INTOXICATED PERSONS)

A dram shop rule (dram shop law or dram shop act) is a civil liability statute that renders a dram shop liable for the harmful acts of its intoxicated customers when the establishment acts negligently in serving the intoxicated customer alcohol, and the customer then causes harm (usually to a third-party victim) as a result of his/her intoxication (examples include drunk driving accidents and bar fights). While most jurisdictions limit liability to only cover harm to third parties, some extend this liability to cover first-party harm, giving a patron a cause of action against the establishment for any injuries the individual may have sustained as a result of his/her own intoxication.

A dram shop is a commercial establishment that sells alcoholic beverages (examples include bars, taverns, and restaurants). While most jurisdictions limit dram shop liability to commercial establishments, some jurisdictions (such as *Maine*) extend liability to social hosts.

Dram shop laws in most jurisdictions establish liability on a negligence (i.e., not strict liability) basis, for serving alcohol to a patron whom the server knows or reasonably should know is intoxicated, or for serving alcohol to someone under the legal drinking age.

CASE REPORT

An intoxicated patron collided with the plaintiff's vehicle, causing serious injuries to himself, the plaintiff, and her child—a passenger in her car. The collision occurred in 1958. Law enforcement considered the driver intoxicated. Serum alcohol was tested at 2248 at a local hospital resulting in 0.127 g/dL. While in treatment with EMS, the intoxicated patron was administered 2 liters of normal saline. While in treatment and transport by/with the air evac, the intoxicated patron was administered 3 liters of normal saline. Intoxicated patron was arrested for felony DUI, pled guilty, and was sentenced to a period of home confinement. Intoxicated patron worked as a cook in the kitchen at the Bar on the day of the accident. He left work at 4:30 pm and returned to the bar at 5:00 PM. He paid for six rum drinks with cash. The tab was paid at 1946. The drinking started at 1700, and the last drink was served at 1720–1730. For purposes of calculating absorption and BACs, it is assumed that the drinks were served at 1700, 1730, 1800, 1830, 1900, and 1920–30, and consumption was continuous. One bartender served the intoxicated patron drinks—6:00 pm and 6:30 pm; another bartender served the last two of the six drinks. A defense toxicologist calculated the amount consumed as the equivalent of nine standard drinks, 1.5-ounce 80 proof alcohol, suggesting that intoxicated patron was over served.

The second bartender testified the intoxicated patron was noticeably intoxicated when leaving. "He went from being fine to what I call a buzz to intoxicated pretty quickly, all of a sudden." She testified that she observed, served, and talked with him for about an hour and a half. She described the intoxicated patron having "glassy eyes, slurred speech, overall motor skills—poor." She testified that she later saw him leaving the back door, followed him out, told him he couldn't drive—"I took your keys"—but apparently the intoxicated patron had a second set of keys in this vehicle, which allowed him to drive his vehicle. She described him as "definitely not walking straight, stumbling a little bit, he had the appearance of someone that was intoxicated." He crashed approximately 10 minutes later. This bartender served the intoxicated patron his fifth drink ~ 7:00 pm and his last drink at approximately 7:30 PM.

The Bar was sued for serving alcohol to a person who was "visibly intoxicated," over serving, failure to count and pace drinks, failure to mitigate, and failure to prevent a "visibly intoxicated" patron from driving a vehicle.

Based upon the evidence in this case, the case required expert opinion on:

1. The approximate BAC at the time the intoxicated patron was served his sixth drink.
2. The likelihood that the intoxicated patron was visibly intoxicated by alcohol at the time the sixth drink was served to him.
3. The alcohol-induced impairments expected by the intoxicated patron's consumption.
4. Evaluation and critique of the defense toxicologist's methodology and calculations of the intoxicated patron's BAC at the time the sixth drink was served.

OPINIONS

1. If only six drinks were consumed per the cash receipt, that each drink must have had an additional 50% volume, 2.25 ounce instead of 1.5 ounce.
2. Retrograde extrapolation from the time of the alcohol test, 2248, could not be performed to the time the last drink was served, 1930.
3. Calculated the BAC at the time of serving the sixth drink with a goal of determining if the calculated BAC is above or below 150 mg/dL (0.150 g/dL), that concluded that greater than 50% of subjects would be visibly intoxicated with a BAC of 0.150 g/dL (The data for the 0150 g/dL includes subjects whose BACs ranged from 141–160 g/dL). This discussion and BAC level has been repeated several times in subsequent years, including statements like "this definition is set at an alcohol concentration at which there is no doubt of obvious intoxication (excess of 50%)."
4. Used certain parameters on serum alcohol to blood-alcohol conversions, metabolic rate, and absorption rates. Toxicologist opined that since the Sprite mixer in the rum drink contains sugar, that the scientific consensus describing rapid transit time from the stomach to the small intestine (through the pyloric valve) did not apply, and that the expected rapid absorption time of an empty stomach would not apply.
5. Cited two published papers evaluating the effect of sugar versus no sugar on the BAC on absorption rates. One studied 16 subjects and found breath alcohol measures were higher in the diet drinks compared to regular sugar mixtures. A second researcher studied eight male subjects and concluded that the substitution of artificial sweeteners for sugars in mixed alcoholic drinks potentially has a profound impact on BAC. The implications expressed by the toxicologist in his deposition is that sugar in the mixer slows gastric emptying and thus slows absorption rate, similar to the fed state.
6. Dismissed the potential dilution and BAC lowering effect of the three liters of normal saline and used a standard volume of distribution of 0.65 L, not the usual Widmark V_d (0.7 L/kg) applied to males.
7. Calculated/estimated the BAC at the time of the fifth drink (~1900) as a range from 0.111 to 0.121 g/dL. He referred to a "Dram shop model" that calculated the intoxicated patron's BAC concentration at the time of the serving of his sixth (final) drink—1920–1930, at 0.129–0.144 g/dL.) The range is caused by substituting different *beta* factors (metabolic rates) 0.015–0.020, with an average of 0.017 g/dL, thus different results.
8. Opined that "Nonetheless, it is clear that when the intoxicated patron was served his last drink at the Bar, his BAC would have been lower than the level reported to consistently cause outward signs of impairment in at least 50% of the population[27] . . . his BAC was never above the point at which impairment is observed in more than 50% of the population."
9. Opined alcohol produces well-documented effects in humans that become more predictable as the amount of alcohol consumed rises. Also, it is unquestionable that alcohol impairs many different sensory and motor skills essential to operating any motor vehicle, and it does so in a dose-dependent fashion.
10. Had no opinion on whether the intoxicated patron was visibly intoxicated at the time of the serving of the sixth drink. "I don't know how to answer that question."
11. Opined that the intoxicated patron was solely responsible for his alcohol consumption.
12. Testified "There's not enough information for me to determine whether or not he is a social drinker or whether he's a binge drinker or whether he's a constant drinker."

13. Referred to a "peer-reviewed dram shop model"; he testified that he developed the model and presented it at a conference; he considered it to be "peer-reviewed" based on the fact that it was presented at a conference.
14. Discounted any effect of marijuana on the intoxicated patron, based on the urine toxicology screen positive at the medical center after the accident.

A pharmacologist (JTOD) retained by the plaintiff, testified (deposition) to the following opinions, facts, and analyses:

1. The intoxicated patron was intoxicated at the following times:
   - He was so visibly intoxicated prior to leaving the bar that the server took his keys. He was visibly intoxicated at or before the serving of the sixth drink. This is based upon my review of the undisputed testimony of the server.
   - Ten minutes after he left the bar, he lost control of his vehicle and crashed into the plaintiff and her 6-year-old daughter. He was intoxicated based upon his blood alcohol of 0.127, which was measured 2 hours and 50 minutes after the collision at a local hospital.
   - Serving a gentleman of the size and weight of the intoxicated patron, it is expected that after four drinks, he would be intoxicated (supported by well-known scientific research and literature).
   - To a reasonable prudent server of alcohol, an intoxicated patron would have been visibly intoxicated by the ingestion of alcohol at the subject bar prior to the fifth and sixth drinks he was served.
2. The intoxicated patron was certainly visibly intoxicated at the time the last drink was served. One bartender described an instant change in sobriety to intoxication state while talking with the intoxicated patron for an hour and a half. "He went from being fine to what I call a buzz to intoxicated pretty quickly—all of a sudden—probably within the hour and a half we were talking. He had glassy eyes, slurred speech, overall motor skills were poor." This bartender's testimony is pharmacologically impossible. Alcohol actions are dose related. The higher the dose, the higher the BAC, the more manifestations consistent with the anticipated BAC. They do not appear "all of a sudden." This is a basic concept. This bartender's testimony of the intoxicated patron's obvious visible intoxication would have been present at the time of the serving of the sixth drink, and most likely before (the fifth drink).
3. The intoxicated patron rarely drank alcohol, twice a year according to his deposition. He would not have developed any type of tolerance to the effects of alcohol or adjusting the effects of alcohol as suggested. Therefore, any suggestion by the toxicologist that the intoxicated patron had tolerance or behavioral tolerance and was able to mask outward signs of alcohol intoxication is not relevant; indeed, it is scientifically inaccurate. The toxicologist testified that he had insufficient information to determine social, binge, or constant drinking status.
4. Based on the intoxicated patron's testimony, I consider him a "social drinker." As such, "6 drinks" over 2 hours (4 × 2.25 oz), in my opinion, would more likely than not cause 'visible intoxication' in the intoxicated patron—the serving of the fifth drink.
5. A few months earlier at the same Bar, the intoxicated patron was "cut off," no more alcohol was served by a bartender on duty. Same bar, same drink, same person, same amount of alcohol. Therefore, it is more likely than not that his visible intoxication at the prior "cut-off" experience would manifest at five drinks on June 5.
6. As a novice drinker, assuming that all the alcohol in the first four drinks was absorbed, it is my opinion that the intoxicated patron would manifest visible signs of intoxication. This would be apparent at 7 pm (the fifth drink).
7. The intoxicated patron was administered 2000 milliliters of normal saline by EMS, and 3000 milliliters by air evac, a total of 5000 milliliter fluid boluses. Physiologically, his blood had to be diluted to some extent, thus lowering the reported alcohol concentration result. Absent mass dilution, the intoxicated patron's BAC at the medical center at 2248 would have been higher than the 127 mg/dL reported. For the same physiological reasons, the volume of distribution would be larger. Five liters of normal saline represents a 6–7% increase in the total body water (incidentally the volume of distribution of alcohol). The intoxicated patron had a low hematocrit shortly after admission to the medical center. Low hematocrits imply greater water content in the blood. Any calculations or conversions of the hospital serum tests would be affected by this artificial dilution effect.
8. The toxicologist's calculations using a delayed food effect time of one hour caused by Sprite regular is *new and novel* and not a consensus in the scientific community. While two studies were provided and discussed the delaying absorption effects on a total of 24 subjects, this does not change the science. The alcohol toxicology community, and consensus literature in that community, is silent on "sugared

mixer" slowing gastric emptying and thus absorption. The current discussion in Garriott's *Medical Legal Aspects of Alcohol* describes gastric transit time and subsequent absorption rapidly and does not differentiate based on sugar-containing beverages. An empty stomach or full stomach and the type of food are the major determinants of the rate of absorption. *Garriott* excerpts may be found on page 217 of the 6th edition. Absorption through the stomach wall is slow whereas absorption from the small intestine is rapid. Therefore, anything that delays the emptying time of the stomach will slow the absorption of alcohol. The rate of flow from the stomach to the small intestine is controlled by the pyloric valve, situated at the base of the stomach, which opens and closes to control the passage of solids, semi-solids, and liquids. Food in the stomach slows stomach emptying time; hence, absorption of alcohol is delayed. This applies to eating while drinking and to eating shortly before drinking. The blood-alcohol level will have a lower peak and a lower rise to that level following a meal, compared to consumption on an empty stomach. The rate of absorption varies from person to person. Generally, most alcohol is absorbed in 20–30 minutes in a fasting person after a single dose; nearly 90% is absorbed within one hour when drinks are consumed successively over time. The presence of carbon dioxide in carbonated beverages, sparkling wines, and champagne promotes evacuation of the stomach which in turn enhances the absorption of alcohol.

9. The toxicologist's "Peer reviewed Dram Shop Model" is not "peer reviewed." A poster at a scientific meeting does not ordain "peer review."
10. The toxicologist's use of 0.65 L/kg volume of distribution is incorrect. The common "rho" factor (Vd) for alcohol for men is 0.7 L/kg. The figure is 0.6 L/kg women, owing to their high percentage of body fat, and thus less percentage of body water. Since alcohol is distributed to water and not fat, the same alcohol content given to a man and a woman of normal weight for height will result in higher BAC in the woman because the volume of distribution is smaller. The larger the volume of distribution, the lower the BAC; the smaller the V_d, the higher the BAC. Current literature recommends a BMI (Body Mass Index) calculation be made. The mean variable is proportional to fat to lean tissue in the body, which in turn depends on age, gender, and obesity as reflected in the body mass index.
11. The intoxicated patron's calculated V_d is 0.53 L/kg, based on his height and weight (18.5% lower than the 0.65 L/kg Vd used by the toxicologist).
12. The intoxicated patron is not normal weight. He is obese. His height and weight calculated to a BMI equal to 32.3 (obese); thus any "peer reviewed Dram shop calculators" will underestimate the BAC, since the volume of distribution of 0.65 used by the toxicologist is too high for the intoxicated patron. The higher the BMI, the lower the volume of distribution: the lower the volume of distribution, the higher the BAC.
13. The 150 mg (0.150 g/dL) criteria for frank or obvious intoxication of the majority of people tested includes a range of 140–160 mg for that grouping.[28] Thus, even the toxicologist's calculations are in this range (144 mg) and therefore would meet the criteria for a greater than 50% probability of visible intoxication. Brick and Erikson[29] include a description of an alcohol concentration of 0.15 g/dL at which there is no doubt of obvious intoxication.
14. Brick and Bennett[30] published a report on alcohol calculations in emergency and forensic medicine reports subjects who were measured with a peak BAC of approximately 30 minutes post-drinking. If drinking is constant then absorption is also constant, so the peak is not always at the end of the cessation of the drink. Brick and Erikson[31] states, "It's reasonable to expect the intoxicated person would be under the influence as a result of the amount served; this means that servers need to count the drinks."
15. The bartenders failed to count drinks and anticipate intoxication based on the amount and volume and frequency of drinks served—they should have anticipated intoxication and ceased serving.
16. The positive marijuana drug screen at the hospital does not support using marijuana at a particular time. There is no evidence that the intoxicated patron smoked marijuana in the 10–12 minutes after leaving the Bar and the collision with the Plaintiff.
17. Using the corrected V_d and absorption time of 30″, and a metabolic rate of 0.015 g/dL/hour, I calculate the BAC at the time of serving the sixth drink to be a BAC of 0.147.5 g/dL. The metabolic elimination rate of 0.015 g/dL/hour is selected based on the (stated) alcohol history (social drinker) of the intoxicated patron. The 30″ absorption time is justified because of the empty stomach and type of alcoholic beverage.

Subject parameters for the BAC estimation:

Wt = 200 lb = 90.9 kg V_d = 0.5295 L/kg Rate of elimination = 0.015 g/dL/hr Absorption rate = 30 min
21 g ethanol per "drink" 80 proof (40% ABV)

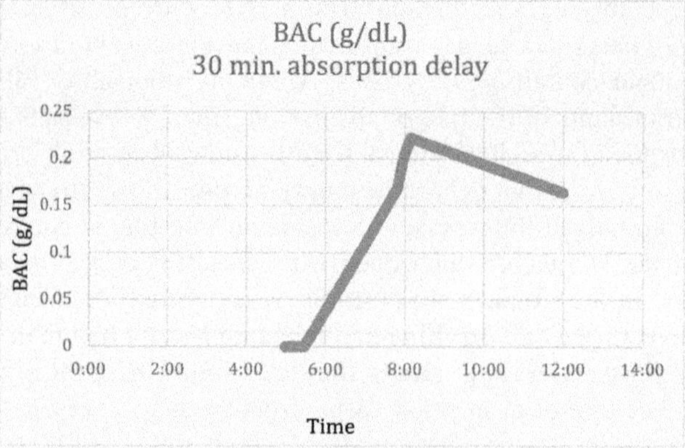

FIGURE 34.1 Conversion of data using Excel software and alcohol absorption curve graphically depicting the 30″ absorption time scenario.

CONCLUSION

The intoxicated patron himself is a good clinical model. At an earlier time—months before—the intoxicated patron was in the defendant's bar and the bartender stopped serving him after five drinks, ostensibly because he was visibly intoxicated. In this case, the intoxicated patron was arrested and pled guilty to driving drunk. The intoxicated patron left the bar at the completion of the sixth drink. Considering all the evidence, in my opinion, the intoxicated patron would have been visibly intoxicated before the sixth drink was served.

(At press time, the case is scheduled for trial.)

34.10 BIOMARKERS FOR ALCOHOL

34.10.1 Family Law

34.10.1.1 Restrictions of Child Visitation Based on Alleged Continued Alcohol Abuse

A young mother has tested positive for the presence of EtG (ethyl glucuronide) and EtS (ethyl sulfate) and biomarkers/metabolites of ethyl alcohol (alcohol). Her most recent "positive" EtG was on May 7, 2012, which, incidentally, was the same day she was examined by a medical toxicologist, whose note states: "No indication of alcohol or ketone odor on her breath." The EtG test ordered on that day was also positive. As a result of her earlier positive tests, her visitation with her daughter is severely restricted (supervised), and she does not enjoy joint custody of her daughter. She denies consumption of alcohol for the relevant periods preceding most of the positive tests. A few tests were ruled "failed" and therefore considered "positive" because the specific gravity and/or creatinine content of the urine was outside the "acceptable" range, according to a court-appointed laboratory broker.

34.10.1.2 Opinions

The EtG test, if positive, should not be considered as the sole basis for any forensic, employment, custodial, or judicial proceeding that results in a restriction of the rights or liberty of the subject tested. A reasonable and prudent scientist or medical review officer must reject the results and thus the validity of the EtG as a single source of proof of alcohol consumption for any forensic proceeding.

A medical toxicologist examined the mother. His medical findings and opinions are included in the Bases for Opinion section of this report. He concurs with my opinions. Indeed, he introduced a resolution to the Illinois State Medical Society recommending "encourage the use of Medical Review Officers when ordering drug testing procedures or results interpretation in non-clinical settings."

The "rejection" criteria for out-of-range specific gravity and creatinine are not proof of urine adulteration. Common clinical conditions, including liberal water consumption, pregnancy, and urinary tract infections, may result in these tests being out of range. Further, the specific gravity "ranges of normal" varies from laboratory to laboratory. For example, this woman's test at the physician's office shows a lower range of 1.002; the laboratory's lower range is 1.003. Common clinical references for urine-specific gravity are as low as 1.001. Since her test recorded 1.002 in a broker's test, her test was rejected, and for the purposes for which it was ordered, it was considered a "positive," an inappropriate punitive consequence based on a very inexact science used by the broker. The EtG test is not accepted in the scientific community as the sole basis for proof of alcohol consumption.

On September 25, 2006 (and updated in 2012), the U.S. Department of Health and Human Services (SAMHSA—Substance Abuse and Mental Health Services Administration) released the Substance Abuse Treatment Advisory entitled: "The Role of Biomarkers in the Treatment of Alcohol Use Disorders."[32]

The Advisory contains the following guidance: (emphasis added)

The most extensively studied (bio)marker, EtG, has been tested primarily in one laboratory in Europe. Although the results published by this laboratory show promise, it is prudent to await replication of results from another independent investigator. Furthermore, it is not known at this time how the test results might be affected by the presence of physical diseases, ethnicity, gender, time, or the use of other drugs. Until considerable more research has occurred, use of these markers should be considered experimental.

Currently, the use of an EtG test in determining abstinence lacks sufficient proven specificity for use as primary or sole evidence that an individual prohibited from drinking, in a criminal justice or a regulatory compliance context, has truly been drinking. Legal or disciplinary action based solely on a positive EtG, or other test discussed in this Advisory, is inappropriate and scientifically unsupportable at this time. These tests should currently be considered as potential valuable clinical tools, but their use in forensic settings is premature.

Biomarkers (EtG and EtS) provide an important indication of drinking status when used appropriately, but they must always be used with a clear understanding of their strengths and potential weaknesses. This is especially true when the consequences of misidentification of alcohol consumption are grave, such as for a healthcare provider whose license, livelihood, and reputation depend on demonstration of abstinence or for an individual who will be ordered to return to jail because of a positive test.

EtG and EtS tests may become positive shortly after even low level exposure to alcohol and may remain detectable in urine for several days. Because of the purported high sensitivity of these tests, exposure to alcohol that is present in many daily use products might also result in a positive laboratory test for these biomarkers. EtG is becoming widely available in the United States, and some laboratories have also begun to test for EtS. At the current time, EtG and EtS testing may have a supportive role in therapeutic interventions in an environment where breath or blood-alcohol tests are used to monitor abstinence. However, until further research has been conducted, the high sensitivity of the EtG and EtS tests does not permit the distinction between alcohol exposure and alcohol consumption at lower levels of possible biomarker detection.

The science of EtG testing—the capability to employ highly sensitive testing procedures to detect recent ethyl alcohol exposure—has outpaced the ability to appropriately interpret the test results in a forensically defensible manner. The conclusions expressed by SAMHSA are not the result of inherent flaws in the testing science for EtG, but rather in the inability to interpret those results in a way that allows the reliable differentiation as to the source of the alcohol—consumption versus unintended exposure. CSAT, through its National Advisory Council, has concluded that there is inadequate research data about the populations being tested to evaluate an "individual's likely exposure to products containing non-beverage alcohol, and the consequences for the individual and society of the individual's being erroneously labeled."[33]

Ethyl alcohol is ubiquitous in our environment. A very brief list of sources—medicines, foods, beverages, personal care products, cleaners, herbal preparations, and so on. There is currently insufficient information to assess the degree to which any one of these sources (or a combination of sources) can result in incidental exposure to ethyl alcohol and the subsequent production and identification of EtG in urine.

Ethyl alcohol is also manufactured de novo in the human body, and many laboratories accommodate for this by reporting lower levels as "less than 10 mg/dL" ethyl alcohol, which accommodates biosynthesis in the patient's body. Any alcohol synthesized in the body will go through EtG and EtS metabolism, and thus contribute to a "positive EtG" alcohol biomarker.

Further, there are no clear thresholds that can be used to distinguish between alcoholic beverage consumption and alcohol exposure from food and drugs (similar to the thresholds that are established in poppy seed/opiate tests). Thus, even with "high" levels, there is insufficient scientific basis to support a definitive and defensible "positive EtG."

34.10.1.3 Summary

The young mother denied continued use of any alcoholic beverages for most EtG positives. The medical toxicologist opined that she is likely "hypersensitive"—unpredictably forming excessive EtG with no alcohol consumption and that her usual and customary voluminous water consumption explains that "rejections" due to low creatinines or low specific gravity. Indeed, despite knowing when she was going to be tested, the mother was tested "positive" by the toxicologist and by the (testing) broker. Since she knew she was going to see the physician and that she would be tested, it is highly improbable that she would have voluntarily consumed alcohol. These circumstances strongly support the medical toxicologist's (and my) opinion that "she is likely hypersensitive."

Any forensic actions, such as restriction of visitation, based solely upon positive EtG or EtS biomarkers for alcohol metabolism are scientifically unsound. SAMHSA is the top scientific drug abuse agency of the federal government, charged with developing and monitoring substance abuse drug testing use in the United States. The advisory of SAMHSA should be considered in this matter by the Court. (Unfortunately for the young mother, the Judge did not change the custody restrictions.)

34.10.2 False-Positive Alcohol Biomarkers in Diabetes

34.10.2.1 EtG/EtS Alcohol Metabolites: False-Positive Urine Alcohol in Diabetes Patient

A defendant tested positive for urine alcohol and negative for alcohol metabolites (EtS and EtG) and now was facing revocation of his Deferred Prosecution of a DUI by allegedly consuming alcohol. Is there any reasonable scientific explanation for how urine alcohol could be present absent from consuming (ethyl) alcohol?

34.10.2.2 Testing Results and Methodology

Urinalysis//Sample: urine Ethanol: positive, quantified at 454 mg/dL

—GCFID (Gas Chromatograph Flame Ionization Detector), 20 mg/dL LOQ (limit of quantification)
EtG/EtS—Ethyl glucuronide screen. *Negative*
—EIA (enzyme immunoassay)
—500 ng/mL LOQ

34.10.2.3 Medical History

Diabetes Mellitus—Type II (uncontrolled) treated with two (2) different insulins (Humalog and Lantus) and metformin.

34.10.2.4 Opinions

1. Ethyl glucuronide (EtG) and ethyl sulfate (EtS) are minor metabolites of ethanol that are used to detect ethanol use.
2. Ethanol appears in the urine before its metabolites. As a result, if a subject drinks within an hour or two of the test, they may test positive for ethanol but not the metabolites.
3. The detection windows for EtG and EtS in urine are much longer than that of ethanol.
4. Based on point #3, after sufficient time has elapsed (1 hr) for the ethanol to metabolize, it is metabolically impossible that a urine test will be positive for ethanol and negative for EtG and/or EtS.
5. The positive urine alcohol was caused by the defendant's diabetes, not by consumption of alcoholic beverages by mouth. Fermentation is a metabolic process that produces chemical changes in organic substrates through the action of enzymes. Given the marked glucosuria and the presence of bacteria in the urine, urine fermentation occurs and produces alcohol in the urine.[34] Glucosuria is produced by Type II diabetes. In fact, before the routine use of blood glucose testing in the home (and in hospitals), diabetes control and the dosing of insulin was based on a urine "dipstick" that provided semi-qualitative results (1+ to 4+)—measurements of glucose (sugar)—in the urine.
6. Since this patient has Type II diabetes whose diabetes is described as "uncontrolled," the positive urine ethanol test and negative EtG and EtS test is probably due to glucosuria and subsequent fermentation of glucose, not alcohol consumption.
7. The 500 mg/dL LOQ employed here is an accepted cut-off (LOQ) to use for urinary EtG and EtS detection to rule out sources of ethanol other than alcohol consumption.
8. Urine alcohol levels following alcohol beverage consumption are not commonly tested, as they are subject to variation, but there is a correlation with concomitant BAC. Generally, the amount of alcohol in a person's urine bears a proportional relationship to the amount of alcohol in the person's blood. On average, the level of alcohol in urine is about 1.3 times the amount of alcohol in the blood.[35] Conversion to BAC = 434/1.3 = 349 mg/dL (0.349 g/dL) blood alcohol.
9. Given the extremely high blood-alcohol conversion, it is scientifically impossible to have positive urine alcohol (especially a high one) and negative EtG and EtS, the metabolites of alcohol.

There is a report/discussion in the Laboratory Medicine literature describing a positive urine alcohol in a documented alcohol abstainer.[36] Although laboratory screening for urine ethanol (alcohol) is highly specific and sensitive, the source of the ethanol can sometimes be unclear. This case report describes a 44-year-old male with positive urine ethanol results who reported having abstained from alcohol. A test for urine EtG and EtS was used to validate the information in the patient history stating that the patient had not consumed alcohol for one year. Evaluation of the urinalysis results from the patient revealed fermentation in the context of glucosuria as the source of the urine ethanol.

If alcohol is consumed, EtG and EtS, metabolites of alcohol will form, and, if tested, will be detected. The following information is excerpted from several authorities documenting the detectability periods for EtG and EtS.

Alcohol testing company website: https://premierbiotech.com/innovation/etg-article/

> "EtG may be detectable (in urine) as soon as 2 hours after use and up to 80 hours past consumption."
> "Urinary Ethyl glucuronide (EtG) and Ethyl sulfate (EtS) are established markers of alcohol consumption."[37]
> "Value of Ethyl Glucuronide and Ethyl Sulfate in Serum as biomarkers of Alcohol Consumption"
> Cut-off for Ethyl glucuronide in urine.
> "An EtG-I cutoff of 100 ng/mL is most likely to detect heavy drinking for up to five days and any drinking during the previous two days. Cutoffs of ≥ 500 ng/mL are likely to only detect heavy drinking during the previous day."
> A 500 ng/L LOQ (cut-off) was used in the toxicological analysis of the Defendant. As such, this is likely to detect heavy drinking during the previous day.
> "A heavy drinking day is defined as over three standard drinks for women and over four standard drinks for men."[38,39]

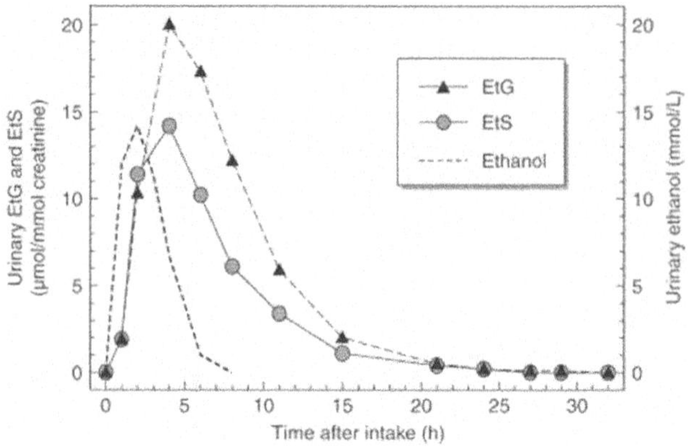

FIGURE 34.2 Urinary Ethanol, EtG, and EtS Appearance Time After Intake.

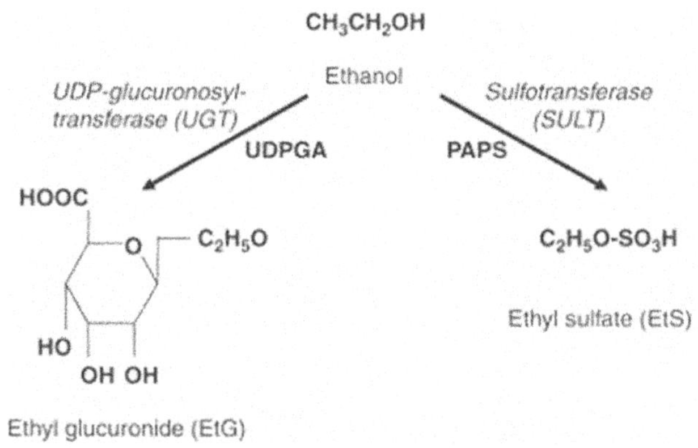

FIGURE 34.3 Alcohol Metabolism to EtG and EtS.

In controlled experiments with oral administration of ethanol to healthy volunteers, a detection time for EtG of 24–48 h after ingestion has been observed.

False positives for EtG, EtS.

Although ethyl glucuronide and ethyl sulfate are widely used as direct biomarkers of alcohol consumption, false-positive results are encountered, probably more often with ethyl glucuronide analysis.

34.10.2.5 Summary

Urine alcohol positive with negative alcohol metabolites (EtG and EtS) in a diabetic person is caused by "de novo" endogenous alcohol fermentation through the well-described scientific process of fermentation. The defendant's "positive" alcohol test should be discarded. The conclusion made in the absence of positive EtS and EtG is scientifically impossible.

The prosecutor dismissed the violation of the Delayed Prosecution after the expert report was submitted.

34.11 MISCELLANEOUS TOPICS REPORTS

34.11.1 Retrograde Extrapolation (See Also Legal Cases *Floyd* and *Cuellar* Earlier in This Chapter)

34.11.1.1 Automobile Turns Left in Front of Speeding Motorcyclist

The (deceased) motorcyclist collided with the side of the defendant's Jeep while the defendant was turning left at 1613 (4:13 pm). The motorcyclist was declared deceased at the scene. The defendant was taken to a local hospital where blood and urine samples were taken at 1838 (6:38 pm). The regional Crime Lab analyzed the blood and reported a BAC of 0.073 g/100 ml (73 mg%). The blood sample was drawn at 1638.

The Responsible Officer at the scene noted "I met with both the decedent's friend (who drove another vehicle but was not involved in the collision) and the defendant and I did not see any signs of impairment."

The defendant was charged with Homicide by Intoxication.

Materials Reviewed:

1. Laboratory Report State Crime Laboratory
   a. Report of, Toxicology-Technical Unit Leader—retrograde extrapolation
   b. Blood/urine analysis alcohol 0.073 g/100 ml (±0.005 g/100 ml); sample drawn in 1838 5/22/20
2. County Sheriff's Department—Incident
   a. Motor Vehicle Fatality Report Form
   b. Written Statement forms
3. Village Police Department Traffic Accident Statement
4. State Motor Vehicle Crash Report
   a. Fatal Supplement Report
   b. Collision Analysis and Reconstruction Report
   c. Supplemental Reconstruction Report (1–2 and scene sketches); CDR reports
5. Private Investigator (Defense)—Statement transcripts/summaries of witnesses to defendant's drinking and behavior at the bar before the fatal accident
6. Scientific literature describing the pharmacology, toxicology, and pharmacokinetic effects of alcohol

I also interviewed the defendant on the telephone.

34.11.1.2 Toxicology Reports

The county toxicologist prepared a report extrapolating the defendant's BAC from 0.073 g/100 ml (time of the test) to a range of 0.097–0.133 at 1613 (time of the accident), depending on a range of metabolic rates. The toxicologist made two assumptions: (1) "All consumed ethanol was fully absorbed at 4:13 pm on May 22, 2020," and (2) "No ethanol was consumed thereafter."

34.11.1.2.1 Interview of the Defendant

The defendant reported his weight as 215 lb. and height as 5′10″. He ran errands that day and had lunch—a sandwich—between 1:00 and 2:00 pm. He went to a car dealer and then stopped at the bar, where he stayed until a few minutes before 4 pm. While at the bar, he drank two bourbons and Coke, finishing the second drink just before leaving. The defendant stated that the accident occurred "minutes" after leaving the bar. He denied experiencing any effects of the alcohol (intoxication or impairment) before or after the accident.

Statements (Excerpts) of Witnesses to the Defendant's Alcohol Consumption by a Private Investigator for the Defense

1. Acquaintance 1. "He came in shortly after opening (3:00 pm) and stayed until approximately 4:00 pm. He had two drinks (short glasses) of bourbon and Coke. He has never seen the defendant intoxicated and that the most he has ever seen him drink is two mix drinks."

2. Acquaintance 2. "She was seated at the bar and that the defendant came in and sat next to her right after the bar opened at 3:00 pm. She stated that when he sat next to her, she did not smell any odor of alcohol emanating from him She stated that he appeared to be sober and lucid. She stated that he had two mix drinks, but she didn't know what kind. She stated that he stayed at the bar for approximately one hour and left at approximately 4:00 pm."
3. Bar manager. "When the bar opened at 3:00 pm, he and the defendant went inside, and the defendant sat down at the bar next to his (bar manager's) wife and ordered a drink. The defendant stayed at the bar for approximately one hour and had two mixed drinks (Bourbon and Coke)."
4. Current bar manager. "Defendant was at the bar at 3:00 pm. He only stayed for about an hour and had one or two (short glass) mix drinks. He did not appear to be intoxicated or under the influence of alcohol."

34.11.1.3 Opinions

My opinions are expressed with reasonable pharmacologic certainty.

1. The toxicologist's first assumption ("all consumed ethanol was fully absorbed at 4:13 pm") is invalid, thus her projected extrapolations (0.097–0.133 g/100 ml) of the defendant's BAC are invalid. Thus, retrograde extrapolation cannot be performed in this case.
2. Based upon the witnesses to the defendant's drinking and time of the bar, the two drinks of bourbon and Coke would not have been completely absorbed by the time (4:13 pm); the BAC curve was rising at the time of the accident. In other words, the alcohol consumed was in the absorption stage, had not peaked, and was going up at the time of the accident.
3. The defendant's BAC would have been below 0.08 g/100 ml at the time of the accident. Based upon the time and amount of consumption of alcohol and the recent meal, the defendant's BAC was more likely than not below 0.05 g/100 ml.
4. The defendant was not intoxicated, impaired, or under the influence of alcohol at the time of the accident.

34.11.1.4 Summary

No observed, chemical, or scientific evidence exists in this matter supporting a conclusion that the BAC was at or above the prohibited level of 0.08 g/100 ml, or that the defendant was intoxicated or impaired by alcohol at the time of the accident (at press time, the case is scheduled for Trial).

34.11.2 Appellate Court Reverses Trial Court Barring of BAC

Extrapolation Not Allowed—Remote BAC Allowed

34.11.2.1 Opinion

PEOPLE V EPSTEIN (2021 IL App (2d) 191059-U No. 2–19–1059 Order filed September 21, 2021) Discusses admissibility of blood alcohol tests where retrograde extrapolation cannot be performed (based on *People v. Floyd*, discussed elsewhere in this Chapter). Excerpts of the Illinois Appellate Court Opinion are provided.

THE PEOPLE OF THE STATE (Appeal from the Circuit Court OF ILLINOIS), of Boone County.) Plaintiff-Appellant)) v.) No. 18-CF-89) LAURA A. EPSTEIN) Honorable), John H. Young, Defendant-Appellee.) Judge, Presiding. JUSTICE JORGENSEN delivered the judgment of the court. Justice Schostok concurred in the judgment. Justice McLaren dissented in the judgment. ORDER 1 Held: In a prosecution for driving under the influence, the trial court wrongly excluded evidence of defendant's BAC of 0.107 measured four hours after the traffic stop. Neither the absence of extrapolation evidence nor the length of the delay between the stop and the BAC test rendered the result inadmissible. 2 The State appeals from an order of the circuit court of Boone County excluding evidence of defendant, Laura A. Epstein's, BAC, based on analysis of blood drawn approximately four hours after she was stopped for driving under the influence of alcohol (DUI). 2021 IL App (2d) 191059-U—2—Because the trial court abused its discretion in excluding the BAC evidence, we reverse and remand. 3 I. BACKGROUND 4 Defendant was indicted on one count of aggravated DUI based on her transporting a person under 16 years old and having previously committed a DUI offense (625 ILCS 5/11-501(d)(1)(K) (West 2016)), one count of aggravated DUI with a BAC of 0.08 or more while transporting a person under 16 years old and having previously committed a DUI offense (id. § 11-501(d)(1)(K)), and one count of aggravated DUI based on her driving while there was any amount of drug, substance, or compound or combination thereof in her breath or blood while transporting a person under 16 years old and having previously committed a DUI offense (id.). 5 Defendant filed a pretrial motion to exclude the BAC test result from her blood drawn pursuant to a search warrant. She contended that (1) because a retrograde extrapolation could not be performed on the test result to establish her BAC at the time she drove, the prejudicial effect of admitting the BAC test result substantially outweighed any probative value; and (2) there was a defective chain of custody. 6 At the hearing on defendant's motion to exclude, Deputy Rhonda Moore of the Boone County Sheriff's Department testified for the State that she mailed the blood sample taken from defendant to the state crime lab in Chicago. She explained that, although the computer-generated lab submittal form showed that the sample was sent to the crime lab in Rockford, she had merely neglected to prompt the computer to show that the sample was, in fact, mailed to the Chicago lab. 7 Dr. James O'Donnell testified for defendant. Dr. O'Donnell, a licensed pharmacist, had been qualified over 100 times in Illinois courts as an expert on alcohol effects, interpretation of 2021 IL App (2d) 191059-U—3—BAC test results, and alcohol-impaired driving. The trial court found him to be an expert in pharmacology and the effects of alcohol on the human body. 8 Dr. O'Donnell has conducted retrograde extrapolation hundreds of times. He described it as a method to determine a BAC earlier in time from a known BAC. Here, Dr. O'Donnell explained the extrapolation process and why it is necessary to know certain facts. In the absence of those known facts here, it was not possible to perform a reliable retrograde extrapolation and, therefore, not possible to determine defendant's BAC at the time she was driving four hours earlier. 9 Dr. O'Donnell reviewed the video of the traffic stop, the interaction between defendant and the arresting officer, the field sobriety tests, and the video of defendant sitting in the back seat of the squad car. Dr. O'Donnell also interviewed defendant. 10 Dr. O'Donnell testified that, according to the records provided to him, defendant was stopped at approximately 10 p.m., arrested at approximately 10:30 p.m., and her blood was drawn between 2 and 2:30 a.m. He opined that retrograde extrapolation could not be performed in this case, because some of the most critical information "necessary to do a full analysis [was] not available." Critically, it was not possible to determine when defendant's alcohol absorption peaked, and alcohol elimination began. According to Dr. O'Donnell, based on when defendant said she last consumed alcohol, and how she acted on the video, her alcohol absorption was not complete at the time of the traffic stop. He added that the BAC test result four hours later proved only that defendant consumed alcohol but could not prove defendant's BAC level when she was stopped four hours earlier. 11 According to Dr. O'Donnell, at 10 p.m., when defendant was stopped, she was able to stand and walk without losing her balance and speak without slurring. At 10:30 p.m., defendant was exhibiting "obvious manifestations of intoxication," such as slurred speech, altered balance, and 2021 IL App (2d) 191059-U—4—poorly performed field sobriety tests. Dr. O'Donnell opined that defendant was still absorbing alcohol when she was stopped and that her peak absorption did not occur until sometime after 10:20 p.m. Dr. O'Donnell concluded there was no way to determine whether defendant's BAC was above or below 0.08 at 10 p.m., and he would "challenge any expert to [do so] with the facts in this case." 12 The State moved for a directed finding on defendant's motion to exclude. The trial court granted the State's motion as to the chain-of-custody issue but denied it as to the extrapolation issue. 13 In denying the State's motion for a directed finding, the trial court found that defendant's blood had been drawn between 2:01 a.m. and 2:30 a.m. The test showed that defendant's BAC was 0.107. The court further found that the traffic stop occurred at approximately 10 p.m. 14 The trial court found that, because it was above the statutory limit of 0.08, the BAC test result had probative value. However, relying on People v. Floyd, 2014 IL App (2d) 120507, the court found that, because retrograde extrapolation would be inherently unreliable, the prejudicial effect of the BAC test result substantially outweighed any probative value. Thus, the court denied the State's motion for a directed finding on that issue. 15 The State did not present evidence. In argument, the State stated that it was not planning to introduce any retrograde extrapolation evidence at trial. Accordingly, the State asserted that defendant's challenge to the BAC test result went to its weight, not its admissibility. Defendant conceded the BAC result itself was reliable. However, defendant argued, absent her ability to challenge the BAC with evidence of reliable retrograde extrapolation, the probative value of the result obtained four hours after the traffic stop was substantially outweighed by its prejudicial effect. 2021 IL App (2d) 191059-U—5–16 In granting defendant's motion to exclude, the trial court noted that it was not finding that the four-hour delay in obtaining the blood sample was unreasonable. The court reiterated that the BAC test result was probative. However, the court, relying on its earlier findings in denying the State's motion for a directed finding, ruled that the BAC test result was not admissible, because its prejudicial effect substantially outweighed its probative value. 17 The State filed a motion to reconsider, which the trial court denied. The State, in turn, filed this timely appeal. 18 II. ANALYSIS 19 On appeal, the State contends that, notwithstanding defendant's inability to present extrapolation evidence, the BAC test result was admissible, subject only to whatever weight the trier of fact might give it. Defendant responds that, because no retrograde extrapolation could be conducted, the BAC test result obtained four hours after defendant was stopped was so prejudicial that it substantially outweighed any probative value.

34.13 SUMMARY AND CONCLUSIONS

Since alcohol continues to be the world's most abused drug and alcohol intoxication and impairment increases the risk of injuries of all types, consideration of the use and interpretation of alcohol tests and impairment will continue to frequent the civil and criminal courts. Scientific principles related to the pharmacodynamics, pharmacokinetics, and toxicology of alcohol provide the basis for the testimony of experts who address these topics in alcohol civil and criminal litigation.

NOTES

1 United Nations. Sustainable development goals. http://www.un.org/sustainabledevelopment/sustainable-development-goals/. Accessed 6 May 2018.

2 National Institute on Alcohol Abuse and Alcoholism. Alcohol use disorder: A comparison between DSM-IV and DSM-5. 2016. https://www.niaaa.nih.gov/publications/brochures-andfact-sheets/alcohol-use-disorder-comparison-between-dsm.

3 National Institute on Alcohol Abuse and Alcoholism. Alcohol facts and statistics. 2018. http://www.niaaa.nih.gov/.

4 Grucza RA, Sher KJ, Kerr WC, Krauss MJ, Lui CK, McDowell YE, Hartz S, Virdi G, Bierut LJ. Trends in adult alcohol use and binge drinking in the early 21st-century United States: A meta-analysis of 6 national survey series. Alcohol Clin Exp Res. 2018;42(10):1939–1950. https://doi.org/10.1111/acer.13859.

5 Alcohol Research: Current Reviews 2 Vol 40 No 2|2020.

6 Bardach AE, Alcaraz AO, Ciapponi A, Garay OU, Riviere AP, Palacios A, Cremonte M, Augustovski F. Alcohol consumption's attributable disease burden and cost-effectiveness of targeted public health interventions: A systematic review of mathematical models. BMC Public Health. 2019;19:1378.

7 https://www.uptodate.com/contents/risky-drinking-and-alcohol-use-disorder-epidemiology-pathogenesis-clinical-manifestations-course-assessment-and-diagnosis.

8 https://www.uptodate.com/contents/risky-drinking-and-alcohol-use-disorder-epidemiology-pathogenesis-clinical-manifestations-course-assessment-and-diagnosis.
9 Statistics. Mothers against drunk driving organization. https://www.madd.org/statistics.
10 NHTSA Traffic Safety Fact Sheet. 2013 State alcohol-impaired driving estimates (DOT HS 812 188).
11 Friedmann PD. Alcohol use in adults. N Engl J Med. 2013;368:365–373.
12 Bouchery EE, Harwood HJ, Sacks JJ, Simon CJ, Brewer RD. Economic costs of excessive alcohol consumption in the U.S., 2006. Am J Prev Med. 2011;41: 516–524.
13 https://www.who.int/news-room/fact-sheets/detail/alcohol.
14 Caplan YH, Goldberger BA, Aguayo EH. Garriott's medicolegal aspects of alcohol, 2015. Print.
15 NHTSA. Traffic safety facts 2004 (DOT HS 809 911).
16 Carvey PC. Drug Action in the Central Nervous System. Oxford University Press, New York, 1988.
17 Giancola PR. Alcohol-related aggression during the college years: Theories, risk factors and policy implications. J Stud Alcohol Suppl. 2002;14:129–139.
18 Abbey A. Alcohol-related sexual assault: A common problem among college students. J Stud Alcohol Suppl. 2002;14:118–128.
19 Lundholm L, Haggård U, Möller J, Hallqvist J, Thiblin I. The triggering effect of alcohol and illicit drugs on violent crime in a remand prison population: A case crossover study. Drug Alcohol Depend. 2013;129(1–2):110–115.
20 Pich J, Hazelton M, Kable A. Violent behaviour from young adults and the parents of paediatric patients in the emergency department. Int Emerg Nurs. 2012;21: 1755–1759.
21 Cherpitel CJ. Alcohol and casualties: A comparison of emergency room and coroner data. Alcohol Alcohol. 1994;29(2):211–218.
22 Michael Petraski, Guardian of the Estate of Margaret Petraski, a Disabled Person, Plaintiff–Appellee, v. Deborah THEDOS, Individually and as Agent/Employee of the Sheriff of Cook County, and Michael Sheahan, Sheriff of Cook County, Defendants–Appellants. https://caselaw.findlaw.com/il-court-of-appeals/1589277.html.
23 People v. Floyd, 2014 IL App (2d) 120507—Illinois Courts.
24 Robinson A, Ketchum CH, Colburn N, Meyer R. Effect of ethyl alcohol on reaction times as measured on a motorcycle simulator. Clin Chem. 1990;36:1170.
25 Colburn N, Meyer RD, Wrigley M, Bradley EL. Should motorcycles be operated within the legal alcohol limits for automobiles. J Trauma. 1993;35(2):183–186.
26 Watson WA, Garriott JC. Alcohol and motorcycle riders: A comparison of motorcycle and car/truck DWIs. Vet Hum Toxicol. 1992;34:213–215.
27 Brick J, Erikson C. Intoxication is not always visible: An unrecognized prevention challenge. Alcohol Clin Exp Res. 2009;33(9):1489–1507.
28 Brick J, Erikson C. Intoxication is not always visible: An unrecognized prevention challenge. Alcohol Clin Exp Res. 2009;33(9):1489–1507.
29 Brick J, Erikson C. Intoxication is not always visible: An unrecognized prevention challenge. Alcohol Clin Exp Res. 2009;33(9):1489–1507.
30 Brick J, Bennett W. Alcohol calculations in emergency and forensic medicine. J Addict Med Therapeut Sci. 2017;3(3):24–29.
31 Brick J, Erikson C. Intoxication is not always visible: An unrecognized prevention challenge. Alcohol Clin Exp Res. 2009;33(9):1489–1507.
32 HHS Publication No. (SMA) 12-4686, The Role of Biomarkers in the Treatment of Alcohol Use Disorders, 2012 Revision.
33 HHS Publication No. (SMA) 12-4686, The Role of Biomarkers in the Treatment of Alcohol Use Disorders, 2012 Revision.
34 https://academic.oup.com/labmed/article/49/3/276/4951361?login=true.
35 http://www.clinlabnavigator.com/alcohol-urine.html.
36 Foley KF. A positive urine alcohol with negative urine ethyl-glucuronide. Lab Med. 2018;49(3):276–279. https://doi.org/10.1093/labmed/lmy008.
37 Shukla L, Sharma P, Ganesha S, Ghadigaonkar D, Thomas E, Kandasamy A, Murthy P, Benegal V. Value of ethyl glucuronide and ethyl sulfate in serum as biomarkers of alcohol consumption. Indian J Psychol Med. 2017 Jul–Aug;39(4):481–487.
38 McDonell MG, Skalisky J, Leickly E, McPherson S, Battalio S, Nepom JR, Srebnik D, Roll J, Ries RK. Using ethyl glucuronide in urine to detect light and heavy drinking in alcohol dependent outpatients. Drug Alcohol Depend. 2015;157:184–187. https://doi.org/10.1016/j.drugalcdep.2015.10.004.
39 Medical University of South Carolina College of Medicine. About urine ethylglucuronide (EtG) testing. https://medicine.musc.edu/departments/psychiatry/divisions-and-programs/programs/cnl/heavy-alcohol-testing/etg.

35 Cocaine

James C. Norris and Rodney G. Richmond

SYNOPSIS

35.1 HISTORICAL BACKGROUND

The source of cocaine is coca plants found in the northern Andes Mountains of South America and in a few areas in India, South Africa, and Indonesia. Historically, the indigenous people of South America have used coca leaves as a stimulant for over 2000 years. The leaves were chewed in their religious ceremonies and then as part of their daily activities. This latter usage was most apparent during the Spanish occupation when the Peruvian Indians could not accomplish the heavy labor required in the mines without access to the coca leaves (Isenschmid, 2002; EMC, 2015).

Cocaine is removed from coca leaves (dried leaves contain as much as 1% cocaine) by moistening them with an alkali solution, and then kerosene is used to extract the cocaine. Sulfuric acid is added to absorb and form cocaine sulfate. This solution is neutralized causing a precipitation into a cocaine paste. This paste is again redissolved in sulfuric acid and potassium permanganate to eliminate cinnamoylcocaine (methylecgonine cinnamate) and other impurities. After filtration, this solution is neutralized, resulting in the precipitation of free base cocaine. Organic solvents are used to dissolve the paste. Highly concentrated hydrochloric acid is added to the organic solvent, thereby producing a precipitate of cocaine hydrochloride (EMC, 2015).

Crack is cocaine base and is produced by mixing cocaine hydrochloride with sodium bicarbonate, followed by heating to allow the precipitation of the base. This results in small lumps (rocks) of the cocaine base (EMC, 2015; NIDA, 2015a).

Street names are blow, coke, crack, dust, flake, gold dust, happy dust, lady, nose candy, rock, snow, stardust, toot, and white. Mixtures with other drugs are known as "speedball" when mixed with heroin, and it is "tick" when mixed with phencyclidine (Isenschmid, 2002).

35.2 MEDICAL USAGES OF COCAINE

Cocaine is listed as a DEA Schedule II drug. It is primarily used in dental procedures and head and neck surgeries. Examples of procedures and surgeries are nasal septum and palate, gingival lesions, and erosion of tooth surfaces (Blanksma and Brand, 2005). Cocaine's properties which are beneficial in these procedures are the combination of local anesthetic and vasoconstriction.

35.3 ILLEGAL USAGE OF COCAINE

Cocaine is the third-most used illicit drug in the United States (Tang et al., 2014). Its usage, however, previously was reduced in recent years. For example, in 2013, the number

DOI: 10.1201/9781003615323-39

of users was 1.5 million, while in 2002 to 2007, the number ranged from 2 to 2.4 million (NIDA, 2015b).

However, the 2019 Annual Surveillance Report of Drug-Related Risks and Outcomes by the Centers for Disease Control and Prevention found that in 2018, an estimated 5,529,000 persons aged 12 years and older (2.0% of the population) reported cocaine use in the past year, including 757,000 persons (0.3% cent of the population) who used crack cocaine. In 2018, an estimated 977,000 (0.4%) persons aged 12 years and older reported a substance use disorder in the past year involving cocaine (*https://www.cdc.gov/drugoverdose/pdf/pubs/2019-cdc-drug-surveillance-report.pdf*).

A percentage of 5.4% of pregnant women aged 14 to 44 years old were current illicit drug users (SAMHSA, 2014). Additionally, 28% of these women were pregnant for an average of 2.5 months before they were aware of their pregnancy. Over 75 million US children have been exposed to cocaine prenatally (Chae and Covington, 2009).

35.4 ROUTES OF ADMINISTRATION

The most common way of cocaine administration is by snorting and smoking. Snorting involves the inhaling of cocaine hydrochloride, typically laid out in a line on a flat surface, through a tube (e.g., rolled-up currency bill) into the nose. Intranasal absorption can be limited by the cocaine-induced vasoconstriction and surface area in the nasal mucosa. Smoking of cocaine involves the free base cocaine lumps/rocks. These lumps/rocks produce a cracking sound when heated—hence the name of "crack." The vapors released from the heating of the lumps/rocks (in a pipe) are inhaled and absorbed into the blood stream (EMC, 2015; NIDA, 2015a). Intravenously injected cocaine hydrochloride is another route of administration, but it is less common (EMC, 2015).

Bioavailability of cocaine is limited to 10 to 20 percent when administered by smoking, in comparison to oral and nasal administration which has 30 to 40 percent bioavailability (Jones, 1997). The rapid onset and intensity of cocaine's euphoria coupled with its short half-life (0.7–1.5 hours) lead the users to repeat their dosing in short sequences of time (Romanoki, 1996). This can result in binge usage of cocaine.

In a study comparing the behavioral responses of users who injected cocaine intravenously with those who smoked it, the administered doses of cocaine were 25 mg, IV, or 42 mg (free base), smoked (Cone, 1995). The smoked cocaine resulted in higher behavioral responses than those achieved by an intravenous route of administration.

In a survey of cocaine users, a trend was uncovered among the cocaine users in that there was a movement from injected cocaine to crack cocaine. Three reasons were determined to promote this change: (1) It was less expensive, (2) the quick and stimulating effects in comparison to the injection form, but (3) the main reason may be the fact that their friends and companions suggested crack cocaine usage, or they were using crack. These authors noted that a benefit for this trend is the decrease of infective diseases among the users with the absence of needle usage (de Carvalho and Seibel, 2009).

Additionally, as a delivery method, smoking crack cocaine offers a very quick delivery to the brain after being presented to the blood through the lungs. The smoking of crack cocaine occurs at a low temperature (98°C) which does not cause the thermal decomposition of the cocaine. Thus, the cocaine is not wasted via the delivery system (Morton, 1999).

35.5 EFFECTS OF COCAINE

Cocaine is a central nervous system stimulant drug which produces short-term euphoria, energy, and talkativeness (NIDA, 2015a). Physiological effects are dilated pupils and increased heart rate, blood pressure, body temperature, and respiration rate. Increased heart rate, blood pressure, and constricted arteries supplying the heart can lead to myocardial infarction. Additionally, an increased risk of stroke, cerebral atrophy, and sudden cardiac death are associated with cocaine use (Schaumburg and Spencer, 2000).

Rhabdomyolysis is also a possible finding with cocaine usage (Hosseinnezhad et al., 2011). This is due to a direct effect on the muscle tissue by inducing vasoconstriction and ischemia (Emadian et al., 1996). Additionally, cocaine can cause the leakage of creatinine kinase (CK) from skeletal muscle myocytes (Ruttenber et al., 1999). Hyperthermia and hyperactivity associated with cocaine usage will also attribute to rhabdomyolysis by increasing energy requirements and depleting the body's energy resources (Curry et al., 1989).

In 2011, there were 1.3 million emergency department visits related to drug misuse or abuse, with cocaine being the implicated drug in 505,224 of those cases (NIDA Cocaine Research Report, 2016). These patients can present with pulmonary issues (also labeled as "Crack Lung"), acute kidney failure, thrombocytopenia, and acute hepatitis (Bontempo et al., 2017; Hosseinnezhad et al., 2011). Almost 41% of Emergency-Department-presenting patients had pleuritic chest pain, and more than half had an elevated creatine phosphokinase concentration (Bontempo et al., 2017). Forrester et al. (1990) noted that crack-related pulmonary injury could present as acute, diffuse, alveolar infiltrates with or without hemoptysis. They recommended that patients with persistent respiratory failure—where infections or immune-mediated pulmonary disorders have been ruled out—and whose pulmonary histopathology shows prominent inflammatory cell infiltrates, could benefit from a short course of corticosteroids. "Crack lung" has also been described as diffuse alveolar damage and hemorrhagic alveolitis that occurred within 48 hours of smoking crack. Dyspnea, fever, cough, or hemoptysis were part of the clinical picture and might progress to respiratory failure. The radiographic findings included diffuse alveolar infiltrates and ground-glass opacities (Dolapsakis and Katsandri, 2019).

Toxicological manifestations associated with acute cocaine usage include the stimulation of the central nervous system with associated psychosis, grand-mal convulsions, ventricular arrhythmias, and respiratory dysfunction with Cheyne–Stoke breathing and respiratory paralysis. Mydriasis, hypertension followed by hypotension, small muscle twitching, and constriction of blood vessels are additional effects exhibited by cocaine usage. Cardiotoxicity is a well-known cocaine effect and can be associated with therapeutic doses. Another serious effect is hyperthermia which can then lead to a coma (Isenschmid, 2002; NIDA, 2015a). Binge usage of cocaine produces a decreased sensitivity to cocaine's euphoric effect as the user progresses through the binge. This is related to the acute tolerance to cocaine. Subjects have experienced depression once their cocaine has been consumed, and this depression can be manifest within 15 to 30 minutes after having finished their last amount of cocaine (Gawin and Kleber, 1986).

The recreational use of cocaine has been linked with the impairment of cognitive flexibility, such as the inability to rapidly adjust one's behavior (Colzato et al., 2009). Shifting between tasks and mental sets was another description of this cognitive flexibility which is impaired (Friedman and Miyake, 2004; Friedman et al., 2006; Miyake et al., 2000). These investigators also suggested that the inhibition of unwanted responses was affected; however, the maintenance of information in the working memory was not impaired in recreational users (Colzato et al., 2009).

Chronic users exhibit rhinitis (possibly in conjunction with nasal septum perforation), shortness of breath, cold sweats, tremors, tachycardia, tachypnea, and dyspnea. Additionally, their abilities of concentrating and memory are impaired (Isenschmid, 2002). Other effects include anxiety, confusion, hyperactivity, irritability, intense depression, and loss of appetite.

Psychiatric disturbance is observed with chronic cocaine users as well as violent protective behavior, distorted perception, and hyperkinetic behavior. A psychological dependence is largely the result of cocaine's ability to stimulate unusually high rewarding effects. This drive can result in a psychological change which is termed being "cokedout" (Isenschmid, 2002).

These individuals can become aggressive, have paranoia events, and have panic attacks. Short temperedness and suspiciousness are part of the effects which can develop into the schizophrenic psychosis. Hallucinations (auditory, visual, and tactile) are among other CNS complications (Isenschmid, 2002).

Cocaine-induced agitated delirium is a rare condition which is characterized by severe cardiopulmonary dysfunction, hyperthermia, and acute neurologic changes (Plush et al., 2015). Bizarre violent behavior, running around, and physically aggressive actions are manifestations of these individuals. This condition predominately leads to death (Menaker et al., 2011). Two associated neurological findings in contrast to chronic cocaine users have been identified: (1) A lack of elevated striatal dopamine transporters (Staley et al., 1995) and (2) a different phenotype of the serotonin transporter in the dopaminergic areas of the brain (Bell, 2008). Chronic symptomatology displayed by cocaine abusers can be dysthymic, major depressive, cyclothymic, or attention-deficit disorder (ADD). These symptoms result in the abuse to self-medicate with cocaine to reverse dysphoric episodes, extend hypomanic episodes in cyclothymic disorder, ease the chronic dysphoric of depressive episode, and alleviate the symptoms of ADD (Gawin and Kleber, 1986).

The need for a supply of crack cocaine by the daily crack users has been related to their illicit and criminal activities (Miller et al., 1991).

35.6 PSYCHOTIC DISORDERS INDUCED BY COCAINE

Cocaine is associated with a transient psychotic syndrome (described as paranoia or hallucinations). The most frequent cocaine-induced psychotic symptoms are paranoid beliefs and suspiciousness. If the psychotic symptoms occur within a month of cocaine intoxication or withdrawal, the diagnosis is cocaine-induced psychotic disorder (CIPD) (Tang et al., 2014). The three factors related to this effect are the amount of cocaine, the presence of antisocial personality disorder, and a history of cannabis dependence (Roncero et al., 2013). Additionally, significant differences among the CIPD individuals are the age of onset of dependence, lifetime cannabis abuse or dependence, and imprisonment (Roncero et al., 2014).

Suspiciousness, distrust, and paranoia have been reported in 62% of cocaine smokers (Siegel, 1982). In another study, individuals were given an IV loading dose of 40 or 80 mg cocaine. This was followed by a low-dose IV of cocaine. Suspiciousness of these subjects correlated with the loading dose and not the cocaine plasma concentration (Sherer et al., 1989). It has been suggested that these effects have resulted in high-speed chases with police (Weitli and Fishbain, 1985). Other disorders can be present in cocaine users, such as mood disorders, anxiety disorders, sexual dysfunction, and sleep disorder (Morton, 1999).

35.7 ADDICTION

Generalizations about addictive drugs, such as cocaine, are (1) that their behavior is increasingly directed toward obtaining and using these drugs of abuse and developing less of an ability to stop using in spite of the interferences with their life; (2) the addicted have altered learning and memory; and (3) the addictive drugs create artificial learning signals which are greater in magnitude and duration than the response to natural events (Torregrossa et al., 2011).

35.8 COGNITIVE DEFICITS

A review of the literature was conducted as to whether the chronic usage of cocaine results in broad cognitive deficits to include domains of executive function, memory, language, and psychomotor speed (Frazer et al., 2018). The authors concluded that broad cognitive deficits with chronic cocaine users were not found.

Fifteen poly-users were administered a single dose of cocaine (300 mg) to determine its effect on their memory (Hutten et al., 2018). Their conclusion was that the cocaine enhanced the users' prospective memory, attention, and arousal. However, the prospective memory performance was only weakly positively associated to measures of attention and arousal. Their conclusion was that the enhanced prospective memory performance was not fully due to a direct change in the neural network which supports the prospective memory.

35.9 PRENATAL COCAINE EXPOSURE (PCE)

In a review of the literature (Martin et al., 2017), the authors concluded that PCE children displayed long-term deficits in arousal and attention, emotional reactivity, and reward systems. They also noted that longitudinal studies of young adults who had been exposed prenatally to cocaine demonstrated persistent behavioral and cognitive deficits.

In a meta-analysis study, children through six years of age have shown no long-term direct effects of prenatal cocaine exposure (PCE) on their physical growth, developmental test scores, or language outcomes (Ackerman et al., 2010). Small changes were noted in the growth, cognitive ability, academic achievement, and language functioning; however, environmental variables modified these changes. For sustained attention and behavioral self-regulation, no association was found from this age group. PCE-related changes in the brain structure and function were limited by the methodologies' inconsistencies.

The impact of PCE on the language development of children aged 10 years old was investigated (Lewis et al., 2011). The authors concluded that subtle effects on specific aspects of language development and phonological processing occurred for these children. The researchers noted these results considered for confounding variables.

A study on language development in 12-year-old children was conducted (Lewis et al., 2013). The findings suggest that PCE continues to have small, subtle effects on specific aspects of language at age 12 years. Significantly impact on the phonological processing skills (i.e., the reading outcomes of the letter–word identification, reading fluency, and reading comprehension) was observed. These were small but lasting effects on the language skills that are related to later literacy skills.

A longitudinal study of 219, 15-year-olds was conducted starting from their fourth gestational month (Richardson et al., 2015). Their findings were: The first trimester PCE was significantly related to adolescent displaying delinquent behavior; poorer problem solving and abstract reasoning; and reduced weight, height, and head circumference at 15 years. An additional impact was the exposure to violence which partially mediated the effect of PCE on delinquent behavior.

Another meta-analysis review of 27 studies, involving adolescents with ages between 11 and 19, was conducted (Buckingham-Howe et al., 2013). In six studies, those authors reported significantly lower scores on language and memory tasks among adolescents with PCE; for eight studies, those authors examined brain structure/function and reported morphologic differences with few functional differences; and for three studies, those authors examined physiologic responses with divergent findings. The meta-analysis authors concluded that while the vulnerability of language continued into adolescence, the effects were small. They also suggested that these small effects were of questionable clinical importance.

35.10 VIOLENCE

Violence is also associated with cocaine usage. In New York City from 1990 to 1991, 31.3% of homicide perpetrators tested positive for cocaine or benzoylecgonine; and 28% of the homicide victims from Detroit in 2000 had cocaine in their blood (Isenschmid, 2002).

An evaluation of crack users revealed an association with violence, while verbal arguments and physical fights were related to alcohol and crack when examined separately. An association of both verbal and physical fights was found for users reporting more than one drug. Theft and death threats were also related to the use of crack cocaine. The extreme type of violence involved death with 80% being friends and acquaintances, as well as victimization and intimate partner violence (de Carvalho and Seibel, 2009).

Evaluations were taken on 101 patients of both sexes for over 12 months to investigate an association between the routes of cocaine administration and the level of displayed violence (Giannini et al., 1993). The evaluations were obtained by a structured questionnaire, and the routes of administration were free base/crack smoking (FB), intravenous injection (IV), and nasal insufflation (NS). FB and IV routes produced more violence than NS; and FB and IV resulted in approximately the same level of violence for most of the measurements. The violent actions associated with sustained activity (such as rape, burglary, and armed robbery) did not display a relationship with the routes. Between men and women, the different levels of violence were related to the circumstances and not the route.

35.11 TOLERANCE

Tolerance (the need for higher doses to achieve euphoric effects) is common in chronic users. Tolerance to cocaine in non-chronic users has been observed, and some chronic tolerance may occur. However, in the latter scenario, the extent may not be similar to alcohol and opiate tolerance (Gawin and Kleber, 1986).

35.12 WITHDRAWAL OR ABSTINENCE EFFECTS

After a cocaine binge, the abuser can transition through three phases:

1. Crash (nine hours to four days)
2. Withdrawal (1 to 10 weeks) and
3. Extinction (indefinite)

The first phase is the crash phase. There are three parts which have the following associated symptoms:

1. Early (agitation, depression, anorexia, high cocaine craving)
2. Middle (fatigue, depression, no cocaine craving, and insomnia coupled with an increasing longing for sleep)
3. Late (exhaustion, hypersomnolence, hyperphagia, and no cocaine craving)

The second phase of withdrawal also has three parts and contains the following symptoms:

- Early (normalized sleep, euthymic mood, low cocaine craving, and low anxiety)
- Middle and late (anhedonia, anergia, anxiety, high cocaine craving, and conditioned cues)

In the third phase of extinction, the abuser can exhibit normal hedonic response, euthymic mood, episodic craving, and conditioned cues (Gawin and Kleber, 1986).

According to other investigators, a gradual recovery with no associated tri-phasic recovery occurs during cocaine abstinence for both cocaine-addicted and nonaddicted control individuals (Weddington et al., 1990).

35.13 MECHANISMS OF ACTION

The euphoric feeling and addictive properties are principally associated with the blockage of the dopamine reuptake (Giros et al., 1996). Dopamine is also increased in the synaptic area by being released from the storage vesicles. Additional central nervous system actions include the blockage of the synaptic reuptake transporters for norepinephrine and serotonin.

The pharmacology of cocaine is more complex than just three neurotransmitters. For example, cocaine also binds to muscarinic acetylcholine receptors in the heart and brain in rats and with sigma receptors in rat cerebellum (Sharkey et al., 1988a, 1988b). The significance of these findings in part is further emphasized in that the binding of cocaine has been also demonstrated with human muscarinic receptors (Flynn et al., 1992). With regard to the local anesthetic effect of cocaine, it binds to several voltage-gated ion channels. This interaction causing the local anesthetic effect may also be responsible for cocaine-induced cardiotoxicity (Heard, 2008). It is the combination of these receptors being bound by cocaine that contributes to its euphoric and toxicological effects.

35.14 METABOLISM

The principal metabolites for cocaine are benzoylecgonine (BE) and ecgonine methyl ester (EME) (Isenschmid, 2002). Each of these metabolites have different pathways. BE is produced by liver methylesterase and chemical hydrolysis; whereas EME is the result of metabolism by liver benzoylesterase and plasma pseudocholinesterase (Isenschmid, 1999a).

These two predominant metabolites have been investigated for their relative production. For example, human pharmacokinetic data have been collected from 10 volunteers with several administrations of cocaine as many users take multiple doses in a short time frame (i.e., binge). The principal two metabolites of cocaine were as expected (i.e., EME and BE). However, as EME was approximately 5% of BE, BE is the primary metabolite of cocaine (Isenschmid et al., 1992).

Cocaine is metabolized into benzoylecgonine in the plasma through the activity of plasma butyrylcholinesterase, which also leads to the formation of ethyl methylecgonidine (EME) (Isenschmid et al., 1989). Adding sodium fluoride for the inhibition of this enzymatic hydrolysis does not prevent the independent hydrolysis of cocaine to BE. In fact, cocaine is hydrolyzed to BE only in a phosphate buffer. This hydrolytic process is also accelerated at a higher temperature and pH (Isenschmid et al., 2002).

Another metabolite, ethylcocaine, becomes prominent in the presence of ethanol and is generated by liver methylesterase. This metabolite is also produced by the hepatic methylesterase but occurs 3.5 times faster than the conversion to BE (Brzezinski et al., 1994). Additionally, the consumption of alcohol with cocaine usage will result in a metabolite called cocaethylene. This metabolite can be found in the blood and urine. Cocaethylene has similar effects on the cardiovascular system as cocaine (Hosseinnezhad et al., 2011). This metabolite can also be found in hair (Gambelunghe et al., 2017).

35.15 BLOOD LEVELS

The intravenous administration of 0.6 mg/kg of cocaine resulted in a peak plasma cocaine concentration of approximately 540 ng/mL, and it occurred very shortly after the time of administration. Intranasal administration of 2 mg/kg produced approximately 340 ng/mL of cocaine at around 60 minutes. Oral ingestion of 2 mg/kg resulted in 300 ng/mL of cocaine at 80 minutes. Smoking 100 mg of cocaine yielded 220 ng/mL of cocaine within a similar time as an intravenous injection (Jones, 1997). Cocaine peak plasma levels were highest for the oral administration of 2 mg at 650 ng/mL, occurring at approximately 100 minutes. Intranasal administration of 2 mg/kg yielded 500 ng/mL of cocaine at approximately 120 minutes. An intravenous injection of 0.6 mg/kg had 260 ng/mL of cocaine at 90 minutes; while smoking 100 mg of cocaine peaked at 170 ng/mL of cocaine at about 100 minutes (Jones, 1997).

Multiple and rapid uses of cocaine occur with users (binge usage) to maintain their high. Thus, to obtain pharmacokinetic data, individuals were administered cocaine via smoking or intravenously within four minutes. After smoking 25 mg of cocaine, the cocaine plasma concentration was 0.14 mg/L at 4 minutes. Fourteen minutes after the first 25 mg of cocaine, an additional 25 mg of cocaine was smoked. This resulted in a cocaine plasma concentration of 0.21 mg/L at 4 minutes later which declined to 0.15 mg/L at 16 minutes from the second ingestion. The double smoking of 50 mg of cocaine resulted in 0.22 mg/L of cocaine at 4 minutes after the first ingestion, 0.38 mg/L at 4 minutes after the second ingestion, and 0.28 mg/L of cocaine at 16 minutes after the second ingestion. The final time point of 90 minutes revealed 0.06 mg/L of cocaine for the 25-mg usage and 0.12 mg/L for the 50-mg usage (Isenschmid et al., 1992).

The double intravenous administration of 16 and 32 mg with the same time points as above yielded cocaine plasma concentrations of 0.12 and 0.26 mg/L, respectively, at the first 4-minute time points, 0.23 and 47 mg/L at the second 4-minute time points, and 0.18 and 37 mg/L at 16-minute time points. The final time point of 90 minutes revealed 0.07 mg/L for the 16-mg usage and 0.14 mg/L for the 32-mg usage (Isenschmid et al., 1992).

35.16 URINE LEVELS

Urine concentrations from six humans who had nasally inhaled cocaine (1.5 mg/kg of body weight) were determined. Within the first hour, the cocaine concentration ranged from 0.3 to 24.1 μg/mL with a mean of 6.7 μg/mL. Five of the six individuals did not have any detected cocaine after 12 hours with a mean of 0.4 μg/mL during the 8-to-12-hour time slot. In the first hour, the benzoylecgonine mean concentration was 13.4 μg/mL with a range of 0 to 37.4 μg/mL. After 48 to 72 hours, five of the six urine samples did not have any benzoylecgonine. However, between 96 to 168 hours, two individuals tested positive for benzoylecgonine at 0.1 to 0.4 μg/mL (Hamilton et al., 1977).

After receiving an oral dose of 25 mg of cocaine, a single volunteer had a peak urinary cocaine concentration of 269 ng/mL at 1 hour and a peak benzoylecgonine concentration of 7,940 ng/mL at 12 hours (Baselt and Chang, 1987). The short half-life of cocaine leads to repeated usage within a short time frame. This can result in high urine benzoylecgonine concentrations.

35.17 IMPAIRMENT

In general, stimulants, such as cocaine, can enhance psychomotor performance and increase alertness; however, the improved psychomotor performance is more closely related to relatively simple tasks, and the improvement is lost as the task complexity increases. As hyperexcitability becomes more evident, stimulant users' driving ability diminishes (Ellinwood and Nikaido, 1987).

Studies have demonstrated that the sleep-deprivation-induced reaction time had been reversed with 96-mg intranasal administration of cocaine (Fischman and Schuster, 1980), and motor abilities in field sobriety test results were improved after an IN dose of cocaine compared to marijuana (Heishman and Crouch, 1997).

The combination of cocaine with other drugs has been investigated in which cocaine was shown to either reverse or have no effect on the ethanol-induced effects (Farré et al., 1993; Fotlin and Fischman, 1989; Fotlin et al., 1993; Higgins et al., 1992; Higgins et al., 1993). Conversely, ethanol reversed some of the cocaine-induced effects. Additionally, no greater impairment was noted when comparing ethanol alone versus the combination of ethanol and cocaine.

However, the combination of ethanol and cocaine may give the user a feeling of elevated mental and physical abilities which could lead to increased risk-taking behaviors (Byck, 1987).

Cocaine users have reported that cocaine alters their vision, i.e., they have increased sensitivity to light, halos surrounding bright objects, difficulty in focusing, blurred vision, glare recovery problems, and loss of blue–yellow vision (Siegel, 1978, 1982, 1987).

Impairment has also been reported by cocaine users during the crash phase of recovery from cocaine usage (Siegel, 1987). Other studies dealing with subjects who have a history of daily usage have noted only modest changes in mood and craving after a cocaine binge (Fotlin and Fischman, 1997a, 1997b). The reaction times (visual and auditory suppression tasks) of cocaine users were assessed in cocaine-dependent individuals and were found to be slower than control subjects who were not drug dependent; however, their response accuracy was not affected.

35.18 ASSOCIATED DEATHS WITH COCAINE USAGE

In 253 motor vehicular fatalities, 25 (10%) of the victims had cocaine or a metabolite in their blood (Isenschmid, 1999b). Additional findings were that in 14 of the 25 (56%), ethanol was detected. Cocaine and ethanol were detected in those victims of accidents associated with the loss of vehicular control. The Center for Disease Control and Prevention (CDC) reports that overdose deaths from cocaine use are rising, with more than 16,000 people dying in 2019 (*https://www.drugabuse.gov/drug-topics/cocaine*).

35.19 SUMMARY AND CONCLUSIONS

Despite the cavalier and widespread use of cocaine by large numbers of the population, cocaine certainly is a physiologically dangerous drug. The chapter documents the risks and circumstances in which risks are increased. There are many legal risks associated with cocaine usage: Aggravated DUI when any cocaine metabolite is detected; prosecution for possession; and, of course, greater penalties for distribution and sale.

REFERENCES

Ackerman, J.P., Riggins, T. and Black, M.M. 2010. A review of the effects of prenatal cocaine exposure among school-aged children. Pediatrics. 125(3): 554–565.

Baselt, R.C. and Chang, R. 1987. Urinary excretion of cocaine and benzoylecgonine following oral ingestion in a single subject. J Anal Toxicol. 11: 81–82.

Bell, M.D. 2008. Disorders of the central nervous system. In: *Pathology, Toxicogenetics, and Criminalistics of Drug Abuse*, edited by Steven Karch, p. 140. Taylor and Francis.

Blanksma, C.J. and Brand, H.S. 2005. Cocaine abuse: Orofacial manifestations and implications for dental treatment. Int Dent J. 55(6): 365–369.

Bontempo, L.J., Magidson, P.D., Hayes, B.D. and Martinez, J.P. 2017. Acute pulmonary injury after inhalation of free-base cocaine: A case report. J Acute Med. 7(2): 82–86.

Brzezinski, M.R., Abraham, T.L., Stone, C.L., Dean, R.A. and Bosron, W.F. 1994. Purification and characterization of a human liver cocaine carboxylesterase that catalyzes the production of benzoylecgonine and the formation of ethylcocaine from ethanol and cocaine. Biochem Pharm. 48: 1747.

Buckingham-Howe, S., Berger, S.S., Scaletti, L.A. and Black, M.M. 2013. Systematic review of prenatal cocaine exposure and adolescent development. Pediatrics. 131(6): e1917–e1936.

Byck, R. 1987. The effects of cocaine on complex performance in humans. Alchol Drug Driv. 3: 9.

Chae, S.M. and Covington, C.Y. 2009. Biobehavioral outcomes in adolescents and young adults prenatally exposed to cocaine: Evidence from animal models. Biol Res Nurs. 10: 318–330.

Colzato, L.S., Huizinga, M. and Hommel, B. 2009. Recreational cocaine polydrug use impairs cognitive flexibility but not working memory. Pschopharmacology. 207: 225–234.

Cone, E. J. 1995. Pharmacokinetics and pharmacodynamics of cocaine. Journal of Analytical Toxicology, 19: 459–478.

Curry, S.C., Chang, D. and Connor, D. 1989. Drug- and toxin-induced rhabdomyolysis. Ann Emerg Med. 18: 1068–1084. [Ref 5 in Coco Klasner 2004].

de Carvalho, H.B. and Seibel, S.D. 2009. Crack cocaine use and its relationship with violence and HIV. Clinics. 64(9): 857–866.

Dolapsakis, C. and Katsandri, A. 2019. Crack lung: A case of acute pulmonary cocaine toxicity. Lung India. 36(4): 370–371.

Ellinwood, E.H. and Nikaido, A.M. 1987. Stimulant induced impairment: A perspective across dose and duration of use. Alcohol Drugs Driv. 3(1): 19–24.

Emadian, S.M., Caravati, E.M. and Herr, R.D. 1996. Rhabdomyolysis: A rare adverse effect of diphenhydramine overdose. Am J Emerg Med. 14: 574–576.

European Monitoring Centre (EMC). 2015. Cocaine and crack drug profile. http://www.emcdda.europa.eu/publications/drug-profiles/cocaine#pharmacology.

Farré, M., Llorent, D.L.T., Ugena, B., Segura, J. and Cami, J. 1993. Alcohol and cocaine interactions in humans. J Pharmacol Exp Ther. 266: 1364.

Fischman, M.W. and Schuster, C.R. 1980. Cocaine effects in sleep-deprived humans. Psychopharmacology (Berlin). 72: 1.

Flynn, D.D., Vaishnav, A.A. and Mash, D.C. 1992. Interactions of cocaine with primary and secondary recognition sites on muscarinic receptors. Mol Pharmacol. 41: 736–742.

Forrester, J.M., Steele, A.W., Waldron, J.A. and Parsons, P.E. 1990. Crack lung: An acute pulmonary syndrome with a spectrum of clinical and histopathologic findings. Am Rev Respir Dis. 142(20): 462–467.

Fotlin, R.W. and Fischman, M.W. 1989. Ethanol and cocaine interactions in humans: Cardiovascular consequences. Pharmacol Biochem Behav. 31: 877.

Fotlin, R.W. and Fischman, M.W. 1997a. A laboratory model of cocaine withdrawal in humans: Intravenous cocaine. Exp Clin Psychopharmacol. 4: 404.

Fotlin, R.W. and Fischman, M.W. 1997b. Residual effects or repeated cocaine smoking in humans. Drug Alcohol Depend. 47: 117.

Fotlin, R.W., Fischman, M.W., Pippen, P.A. and Kelly, T.H. 1993. Behavioral effects of cocaine alone and in combination with marihuana in humans. Drug Alcohol Depend. 32: 93.

Frazer, K.M., Richards, Q., Keith, D.R. 2018. The long-term effects of cocaine use on cognitive functioning: A systemic critical review. Behav Brain Res. 348: 241–262.

Friedman, N.P., Miyake, A. 2004. The relations among inhibition and interference control functions: A latent-variable analysis. J Exp Psychol Gen. 133: 101–135.

Friedman, N.P., Miyake, A., Corley, R.P., Young, S.E., DeFries, J.C. and Hewitt, J.K. 2006. Not all executive functions are related to intelligence. Psychol Sci. 17: 172–179.

Gambelunghe, C., Rossi, R., Aroni, K., Gili, A., Bacci, M., Pascali, V. and Fucci, N. 2017. Norcocaine and cocaethylene distribution patterns in hair samples from light, moderate, and heavy cocaine users. Drug Test Anal. 9: 161–167.

Gawin, F.H. and Kleber, H.D. 1986. Abstinence symptomatology and psychiatric diagnosis in cocaine abusers. Arch Gen Psychiat. 43: 107–113.

Giannini, A.J., Miller, N.S., Losielle, R.H. and Turner, C.E. 1993. Cocaine-associated violence and relationship to route of administration. J Subst Abuse Treat. 10: 67–69.

Giros, B., Jaber, M., Jones, S.R., Wightman, R.M. and Caron, M.G. 1996. Hyperlocomotion and indifference to cocaine and amphetamine in mice lacking the dopamine transporter. Nature. 379: 606–612.

Hamilton, H.E., Wallace, J.E., Shimek, E.L., Land, P., Harris, S.C. and Christenson, J.G. 1977. Cocaine and benzoylecgonine excretion in humans. J Forensic Sci. 22(7): 697–707.

Heard, K., Palmer, R. and Zahniser, N. 2008. Mechanisms of acute cocaine toxicity. Open Pharmacol J. 2(9): 70–78.

Heishman, S.J. and Crouch, D.J. 1997. Pharmacokinetic-pharmacodynamic relationships following acute marihuana and cocaine administration. Presentation—: Society of Forensic Toxicologists Annual Meeting, Snowbird, UT, October.

Higgins, S.T., Rush, C.R., Bickel, W.K., Hughes, J.R., Lynn, M. and Capeless, M.A. 1993. Effects of cocaine and alcohol, alone and in combination, on humans. Psychopharmacology (Berlin). 111: 285.

Higgins, S.T., Rush, C.R., Hughes, J.R., Bickel, W.K., Lynn, M. and Capeless, M.A. 1992. Effects of cocaine and alcohol, alone and in combination, on human learning and performance. J Exp Anal Behav. 58: 87.

Hosseinnezhad, A., Vijayakrishnan, R. and Farmer, M.J.S. 2011. Acute renal failure, thrombocytopenia, and elevated liver enzymes after concurrent abuse of alcohol and cocaine. Clin Pract. 1(e35): 65–66.

Hutten, N.R.P.W., Kuypers, K.P.C., Wel, J.H.P., Theunissen, E.L., Toennes, S.W., Verkes, R-J. and Ramaekers, J.G. 2018. A single dose of cocaine enhances prospective memory performance. J Psychopharmacol. 32(8): 883–892.

Isenschmid, D.S. 1999a. Cocaine. In: *Principles of Forensic Toxicology*, edited by B. Levine, p. 221. Washington, DC: AACC Press.

Isenschmid, D.S. 1999b. Unpublished data [cited in Isenschmid, D.S. 2002].

Isenschmid, D.S. 2002. Cocaine: Effects on human performance and behavior. Forensic Sci Rev. 14: 61–100.

Isenschmid, D.S., Fischman, M.W., Foltin, R.W. and Caplan, Y.H. 1992. Concentration of cocaine and metabolites in plasma of humans following intravenous administration and smoking cocaine. J Anal Toxicol. 16: 311–314.

Isenschmid, D.S., Levine, B.S. and Caplan, Y.H. 1989. A comprehensive study of the stability of cocaine and its metabolites. J Anal Toxicol. 13: 250.

Jones, R.T. 1997. Pharmacokinetics of cocaine: Considerations when assessing cocaine use by urinalysis. NIDA RES Monogr. 175: 221–234.

Lewis, B.A., Minnes, S., Short, E.J., Min, M.M., Wu, M., Lang, A., Weishampel, P. and Singer, T. 2013. Language outcomes at 12 years for children exposed prenatally to cocaine. J. Speech Lang Hear Res. 56(5): 1662–1676.

Lewis, B.A., Minnes, S., Short, E.J., Weishampel, P., Satayathum, S., Min, M.O., Nelson, S. and Singer, L.T. 2011. The effects of prenatal cocaine on language development at 1 years of age. Neurotoxicol Teratol. 33(1): 17–24.

Martin, E.M., Longstreth, L.E., & Coohey, C. 2017. Effects of prenatal cocaine exposure: An integrative analysis of findings from animal and human studies. Am J Drug Alcohol Abuse, 43(4), 410–418. https://doi.org/10.1080/00952990.2016.1236464

Menaker, J., Farcy, D.A., Boswell, S.A., Stein, D.M., Dutton, R.P., Hess, J.R. and Scalea, T.M. 2011. Cocaine-induced agitated delirium with associated hyperthermia: A case report. J Emerg Med. 41(3): 49–53.

Miller, N.S., Gold, M.S., Mahler, J.C. 1991. Violent behaviors associated with cocaine use: Possible pharmacological mechanisms. Int J Addict. 1991 Oct;26(10): 1077–1088.

Miyake, A., Friedman, N.P., Emerson, M.J., Witzki, A.H., Howerter, A. and Wager, T. 2000. The unity and diversity of executive functions and their contributions to complex "frontal lobe" tasks: A latent variable analysis. Cogn Psychol. 41: 49–100.

Morton, W.A. 1999. Cocaine and psychiatric symptoms. Prim Care Companion J Clin Psychiatry. 1: 109–113.

National Institute on Drug Abuse (NIDA). 2015a. Drug facts. http://www.drugabuse.gov/publications/drugfacts/cocaine.

National Institute on Drug Abuse (NIDA). 2015b. Drug facts: Nationwide trends. http://www.drugabuse.gov/publications/drugfacts/nationwide-trends.

National Institute on Drug Abuse (NIDA). 2016. Cocaine research report, February 2021. https://www.drugabuse.gov/publications/research-reports/cocaine/what-cocaine.

Plush, T., Shakespeare, W., Jacobs, D. Ladi, L., Sethi, S. and Gasperione, J. 2015. Cocaine-induced agitated delirium: A case report and review. J Intensive Care Med. 30(1): 49–57.

Richardson, G.A., Goldschmidt, L., Larkby, C. and Day, N.L. 2015. Effects of prenatal cocaine exposure on adolescent development. Neurotoxicol Teratol. 49: 41–48.

Romanoki, A.J. 1996. Alcohol and drug dependence. In: *The Principles and Practices of Medicine*, 23rd ed. Stanford, Connecticut: Appleton and Lange.

Roncero, C., Comin, M., Daigre, C., Grau-López, L., Martónez-Luna, N., Eiroa-Orosa, F.J., Barral, C., Torrens, M. and Casas, M. 2014. Clinical differences between cocaine-induced psychotic disorder and psychotic symptoms in cocaine-dependent patients. Psychiatry Res. 216(3): 398–403.

Roncero, C., Daigre, C., Gonzalvo, B., Valero, S., Castells, X., Grau-López, L., Eiroa-Orosa, F.J. and Casas, M.

2013. Risk factors for cocaine-induced psychosis in cocaine-dependent patients. Eur Psychiatry. 28(3): 141–146.

Ruttenber, A.J., McAnally, H.B. and Wetli, C.V. 1999. Cocaine-associated rhabdomyolysis and excited delirium: Different stages of the same syndrome. Am J Forensic Med Pathol. 20: 120–127.

SAMHSA. 2014. Results from the 2013 National Survey on Drug Use and Health: Summary of national findings, NSDUH Series H-48, HHS Publication No (SMA) 14-4863. Rockville, MD: Substance Abuse and Mental Health Services Administration.

Schaumburg, H.H. and Spencer, P.S., eds. 2000. *Experimental and Clinical Neurotoxicology*, 2nd ed. New York: Oxford University Press.

Sharkey, J., Glen, K.A., Wolfe, S. and Kuhar, M.J. 1988b. Cocaine binding at sigma receptors. Eur J Pharmacol. 149: 171–174.

Sharkey, J., Ritz, M.C., Schenden, J.A., Hanson, R.C. and Kuhar, M.J. 1988a. Cocaine inhibits muscarinic cholinergic receptors in heart and brain. J Pharmacol Exp Ther. 246: 1048–1052.

Sherer, M.A., Kumor, R.A., Cone, E.J. and Jaffe, J.H. 1989. Suspiciousness induced by four-hour intravenous infusions of cocaine: Preliminary findings. Arch Gen Psychiatry. 45: 1152.

Siegel, R.K. 1978. Cocaine hallucinations. Am J Psychiatry. 135: 309.

Siegel, R.K. 1982. Cocaine smoking. J Psychoactive Drugs. 14: 271.

Siegel, R.K. 1987. Cocaine use and driving behavior. Alcohol Drug Driv. 3: 1.

Staley, J.K., Wetli, C.V., Ruttenbar, A.J., Hearn, W.L. and Mash, D.C. 1995. Altered dopaminergic synaptic markers in cocaine psychosis and sudden death: In: *Problems of Drug Dependence 1994—Proceedings of the 56th Annual Scientific Meeting: The College on Problems of Drug Dependence, Inc., Vol II—Abstract: NIDA Research Monograph Series 153*. Rockville, MD: Department of Health and Human Services, p. 491.

Tang, Y., Martin, N.L. and Cotes, R.O. 2014. Cocaine-induced psychotic disorders: Presentation, mechanism, and management. J Dual Diagn. 10(2): 98–105.

Torregrossa, M.M., Corlett, P.R. and Taylor, J.R. 2011. Aberrant learning and memory in addiction. Neurobiol Learn Mem. 96(4): 609–623.

Weddington, W.W., Brown, B.S., Haertzen, C.A., Cone, E.J., Dax, E.M., Herning, R.I. and Michaelson, B.S. 1990. Changes in mood, craving, and sleep during short-term abstinence reported by male cocaine addicts: A controlled residential study. Arch Gen Psychiatr. 47: 861–868.

Weitli, C.V. and Fishbain, D.A. 1985. Cocaine-induced psychosis and sudden death in recreational cocaine users. J Forensic Sci. 30: 873.

36 Marijuana
Pharmacology, Toxicology, and Forensic Issues

Stephanie E. Tedford, James T. O'Donnell, and James J. O'Donnell III

The authors would like to thank John P. Bederka, Jr. (Ph.D.) (deceased) for his past contributions to this chapter in prior editions of the book.

SYNOPSIS

DOI: 10.1201/9781003615323-40

36.1 INTRODUCTION

Marijuana (cannabis) is the third most-used addictive drug in the United States following tobacco and alcohol use.[1] In 2020, approximately 49.6 million people aged 12 and older reported using marijuana in the previous year, and 5.1% (14.2 million people) met the criteria for a marijuana use disorder.[2] Despite its widespread use, the legality of its use presents with confusion and challenges across the nation. Over 50% of states have reformed their marijuana laws by allowing medical marijuana use, reducing legal ramifications with regard to marijuana possession, and by making marijuana recreationally available for adult use. The majority of Americans support making marijuana use legal and overwhelmingly support allowing medical marijuana use. Consequently, lawmakers are increasingly realizing that the public is open to marijuana policy reforms. As such, marijuana legality continues to gain acceptance in a number of state legislatures, and supporters promise more to follow. Recreational use is gaining legal acceptance at a slower pace than medical use. Marijuana is still illegal at the federal level as a Schedule I drug under the federal Controlled Substances Act. However, states continue to take action to legalize marijuana medically and recreationally through state-invoked legislation and ballot initiatives.

Medical marijuana may be prescribed as a treatment for a variety of medical conditions including neuropathic pain, Parkinson's disease, nausea and vomiting related to chemotherapy, anxiety disorder and depression, sleep disorders, Tourette's syndrome, and Crohn's disease.[3] Those presenting with a qualifying condition are able to obtain medical marijuana prescriptions in the 36 states and 4 territories in the United States that allow it. The laws surrounding medical marijuana vary by state, including which medical conditions qualify for its use.

36.2 FEDERAL LAW VERSUS STATE LAW

A conflict exists between federal and state regulation of marijuana. State laws may allow the use of marijuana for medicinal or recreational purposes; however, federal law does not. Though many states have approved marijuana for medical use, at the federal level, marijuana remains classified as a Schedule I substance under the Controlled Substances Act. As such, marijuana as a Schedule I substance is considered to have a high potential for dependency and no accepted medical use, making the distribution of marijuana a federal offense. Due to conflicting legislation between federal and state law, residents may find themselves using marijuana in compliance with state law while simultaneously violating the federal law.

California paved the way for medicinal use of marijuana by becoming the first state to legalize medical marijuana in 1996. California released on the ballot the California Proposition 215, also known as the Medical Marijuana Initiative. This would later be termed the "Compassionate Use Act" and was approved on November 5, 1996, with 55.58% approval of the vote. This act exempted patients and authorized caregivers in possession of marijuana for medical treatment (as recommended by a physician) from criminal laws prohibiting its possession. Following California's passage of the Compassionate Use Act, Raich and Monson[4] were charged with and found guilty under Federal DEA laws at the time. The Defendant sued the US Attorney General arguing that Congress had exceeded their interstate commerce clause authority in legislating the behavior of a local citizen, consuming a locally grown herb in her own home. The issue in the case was whether Congress can regulate homegrown medical marijuana consumed at home pursuant to the interstate commerce clause. The Court upheld the law, deciding that Congress' Commerce Clause authority includes the power to prohibit the local cultivation and use of marijuana in compliance with California law. Congress may regulate intrastate activity where the behavior, in the aggregate, can impact interstate commerce. The court should not necessarily look for a substantial impact but should only require that a "plausible story" be told to uphold congressional action pursuant to the Commerce Clause. The plausible story in this case is that the federal government cannot rightly distinguish between marijuana grown in one's own home and the marijuana sold in interstate commerce (clearly a constitutionally authorized regulation, according to the Court). In order to regulate the latter, Congress must be able to regulate the former (grown in one's own home). The full case opinion is openly available.[5]

In October of 2009, the Obama Administration sent a memo to federal prosecutors encouraging them not to prosecute people who distribute marijuana for medical purposes in accordance with state law. In August 2013, the U.S. Department of Justice (USDOJ) announced an update to their marijuana enforcement policy. While marijuana remains illegal federally, the USDOJ expects states which have legalized marijuana to create "strong, state-based enforcement efforts . . . and will defer the right to challenge their legalization laws at this time." The department also reserves the right to challenge the states at any time they feel it necessary.[6]

Federal law enforcement would instead focus efforts on the following:

- Revenue that appears to fund violence and gangs
- Distribution of marijuana to minors
- Interstate transportation of marijuana to states where it is illegal
- Money laundering
- Violence and firearm use in growing or distribution of marijuana
- Driving under the influence and/or other public health consequences of using marijuana, and
- Marijuana possession or use on federal property

In 2018, the USDOJ terminated this policy under new presidential administration and announced that federal prosecutors can pursue criminal cases whenever state and federal marijuana laws collide.

36.2.1 Harrison Narcotics Tax Act

The first meaningful federal law enacted to regulate and tax opioids and coca products was the Harrison Narcotics Tax Act (Ch. 1, 38 Stat. 785). The Act was proposed by Rep. Francis Burton Harris of New York and was approved on December 17, 1914. The Act regulated and taxed the production, importation, and distribution of opiates and coca products (from which cocaine is extracted).

The Act provided for the

> [R]egistration of, with collectors of internal revenue, and to impose a special tax upon all persons who produce, import, manufacture, compound, deal in, dispense, sell, distribute, or give away opium or coca leaves, their salts, derivatives, or preparations, and for other purposes.

The courts interpreted this to mean that physicians could prescribe narcotics to patients in the course of normal treatment but not for the treatment of addiction.

36.2.2 Comprehensive Drug Abuse Control and Prevention Act

In 1970, the Harrison Narcotics Act was superseded when Congress enacted the Comprehensive Drug Abuse Prevention and Control Act of 1970 and repealed the Harrison Narcotics Act of 1916 and its 1965 amendment. The Comprehensive Drug Abuse Prevention and Control Act of 1970, commonly referred to as the Controlled Substances Act (CSA) of 1970 (1), set forth a uniform system of classifying all drugs with a potential for abuse and (2) required registration and recordkeeping sufficiently detailed to provide an accurate accounting of the distribution of such drugs by the registrant.

According to the Comprehensive Drug Abuse Prevention and Control Act of 1970, scheduled drugs are assigned to one of four categories (often called classes or schedules), which are labeled with a capital letter C followed by a Roman numeral, e.g., C-I, C-II, C-III, or C-IV or an encircling of the schedule number.

According to the Controlled Substances Act (CSA) of 1970, Schedule I drugs have no accepted medical use, have the greatest potential for abuse, and even when used under medical supervision, the drug lacks an acceptable level of safety.

Schedule I

A. The drug or other substance has a high potential for abuse,
B. The drug of other substance has no currently accepted medical use in treatment in the United States,
C. There is a lack of accepted safety for the use of the drug or other substance under medical supervision.

Schedule I is the class in which both heroin and marijuana were placed. According to the federal system, marijuana is still a Schedule I drug, despite its reclassification to a lower schedule in states that have approved marijuana for medical and recreational use.

Other Schedule I drugs include:

- LSD (lysergic acid diethylamide)
- Mescaline
- Ecstasy (MDMA—methylenedimethoxymethamphetamine)
- Date rape drugs: E.g., gamma-hydroxybutyrate (GHB); a medical GHB product has been approved by the FDA for the treatment of narcolepsy. Accordingly, this GHB product [sodium oxybate (Xyrem), a sodium salt of GHB] is Schedule III.[7]
- Rohypnol ® (flunitrazepam), a potent hypnotic benzodiazepine that is not marketed in the United States, is classified as a C-IV drug in Massachusetts. However, penalties for possession and dealing are similar to heroin (considered "Class A" narcotics). At least eight other states classify flunitrazepam as C-I.

36.2.3 Marijuana Drug Laws at the State Level

As of May 18, 2021, 36 states and 4 territories allowed for the medicinal use of marijuana products. As of November 29, 2021, 18 states, 2 territories, and the District of Columbia have enacted legislation to regulate marijuana for nonmedical use.[8] There are a number of different options available to a state that wishes to make marijuana available to patients for medical purposes. These policies, described below, include:

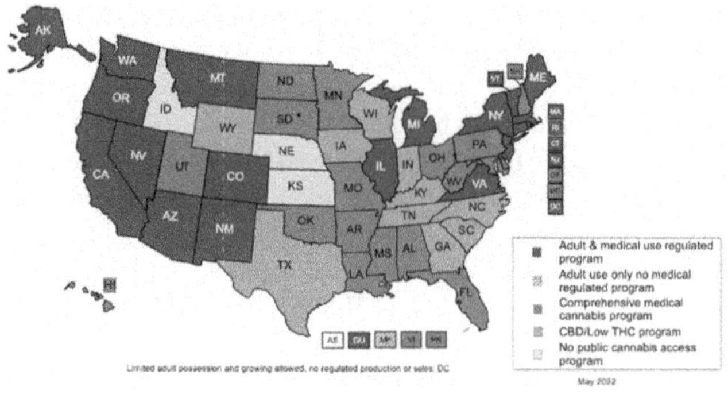

FIGURE 36.1 State-Regulated Cannabis Programs.

*** = Measures approved by voters in Mississippi for medical use and South Dakota for non medical use were overturned in 2021. The Mississippi legislature passed new medical cannabis legislation which the governor signed on Feb. 2, 2022.**
Please see Table 1 below for more information.

1. Legalization,
2. Decriminalization,
3. Controlled prescribing and distribution for medical purposes only, and
4. Unregulated use of marijuana for recreational purposes.

The geographic distribution of marijuana legal status, e.g., legalization, decriminalization, medical marijuana, or recreational marijuana, is shown in Figure 36.1.

36.2.4 Legalization

Legalization refers to the possession of marijuana that cannot be prosecuted or punished by state law. The fact that the substance is legal does not mean the person cannot be prosecuted for crimes related to being impaired by the drug. Nor does it permit them to smoke marijuana in the streets or in restaurants, bars, or public places where cigarette smoking is permitted. It simply means that if law enforcement catches an individual in possession or use of marijuana, he or she cannot be prosecuted under state law.

The marijuana plant may contain 400 or more cannabinoid derivatives.[9] Only some of these derivatives are psychoactive so some states have enacted specialized laws which permit the use of the nonpsychoactive cannabinoid, cannabidiol (CBD), which is shown to be clinically effective for medical use in patients with intractable seizures or epilepsy.[10]

Utah is one state that has passed this type of law in 2014. The law, HB 105, known as "Charlee's Law" was signed by Utah Gov. Gary Herbert on March 21, 2014. "Charlee's Law" allowed for the use and possession of marijuana extract (CBD only), under certain conditions, by people with intractable epilepsy who have a statement signed by a neurologist. The CBD-containing extract must contain less than 0.3% THC, must have at least 15% CBD by weight, and may not contain any of the psychoactive substances. The law went into effect on July 1, 2014. The CBD medicinal extract must be obtained in a sealed container from a laboratory that is licensed by the state where it was produced with a label stating the extracts ingredients and origin. The program is monitored by the Utah Department of Health.

Some will recall that Dr. Sanjay Gupta on CNN featured this little girl, Charlee, on several of his TV shows and demonstrated how her seizures and limb movements stopped after she received the CBD extract.[11] Some parents with children with seizure disorders, who were not able to obtain CBD legally, moved to another state so their child could benefit from more progressive laws regarding CBD use.

In 2018, 53% of Utah voters approved the Medical Cannabis Act which allows the use of marijuana for select medical conditions. Recreational use of marijuana is not legal, and marijuana possession is not decriminalized.[12]

36.2.5 Decriminalization

Decriminalization differs from legalization from the perspective that people who use marijuana can be punished under state law but only by some means other than imprisonment. Under the new enforcement, some without any changes in any law, typically, offenders receive a violation similar to a traffic ticket and may have to pay a fine.[13] In Massachusetts, individuals in possession of one ounce or less of marijuana can be cited by law enforcement and required to pay a fine of $100.

36.2.6 Marijuana Policy Project

The Marijuana Policy Project (MPP) is an organization dedicated to changing federal law to allowing states to determine their own marijuana policies without federal interference.[14] The MPP has been integral to the enactment of medical marijuana laws, and it has run winning campaigns and legislative efforts in many now legalized states. The MPP has released a new report on tax revenue generated from state-legal, adult-use marijuana since 2014 when sales began in Colorado and Washington state. As of December 2021, states reported a combined total of $10.4 billion in tax revenue from legal, adult-use marijuana sales highlighting the significant impact of revenue on legal marijuana sales.[15]

36.3 CONTROLLED PRESCRIPTION AND DISTRIBUTION OF MEDICAL MARIJUANA

The simplest legal way of obtaining smoke-able or edible marijuana products for medical purposes is by obtaining an authorization from a doctor. A patient either requests an authorization for medical marijuana from their primary care physician or other healthcare provider or can make an appointment to see a physician who specializes in providing authorizations for medical marijuana. If the patient goes to see a physician who has not been caring for them, but specializes in prescribing medical marijuana, the patient brings his or her medical records and documentation of his/her

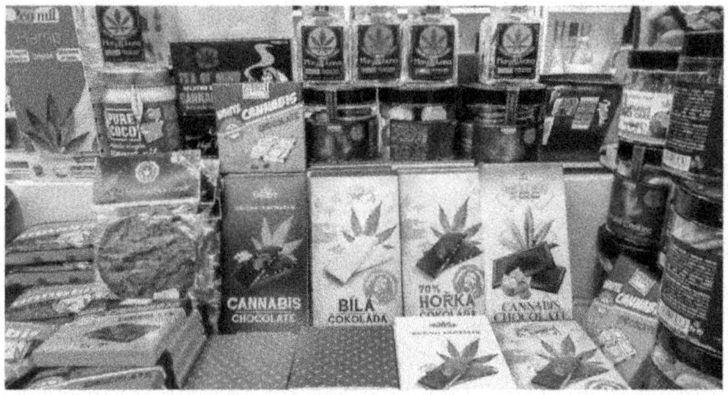

FIGURE 36.2 Edible Marijuana Products.

diagnosed condition and requests the prescribing physician to issue the required authorization for medical marijuana. Proof of the physician prescription and registration with the state's medical marijuana registry are commonly necessary to access medical marijuana from a dispensary which is licensed by the state. Once approved, patients have access to a variety of marijuana products including oral solutions, topical creams or applications, pills, oils for vaporizing, dried-out leaves for smoking, and sprays (Figure 36.2). In states where recreational use is legal, customers can also obtain products from these licensed venues.

The patient does not go to a pharmacy to obtain marijuana. Instead, the patient goes to a licensed marijuana dispensary which is regulated by the state and is entitled to sell marijuana products to a patient in possession of a valid authorization from a physician or other licensed healthcare provider.

36.3.1 Medical Conditions Approved for Treatment with Medical Marijuana

The types of conditions approved for treatment with medi cal marijuana vary from state to state. However, there is a similarity among many of the states, and a core group of conditions are often listed in the states' statute. For the most part, the logical categories for the medical use of marijuana are not based on particular diseases so much as symptoms of conditions—such as pain, nausea and vomiting, appetite stimulation, increased intraocular pressure in glaucoma, and for neurological symptoms including muscle spasticity.

The Institute of Medicine (IOM) study team received reports of more than 30 different medical uses of marijuana. For most of the infrequently mentioned medical uses of marijuana, there are only a few anecdotal reports.[16] This report[17] acknowledges the potential benefits of smoking marijuana in stimulating appetite, particularly in patients with AIDS, wasting syndrome, chemotherapy-induced nausea and vomiting, severe pain, and some forms of spasticity.

In Alaska, approved conditions include cachexia, cancer, chronic pain, epilepsy, and other disorders characterized by seizures. Glaucoma, HIV or AIDS, multiple sclerosis, and other disorders characterized by muscle spasticity are also included. Nausea, as a result of chemotherapy, is a common symptom included in a state's list of treatable conditions. Connecticut has added Parkinson's disease; damage to the nervous tissue of the spinal cord with objective neurological indication of intractable spasticity; Crohn's disease; post-traumatic stress disorder (PTSD); or any medical condition, medical treatment, or disease approved by the Department of Consumer Protection. Delaware includes decompensated cirrhosis (hepatitis C), Lou Gehrig's disease (ALS), and Alzheimer's disease. The conditions mentioned in this section are just examples of what a few states have included in their statutes and are not meant to comprise an exhaustive list.

Supporting scientific evidence and comprehensive data for marijuana's efficacy across various medical conditions is lacking. An analysis of state registry data provides nationwide estimates on qualifying conditions for which patients are licensed to use medical marijuana. Chronic pain remains the most common condition reported (67.5% of patients). Registry data also suggests that 85.5% of patient-reported qualifying conditions had either substantial or conclusive evidence of treatment efficacy. As medical marijuana use continues to increase, nationwide patient registries will assist in furthering our understanding of use trends, safety, and efficacy data.[18]

In 2017, a comprehensive review of the literature was undertaken by the Committee of Health Effects of Marijuana of the National Academy of Sciences, Engineering, and Medicine (NASEM) to evaluate the strength of evidence, supporting the use of cannabinoids as medical treatment for various diseases.[19] The report concluded that there was "conclusive or substantial evidence that cannabis or cannabinoids are effective" for treatment of the following conditions: Chronic pain, chemotherapy-induced nausea/vomiting if refractory to other antiemetics, and spasticity (as reported by patient) in multiple sclerosis. They concluded that there was moderate evidence that can nabis/cannabinoids improve sleep outcomes in those with sleep disturbance associated with obstructive sleep apnea, fibromyalgia, chronic pain, and multiple sclerosis. Among other conditions in which cannabinoids have been claimed to be beneficial, there was insufficient or no evidence supporting their use for treatment of the following conditions: Cancer, anorexia and weight loss associated with HIV, irritable bowel syndrome, epilepsy, Tourette's Syndrome, ALS, Huntington's disease, Parkinson's disease, dystonia, dementia, glaucoma, traumatic brain injury, addiction, anxiety, depression, sleep disorders, PTSD, schizophrenia, and other psychoses. Since this report was issued, a cannabinoid (cannabidiol—Epidiolex) was approved for the treatment of seizures in a small subset of seizure-inducing conditions (see Section "Marijuana and Epilepsy"). Clearly, claims that marijuana is a panacea are unwarranted or at least premature.

36.3.2 Marijuana and Epilepsy

Mounting anecdotal evidence, preclinical data, and mechanistic insights support the interest in cannabinoids as a treatment for epilepsy. The stratospheric rise of medical marijuana highlights the sharing of personal stories on the internet and social media, according to a leading expert in the field. Daniel Friedman, MD, New York University (NYU) Langone School of Medicine, is a coauthor of, "Cannabinoids in the Treatment of Epilepsy," published in the September 10, 2015 issue of *The New England Journal of Medicine*.[20] In this review article, the author identifies cannabidivarin as the propyl variant of the cannabinoid—cannabidiol. It emphasized the anti-seizure effects of cannabidivarin, noting,

> Like cannabidiol, cannabidivarin has anti-seizure effects that are independent of the endocannabinoid system and may function by means of its influence on TRP (transient receptor potential) channels or by lowering 2-AG (2-arachidonoylglycerol) synthesis through the inhibition of DAGL-α (diacylglycerol lipase alpha).[21]

In an interview conducted by *Medscape*,[22] Friedman commented,

> It is a very interesting mix of science, politics, and social phenomena which has moved medical marijuana to the forefront of treatment for severe drug-resistant epilepsy/ Two years ago the epilepsy community wasn't really seriously considering this as an option. But it has now really taken off.

Dr. Friedman noted that the idea that marijuana may be useful for epilepsy has been around for centuries.

> It was used medicinally in ancient China and by Victorian neurologists for seizures, but it has never been properly scientifically studied. That is now happening. This has come about because individuals have shared anecdotal experiences about its effectiveness in children with severe intractable epilepsy on the Internet and these have spread across the globe.

Friedman added, "Once it became 'out there,' families have been clamoring for access to the product and we have had to pay attention. That is why medical marijuana is being legalized and studies are finally being done."

In the review, the authors caution that it is of the utmost importance that science be backed by double-blind, randomized studies. They write,

> The use of medical cannabis for the treatment of epilepsy could go the way of vitamin and nutritional supplements, for which the science never caught up to the hype and was drowned out by unverified claims, sensational testimonials, and clever marketing.[23]

In 2013, Epidiolex (cannabidiol) was the first CBD product to be evaluated in a phase I clinical trial which showed positive efficacy outcomes. Subsequent randomized controlled trials showed significant improvements in efficacy, safety, and tolerability outcomes for the treatment of drug-resistant epilepsies. Positive results of these trials led to the drug's 2018 and 2019 FDA and EMA approval. Epidiolex is the only FDA-approved CBD product. It is approved for the treatment of seizures associated with Lennox–Gastaut syndrome (LGS), Dravet syndrome, or tuberous sclerosis complex (TSC) in patients one year of age and older.[24]

36.3.3 Marijuana and Endometriosis

Pain management has long been a condition for which marijuana has been utilized as a treatment. Endometriosis is a reproductive disease of women characterized by infertility, reproductive failure, and chronic pain. Information on the use and effectiveness of marijuana against endometriotic pain is lacking; however, a recent study suggests its benefit. Expression of cannabinoid receptors 1 and 2 (CB1 and CB2) were detected in the epithelial cells in ovarian endometriotic lesions. These findings suggest that ovarian endometriotic lesions expressing CB1 and CB2 receptors may respond to cannabinoids as pain medication. Further foundational studies are necessary to determine the efficacy.[25]

36.4 PHARMACOLOGICAL PROPERTIES OF MARIJUANA

36.4.1 Active Compounds and Overview of Pharmacology

Ingestion of marijuana (leaves and flowering tops) or ganja (resin) results in an intoxication characterized by sedation, cognitive dysfunction, failure to consolidate short-term memory, alteration in time assessment, perceptual changes, motor incoordination, and poor executive function.

Marijuana (cannabis) contains over 400 chemical components, of which, more than 60 are cannabinoid compounds.[26] Cannabinoids exert their effects by binding to cannabinoid receptors in the central and peripheral nervous system. The most common receptors include the CB1 and CB2 receptors. CB1 is widely expressed throughout the body, including the Central Nervous System (CNS) and Peripheral Nervous System.[27] CB2 is primarily expressed on immunomodulatory cells, and in disease states, CB2 expression is upregulated in microglia in the CNS.[28] Most of the physiological effects attributed to marijuana work through the stimulation of the CB1 receptor, including euphoria, cognitive impairment, and tachycardia. Among cannabinoid compounds, delta-9-tetrahydrocannabinol (THC) and cannabidiol (CBD) remain the most well known. THC is the main psychoactive ingredient in marijuana known for producing dose-dependent psychotropic effects. CBD is not a psychoactive compound and thus does not produce any psychotropic effects commonly associated with marijuana. In contrast, CBD displays anticonvulsant, anxiolytic, and antipsychotic effects making it a compound of interest for further exploration in many medical conditions for clinical benefit.[29,30]

A recent review on CBD revealed only eight publications which report pharmacokinetic parameters after administering CBD on its own and only one study on the bioavailability of CBD in humans.[31] These papers came to the following conclusions:

1. CBD peak plasma concentrations are dose-dependent and show minimal accumulation
2. Cmax is increased and reached faster following IV smoking or inhalation
3. Cmax is increased and reached faster after oral administration in a fed state or in a pro-nanolipo-sphere formulation
4. Tmax does not appear to be dose-dependent
5. Half-life depends on dose and route of administration

Overall, considerable variation was noted among the CBD studies highlighting the need for further research. Continued discussions on marijuana pharmacology will place the focus on THC as more pharmacologic evidence exists.

As with most drugs, the effects of marijuana vary depending upon the potency of the marijuana and the route of administration (e.g., smoking versus vaporizing versus oral ingestion). Almost immediately after smoking, there is a rapid increase in the plasma levels of THC, followed by a rapid decline. This decline is due to a redistribution of the THC from the plasma into a peripheral storage compartment for lipophilic drugs. The THC is rapidly metabolized to the psychoactive 11-OH-THC metabolite, which is further metabolized to the inactive compound THC-COOh (acid). THC-COOH appears in both blood and urine and is usually the compound targeted in urine drug screens for marijuana.

36.4.2 Variability in Marijuana Regulation and Content Uniformity

Over the past few decades, increasing marijuana potency has been observed. Marijuana potency is proportional to THC content. Hybridization of plant species, processing of marijuana plants, and preparation techniques have led to the development of available products containing higher levels of THC. Current commercialized products may contain 20–40% THC, while in the 1980s, concentration was less than 2%. This 10–20-fold increase in potency does not include other formulations such as oils, waxes, and dabs, which can reach 80–90% THC.[32,33] This increase in the potency is also due to changes to the ratio between the two primary components (THC and CBD) toward a higher proportion of THC and may contribute to increased associations of psychiatric events linked to marijuana use.

The unregulated manufacturing of drugs may lead to the inclusion of other various pharmacologically active compounds, in addition to the target substance. An adulterant is a substance found within other compounds such as pharmaceuticals, which compromises the safety or effectiveness of the compound. Adulterants can impose a wide range of toxic effects when ingested alone or in combination with other drugs. The presence of these adulterants in drugs contributes to the complexity of understanding the precise pharmacological and safety profiles. Identifying adulterants is complicated by analysis limitations as most commercially available toxicology analyses identify only a limited number of known adulterants in drug samples. Consequently, adulterants often go undetected, and their presence tends to be underreported or unknown.[34]

THC and CBD-containing products purchased legally in the United States may contain harmful substances. It is difficult to know product specifics as full ingredient lists are typically not available. This is even more ambiguous in products purchased illegally or from unknown sources. The marijuana concentrate hashish has an extensive history of containing adulterants. A recent analysis of hashish in Madrid found that 18% of products show contamination with glucose, sucrose, and/or abietic acid (a principal component of pine rosin).[35] Pine rosin has also been identified as a hashish adulterant in Italy, Israel, and the Czech Republic. Pine rosin (colophony) has been identified as a potentially new adulterant in marijuana oil. Its significant inhalation toxicity poses a significant health concern to users. Pine rosin is typically used as an ingredient in industrial products such as varnishes, adhesives, soldering fluxes, and sealing wax. Due to the significant toxicity, adulterated marijuana oil is of concern to the health status of users.[36]

Commercially available e-liquid formulations are not regulated by the FDA and have been shown to contain inaccurate dosing and product specifics that differ from labeling. For example, an evaluation of two commercial CBD e-liquids showed that they contained 3.3 mg/mL of CBD as the active ingredient. These products were found to contain 6.5 and 7.6 mg/mL of CBD in propylene glycol and vegetable glycerin with a variety of flavoring agents. In an evaluation of nine CBD-labeled e-liquids, THC, synthetic cannabinoid 5F-ADB, and dextromethorphan (DXM) were also found. All the e-liquids were determined to contain CBD. Upon substance analysis, two contained THC, four contained 5F-ADB, and one contained DXM. The synthetic cannabinoid 5-fluoro MDMB-PINACA (5F-ADB) is a cannabimimetic that has psychoactive effects similar to THC through the activation of CB1 and/or CB2 receptors. 5F-ADB has been linked to clinical intoxications after smoking of "Spice" or "herbal preparations" in which subjects presented with anxiety, confusion, psychomotor agitation, psychosis, and tachycardia.[37] In 2014, 5F-ADB was linked to 2,311 incidents involving medical intervention or death which resulted in a drug status change to a Schedule I drug designation in 2017. Dextromethorphan (DXM) is an antitussive, or cough suppressing, medication with known abuse liability. DXM is associated with agitation, ataxia, hypertonic, and sedation and may produce dissociative hallucinations at high doses.

Other studies have similarly reported inaccuracies in labeling and additions of other substances in CBD e-liquids.[38,39] An evaluation of 84 CBD products yielded a wide range of CBD concentrations inconsistent with product labeling. In the analysis, THC was detected in 18 of the 84 samples tested, cannabidiolic acid in 13 of the 84 samples tested, and cannabigerol (CBG) in 2 of the 84 samples tested.[40] Inaccurate dose specifications and the addition of other chemical substances in e-liquids (e.g., THC, 5F-ADB and DXM) further demonstrate quality control issues that occur in an unregulated market and can impact significantly on user health outcomes.[41]

36.4.3 Routes of Administration

Marijuana can be taken by smoking and sublimation through a vaporizer; by sublingual or buccal administration; by extraction into lipophilic solvents and subsequent ingestion; or by ingestion of marijuana-infused baked goods, candy, or liquids. Vaporizers or "Vapes" have become popular, which include pyramid pens, a selected type of vaping tool. Both vaping and pyramid pens heat marijuana to a point where it vaporizes or sublimes into a gaseous form; it can then be collected in a cellophane bag on top of the pyramid or inhaled from a vape. Less smoke is produced, and the potential to inhale only THC vapor instead of smoke from the entire plant is desirable.

Smoking has historically been the gold standard for ingestion of marijuana. However, after the identification of the cannabinoids as the principal unique chemicals in marijuana, objective scientific studies related to marijuana became a reality. In the last 60 years, extraction and identification methodologies for very small amounts of chemicals in diverse specimens have been developed. The published reports of such efforts have afforded tentative dose-response information relative to drugs in general and cannabinoids in particular. Even though most interest in marijuana use has focused on the legality of recreational marijuana use, some early studies in the 1970s referred to human health conditions such as epilepsy as possible therapeutic avenues for marijuana and cannabinoids. Even in consideration of positive avenues for cannabinoid-related therapies, the primary difficulty was that smoking was not usually the desired route for administration for medicinal use. Thus, for about 50 years, the literature on the oral route for the administration of cannabinoids has been accumulating.[42] Due to legalization and commercial efforts surrounding marijuana, actual and perceived use of the ingestion and oromucosal routes of marijuana-based products have seen an upswing.

36.4.4 Pharmacokinetics—Time Course of THC and Metabolites

Smoking of THC in marijuana produces very low blood levels of the active 11-OH-THC metabolite, which is rapidly converted to the inactive water-soluble acid THC-COOH. This acid subsequently appears in both blood and urine and is the compound that urine drug screens are testing for, not THC itself. THC in marijuana edibles or beverages is absorbed from the gastrointestinal tract, through the hepatic portal vein, and returned to the liver, where the THC is converted to the 11-OH-THC in far greater amounts than when marijuana is smoked. This difference in the route of administration leads to an accumulation of the active 11-OH-THC metabolite, which, in conjunction with THC, is most likely responsible for producing many of the psychotomimetic effects associated with the oral ingestion of marijuana, which cause users to go to the emergency room or require acute psychiatric care.[43]

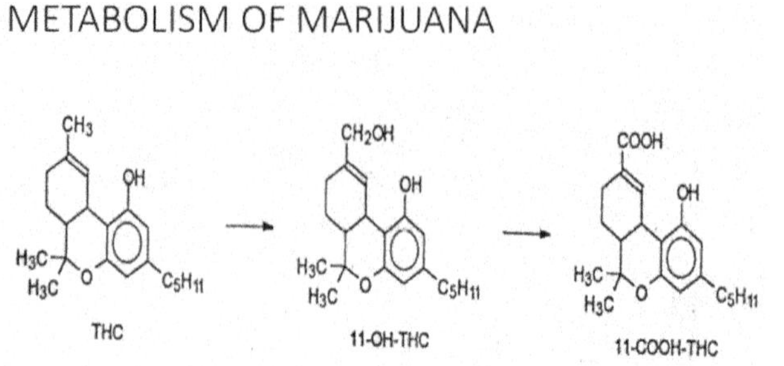

FIGURE 36.3 Marijuana Structural Composition and Metabolism.

Figure 36.3 shows the chemical structures and metabolism of marijuana key cannabinoids. These and other cannabinoids may show additive and/or inhibitory effects by interacting at the diverse psychologic, physiologic, metabolic, and excretory processes. The addition of only one atom of oxygen changes THC into 11-hydroxy-THC, both of which are considered to be equally psychoactive. However, given the differences in plasma levels for perceived psychoactivity, 11-hydroxy-THC may be the more potent of the two. The further addition of oxygen to 11-hydroxy-THC produces the THC-COOH, which has no known psychoactivity and is the molecule found in the most abundance in the urine. After smoking marijuana for a few minutes, the brain is accumulating only THC for about five minutes, and then THC and 11-Hydroxy-THC plus other cannabinoids are present in the brain for minutes to hours during the experiencing of the "high" as shown in Table 36.1.

Despite the rapid increase in THC blood levels following the smoking of marijuana, there is a latency period before a subjective euphoric effect is experienced by the user. With the smoking of marijuana, a peak euphoric high is not experienced for approximately 0.2 hours (12 minutes). This most likely is due to the time required to distribute the THC from the blood into the central nervous system (CNS). In contrast to smoking, oral ingestion of marijuana requires a much longer time for absorption from the gastrointestinal track into the bloodstream, with subsequent distribution through the blood–brain barrier into the CNS. Moreover, oral ingestion involves absorption through the hepatic portal vein, with delivery of the THC to the liver and subsequent conversion to the active 11-OH-THC metabolite.[44]

TABLE 36.1
Time-Course of Plasma Cannabinoids.

Time (Minutes)	THC	11-Hydroxy-THC	8-Alpha-Hydroxy-THC	8-Beta-Hydroxy-THC	8,11-Dihydroxy-THC
4–5 mg IV					
5	33	0.8	0.26	0.8	0.3
15	51	2.3	0.34	1.8	0.6
30	36	2.8	0.79	2.2	1.0
60	12	1.7	0.70	1.8	1.0
90	8.6	1.4	0.68	1.3	1.0
20 mg PO (Orally)					
60	3.8	3.4	–	–	2.0
90	5.7	4.7	–	–	3.8
120	4.3	7.2	–	–	6.0
180	7.1	8.5	–	–	6.7

Plasma levels are in nanograms/milliliters (ng/mL)[45]

36.4.5 Pharmacodynamics

Acute intoxication from marijuana is related to both the dose of THC and the route of administration, the latter of which may affect the peak concentration. THC is absorbed more rapidly from marijuana smoking than from orally ingested marijuana compounds. THC stimulates the CB1 and CB2 receptors, although CB1 is the receptor mediating the most clinically observable CNS effects such as intoxication, euphoria, and cognitive impairment as well as peripheral physiological effects such as tachycardia. Acute marijuana intoxication may produce a perception of relaxation and mild euphoria resembling mild-to-moderate alcohol intoxication. This condition is usually accompanied by some impairment in thinking, concentration, and perceptual and psychomotor function. Higher doses of marijuana may produce more pronounced impairment in concentration and perception, as well as greater sedation. Although the acute effects of marijuana intoxication are relatively benign in normal users, the drug can precipitate severe emotional disorders in individuals who have antecedent psychotic or neurotic problems. Like other psychoactive compounds, both the user's expectations and the environmental context are important determinants of the type and severity of the effects of marijuana intoxication. Chronic users may develop significant tolerance to THC.

36.4.6 Vaping versus Traditional Smoking of Cannabinoids

Technology advancements have led to widespread use of modified electronic cigarettes and unregulated black-market devices to ingest or "vape" nicotine and other drugs like THC. Vaping THC has become popular due to its convenience (e.g., less conspicuous, odorless, ease of use) compared to traditional means of smoking THC. Vaping is also associated with less toxicant exposure (e.g., polycyclic aromatic hydrocarbons) compared to traditional smoking, further increasing the product appeal.[46] However, this method presents novel health concerns including reports of vaping-related lung injuries and increased psychiatric issues. Recent CDC investigations into unexplained vaping-related deaths in the United States highlight how the direct effects of vaping substances versus traditional methods do not run in parallel.

Vaporizers heat concentrated marijuana extracts and/or resins, creating an inhalable aerosol or vapor.[47] Electronic liquids (e-liquids) are formulations used in e-cigarettes or vaporizers, which contain a combination of propylene glycol and vegetable glycerin, the pharmaceutical compound, and typically a flavoring agent. When the e-cigarette is activated, the e-liquid is vaporized, followed by a rapid condensation into an aerosol which is inhaled by the user.[48] The CDC and FDA do not recommend using THC-containing e-cigarettes or vaping products, especially from unregulated sources such as friends, family, or in-person or online dealers.

Several studies directly comparing the acute effects of smoked and vaporized marijuana have generally revealed similar pharmacokinetic profiles. Limitations of these studies include single THC doses, low THC concentrations (1.7%–6.9% THC), small sample sizes, and/or use of uniform smoking protocols that may be inconsistent with realistic profiles and do not account for individual differences impacting on dose delivery. Furthermore, the impact on cognitive and psychomotor impairment has not been systematically evaluated. Spindle et al. evaluated the pharmacological profiles of smoked versus vaporized marijuana in healthy adults. Multiple doses of THC were evaluated across inhalation methods in individuals with infrequent marijuana use patterns. A comprehensive test battery (i.e., subjective drug effects, cognitive and psychomotor performance, and vital signs) was performed. Vaping resulted in significantly higher plasma THC compared to smoking groups. Higher plasma THC was positively correlated with subjective experience, which was increased in the vaping group. Vaping was found to elicit significantly higher paranoia ratings, with similar findings in regard to cognitive impairment. At a THC dose equivalent, this study suggests that vaporizers are a more efficient marijuana and THC delivery method, likely because with traditional smoked preparations, more THC is lost as a result of pyrolysis (combustion) and/or side stream smoke.[49] Therefore, inhaling marijuana through a vaporizer could produce a more pronounced drug effect and impairment than traditional smoking methods. Another recent study also reports that vaping produces greater neurotoxicity versus smoking following acute exposure.[50]

The use of CBD in electronic cigarettes is also widespread. CBD has increased in popularity as an effective treatment devoid of the psychoactive effects of THC. Previously, it was reported that CBD is only partially transformed to THC when consumed through cigarette smoking. Recent evaluation on the pyrolysis of CBD demonstrates a higher conversion to THC when ingested using an e-cigarette. One evaluation of the effect of temperature on the composition of pyrolysis in CBD products investigated product outputs in the operating temperature range of e-cigarettes under both inert and oxidative conditions. Depending on the temperature and atmosphere, 25–52% of CBD was transformed into other chemical substances including Δ9-THC, Δ8-THC, cannabinol, and cannabichromene. THC was the main pyrolysis product at all temperatures under both oxidative and inert conditions. Study findings show that CBD in e-cigarettes may be considered as a precursor of THC and therefore presents all consequences related to THC.[51]

36.4.7 Traditional Smoking versus Ingestion of Cannabinoids

Smoking marijuana, like smoking tobacco, causes local lung toxicity in and of itself, not related to the marijuana or tobacco. When something is burning and producing smoke, inhaling the smoke is logically considered to be harmful. Smoke is a product of combustion. Combustion produces carcinogenic hydrocarbons and hundreds of known toxins—marijuana smoke produces similar products.[52]

The respiratory and gastrointestinal routes for the administration of chemicals into the human body offer dramatic contrasts. Small molecules in the air are generally known to pass into the blood stream very quickly. Breathing is the best example of such a chemical exchange. Absorption from the GI tract, however, is quite another scenario. Time of transport differs between these two routes of administration. Thus, inhalation will produce blood levels of volatile chemicals within seconds to minutes. In fact, the blood in the lungs only has to pass through the left heart and up to the brain in seconds. Since the output from the heart traffics about 20% of the blood to the brain, rapid onset is the norm after inhalation exposures. Continued smoking of a marijuana cigarette thus affords the brain first choice of inhaled cannabinoids with about 50% of the blood first going to the liver (27%) and kidney (23%). Then, the recirculating blood affords more THC and new cannabinoids formed in the liver or other tissue sites.

In contrast, the absorption in the GI tract may require hours to produce significant blood levels of many chemicals. The reasons for this may include gastric emptying time, which depends on food in the stomach and other conditions. The digestion processes in the stomach and intestines may also alter the rate and amount of absorption. Even then, the chemicals must pass through the liver after entering the blood stream. The biotransformations in the liver both create and destroy large amounts of chemicals. The absorbed THC is thus subject to destruction (metabolism) in the liver. The new products of this metabolism are new cannabinoids such as 11-hydroxy-THC and other hydroxy-THCs that may have effects on the brain (psychoactivity) as shown in Figure 36.1.

36.4.8 Pharmacokinetics Applications: Timing of the Peak Euphoric Effect

As an example, consider the 15 minutes' time point and note the levels of each chemical in Table 36.1. The THC value seems to have peaked at about 50 ng/ml. None of the other hydroxylated metabolites of the THC molecule have reached their peak values. Thus, it seems quite logical that the feeling of some aspects of the "high" even during the first deep inhalation must be ascribed almost exclusively to the THC molecules impacting the brain. A more detailed evaluation of the above tabulations affords a molecular view of the effects of marijuana via smoking and IV routes versus the oral route. Thus, at five minutes, the THC level was at 33 ng/ml, whereas the other four cannabinoids were at a total of 2.16. Then at 60 minutes, the levels were THC at 12 versus 5.2 for smoking/IV and 3.8 versus 5.4 for ingestion; however, even at 90 minutes, the THC was the highest after the IV route. Then, at 90 minutes, the metabolites of THC were about equal to or higher than the THC levels after ingestion. These data comparisons allow relative changes whereby the molecules become more concentrated in the blood than the original THC. And several authors have stated that it is the metabolites with psychoactivity that are the agents of the "high" at about one to three hours post marijuana use.[53]

About two hours after ingestion of THC-products, the brain will be almost equally exposed to three or four cannabinoids due to the metabolism of the ingested THC (as noted before and in Table 36.2). Most importantly, this exposure may not begin for one to three hours after ingestion as noted in the time versus effects and plasma levels in Table 36.2. This summary tabulation clearly shows the distinguishing characteristics between the timing of the "high" after inhalation versus ingestion. Moreover, the tabulation affords

TABLE 36.2
Psychometrics after Cannabis Ingestion.

"High"	Smoking* (Minutes)	Ingestion* (Minutes)
Onset	0–10	30–120
Increasing	5–20	30–90
Plateau	15–30	130–300
Decreasing	45–180	60–240
Duration	60–240	240–600
Blood Testing Data		
THC/11-Hydroxy-THC Ratio at Onset	10–20 times	1.0–0.45 times
Cannabinoids Found in Plasma at Onset	THC 11-Hydroxy-THC	THC 11-Hydroxy-THC 8-Hydroxy-THCs 8,11-Dihydroxy-THC
Plasma Levels at Plateau (ng/mL)	THC: 100–200 11-Hydroxy-THC: 5–10	THC: 7.1 11-Hydroxy-THC: 8.5 Dihydroxy-THC: 6.7
Plasma Levels at 1 hour:	THC: 10–15 11-Hydroxy-THC: 3–5	Variable to none

**Source: Modified from EROWID March 24, 2014.*[54]
** Average values from products containing ~20 mg THC.*[55]

some blood testing data that allow a better appreciation of the user's marijuana-effect scenario. In this regard, the seemingly seminal data are for the plasma levels of the cannabinoids near the plateau phase, which may be described as the desired level of "high" for many persons. Thus, it is shown that the total of the plasma levels after both routes of assimilation are very nearly identical at one hour, namely, 13–18 ng/mL for inhalation and 22.3 ng/mL for ingestion. In neither of these conditions would the users be objectively considered impaired even with the plasma levels above 5 ng/mL but less than 30 ng/mL.

From this confluence of time-of-onset of effects and different cannabinoids in the blood during the perception of marijuana effects, as one source intimates, "it may be useful to think of oral marijuana as a different drug than smoked marijuana."[56] Most noteworthy in regard to this comparison of smoking versus ingestion is that the smoker can attain levels of THC up to 200 ng/mL within minutes of starting to smoke, but levels less than 30 ng/mL appear to be attainable via the oral route as noted in the earlier tabulation.

This difference in the cannabinoid levels while "high" is shown with the THC/11-hydroxy-THC ratio. Thus, only after a few minutes of smoking, the THC level is 10 to 20 times the level of 11-hydroxy-THC. However, after ingestion, the THC is less than one-half that of the 11-hydroxy-THC metabolite. Perhaps after reading this chapter, the perceptive reader will conclude that the specifics of assimilation via the different routes do have different objective behavioral consequences.[57]

36.4.9 Bioavailability

The bioavailability is the fraction of a dose which reaches systemic circulation. Table 36.3 presents the bioavailability data on THC from multiple dosage forms. The relatively low oral bioavailability of marijuana products is reflective of the many obstacles to entering the blood that the psychoactive cannabinoids encounter. This is reflected in the increased travel time of about 0.5 to 1.5 hours in oral administration compared with smoking with a travel time of seconds to minutes. Furthermore, given the known facts that the cannabinoids bind very strongly to proteins and are highly selective for fatty tissues, the very biology of the gastrointestinal tract interferes with the passage of the cannabinoids into the blood. This propensity for fatty tissue distribution is proportional to a physiological parameter known as the Volume of Distribution (V_d). Thus, alcohol which is water soluble has a V_d of 0.65 L/kg (45.5 L in a 70 kg individual), which corresponds approximately to the total body water. The V_d for THC is about 10 L/kg, or 700 L in a 70 kg individual. Since this volume exceeds the physical volume of the body, this indicates that there is significant sequestration of THC in peripheral compartments. Drugs with a high V_d are not usually well understood in terms of their effects when plasma level data are used in therapeutic drug-monitoring situations.[58] This V_d-related effect thus well explains the general lack of dose–response relationships with marijuana-related products.

36.4.9.1 Is There a Good Model for Marijuana Ingestion?

Dronabinol (THC, Marinol) may be the most researched of the drug products listed in the bioavailability comparisons noted earlier. Even with an absorption of 90 to 95% of the administered dose of THC, only about 10 20% eventually reaches the circulating blood. Furthermore, the diverse effects of this therapeutically available drug (THC, Marinol, Dronabinol) have been well-documented as both psychological and physiological. One source lists increased heart rate, reddening of the eyes, dry mouth and throat, increased appetite, and vasodilation as most frequently noted.[59] A listing of adverse effects is presented in Table 36.4.

This listing of 35 "events" may seem excessive and/or prejudicial, but similar listings are as follows: Xanax-46, Paxil-35, Cymbalta-30. Most critically, one must consider

TABLE 36.3
Bioavailability Data on THC from Dosage Forms.

Method	% Bioavailability
Smoking	2–56%
Ingestion	4–20%
Dronabinol (Marinol)	10–20%
Sativex (40% THC and 35% cannabidiol)	11–13%
Volcanos	36–61%

TABLE 36.4
Adverse Events after Dronabinol Ingestion.*

Incidence >10%		Incidence <1%
Asthenia	Aberrant thoughts	Conjunctivitis
Facial flush	Nervousness	Hypotension
Palpitations	Ataxis	Myalgias
Tachycardia	Confusion	Diarrhea
Vasodilation	Depersonalization	Fecal incontinence
Abdominal pain	Dizziness	Depression
Nausea	Euphoria	Nightmares
Vomiting	Hallucinations	Speech difficulty
Amnesia		Tinnitus
Paranoia		Flushing of skin/limbs
Somnolence		Vision difficulties
Overdose is Indicated by the Following		
Decreased motor coordination	Seizures	
Slurred speech	Postural hypotension	
Panic	Lethargy	

**Source:* PDR 2007.[60,61]

TABLE 36.5
Pharmacokinetics: Dronabinol in Fasting Persons.*

Twice Daily Dose (mg)	Plasma Levels ng/mL (SD)	Effect (Hours)
2.5	1.32 (0.62)	0.5–4.0
5	2.96 (1.81)	0.5–4.0
10	7.88 (4.54)	0.5–3.5
20 (extrapolated data)	17.0 (9.0 estimated.)	Unknown

**Source:* PDR 2007.[64,65]

that with all drugs, the concept of side effects is obfuscation since they all have multiple effects. A comprehensive listing of these effects is available at EROWID.com.[62] One precautionary event is described as the abstinence syndrome after dronabinol. This phenomenon was noted in a seemingly unique study at a dose of 210 mg/d for 12 to 16 consecutive days.[63] Within about 12 hours of discontinuation of dosing, some of the volunteer subjects exhibited irritability, insomnia, restlessness, hot flashes, sweating, rhinorrhea, loose stools, hiccoughs, and anorexia for up to 48 hours.

As a prescription medication uniquely formulated with THC as the active ingredient, to ask whether Dronabinol is a good model of ingestion seems like a moot question. The Physician's Desk Reference affords quite unique details of dose and response but, more importantly, plasma levels of THC with accompanying text in Table 36.5.

To be specifically noted in this tabulation are the apparent therapeutic levels after the dosages of 10 and 20 mg twice a day. As noted earlier, the generally stated level is 5 ng/mL for impairment relative to the operation of a motor vehicle in several states. Noted under warnings: "Patients . . . should be specifically warned not to drive, operate machinery, or engage in any hazardous activity until it established that they are able to tolerate the drug and to perform such tasks safely." One may be tempted here to ask, "how do I do this safety analysis?"

The most definitive quantitative study with Dronabinol reported plasma levels of THC and 11-hydroxy-THC as well as diverse effects for 12 hours following the ingestion of up to 90 mg of THC in fixed doses from 15 to 90 mg. Thus, at doses of 60, 75, and 90 mg, the plasma THC levels were above 30 ng/mL (25 to 75 ng) for three to five hours. The 11-hydroxy-THC levels never reached 30 ng/mL. Only at the lowest doses of 15 and 30 mg were the levels of THC and 11-hydroxy-THC about equal at between 5 and 15 ng/mL.[66] Previous reports at lower doses show near-equal levels of both these cannabinoids after the administration of THC. These higher levels of THC at the higher doses suggest that the metabolic machinery can be saturated by excess THC. The question then becomes, "what are the behavioral effects of any ratio differences of the levels of cannabinoids with unequal efficacy?"

The studies noted in the Physician's Desk Reference discussed earlier had an analysis of the drug's effects between 30 and 60 minutes with the "high" at 2–4 hours and some psycho stimulation from 4 to 6 hours with the plasma levels at or below 20 ng/mL. Lile et al.[67] report no significant dose-dependent effects on "good drug effect, high, and tired sedated" up to 90 mg doses with blood levels of THC in the 10 to 20 ng/mL range in the first 1 to 2 hours, and levels between 30 and 75 ng/mL during 3 to 5 hours in the regular marijuana users. This comparison of two sets of data suggests, that set-and-setting are prime factors in physiological and psychological effects during can marijuana use. Also documented and discussed in the report was the phenomenon of individual variability. Thus, the highest THC value was 130 ng/mL with an average of about 75; and the highest 11-hydroxy-THC value was 50 with an average value of about 25 ng/mL.

The route of administration of THC affords a different ratio of cannabinoids in the blood of the users over time from the earliest minutes until about one hour post inhalation. Ingestion of THC shows different amounts of the cannabinoids over the three to five hours timeframe. Quantitative comparisons further suggest that the effects after marijuana use cannot be completely described as the direct effect of only THC.

36.4.9.2 Overall Advantages of the Oromucosal Route

Sativex was introduced as an oromucosal spray of a formulated marijuana extract in Canada and the United Kingdom in the treatment of spasticity with multiple sclerosis. Up to 13 cannabinoids and related chemicals have been detected in some samples. In this regard, Sativex can be considered as a mixture not unlike the smoke from a burning reefer. A sample studied by Karschner et al.[68] had a composition of near-equal amounts of THC and CBD that was administered to nine marijuana smokers. They reported that absorption was 92–98% with bioavailability of 11–13%, which are similar parameters noted for Dronabinol. They also interpreted their data to show that there was no significant interference in the disposition of THC in the body due to the presence of CBD. This finding suggests that absorption, distribution, metabolism, and excretion were not integral to any drug–drug interactions of these two cannabinoids. Their data were presented as comparisons of plasma levels of THC after oral THC versus oromucosal (buccal) administration as follows:

As can be noted from this discussion, the levels of both the THC and CBD were about equal from both dosage forms. The times to maximum levels were about equal. The times until detectable effects were 2.0 to 2.5 hours for the two doses, which is not significantly different. The maximum levels for CBD were 1.6 and 6.7 and for THC, they were 5.1 and 15.3 ng/mL between the two doses. The highest level for CBD was 20.5 ng/mL. The 11-hydroxy-THC levels after the spray administration were 4.2 and 8.4 ng/mL for the doses, respectively. Individual variability among the participants was seen as with the Dronabinol reports. Again, note that these therapeutically directed blood levels were above the legal/illegal value of 5 ng/mL.

Given the ability to spray as desired would seem to offer as much control as smoking until one notes the times of effect of an hour or so. That delay would argue that smoking allows the most control toward eliciting the desired effects of marijuana use. The oromucosal route may be second best, with the ingestion route and all of the diverse dosage forms already on the market the least likely to be effectively mastered. One additional caveat needs to be kept in mind regarding the buccal route of administration is that sometimes too much of the material is swallowed. Thus, one has two routes contributing to the blood levels.

36.4.9.3 Can the Effects after the Ingestion of Marijuana Be Made More Objective?

The marijuana smoker has almost total control of the process of assimilation of cannabinoids into the blood stream. Given the spray of Sativex with the oromucosal route, one would think that one would have control of the effects as well. However, the buccal route is not as efficient as was originally postulated as detailed before. This process of controlled application/administration of several prescription medications such as morphine and Xanax is known as titration. In general, one starts with the lowest dose which is readily/rapidly acting, and, depending upon the perceived effect, one can the change the dose or not. In this manner, one can arrive at a dose and time process to afford optimal drug effectiveness. In contrast to the smoking and oromucosal routes, one has the tedious ingestion route of assimilation. In fact, emesis may be the only method to intervene with the effects of the ingestion of the marijuana products.

Unlikely as the probability for effectively interrupting the effects following the ingestion of marijuana seems, a very reasoned process for effective ingestion of marijuana-containing products has been published on the EROWID website which they have entitled "L.E.S.S." Perhaps, this is one instance where LESS is likely more! We further afford an interpretation of this "L.E.S.S." process as follows: A low-percent THC marijuana product is ingested regularly (about every 30 minutes) to establish effects for at least 2 hours, then supplemented slowly. A further note states that marijuana products are drugs and not food.[69] These comestibles are "drug delivery devices" or dosage forms, and not food.

Another listing may be more effective for novices:

- Start low (% THC)
- Establish potency (30 to 60-minute intervals for 4 to 6 hours)
- Slow, be patient (haste makes wasted)
- Supplement as determined from effects at interval ingestions
- Start sober
- Larger batches provide consistency (unless Rx-perientialism is the philosophy)

36.5 MARIJUANA SAFETY

While the potential health benefits of marijuana have been demonstrated, accumulating evidence also shows that marijuana use has its associated risks. Marijuana is often considered to be less hazardous than other controlled drugs and substances; however, very potent forms of marijuana are now available, and concurrent use of marijuana with illicit substances like crack/cocaine and phencyclidine is not uncommon.

When smoked in small amounts, serious adverse effects are quite infrequent. Although there have been reports of people suffering myocardial infarctions after smoking marijuana, this may be due to tachycardia and a pre-existing cardiac condition. Use of high-dose marijuana can produce anxiety and panic attacks, and the user is often in a dissociated state from the marijuana itself. Drug-induced psychosis has been reported and is of concern.[70]

A comprehensive analysis of health outcomes and harms in nonmedical marijuana use within the general population yielded the evaluation of 68 reviews. Evidence of harm was reported in 91% of reviews for mental health disorders, brain changes, cognitive outcomes, pregnancy outcomes, and testicular cancer. Inconclusive evidence was found for 20 of these outcomes (some mental health outcomes, other types of cancers, and all-cause mortality). Harm risk was highest for teenagers, pregnant women, and people with risk factors for mental illness.[71]

36.5.1 Serious Adverse Effects

Adverse effects from marijuana may vary as a function of dose, route of administration, expectation of subject, and individual vulnerability to a certain effect. Despite the influence of these factors, the cannabinoids have been shown to produce a unique syndrome of effects on behaviors of humans and animals. The most prominent feature is an initial period of euphoria and relaxation which is followed by a depressant period. At low doses, cannabinoids produce a period of stimulatory and depressant effects, and at higher doses, they exert predominantly depression. The pleasurable subjective effects of marijuana use, which presumably contribute to its abuse, include, furthermore, the feeling of tranquility and distortions in hearing and vision. The psychoactive, antinociceptive, and antiepileptic effects of cannabinoids are mediated by their action on the central nervous system (CNS).[72] Psychosis is another rare but serious adverse effect of marijuana, as described next.

36.5.2 Risk of Psychosis

Psychosis refers to a composition of clinically observable features that present as part of a syndrome, which impact on an individual's sense of contact with reality. A psychotic episode is characterized by abnormal thoughts and perceptions leading to a loss or difficulty in understanding reality. Symptoms of psychosis include delusions and hallucinations, incoherent or nonsense speech, and behavior that is inappropriate for the situation. A person in a psychotic episode may also experience agitation, anxiety, aggression, pacing, withdrawal from society, depression, sleep problems, lack of motivation, and general difficulty in normal functioning.

Substance-induced psychosis (SIP) refers to hallucinations and/or delusions caused by intoxication or withdrawal from a substance and occurs in approximately 6.5/100,000 persons per year. About 25% of first-episode psychoses are substance-induced.[73] Widespread increases in the use of marijuana, in part due to increased availability and changes in legislation, have highlighted concerns linking marijuana use to psychosis.

Marijuana has known addictive effects and is linked to an increased risk for the development of psychiatric disorders, including episodes of psychosis, schizophrenia, depression, and anxiety.[74,75] A review of relevant literature suggests that marijuana is involved in approximately 50% of psychosis, schizophrenia, and schizophreniform psychosis cases.[76,77,78,79,80] A catalytic role for marijuana is suggested in the onset of psychosis in patients with a first episode of non-affective psychosis and ultra-high-risk patient populations.[81,82] Patients experiencing first-episode psychosis show similar rates of progression to schizophrenia, regardless of whether they have a history of marijuana use or not.[83] While the precise neurological underpinnings are not understood, marijuana is considered a risk factor for schizophrenia and other psychiatric disorders.

The magnitude of the effect of the combined 11-OH-THC and THC has been implicated in reported psychotic reactions. For example, in October 2014, a 19-year-old student ate a marijuana-laced cookie and shortly thereafter began rambling incoherently and subsequently jumped to his death from the balcony of a Denver hotel. The Denver coroner listed marijuana intoxication as a significant factor in his death and reported that he had a blood level of 7.2 ng/ml (equivalent to 14 ng/ml plasma concentration), a concentration that would be found approximately 2 hours after smoking a 3.55% THC marijuana cigarette.[84] Another case involved a man who developed hallucinations and rambling speech after eating marijuana candy with concomitant ingestion of an unidentified prescription medication. Amid an apparent psychotic break, he fatally shot his wife while she was calling 911 for help.

In early September 2014, five high school students in the San Francisco, California area, aged 14–16, became ill after eating brownies that had been laced with marijuana. Three developed nausea and vomiting, and two became unconscious and were hospitalized. The brownies were sold to the students by a classmate. There are no toxicology results indicating if the brownies contained other "drugs" or if they contained only marijuana.

36.5.2.1 Drug-Induced Psychosis: Potential Mechanisms

Substance-induced psychosis is observed following ingestion of many medications and can occur at normal doses, excessive doses, or as a symptom of drug withdrawal. In addition to marijuana, common drugs with linked psychiatric effects include amphetamines, amantadine, anticonvulsants, dronabinol, and ketamine. No single mechanism of action has been identified for the occurrence of SIP. Mechanisms are complex and poorly understood, but psychosis likely manifests due to multi-neural network dysfunctions that impact on a variety of brain regions (and multiple neurotransmitter-specific pathways). Abnormalities at any level can influence the manifestation of psychosis.[85]

Multiple brain regions have been identified in the pathophysiology of psychosis. A link between schizophrenia, schizophrenia-like psychosis of epilepsy, and delusional misidentification syndromes appears to be the involvement of neural limbic structures. In addition to deficits in limbic structures, visual and auditory hallucinations also involve changes in cortical regions subserving normal functioning. Overall, limbic structures play a critical role in the pathology of psychosis with contributions from other frontal and parietal structures further highlighting the complexity of this multifaceted syndrome.[86]

Evidence suggests a prominent role for dopamine, in particular the role for a hyperdopaminergic brain state. Indirect or direct neural activities leading to abnormal dopamine concentration in brain structures located within the mesolimbic system are linked to psychosis. Increased dopamine concentrations in the mesolimbic pathway are often associated with hallucinations, delusions, and paranoia. Furthermore, the administration of dopamine antagonists reduces these clinical psychotic symptoms.[87] Altered serotonin and glutamate systems are also implicated in psychosis. Hallucinogenic substances LSD and psilocybin are associated with psychosis and specifically support a link between these symptoms and activation of the serotonin 5-HT2A receptor. Various types of anti-psychotic medications that target 5-HT and NMDA glutamate receptors impact on these neurotransmitter systems contributing to these theories.[88]

36.5.2.2 Vaping and Associated Risk for Psychosis

Vaping has become increasingly popular among adolescents. An evaluation of 1,542 undergraduates who were self-reported e-cigarette users showed that 7% used the device to consume substances other than nicotine. Within this group, approximately 80% reported the use of a CBD or some derivative of marijuana.[89] Due to the vulnerability of the developmental brain state, the high potency of THC or CBD vaping solutions compounded with the increased use of vaping among adolescents places this population at a higher risk of adverse effects including psychiatric illness.

While marijuana has a known link to the development of psychiatric disorders, the comparative acute effects of smoked versus vaporized marijuana and individual responses to acute exposure have not been sufficiently characterized. Experiential evidence suggests that vaping may be linked to higher rates of psychosis. Due to the high potency of vaping solutions, it is postulated that there is an increased risk for THC-induced psychosis and schizophrenia spectrum disorders. While limited, recent evidence shows that THC vaping produces notably different pharmacodynamic effects and more intense subjective experience in users compared to traditional smoking inhalation.[90]

There are limited studies that have examined the association between vaping and the development of psychotic experiences. One retrospective regression study examined the associations between vaping (within 30 days of ingestion) and psychotic experiences over the past 12 months in 29,232 students (using the Healthy Minds Survey). Approximately 14% of students reported psychotic experiences over the past year, and around 14–15% of students reported vaping over the past month. In the multiple logistic regression model, vaping was significantly associated with psychotic experiences. This association was significant even after adjusting for any cigarette/marijuana use and after adjusting for depression and anxiety.[91]

36.5.3 Pulmonary Function

Significant decrements in pulmonary vital capacity have been found in regular and daily marijuana smokers. Marijuana smoking typically involves deep inhalation and prolonged retention of marijuana smoke. Therefore, marijuana smokers may develop chronic bronchial irritation. The impairment of single-breath carbon monoxide diffusion capacity (DlCO) is greater in persons who smoke both marijuana and tobacco than in tobacco smokers. Marijuana smoking is associated with inflammation of the large airways, increased airway resistance, and lung hyperinflation. These associations align with consistent findings that regular marijuana smokers are more likely to experience chronic bronchitis compared to nonsmokers.[92] However, the long-term effect of low levels of marijuana exposure does not appear to be significant.[93] It is more difficult to estimate the potential effects of regular heavy use in small sample sizes; however, findings do suggest an accelerated decline in pulmonary function with heavy use and a resulting need for caution and moderation when marijuana use is considered.

According to a recent review,

> The effects of long-term marijuana smoking on the risk of lung cancer are unclear. For example, the use of marijuana for the equivalent of 30 or more joint-years (with 1 joint-year of marijuana use equal to 1 cigarette [joint] of marijuana smoked per day for 1 year) was associated with an increased incidence of lung cancer and several cancers of the upper gastro-digestive tract; however, the association disappeared after adjustment for potential confounders such as cigarette smoking. Although the possibility of a positive association between marijuana smoking and cancer cannot be ruled out, the evidence suggests that the risk is lower with marijuana than with tobacco.[94]

Smoked marijuana is absorbed into the pulmonary circulation and returned to the heart through the pulmonary vein. From the heart, it is distributed systemically, without passing through the liver. Orally ingested THC is subject both to transmural metabolism in the gastrointestinal tract and hepatic metabolism as it passes through the liver. As a result, when the THC passes through the gut wall or into the liver, there is a synthesis of a relatively significant amount of 11-OH-THC that can combine its psychotropic affects with those of THC to produce an additive psychotropic affect in the CNS.

36.5.4 Risk of Addiction

Evidence indicates that long-term marijuana use can lead to addiction. Approximately 9% of users who experiment with marijuana become addicted.[95] This statistic goes up to about 17% among those who start using marijuana as teenagers and to 25 to 50% among those who smoke marijuana daily.[96] There is also recognition of a marijuana withdrawal syndrome[97] with symptoms that include irritability, sleeping difficulties, dysphoria, craving, and anxiety. Withdrawal symptoms contribute to difficulties in cessation and relapsing potential.

Volkow et al. write:

> Marijuana use by adolescents is particularly troublesome. Adolescents' increased vulnerability to adverse long-term outcomes from marijuana use is probably related to the

fact that the brain, including the endocannabinoid system, undergoes active development during adolescence. Indeed, early, and regular marijuana use predicts an increased risk of marijuana addiction, which in turn predicts an increased risk of the use of other illicit drugs. As compared with persons who begin to use marijuana in adulthood, those who begin in adolescence are approximately 2 to 4 times as likely to have symptoms of marijuana dependence within 2 years after first use.[98]

36.5.5 Effect on Brain Development

Volkow goes on to state:

> The brain remains in a state of active, experience-guided development from the prenatal period through childhood and adolescence until the age of approximately 21 years. During these developmental periods, it is intrinsically more vulnerable than a mature brain to the adverse long-term effects of environmental insults, such as exposure to tetrahydrocannabinol, or THC, the primary active ingredient in marijuana. This view has received considerable support from studies in animals, which have shown, for example, that prenatal or adolescent exposure to THC can recalibrate the sensitivity of the reward system to other drugs and that prenatal exposure interferes with cytoskeletal dynamics, which are critical for the establishment of axonal connections between neurons.[99]

In 1973, Lemberger demonstrated the psychotropic effects of the 11-OH-THC metabolite when he administered tritiated IV doses of THC, 11-OH-THC (formulated in ethanol), or ethanol, under blinded conditions, to nine casual marijuana users.[100] Following the administration of one mg of 11-OH-THC, a marked tachycardia and euphoric "high" occurred in three to five minutes, and psychologic effects correlated well with 11-OH-THC plasma levels. However, IV administration of 1 mg of THC required a latency period of 10–20 minutes after IV administration, before the peak subjective "high" was reported by the subjects. The authors concluded that these results indicated that the psychologic effects of THC were at least partially mediated through the 11-OH-THC metabolite and that the latency period was indicative of the time required to convert THC to 11-OH-THC.

As THC is metabolized more extensively by the oral route, leading to the synthesis of a much larger amount of 11-OH-THC than is generally formed following smoking, blood levels of the psychopharmacologically active 11-OH-THC metabolite can combine its psychotropic effects with those of THC to produce a more robust psychotropic effect in the CNS. Some investigators postulate that the 11-OH-THC metabolite is four times as psychoactive as THC, and other investigators have postulated an activity up to 17 times that of THC.[101] The magnitude of the effect of the combined 11-OH-THC and THC most likely was the cause of the psychotic reactions and loss of consciousness described in the cases reported before.

36.5.6 Long-Term Behavioral Effects

It is unclear, however, if the established evidence of marijuana effects on cognition is reversible or irreversible. The factors that impact marijuana-related cognitive impairment and recovery of cognitive function include the age of onset of smoking marijuana, the duration of use, and the amount of marijuana used.

Chronic marijuana use has been associated with deficits such as memory impairment,[102,103,104] and changes in brain morphology;[105,106] however, the reversibility of these deficits depends on a number of factors, especially the age of onset and length of abstinence.

36.5.7 Age of Onset of Use

The age of onset of marijuana use is a significant factor in determining if chronic marijuana use will cause permanent cognitive damage. In a study done in 2008 by Brook et al., adolescents who started smoking marijuana between the ages of 14 and 22, and had stopped by age 22, had significantly more cognitive deficits at age 27 than non-marijuana users. Additionally, in contrast to the users who began after age 17, adult marijuana users who began smoking before the age of 17 had significant impairment of executive functioning, abstract reasoning, verbal fluency, and memory compared to nonuser controls.[107] This was also exhibited in a rodent study where cannabinoid exposure during adolescence permanently suppressed the cortical network activity in adult mice.[108]

The relationship between marijuana use by young people and psychosocial harm is likely to be multifaceted, which may explain the inconsistencies among studies. For example, some studies suggest that long-term deficits may be reversible and remain subtle rather than disabling once a person abstains from use.[109]

A review by Schweinsburg et al. came to a similar conclusion after reviewing the cumulative literature on the subject. Humans who initiated the use of marijuana in early adolescence have shown a higher rate of cognitive dysfunction than those who began after adolescence. It is thought that these results are connected to the ongoing neuromaturation during the teen years and that adults who began using marijuana in adolescence are more susceptible to cognitive deficiencies than adults who have not.[110]

36.6 IMPACT OF LEGALIZATION

36.6.1 Hospital Resources

Multiple studies have come out of Colorado, one of the first states to legalize marijuana, assessing the longitudinal impact of legalized marijuana on health outcomes in the state. Colorado approved recreational and medical marijuana use in 2014. Marijuana legalization has contributed to significant mental and behavioral consequences, particularly in patients presenting to emergency departments (ED) and urgent care (UC) facilities in Colorado. Of high concern includes the development of psychosis, suicide, and other substance abuse issues. An increase in fatal motor vehicle collisions, cardiovascular and pulmonary effects, accidental pediatric exposure, marijuana-associated exposure to contaminants and infectious agents, heavy metals, pesticides, and hash-oil burn and lung-related injuries have all been documented.

Following legalization, the frequency of ED visits and hospitalizations related to marijuana has increased. Contributing to ED/UC visits are the increasing potency of marijuana preparations and general use of marijuana. Psychiatric illness represents most marijuana-related visits. A retrospective review of Colorado hospitalizations and ED visits related to marijuana showed a 116% increase from the years 2000 to 2015 (equivalent of 274 to 593 per 100,000 hospitalizations). The prevalence of psychiatric illness determined at diagnosis was five times higher for ED visits and nine times higher for hospital admissions for patients with marijuana-related billing codes compared to others.[111] Subsequent data by the Colorado Public Health Department show significant increases in hospitalizations across each phase of marijuana legalization.[112]

ED/UC visits with marijuana-related International Classification of Diseases (ICD) codes and positive drug screenings for teenagers and young adults have also increased since legalization, with the majority requiring a behavioral health evaluation. Another retrospective study showed 67% of patients (aged 13–21 years) who met the criteria for a marijuana-associated ICD code or positive drug test needed a behavioral health evaluation; a psychiatric diagnosis was made for the majority (71%) of these visits. These data indicate that there has been a significant increase in adolescent/young adult ED/UC visits with marijuana-associated ICD codes or positive urine drug screens.[113]

Annual pediatric marijuana cases increased more than five-fold from 2009 to 2015 in Colorado, highlighting the significant effect on pediatric exposure.[114] Colorado had an average increase in poison control reporting of 34% per year in contrast to an increase of 19% that was observed in other parts of the United States. Despite public health interventions in legislation after 2014 to reduce pediatric exposure (e.g., child-resistant packaging, dose limitations, limiting marketing campaigns, and banning of specific products), the incidence of pediatric hospital visits and poison control calls continued to rise in Colorado with an observed doubling of children's hospital visits in 2017 compared to 2016.[115]

Overall, longitudinal data from Colorado shows that the prevalence of psychiatric health conditions in ED/UC visits with marijuana-related events or diagnostic codes is higher since legalization. This has negatively impacted on pediatric exposure and is of concern among the use of marijuana in adolescents and young adults.

36.6.2 Driving under the Influence of Drugs

The US Dept. of Transportation National Highway Traffic Safety Administration conducted a roadside survey in which driving under the influence of drugs (DUID) was found to be a growing factor in impaired-driving crashes. The 2013–2014 report showed a decreasing trend in alcohol use by drivers between 1973 and 2013–2014. In contrast, the percentage of weekend nighttime drivers who tested positive for marijuana increased from 8.6% in 2007 to 12.6% in 2014. In 2013–2014, 8.3% of weekend nighttime drivers tested positive for alcohol, of which 22.5% had a positive drug oral fluid and/or drug blood test. The survey reviewed drugs with the potential to impair driving skills. The study does highlight that a positive screen for the presence of drugs does not necessarily imply impairment. Drug use among drivers who were fatally injured and tested for drugs rose from 25% in 2007 to 42% in 2016.[116]

36.6.3 Relationship of Marijuana Use and Co-Use with Other Substances

The relationships of marijuana policy liberalization have been questioned with its impact on the use effect trends alone and with other substances, such as alcohol use. Legalization of marijuana has been a key public health concern for many reasons including the impact marijuana liberalization laws might have on alcohol use and alcohol-related outcomes. It is believed by some that marijuana may act as a replacement for alcohol consumption, and, therefore, liberalizing marijuana policies may reduce excessive alcohol use. However, marijuana use is a risk factor for underage drinking, excessive drinking, and vehicle-related fatalities involving alcohol.[117] These findings suggest another train of thought—that liberalizing of marijuana policies may contribute to rises in alcohol use. A narrative review by Pacula et al.[118] focused on evaluating the potential impact of marijuana policy liberalization, and alcohol use, alcohol-related outcomes, and the co-use of alcohol and marijuana were inconclusive. A number of studies with positive, negative, and no correlation were found. In studies that showed a positive correlation between marijuana policy liberalization and decreases in alcohol outcomes, there was no impact of the marijuana policy on marijuana use alone. The lack of a consistent correlation was robust. Safety concerns regarding marijuana use and the impact of consumption of other substances remain unknown. This review was unable to provide a comprehensive interpretation of the scientific evidence to date while considering the rapid influx of articles published in recent years following the legalization of marijuana in many states. Further studies are necessary to determine this impact.

Marijuana policy liberalization may lead to changes in prescription drug intake and use as well. A preliminary study presented at the American Academy of Orthopedic Surgeons showed a reduction in opioid use with access to medical marijuana in patients with back pain. In patients with chronic back pain, daily morphine significantly reduced, and more than one-third of patients (38.7%) stopped taking morphine after starting medical marijuana treatment. The authors also found that medical marijuana reduced opioid use in patients with osteoarthritis by 46.3%. The percentage of patients who stopped using opioids was 37.5%.[119] Considering the known abuse liability of opioids, marijuana may provide an alternative for pain management in a variety of indications that can reduce opioid intake.

36.7 ANALYSIS AND TESTING FOR MARIJUANA USE

The challenge of new and increasing prevalence of marijuana use requires effective evaluation by businesses, governments, legal entities, and scientists to position marijuana use into a positive functional societal role. Having expertise as slaboratory scientists and consultants and in small businesses, the authors afford this brief review of some of the scientific studies in the marijuana arena. In doing so, we evaluate the logic of a 5 ng/mL level of blood THC in assessing the psychomotor functionality of a marijuana user. For context, the marijuana smoker attains a plasma THC level up to about 250 ng/mL that decreases to less than 10 ng/mL in the 1 hour from the beginning of a 10–15-minute smoking session. Even more confounding are the results of 2, 7-day abstinence studies in which THC-positive plasma test results even after the 7-day washout period show THC up to 5.5 ng/mL.[120,121] Even more absurd is the 2006 report which recommended a THC level of 0.5 ng/mL as the cut-off for psychomotor functionality.[122] One author (Bederka) proposes a plasma THC level of 30 ng/mL as an objective value toward assessing impairment related to marijuana smoking in accident/incident conditions. In 2015, then Governor Rauner rom Illinois was presented with a bill setting the "per se" blood level at 15 ng/mL. Unfortunately, after political pressure from the International Association of Police Chiefs, the Governor set the "per se" level at 5 ng/mL, a level that is too low and is not based on scientific facts supporting impairment. Indeed, a published study[123] provides that a THC level of 13 ng/mL is similar to that of an alcohol blood concentration of 0.08 g/dL.

36.8 SCIENTIFIC DATA RELATING TO THC

36.8.1 Blood THC versus Brain THC: Any Relationships?

Given the effects of cannabinoids in the brain, it is appropriate that early studies attempted to measure the precise concentrations that induce selected effects.[124,125,126] Animals were of necessity in those quantitative studies such as mice, rats, and pigs, which afforded consistent comparable results. A 1972 study with radioactive-labeled THC found that brain levels were at their maximum 15 minutes after IV administration.[127] The two cannabinoids were THC and hydroxy-THC, and the effects paralleled the brain cannabinoid levels over 1.5 to four hours.[128] A similar study with mice noted that relative cannabinoid levels in the smoke were the same as relative levels in the brain for three cannabinoids.[129] They further showed that no hydroxy-THC was in the smoke condensate but was found in the brain. Other studies have proposed that THC is metabolized in the lung and liver, but no definitive data is available as to metabolism in either brain tissue or brain blood vessels. The evidence is that both THC and hydroxy-THC easily penetrate into brain tissue, with hydroxy-THC most easily accumulating in the brain. Likewise, a study with eight cannabinoids noted that all effects correlated with their brain/plasma level ratios.[130]

36.8.2 Relationships between Percent Plant-THC and Plasma-THC

In general, reports show marijuana potency in the range of 1.3–13% THC per cigarette. However, as mentioned previously, potency has increased considerably over the past decades. The free molecules of THC in the marijuana plant are not the defining number as to the potential blood level of THC in the user. New molecules of THC are created during smoking, while some THC is destroyed during smoking.[131] Thus, only 10–60% of the potential THC in the plant is actually delivered to the user. Further of note is the use of the word "blood" in some of the studies. Blood is normally used to denote whole blood, rather than the derived fractions known as plasma and serum. Given that plasma is about 55% of the whole blood and that THC and other cannabinoids are about 90% bound to proteins in the plasma, the specimen of choice for marijuana studies is plasma from the living humans.[132]

36.8.3 Is There a Relationship between Percent THC in the Smoked Cigarette and Plasma THC?

There seems to be no direct relationship of increasing plasma levels with increasing the percentage of THC in the plant. The true variable is likely the user, whereby a level of effect is personally attained by adjustments in smoking to obviate the variable amount of THC in the cigarette. Another logical conclusion could be that even with marijuana at 25% THC or higher, users will not increase their maximum plasma THC levels. With more THC per puff, one could expect that total intake of THC will not increase because the user may stop smoking once the desired high is achieved—that is, they titrate their dose to the desired effect.

36.8.4 Relation between Degree of "High" and Plasma THC

One learns to smoke and to get to a "high" that is likely unique to the person. As suggested in the following tabulation, with no dose–response relationship, some persons report a perception of a "high" from marijuana cigarettes with little-to-no THC. The "personalization" of this phenomenon, "the high," seems to be well illustrated.

An analysis of the tabulated results before allows one to conclude that there is no direct relationship between the degree of "high" and plasma THC level. An analysis of the range of the maxima for the range of plasma levels affords an average of 214.1 with a standard deviation of 55.9. For the percent THC, we note only a variation of 26% when the "degree of high" changed by more than 1,000%. The first entry in the table shows that the "high" was experienced by no one, even at a plasma level of 190, and some noted a maximum "high" of 10 with a Plasma THC of only 5. It seems that the true variable is the user.

As reported by Heustis, the peak plasma level can occur in 5 minutes while smoking, or up to about 15 minutes post-smoking even after the IV administration of THC.[133] The peak level is usually found before the perception of the "high." It is also noted that the plasma level of THC decreased from about 150 ng/mL to less than 10 ng/mL within 50 minutes after starting to smoke.[134] The practiced user will usually experience the "high" earlier than the occasional user under the same conditions, as does the alcohol drinker at low blood alcohol levels. In general, it is accepted that there is a poor correlation between plasma THC concentration and effects such as euphoria and cognitive impairment. This contrasts alcohol, for which there is a more predictable relationship between concentration and symptoms.

36.8.5 Occasional Marijuana Users versus Practiced Users

The practiced marijuana user is additionally distinguishable from the occasional user by at least the following points:[135]

1. Achieves a "high" about five minutes earlier than the occasional user.
2. Achieves a plasma THC level about twice as high as the occasional user when smoking equal cigarettes as shown in Table 36.6 at 5 minutes post smoking at a dose of 500 micrograms (μg) THC per kilogram body mass.
3. On the first day of a 7-day forced abstinence study, heavy users had residual plasma-THC levels from 7.0 to 9.0 ng/mL.
4. Even after a 7-day forced abstinence, heavy/practiced users can have plasma THC levels of 1.2 to 5.5 ng/mL. More importantly, the change over time of the THC level was not continuously decreasing; however, some days showed an increased level from the previous day's level.[137]
5. At 5 to 15 minutes post smoking of a single marijuana cigarette, as shown in the table, the heavy user can achieve a plasma THC of up to 250 ng/mL.
6. One study with 6.8 percent plant-THC found no adverse behavioral effects in heavy users at 15 minutes post smoking with plasma levels of THC of 13 to 63 ng/mL.[138]

TABLE 36.6
Plasma THC Levels* Occasional versus Practiced Users:

Occasional Users	(Plasma Levels)	Practiced Users
1.9–134 ng/mL	Range	7.9–244.8 ng/mL
After Smoking 13% THC at the Two Doses:[136]		
250 μg/mL		500 μg/mL
57.3 ± 48.9 ng/mL		93.6 ± 63.9 ng/mL
58.0 ± 47.7 ng/mL		95.1 ± 63.2 ng/mL

**These two groups show a dose–response of about 2 when the amount of THC was doubled from 250 to 500 μg/mL. This seeming dose–response relationship was not seen in population studies noted in the foregoing tabulations of "percent THC" and "degree of high" relative to plasma levels of THC.*

36.8.6 Is THC the Only Psychoactive Cannabinoid?

One of the earliest studies with carbon-14-labeled (radioactive) THC concluded that the peak of the "high" was between 10 to 140 minutes.[139] The other key finding was that the peak effects coincided with peak levels of THC-metabolites. The study further identified two of these metabolites as 11-hydroxy-THC and 8,11-dihydroxy-THC. Early studies conclude that the whole marijuana experience is due to the diverse cannabinoids formed in the plant, the smoke, and the user. Consistent with these early observations, more recent analytical reports show how rapidly the metabolites are found in the blood either after smoking or IV administration of THC. For example, after having smoked a cigarette with 15.8 milligrams of THC, a peak THC plasma level occurred at 8.4 minutes during smoking. A peak level of 11-hydroxy-THC occurred at 15 minutes post smoking.[140]

A further study after IV injection of 4 to 5 mg THC afforded the following:[141]

- THC peak level at 20 minutes with 63.0 ng/mL
- 11-hydroxy-THC peak level at 25 minutes with 3.0 ng/mL
- Beta-hydroxy-THC peak level at 25 minutes with 4.0 ng/mL

TABLE 36.7
Times to Peak Cannabinoid Plasma Levels.

Time (Minutes)	THC (ng/mL)	11-Hydroxy-THC (ng/mL)
0	7.1	2.9
15	101.0*	17.5
30	47.4*	15.2
60	22.1	10.8
240	8.0	4.7

**Source:* From these and the corresponding times of measurement, one can note the plasma half-life or half-time for elimination. Thus, the decrease from 101.0 to 47.4 ng/mL is about a 50% drop in 15 minutes—an initial half-life.

THC, 11-hydroxy-THC, and beta-hydroxy-THC are all psychoactive substances. In this study, the heavy user was back to near pre-smoking THC level after 4 hours (7.1 ng/mL versus 8.0 ng/mL) but not the metabolite level (2.9 ng/mL versus 4.7 ng/mL). As noted in the seven-day abstinence study, one can tentatively conclude that the heavy user will have an elevated level of THC and at least one active metabolite at some time even if not having recently smoked. The metabolite did not decrease in concentration in the blood as rapidly as did the THC. The delay is likely due to the time of metabolism from THC to the 11-hydroxy-THC metabolite. This property of the half-time (half-life) for elimination is an individual characteristic for redistribution to tissues and metabolic efficiency and is a measure of the time for the level to decrease by 50%. There is an initial half-life of 15 to 30 minutes and a terminal half-life of hours to weeks at levels below 10 ng/mL. THC is reported to decrease by about 50% in about 0.3 to 1.6 hours, and 11-hydroxy-THC in 2–3.1 hrs. This infers that after a single cigarette, an occasional user would likely have a plasma THC level less than 1.0 ng/mL at six hours post smoking.[142,143,144]

In contrast to the above numbers for the living patient, the postmortem values have been noted to have much higher 11-hydroxy-THC values of 2.5–85, with THC levels of 1.4–20.0.[145,146] The conclusion here could be that the user involved in an auto accident had smoked some hours prior to an accident. The autopsy condition affords another complication in the impairment question in that postmortem redistribution of THC from the lung has been demonstrated affording higher blood levels than premortem.[147]

36.8.7 Urine Testing for Cannabinoids: Clinical or Evidentiary Value?

Current laws/statutes of some states note that any amount of a marijuana-related substance (i.e., THC-COOH) in urine affords that you are under the influence and impaired.

What is a different science-based reality for tomorrow's laws/statutes?

- Two studies of "long-term heavy cannabis users" maintained in a research unit for a seven-day period of marijuana absence reported that all 43 had measurable plasma THC-COOH at day seven. The amounts were between 2.8 and 45.6 ng/mL. Although limited urinary data were collected, it is well recognized that some substances are concentrated in the urine relative to their blood levels. THC-COOH is used as the abbreviation for the principal nonpsychoactive metabolite of THC that is found in blood, urine, and elsewhere after THC is metabolized in some form.[148,149]
- Importantly, a 1992 study concludes that "No correlation was found between blood THC and blood or urine THC-Acid concentrations."[150]
- A 2001 article that focused on urine THC for an eight-hour period after smoking concluded that urine-THC peaked after about two hours post-smoking. They then positively concluded that a urine THC value greater than 1.5 ng/mL "suggests" use in the previous eight-hour period. These authors also positively concluded for THC-COOH that "this metabolite cannot be employed as a chemical marker in urine for recent use." Passive inhalation or false positive test results further complicate the interpretation of the urine test data for THC-COOH.[151,152]
- The issue of *new* use of THC, as opposed to residual THC remaining from previous usage, may be important for a person on a periodic drug-testing program as a result of a previous violation. Marijuana pharmacologist Dr. Heustis weighed in on this issue, insisting that if there is any consequence to a positive result indicating new use, the ratio of normalized THC-COOH concentrations for two time points should exceed 1.5.[153] For example, if someone is going to lose a child custody case or be put in jail for new THC use, the ratio one should use as the criterion should be a THC-COOH ratio over 1.5 (THC-COOH concentrations should be normalized to creatinine, an endogenous substance produced by the body that is unrelated to THC). The false positive rate was found to be only 0.1% in identifying new THC usage when the ratio is 1.5.[154] A lower bar may be used if there is no penalty for usage; for instance, if this test is being used as part of a drug treatment program and there are no legal punishment for testing positive.
- The presence of THC-COOH cannot be used as evidence of new THC usage because it is long lived. Other cannabinoids may be used for this purpose. Cannabinol (CBN) and THC glucuronide, both derivatives of THC, may both be used to indicate new usage of THC.[155] One study showed that these cannabinoids were eliminated by an hour after THC usage, so not finding detectible

levels of these metabolites does not preclude recent use. That is, someone may have used THC recently but may not have detectible CBN or THC-glucuronide. It is not well established to employ cannabidiol (CBD) detection alone as an indicator for new THC use.

- Retrograde extrapolation, a method of predicting blood alcohol concentration at the time of a crash from the measured concentration at the time of blood sampling, is a staple of DUI analysis. The pharmacokinetics of THC/marijuana is much more complicated than that of alcohol or other drugs of abuse for that matter.[156] THC is lipophilic and will distribute into body fat, from where it may leech out into the blood to replenish blood THC lost to elimination. The elimination curve for THC blood concentration would not be expected to be a simple elimination curve (e.g., first order), and thus it is not possible to predict a previous THC concentration from a later time point. Scientific consensus among pharmacologists is that retrograde extrapolation is not scientifically valid for marijuana/THC.[157] Therefore, this analytical method should not be used for THC in legal cases.
- Ellis et al. found that one person had a positive test for urine THC-COOH up to day 77 post use before the test became negative at the 20 ng/mL cut-off level.[158]
- Concurring with the manufacturer of the Emit II screening test kit statement relative to a positive result, "does NOT indicate or measure intoxication." Leiken and Paloucek assert that "urine drug levels are NOT directly related to toxic symptoms seen clinically."[159,160,161]
- A positive urine test result for THC-COOH after a single smoking event does not repeatedly retest as positive on consecutive days and does not relate to a plasma level of any psycho-active cannabinoid. A positive test result for urinary THC-COOH should *not* be used to predict either the time-of-use of marijuana or the condition of the user at the time of presentation of the specimen.[162]

36.8.8 Impairment and Marijuana: Laboratory and On-Road Driving Performance Data

The behavioral effects of marijuana include forgetfulness, distractibility, attention, concentration, transient awareness lapses (getting stuck), short-term memory, tympanic awareness of cardiac effects, heightened senses, anxiety/panic, sleepiness, munchies (hunger), giggles, uncontrolled (collective) laughter, increased sociability, need for physical activity, and relaxation, among others. These effects can drastically influence the physical, cognitive, and executive performance of users and therefore can impair driving capacity. Challenges exist, however, when objectively determining the correlation between use and impairment.

Thus, we begin with a quote from O'Kane et al. in 2002:[163] "The purpose of measuring active THC levels can only be to detect recent use, or estimate the time of use, rather than directly measure the degree of intoxication." They further note that after a single cigarette, the perceived effects last about 45 minutes; and a meta-analysis indicated that THC-related impairment is concentrated in the first two hours after smoking. Kurzthaler et al. noted, "very important parameters of driving ability seem to be impaired immediately after cannabis consumption," and "physiological, emotional and perceptual changes rarely last longer than 2–3 hours after consumption of a single cigarette."[164] More specifically, the report by Solowij et al. notes that laboratory tasks and flight simulators may not be realistic in modeling actual driving performance.[165] A review by Iverson et al. states, "marijuana users, however, seem to be aware that their driving skills may be impaired and they tend to compensate by driving more slowly, keeping some distance away from the vehicle ahead and in general taking less risks."[166] These authors also note that some drug-experienced subjects show no deficits in cognitive and motor functions at all with heavy marijuana use, whereas naïve users were very much affected.[167] A study by Klonoff et al. showed that 23% of subjects showed comparative improvement, and 14% significant improvement in a high-dose condition with on-road driving.[168] Under an emergency situation, the seeming ability of the marijuana user to compensate is decreased.[169]

The following studies provide evaluations and expert opinion on impairment with marijuana use:

1. Schwope et al. evaluated the performance and observable signs of ten chronic, heavy marijuana users for six hours after having smoked a 6.8% cigarette (58 mg THC). A summary of their findings is as follows:[170,171]
   - Peak "high" and heart rate were noted at about 15 minutes from the beginning of the ten-minute smoking period. Blood pressure and respiration were not affected.
   - At five minutes post-smoking with plasma THC levels of 13 to 63 ng/mL, "little psychomotor impairment was observed, although there were robust cardiovascular and subjective responses."
   - Blood THC concentrations decreased rapidly during the hour after smoking; however, subjective effects persisted and decreased linearly for one to six hours post-smoking. Good subjective effects included good drug effect, stoned, high, stimulated, and sedated.
2. Bosker et al. studied the possibility of using Standardized Field Sobriety Testing (SFST) for evaluating the effect on performance in 20 heavy users. They concluded that SFSTs were mildly sensitive to impairment from marijuana in heavy users, mirroring the results of a similar study by Papafotiou *et al.* in 2005. Both of these studies

showed a 30 to 50 percent probability of indicating impairment. These results are about as ineffective as the breath test to blood test relationship and FSTs at alcohol levels below about 0.125.[172,173,174]

3. Bramness et al. employed the Norwegian Clinical Test for Impairment (CTI) consisting of some 20 subtests. They apparently concluded from a study of 589 drivers that "No relationship was found between blood THC and most of the CTI tests." The study seemed to allow between a 5 to 53 percent probability of indicating impairment using CTI data. They did conclude that blood THC was related to conjunctival injection, pupil dilation, pupil reaction to light, and the overall risk of being judged impaired. Clearly, the variable results seem to be highly subjective, as with FSTs of DUI-related suspects.[175]
4. Ramaekers et al. tried 3 performance test protocols with 20 marijuana users. Only at serum THC levels greater than 30 ng/mL did they find impairments for about the first hour.[176] They noted that the suggestions of impairment were noted between two to five ng/mL. The dose–response plots of performance versus THC afforded correlations of 3 to 14%; thus, not supporting their conclusions. A similar study by Barnett et al. indicated impairment at 25 ng/mL. However, no linear plots were provided, so no statistical analysis was possible.[177]
5. An on-the-road study report by NHTSA noted that a dose of 100 µg/kg: "Significantly impaired performance" and "performance deficits were minor."[178]
6. Ramaekers et al. evaluated 20 "light users" with 13% plant-THC cigarettes at 250 and 500 µg/kg and showed a serum THC of 93.6 ng/mL at 5 minutes and 10.61 ng/mL at 60 minutes post-smoking. Major impairments were observed from 15 to 90 minutes for cognition, impulse control, and psychomotor function.[179]
7. Heishman et al. evaluated a lesser THC concentration in moderate users and found no significant impairment in a circular lights task, a tracking task, and DSST at times up to 135 minutes post-smoking.[180,181]
8. N. Solowij stated that "A clear relation between blood levels of THC or its metabolites and degree of either impairment or subjective intoxication has not been demonstrated."[182]

36.8.9 Hospital and Provider Considerations

The following is excerpted (with permission) from a 2019 article in the *Pharmacy and Therapeutics* (*P&T*) journal.[183]

> For health plans or self-funded plan sponsors (employers, municipalities, unions), the advent of state legalized marijuana along with wide availability of CBD products has created not only a health care benefits issue but a legal conundrum around workplace safety or employment policy compliance.
>
> CBD products are not considered a prescription product nor sold exclusively in a pharmacy so benefit coverage itself is not an issue. However, CBD can be detected in routine and mandatory workplace safety or employment screenings of employees. This remains a murky area of law depending on the state and issue of Federal law or workplace policies and procedures effected.
>
> Medical marijuana, other than the prior list of prescription products, has similar issues as CBD. Since ERISA (Employee Retirement Income Security Act of 1974) as federal law covers self-insured employer plans, federal law impacts coverage provisions available to these healthcare benefit plans. For state licensed health plans, healthcare benefit plan rules—if any—may be determined under applicable state law. For commercial insurance plans, medical marijuana coverage remains limited due to the current standing of Federal law and Department of Justice position on this matter. Hospitals, as an employer and a place of healthcare, create a dual perspective on this matter that effect deliberations by their internal teams, including insurance, pharmacy and therapeutics committees.
>
> *WHAT IS A P&T (Pharmacy & Therapeutics Committee) TO DO?*
>
> With the fast-changing landscape surrounding marijuana use and legality, hospitals and other healthcare facilities must update their policies and procedures regarding medical marijuana use in their facilities. While legal in certain states, marijuana is still classified by the federal government as a schedule I controlled substance making these discussions quite challenging. The impact of state-specific regulations of marijuana accounts for the wide range of policies and procedures addressing the use and possession of medical marijuana. These policies range from tightly controlled use to sanctioned self-therapy during hospital stays. Hospitals are now forced to present their philosophy (either from a political or medicinal perspective) on medical marijuana and its place in their facility.
>
> Considerations should also include discussions on patient demographics, i.e., does the hospital treat a particular demographic with a higher rate of medical marijuana use, specialization in indications that would qualify for medical marijuana use, and if the facility receives federal funding that could be impacted by permitting the use of medical marijuana? Nearly all hospitals in the US contract with the federal government through federal-state jointly funded programs as Medicare providers and/or with states as Medicaid. While illegal federally, any program designed to allow patients to use medical marijuana (and any program that gives a facility possession of medical marijuana) violates Medicare participation and could invite sanctions.
>
> Further considerations include, will the hospital allow smoking (most ban any use of tobacco products, fire and health hazard), and many ban/severely limit the use of dietary supplements brought to the hospital by the patient. Will a special exception be granted, the rules changed, to accommodate the growing population who claim that medical marijuana is beneficial to them? And if such an exception is made, what liability and other legal complications (theft of marijuana by staff) will complicate the efforts of

the P&T to guarantee safe and effective use of 'medicine' in hospitals?

As marijuana legalization and use expands cross the US, healthcare systems (hospitals) as a provider of care and employer plan sponsor are struggling to account for changes or trends in regulations or law. Despite state laws to-date, federally determined marijuana and high THC concentration derivatives are still scheduled as a schedule I controlled substance. Hospitals are forced to provide their stance on marijuana use clinically while addressing compliance issues with potentially divergent state and federal law, and the facilities' own financial, operational, and political affiliations. These policies and procedures must also consider patient rights and interests to include when a patient may be an employee.

Due to the federal illegality and other regulatory imposed limitations for use in general, limited evidence for clinical efficacy and the myriad of psychological adverse events including anxiety and psychosis, it is best to proceed with thoughtfulness when establishing or revising policies and procedures regarding marijuana and/or CBD product coverage in managed care organizations or approved use within the continuum of organized care settings.

36.9 FORENSIC CASE REPORTS

CASE REPORT 1: MOTORCYCLIST V. TRUCK

FACTS OF THE CASE

Johnny Motorcyclist (Motorcyclist) collided his motorcycle into the rear trailer rear wheels of a semi-trailer, who was turning left into a USPS driveway entrance to/on a street in an industrial area at approximately 6.39 a.m. on October 5, 2016. EMS came to the scene: Williams was unresponsive, with no vital signs, with a Glasgow Coma Score of 0. Approximately, 1,500 ml (1.5 L) of fluids was administered intravenously at the scene and en-route to the hospital. He was taken to Emergency Department (ED), pulseless, in full arrest; resuscitative efforts were unsuccessful.

Another eyewitness told police that he saw the motorcycle "a block away." One pedestrian eyewitness testified that he was (traveling at a high rate of speed) "maybe 50 or 60 (mph)" "in excess of the speed limit." Another eyewitness motorist testified that Mr. Motorcyclist was weaving in traffic, driving at a high rate of speed (50 mph or more), and drove between her SUV and another SUV (weaving) in the next traffic lane. The eyewitness further testified that Mr. Motorcyclist applied his brakes after he passed her and (attempted to stop abruptly) was unable to stop or avert the truck—his motorcycle slid into the truck. She further testified that, based on her speed (~ 30mph), "the truck would have been fine going past without me having to actually stop." This eyewitness testified that the "motorcyclist was driving somewhat unsafe when he was doing that maneuver (came between two cars)." Two other witnesses at the scene (in another vehicle) told police that they observed the motorcycle traveling at a high rate of speed while swerving through traffic. They further stated that the motorcyclist was unable to stop and began sliding/skidding, before striking the rear of the truck.

The motorcyclist's body was taken to the Coroner's Office where the forensic pathologist performed an autopsy. The medical examiner ruled the cause of death (minutes after the collision) as multiple blunt trauma. During the autopsy, several body fluids were taken for toxicology testing. Toxicology findings on blood noted Delta-9 THC (active marijuana) levels to be 21 ng/ml, 11-hydroxy Delta 9 THC (active THC metabolite) to be 1.8ng/ml, and Delta 9—Carboxy-THC (inactive metabolite) to be 11ng/ml.

OPINIONS

1. The motorcyclist was intoxicated and impaired by marijuana at the time of the collision with the truck, and the THC in his body impaired his ability to operate his motorcycle safely at the time of the accident. This opinion is based upon the Delta 9 THC level and the witnesses' testimony of erratic driving.
2. Based upon the levels of the Delta 9 THC, 11-hydroxy THC, and the carboxy THC, the marijuana use was recent, with an hour or two prior to the collision.
3. The administration of IV fluids (1,500 ml) and blood products (packed RBCs) (600 ml) most likely diluted the toxicology findings, meaning that the levels would have been higher when he was alive.
4. The motorcyclist was following and drove between two SUVs, which may have blocked his vision of the truck (which was visible to an eyewitness, the driver of one of the SUVs). Thus, his abrupt braking on passing and exceeding the eyewitness's speed on his first vision of the truck.

CASE CONCLUSION

The case was resolved/settled, favorably, by the defendant trucking company, based primarily on the marijuana intoxication of the motorcyclist.

CASE REPORT 2: CRIMINAL SEXUAL ASSAULT ("SHE SAID/HE SAID"—EFFECTS OF THC)

FACTS OF THE CASE

A 16-year-old high school girl accused a 16-year-old boy classmate of uninvited fondling her breasts and rape with vaginal penetration during a "date" at the boy's home. She told Police and a Prosecutor that the boy gave her a marijuana cookie which caused her to go to sleep, and when she awoke, the boy was penetrating her vagina with his penis. The girl went to a local hospital where she was examined by medical personnel and police officers. Relevant clinical notes (PD, MD) include:

1. "Patient is a 15-year-old female presenting with Unplanned Sexual Encounter . . . sexual assault patient was exposed to food (marijuana cookie) then woke up with boyfriend on top of her. She began to feel lightheaded and dizzy. Patient came to ED for eval. No pain currently. . . . She previously had sexual intercourse 6 months prior with another male."
2. "She has tried ETOH once; she has never tried other illicit drugs." Chlamydia and Neisseria tests were negative. Prophylaxis for STDs, including HIV, was administered and prescribed for discharge use.

POLICE REPORT

The girl told a police detective that she ate half of what she understood was a marijuana cookie while at the boy's home. While watching a movie, she stated that she was having problems seeing—like everything was slowing down, she began to see different shapes, and she was shaking a lot. She later stated that she was starting to freak out because she was aware of the time, and she needed to be home by 10:00 pm. She began to shake violently, and she began to feel like she could not breathe—she was cold. She tried to fall asleep, and while doing so, the boy started "spooning her," touching her chest, and moving his hand down toward her underwear. She stated she passed out, and when she woke up at around 9:45 hours, she saw and felt the offender "thrusting" her from behind, meaning that the offender was penetrating her vagina with his penis; (she said) she black(ed) out again.

EXPERT INTERVIEW OF DEFENDANT BOY

They had had oral sex several times over the months that they were boyfriend/girlfriend. They had frequently consumed alcohol together. They had discussed to have sexual intercourse when the opportunity presented. She told him that she had had intercourse; he told her that he had not. When they discovered that his parents were out for the evening, they planned the intercourse. They both wanted to have intercourse. After they disrobed, he was unable to maintain an erection—twice. They decided to eat and watch a movie. The girl asked him for the marijuana. She had not used marijuana before; the boy had (from his father's edible THC cookies). The boy also had prior experience smoking marijuana. The boy said that the marijuana cookie was stronger than on his previous experience but no different that smoking a marijuana cigarette.

After eating the marijuana cookie, "She 'slowed down, acting weird, time." Both were high; she worried effects last too long. They both laid down together, trying to sleep. He was trying to comfort and calm her down. Later, he noticed his penis was erect and showed it to her. "She freaked out." The boy denied doing anything sexual without her permission and/or consensus.

OPINIONS

1. The girl was severely intoxicated and impaired by marijuana at the time of the alleged sexual assault.
2. She reported visual and perceptual disturbances, consistent with hallucinations. She reported significant central nervous depression signs, consistent with marijuana intoxication.
3. She consumed marijuana as an edible; that is, she swallowed the marijuana in a cookie. The metabolism of marijuana consumed by mouth is quite different than when smoked; an abundance of a psycho-toxic active metabolite (11-OH-THC) is formed by the liver metabolism that is absent in smoking. Psychiatric toxicities are greater with edibles/oral that are absent in smoking. Adolescents, especially naïve users, are subject to greater psychiatric toxicity and effects of marijuana than adults.
4. Marijuana psycho-toxicity causes distorted perceptions of reality, makes memory formation difficult, and alters the thought and deliberation processes of the marijuana-intoxicated person.
5. The girl herself describes her symptoms and experiences which are textbook signs of marijuana intoxication. Given this well-documented toxicity, based on her description of the effects, her memory and recollections of the events of the evening are highly suspect and subject to substantial doubt.

There is direct contradiction between what she says happened sexually and what he recalled. She claims vaginal intercourse. There is no DNA or physical acute evidence of vaginal intercourse. He denies any penile penetration. She claims she did not consent and never talked about intercourse; he claims they did. She claims that he pressured her to eat the cookie; yet, she agrees that she did eat the cookie. He states she asked for the marijuana cookie when they saw it in the freezer while looking for a frozen pizza. By her own description, she had significant marijuana intoxication, hallucinations, distortions, confusion, sleep, blackout (?). She cannot know if her memory was accurate or distorted. Marijuana can impair and distort memory; thus, her recollection is suspect and subject to doubt.

CASE CONCLUSION

The case was tried to a Judge in a Juvenile Court. The Judge found the boy Not Guilty.

CASE REPORT 3: TRUCK DRIVER REAR-ENDS SEVERAL VEHICLES

FACTS OF THE CASE

The defendant's semi-tractor truck/trailer crashed into several vehicles on an interstate highway at 4:30 am on 10/22/16. When interviewed by state patrol officers, the driver stated that his phone dropped to the floor of the truck cab, and he looked down "for a few seconds" and then when he looked up "didn't have time to react"; it was too late to avoid the collisions—although he did swerve to the left in an attempt to avoid the first rear-end collision. The driver admitted he smoked a joint approximately 20 hours before the crash.

The Investigative Summary of the Trooper stated:

> An analysis completed on a blood sample collected from Mr. Bartlett several hours (7:45 am) after the crash showed he had a 3.4 ng/ml of Delta-9-THC. The Delta-9 THC in the truck driver's system was a major causal factor in this crash likely causing his drowsiness and inattentive driving. The fact sample was obtained more than 3 hours after the crash occurred strongly suggests that the amount of Delta-9-THC in Bartlett's system would have been higher at the time of the crash.

OPINIONS

1. A THC blood level of 3.4 ng/ml is consistent with use 20 hours earlier by a chronic user of marijuana.
2. No impairments are associated with marijuana use 20 hours after use.
3. No scientific literature describes or supports marijuana impairment in a chronic user at a level of 3.4 ng/ml. This may be different for an occasional user; however, conventional wisdom requires a clinical correlation with the blood level to determine impairment. (NHTSA Fact Sheet—Marijuana)
4. Marijuana has very complicated nonlinear kinetics, making extrapolation difficult and quite non-reliable. Thus, you cannot take a level at 7:45 and reliably estimate a level at 4:30 with any certainty.
5. The Trooper's comment that "the level would have been higher at the time of the crash" and "was a major causal factor in this crash likely causing his drowsiness and inattentive driving" is baseless. A 20-hour interval following marijuana use is not associated with any impairments, even in an occasional marijuana user. Twenty hours after use, a THC elimination curve is relatively flat (very little slope), nonlinear, and, as stated earlier, extrapolation is difficult and quite non-reliable.

Reaching for a dropped item is not evidence of drowsiness.

CASE CONCLUSION

The civil case was resolved favorably by the trucking company due to the lack of proof of marijuana impairment in their truck driver. The outcome of the criminal case against the driver is unknown.

CASE REPORT 4: MOTORCYCLIST KILLED IN TRUCK COLLISION; DEFENSE CLAIMS HE WAS HIGH ON THC

FACTS OF THE CASE

A motorcyclist died in a collision when a truck turned left in front of him. Toxicology findings on iliac blood noted the THC level of 4ng/ml and THC-COOH level of 5.3 ng/ml. The medical examiner ruled the cause of death as multiple blunt trauma. No attribution was made to marijuana. An inventory of his personal effects failed to identify any marijuana or paraphernalia for marijuana or drug use.

A toxicologist for the defendant truck company opined that:

> Correlation of behaviors with THC concentration is complicated in that there is not a linear relationship between behavior and concentration as one may find with alcohol. However, the presence of THC in the blood indicates recent usage and correlates with impairment of certain functions important to operation of motor vehicles. THC causes dose-related impairment in attention, perception, tracking behavior, information processing, decision making, reaction time, coordination, and motor performance, all of which can significantly impair one's ability to operate a motor vehicle.
>
> It is thus my opinion to a reasonable degree of scientific certainty that the motorcyclist had recently used marijuana at the time of his death, was under the influence of THC at the time of his death, and that the THC in his body impaired his ability to operate his motor vehicle at the time of the accident. This opinion is based upon the postmortem toxicology results concerning iliac blood sample. While postmortem THC concentrations can differ somewhat from premortem THC concentration, the scientific literature is in agreement that the difference is not of a magnitude to explain the concentration of THC in the postmortem blood sample from the decedent.

A coworker testified that he has known the decedent since childhood and had worked in outside shipping on the "graveyard" shift—nightshift—7:30 pm to 6:00 am. They socialized together outside of work. He knew that the decedent would smoke marijuana at home after he got off work but did not see him smoke marijuana any time on his breaks or anything. They visited in the parking lot for about five minutes before leaving for home. He did not observe Blake smoking anything in the parking lot.

OPINIONS

1. I do not disagree with the defense toxicologist's description of the potential impairing effects of THC. However, the facts in this case argue against any significant recent marijuana use and any signs of impairment. Epidemiological studies have been inconclusive regarding whether marijuana use causes an increased risk of accidents; in contrast, unanimity exists that alcohol use increases crash risk.
2. I strongly disagree with the defense toxicologist's opinion that the motorcyclist was impaired by THC at the time of the collision and that THC impairment contributed to the crash. There is no clinical evidence of impairment, or evidence of relevant recent use, and such a conclusion goes against the current consensus in marijuana scientific literature.
3. I strongly disagree with the defense toxicologist's statement, "However, the presence of THC in the blood indicates recent usage and correlates with impairment of certain functions important to operation of motor vehicles." He does not define "recent use." He relies only on the finding of THC in postmortem blood with impairment at the time the truck turned in front of the motorcycle and killed him. This is a critical flaw in his opinion. Literature defines both the period of time that impairment continues after use (a few to several hours) and remote samples that noted THC in the blood, and that finding "Correlation of behaviors with THC concentration is complicated in that there is not a linear relationship between behavior and concentration," in the toxicologist's own words! In other words, one cannot opine that an individual is impaired simply on the basis of a blood THC level!
4. There is no evidence that the motorcyclist used/smoked marijuana from the time he arrived at work, at any time through the night, after work, or on the short drive home (< 5 minutes) until the time he was fatally injured by the truck. In contrast, there is at least one witness, the coworker, who testified that the decedent did not appear impaired, did not take smoke breaks, and that he closely followed his car on the way home.
5. Marijuana is subject to postmortem redistribution[184]. Studies have shown up to a three times level increase in postmortem blood compared to premortem levels.[185] Marijuana is highly bound to fat in the body,[186] as evidenced by its high volume of distribution ($V_d = 4 - 14$ L/kg).[187] Extensive blunt trauma (crush injuries) would liberate THC from damaged muscle tissues surrounding the iliac vein, raising the postmortem levels higher than normally found following nontraumatic deaths. Marijuana also has complicated nonlinear elimination kinetics.[188] Thus, the premortem levels were probably substantially lower than the postmortem findings.
6. Marijuana blood (or urine) levels cannot predict impairment levels,[189] the dose–response relationship is not linear, and the effects vary from person to person at the same or similar levels.[190]
7. Prolonged marijuana use can result in elevated levels, despite abstaining from marijuana.[191,192,193,194]

CASE CONCLUSION

The decedent's (plaintiff's) attorney petitioned the Court to exclude the testimony of the defense toxicologist. After a Daubert Hearing, the Judge excluded any reference to marijuana. The case was resolved/settled shortly thereafter.

CASE REPORT 5: EPILEPTIC DRIVER CHARGED WITH AGGRAVATED DUI BASED ON THC BLOOD LEVELS

FACTS OF THE CASE

A 52-year-old driver was involved in a multi-vehicle accident on June 11, 2017. He was described as driving at a high rate of speed through at least one red light and one stop sign and crashed into another vehicle causing a chain reaction. One person was killed, and one person was seriously injured. A witness at the scene told Police that the driver was shouting, "I think I'm having a heart attack." The Police described the driver as disoriented and belligerent at the scene. EMS immobilized him, and while placing him in the ambulance, the driver started seizing. Narcan (an opiate reversal agent) was administered in the ambulance. No anti-convulsant medications were noted in the EMS record. On arrival at the hospital, the driver was described as seizing. Ativan and, later, Keppra were administered—both anticonvulsants—to control seizure. Blood drawn for blood type at 11:30 am was later given to Police after a subpoena was issued. The state toxicology lab reported 5.5 ng/mL ± 0.5 ng/mL THC. A urine drug screen reported Positive for Cannabinoids (marijuana). The driver has a history of seizure (epilepsy—convulsive disorder).

Illinois Law (SB 2228) makes it a violation to drive or be in actual physical control of a motor vehicle with 5 ng THC per ml (or more) of whole blood. The driver was charged with Aggravated DUI Drugs as well as other traffic violations.

An expert neurologist reviewed the case and examined the defendant and opined that the driver was in a prodrome or seizing at the time of the crash.

OPINIONS

1. There is a lack of certainty, a reasonable doubt, that the laboratory value of Delta 9 THC is five ng/ml or above. The THC level in the driver's blood was most likely less than the legal threshold or five ng/ml, and therefore there is no DUI violation. The value and error for the THC concentration measurement was given as 5.5 ng/mL ± 0.5 ng/mL, with a 99.7% confidence level that the true level was between 5.0 ng/mL and 6.0 ng/mL. Taking this at face value, this would imply that there is a 0.15% probability that the THC concentration was lower than 5.0 ng/ml. However, the cited error presumably does not take into account other factors such as the selection of the peak in the spectra, the unevenness of the baseline, and inclusion of part of contaminant or other peaks in the THC peak area. Concentration of a substance is calculated by selecting the (chromatogram spectral) peak corresponding to that substance, finding the peak area, and then converting that to concentration. If the baseline is horizontal and there are no other obscuring peaks corresponding to other substances, then this is a simple task. However, an examination of the spectra shows that the baseline is not level, and the peak is small and surrounded by other peaks of similar size presumably due to contaminants or unrelated substances. In fact, the baseline for a different part of the graph appears to be slightly higher than the THC peak itself. The fact that there are peaks of similar size nearby raises the question of whether there are other substances which contribute to the peak area; hence, the calculated THC concentration would be an overestimate. The fact that the baseline is not horizontal also introduces error into the peak selection. Typically, analysis software will draw a baseline by connecting the beginning of the peak to the end of the peak. The peak area is calculated from the region over the baseline between the beginning and end points, and the area under the baseline is assumed to be a signal which is not due to the substance. However, the baseline is not likely to be exactly a straight line; if it is convex, then the calculated concentration will be an overestimate. In the cases of large peaks, these sources of error are not important. However, because the peak is so small and the separation between legality and illegality (five ng/mL) is razor thin, these sources of error make it possible that the THC level may have been under five ng/mL. With no way of quantifying the other sources of error and given the thin margin between the measured value and the five ng/mL cut-off, it cannot be proven that the THC concentration is five ng/mL or above. Of note, there were three triplicate measurements of the same sample, with the lowest one being five ng/mL and with a range of over one ng/mL.
2. No competent scientific evidence exists that the driver was impaired by or was under the influence of marijuana at the time of the collision. Marijuana levels are not predictive of or correlated with impairment. Marijuana users are usually docile and noncombative—not "combative" as described in the police report.

CASE CONCLUSION

With anticipated testimony raising doubt of the precision of the THC blood level as well as the neurologist's opinion, the Aggravated DUI charges were dropped, and the case was resolved without a trial.

36.10 SUMMARY AND CONCLUSIONS

All healthcare professionals as well as legal and law enforcement must be prepared to understand the beneficial and toxic effects of marijuana, because, predictably, the use of THC will continue to increase as the remaining states implement changes to legislature, allowing for medical and recreational use of or decriminalization of marijuana. The pharmacology of marijuana remains challenging. However, continued research provides potential for advancing our understanding and key metrics for assessment. Enhancing and consequent effects of marijuana will be seen, and expert analysis in drugged driving and other cases that consider cognitive impairment will be needed to a greater extent.

NOTES

1 NIDA. 2021, December 22. What is the scope of cannabis (marijuana) use in the United States? https://www.drugabuse.gov/publications/research-reports/marijuana/what-scope-marijuana-use-in-united-states. Accessed 10 January 2022.
2 2020 National Survey on Drug Use and Health. Accessed 10 January 2022.
3 Turner AR. Agrawal S. Marijuana. Updated 29 August 2021. In: StatPearls [Internet]. Treasure Island, FL: StatPearls Publishing; 2021. https://www.ncbi.nlm.nih.gov/books/NBK430801/.
4 https://www.law.cornell.edu/supremecourt/text/03-1454. Accessed 22 January 2022.
5 GONZALES v. RAICH [03-1454]. http://caselaw.lp.findlaw.com/scripts/getcase.pl?court=us&vol=000&invol=03-1454. Accessed 11 January 2022.
6 State Medical Cannabis Laws. http://www.ncsl.org/research/health/state-medical-marijuana-laws.aspx#Table. Accessed 11 January 2022.
7 Xyrem (sodium oxybate) information. Food and Drug Administration. https://www.fda.gov/drugs/postmarket-drug-safety-information-patients-and-providers/xyrem-sodium-oxybate-information#:~:text=GHB%20has%20not%20been%20approved,under%20the%20Controlled%20Substances%20Act. Accessed 6 July 2022.
8 State Medical Cannabis Laws. https://www.ncsl.org/research/health/state-medical-marijuana-laws.aspx. Accessed 10 January 2022.
9 Atakan Z. Cannabis, a complex plant: Different compounds and different effects on individuals. Ther Adv Psychopharmacol. 2012 Dec;2(6):241–254.
10 State Medical Cannabis Laws. http://www.ncsl.org/research/health/state-medical-marijuana-laws.aspx#Table. Accessed 11 January 2022.
11 Marijuana stops child's severe seizures. https://www.cnn.com/2013/08/07/health/charlotte-child-medical-marijuana/. Accessed 11 January 2022.
12 Map of marijuana legality by state. https://disa.com/map-of-marijuana-legality-by-state. Accessed 16 January 2022.
13 See, e.g., Conn. Stat. 16 § 4764.
14 Marijuana Policy Project. https://www.mpp.org/about/. Accessed 10 January 2022.
15 Cannabis tax revenue in states that regulate cannabis for adult use. https://www.mpp.org/issues/legalization/cannabis-tax-revenue-states-regulate-cannabis-adult-use/. Accessed 10 January 2022.
16 O'Donnell JT, O'Donnell JJ. Pharmacology of marijuana. In Tiftickjian J, Ed., Colorado Marijuana Law. Tucson: Lawyers & Judges, 2015.
17 Joy JE, Watson SJ, Benson JA. Marijuana and Medicine: Assessing the Science Base. Washington, DC: National Academy Press, 1999.
18 Boehnke KF, Gangopadhyay S, Clauw DJ, Haffajee RL. Qualifying conditions of medical cannabis license holders in the United States. Health Affairs (Project Hope). 2019;38(2):295–302. doi:10.1377/hlthaff.2018.05266.
19 National Academies of Sciences, Engineering, and Medicine; Health and Medicine Division; Board on Population Health and Public Health Practice; Committee on the Health Effects of Marijuana: An Evidence Review and Research Agenda. The Health Effects of Cannabis and Cannabinoids: The Current State of Evidence and Recommendations for Research. Washington, DC: National Academies Press (US), 12 January 2017: 4, Therapeutic Effects of Cannabis and Cannabinoids. https://www.ncbi.nlm.nih.gov/books/NBK425767/.
20 Friedman D, Devinsky O. Cannabinoids in the treatment of epilepsy. N Engl J Med. 2015;373:1048–1058.
21 Friedman D, Devinsky O. Cannabinoids in the treatment of epilepsy. N Engl J Med. 2015;373:1048–1058.
22 Hughes S. Stratospheric rise of medical marijuana in epilepsy. *Medscape Medical News >Neurology*, 10 September 2015. http://www.medscape.com/viewarticle/850805?nlid=88228_2981&src=wnl_edit_dail&uac=242394CR&impID=820586&faf=1.
23 Friedman D, Devinsk O. Cannabinoids in the treatment of epilepsy. N Engl J Med. 2015;373:1048–1058.
24 Nabbout R, Thiele EA. The role of cannabinoids in epilepsy treatment: A critical review of efficacy results from clinical trials. Epileptic Disord. 2020 January 1;22(S1):23–28.
25 Allam S, Paris E, Lazcano I, Bitterman P, Basu S, O'Donnell J, Barua A. Detection of cannabinoid receptor expression by endometriotic lesions in women with endometriosis as an alternative to opioid-based pain medication. J Immunol Res. 2022 Jun 2;2022:4323259.
26 Atakan Z. Cannabis, a complex plant: Different compounds and different effects on individuals. Ther Adv Psychopharmacol. 2012 Dec;2(6):241–254.
27 Kendall DA, Yudowski GA. Cannabinoid receptors in the central nervous system: Their signaling and roles in disease. Front Cell Neurosci. 2017 Jan 4;10:294.
28 Kendall DA, Yudowski GA. Cannabinoid receptors in the central nervous system: Their signaling and roles in disease. Front Cell Neurosci. 2017 Jan 4;10:294.

29 Atakan Z. Cannabis, a complex plant: Different compounds and different effects on individuals. Ther Adv Psychopharmacol. 2012;2(6):241–254.

30 Amin MR, Ali DW. Pharmacology of medical cannabis. Adv Exp Med Biol. 2019;1162:151–165.

31 Millar SA, Stone NL, Yates AS, O'Sullivan SE. A systematic review on the pharmacokinetics of cannabidiol in humans. Front Pharmacol. 2018;9:1365. doi:10.3389/fphar.2018.01365.

32 Karschner EL, Schwilke EW, Lowe RH, Darwin WD, Pope HG, Herning R, Cadet JL, Huestis MA. Do Delta9-tetrahydrocannabinol concentrations indicate recent use in chronic cannabis users? Addiction. 2009 Dec;104(12):2041–2048.

33 Lafaye G, Karila L, Blecha L, Benyamina A. Cannabis, cannabinoids, and health. Dialogue Clin Neurosci. 2017 Sep;19(3):309–316.

34 Singh VM, Browne T, Montgomery J. The emerging role of toxic adulterants in street drugs in the US illicit opioid crisis. Public Health Rep. 2020 Jan;135(1):6–10.

35 Pérez-Moreno M, Pérez-Lloret P, González-Soriano J, Santos-Álvarez I. Cannabis resin in the region of Madrid: Adulteration and contamination. Forensic Sci Int. 2019 May;298:34–38.

36 Meehan-Atrash J, Strongin RM. Pine rosin identified as a toxic cannabis extract adulterant. Forensic Sci Int. 2020 Jul;312:110301.

37 Barceló B, Pichini S, López-Corominas V, Gomila I, Yates C, Busardò FP, Pellegrini M. Acute intoxication caused by synthetic cannabinoids 5F-ADB and MMB-2201: A case series. Forensic Sci Int. 2017;273:e10–e14.

38 Vandrey R, Raber JC, Raber ME, Douglass B, Miller C, Bonn-Miller MO. Cannabinoid dose and label accuracy in edible medical cannabis products. JAMA. 2017;313:2491.

39 Peace MR, Stone JW, Poklis JL, Turner JB, Poklis A. Analysis of a commercial marijuana e-cigarette formulation. JAT. 2016;40:374–378.

40 Bonn-Miller MO, Loflin MJE, Thomas BF, Marcu JP, Hyke T, Vandrey R. Labeling accuracy of cannabidiol extracts sold online. JAMA. 2017;318(17):1708–1709.

41 Poklis JL, Mulder HA, Peace MR. The unexpected identification of the cannabimimetic, 5F-ADB, and dextromethorphan in commercially available cannabidiol e-liquids. Forensic Sci Int. 2019 Jan;294:e25–e27.

42 Lemberger L, Weiss JL, Watanabe AM, Galanter IM, Wyatt RJ, Cardon PV. Delta-9-tetrahydrocannabinol: Temporal correlation of the psychologic effects and blood levels after various routes of administration. N Engl J Med. 1972 Mar 30;286(13):685–688.

43 Amin MR, Ali DW. Pharmacology of medical cannabis. Adv Exp Med Biol. 2019;1162:151–165.

44 Amin MR, Ali DW. Pharmacology of medical cannabis. Adv Exp Med Biol. 2019;1162:151–165.

45 Ohlsson A, Lindgren JE, Wahlen A, Agurell S, Hollister LE, Gillespie HK. Plasma delta-9 tetrahydrocannabinol concentrations and clinical effects after oral and intravenous administration and smoking. Clin Pharmacol Ther. 1980 Sep;28(3):409–416.

46 Lee DC, Crosier BS, Borodovsky JT, Sargent JD, Budney AJ. Online survey characterizing vaporizer use among cannabis users. Drug Alcohol Depend. 2016;159:227–233.

47 Budney AJ, Sargent JD, Lee DC. Vaping cannabis (marijuana): Parallel concerns to e-cigs? Addiction. 2015;110(11):1699–1704.

48 Poklis JL, Mulder HA, Peace MR. The unexpected identification of the cannabimimetic, 5F-ADB, and dextromethorphan in commercially available cannabidiol e-liquids. Forensic Sci Int. 2019;294:e25–e27.

49 Pomahacova B, Van der Kooy F, Verpoorte R. Cannabis smoke condensate III: The cannabinoid content of vaporised cannabis sativa. Inhal Toxicol. 2009;21(13):1108–1112.

50 Alchin DR. 'Vaping psychosis': Ultra-acute onset of severe, persisting and unusual psychotic symptoms following first-time cannabis vaping in a previously well individual. Australian & New Zealand Journal of Psychiatry. 2020;54(8):848.

51 Czégény Z, Nagy G, Babinszki B, Bajtel Á, Sebestyén Z, Kiss T, Csupor-Löffler B, Tóth B, Csupor D. CBD, a precursor of THC in e-cigarettes. Sci Rep. 2021 Apr 26;11(1):8951.

52 LaBenne, L. Smoke marijuana is not good medicine. Drug Topics: Voice of the Pharmacist, 6 July 2004.

53 Ohlsson A, Lindgren JE, Wahlen A, Agurell S, Hollister LE, Gillespie HK. Plasma delta-9 tetrahydrocannabinol concentrations and clinical effects after oral and intravenous administration and smoking. Clin Pharmacol Ther. 1980 Sep;28(3):409–416.

54 Lemberger L, Martz R, Rodda B, Forney R, Rowe H. Comparative pharmacology of Delta9-tetrahydrocannabinol and its metabolite, 11-OH-Delta9-tetrahydrocannabinol. J Clin Invest. 1973 Oct;52(10):2411–2417.

55 Ohlsson A, Lindgren JE, Wahlen A, Agurell S, Hollister LE, Gillespie HK. Plasma delta-9 tetrahydrocannabinol concentrations and clinical effects after oral and intravenous administration and smoking. Clin Pharmacol Ther. 1980 Sep;28(3):409–416.

56 Wall ME, Perez-Reyes M. The metabolism of delta 9-tetrahydrocannabinol and related cannabinoids in man. J Clin Pharmacol. 1981 Aug–Sep;21(8–9 Suppl):178S–189S.

57 Lemberger L, Martz R, Rodda B, Forney R, Rowe H. Comparative pharmacology of Delta9-tetrahydrocannabinol and its metabolite, 11-OH-Delta9-tetrahydrocannabinol. J Clin Invest. 1973 Oct;52(10):2411–2417.

58 Heustis, M. ACannabis (marijuana): Effects on human behavior and performance. Forensic Sci Rev. 2002;14(2):15–60.

59 Turner CE, Elsohly MA, Boeren EG. Constituents of Cannabis sativa L. XVII. A review

of the natural constituents. J Nat Prod. 1980 Mar–Apr;43(2):169–234.
60 Lile JA, Kelly TH, Charnigo RJ, Stinchcomb AL, Hays LR. Pharmacokinetic and pharmacodynamic profile of supratherapeutic oral doses of Δ(9)-THC in cannabis users. J Clin Pharmacol. 2013 Jul;53(7):680–690.
61 Goodwin RS, Gustafson RA, Barnes A, Nebro W, Moolchan ET, Huestis MA. Delta(9)-tetrahydrocannabinol, 11-hydroxy-delta(9)-tetrahydrocannabinol and 11-nor-9-carboxy-delta(9)-tetrahydrocannabinol in human plasma after controlled oral administration of cannabinoids. Ther Drug Monit. 2006 Aug;28(4):545–551.
62 EROWID cannabis (marijuana) vault, cannabis effects, 4 June 2014, 6 pages.
63 Physicians Desk Reference, 61st ed. Thomson PDR Copyright, 2007.
64 Lile JA, Kelly TH, Charnigo RJ, Stinchcomb AL, Hays LR. Pharmacokinetic and pharmacodynamic profile of supratherapeutic oral doses of Δ(9)-THC in cannabis users. J Clin Pharmacol. 2013 Jul;53(7):680–690.
65 Goodwin RS, Gustafson RA, Barnes A, Nebro W, Moolchan ET, Huestis MA. Delta(9)-tetrahydrocannabinol, 11-hydroxy-delta(9)-tetrahydrocannabinol and 11-nor-9-carboxy-delta(9)-tetrahydrocannabinol in human plasma after controlled oral administration of cannabinoids. Ther Drug Monit. 2006 Aug;28(4):545–551.
66 Lile JA, Kelly TH, Charnigo RJ, Stinchcomb AL, Hays LR. Pharmacokinetic and pharmacodynamic profile of supratherapeutic oral doses of Δ(9) -THC in cannabis users. J Clin Pharmacol. 2013 Jul;53(7):680–690.
67 Lile JA, Kelly TH, Charnigo RJ, Stinchcomb AL, Hays LR. Pharmacokinetic and pharmacodynamic profile of supratherapeutic oral doses of Δ(9)-THC in cannabis users. J Clin Pharmacol. 2013 Jul;53(7):680–690.
68 Karschner EL, Darwin WD, Goodwin RS, Wright S, Huestis MA. Plasma cannabinoid pharmacokinetics following controlled oral delta9-tetrahydrocannabinol and oromucosal cannabis extract administration. Clin Chem. 2011 Jan;57(1):66–75.
69 EROWID Cannabis (marijuana) vault, Cannabis Effects, 4 June 2014, 6 pages.
70 Benjamin DM. Toxic ingestions of marijuana (THC). Presented at the Second International Conference on Neu Psyco, Havana, Cuba, 18 November 2014.
71 Memedovich KA, Dowsett LE, Spackman E, Noseworthy T, Clement F. The adverse health effects and harms related to marijuana use: An overview review. CMAJ Open. 2018 Aug 16;6(3):E339–E346.
72 Ameri A. The effects of cannabinoids on the brain. Prog Neurobiol. 1999;58(4):315–348.
73 Martinotti G, De Risio L, Vannini C, Schifano F, Pettorruso M, Di Giannantonio M. Substance-related exogenous psychosis: A postmodern syndrome. CNS Spectrums. 2021;26(1):84–91.
74 Diamond G, Panichelli-Mindel SM, Shera D, Dennis M, Tims F, Ungemack J. Psychiatric syndromes in adolescents with marijuana abuse and dependency in outpatient treatment. J Child Adolesc Subst Abuse. 2006;15(4):37–54.
75 Di Forti M, Quattrone D, Freeman TP, Tripoli G, Gayer-Anderson C, Quigley H, Rodriguez V, Jongsma HE, Ferraro L, La Cascia C, La Barbera D. The contribution of cannabis use to variation in the incidence of psychotic disorder across Europe (EU-GEI): A multicentre case-control study. Lancet. 2019;6(5): 427–436.
76 Baldacchino A, Blair H, Scherbaum N, Grosse-Vehne EV, Riglietta M, Tidone L, Criaco C, Marelli MC, Sommer B, Tan L, Little H. Drugs and psychosis project: A multi-centre European study on comorbidity. Drug Alcohol Rev. 2009;28:379–389.
77 Varma LP. Cannabis psychosis. Indian J Psychiatry. 1972;14:241–255.
78 Moore TH, Zammit S, Lingford-Hughes A, Barnes TR, Jones PB, Burke M, Lewis G. Cannabis use and risk of psychotic or affective mental health outcomes: A systematic review. Lancet. 2007;370:319–328.
79 Chen CY, Lin KM. Health consequences of illegal drug use. Curr Opin Psychiatry. 2009;22:287–292.
80 Gregg L, Barrowlough C, Haddock G. Reasons for increased substance use in psychosis. Clin Psychol Rev. 2007;27:494–510.
81 Barrigón ML, Gurpegui M, Ruiz-Veguilla M, Diaz FJ, Anguita M, Sarramea F, Cervilla J. Temporal relationship of first-episode non-affective psychosis with cannabis use: A clinical verification of an epidemiological hypothesis. J Psychiatr Res. 2010 May;44(7): 413–420.
82 de la Serna E, Mayoral M, Baeza I, Arango C, Andrés P, Bombin I, González C, Rapado M, Robles O, Rodríguez-Sánchez JM, Zabala A, Castro-Fornieles J. Cognitive functioning in children and adolescents in their first episode of psychosis: Differences between previous cannabis users and nonusers. J Nerv Ment Dis. 2010 Feb;198(2):159–162.
83 Sewell RA, Skosnik PD, Garcia-Sosa I, Ranganathan M, D'Souza DC. Behavioral, cognitive and psychophysiological effects of cannabinoids: Relevance to psychosis and schizophrenia. Rev Bras Psiquiatr. 2010;32(Suppl 1):S15–S30.
84 Marijuana treats pose hidden dangers. Trevor Hughes. *USA Today Weekend*, 1A–2A, May 9–11, 2014.
85 Kesby JP, Eyles DW, McGrath JJ, Scott JG. Dopamine, psychosis and schizophrenia: The widening gap between basic and clinical neuroscience. Transl Psychiatry. 2018 Jan 31;8(1):30.
86 Oyebode F. The neurology of psychosis. Med Princ Pract. 2008;17(4):263–269.
87 Goren JL. "Psychosis" drug-induced diseases: Prevention, detection and management. In Tisdale JE, Miller DA, Eds., American Society of Health System Pharmacists, 2nd ed., 2010:344–356.
88 Goren JL. "Psychosis" drug-induced diseases: Prevention, detection and management. In Tisdale JE,

Miller DA, Eds., American Society of Health System Pharmacists, 2nd ed., 2010:344–356.
89 Kenne DK, Fischbein RL, Tan ASL, Banks M. The Use of Substances Other Than Nicotine in Electronic Cigarettes Among College Students. Substance Abuse, 2017.
90 Spindle TR, Cone EJ, Schlienz NJ, Mitchell JM, Bigelow GE, Flegel R, Hayes E, Vandrey R. Acute effects of smoked and vaporized cannabis in healthy adults who infrequently use cannabis: A crossover trial. JAMA Netw Open. 2018 Nov 2;1(7):e184841.
91 Oh H, Banawa R, Jungeun OL, Zhou S, Huh J. Vaping and psychotic experiences among college students in the United States. Drug Alcohol Depend. 2021;227(1):1–5.
92 Tashkin DP. Effects of marijuana smoking on the lung. Ann Am Thorac Soc. 2013;10:239–247.
93 Pletcher MJ, Vittinghoff E, Kalhan R, Richman J, Safford M, Sidney S, Lin F, Kertesz S. Association between marijuana exposure and pulmonary function over 20 years. JAMA. 2012;307:173–181.
94 Volkow ND, Baler RD, Compton WM, Weiss SR. Adverse health effects of marijuana use. N Engl J Med. 2014;370:2219–2227.
95 Lopez-Quintero C, de los Cobos JP, Hasin DS, Okuda M, Wang S, Grant BF, Blanco C. Probability and predictors of transition from first use to dependence on nicotine, alcohol, cannabis, and cocaine: Results of the National Epidemiologic Survey on Alcohol and Related Conditions (NESARC). Drug Alcohol Depend. 2011 May 1,115(1–2):120–130. doi:10.1016/j.drugalcdep.2010.11.004. Epub 8 December 2010.
96 Hall W, Degenhardt L. Adverse health effects of non-medical cannabis use. Lancet. 2009;374:1383–1391.
97 Gorelick DA, Levin KH, Copersino ML, Heishman SJ, Liu F, Boggs DL, Kelly DL. Diagnostic criteria for cannabis withdrawal syndrome. Drug Alcohol Depend. 2012;123:141–147.
98 Volkow ND, Baler RD, Compton WM, Weiss SR. Adverse health effects of marijuana use. N Engl J Med. 2014;370:2219–2227.
99 Volkow ND, Baler RD, Compton WM, Weiss SR. Adverse health effects of marijuana use. N Engl J Med. 2014;370:2219–2227.
100 Lemberger L, Martz R, Rodda B, Forney R, Rowe H. Comparative pharmacology of Δ9-tetrahydrocannabinolanditsmetabolite, 11-OH-Δ9-tetrahydrocannabinol. J Clin Investig. 1973;52: 2411–2417.
101 McPartland J. Advantages of pharmaceutical herbal cannabis compared to single-ingredient, synthetic tetrahydrocannabinol. Presented at The Third International Symposium: Bioresource Hemp, Wolfsburg, Germany, 13–16 September 2000.
102 Solowij N, Battisti R. The chronic effects of cannabis on memory in humans: A review. Curr Drug Abuse Rev. 2008;1(1):81–98.
103 Solowij N, Stephens RS, Roffman RA, Babor T, Kadden R, Miller M, Christiansen K, McRee B, Vendetti J, Marijuana Treatment Project Research Group. Cognitive functioning of long-term heavy cannabis users seeking treatment. JAMA. 2002;287(9):1123–1131.
104 Battisti RA, Roodenrys S, Johnstone SJ, Respondek C, Hermens DF, Solowij N. Chronic use of cannabis and poor neural efficiency in verbal memory ability. Psychopharmacology. 2010;209(4):319–330.
105 Lorenzetti V, Lubman DI, Whittle S, Solowij N, Yücel M. Structural MRI findings in long-term cannabis users: What do we know? Subst Use Misuse. 2010;45:1787–1808.
106 Tzilos GK, Cintron CB, Wood JB, Simpson NS, Young AD, Pope Jr HG, Yurgelun-Todd DA. Lack of hippocampan volume change in long-term heacy cannabis users. Am J Addict. 2005;14:64–72.
107 Pope HG Jr, Gruber AJ, Hudson JI, Cohane G, Huestis MA, Yurgelun-Todd D. Early-onset cannabis use and cognitive deficits: What is the nature of the association? Drug Alcohol Depend. 2003;69:303–310.
108 Friedman D, Devinsky O. Cannabinoids in the treatment of epilepsy. N Engl J Med. 2015;373:1048–1058.
109 Macleod J, Oakes R, Copello A, Crome I, Egger M, Hickman M, Oppenkowski T, Stokes-Lampard H, Smith GD. Psychological and social sequelae of cannabis and other illicit drug use by young people: A systematic review of longitudinal, general population studies. Lancet. 2004;363:1579–1588.
110 Tapert SF, Schweinsburg AD, Brown SA. The influence of Marijuana use on neurocognitive functioning in adolescents. Curr Drug Abuse Rev. 2008;1(1):99–111.
111 Wang GS, Hall K, Vigil D, Banerji S, Monte A, VanDyke M. Marijuana and acute health care contacts in Colorado. Prev Med. 2017;104:24–30.
112 Marijuana legalization in Colorado: Early findings. A report pursuant to Senate Bill 13-283, 2016. Accessed 6 January 2022.
113 Roberts BA. Legalized cannabis in Colorado emergency departments: A cautionary review of negative health and safety effects. West J Emerg Med. 2019;20(4):557–572.
114 Wang GS, Le Lait MC, Deakyne SJ, Bronstein AC, Bajaj L, Roosevelt G. Unintentional pediatric exposures to marijuana in Colorado, 2009–2015. JAMA Pediatr. 2016;170(9):e160971.
115 Wang GS, Hoyte C, Roosevelt G, Heard K. The continued impact of marijuana legalization on unintentional pediatric exposures in Colorado. Clin Pediatr (Phila). 2019;58(1):114–116.
116 US Department of Transportation National Highway Traffic Safety Administration. Results of the 2013–2014 national roadside survey of alcohol and drug use by drivers. DOT HS 812 118, February 2015.
117 National Academies of Sciences, Engineering, and Medicine. The Health Effects of Cannabis and Cannabinoids: The Current State of Evidence and

Recommendations for Research. Washington, DC: The National Academies Press, 2017.
118 Pacula RL, Smart R, Lira MC, Pessar SC, Blanchette JG, Naimi TS. Relationships of cannabis policy liberalization with alcohol use and co-use with cannabis: A narrative review. Alcohol Res Curr Rev. 2022;42(1):1–18.
119 American Academy of Orthopaedic Surgeons (AAOS). 2022 Annual Meeting. Abstract 80 and Abstract 85. Presented 22 March 2022.
120 Karschner EL, Schwilke EW, Lowe RH, Darwin WD, Herning RI, Cadet JL, Huestis MA. Implications of plasma Delta9-tetrahydrocannabinol, 11-hydroxy-THC, and 11-nor-9-carboxy-THC concentrations in chronic cannabis smokers. J Anal Toxicol. 2009 Oct;33(8):469–477.
121 Karschner EL, Schwilke EW, Lowe RH, Darwin WD, Pope HG, Herning R, Cadet JL, Huestis MA. Do Delta9-tetrahydrocannabinol concentrations indicate recent use in chronic cannabis users? Addiction. 2009 Dec;104(12):2041–2048.
122 Mura P, Brunet B, Favreau F, Hauet T. [Cannabis and road crashes: A survey of recent French studies]. Ann Pharm Fr. 2006 May;64(3):192–196.
123 Hartman RL, Brown TL, Milavetz G, Spurgin A, Gorelick A, Gaffney GR, Huestis MA. Effect of blood collection time on measured δ9-tetrahydrocannabinol concentrations: Implications for driving interpretation and drug policy. Clin Chem. 2016;62:2367–2377.
124 Lawrence DK, Pertwee RG. Brain levels of Δ1-tetrahydrocannabinol and its metabolites in mice tolerant to the hypothermic effect of Δ1-tetrahydrocannabinol. Br J Pharmacol. 1973 Oct;49(2):373–375.
125 Lemberger L, Weiss JL, Watanabe AM, Galanter IM, Wyatt RJ, Cardon PV. Delta-9-tetrahydrocannabinol: Temporal correlation of the psychologic effects and blood levels after various routes of administration. N Engl J Med. 1972 Mar 30;286(13):685–688.
126 Ohlsson A, Widman M, Carlsson S, Ryman T, Strid C. Plasma and brain levels of delta 6-THC and seven monooxygenated metabolites correlated to the cataleptic effect in the mouse. Acta Pharmacol Toxicol (Copenh). 1980 Oct;47(4):308–317.
127 Lawrence DK, Pertwee RG. Brain levels of Δ1-tetrahydrocannabinol and its metabolites in mice tolerant to the hypothermic effect of Δ1-tetrahydrocannabinol. Br J Pharmacol. 1973 Oct;49(2):373–375.
128 Poklis JL, Thompson CC, Long KA, Lichtman AH, Poklis A. Disposition of cannabichromene, cannabidiol, and δ9-tetrahydrocannabinol and its metabolites in mouse brain following marijuana inhalation determined by high-performance liquid chromatography–tandem mass spectrometry. J Anal Toxicol. 2010 Oct 1;34(8):516–520.
129 Heustis, M. A cannabis (marijuana)-effects on human behavior and performance. Forensic Sci Rev. 2002;14(2):15–60.
130 Ohlsson A, Widman M, Carlsson S, Ryman T, Strid C. Plasma and brain levels of delta 6-THC and seven monooxygenated metabolites correlated to the cataleptic effect in the mouse. Acta Pharmacol Toxicol (Copenh). 1980 Oct;47(4):308–317.
131 Agurell S, Halldin M, Lindgren JE, Ohlsson A, Widman M, Gillespie H, Hollister L. Pharmacokinetics and metabolism of delta 1-tetrahydrocannabinol and other cannabinoids with emphasis on man. Pharmacol Rev. 1986 Mar;38(1):21–43.
132 Giroud C, Ménétrey A, Augsburger M, Buclin T, Sanchez-Mazas P, Mangin P. Delta(9)-THC, 11-OH-Delta(9)-THC and Delta(9)-THCCOOH plasma or serum to whole blood concentrations distribution ratios in blood samples taken from living and dead people. Forensic Sci Int. 2001 Dec 1;123(2–3):159–164.
133 Huestis MA. Human cannabinoid pharmacokinetics. Chem Biodivers. 2007 Aug;4(8):1770–1804.
134 Huestis MA, Henningfield JE, Cone EJ. Blood cannabinoids. I. Absorption of THC and formation of 11-OH-THC and THCCOOH during and after smoking marijuana. J Anal Toxicol. 1992 Sep–Oct;16(5):276–282.
135 Huestis MA, Henningfield JE, Cone EJ. Blood cannabinoids. II. Models for the prediction of time of marijuana exposure from plasma concentrations of delta 9-tetrahydrocannabinol (THC) and 11-nor-9-carboxy-delta 9-tetrahydrocannabinol (THCCOOH). J Anal Toxicol. 1992 Sep–Oct;16(5):283–290.
136 Ramaekers JG, Berghaus G, van Laar M, Drummer OH. Dose related risk of motor vehicle crashes after cannabis use. Drug Alcohol Depend. 2004 Feb 7;73(2):109–119.
137 Karschner EL, Schwilke EW, Lowe RH, Darwin WD, Herning RI, Cadet JL, Huestis MA. Implications of plasma Delta9-tetrahydrocannabinol, 11-hydroxy-THC, and 11-nor-9-carboxy-THC concentrations in chronic cannabis smokers. J Anal Toxicol. 2009 Oct;33(8):469–477.
138 Schwope DM, Bosker WM, Ramaekers JG, Gorelick DA, Huestis MA. Psychomotor performance, subjective and physiological effects and whole blood Δ^9-tetrahydrocannabinol concentrations in heavy, chronic cannabis smokers following acute smoked cannabis. J Anal Toxicol. 2012 Jul;36(6):405–412.
139 Lemberger L, Weiss JL, Watanabe AM, Galanter IM, Wyatt RJ, Cardon PV. Delta-9-tetrahydrocannabinol: Temporal correlation of the psychologic effects and blood levels after various routes of administration. N Engl J Med. 1972 Mar 30;286(13):685–688.
140 Huestis MA, Henningfield JE, Cone EJ. Blood cannabinoids. I. Absorption of THC and formation of 11-OH-THC and THCCOOH during and after smoking marijuana. J Anal Toxicol. 1992 Sep–Oct;16(5):276–282.
141 Agurell S, Halldin M, Lindgren JE, Ohlsson A, Widman M, Gillespie H, Hollister L. Pharmacokinetics and metabolism of delta 1-tetrahydrocannabinol and

other cannabinoids with emphasis on man. Pharmacol Rev. 1986 Mar;38(1):21–43.

142 Lawrence DK, Pertwee RG. Brain levels of Δ1-tetrahydrocannabinol and its metabolites in mice tolerant to the hypothermic effect of Δ1-tetrahydrocannabinol. Br J Pharmacol. 1973 Oct;49(2):373–375.

143 Heustis, M. A cannabis (marijuana): Effects on human behavior and performance. Forensic Sci Rev. 2002;14(2):15–60.

144 Agurell S, Halldin M, Lindgren JE, Ohlsson A, Widman M, Gillespie H, Hollister L. Pharmacokinetics and metabolism of delta 1-tetrahydrocannabinol and other cannabinoids with emphasis on man. Pharmacol Rev. 1986 Mar;38(1):21–43.

145 Giroud C, Ménétrey A, Augsburger M, Buclin T, Sanchez-Mazas P, Mangin P. Delta(9)-THC, 11-OH-Delta(9)-THC and Delta(9)-THCCOOH plasma or serum to whole blood concentrations distribution ratios in blood samples taken from living and dead people. Forensic Sci Int. 2001 Dec 1;123(2–3):159–164.

146 Gerostamoulos J, Drummer OH. Incidence of psychoactive cannabinoids in drivers killed in motor vehicle accidents. J Forensic Sci. 1993 May;38(3):649–656.

147 Brunet B, Hauet T, Hébrard W, Papet Y, Mauco G, Mura P. Postmortem redistribution of THC in the pig. Int J Legal Med. 2010 Nov;124(6):543–549.

148 Mura P, Brunet B, Favreau F, Hauet T. [Cannabis and road crashes: A survey of recent French studies]. Ann Pharm Fr. 2006 May;64(3):192–196.

149 Huestis MA, Cone EJ. Urinary excretion half-life of 11-nor-9-carboxy-delta9-tetrahydrocannabinol in humans. Ther Drug Monit. 1998 Oct;20(5):570–576.

150 Moody DE, Monti KM, Crouch DJ. Analysis of forensic specimens for cannabinoids. II. Relationship between blood delta 9-tetrahydrocannabinol and blood and urine 11-nor-delta 9-tetrahydrocannabinol-9-carboxylic acid concentrations. J Anal Toxicol. 1992 Sep–Oct;16(5):302–306.

151 Huestis MA, Henningfield JE, Cone EJ. Blood cannabinoids II: Models for the prediction of time of marijuana exposure from plasma concentrations of delta-9-tetrahydrocannabinol(THC) and 11-nor-9-carboxy-delta-9-tetrahydrocannabinol(THCCOH). J Anal Tox. 1992;16:283–290.

152 Cone EJ. Marijuana effects and urinalysis after passive inhalation and oral ingestion. NIDA Res Monogr. 1990;99:88–96.

153 Huestis MA. Acute and chronic frequent cannabis intake. American College of Medical Toxicology (ACMT) Seminars in Forensic Toxicology, Denver, CO, 12 September 2015.

154 Huestis MA. Acute and chronic frequent cannabis intake. American College of Medical Toxicology (ACMT) Seminars in Forensic Toxicology, Denver, CO, 12 September 2015.

155 Huestis MA. Acute and chronic frequent cannabis intake. American College of Medical Toxicology (ACMT) Seminars in Forensic Toxicology, Denver, CO, 12 September 2015.

156 Huestis MA. Human cannabinoid pharmacokinetics. Chem Biodivers. 2007 Aug;4(8):1770–1804.

157 American College of Medical Toxicology (ACMT). Seminars in Forensic Toxicology. Denver, CO, 12 September–15 October.

158 Ellis GM Jr, Mann MA, Judson BA, Schramm NT, Tashchian A. Excretion patterns of cannabinoid metabolites after last use in a group of chronic users. Clin Pharmacol Ther. 1985 Nov;38(5):572–578.

159 Diagnostics Reagents, Inc. Cannabinoid (THC) Enzyme Immunoassay, Package Insert, Limitations of the Assay Results, August 1999.

160 Leiken JB, Paloucek FP, eds. Limitations of the urine drug screening assay positive test results. In Poisoning & Toxicology Handbook, 3rd ed, 1201.

161 Cone EJ. Marijuana effects and urinalysis after passive inhalation and oral ingestion. NIDA Res Monogr. 1990;99:88–96.

162 Goodwin RS, Darwin WD, Chiang CN, Shih M, Li S-H, Huestis MA. Urinary elimination of 11-nor-9-carboxy-9-tetrahydrocannnabinol in cannabis users during continuously monitored abstinence. J Anal Toxicol. 2008 Oct;32(8):562–569.

163 O'Kane CJ, Tutt DC, Bauer LA. Cannabis and driving: A new perspective. Emerg Med (Fremantle). 2002 Sep;14(3):296–303.

164 Kurzthaler I, Hummer M, Miller C, Sperner-Unterweger B, Günther V, Wechdorn H, Battista HJ, Fleischhacker WW. Effect of cannabis use on cognitive functions and driving ability. J Clin Psychiatry. 1999 Jun;60(6):395–399.

165 Solowij N, Stephens RS, Roffman RA, Babor T, Kadden R, Miller M, Christiansen K, McRee B, Vendetti J. Marijuana Treatment Project Research Group. Cognitive functioning of long-term heavy cannabis users seeking treatment. JAMA. 2002 Mar 6;287(9):1123–1131.

166 Iversen LL. The Science of Marijuana. Oxford University Press, 2000, 90–92.

167 Logan BK. Marijuana and Driving Impairment (An Overview), 2004, 1–20.

168 Klonoff H. Marijuana and driving in real-life situations. Science. 1974 Oct 25;186(4161):317–324.

169 Smiley A, Noy I, Tostowaryk W. Alcohol, drugs and traffic safety. In Nordic, Roszbach, Eds., The Effects of Marijuana Alone and in Combination With Alcohol on Driving Performance. Elsevier Science Publishers B.V., 1987, 203–206.

170 Diagnostics Reagents, Inc. Cannabinoid (THC) Enzyme Immunoassay, package Insert, Limitations of the assay results, August 1999.

171 Schwope DM, Bosker WM, Ramaekers JG, Gorelick DA, Huestis MA. Psychomotor performance, subjective and physiological effects and whole blood Δ^9-tetrahydrocannabinol concentrations in heavy,

chronic cannabis smokers following acute smoked cannabis. J Anal Toxicol. 2012 Jul;36(6):405–412.

172 Bosker WM, Theunissen EL, Conen S, Kuypers KP, Jeffery WK, Walls HC, Kauert GF, Toennes SW, Moeller MR, Ramaekers JG. A placebo-controlled study to assess Standardized Field Sobriety Tests performance during alcohol and cannabis intoxication in heavy cannabis users and accuracy of point of collection testing devices for detecting THC in oral fluid. Psychopharmacology (Berl). 2012 Oct;223(4):439–446.

173 Oberman S, Compher-Rice S. The Standardized Field Sobriety Tests Validation Myth. DWI, June 2006, 36–42.

174 Bramness JG, Khiabani HZ, Mørland J. Impairment due to cannabis and ethanol: Clinical signs and additive effects. Addiction. 2010 Jun;105(6):1080–1087.

175 Bramness JG, Khiabani HZ, Mørland J. Impairment due to cannabis and ethanol: Clinical signs and additive effects. Addiction. 2010 Jun;105(6):1080–1087.

176 Ramaekers JG, Moeller MR, van Ruitenbeek P, Theunissen EL, Schneider E, Kauert G. Cognition and motor control as a function of Delta9-THC concentration in serum and oral fluid: Limits of impairment. Drug Alcohol Depend. 2006 Nov 8;85(2):114–122.

177 Alcohol combined severely impede driving performance. Ann Emerg Med. 2000 Apr;35(4):398–399.

178 National Highway Traffic Safety Administration (NHTSA) Notes. Marijuana and alcohol combined severely impede driving performance. Ann Emerg Med. 2000 Apr;35(4):398–399.

179 Ramaekers JG, Moeller MR, van Ruitenbeek P, Theunissen EL, Schneider E, Kauert G. Cognition and motor control as a function of Delta9-THC concentration in serum and oral fluid: Limits of impairment. Drug Alcohol Depend. 2006 Nov 8;85(2):114–122.

180 Heishman SJ, Stitzer ML, Bigelow GE. Alcohol and marijuana: Comparative dose effect profiles in humans. Pharmacol Biochem Behav. 1988 Nov;31(3):649–655.

181 Heishman SJ, Huestis MA, Henningfield JE, Cone EJ. Acute and residual effects of marijuana: Profiles of plasma THC levels, physiological, subjective, and performance measures. Pharmacol Biochem Behav. 1990 Nov;37(3):561–565.

182 Solowij N, Stephens RS, Roffman RA, Babor T, Kadden R, Miller M, Christiansen K, McRee B, Vendetti J; Marijuana Treatment Project Research Group. Cognitive functioning of long-term heavy cannabis users seeking treatment. JAMA. 2002 Mar 6;287(9):1123–1131. doi: 10.1001/jama.287.9.1123.

183 O'Donnell JT, Vogenberg FR. Beyond medical cannabis: Considerations for updates to hospital policies and procedures. P&T. 2019 Jul/Aug;44(7).

184 Holland MG. Postmortem redistribution of Delta9-THC. Forensic Sci Int. 2011;212:247–256.

185 Holland MG, Schwope DM, Stoppacher R, Gillen SB, Huestis MA. Postmortem redistribution of Δ9-tetrahydrocannabinol (THC), 11-hydroxy-THC (11-OH-THC), and 11-nor-9-carboxy-THC (THC-COOH). Forensic Sci Int. 2011 Oct 10;212(1–3):247–251.

186 Wang GS. Cannabis (marijuana): Acute intoxication up to date. https://www.uptodate.com/contents/cannabis-marijuana-acute-intoxication. Accessed 8 July 2019.

187 Baselt RC. Tetrahydrocannabinol Monograph: Disposition of Toxic Drugs and Chemicals in Man. Seal Beach, CA: Biomedical Publications, 2014, 1948–1941.

188 Hartman RL, Brown TL, Milavetz G, Spurgin A, Gorelick A, Gaffney GR, Huestis MA. Effect of blood collection time on measured Δ9-tetrahydrocannabinol concentrations: Implications for driving interpretation and drug policy. Clin Chem. 2016;62:2367–377.

189 Drugs and Human Performance. Fact Sheets: Cannabis/Marijuana. National Highway Traffic Safety Administration, Drugs and human Performance Sheets, 13 December 2013. www.nhtsa.gov/people/injury/research/job185drugs/cannabis.htm.

190 Bederka JP. Marijuana-impaired or just cannabinoid positive? In O'Donnell JT, O'Donnell JJ, Eds., O'Donnell's Drug Injury. Tucson: L&J Publ, 2016.

191 Bergamaschi MA, Karschner EL, Goodwin ES, Scheidweiler KB, Hirvonen J, Queiroz RHC, Huestis MA. Impact of prolonged cannabinoid excretion in chronic daily cannabis smokers' blood on per se drugged driving laws. Clin Chem. 2013;59(3):519–526.

192 Odell MS, Frei MY, Gerostamoulos D, Mark Chu M, Lubman DL. Residual cannabis levels in blood, urine and oral fluid following heavy cannabis use. Forensic Sci Int. 2015;249:173–180.

193 Kelly P, Jones RT. Metabolism of tetrahydrocannabinol in frequent and infrequent marijuana users. J. Anal Tox. 1992 Jul/Aug;16.

194 Huestis (Interview). In new era, cannabis testing a mixed bag. *Captodayonline.com*, 18 January 2017.

37 Drug Evaluation and Classification Program

An Evidence-Based Analysis

Fran M. Gengo and Anna G. Mattle

SYNOPSIS

37.1 INTRODUCTION

Driving while impaired due to drugs is a vexing issue in the United States. A recent analysis found that 56.1% of drivers who were seriously injured or killed in motor vehicle accidents in the fourth quarter of 2020 tested positive for at least one of the following: Alcohol, cannabinoids, opioids, stimulants, sedatives, antidepressants, or other drugs.[1] In spite of the potential danger, operation of a motor vehicle while an illegal drug and/or prescription medication is present in the body is prevalent. A survey of weekend nighttime drivers from 2013 to 2014 found that 15.1% tested positive for an illegal drug, and 4.9% tested positive for a prescription or over-the-counter medication.[2] However, as we will detail in this chapter, "testing positive" for any of these drugs is not synonymous with driver impairment. Moreover, even a quantitative report of drug concentrations in the driver's blood is not necessarily proof of impairment. Unlike ethanol, *per se* concentrations of most drugs are not well established and have wide inter and intrasubject variability based on route of administration, concomitant medication use, frequency of drug use, age, gender, and race.[3,4,5]

The Drug Evaluation and Classification (DEC) program was founded by the Los Angeles Police Department in the 1970s to combat the issue of impaired driving. This program has since expanded and focuses on training police officers to become drug recognition evaluators (DREs). To become DRE-certified, police officers attend class instructed by other police officers for a total of 72 hours. The objective

DOI: 10.1201/9781003615323-41

of the DRE certification course is to provide police officers sufficient knowledge to determine: (1) If a person is impaired, (2) the cause of impairment (drug-related versus injury/illness/disease), and (3) the category of drug(s) causing impairment, if applicable.

If an arresting officer suspects a driver is impaired due to a drug other than alcohol, the individual is taken into custody and examined by a certified DRE officer, who follows a standardized examination process.

37.2 THE 12 STEPS OF DRE EXAMINATIONS

DRE officers examine suspects using a 12-step systematic and standardized process that includes interviews, psychophysical tests, and observations:

1. Breath alcohol test
2. Interview of the arresting officer
3. Preliminary examination and initial pulse measurement
4. Eye examination
5. Divided attention tests
6. Second pulse reading, body temperature, and blood pressure measurement
7. Eye examination of pupil size in various lighting conditions
8. Assessment of muscle tone
9. Checking for injection sites and third pulse reading
10. Interview of the subject
11. Opinion is stated by DRE officer regarding if the subject is drug-impaired and, if so, identifies the causative drug category
12. Toxicology sample[6]

First, breath alcohol is measured to determine if the subject's blood alcohol content (BAC) may account for the level of impairment observed by the officer. There is a well-established relationship between BAC and driving impairment, where the level of impairment increases with rising BAC.[7,8,9] DRE officers are expected to recognize when a subject is exhibiting symptoms of impairment beyond what is expected on the basis of measured BAC. This initial BAC measurement is expected to aid the officer in later determining the cause of the subject's impairment as alcohol versus other drugs/injury/illness. For example, if the arresting officer believes that a suspect is acting impaired, but breathalyzer results show there is no alcohol in his/her system, a DRE officer will be called to examine the suspect. Typically, DRE officers are only contacted to examine someone whose breathalyzer results show a BAC less than 0.08%.

Next, DRE officers interview the arresting officer to obtain pertinent information regarding the arrest; this includes the presence of drugs and/or drug paraphernalia. The DRE officer then performs a preliminary examination of the subject, starting with a series of questions:

1) Are you sick or injured?
2) Do you have any physical defects?
3) Are you diabetic or epileptic?
4) Do you take insulin?
5) Are you under a doctor or dentist's care?
6) Are you taking any medications or drugs?

The purpose of these questions is to assess the presence of injuries and/or medical problems. The preliminary examination also includes observations of the subject's face, breath, speech, and an initial eye check and pulse reading. Officers monitor for the following in the initial eye exam: Pupil size, nystagmus, and tracking ability.

Next, the DRE officer performs an eye examination to assess horizontal gaze nystagmus (HGN), vertical gaze nystagmus, and lack of convergence. Subjects must then perform divided attention tests including the modified Romberg balance, walk-and-turn, one-leg stand, and finger-to-nose.

After the divided attention tests, the subject's pulse, body temperature, and blood pressure are measured. A second eye examination is then conducted in three different lighting conditions: Ambient light, low light, and direct light. This is performed to detect pupil changes in response to environmental changes.

DRE officers then assess the subject's muscle tone by firmly grasping the subject's left upper arm and slowly moving down the subject's arm with his/her fingers. This is repeated for the subject's right arm. Officers are expected to identify the subject's muscle tone as rigid, flaccid, or normal during this assessment.

Finally, the DRE officer checks for sites of drug injection, takes a third pulse measurement, and interviews the subject. The officer then states a final opinion regarding if the subject is impaired and, if so, identifies if impairment is due to drugs or injury/illness. Further, the DRE officer determines the class(es) of drug that is (are) causing impairment from a choice of seven classes: Central nervous system (CNS) depressants, CNS stimulants, hallucinogens, dissociative anesthetics, narcotic analgesics, inhalants, and/or cannabis.

Given next is a matrix from the DRE training manual, which is what DRE officers use to distinguish between impairment by different drug classes (Table 37.1):[6]

DRE officers also reference "general indicators"; for example, CNS depressant general indicators include disorientation, droopy eyelids, drowsiness, drunk-like behavior, slow/sluggish reactions, thick/slurred speech, lack of coordination, and unsteadiness when walking. Further, DRE officers reference duration of drug effects, usual methods of administration, and signs of overdose to help in forming their opinion.[6]

TABLE 37.1
Example DRE Matrix.

	CNS Depressant	CNS Stimulant	Hallucinogen	Dissociative Anesthetic	Narcotic Analgesic	Inhalant	Cannabis
HGN	Present	None	None	Present	None	Present	None
VGN	Present (high dose)	None	None	Present	None	Present (high dose)	None
LOC	Present	None	None	Present	None	Present	Present
Pupil size	Normal[a]	Dilated	Dilated	Normal	Constricted	Normal[d]	Dilated[f]
Reaction to light	Slow	Slow	Normal[c]	Normal	Little or none visible	Slow	Normal
Pulse rate	Down[b]	Up	Up	Up	Down	Up	Up
Blood pressure	Down	Up	Up	Up	Down	Up/down[e]	Up
Temperature	Normal	Up	Up	Up	Down	Up/down/ normal	Normal
Muscle tone	Flaccid	Rigid	Rigid	Rigid	Flaccid	Normal or flaccid	Normal

Abbreviations: HGN = horizontal gaze nystagmus, VGN = vertical gaze nystagmus, LOC = loss of convergence
[a]Except Soma, Quaaludes and some antidepressants usually dilate pupils
[b]Except Quaaludes, ethanol and some antidepressants may elevate
[c]Certain psychedelic amphetamines may cause slowing
[d]Normal, but may be dilated
[e]Down with anesthetic gases, up with volatile solvents and aerosols
[f]Pupil size possibly normal

37.3 SCIENTIFIC EVALUATION OF DRE EXAMINATIONS

37.3.1 Step 2: Interview of the Arresting Officer

After DRE officers are called to assess a subject, they interview the arresting officer before performing their full examination. The arresting officer will provide details about the arrest, including drugs and/or drug paraphernalia found at the scene or on the subject.[6] This is problematic in the sense that DRE officers already know what opinion they should be forming before they even examine the subject. If the arresting officer tells the DRE officer that the subject was found with cannabis in the center console of the vehicle, the DRE officer will be primed to find evidence of cannabis "impairment" before they even start their examination.

37.3.2 Step 3: Preliminary Examination and Initial Pulse Measurement

DRE officers must ask subjects certain questions in their preliminary examinations and additional follow-up questions if they deem it necessary.[6] However, it would be common for a subject to answer "no" to all of the preliminary examination questions and still be suffering from an injury or medical condition—for example, a subject who suffers a concussion or traumatic brain injury (TBI). Symptoms of mild TBI and concussion include trouble thinking clearly, problems with short- or long-term memory, and attention/concentration problems, among others.[10] This is likely a common scenario in the circumstance of a motor vehicle accident. Although someone with a TBI is injured, they may have difficulty thinking and remembering and therefore struggle to correctly answer the DRE officer's questions.

There are many other examples when a driver may answer "no" to these questions but still demonstrate signs or symptoms of disease that a DRE officer could interpret as drug-induced impairment. DRE officers have no clinical training to be able to identify disease-related impairment.

The preliminary examination includes observations of the subject's face, breath, speech, eyes (pupil size, nystagmus, tracking ability), and a pulse measurement.[6] There are several reasons why a subject may appear "abnormal" in terms of these measures; perhaps they are nervous from being interrogated by an officer and are sweating with a racing pulse. Another possibility is that they normally take a beta blocker medication and are suffering from withdrawal symptoms because they forgot to take their medication. Symptoms of beta blocker withdrawal may include arrhythmias, increased blood pressure/heart rate, and tremors.[11] All of these effects are listed as symptoms of CNS stimulants in the DRE course; yet, beta blockers are not mentioned at all in the course. It is unfair to expect a DRE officer to be able to differentiate between all of the medical possibilities when they are examining subjects. DRE officers are taught by other police officers in their training course, none of whom possess the medical knowledge necessary to make this distinction.

37.3.3 Step 4: Eye Examination

There are several scenarios where abnormal eye examinations can lead to a DRE officer falsely concluding that a subject is drug-impaired. The DRE training course fails to mention the various other causes of nystagmus apart from drug use. A 2010 review of HGN concluded that the assessment is susceptible to false-positives as a result of various medical conditions, environmental factors, and/or prescription medications.[12] Smooth-pursuit lateral eye movements can be found in patients with schizophrenia and/or even their first-degree relatives who are not diagnosed with the disorder.[13] Nystagmus can be a symptom of several nervous system diseases and even brain lesions,[14] while the failure of the test for a lack of convergence is disease for at least 3.4% to 7.7% of adults with convergence insufficiency—the most common binocular vision disorder.[15] These are only a few of many common scenarios where abnormal eye examinations do not necessarily indicate drug use; yet, DRE officers are expected to use these exams to help identify drug impairment with no background knowledge of other potential medical contributors.

The DRE manual defines the term "impairment" as a physiologic abnormality (e.g., high pulse rate or nystagmus) which is synonymous to driving impairment. Often, we see patients with nystagmus or tachycardia on no medications causing these "impairments." Neither nystagmus nor tachycardia would be expected to compromise driving ability. Patients often have "pinpoint pupils" when chronically treated with therapeutic doses of narcotic analgesics. Neither would have compromised driving, both display "DRE clues," and both are taking medication contained in the DRE drug categories. If either underwent toxicology testing of blood or urine, it would confirm the use of these medications. However, neither the DRE clues nor chemical confirmation are definitive indicators of impaired driving.

37.3.4 Step 5: Divided Attention Tests

Officers are expected to recognize when a subject is exhibiting symptoms of impairment using tools including field sobriety tests. These were developed by the National Highway Traffic Safety Administration to assist officers in making correct arrest decisions in cases involving alcohol. These tests have never been shown to be a valid assessment tool in cases involving drugs other than alcohol, nor are they intended to be a measure of impairment.

One of these divided attention tests is the Modified Romberg Balance. In the medical community, the Romberg Test is a neurological exam to be administered by trained medical professionals, which can aid in the diagnosis of diseases including Parkinson's disease, vitamin B12 deficiency, normal pressure hydrocephalus, and Meniere's disease, among others.[16] This is not the case with the Modified Romberg Balance, which is a non-standardized test that is conducted differently than the medical version and includes no formal scoring or administration guidelines.

The results of the "coordination" tests must be carefully interpreted, taking administration errors, environmental factors (e.g., shoe type), and the subject's age/medical conditions into consideration. DRE officers generally perform the tests in an indoor controlled environment; however, as discussed, DRE training providers the officer with minimal training to discern the signs/symptoms of medical problems from adverse effects of recreational drugs or therapeutic medications.

37.3.5 Step 6: Second Pulse Reading, Body Temperature, and Blood Pressure Measurement

After the divided attention tests, the subject's pulse, body temperature, and blood pressure are measured. The DRE course discusses normal ranges of blood pressure and heart rate for DRE officers to use as a basis of comparison.[6] As previously mentioned, these measurements can appear abnormal for a number of reasons. If a DRE officer finds a subject's blood pressure and pulse to be less than the manual's standard of normal (120/80 mmHg blood pressure, 70 beats per minute pulse), the finding could falsely reinforce the DRE officer's impression that the subject is impaired by a CNS depressant or narcotic analgesic. However, in a subject taking a beta blocker medication, a blood pressure of 110/68 with a pulse of 59 would not concern doctors who understand that these readings are not clinically significant in this patient.

37.3.6 Step 7: Eye Examination of Pupil Size in Various Lighting Conditions

A second eye examination is conducted in three different lighting conditions to assess how eye measures change with light. However, there is no standardization of the intensity of light for each of the three conditions. This likely leads to differing results of these eye exams depending on who administers them and the setting where they are administered.

37.3.7 Step 8: Assessment of Muscle Tone

The muscle tone assessment performed by DRE officers is not the same method employed by medical professionals. Medical doctors examine muscle tone by moving a patient's relaxed limb to determine the amount of involuntary muscle resistance as a measure of muscle tone. Variations in muscle tone can have several different etiologies: For example, increased muscle tone (rigidity) may be due to Parkinson's disease, while decreased muscle tone (flaccidity) may be secondary to polyneuropathy. In instances where patients are unable to relax their muscles during the muscle tone examination (e.g., anxiety/nervousness), it is difficult even for medical professionals to evaluate.[17] The simplified DRE muscle tone assessment is not supported by medical evidence.

37.3.8 Step 11: DRE Officer Opinion Statement

There are several issues with how the drugs within the DRE classes are described in the DRE course, resulting in DRE officers lacking the proper education to correctly form an opinion. The CNS depressants category in the DRE manual includes the following subcategories: Barbiturates, non-barbiturates, antianxiety tranquilizers (includes benzodiazepines), antidepressants, and antipsychotic tranquilizers.[6] "Clumping" many of these drugs together in one class and describing them identically pose several issues and ill-prepare DRE officers to correctly identify the etiology of drug impairment. The CNS depressants category is especially problematic, including drugs with widely varying potencies and mechanisms of action and characterizing them altogether. In pharmacology, potency describes the relationship between the dose of a drug and the magnitude of its effect.[18] The mechanism of action of a drug describes how a drug produces its effect.

For example, when comparing clonazepam (a benzodiazepine) and venlafaxine (an antidepressant), clonazepam is much more potent with an increased risk for CNS side effects at therapeutic doses. Patients who take clonazepam experience drowsiness, impaired coordination, and dizziness at reported rates of 50%, 30%, and 5–12%, respectively.[19] Meanwhile, those who take venlafaxine may experience drowsiness and dizziness at much lower rates (15% and 16% respectively), and impaired coordination was reported only in post-marketing studies with unknown incidence.[20]

These drugs have vastly different side effect profiles which are supported by their varying mechanisms of action; clonazepam is believed to enhance the activity of the GABA neurotransmitter, while venlafaxine increases levels of different neurotransmitters altogether (serotonin, norepinephrine, and dopamine). DRE officers are trained to identify the impairment due to these drugs as identical when they are not, which likely results in falsely forming the opinion that someone who admits to being prescribed venlafaxine is impaired.

Further, overdoses on these two drugs produce different symptom profiles; while clonazepam overdose often results in sedation, slurred speech, and/or impaired coordination with normal or near-normal vitals, venlafaxine overdose symptoms may include increased pulse rate, seizures, arrhythmias, and/or vomiting.[21,22] However, DRE officers are instructed in their course that, "overdoses of the CNS depressants produce symptoms essentially identical to those of alcohol overdoses," listing symptoms including drowsiness, rapid/weak pulse, shallow breathing, cold/clammy skin, and potential respiratory failure. While there is some overlap in these symptoms, DRE officers do not possess sufficient knowledge to correctly discern that these two differing clinical presentations are both that of CNS depressant overdose and not of other categories; this must be left to medical doctors trained in differential diagnoses.

The determination of a drug class is a straightforward process. The DRE officer records their observations from the evaluation and compares them to the DRE matrix, selecting the drug category that aligns most closely with the observed indicators. Often, the officer arbitrarily chooses which nonmatching observations to ignore in making his/her choice.

A footnote at the bottom of the matrix acknowledges that "These indicators are the most consistent with the category, keep in mind that there may be variations due to individual reaction, dose taken and drug interactions."[23] However, DRE officers do not possess the clinical skills necessary to take these variations into consideration when forming their opinion, considering many subjects may be taking multiple therapeutic medications and have several different health conditions. Making this distinction requires years of medical training.

There are no studies validating the DRE process for subjects with underlying neurologic or other diseases which may complicate their assessment. The DRE course attempts to distinguish between DRE officers and medical professions by stating:

> As a DRE, when you complete an evaluation and decide whether the person is impaired, whether the impairment is a result of a medical problem or drugs, and if drugs, what drug category or categories is/are causing the impairment, you are rendering an OPINION. You are NOT making a diagnosis.[6]

According to Merriam-Webster dictionary, the definition of a diagnosis is: "Investigation or analysis of the cause or nature of a condition, situation, or problem."[24] Clearly, DRE officers are being asked to diagnose the cause of a subject's impairment, despite assertions in the DRE course that this is not the case.

In health care, physicians are the only professionals licensed to diagnose a patient based on their entire clinical picture: Preexisting diseases, medications, medical and surgical history, etc.[25] Physicians earn the ability to diagnose only after completing several years of classroom and clinical training. Pharmacists, with several years of training specifically in pharmacology and related fields, are equipped to identify medication-related symptoms other providers may misdiagnose.[26] Despite this, the DRE course states that "doctors . . . receive little training in the recognition of specific signs of drug impairment, particularly at street-level doses."[6] This is blatantly untrue; providers and pharmacists are trained to assess patients for drug versus disease-related impairment, and both receive several years of classroom and clinical training to do so. Professionals working in emergency departments are regularly exposed to drug-impaired patients and must uncover the etiology of any complications the patient is suffering, taking their medical history and concomitant medications into consideration.

There is a reason that even registered nurses receiving multiple years of health care education cannot diagnose a patient; it is because it takes more than this amount of time to properly train someone on every possible cause of a patient's signs and symptoms. The idea that a seven-day training course led by police officers can prepare DRE officers to differentiate between disease/injury/illness symptoms and drug impairment sets well-meaning officers up to fail. This will be evident in the discussion of the DRE validation studies.

37.3.9 Step 12: Toxicology Sample

The DRE course states that "toxicology supports the DRE's opinion, it does not confirm it."[6] However, it is important to recognize that the DRE course discusses toxicology results as if all are considered interchangeable—there is no mention of qualitative versus quantitative assays, drug versus metabolite measurements, or blood versus urine versus oral fluid samples. Qualitative assays will give the interpreter a yes/no answer of whether or not a particular drug is present in a sample. Quantitative assays are able to determine the exact amount of a particular drug present in a sample. This is important to distinguish when interpreting toxicology results because quantitative analyses may offer more information about whether a drug was psychoactive at the time of sample procurement, depending on the drug.

Toxicology results must take into consideration whether the drug itself or its metabolites are being measured in a sample, in addition to the psychoactivity of the drug and its metabolites. For example, tetrahydrocannabinol (THC) is the psychoactive cannabinoid in cannabis and is metabolized to hydroxy-THC and carboxy-THC in the body. While hydroxy-THC is psychoactive, carboxy-THC is not.[27] Therefore, a toxicology sample testing positive for only carboxy-THC without THC or hydroxy-THC would indicate a lack of psychoactive drug effects at the time the sample was procured.

Blood, urine, and oral fluid toxicology results must also be interpreted carefully. A drug concentration that is measured in oral fluid does not necessarily translate to the same blood drug concentration, and the translation may vary widely between subjects.[28] A urine sample testing positive for a drug or metabolite must take the clinical picture and pharmacology of the drug into consideration when interpreting the results. For example, urine samples may test positive for carboxy-THC long after the psychoactive effects of cannabis have ended.[29]

Unfortunately, practices surrounding the toxicology analyses of driving-impaired subjects are highly variable. A report published by the *Journal of Analytical Toxicology* recommends more uniform analytical toxicology practices to support the collection of more robust data concerning drug use among impaired drivers.[30]

37.4 LITERATURE EVALUATIONS AND CRITIQUES OF DRE

A consensus paper was published in the *Journal of the American Medical Association* (*JAMA*) in 1985 which put forth five criteria that would be needed to properly identify drug-impaired drivers; despite its year of publication over 30 years ago, the concepts remain valid.[31] These criteria were:

1. Laboratory studies produce dose-related driving impairment (and/or impairment of related psychomotor skills).
2. Concentration of the active drug and/or metabolite in body fluids can be quantitatively measured and correlated to degree of impairment.
3. Impairment is confirmed by actual driving experience.
4. Simple behavioral tests can be done at the roadside by trained police officers, which can indicate the presence of impairment.
5. A range of drug concentrations can be incorporated into laws relating to impaired driving as *ipso facto* evidence.[31]

The first criterion requires that laboratory studies show a dose-related impairment of driving skills. Studies have analyzed the relationship between drugs and driving impairment using dual-controlled cars with computerized sensors in the car and on the road to sense lateral car movement. Data from these studies show that some drugs categorized as CNS depressants do not impair driving.[32]

Studies have shown dose-related impairment effects for certain drugs, but these results often cannot be applied to real-world scenarios. For example, Jongen et al. (2018) evaluated the effects of diazepam and oxazepam (CNS depressants) on driving in a highway driving test in a double-blind, placebo-controlled, randomized study.[33] Participants were healthy with no history of drug/alcohol abuse and were dosed with placebo, oxazepam, or diazepam prior to performing in the driving test. Results showed dose-related impairment of driving skills, where low-dose oxazepam caused minor impairment, while high-dose oxazepam caused severe impairment. However, the study used drug-naïve participants, so results do not necessarily apply to chronic users of these medications. Further, the results of the Jongen et al. (2018) study cannot be generalized to all CNS depressants, given their varying mechanisms of action.

Often, CNS depressant drug effects are strongest initially and decline with chronic use. A 1987 study showed that the effects produced by specific concentrations of alprazolam following the first dose produced significantly greater effects than the same concentration after subjects had been taking alprazolam for consecutive days; in fact, after the development of tolerance, the previously impairing concentrations produced effects no different from placebo.[34]

A double-blind study looked at the effects of placebo, alprazolam (CNS depressant), and/or hydrocodone-acetaminophen (narcotic) on performance in a simulated driving protocol in eight healthy participants.[35] Subjects who took alprazolam, with or without hydrocodone, showed significantly worse driving performance compared to placebo. Interestingly, hydrocodone alone was not shown to impact driving performance. When alprazolam and hydrocodone were taken in combination, results indicate that the negative impact on driving was primarily due to alprazolam, and there was no evidence of a drug–drug interaction or synergistic effect.[35] Results of this study demonstrate the complicated interplay between drugs and how they impact driving performance. Despite the notorious reputation of narcotics and their cognitive effects, this study does not support the notion that typical therapeutic doses of narcotics impair driving performance, even when given to drug-naïve individuals.

The second criterion requires that the drug can be accurately measured in a body fluid sample and that measured concentrations are related to the magnitude of driving impairment. The current DRE process does not measure up to this standard on several counts. First, the DRE process considers qualitative urine screens and quantitative serum drug concentrations as interchangeable. As previously discussed, this is simply incorrect; a qualitative test result of "positive" gives no measurement of the amount of drug present in the body. Many drugs and/or their active metabolites are found in the urine or blood long after impairing effects have resolved. Cannabis is a good example of this phenomenon. A study serially tested 86 chronic cannabis users who discontinued the use for toxicological evidence of cannabis for ten days after the first negative test.[36] It was found that 60.6% tested positive at least 21 days, 32.7% tested positive for at least 30 days, and 4.7% tested positive for at least 60 days. Still, the current DRE process considers a positive qualitative cannabinoid metabolites urine test as supporting DRE officer opinion of drug impairment.

The second criterion also requires that measured drug concentrations are related to the degree of driving impairment. A 2018 review examined the current literature on the relationship between various drugs and driving impairment.[37] This review shows that while some studies suggest cannabis impairs driving at THC blood levels of at least 2 to 5 ng/mL, due to the wide interindividual variability in THC metabolism and drug effects, the relationship between THC blood level and driving impairment remains unclear. This is consistent with the findings of a 2021 study by Spindle et al., which revealed inconsistency in the relationship between THC concentrations and effects.[3] Further, the route of administration of THC (ingestion versus inhalation) has been found to significantly impact the concentration–time relationship.[3]

The 2018 review was inconclusive regarding opioid use and driving impairment, with studies highlighting the differences between opioid-naïve users and chronic opioid users.[37] According to the review, studies have shown moderate psychomotor impairment due to opioids which are most pronounced when first initiating therapy and decline as tolerance develops. No clear dose–effect relationship has been shown between single-dose morphine (up to five mg) and driving performance. With regard to cocaine, the review comments on different responses with varying routes of administration, the complexity of the drug–drug interaction with alcohol where concomitant alcohol use may actually decrease cocaine-induced psychomotor impairment, and lack of a correlation between oral fluid and blood cocaine concentrations. Ultimately, the influence of cocaine on driving is understudied due to ethical concerns of administering a highly addictive schedule I substance to participants. The review also discusses the current literature pertaining to amphetamines/amphetamine-like substances and impaired driving. One study found a significant concentration–effect relationship between blood amphetamine levels and driving impairment.[38] However, other studies had mixed results; amphetamines remain difficult to study at the high doses which may impact driving performance due to ethical concerns for study participants. The 2018 review concluded that, "a wider knowledge on concentration/impairment relationship is still missing."[37] Clearly, there is no scientific consensus regarding the relationship between measured drug levels and impairment for several DRE-classified drugs.

The third criterion requires that impairment is confirmed by actual driving experience. The necessity of this criterion is supported by findings of a 2018 study, which concluded that "no neurocognitive test can replace the on-the-road highway driving test" in the context of assessing drug-induced driving impairment.[37] Drug-induced driving impairment has been confirmed for some drugs in specific circumstances but not for all drugs that are specified in the DRE training course. For example, a 2019 clinical trial on the effects of methadone and buprenorphine on driving found large interindividual variations for both drugs; overall, methadone impaired cognition but not driving performance, while buprenorphine mildly impaired driving and cognition.[39] Similarly, a study was published in 2016 which examined the relationship between prescribed drugs and crash risk in fatally injured drivers.[40] This study concluded that even if medicinal drugs are potentially impairing, medicinal drug use alone is unlikely to increase crash risk significantly. The DRE course does not specify the differences between drugs within a class and how likely they are to cause driving impairment; instead, all drugs within a class are treated identically in terms of causing impairment. This assertion is not supported by scientific data whatsoever.

The fourth criterion states that simple behavioral tests can be done at the roadside by trained police officers, which can indicate the presence of impairment. Standardized field sobriety tests have been validated for alcohol, but the same is not true for other drugs. A 2012 study of heavy cannabis users found that standardized field sobriety tests were only mildly sensitive to the effects of cannabis; a dose of 400 μg/kg THC increased the percentage of participants displaying impairments in the one-leg stand from 21% to 50%, but there was no significant difference in performance on the walk-and-turn or overall standardized field sobriety test performance.[41] A 2019 literature review of the detection of cannabis-impaired driving highlighted that it is difficult to assess impairment due to the lack of a validated field test to do so.[42]

The fifth criterion required by the *JAMA* consensus paper is that a range of various drug concentrations can be incorporated into law as causing impairment. Drug concentration ranges associated with impairment should not be codified into law due to the numerous clinical variables that influence how a given concentration affects each individual driver. These include variability in tolerance based on chronicity of drug use and intersubject variability in absorption, distribution, metabolism, and elimination rates.

37.5 CANNABIS

Cannabis has been the focus of recent efforts by law enforcement concerned with impaired driving. Despite robust scientific evidence of tolerance and intersubject variability in studies of cannabis use, some states have enacted *per se* laws which establish cannabis concentrations above which drivers are deemed "impaired."[43] For example, a 2006 study recommended a lower threshold of cannabis impairment between two and five ng/mL serum concentration despite results showing that participants with concentrations in that range performed no differently at tasks measuring motor impulsivity or cognitive function compared to control.[44] Another 2006 study found that at similar THC concentrations, chronic cannabis users were less often judged "impaired" by physicians after cannabis use compared to those who did not regularly use cannabis, supporting the notion that chronic users become tolerant to the impairing effects of cannabis.[45] In fact, evidence of cannabis use may be detected in blood for up to one month after cessation in chronic cannabis users.[46] There is no scientific basis for establishing a range of drug concentrations that cause impairment even for cannabis, one of the most widely studied recreational drugs.

37.6 STATISTICAL VALIDITY AND OVERALL STRENGTH OF DRE STUDIES

The DRE evaluation is a "test" given to a driver for the DRE officer to opine whether the driver is impaired. This is analogous to a test given to a patient in order for a physician to diagnose if the patient has a certain illness. No medical test is perfect. It becomes important for the physician and the patient to know how often the test indicates the patient has the diagnosis, where the patient does not (false positive), and how often the test indicates the patient does not have the diagnosis but the patient actually has the disease (false negative). In general, a test is not considered medically reliable unless it has a false positive rate of 5% or less and a false negative rate of 5% or less. In the same way, it is important to know the rate of false positives and false negatives for the DRE evaluation.

Several studies have been published which discuss the outcomes of evaluations using the DRE protocol. These studies have been evaluated for statistical endpoints to determine their validity in supporting the DRE program. Where possible, each study has been analyzed for rate of false positives, true positives, false negatives, true negatives, and prevalence of the population, given a drug. These then allow the calculation of sensitivity and specificity.

Prevalence of the population, given a drug, in these studies is an important metric to quantify. If prevalence rates in these studies are higher than rates seen in real-life scenarios, these studies cannot be reliably compared to how DRE officers will perform in the field. Higher prevalence rates in these studies can lead to a false improvement in DRE officer performance.[47] As previously stated, data show that around 15% of drivers test positive for an illegal drug, while around 5% of drivers test positive for a prescription or over-the-counter medication.[2] Studies with prevalence rates significantly higher than these percentages cannot be reliably translated to real-life DRE performance.

True positives (TP) represent the number of cases where DRE officers identified subjects as drug-impaired, and these subjects were found to have drugs in their system. False positives (FP) are cases where DRE officers identified subjects as drug-impaired, but these subjects did not have any drugs in their system. True negatives (TN) include cases where DRE officers correctly identified subjects as not drug-impaired, and the subjects had not taken any drugs. False negatives (FN) represent cases where DRE officers determined subjects were not drug-impaired, but the subjects were found to have taken a drug.

Sensitivity and specificity are statistical endpoints calculated from the number of TP, FP, TN, and FN. Sensitivity represents the proportion of subjects dosed with a drug, who were subsequently identified as drug-impaired by DRE officers, while specificity is the proportion of drug-free subjects correctly identified as not being drug-impaired by DRE officers.[47]

Next, Table 37.2 shows the results of published DRE validation studies regarding the ability of an officer to distinguish between drug-impaired and unimpaired, regardless of which drug class was administered to the subject and which class the officer identified. In other words, if a subject had taken a narcotic and the DRE officer determined that the subject had taken a CNS depressant, this was still counted as a TP as given in the table. These statistical endpoints were previously described in detail in "A Critical Evaluation of the Scientific and Statistical Validity

TABLE 37.2
Statistical Endpoints of DRE Studies—Impaired versus Unimpaired (Any Drug).

Study	n	Prev. (%)	TP (n [%])	FP (n [%])	TN (n [%])	FN (n [%])	Sens. (%)	Spec. (%)
Bigelow 1985[49]	320	88	155 [48]	2 [1]	38 [12]	125 [39]	55	95
Heishman 1996[50]	158	66	59 [37]	22 [14]	32 [20]	45 [28]	57	59
Heishman 1998[51]	280	67	85 [30]	27 [10]	66 [24]	102 [36]	45	71
Smith 2002[52]	1259	93	1108 [88]	31 [2]	59 [5]	61 [5]	95	66
Shinar 2005[53]	300	66	143 [48]	58 [19]	44 [15]	55 [18]	72	43

Abbreviations: n = sample size, Prev. = prevalence, TP = true positives, FP = false positives, TN = true negatives, FN = false negatives, Sens. = sensitivity, Spec. = specificity

of the Drug Recognition Evaluation (DRE) Program" by Drs. Gengo, Kirsch, and Janofsky.[48]

Study results shown in Table 37.2 display the wide variation in outcomes. For all studies, the prevalence of drug use is significantly higher than the prevalence of drug use DRE officers see in the field (~15%), which may falsely elevate DRE officer performance and certainly makes it difficult to translate study results to real-world application.[2] Sensitivity ranges from 45% to 95%, and specificity from 43% to 95%.

37.7 DRE SUPPORT LITERATURE

37.7.1 Bigelow et al. 1985 Study

In the double-blind Bigelow et al. 1985 study, 80 subjects were administered diazepam (a CNS depressant), d-amphetamine (a CNS stimulant), secobarbital (a CNS depressant), cannabis, or placebo.[49] All participants were healthy adult males who passed a physical and psychiatric examination and did not have a history of illicit drug use (other than marijuana). In the field, DRE officers must discriminate between drug-induced impairment and injury/illness; as all participants were healthy, results of this study cannot be reliably translated to real-life situations. Additionally, this study assessed drug-naïve subjects given diazepam/d-amphetamine/secobarbital doses three to six times greater than therapeutic doses. This does not account for those in the field who are chronic drug users and/or those who are taking regular therapeutic doses of these medications, all of which the DRE officer must distinguish between.

Results from the Bigelow et al. 1985 study show a high specificity of 95%.[49] This value is likely inflated due to the study design characteristics described earlier, as well as the fact that DRE officers only had to select between four different drug classes (not seven as described in the DRE manual): Opiate, sedative, stimulant, or marijuana. Officers also did not have to worry about drug combinations and only determined a single drug class per subject, further simplifying the procedure in this study compared to real-world application.

37.7.2 Heishman et al. 1996 and 1998 Studies

The Heishman et al. 1996 and 1998 studies both utilized a randomized, double-blinded design and were published in peer-reviewed journals.[50,51] Overall, these studies were designed to capture DRE performance in a more realistic capacity compared to the Bigelow et al. 1985 study. In the Heishman et al. 1996 study, 18 frequent drug users were each given placebo, low, or high doses of each study drug in nine separate sessions: Ethanol, cocaine, or marijuana.[50] DRE officers were told that the subjects could have been given no drugs, a combination of drugs, or one of the following: Alcohol, cannabis, depressant, narcotic, stimulant, or phencyclidine. The DRE protocol was followed, but a complete interview was not performed to prevent confirmation bias. Sensitivity and specificity were low at 57% and 59%, respectively.

The Heishman et al. 1998 study included 48 frequent drug users equally divided into four test groups mirroring their drug use history.[51] Participants with a history of CNS depressant use were assigned to receive alprazolam; those with a history of cocaine use received d-amphetamine; those with a history of heroin use received codeine; and those with a history of marijuana use received marijuana. Each participant was dosed with placebo and low or high dose of the test drug twice. DRE officers were told that the subjects could have been given no drugs, a combination of drugs, or one of the following: Alcohol, cannabis, depressant, narcotic, stimulant, or phencyclidine. Results of this study are similar to the Heishman et al. 1996 study, with a low sensitivity (45%) and specificity (71%). The Heishman et al. 1996 and 1998 studies demonstrate the inability of DRE officers to identify drug use, contrasting the artificially inflated results of the Bigelow et al. 1985 study.[49,50,51]

37.7.3 Smith et al. 2002 Study

The Smith et al. 2002 study describes 70 cases of subjects previously evaluated by DRE officers.[52] These were all cases where a DRE officer had originally evaluated the subject, determined evidence of a particular drug class, and the presence of this drug class in the subject was verified by toxicology results. Observational reports, physiological test results, and psychophysical test results of these cases were provided to 18 DRE officers for evaluation. It is clear that results of this study would be biased to represent more cases with easier distinction between drug classes, as these cases had already been matched on the basis of original DRE officer opinion and toxicology results. Sensitivity is high at 95%, likely due to the study design issue described, while specificity is low at 66%.

37.7.4 D. Shinar and Schechtman 2005 Study

Shinar and Schechtman's 2005 study included 54 participants dosed on six separate occasions with placebo, codeine (narcotic), alprazolam (CNS depressant), d-amphetamine (stimulant), or marijuana.[53] This study had a randomized, double-blinded design and was published in a peer-reviewed journal. The procedure was similar to that of Heishman et al. 1998, where subjects were placed in the drug group that matched their drug use history.[51] The officers were told that the subjects may be impaired by any of five drug classes, including the ones given and phencyclidine, a combination of the drugs, or no drug at all. Results showed a low sensitivity (72%) and specificity (43%).

Overall, the current literature examining the ability of a DRE officer to discriminate between impaired and unimpaired is limited. Existing studies show varying results, with a trend of more well-designed studies resulting in poorer DRE officer performance. To the knowledge of the authors, there have been no further studies examining the ability of DRE officers to identify drug-impaired versus unimpaired individuals since 2005.

37.7.5 E. Specific Identification of Drug Class by DRE Officers in Validation Studies

The ability of DRE officers to opine the exact class that subjects were dosed with in these validation studies was assessed. Table 37.3 displays the accuracy of DRE officers' impairment evaluation when subjects were administered only a CNS depressant in these studies. TP represents the percentage of cases where an officer correctly identified at least one drug class that a subject had taken (e.g., CNS depressant was at least one of the drug classes identified by the DRE officer). FN is the percentage of cases where an officer determined that a subject was not drug-impaired when a CNS depressant was taken by the subject. Incorrect class displays the percentage of cases where a DRE officer determined a subject was impaired but identified the wrong drug class. Exact identification represents the percentage of cases where the DRE officer identified exactly which drug classes a subject had taken; for example, the officer did not determine that a subject had used other drugs in addition to a CNS depressant.

The results are highly variable across studies and show that between 9% and 74% of subjects who took only a CNS depressant were correctly identified by a DRE officer as impaired only by a CNS depressant. As discussed previously, the Bigelow et al. 1985 study results are likely falsely elevated as officers only selected one drug class per case (as opposed to real life, where subjects may be impaired by multiple agents) and were only choosing between four different drug classes (instead of seven).[49] It is clear from the discrepancies between the TP and exact identifications in the Heishman et al. 1998 and Smith et al. 2002 studies that an exact identification of a drug class is much more difficult for officers than happening to include the correct drug class as one out of a multi-drug combination.[51,52] For example, in the Smith et al. 2002 study, of the subjects who took only a CNS depressant, officers included a CNS depressant as at least one of the identified drugs in 77% of cases but correctly identified a CNS depressant alone in just 46% of cases.[52]

Table 37.4 shows the ability of DRE officers to correctly identify impairment and drug class in subjects who took only a CNS stimulant.

It appears that the ability of DRE officers to identify CNS stimulant impairment was lower in some studies compared to their ability to identify CNS depressants. Zero to 55% of cases where subjects took a CNS stimulant were correctly identified by DRE officers as stimulant-impaired.

Table 37.5 shows the results of DRE validation studies regarding the ability of an officer to determine impairment and identify drug class for subjects administered cannabis only.

Subjects who took cannabis were correctly identified by DRE officers in 11% to 70% of cases. In the studies with

TABLE 37.3
Statistical Endpoints of DRE Studies—CNS Depressants.

Study	n	TP (%)	FN (%)	Incorrect Class (%)	Exact Identification (%)
Bigelow 1985[49]	120	74	23	3	74
Heishman 1998[51]	46	39	24	37	9
Smith 2002[52]	226	77	7	16	46
Shinar 2005[53]	49	43	10	47	43

Abbreviations: n = sample size, TP = true positives, FN = false negatives.

a more realistic design (Heishman et al. 1996 and 1998, Shinar & Schechtman 2005), the rate of correct cannabis identification cases falls to 11% to 31%.[50,51,53]

Table 37.6 shows the ability of DRE officers to detect impairment in subjects who took only a narcotic. The rates of exact identification are very low, ranging from 9% to 57%.

Table 37.7 displays the ability of a DRE officer to correctly identify which drug class a subject had in their system out of those subjects who took only one drug.

TABLE 37.4
Statistical Endpoints of DRE Studies—CNS Stimulants.

Study	n	TP (%)	FN (%)	Incorrect Class (%)	Exact Identification (%)
Bigelow 1985[49]	80	20	78	3	20
Heishman 1996[50]	36	14	61	25	11
Heishman 1998[51]	48	4	71	25	0
Smith 2002[52]	337	79	5	16	55
Shinar 2005[53]	51	8	41	51	8

Source: n = sample size, TP = true positives, FN = false negatives.

TABLE 37.5
Statistical Endpoints of DRE Studies—Cannabis.

Study	n	TP (%)	FN (%)	Incorrect Class (%)	Exact Identification (%)
Bigelow 1985[49]	80	49	45	6	49
Heishman 1996[50]	26	53	22	25	28
Heishman 1998[51]	46	35	52	13	11
Smith 2002[52]	355	82	5	13	70
Shinar 2005[53]	49	31	24	45	31

Abbreviations: n = sample size, TP = true positives, FN = false negatives.

TABLE 37.6
Statistical Endpoints of DRE Studies—Narcotics.

Study	n	TP (%)	FN (%)	Incorrect Class (%)	Exact Identification (%)
Heishman 1998[51]	47	19	70	11	9
Smith 2002[52]	215	94	4	2	57
Shinar 2005[53]	49	37	35	29	37

Abbreviations: n = sample size, TP = true positives, FN = false negatives.

TABLE 37.7
Statistical Endpoints of DRE Studies—Correct Identification of Drug Class.

Study	n	TP (%)	FN (%)	Incorrect Class (%)	Exact Identification (%)
Bigelow 1985[49]	280	51	45	4	51
Heishman 1996[50]	72	33	42	25	19
Heishman 1998[51]	187	24	55	21	7
Smith 2002[52]	1133	82	5	12	59
Shinar 2005[53]	198	29	28	43	29

Abbreviations: n = sample size, TP = true positives, FN = false negatives.

When the results are presented altogether, it is clear that DRE officers lack the ability to correctly identify the drug class of impairment. Exact identification of any drug class, in those who took only one drug, ranges from just 7% to 59%. It is important to remember that these studies are difficult to translate to real life due to their designs which likely inflate DRE officer performance. Therefore, DRE officer's ability to identify the drug class of impairment in the field may be even poorer than is shown here. In addition, none of the previously mentioned studies included inhalants or hallucinogens, so the ability of DRE officers to examine subjects impaired with these agents is unknown. These data represent the most simplistic possible scenarios for DRE officers; subjects took only one drug (not a combination), and DRE office performance was still poor. Further studies, with realistic designs which allow for the calculation of validity statistics, are needed to discern the legitimacy of the DRE certification course.

37.8 OTHER DRE VALIDATION STUDIES

The DRE training manual cites several reports that attempt to validate the program. However, these reports are not published or peer reviewed and are missing necessary data to enable calculations of statistical validation endpoints. The field evaluation of the Los Angeles Police Department Drug Detection Program (LAPD-DDP) was released in 1986.[54] The LAPD-DDP not only differs from the standardized DRE protocol but also does not include any data on unimpaired subjects; therefore, the calculation of false positives and true negatives is impossible. Additionally, the DRE program cites the 1993 Minnesota Corroboration Study for validation.[55] This study also does not provide data for subjects determined to be unimpaired, so validity statistics cannot be calculated. The same is true for the 1994 Arizona DRE Validation Study cited in the DRE training manual.[56]

Studies have been conducted recently which were not designed to assess the validity of the DRE program; each was designed to investigate a different endpoint but mentioned the opinions of DRE officers as part of the dataset. Hartman et al. (2016) looked at 302 cases where DRE officers determined that the subject was impaired by cannabis only, and this was confirmed toxicologically.[57] The goal of this study was to compare DRE evaluation results of these cases with control cases (no drug use) to identify which metrics of the DRE examination are indicative of cannabis impairment. While this information may be useful to modify the DRE course in the future, this study is not designed to assess DRE officer performance. The study reports diagnostic statistics for each of the detected signs that correspond to cannabis impairment; these statistics do not apply to the DRE program itself.

Similarly, Declues et al. 2017 evaluated the relationship between cannabis impairment and several measurements obtained during DRE examination such as objective signs, eye changes, and physiologic indicators.[58] Additionally, a 2019 study by Porath and Beirness looked at cases of CNS depressant, CNS stimulant, narcotic, or cannabis impairment to analyze correlations between DRE exam measures and impairing substance.[59] DRE performance was not assessed in any of these studies.

Edwards et al. (2017) examined the utility of a handheld drug-screening device measuring drug concentrations in oral fluid compared to standard blood toxicology results in subjects arrested for driving while impaired.[60] DRE evaluation results are reported for 16 subjects in this study as well as corresponding oral fluid and blood toxicology results. Using blood toxicology results as the standard of comparison, the validity statistics of DRE officer performance were as follows: 88% prevalence, 13 TP, 1 FP, 1 FN, 1 TN, 93% sensitivity, 50% specificity. This study included a very small number of DRE officer opinions and was not designed to examine DRE officer performance as an endpoint; therefore, it is difficult to draw firm conclusions from these data.

A study by Truver et al. in 2019 was conducted to compare urine toxicology results and oral fluid toxicology results in those undergoing DRE examination.[61] The study also reports DRE officer opinions for 18 of the 20 subjects in the study. Validity statistics cannot be calculated for DRE performance because there were no true negatives; 100% of the subjects examined were found to have evidence of drugs in their system.

It is important to recognize that the DRE validation studies do not use a subject's actual driving impairment as its standard of comparison. In the Bigelow et al. 1985 study, the Heishman et al. 1996 and 1998 studies, and the Shinar and Schechtman 2005 study, the administration of the known drugs to human subjects was equated to impairment.[49,50,51,53] The standard of comparison used in the LAPD-DDP 1986, Arizona 1994, and Minnesota 1993 studies was laboratory analysis of subjects' urine; however, urine toxicology results cannot determine whether a drug was active in a subject's blood or brain.[54,55,56] In none of these studies did subjects actually operate a motor vehicle.

Despite a lack of evidence supporting the ability of DRE officers to differentiate between impaired and unimpaired subjects or identify the class of drug causing impairment, the DRE program has continued to expand across the United States and to other countries around the world.[62]

37.9 SUMMARY AND CONCLUSIONS

The current DRE process has not been shown to accurately discriminate between impaired and unimpaired drivers or to discriminate between drug-induced impairment and impairment caused by medical conditions. This is expected on the basis of our current robust knowledge of the complexity of drug effects and the interplay between drugs and diseases in a patient.

Further, the current DRE process has not been able to accurately identify the category of drug causing driving impairment. Officers are not equipped with the pharmacologic knowledge to be able to recognize the different pharmacodynamic effects a single drug may have in different people, making it extremely difficult for them to categorize these differing clinical presentations as being caused by the same drug class. Current data do not support the DRE program as the basis for an expert opinion in a court of law regarding whether a driver was impaired by drugs.

Police officers do not possess the necessary clinical training to form an educated opinion about driver impairment using the current tools provided to them by the DRE training program. Well-meaning DRE officers are at high risk of incorrectly opining that someone with a neurologic condition or taking therapeutic medications is impaired while driving. The current DRE examination process risks incarceration of innocent drivers and must be updated to match the scientific community's modern understanding of the many factors surrounding drug-induced driving impairment.

NOTES

1 Office of Behavioral Safety Research. (2021, June). Update to special reports on traffic safety during the COVID-19 public health emergency: Fourth quarter data (Report No. DOT HS 813 135). National Highway Traffic Safety Administration.
2 Berning, A., Compton, R., & Wochinger, K. (2015, February). Results of the 2013–2014 National Roadside Survey of alcohol and drug use by drivers (Traffic Safety Facts Research Note, Report No. DOT HS 812 118). Washington, DC: National Highway Traffic Safety Administration.
3 Spindle, T. R., Martin, E. L., Grabenauer, M., Woodward, T., Milburn, M. A., & Vandrey, R. (2021). Assessment of cognitive and psychomotor impairment, subjective effects, and blood THC concentrations following acute administration of oral and vaporized cannabis. Journal of Psychopharmacology, 35, 786–803.
4 Irwin, C., Iudakhina, E., Desbrow, B., & McCartney, D. (2017). Effects of acute alcohol consumption on measures of simulated driving: A systematic review and meta-analysis. Accident Analysis & Prevention, 102, 248–266.
5 Arkell, T. R., Spindle, T. R., Kevin, R. C., Vandrey, R., & McGregor, I. S. (2021). The failings of per se limits to detect cannabis-induced driving impairment: Results from a simulated driving study. Traffic Injury Prevention, 22(2), 102–107.
6 Transportation Safety Initiative. (Rev. 2018, February). Drug Recognition Expert Course Participant Manual. National Highway Traffic Safety Administration.
7 Yadav, A. K., & Velaga, N. R. (2019). Laboratory analysis of driving behavior and self-perceived physiological impairment at 0.03%, 0.05% and 0.08% blood alcohol concentrations. Drug and Alcohol Dependence, 205, 107630.
8 Jongen, S. (2013, August). Measuring the impairment of different doses of alcohol on car driving related skills: A calibration study. In 20th International Conference on Alcohol, Drugs and Traffic Safety (T2013), Brisbane, Queensland, Australia.
9 Martin, T. L., Solbeck, P. A., Mayers, D. J., Langille, R. M., Buczek, Y., & Pelletier, M. R. (2013). A review of alcohol-impaired driving: The role of blood alcohol concentration and complexity of the driving task. Journal of Forensic Sciences, 58(5), 1238–1250.
10 Centers for Disease Control and Prevention. (2021, May). Symptoms of Mild TBI and Concussion. National Center for Injury Prevention and Control. https://www.cdc.gov/traumaticbraininjury/concussion/symptoms.html.
11 Rangno, R. E., & Langlois, S. (1981). Comparison of withdrawal phenomena after propranolol, metoprolol and pindolol. In Catecholamines and the Heart (pp. 313–324). Springer, Berlin, Heidelberg.
12 Rubenzer, S. J., & Stevenson, S. B. (2010). Horizontal gaze nystagmus: A review of vision science and application issues. Journal of Forensic Sciences, 55(2), 394–409.
13 Kathmann, N., Hochrein, A., Uwer, R., & Bondy, B. (2003). Deficits in gain of smooth pursuit eye movements in schizophrenia and affective disorder patients and their unaffected relatives. American Journal of Psychiatry, 160(4), 696–702.
14 Strupp, M., Hüfner, K., Sandmann, R., Zwergal, A., Dieterich, M., Jahn, K., & Brandt, T. (2011). Central oculomotor disturbances and nystagmus: A window into the brainstem and cerebellum. Deutsches Ärzteblatt International, 108(12), 197.
15 Alvarez, T. L., Scheiman, M., Morales, C., Gohel, S., Sangoi, A., Santos, E. M., Yaramothu, C., d'Antonio-Bertagnolli, J. V., Li, X., & Biswal, B. B. (2021). Underlying neurological mechanisms associated with symptomatic convergence insufficiency. Scientific Reports, 11(1), 1–10.
16 Forbes, J., & Cronovich, H. (2020). Romberg Test. StatPearls [Internet]. Accessed September 3, 2021.
17 Merck Manual. (Rev. 2021, July). Neurologic Examination [Internet]. Merck Sharp & Dohme Corp. https://www.merckmanuals.com/home/brain,-spinal-cord,-and-nerve-disorders/diagnosis-of-brain,-spinal-cord,-and-nerve-disorders/neurologic-examination.
18 Currie, G. M. (2018). Pharmacology, part 1: Introduction to pharmacology and pharmacodynamics. Journal of Nuclear Medicine Technology, 46(2), 81–86.
19 Clonazepam (Lexicomp Online). Waltham, MA: UpToDate, Inc. https://online.lexi.com. Accessed August 14, 2021.
20 Venlafaxine (Lexicomp Online). Waltham, MA: UpToDate, Inc. https://online.lexi.com. Accessed August 14, 2021.

21 Kang, M., Galuska, M. A., & Ghassemzadeh, S. (Rev. 2021, July). Benzodiazepine toxicity. In StatPearls [Internet]. Treasure Island, FL: StatPearls Publishing. https://www.ncbi.nlm.nih.gov/books/NBK482238/.
22 Effexor XR [Package Insert]. Pfizer, Rev. 2021, July. https://www.pfizermedicalinformation.com/en-us/effexor-xr/overdose.
23 Minnesota Department of Public Safety. (Rev. 2018, February). Indicators consistent with drug categories [Internet]. https://dps.mn.gov/divisions/msp/about/Documents/dre-drug-category-matrix.pdf.
24 Diagnosis. Merriam-Webster [Internet]. https://www.merriam-webster.com/dictionary/diagnosis. Accessed September 3, 2021.
25 Types of healthcare providers. Medline Plus [Internet]. https://medlineplus.gov/ency/article/001933.htm. Accessed September 3, 2021.
26 Graber, M. L., Grice, G. R., Ling, L. J., Conway, J. M., & Olson, A. (2019). Pharmacy education needs to address diagnostic safety. American Journal of Pharmaceutical Education, 83(6).
27 Amin, M. R., & Ali, D. W. (2019). Pharmacology of medical cannabis. Recent Advances in Cannabinoid Physiology and Pathology, 1162, 151–165.
28 Desrosiers, N. A., & Huestis, M. A. (2019). Oral fluid drug testing: Analytical approaches, issues and interpretation of results. Journal of Analytical Toxicology, 43(6), 415–443.
29 Lowe, R. H., Abraham, T. T., Darwin, W. D., Herning, R., Cadet, J. L., & Huestis, M. A. (2009). Extended urinary Δ9-tetrahydrocannabinol excretion in chronic cannabis users precludes use as a biomarker of new drug exposure. Drug and Alcohol Dependence, 105(1–2), 24–32.
30 Logan, B. K., Lowrie, K. J., Turri, J. L., Yeakel, J. K., Limoges, J. F., Miles, A. K., Scarneo, C. E., Kerrigan, S., & Farrell, L. J. (2013). Recommendations for toxicological investigation of drug-impaired driving and motor vehicle fatalities. Journal of Analytical Toxicology, 37(8), 552–558.
31 Consensus Development Panel. (1985). Consensus report, drug concentrations and driving impairment. JAMA, 254, 2618–2621.
32 Verster, J. C., Veldhuijzen, D. S., Patat, A., Olivier, B., & Volkerts, E. R. (2006). Hypnotics and driving safety: Meta-analyses of randomized controlled trials applying the on-the-road driving test. Current Drug Safety, 1(1), 63–71.
33 Jongen, S., Vuurman, E. F. P. M., Ramaekers, J. G., & Vermeeren, A. (2018). Comparing the effects of oxazepam and diazepam in actual highway driving and neurocognitive test performance: A validation study. Psychopharmacology, 235(4), 1283–1294.
34 Smith, R. B., & Kroboth, P. D. (1987). Influence of dosing regimen on alprazolam and metabolite serum concentrations and tolerance to sedative and psychomotor effects. Psychopharmacology, 93(1), 105–112.
35 Brown, T. L., Milavetz, G., Gaffney, G., & Spurgin, A. (2018). Evaluating drugged driving: Effects of exemplar pain and anxiety medications. Traffic Injury Prevention, 19(sup1), S97–S103.
36 Ellis Jr, G. M., Mann, M. A., Judson, B. A., Schramm, N. T., & Tashchian, A. (1985). Excretion patterns of cannabinoid metabolites after last use in a group of chronic users. Clinical Pharmacology & Therapeutics, 38(5), 572–578.
37 Paolo Busardo, F., Pichini, S., Pellegrini, M., Montana, A., Fabrizio Lo Faro, A., Zaami, S., & Graziano, S. (2018). Correlation between blood and oral fluid psychoactive drug concentrations and cognitive impairment in driving under the influence of drugs. Current Neuropharmacology, 16(1), 84–96.
38 Gustavsen, I., Mørland, J., & Bramness, J. G. (2006). Impairment related to blood amphetamine and/or methamphetamine concentrations in suspected drugged drivers. Accident Analysis & Prevention, 38, 490–495. https://doi.org/10.1016/j.aap.2005.11.005.
39 Strand, M. C., Vindenes, V., Gjerde, H., Mørland, J. G., & Ramaekers, J. G. (2019). A clinical trial on the acute effects of methadone and buprenorphine on actual driving and cognitive function of healthy volunteers. British Journal of Clinical Pharmacology, 85(2), 442–453.
40 Drummer, O. H., & Yap, S. (2016). The involvement of prescribed drugs in road trauma. Forensic Science International, 265, 17–21.
41 Bosker, W. M., Theunissen, E. L., Conen, S., Kuypers, K. P. C., Jeffery, W. K., Walls, H. C., Kauert, G. F., Toennes, S. W., Moeller, M. R., & Ramaekers, J. G. (2012). A placebo-controlled study to assess Standardized Field Sobriety Tests performance during alcohol and cannabis intoxication in heavy cannabis users and accuracy of point of collection testing devices for detecting THC in oral fluid. Psychopharmacology, 223(4), 439–446.
42 Ginsburg, B. C. (2019). Strengths and limitations of two cannabis-impaired driving detection methods: A review of the literature. The American Journal of Drug and Alcohol Abuse, 45(6), 610–622.
43 Hartman, R. L., Brown, T. L., Milavetz, G., Spurgin, A., Gorelick, D. A., Gaffney, G. R., & Huestis, M. A. (2016). Effect of blood collection time on measured Δ9-tetrahydrocannabinol concentrations: Implications for driving interpretation and drug policy. Clinical Chemistry, 62(2), 367–377.
44 Ramaekers, J. G., Moeller, M. R., van Ruitenbeek, P., Theunissen, E. L., Schneider, E., & Kauert, G. (2006). Cognition and motor control as a function of Δ9-THC concentration in serum and oral fluid: Limits of impairment. Drug and Alcohol Dependence, 85(2), 114–122.
45 Khiabani, H. Z., Bramness, J. R. G., Bj∅ rneboe, A., & M∅ rland, J. R. (2006). Relationship between THC concentration in blood and impairment in

apprehended drivers. Traffic Injury Prevention, 7(2), 111–116.

46 Bergamaschi, M. M., Karschner, E. L., Goodwin, R. S., Scheidweiler, K. B., Hirvonen, J., Queiroz, R. H., & Huestis, M. A. (2013). Impact of prolonged cannabinoid excretion in chronic daily cannabis smokers' blood on per se drugged driving laws. Clinical Chemistry, 59(3), 519–526.

47 Parikh, R., Mathai, A., Parikh, S., Sekhar, G. C., & Thomas, R. (2008). Understanding and using sensitivity, specificity and predictive values. Indian Journal of Ophthalmology, 56(1), 45.

48 Gengo, F. M., Kirsch, J. M., Janofsky, J. S. (2012). A critical evaluation of the scientific and statistical validity of the drug recognition evaluation (DRE) program. In Inside the Minds: Understanding DUI Scientific Evidence (pp. 139–170). Aspatore Books.

49 Bigelow, G. E., Bickel, W. E., Liebson, I. A., & Nowowieski, P. (1985). Identifying types of drug intoxication: Laboratory evaluation of a subject-examination procedure (No. DOT-HS-806-753). United States. National Highway Traffic Safety Administration.

50 Heishman, S. J., Singleton, E. G., & Crouch, D. J. (1996). Laboratory validation study of drug evaluation and classification program: Ethanol, cocaine, and marijuana. Journal of Analytical Toxicology, 20(6), 468–483.

51 Heishman, S. J., Singleton, E. G., & Crouch, D. J. (1998). Laboratory validation study of drug evaluation and classification program: Alprazolam, d-amphetamine, codeine, and marijuana. Journal of Analytical Toxicology, 22(6), 503–514.

52 Smith, J. A., Hayes, C. E., Yolton, R. L., Rutledge, D. A., & Citek, K. (2002). Drug recognition expert evaluations made using limited data. Forensic Science International, 130(2–3), 167–173.

53 Shinar, D., & Schechtman, E. (2005). Drug identification performance on the basis of observable signs and symptoms. Accident Analysis & Prevention, 37(5), 843–851.

54 Compton, R. (1986). Field Evaluation of the Los Angeles Police Department Drug Detection Program. Washington, DC: National Highway Traffic Safety Administration.

55 Hardin, M., & Juejurikar (1993). Minnesota Corroboration Study: DRE Opinions and Toxicology Evaluations (Minn Bureau of Crim). Apprehension.

56 Adler, E. V., & Burns, M. (1994). Drug Recognition Expert (DRE) Validation Study: Final Report to Governor's Office of Highway Safety. State of Arizona.

57 Hartman, R. L., Richman, J. E., Hayes, C. E., & Huestis, M. A. (2016). Drug Recognition Expert (DRE) examination characteristics of cannabis impairment. Accident Analysis & Prevention, 92, 219–229.

58 Declues, K., Perez, S., & Figueroa, A. (2017). A two-year study of D 9 tetrahydrocannabinol concentrations in drivers; part 2: Physiological signs on drug recognition expert (DRE) and non-DRE examinations. Journal of Forensic Sciences. https://doi.org/10.1111/1556-4029.13550.

59 Porath, A. J., & Beirness, D. J. (2019). Predicting categories of drugs used by suspected drug-impaired drivers using the Drug Evaluation and Classification Program tests. Traffic Injury Prevention, 20(3), 255–263.

60 Edwards, L. D., Smith, K. L., & Savage, T. (2017). Drugged driving in Wisconsin: Oral fluid versus blood. Journal of Analytical Toxicology, 41(6), 523–529.

61 Truver, M. T., Palmquist, K. B., & Swortwood, M. J. (2019). Oral fluid and drug impairment: Pairing toxicology with drug recognition expert observations. Journal of Analytical Toxicology, 43(8), 637–643.

62 The International Association of Chiefs of Police [Internet]. https://www.theiacp.org/states-and-countries-with-dres. Accessed September 3, 2021.

38 Involuntary Intoxication

James T. O'Donnell, James J. O'Donnell III, and William Vaughn

SYNOPSIS

38.1 INTRODUCTION

A pharmacologist is a drug expert who provides aid in legal settings by assisting the attorney, examining the defendant, and providing expert opinion and testimony on a multitude of cases involving criminal behaviors influenced by drug use. Defense lawyers are no stranger to complex cases involving criminal acts of violence and substance abuse. Many cases demonstrate the strong relationship between drugs and violent activity. For example, in one widely publicized case, an individual (referred to as MM) brandished a knife and attacked police, firefighters, and their vehicle, following the ingestion of an illegal drug. His violent advances led an officer to fire, resulting in the loss of his life. The autopsy determined that MM had ingested the illegal substance cocaine. MM's family brought an excessive force charge against the city; however, the jury found the city not liable due to the evidence of high levels of cocaine in MM's blood and expert testimony provided from one of the authors (JTOD) of how cocaine may cause drug-induced psychosis. Another important factor in the outcome of this case is that MM had voluntarily ingested the drug. A similar defense can be used in criminal cases in which the victim is significantly intoxicated, acting psychotic, threatening others, or who acts in self-defense and find themselves defending criminal charges as a result. Cases like this highlight the ever-growing association between drug use and altered behavior leading toward violent acts.

38.2 LEGAL DEFENSE CONSIDERATIONS FOR A VIOLENT CRIME

"The drugs made me do it."

Many criminal defense lawyers find themselves hearing this statement from clients who committed violent acts while under the influence of a drug. Alternatively, the client/defendant may maintain that they were acting in self-defense against crazed drug-induced actions by a "victim" who was under the influence. Clients who were under the influence of drugs at the time of an alleged crime may maintain that their behavior was well outside of their normal range and capacity. Many individuals report no recollection of the event. Certain classes of drugs are well known to cause "blackouts" or amnesia (e.g., alcohol and benzodiazepines), which disrupts memory formation processes resulting in significant lapses in memory recall.[1]

Generally, the judicial system is not lenient on offenders who commit crimes under the influence of voluntarily consumed recreational or illegal substances and holds defendants criminally responsible for their actions.[2] In the federal court system, voluntary ingestion of a drug eliminates any potential use of the insanity defense.[3] Voluntary consumption implies that the individual was sufficiently aware that the intake of the substance would lead to impairment, whereas involuntary intoxication means that the person was unknowingly given the substance (e.g., a drink was spiked with a drug) or became impaired by physician-prescribed medication.[4] In certain jurisdictions, if the drug ingestion and subsequent effect on the user were severe enough to raise a reasonable doubt about the capacity of the defendant to formulate specific intent of the crime, the accused may be convicted of a reduced offense. Involuntary intoxication, where applicable, generally excuses more behaviors but may not result in complete exoneration. Laws on involuntary intoxication vary from state to state. In certain jurisdictions, mitigating factors such as severe intoxication or diminished capacity may aid in receiving a reduced sentencing. Defense attorneys should pay particular attention to the applicable involuntary intoxication statutes and case law in their jurisdictions.

Defending clients with drug-induced violent offences proves difficult as many factors contribute to the legal outcome. Contributing factors include the voluntary or involuntary ingestion of the drug, the indication of the drug and whether it was prescribed by a physician, whether the drug is consumed in the prescribed dosing regimens, multi-drug

DOI: 10.1201/9781003615323-42

use and drug–drug interactions, and, finally, the client medical history of substance abuse and mental health status. All of these factors should be considered when evaluating a case involving drug-induced violence. These factors are important in determining if involuntary intoxication is a viable defense. If a person unknowingly consumes an intoxicant (e.g., spiked drink), or becomes intoxicated and/or violent as a result of the use of a prescribed medication, then the defense of involuntary intoxication may be considered, depending on jurisdiction. In one case example, a man (CG) faced charges for first degree murder of his wife. A Federal Defender in the habeas corpus court was recently appointed to represent the defendant in a claim of ineffective assistance of counsel. The claim is based on the trial counsel's failure to present an involuntary intoxication defense during the case in chief. Trial counsel did introduce the topic after the conviction as mitigation before sentencing. Prior to the murder, the defendant attempted to check into a Mental Health Hospital but was denied because of insurance. He was then prescribed Xanax (anti-anxiety), Pristiq (antidepressant), and Lamictal (mood stabilizer) by his child's psychiatrist to handle his acute needs until he could be seen during a scheduled appointment the next week. The defendant had a medical history that included the psychiatric condition of bipolar disorder. On the day of the murder, the defendant was found wandering near a vehicle crash site where he had attempted suicide by crashing his wife's vehicle into a bridge wall. His wife was later found stabbed to death at their home. The defendant displayed an altered mental status and serious psychotic behaviors and had no recollection of stabbing his wife. A pharmacologist expert, retained by the Federal Defender, determined that the defendant was involuntarily intoxicated and impaired by the prescribed Xanax at the time of the murder of his wife. This intoxication severely impaired his brain; causing delusions; triggering psychotic, aggressive, violent, and erratic behavior; and causing amnesia. The defendant displayed drug-induced psychosis which is time-limited—until the drug wears off (as it did in this case).[5] An evidentiary hearing to determine if a new trial should be granted was held. The Federal Defender advised that the new trial was not granted at the district level, appealed, and also denied in the court of appeals. The Federal Defender is planning to file for a certiorari petition in the supreme court, as well as a petition for a writ of habeas corpus.[6]

38.3 CONFIRMING THAT DRUGS ARE INVOLVED IN A VIOLENT CRIME

Determining if a drug is involved in a violent offense first requires a confirmation through various routes of drug testing. Drug tests may be performed on samples extracted from various tissues or secretions of the body including blood, urine, saliva (oral), hair, and sweat. Each test varies in its specificity for the drug or its metabolites (the compounds the drug is broken down into by the body) and the detection window. Immediate testing following a crime allows for the best interpretation of drug status in an individual; however, this may not be feasible in certain cases. Confirming that a drug was involved several days following a crime presents many challenges. Depending on the drug in question, detection windows for accurately measuring a drug vary among the different classes. Urine analysis is the most commonly employed screen for drugs and the most thoroughly studied along with the analysis of the blood. Sampling of the urine is less invasive, and there is a longer detection window compared to blood. Drugs may be detected in the urine up to 30 days following ingestion; however, specific drugs have different detection windows. For example, marijuana may be detected up to 30 days (or longer in heavy cannabis users) in urine compared to methamphetamine which is only detectable up to 5 days in the urine.[7] While urine screens are less invasive and have longer detection windows in urine for the drugs in comparison to blood, screens only indicate that the drug has been ingested sometime in the past (within the detection window). Only detection and quantification of drug in blood can be used to infer impairment *at the time* of a criminal act. This is the Achilles' heel of urine drug tests, and this may be exploited by prosecutors to argue against drug impairment.

Because of the variability in detection windows for different drugs, it is best to collect the urine or blood sample to test for drug involvement immediately after a crime has been committed. This typically is accomplished when an individual is arrested on site after an incident has occurred. In one Cook County, Illinois case, a man (JG) was charged with firing a weapon at police officers. JG was apprehended immediately at the scene and taken to a police station. A urine drug test confirmed the presence of PCP (phencyclidine) and amphetamine. JG was noted as being disoriented and having an altered mental status. He was hospitalized and diagnosed with PCP intoxication, and blood tests demonstrated intoxicating levels of PCP. Further investigation revealed that JG had unknowingly ingested these substances at a party and had no intent of ingesting or becoming intoxicated from these drugs. A pharmacologist gave expert testimony opining that JG was involuntarily intoxicated by PCP and that JG would have been deprived of substantial capacity either to appreciate the criminality of his conduct or to conform his conduct to the requirements of law. In this case, the defense attorney argued for involuntary intoxication.[8,9]

Immediate drug testing is encouraged when a crime is committed by individuals whose behavior dramatically differs from their baseline (normal) behavior. Another example case involves an individual (JB) who attended a hockey game with his family and then went out with friends to a bar. His friends noted extremely abnormal and irrational behavior from JB toward the end of the night. JB was arrested by police, responding to 911 calls of a man banging on their door at approximately 2 am in the morning and yelling he was with "NYPD." When police arrived, JB had kicked in the back door of the residence and was physically threatening the occupant. He was tested for the usual drugs of abuse when he was released on bond 40 hours later. JB screened negative for drugs on both tests. The Emergency Department physician posed that while no drugs were detected in JB's urine, many designer drugs, such as the date rape drugs, hallucinogens, and anesthetics, can be cleared out of a person's system in about six hours, leaving them undetectable. JB's drug test was conducted approximately 40 hours after he was at the bar. All drug testing came up negative (panel of usual drugs of abuse); yet, the defendant was obviously seriously intoxicated, impaired, and experiencing a drug-induced psychosis in the assault. In this case, JB was involuntarily intoxicated by an unknown substance. He was acquitted of all charges at the conclusion of his criminal trial. Citations to two court opinions in the Hari case in Illinois regarding involuntary intoxication are available.[10,11]

When an individual experiences drug-induced psychosis, they are not aware nor can they control their actions due to the acute effects of a mind-altering drug at the time of the criminal act. An association exists between Central Nervous System (CNS)-acting drugs and the development of a wide range of behavioral changes. However, the clinical manifestation of drug-induced psychosis is complicated by the underlying brain pathology, which may contribute to behavioral manifestations leading to crime. Currently, the legal ramifications for offenses committed by those exhibiting psychotic symptoms draw a distinction when assigning criminal responsibility between those who experience symptoms related to their innate mental status (i.e., underlying mental illness) versus psychotic symptoms resulting from the effects of an ingested drug. However, drawing this distinction between drug use and mental status is problematic and difficult to determine. Thus, a defense that includes mental instability or illness as a contributor, if applicable, may aid in obtaining an acquittal or reduced sentencing.

Chronic drug use may also predispose an individual to psychotic symptoms.[12] This is the basis for a "settled" insanity defense where voluntary intoxication for extended periods of time results in psychosis that is independent from the acute effects of the drug. Psychotic symptoms that persist for periods long after drug use and beyond the time a drug test finds them detectable in the body provide evidence for an underlying mental illness and against a drug-induced psychosis. A drug-induced psychosis corrects quite quickly—within a day or so. Non-drug psychosis persists.

38.4 BEYOND PHARMACOLOGY: THE MULTIFACTORIAL ROLE OF DRUGS IN AGGRESSION AND VIOLENCE

There are many ways to categorize aggression. One common method is to classify aggression into premeditated (predatory) or impulsive (affective) aggression. Predatory aggression involves planning, is not an immediate response to a frustration, and has clear goals in mind. Impulsive aggression involves little-to-no planning, precipitation by an immediate frustration, and a lack of clear goals in mind. The violence from impulsive aggression is often an overreaction to environmental stressors or a perceived threat. With impulsive aggression, the person may disregard or not consider the consequences of the violence.[13] According to the FBI's Uniform Crime Reporting Program, violent crimes are offenses that involve force or the threat of force and are categorized into four different types of offences: Murder and nonnegligent manslaughter, rape, robbery, and aggravated assault.[14]

Drugs contribute to crimes and injuries in many ways. Individuals abusing addictive drugs can have severe withdrawal reactions which may lead to crimes such as armed robbery or burglary to obtain funding for additional drugs. Drug dealers may also use deadly force as a strategy to eliminate competition. While commonly associated with crime related to the possession, manufacturing, or distribution of illicit substances, certain drugs may more directly influence criminal behavior by causing the person who has ingested the substance to act out in a violent or criminal manner. Many criminal cases involve the use of illicit and prescription drugs which precede the criminal activity. Intoxication can impair a person and cause them to lose control of themselves and disable their judgment of differentiating right from wrong. Drug-induced violence is incompletely understood, but evidence demonstrates that certain drug classes interfere with an individual's behavior such that they engage in actions or precipitated events that otherwise would not occur had they not been impaired by drugs.

38.5 ASSOCIATION OF DRUGS WITH AGGRESSION AND VIOLENCE

Approximately 80% of criminal activities resulting in incarceration in the United States are committed by offenders who abuse drugs or alcohol, while 60% of those arrested for the majority of crimes test positive for an illicit substance at the time of arrest.[15] Approximately 50% of inmates who had committed a violent crime against a spouse, boyfriend, or girlfriend had been drinking alcohol or using drugs when the offense occurred.[16] A survey conducted in state and federal correctional facilities reports that 32% of state prisoners committed their offense under the influence of drugs, with the highest incidence of drug use at the time of the criminal offense reported among drug offenders (44%) and property offenders (39%). Among federal prisoners, violent offenders (24%) and drug offenders (32%) were most likely to be under the influence of drugs at the time of their offense.[17] Clearly, there is a strong association between drug or alcohol use and serious crime, including violent crime.

A key question of association versus causality remains: Is drug and alcohol use contributing to the criminal behavior or is it merely a characteristic of those who commit crime? This question of whether drugs or alcohol definitively cause the criminal behavior has important legal implications. The difficulty in determining the causality of drug-induced behaviors arises from the involvement of many influences including biological, psychological, social, economic, and environmental factors. Biologic and psychologic factors include differences in drug metabolism and the way a person responds to being on a drug, whereas the social, economic, and environmental factors are unique among individuals and can influence a drug user's behavior in various ways, depending on the situational use of the drug. Thus, the answer to this question must be evaluated on a case-by-case basis.

While particular cases must be evaluated on an individual basis to determine the contribution of drugs, certain drug classes are linked to increases in violence and aggression. Drug use can contribute to a wide range of behaviors from irritation and hostility to domestic violence, assault, and homicide. Significant behavioral changes resulting in violent actions are seen with both prescription and illicit substance use.

Violence-related symptoms are evident in many drug-induced adverse event cases reported to the FDA. A review of MedWatch, the FDA's adverse event reporting system, revealed 14,773 reports of violent adverse events associated with psychiatric drugs from 2004 to 2012. The review included 1,531 cases of homicidal ideation/homicide, 3,287 cases of mania, and 8,219 cases of aggression.[18] The FDA has mandated labeling of certain medications to include warnings of violent actions and recommends that changes in behavior be monitored closely. These precautions include labeling of irritability, impulsivity, aggressiveness, agitation, hostility, and changes in behavior and mood. When a violent crime occurs, it is worthwhile reviewing the drug in question to see if reports linking its use to violence are known, or if limited reports have emerged in MedWatch.

38.6 MECHANISMS OF DRUG-INDUCED VIOLENCE

Drugs that have known associations with violent behavior are all substances that act in the central nervous system (CNS) and affect the brain. The brain's limbic system is responsible for regulating emotions (e.g., anger) and connects to other parts of the brain that act to inhibit what we would consider inappropriate behavior driven by these emotions.

Drugs can be divided into groups based on their influence on the activity of specific molecules in the brain called neurotransmitters. There are multiple groups of drugs that influence violence, highlighting the complicated nature of this behavioral manifestation. These groups include stimulants (e.g., Cocaine, Methamphetamine, Bath salts); hallucinogens (e.g., PCP, LSD (lysergic acid); antidepressants (e.g., Prozac, Zoloft, Lexapro), anabolic steroids (e.g., Testosterone, Androstenedione); smoking cessation (e.g., Chantix[r]—varencline); and antimalarial (e.g., Larium[r]—mefloquine) drugs (Table 38.1). Drugs most commonly associated with violence activate dopamine and serotonin neurotransmitter systems in the brain. Physiological changes subsequent to drug use may prime the individual for violence through direct or indirect activation of the sympathetic nervous system which facilitates "fight or flight" responses—a set of physiological effects in various organs throughout the body that collectively aim to promote enhanced physical and mental capacity. The body is thus "primed" for action and ready to engage. Specific drug effects that may contribute to violence include increased physical energy, alertness and concentration, heart rate, metabolic function, and reduced pain sensitivity and fatigue. Supplemental cognitive effects such as feelings of invincibility and elevated self-confidence may also contribute to the overall elevated profile for engaging in violence.[19,20,21]

TABLE 38.1
Common Drugs Associated with Violence.

Drug Group	Examples
Stimulants	Cocaine, Amphetamines (Methamphetamine, Adderall), Bath Salts (Mephedrone, MDPV and Methylone), Spice (Synthetic Marijuana)
Hallucinogens	PCP, LSD
Antidepressants	Prozac, Zoloft, Lexapro
Benzodiazepines	Xanax, Valium
Antimalarial drugs	Lariam
Anti-smoking drugs	Chantix
Anabolic steroids	Testosterone, Propionate, Insulin
Hypoglycemic drugs	Insulin, Lopressor

Source: Adapted from References[22,23]

38.7 INTOXICATION OF VICTIM DEFENSE

A recent engagement by defense counsel in a murder trial identified a toxic level of a hallucinogenic psychostimulant (bromantane) in the blood of the murder victim. Over objections by the prosecutor, the Court allowed testimony by the retained expert pharmacologist (JTOD) to explain to the Jury the significance of the toxicology findings. Defense counsel then argued that his client, a tow truck driver, was acting in self-defense from the erratic driving of a semi-truck driver (the victim) in a road rage incident.

Bromantane, also known as Ladasten or NP-160, is an atypical psychostimulant drug. Bromantane is also referred to as an actoprotector. These drugs comprise a class of pharmacologically active substances that improve physical and mental efficiencies in humans, after initial investigations were conducted at the Military Medical Academy (then Leningrad, USSR—now, St. Petersburg, Russia) Department of Pharmacology. These drugs were used in preparing individuals for sports competitions, most notably the Olympics, and in various military operations due to their enhancement of physical and mental capacities. Due to anti-doping regulations, bromantane and other actoprotectors have been prohibited for use in sports. Bromantane is currently used in Russia for the treatment of neurasthenia. Bromantane is not approved by the FDA for use in humans in the United States for any indication.

The mechanism of action (MOA) of bromantane is uncertain. As an actoprotector, bemitil is considered the prototype drug. The MOA of bemitil is attributed to a complex mechanism entailing cell genome activation, optimization of mitochondrial oxidation, oxidative stress reduction, and stimulation of cellular immune response.[24,25] At the molecular level, studies suggest that bromantane delays an increase in 5-HT and 5-HIAA content in subcortical brain regions, increases content in the frontal cortex, and decreases levels in the cerebellum. Bromantane also affected the DA parameters of the brain. These findings suggest a key role of dopaminergic system activity in the key effects of bromantane.[26]

Preclinical studies show behavioral effects of bromantane associated with the stimulation of the central dopamine and the suppression of muscarinic and nicotinic cholinergic structures. Spontaneous motor activity increased after treatment with bromantane (30–300 mg/kg), but no effect was observed at 600 mg/kg. Motor activity was inhibited at doses more than 600 mg/kg. At a dose range of 300–600 mg/kg, bromantane reduced the pain sensitivity threshold and elevated the pain threshold, tactile sensitivity, and reaction to knock in doses above 600 mg/kg. Bromantane induced mydriasis in all studied doses; in doses above 10 g/kg, the preparation induced blepharoptosis. In doses above five g/kg, bromantane slightly increased the respiration rate and depth (Kussmaul-like respiration). In some animals, bromantane in high doses induced regurgitation, diarrhea, and polyuria.[27] Quantitative pharmaco-electroencephalographic (EEG) evaluation in rats suggests that bromantane has more profound and prolonged stimulant properties than other adamantane-derived psychostimulants.[28] Additional studies show psychostimulating activity in animals across multiple measures (e.g., increases in motor and EEG).[29,30] Limited research exists on bromantane. Most studies have been conducted on rodents (most in Russian and unavailable in full documents), and it does not appear that any clinical trials have been conducted on humans. Therefore, the safety of bromantane in humans is uncertain.

Stimulants are a class of psychoactive drugs that increase neural activation providing temporary increases in physical and/or mental output. Stimulants (e.g., cocaine, amphetamine) are often implicated in aggressive behaviors and violence. While presumably associated, a defined relationship between substances and the development of aggression is lacking. More specifically, blood–drug concentration thresholds which show high levels of intoxicated aggression are not known. Psychostimulant use can lead to a wide range of behaviors from irritation and hostility to domestic violence, assault, and homicide. Drugs that have known associations with violent behavior are all substances that act on the central nervous system (CNS) and affect the brain. The brain's limbic system is responsible for regulating emotions (e.g., anger) and connects to other parts of the brain that act to inhibit what we would consider inappropriate behavior driven by these emotions. Many molecules in the brain are involved in regulation of these activities.

There are multiple groups of drugs that are associated with violence and aggressive behaviors. These groups include stimulants, with bromantane classified as such due to its known pharmacologic actions and observed behavioral effects. The drugs most commonly associated with violence reported to the FDA MedWatch system activate the dopamine and serotonin neurotransmitter systems in the brain. Physiological changes subsequent to drug use may prime the individual for violence through direct or indirect activation of the sympathetic nervous system which facilitates "fight or flight" responses. Excitation of the adrenal system releases adrenaline and initiates a cascade of biological events that aim to promote enhanced physical and mental capacity. The body is thus "primed" for action and ready to engage. Specific drug effects that may contribute to violence include increased physical energy, alertness and concentration, heart rate, metabolic function, and reduced pain sensitivity and fatigue. Supplemental cognitive effects such as feelings of invincibility and elevated self-confidence may also contribute to the overall elevated profile for engaging in violence.[31,32,33]

Psychostimulants are a risk factor for violence perpetration and victimization in the general population. Specific studies show that a history of methamphetamine use is associated with an increased adjusted risk of violence perpetration (OR 1.60; 1.01–2.54), intimate partner violence perpetration (OR 1.55, 95 % CI 1.04–2.30), and violence victimization (OR 1.57, 1.00–2.47). A dose–response relationship was observed in those who demonstrated chronic use (i.e., methamphetamine at least weekly at any time from age 18 to 35 years), whereas they had substantially elevated adjusted odds of violence involvement compared to people who used less frequently or had never used.[34]

A global review on the harms of psychostimulant use evaluated the impact on measures of violence. Stimulant use is associated with poor mental health including suicidality, psychosis, depression, and violence. Any use of amphetamines was associated with higher odds of psychosis (odds ratio [OR] = 2.0, 95%CI 1.3–3.3) and violence (OR = 2.2, 95%CI 1.2–4.1; adjusted OR [AOR] = 1.4, 95%CI 0.8–2.4). Overall, any use of amphetamines was associated with 2.2 times the odds of violence. Differences were observed in the strength of the association depending on the measure of violence used. Unadjusted odds ratios were large and consistent for violent behavior (OR 3.7, 95% CI 3.1–4.5, $p < 0.001$; 2 – 34, $p = 0.163$). Longitudinal studies provided evidence for increased violent behavior during periods of when amphetamines were being used (which persisted after adjustment for contemporaneous changes in other substance use)[35] and higher rates of recidivism for violent offences among forensic inmates with an amphetamine use disorder post their release.[36,37]

Overall, evidence suggests that bromantane is a psychostimulant drug that shows molecular and behavioral effects similar to other stimulant drugs. Limited research exists on the effects of bromantane, and no clinical trials appear to have ever been conducted although its use has been discussed for the enhancement of mental and physical output in sports and military settings outside the United States. Evidence from the manifestation of aggression and violence observed with other psychostimulants likely translates to a potential harmful effect with bromantane use.

38.8 SUMMARY AND CONCLUSIONS

The strong association between drug use, violence, and crime ensures that defense lawyers will likely continue to defend a wide range of drug-induced violent offences. Consequently, lawyers need to consider if the intoxication was involuntary, which would be exculpatory, or whether voluntary intoxication may be useful in mitigation. Alternatively, the intoxication may be in the victim, and thus it provides an explanation for the actions of a defendant. These types of crimes can necessitate very complicated defense organization that requires lawyers to understand critical components of scientific/medical methodology and fact. Many abusable illicit and prescription drugs can significantly affect brain processes, leading to the development of violent or aggressive behavior. Definitive proof of drug influence lies in a variety of scientific and clinical assessments that evaluate drug effects and/or concentrations. If drugs are suspected in a violent case, an experienced defense attorney should consider a number of factors while developing a successful defense, including drug pharmacology, the client's mental status, and history of drug use. A pharmacologist is an appropriate expert to assist the attorney, examine the defendant, and provide expert opinion and testimony in these matters.

NOTES

1. Baughman SB. Drugs and Violence. University of Utah College of Law Research Paper No. 75, 2014, 88.
2. Weinstock R. Drug and Alcohol Intoxication: Mens Rea Defenses. American Academy of Psychiatry and the Law. 1999;24(1).
3. Wolber JFG. Intoxication and Settled Insanity: A Finding of Not Guilty by Reason of Insanity. Journal of the American Academy of Psychiatry and the Law Online. 2007;35:172–182.
4. Murray PE. In Need of a Fix: Reforming Criminal Law in Light of a Contemporary Understanding of Drug Addiction. UCLA Law Review. 2013;60:1006.
5. Cone EJ, Huestis MA. Interpretation of Oral Fluid Tests for Drugs of Abuse. Annals of the New York Academy of Sciences. 2007;1098:51–103.
6. Gish v. Hepp, 955 F.3d 597 (7th Cir. 2020).
7. Hadland SE, Levy S. Objective Testing: Urine and Other Drug Tests. Child and Adolescent Psychiatric Clinics of North America. 2017;25(3):549–565.
8. Wolber JFG. Intoxication and Settled Insanity: A Finding of Not Guilty by Reason of Insanity. Journal of the American Academy of Psychiatry and the Law Online. 2007;35:172–182.
9. Murray PE. In Need of a Fix: Reforming Criminal Law in Light of a Contemporary Understanding of Drug Addiction. UCLA Law Review. 2013;60:1006.
10. 2014 IL App (1st) 120531. The People of the State of Illinois, Plaintiff-Appellee, v. Oscar Orozco, Defendant-Appellant. No. 1-12-0531. Appellate Court of Illinois First Judicial District Sixth Division, March 14, 2014.
11. 33.843 N.E.2d 349 218 Ill.2d 275. The People of the State of Illinois, Appellee, v. David A. HARI, Appellant. No. 100055. Supreme Court of Illinois, January 20, 2006.
12. Dixon L, Haas G, Weiden PJ, Sweeney J, Frances AJ. Drug Abuse in Schizophrenic Patients: Clinical Correlates and Reasons for Use. The American Journal of Psychiatry. 1991;148(2):224–230.
13. PA. Drug Induced Aggression and Violence, 4th ed. Tucson: L&J Publ; 2016.
14. FBI:UCR. Violent Crime. https://ucr.fbi.gov/crime-in-the-u.s/2015/crime-in-the-u.s.-2015/offenses-known-to-law-enforcement/violent-crime.
15. Dependence NCoAaD. Alcohol, Drugs and Crime [Cited May 29, 2018]. https://www.ncadd.org/about-addiction/alcohol-drugs-and-crime.
16. Fox JA. Violence by Intimates: Analysis of Data on Crimes by Current or Former Spouses, Boyfriends, and Girlfriends. Bureau of Justice Statistics; 1998.
17. Mumola CJ, Karberg JC. Drug Use and Dependence, State and Federal Prisoners. Bureau of Justice Statistics; 2004.
18. International CCoHR. Psychiatric Drugs: Regulatory Warnings on Violence, Mania, Psychosis, Homicide [Cited May 16, 2018]. https://www.cchrint.org/psychiatric-drugs/drug_warnings_on_violence/.
19. Knopp WD, Wang TW, Bach BR Jr. Ergogenic Drugs in Sports. Clinics in Sports Medicine. 1997;16(3):375–392. Epub July 1, 1997. PubMed PMID: 9209817.
20. Juhn M. Popular Sports Supplements and Ergogenic Aids. Sports Medicine (Auckland, NZ). 2003;33(12):921–939.
21. Marsden CD, Meadows JC. The Effect of Adrenaline on the Contraction of Human Muscle. The Journal of Physiology. 1970;207(2):429–448.
22. International CCoHR. Psychiatric Drugs: Regulatory Warnings on Violence, Mania, Psychosis, Homicide [Cited 2018 May 16]. https://www.cchrint.org/psychiatric-drugs/drug_warnings_on_violence/.
23. Moore TJ, Glenmullen J, Furberg CD. Prescription Drugs Associated With Reports of Violence Towards Others. PLoS One. 2010;5(12):e15337.

24 Shabanov PD. Clinical Pharmacology of Metaprot, a New Antiasthenic Drug With Psychoactivating Properties. Obzori po klinichaskoi farmakologii i lekarstvennoi terapii (Reviews on Clinical Pharmacology and Drug Therapy) (St.Petersburg). 2009;7:48–81.
25 Oliynyk S, Oh S. The Pharmacology of Actoprotectors: Practical Application for Improvement of Mental and Physical Performance. Biomolecules & Therapeutics. 2012;20(5):446–456.
26 Kudrin VS, Sergeeva SA, Krasnykh LM, Miroshnichenko II, Grekhova TV, Gaĭnetdinov RR. Vliianie bromantana na dofamin-i serotoninergicheskie sistemy mozga krys [The Effect of Bromantane on the Dopamin- and Serotoninergic Systems of the Rat Brain]. Eksp Klin Farmakol. 1995 July–August;58(4):8–11. Russian.
27 Iezhitsa IN, Spasov AA, Bugaeva LI, Morozov IS. Toxic Effect of Single Treatment With Bromantane on Neurological Status of Experimental Animals. Bulletin of Experimental Biology and Medicine. 2002 April;133(4):380–383.
28 Krapivin SV, Sergeeva SA, Morozov IS. Kolichestvennyĭ farmako-élektroéntsefalograficheskiĭ analiz deĭstviia bromantana [A Quantitative Pharmaco-Electroencephalographic Analysis of the Action of Bromantane]. Bulletin of Experimental Biology and Medicine. 1993 November;116(11):515–518. Russian.
29 Morozov IS, Klimova NV, Karpova TD, Shestopalov SS. Kharakteristika neĭropsikhotropnoĭ aktivnosti bromantana u laboratornykh zhivotnykh [The Characteristics of the Neuropsychotropic Activity of Bromantane in Laboratory Animals]. Eksp Klin Farmakol. 1999 March–April;62(2):3–6. Russian.
30 Iëzhitsa IN, Bugaeva LI, Spasov AA, Morozov IS. Vliianie bromantana na nevrologicheskiĭ status krys pri dvukhmesiachnom vvedenii [Effect of Bromantane on the Rat Neurologic Status in Two Month Course]. Eksp Klin Farmakol. 2000 September–October;63(5):13–17. Russian.
31 Knopp WD, Wang TW, Bach BR Jr. Ergogenic Drugs in Sports. Clinics in Sports Medicine. 1997;16(3):375–392. Epub July 1, 1997.
32 Juhn M. Popular Sports Supplements and Ergogenic Aids. Sports Medicine (Auckland, NZ). 2003;33(12):921–939. Epub September 17, 2003.
33 Marsden CD, Meadows JC. The Effect of Adrenaline on the Contraction of Human Muscle. The Journal of Physiology. 1970;207(2):429–448. Epub April 1, 1970.
34 Foulds JA, Boden JM, McKetin R, Newton-Howes G. Methamphetamine Use and Violence: Findings From a Longitudinal Birth Cohort. Drug and Alcohol Dependence. 2020 February 1;207:107826.
35 Sekine Y, Ouchi Y, Takei N, Yoshikawa E, Nakamura K, Futatsubashi M, Okada H, Minabe Y, Suzuki K, Iwata Y, Tsuchiya KJ. Brain Serotonin Transporter Density and Aggression in Abstinent Methamphetamine Abusers. Archives of General Psychiatry. 2006;63:90–100.
36 Miczek KA, Tidey JW. Amphetamines: Aggressive and Social Behaviour. In: Pharmacology and Toxicology of Amphetamine and Related Designer Drugs Research Monograph 94. Rockville, MD: NIDA; 1989:68–100.
37 Farrell M, Martin NK, Stockings E, Bórquez A, Cepeda JA, Degenhardt L, Ali R, Tran LT, Rehm J, Torrens M, Shoptaw S. Responding to Global Stimulant Use: Challenges and Opportunities. Lancet (London, England). 2019;394(10209):1652–1667.

39 Drug-Induced Aggression and Violence

Peter D. Anderson

SYNOPSIS

39.1 CLASSIFICATION OF AGGRESSION

Violence is recurrently seen in both criminal and civil litigation. Hoaken and Stewart define aggression as "any form of behavior directed toward the goal of harming or injuring another being who is motivated to avoid such treatment."[1] In everyday language, the words aggression and violence are often used interchangeably. Conversely, violence can be considered overt physical aggression.[2] The term aggression tends to be used in animal-based laboratory studies or clinical practice. In the criminal justice system or the forensic literature, the term violence tends to be used.[3] Agitation refers to a pathologically intense emotional arousal and motor restlessness.[2] Irritability is an abnormally low frustration tolerance in which the individual is readily provoked to anger and hostility.

There are many ways to categorize aggression. One common method is to classify aggression into predatory (premeditated) or impulsive (affective) aggression.[4,5] Predatory aggression involves planning, is not an immediate response to a frustration, and has clear goals in mind. Impulsive aggression involves little-to-no planning, precipitation by an immediate frustration, and a lack of clear goals in mind. Impulsive aggression involves the fight or flight response to a perceived threat. The violence from impulsive aggression is often an overreaction to environmental stressors or a perceived threat. With impulsive aggression, the person may disregard or not even think about the consequences of their actions. See Table 39.1 for a comparison of impulsive and predatory aggression. The distinction of predatory and impulsive aggression is not always clear cut. A specific transaction of violence may possess characteristics of both predatory and impulsive aggression. For example, an individual robs a bank and utilizes a firearm. The robbery involves planning—this is predatory aggression. However, the culprit shoots a teller that does not fully comply or is perceived not to fully comply with the instructions; this would be the impulsive part of the transaction. Sexual-based aggression is predominately a predatory aggression.

Predatory aggression is often associated with antisocial personality disorder.[6] Features of antisocial personality disorder include a disregard of laws and moral standards, manipulative behavior, lack of empathy, shallow effect, and pathological lying.[4] This is not to say persons with antisocial personality disorder cannot have episodes of impulsive aggression, as impulsive episodes are common with antisocial personality disorder. Delusional or psychotic features are not part of antisocial social personality disorder diagnosis, as it is with schizophrenia or bipolar disorder. The

DOI: 10.1201/9781003615323-43

TABLE 39.1
Predatory versus Impulsive Aggression.

Predatory Aggression or Premeditated Aggression	Impulsive Aggression or Affective Aggression
More cognitive	More emotional
Planning involved	Little-to-no planning
Not an immediate response to a frustration or perceived threat	An immediate response to a frustration or a perceived threat
More organized.	Less organized.
Clear goals in mind.	No clear goals in mind.
Material gain is sought (money, power, sexual gratification).	No material gain is sought.
No or minimal surge in sympathetic nervous system.	Surge in sympathetic nervous system (fight or flight response)
Remorse is rare.	Remorse is relatively common.
May have evolved as a hunting mechanism for acquiring food.	May have evolved as a protective mechanism against environmental hazards and predators.
Not induced by drugs or medical illness.	Can be induced by drugs or medical illness.
Resistant to pharmacotherapy.	May be responsive to pharmacotherapy.

Note: A common way of categorizing aggression is by predatory versus impulsive aggression. A given transaction of violence may have characteristics of both impulsive and predatory aggression.

potential does exist for a coexisting psychotic or mood disorder with antisocial personality disorder.

Another method of classifying violence is on the bases of hostility or instrumentality.[7] Hostile violence is where physical injury is the primary goal of the transgression. In instrumental violence, the goal is materialistic (e.g., money), and any harm to the individual is secondary or incidental.[7] Furthermore, aggression can be sorted on the basis of the type of victim (e.g., spousal abuse, patient abuse, elder abuse, animal cruelty) or type of harm (e.g., physical, emotional, and so forth).

39.2 CAUSES OF AGGRESSION AND VIOLENCE

The causes of violence are far from being completely understood but are multifactorial and involve biological, psychological, political, religious, sociological, economic, and environmental factors.[8] Biological causes comprise genetics, hormones, disease states, sleep deprivation, poor nutrition, drugs, head trauma, seizures, and tumors. Psychological causes include major mental illness and a history of abuse. Sociological factors include gang-related activity and peer attitudes toward violence. Economic factors consist of unemployment or a lack of financial resources. Environmental contributors include crowding, excessive noise, or other external stimulation.

39.2.1 Neurobiology of Aggression

The two divisions of the brain most relevant to aggression are the limbic system and the frontal lobe. The limbic system of the brain is responsible for emotions including reward, happiness, fear, and anger. The limbic system contains the hippocampus, the amygdala, and the temporal lobes. Overactivity of the limbic system can result in aggression.[9] The frontal lobe, more specifically the prefrontal cortex, is responsible for executive functions including impulse control. A properly functioning prefrontal cortex inhibits inappropriate impulses from the limbic system. Impairment of the frontal lobe results in disinhibition, a mental state where the person's capacity for preemptive review and restraint of behavioral responses is decreased or absent.[2] Thus, a decreased activity of the prefrontal lobe can result in impulsive aggression.

Neurotransmitters are biochemical messengers the nerve cells use for communication. The neurotransmitters involved with aggression include serotonin, epinephrine, norepinephrine, dopamine, GABA, glutamate, substance P, and acetylcholine.[1,4,10] Serotonin is the neurotransmitter with the most evidence linked to violence. In general, serotonin inhibits aggression, and a decrease in serotonergic activity leads to impulsive aggression.[3] Psychotropic medications and drugs of abuse work by altering the activity of neurotransmitters.

Genetics play a role in aggression. Specific variants on the cadherin 13 gene or the MAO-A gene (the "warrior gene") are a risk factor for violence. The former is located on chromosome 16 and involved with nerve cell circuitry. The latter is located on the X chromosome and involved with producing enzymes that metabolize epinephrine, dopamine, norepinephrine, and serotonin. Genetic variations impacting the cytochrome P450 system, the primary metabolic pathway for drugs in the liver, that result in slower drug metabolism increase the risk of drug-induced violence.

39.2.2 Medical and Psychiatric Causes of Aggression

Numerous medical, psychiatric, and neurologic conditions can cause or contribute to aggression. Medical conditions that can cause aggression include thyroid malfunction, vitamin B_{12} deficiency, hypoglycemia, delirium, dementia, temporal lobe epilepsy (complex partial seizures, aka focal seizures with impaired awareness), and head trauma.[11–21] Various disease states contribute or cause aggression by inducing psychosis, precipitating mania, producing confusion, or leading to depression. Regardless of etiology, most persons with mental illness are not violent.

Psychiatric disorders that can cause violence include schizophrenia, schizoaffective disorder, bipolar disorder, delirium, paraphilias, conduct disorder, posttraumatic stress disorder, delusional disorder, and certain personality disorders such as antisocial personality disorder, borderline personality disorder, and narcissistic personality disorder.

39.3 THE ROLE OF DRUGS AS A CAUSE OF VIOLENCE

39.3.1 Introduction

This chapter uses the pharmacological definition of a drug, which is "drugs are substances other than food that alter the function of the body via chemical means." Drugs contribute to crimes in many ways.[22] For example, it is unlawful to manufacture, possess, or use a controlled substance unless for legitimate use as regulated by the Food and Drug Administration (FDA) and Drug Enforcement Administration. Individuals abusing addicting drugs can have severe withdrawal reactions which may lead to crimes such as armed robbery or burglary to obtain funding for additional supplies. Drug dealers may also engage deadly force as a strategy to eliminate competition. Charles Manson gave lysergic acid diethylamide to his followers for indoctrination with his perverted philosophy. This eventually led to Tate–LaBianca murders.[23]

This chapter focuses on how drugs induce violence in defendants and, more specifically, on interpersonal violence facilitated by the direct pharmacological effects of drugs—that is how intoxication impairs a person and causes them to lose control of themselves. In other words, an individual falsely perceived that what he or she did was not wrong or was unable to control their actions. The spectrum of drug-induced violence is wide and involves anything from bar fights, road rage, domestic abuse, to murder.[24,25]

A variety of chemicals can alter human behavior including over-the-counter products, prescription medications, herbal supplements (e.g., ephedra, Jimson weed, and so forth), drugs of abuse, and environmental toxicants. Drug-induced behavioral changes and violence have been used as a defense in criminal trials ranging from drug-induced insanity to being a mitigating factor in sententing.[26] Mechanisms of drug-induced aggression include impairing inhibiting mechanisms (e.g., decreasing frontal lobe activity) and causing temporal lobe seizures, hallucinations, akathisia (an inner sense of restlessness), dysphoric or mixed manic episode, depression, distorted perception, paranoia, or combination of these factors.[27,28] Other pharmacological properties that promote aggression are pain relief, anxiety-provoking traits, withdrawal reactions, and hypoglycemia.[3] Specific drugs or drugs classes associated with aggression include ethanol, antidepressants, benzodiazepines, mefloquine, phencyclidine, lysergic acid diethylamide (LSD), insulin, cocaine, amphetamines, varenicline, antipsychotics, antiparkinsonian medications, zolpidem, antiepileptics (especially levetiracetam and perampanel), and volatile substances (inhalants).[3,28]

39.3.2 Problems with the Literature

The vast majority of data regarding drug-induced violence are from case reports rather than controlled clinical studies. These case reports are often not published in scientific journals but presented in case law or in the public media. As with any case report, there are problems with recall bias, confounding factors, and no controlled environment. Furthermore, with forensic case reports, there is often additional bias because the defendant and the defense attorney desire a finding of not guilty, which may slant the ways facts and opinions are presented.

Numerous epidemiological studies suggest that drugs can induce aggression, and, unfortunately, several fundamental limitations exist in these studies linking crime to drugs. As discussed earlier, most crimes result from a combination of factors including economic, cultural, biological, environmental, and interpersonal.[22,29,30] Even in situations where the drug is the cause, it is one of many factors that played a part in the event.[3,22] The definition of "drug related" differs among studies and professional opinion. Urine testing for drugs of abuse is the standard for many epidemiological studies. Standard urine drug tests are effective but detect only a few of the many chemicals.[31] Particular substances, such as LSD, are difficult to detect by standard urine drug-testing protocols. Synthetic cannabinoids are not routinely tested for in forensic urine tests. Reports by offenders may aim to minimize or exaggerate the specific contribution of drugs to a given crime, leading to inaccuracies in reports. Most forensic cases involve illicit drugs rather than prescription medications, so the purity and authenticity of these products are not certain. Direct human studies related to drug-induced aggression are limited, but animal studies may provide the background information as to whether a drug induces aggression; for example, cocaine.[32]

39.3.3 Specific Drugs or Drug Classes that Cause Aggression

39.3.3.1 Ethanol

Ethanol or drinking alcohol is the most common social drug, and the evidence linking alcohol to violence is overwhelming.[3] Ethanol has a broad range of effects including incoordination, altered perceptions, sedations, and decreased inhibitions. Alcohol contributes to aggression in many ways including increased sensation seeking and impulsive behaviors.[3] Ethanol also reduces fear via its mechanisms on the GABAergic system. Fear typically has an inhibitory effect on a person's behavior, and by minimizing an individual's inhibitory response, a person in a stressful situation may overreact to the event. Alternatively, if the inhibitory functions are still present and unimpaired, the individual might seek a more diplomatic or constructive method of resolving the problem rather than a violent one. Alcohol decreases activity in the frontal lobe of the brain, which is needed for executive functions such as organizing and planning. The decreased activity of the frontal lobe leads to impulsivity. A case-crossover study by Haggård-Grann et al. found an increased risk of violence of 13.2 (95% confidence interval, 8.2–21.2) after consuming alcohol.[33]

39.3.3.2 Lysergic Acid Diethylamide

Lysergic acid diethylamide (LSD) was first synthesized in 1938, and its mind-altering effects were discovered five years later. Its actions include stimulation of affect, enhanced introspection, and numerous perceptual changes such as illusions and pseudohallucinations.[3] Beginning in the 1960s, LSD became a popular drug of abuse for "tripping." The primary targets in the brain for LSD appears to be 5-HT_{2a} and the 5-HT_{2B} receptors both of which involve serotonin.[34] Serotonin's primary role in the brain is that of an inhibitory neurotransmitter and protects the mind from sensory overload.

A 22-year-old male undergraduate student had a previous history of LSD use.[35] He drank a glass of beer, smoked one marijuana cigarette, and ingested two tablets of LSD of unknown dose. He then attacked his girlfriend with a knife causing superficial injuries. The police arrested him, and he was sent for a psychiatric evaluation, which found moderate depression, no evidence of psychosis, and mildly abnormal brain waves. The only abnormal behavior he displayed, during the hospital stay, was a lack of socialization with other patients and staff. He appeared to lack remorse for conducting the assault. The discharge diagnosis was substance abuse and an unspecified personality disorder. He was referred to outpatient substance abuse treatment. Three days after discharge, he fatally shot another girlfriend. He was reported smoking much marijuana and taking LSD two days prior to the murder. The defendant later admitted to concealing delusional thoughts from the staff at the earlier hospital admission. This case illustrates the difficulties with interpreting forensic cases. The subject may not be forthcoming with information or lie in order to avoid punishment.

Valerie Dawn Kelly started abusing drugs when she was 15 years of age. Three years later, she began abusing mescaline and LSD. On December 7, 1970, Kelly stabbed her mother with kitchen knives. She was charged with assault with a deadly weapon and intent to commit murder. The defendant claimed to have used LSD and mescaline 50 to 100 times in the months preceding the attacks. Kelly pleaded not guilty by reason of insanity claiming drugs of abuse as the cause. A trial by jury was waived, and she underwent a trial by judge. The court agreed that the Kelly was psychotic during the assault and incapable of understanding that her actions were wrong but found guilty and sane. This case provides an example of where a defendant may be considered mentally ill but still be sane. The court felt that this case of insanity "was not of a settled and permanent nature" and that the ingestion was voluntary, so rejected the insanity defense. Kelly received a suspended sentence and granted probation. The case was appealed to the California Supreme Court, which reversed the decision of the lower court and ruled that a permanent state is not required for settled insanity.[36]

39.3.3.3 Phencyclidine and Ketamine

Phencyclidine (PCP) was previously used as an animal tranquilizer. PCP was studied as an anesthetic in humans and initially showed clinical promise because of a lack of hypotension and low respiratory depression, common problems associated with many anesthetic agents.[37] Clinical studies were stopped after agitation, hallucinations, and disorientations manifested as common reactions.[38] The street name for PCP powder is "angel dust," and the liquid form is referred to as "whack." The most common route of administration is inhalation, although it has been taken orally, intranasally, intravenously, and subcutaneously. The classic picture of PCP intoxication includes violence, nystagmus, hypertension, and analgesia. Hypersalivation (excessive drooling) is another common side effect of PCP. At higher doses, seizures, hypertonic muscle activity, hyperthermia, and ataxia can occur. PCP works primarily by blocking glutamate, the predominate excitatory neurotransmitter in the body, at the N-methyl-D-aspartate receptors in the hippocampus, neocortex, basal ganglia, and limbic system. PCP has numerous other pharmacological reactions including inhibiting the reuptake of dopamine, serotonin, and norepinephrine; increased production of norepinephrine and dopamine; and various effects at opioid receptors.

Ketamine is a derivative of PCP with less potent activity and has the street name "special K."[39] Ketamine is commonly used in veterinary medicine and in human medicine, especially in emergency departments for conscious sedation, rapid-sequence intubation, and as a chemical restraint. Ketamine can also cause violent reactions but not to the degree of PCP.

39.3.3.4 Anabolic Steroids

Androgenic anabolic steroids refer to testosterone and its derivatives.[40] For the rest of this chapter, the phrase "anabolic steroids" is used. Anabolic steroids possess both anabolic (muscle building) and androgenic (masculinizing) properties. These drugs increase muscle mass, cause nitrogen retention, and increase lean body weight. Medical uses of anabolic steroids include replacement therapy for testosterone deficiency and the treatment of wasting syndrome associated with acquired immunodeficiency syndrome in adults. Additionally, anabolic steroids have been studied as a treatment for depression in men. Toxic effects of anabolic steroids, specifically orally ingested products, include cardiovascular, hepatic (liver), endocrine, and psychiatric reactions. Cardiovascular side effects include a lowering of high-density lipoprotein (HDL) cholesterol, elevations of low-density lipoprotein (LDL) cholesterol, and impairing the contractile functions of the heart. Psychiatric adverse effects include distractibility, delirium, psychosis, hypomania and mania, insomnia, hostility, and mood liability.[40] Withdrawal effects, such as hypogonadism and depression, may occur with anabolic steroid use. Addiction has been reported with anabolic steroids. Research studies and case reports suggest that exogenous anabolic steroids cause aggression, although the concise correlation between anabolic steroids and aggression is not well defined. However, an observational study found a nine-fold increase in risk of imprisonment with use of anabolic steroids compared with controls in the general population.[41]

The use of anabolic steroids as a criminal defense has been reported in the lay media. For example, Horace Williams was charged with a deadly beating of a hitchhiker in West Palm Beach, Florida.[42] Williams administered anabolic steroids obtained on the black market. Williams and William Whitmore, another defendant, tied the hitchhiker between two posts and fatally beat him. Defense counsel argued that the anabolic steroids induced the violence leading to the homicide. The jury disagreed and convicted Williams of murder. Whitmore did not use the "steroid rage" as a defense. Planning was used in the murder so it may have made the insanity defense less plausible to the jury. The violence in this case was predatory as opposed to impulsive.

39.3.3.5 Insulin

Insulin is a hormone produced by the pancreas and lowers blood glucose. Exogenous insulin and sometimes endogenous insulin can produce hypoglycemia, which is subnormal glucose levels in the blood. Certain other drugs can induce hypoglycemia such as sulfonylureas (e.g., glipizide, glyburide) which increase insulin secretion from the pancreas and are used as a treatment for diabetes mellitus type 2. Signs and symptoms of hypoglycemia include tachycardia (elevated heart rate), diaphoresis, hunger, incoherent speech, confusion, behavioral changes, and seizures. Other causes of hypoglycemia include growth hormone deficiency, renal failure, adrenal insufficiency, and pancreatic tumors.[42] The clinical features of hypoglycemia can be categorized as either adrenergic or neuroglycopenic.[43] Adrenergic symptoms, including sweating and tachycardia, result from counter regulatory hormones such as epinephrine, glucagon, cortisol, and growth hormone. The neuroglycopenic symptoms result from a prolonged hypoglycemia. Neuroglycopenic manifestations include ataxia, confusion, and psychiatric changes. The psychiatric effects of hypoglycemia have been known for decades.[44–46] Psychological effects of hypoglycemia include bizarre behavior, anxiety, reckless driving, hallucinations, aggression, and violence.[13,14,43,44] Mechanisms of aggression include a decrease in overall brain activity leading to the inhibition of negative feedback control, adrenergic response to hypoglycemia, or temporal lobe seizures.[13,14] Decreased non-oxidative glucose metabolism (glycogen production) may contribute to impulsive aggression in individuals with antisocial personality disorder.[15] Diminished glycogen storage in the brain is problematic because the brain cannot tolerate milder hypoglycemic episodes.

Hypoglycemia has been used as a defense in criminal cases from shoplifting to homicide. Evidence supporting such a claim include behaviors that are out of character for the affected individual. Hypoglycemic related criminal events typically have these themes: No apparent motive of the crime; the presence of circumstances consistent with a hypoglycemia event (missing a meal, medication errors, and so forth); a rapid and substantial change in behavior when given sucrose, glucose, or other sugar; and a true amnesia preceding, during, and after the crime.[46] In 2005, the Colorado Supreme Court ruled that hypoglycemia qualifies as an affirmative defense of involuntary intoxication in criminal cases.[47]

39.3.3.6 Psychostimulants

Cocaine is a stimulant drug and topical anesthetic. Cocaine elevates levels of dopamine and norepinephrine in the brain, producing a number of behavioral symptoms including agitation, paranoia, violence, and hallucinations. Rates as high as 84% of persons using cocaine experience paranoia.[47] Approximately 65% of individuals who have psychiatric symptoms from cocaine exhibit violent behavior.[48] Co-ingestion of cocaine and alcohol in the body results in the biosynthesis of cocaethylene, a metabolite which has a longer duration than cocaine.

Amphetamines possess pharmacological effects similar to cocaine, producing increases in dopamine and norepinephrine, but lack anesthetic actions. The abuse of amphetamines can lead to aggression and violence. When used therapeutically, amphetamines enhance frontal lobe activity, thus decreasing impulsive behavior such as violence.[49] Amphetamines have been reported to cause manic episodes in susceptible individuals, even at therapeutic doses.[49] A minority of cases of manic episodes can produce violent behavior. Amphetamines, via an increase in dopamine, can create paranoia and visual hallucinations also resulting in violence. Methylphenidate, a drug used for attention-deficit/hyperactivity disorder and narcolepsy, is pharmacological and chemically related to the amphetamines.

39.3.3.7 Benzodiazepines

Benzodiazepines are a group of psychoactive drugs that consist chemically of a benzene ring attached to a diazepine ring and work by increasing the action of the GABA neurotransmitter at the $GABA_A$ receptor. GABA is the primarily inhibitory neurotransmitter. Benzodiazepines have antianxiety, sedative, muscle-relaxant, memory-suppressive, and antiseizure activities. Benzodiazepines are used clinically to treat conditions including generalized anxiety, phobias, bipolar disorder, insomnia, preoperative sedations, seizure disorders, and muscle spasms and as a chemical restraint. Benzodiazepines are generally considered to have calming effects. Nevertheless, paradoxical reactions frequently result from benzodiazepines.[50]

Gaillard and Hemras report a case of a woman who murdered her husband with a chopper.[51] She was taking an unspecified benzodiazepine to treat the negative symptoms of schizophrenia. The woman had damage to the frontal lobe of the brain which likely made her prone to the paradoxical reaction. The mechanism of the paradoxical reactions often results from disinhibition because benzodiazepines interfere with the anxiety/threat detection system. In other words, the individual is not immediately worried about the consequences of their aggression. Risk factors for disinhibition include brain damage (e.g., the frontal lobe) and preexisting high levels of underlying hostility.

Daderman and colleagues describe a case series of five persons who became violent after taking flunitrazepam.[52] All of the cases involved murder or attempted murder. One case consisted of armed robbery which was motivated by financial troubles. In two of the cases, the victims were stabbed in the eye, suggesting intense rage. Four of the cases involve co-ingested substances other than benzodiazepines. Two of the perpetrators used cannabis and amphetamines, and another two individuals combined flunitrazepam with alcohol. Three of the cases describe impulsive activity, two of the cases had depression listed as a diagnosis, and one perpetrator showed signs of paranoia. Limitations of this study include a small study sample, multiple confounding factors, and retrospective bias.

39.3.3.8 Selective Serotonin Reuptake Inhibitors

The selective serotonin reuptake inhibitors (SSRIs) are a class of drugs that increase serotonin activity in the brain. Serotonin has many functions in the body including increasing stress tolerance, stabilizing mood, modulating other neurotransmitters, regulating appetite and sleep, and impulse control. Clinical uses of SSRIs include depression, obsessive-compulsive disorder, posttraumatic stress disorder, generalized anxiety, panic attacks, and aggressive behavior. A deficit in serotonin can lead to impulsive violence.[3] However, SSRIs can cause violence.[53] A cohort study of the Swedish Prescribed Drug Register reported an increased risk of 1% for violent crime convictions in individuals aged 15 to 24 years of age but not for older age groups.[54] The mechanisms by which SSRIs cause violence include an induction of a dysphoric manic episode, disinhibition, akathisia (an inner sense of restlessness), or serotonin syndrome.[53] Serotonin syndrome is a toxic syndrome resulting from excessive serotonergic activity in the brain and body. Serotonin syndrome is characterized by the triad of altered mental status, dysfunction of the automatic functions of the nervous system, and neuromuscular abnormalities.[55] Serotonin syndrome most often results from the drug interaction of two or more drugs with serotonergic activity or much less commonly from the overdose of a single serotonergic drug.[56] The Swedish study indicates that risk of violence appears more likely with citalopram or paroxetine than other SSRIs such as fluoxetine and sertraline.[54] Citalopram and paroxetine have shorter half-lives than other SSRIs such as sertraline and fluoxetine. Fluvoxamine has a shorter half-life than paroxetine but not evaluated in the study. An analysis of the FDA MedWatch database found fluoxetine to be associated with more violence than paroxetine.[57]

39.3.3.9 Varenicline

Varenicline is a drug used in smoking cessation and works by binding to the $\alpha_4\beta_2$ nicotinic receptor in the brain. Varenicline has a black-box warning informing of psychiatric side effects such as agitation, hostility, depression, or changes in thinking or behavior. A study published in January 2011 PLoS One examined prescription drugs believed to cause violence.[57] The researchers reviewed the FDA database covering a 69-month period. This inquiry comprised the key words homicide, physical assault, physical abuse, homicidal ideation, and violence-related symptoms. The most common prescription drug associated with violence was varenicline.

On May 17, 2009, Sean Wain, a 34-year-old man, fatally shot his wife Natalie Wain and then aimed the shotgun in his own mouth and fired.[58] The crime took place in Economy, Pennsylvania. The Beaver County Coroner ruled the deaths a murder/suicide. Sean Wain had been taking varenicline for one to two weeks prior to the incident. The estates of Sean and Natalie Wain filed a product liability lawsuit against Pfizer in U.S. District Court for Western District of Pennsylvania. The plaintiff alleged that Pfizer failed to adequately warn about the potential psychiatric reactions.[59]

39.3.3.10 Environmental Chemicals

Numerous environmental chemicals have been reported to alter behavior. Lead exposure during childhood has been linked to criminal behavior.[60] Mercury poisoning has been reported to cause irritability and excitability.[61] Solvent abuse can produce depression, anxiety, mood swings, hallucinations, delusions, and violence. Solvents include gasoline, correction fluid, paint thinner, aerosol propellants, modeling glue, and rubbing alcohol. Airborne exposure to manganese has been reported to cause aggression, loss of impulse control, psychosis, and emotional instability.[62]

39.4 THE DRUG-INDUCED INSANITY DEFENSE

Individuals using the phrase "the drug made me do it" as it relates to drug-induced intoxication as a defense is far from new. In 1857, in a murder trial, the defense claimed that the defendant was insane because he overdosed on chloroform.[63] The case was prosecuted by Abraham Lincoln, and the lead defense attorney was Leonard Swett. The defendant, Isaac Wyant, was accused of shooting to death Anson Rush. Wyant and Rush feuded over a land boundary for months. Eventually, members of both families got into a fight in June 1855. Wyant needed to have his arm amputated after the struggle. Chloroform was used as the anesthetic. On October 12, 1885, Wyant shot Rusk in the head and the shoulder, leading to his death. An indictment was handed down to Wyant one week later with attorney Swett claiming insanity. Numerous expert witnesses testified for the defense, and lay witnesses provided specific examples of odd behavior by Mr. Wyant. Attorney Lincoln presented rebuttal expert witnesses and lay witnesses. The jury acquitted the defendant. Three years later, Lincoln was elected President of the United States.

In a review article, **Spiegel** and Suskind suggest that Lincoln was unaware of much of the medical literature on chloroform.[63] Medical literature at the time considered chloroform safe, especially when contrasted to ether. Wyant had a well-known track record of hostility against Rusk which provides motive. Planning was clearly used in the murder of Rusk. Today, this would likely be used in an attempt to rebut the insanity claim. Modern pharmacokinetics did not exist at the time. The half-life of chloroform (by inhalation) is eight hours. Chloroform was obviously eliminated from the body between June and October of the same year. One would need to demonstrate that the chloroform causes permanent brain damage. Motive was present in the crime which is inconsistent with drug-induced violence. If this case was tried today, it would likely be a different verdict.

Senay and Wettstein report of 24 cases of homicides committed by individuals who previously ingested psychoactive drugs.[64] They found the following characteristics of the homicide: 1) No plan or a poorly thought out plan, 2) no plan for escape, 3) a frequent confession to the crime, and 4) showing of remorse.

Numerous factors add to the difficulty in obtaining an acquittal relating to drug-induced violence. Utilizing drug-induced insanity is less likely to be a successful defense if the intoxication was voluntary versus a prescribed drug or nonprescription medication. In fact, many jurisdictions will not permit an insanity defense in a voluntary intoxication. An exception may occur if the defendant had a mental illness which contributed to the effects of the drug.[65] In addition, the psychiatric condition must also be able to independently account for the insanity.[65] A number of jurisdictions allow for a "settled insanity." This is when a voluntary intoxication on a long-term basis causes insanity that is independent from the acute intoxication of the drug.[62] A defense of insanity, in general, regardless if a drug is claimed to be the causative, is less likely to be effective if the defendant shows that he/she was organized, had a motive, or attempted to cover up the crime.[3]

The insanity defense requires that the person did not know or comprehend what they did was outside the confines of the law.[66] A defendant found not guilty by insanity is legally excused from his or her acts.[66] A plea of insanity usually is not entered in minor crimes. The reason being a finding of not guilty of reason of insanity usually results in a commitment to a psychiatric hospital. The commitment is considered for the safety of the public and the patient rather than a punishment. Therefore, it can fairly easily be renewed. The time spent in a locked psychiatric facility may be months or years longer than a prison sentence. Therefore, most attorneys will not seek an insanity defense for a minor crime.[67]

Drug-induced insanity is not commonly used as a criminal defense. A more typical situation is an argument that a drug caused diminished capacity.[68] Numerous differences exist between diminished capacity and insanity. A finding of insanity in most states will result in acquittal of the defendant although this almost always results in commitment to a mental institution.[67] A finding of diminished capacity results in the defendant being found guilty and convicted of a lesser charge.[69] For example, a defendant may be convicted of manslaughter rather than murder. The argument being that the defendant lacked the mental capacity to intent to murder but acted recklessly, resulting in the death.

39.5 SUMMARY AND CONCLUSIONS

Medications, herbal products, drugs of abuse, and environmental toxicants can sometimes cause or contribute to violence, especially impulsive or affective violence. Drugs interfere with numerous pathways in the brain thus altering behavior. Crimes involving drug-induced violence typically show an absence of planning and no clear motive. Diminished capacity is more likely to be used than an insanity defense in drug-induced violence cases.

REFERENCES

1. Hoaken PNS, Stewart SH. "Drugs of abuse and elicitation of human aggressive behavior." *Addict Behav.* 2003; 28 (9): 1533–1544.
2. Wise EA, Lyketsos CG, Onyike CU. "Aggression and violence." *In JL Levenson, ed. Textbook of psychosomatic medicine and consultation-liaison psychiatry.* Washington, DC: American Psychiatric Publishing, 2019, 165–191.
3. Anderson PD, Bokor G. "Forensic aspects of drug-induced violence." *J Pharm Pract.* 2012; 25 (1): 41–49.
4. Siever LJ. "Neurobiology of aggression and violence." *Am J Psychiatry.* 2008; 165 (4): 429–442.
5. Kockler T, Melory JR. "The application of affective and predatory aggression to psycholegal opinions." In RC Brown, ed. *Forensic psychiatry research trends.* Hauppauge, NY: Nova Science Publishers, Inc., 2007, 62–83.
6. Meloy JR. http://drreidmeloy.com/wp-content/uploads/2015/12/2007_AntisocialPerso.pdf. Last accessed July 20, 2021.

7. Anonymous. http://law.jrank.org/pages/2291/Violence-Classification.html. Last accessed July 20, 2021.
8. Monahan J. "The causes of violence." *FBI Law Enforcement Bull.* 1994; 63: 11–15.
9. Lane SD, Kjome KL, Moeller FG. "Neuropsychiatry of aggression." *Neurol Clin.* 2011; 29 (1): 49-vii.
10. Katsouni E, Sakkas P, Zarros A, Skandali N, Liapi C. "The involvement of substance P in the induction of aggressive behavior." *Peptides.* 2009; 30 (8): 1586–1591.
11. Peiris AN, Oh E, Diaz S. "Psychiatric manifestations of thyroid disease." *South Med J.* 2007; 100 (8): 773–774.
12. Chen TS, Wen MJ, Hung YJ, Hsieh CH, Hsiao FC. "A rare storm in a psychiatric ward: Thyroid storm." *Gen Hosp Psychiatry.* 2012; 34 (2): 210.e1–210.e4.
13. Buckley RE. "Hypoglycemia, temporal lobe disturbance, and aggressive behavior." *J Orthomol Psychiatry.* 1979; 8 (3): 188–192.
14. Messer SC, Morris TL, Gross AM. Hypoglycemia and psychopathology: A methodological review. *Clin Psychol Rev.* 1990; 10 (6): 631–648.
15. Virkkunen M, Rissanen A, Franssila-Kallunki A, Tiihonen J. "Low non-oxidative glucose metabolism and violent offending: An 8-year prospective follow-up study." *Psychiatry Res.* 2009; 168 (1): 26–31.
16. Epilepsy therapy project. http://www.epilepsy.com/epilepsy/epilepsy_temporallobe. Last accessed July 20, 2021.
17. Blair RD. "Temporal lobe epilepsy semiology." *Epilepsy Res Treat.* 2012. doi: 10.1155/2012/7151510.
18. Van Elst LT, Woermann FG, Lemieux L, Thompson PJ, Trimble MR. "Affective aggression in patients with temporal lobe epilepsy: A quantitative MRI study of the amygdala." *Brain. 2000*; 123 (Pt 2): 234–243.
19. Haut S. "Frontal lobe epilepsy." http://emedicine.medscape.com/article/1184076-overview. Accessed July 20, 2021.
20. Grafman J, Schwab K, Warden D, Pridgen A, Brown HR, Salazar AM. "Frontal lobe injuries, violence, and aggression: A report of the Vietnam head injury study." *Neurology.* 1996; 46 (5): 1231–1238.
21. Rao V, Rosenberg P, Bertrand M, Salehinia S, Spiro J, Vaishnavi S, Rastogi P, Noll K, Schretlen DJ, Brandt J, Cornwell E. "Aggression after traumatic brain injury: Prevalence and correlates." *J Neuropsychiatry Clin Neurol.* 2009; 21 (4): 420–429.
22. Spiess M, Fallow D. *Executive office of the president: Office of national drug control policy.* ONDCP Drug Policy Information Clearinghouse Fact Sheet, March 2000.
23. Muggleton W. *https://www.dailystar.co.uk/news/world-news/charles-manson-family-reveal-death-16888070.* Accessed July 20, 2021.
24. Fierro I, Morales C, Alvarez FJ. "Alcohol use, illicit drug use, and road rage." *J Stud Alcohol Drugs.* 2011; 72 (2): 185–193.
25. Beech DJ, Mercadel R. "Correlation of alcohol intoxication with life threatening assaults." *J Nat Med Assoc.* 1998; 90 (12): 761–764.
26. Anderson PD. "The broad field of forensic pharmacy." *J Pharm Pract.* 2015; 22 (1): 7–12.
27. Albert HJ. "Addiction, intoxication, criminal law and criminal justice: An introduction." *Eur Addict Res.* 1998; 4 (3): 85–88.
28. Ferner RE. "Effects of drugs on behavior." *In Forensic pharmacology: Medicines, mayhem, and malpractice.* Oxford/New York, NY: Oxford University Press, 1996, 73–78.
29. Schmitt JA, Lamers CT, Kuypers KP, Ramaekers JG, Riedel WJ. "Performance and behavioral effects of illicit drugs." In M Burns, ed. *Medical-Legal Aspects of Drugs.* Tucson, AZ: Lawyers and Judges Publishing Company, 2003, 133–167.
30. Morris SC. The causes of violence and the effects of violence on community and individual health. https://www.cugh.org/sites/default/files/62_Causes_Of_Violence_and_Violence_%20Effects_on_Community_and_Individual_Health_FINAL.pdf. Accessed December 29, 2015.
31. Anderson PD, Naik K, Kinemond C, ImObersteg A. "Forensic testing for drugs of abuse." *J Pharm Pract.* 2000; XIII (3): 226–235.
32. DeLeon KR, Grimes JM, Connor DF, Melloni RH Jr. Adolescent cocaine exposure and offensive aggression-involvement of serotonin neural signaling and innervations in male Syrian hamsters. *Behav Brain Res.* 2002; 133 (2): 211–220.
33. Haggård-Grann U, Hallqvist J, Långström N, Möller J. "The role of alcohol and drugs in triggering criminal violence: A case crossover study." *Addiction.* 2006; 108 (1): 100–108.
34. Wacker D, Wang S, McCorvy JD, Betz RM, Venkatakrishnan AJ, Levit A, Lansu K, Schools ZL, Che T, Nichols DE, Shoichet BK. "Crystal structure of an LSD-bound human serotonin receptor." *Cell.* 2017; 68 (3): 377–389.
35. Klepfisz A, Racy J. "Homicide and LSD." *JAMA.* 1973; 223 (4): 429–430.
36. People vs. Kelly. 516 P 2d 875-Cal Supreme Court 1973. http://law.justia.com/cases/california/supreme-court/3d/10/565.html. Last accessed December 3, 2015.
37. Burns RS, Lerner SE, Corrado R. "Phencyclidine-states of abuse acute intoxication and fatalities." *West J Med.* 1975; 123 (5): 345–349.
38. Bey T, Patel A. "Phencyclidine intoxication and adverse effects: A clinical and pharmacological review of an illicit drug." *Cal J Emerg Med.* 2007; 8 (1): 9–14.

39. Bokor G, Anderson PD. "Ketamine: An update on its abuse." *J Pharm Pract.* 2014; 27 (6): 582–586.
40. Kanayama G, Hudson JI, Pope HG. "Illicit anabolic-androgenic steroid use." *Horm Behav.* 2010; 58 (1): 111–121.
41. Christoffersen T, Andersen JT, Dalhoff KP, Horwitz H. "Anabolic-androgenic steroids and the risk of imprisonment." *Alcohol Dep.* 2019; 203: 92–97.
42. Greenbaum K. Steroid defense rejected jury finds suspect guilty. http://articles.sun-sentinel.com/1988-06-08/news/8802030649_1_insanity-defense-horace-williams-violent-behavior. Accessed December 3, 2015.
43. Ferry R. Hypoglycemia. http://www.emedicinehealth.com/low_blood_sugar_hypoglycemia/page2_em.htm. Accessed July 20, 2021.
44. Smith KC, Barish J, Correa J, Williams RH. "Psychiatric disturbance in endocrinologic disease." *Psychosom Med.* 1972; 34 (1): 69–86.
45. Romano J, Cood GP. "Physiologic and psychogenic studies in spontaneous hypoglycemia." *Psychosom Med.* 1942; 4: 283–300.
46. Marks V. "Hypoglycaemia: Insulin and conflicts with the law." *Br J Diabetes Vasc Dis.* 2006; 6 (6): 281–285.
47. Colorado Bar Association. No. 03SC675, People v. Garcia, Jr.- June 13, 2005. Colorado Supreme Court Opinion. http://www.cobar.org/opinions/opinion.cfm?OpinionID=5170. Accessed December 26, 2015.
48. Morton WA. "Cocaine and psychiatric symptoms." *Prim Care Companion J Clin Psychiatry.* 1999; 11 (4): 109–113.
49. Bokor G, Anderson PD. "Attention-deficit/hyperactivity disorder." *J Pharm Pract.* 2014; 27 (4): 336–349.
50. Mancuso CE, Tanzi MG, Gabay M. "Paradoxical reactions to benzodiazepines: Literature review and treatment options." *Pharmacotherapy.* 2004; 24 (9): 1177–1185.
51. Gaillard R, Hemras A. "Cognitive facilitation and behavioral disinhibition with benzodiazepine: A case report." *J Clin Psychiatry.* 2007; 68 (8): 1305–1306.
52. Dåderman AM, Fredriksson B, Kristiansson M, Nilsson LH, Lidberg L. "Violent behavior, impulsive decision-making, and anterograde amnesia while intoxicated with flunitrazepam and alcohol or other drugs: A case study in forensic psychiatric patients." *J Am Acad Psychiatry Law.* 2002; 30 (2): 23–51.
53. Breggin PR. "Suicidality, violence and mania caused by selective serotonin re-uptake inhibitors (SSRIs) a review and analysis." *Int J Risk Safety Med.* 2003/2004; 16 (1): 31–49.
54. Molero Y, Lichtenstein P, Zetterqvist J, Gumpert CH, Fazel S. "Selective serotonin reuptake inhibitors and violent crime: A cohort study." *PLoS Med.* http://journals.plos.org/plosmedicine/article?id=10.1371/journal.pmed.1001875. Accessed December 28, 2015.
55. Martin TG. "Serotonin syndrome." *Ann Emerg Med.* 1996; 28 (5): 520–526.
56. Anderson PD. "Forensic aspects of drug interactions, part II." *Forensic Exam.* 1999; 8 (11&12): 13–16.
57. Moore TJ, Glenmullen J, Furberg CD. "Prescription drugs associated with reports of violence towards others." *PLoS One.* 2010; 5 (12): 1–5.
58. Blazer N. Product liability monitor: Murder/suicide allegedly linked to anti-smoking drug. estate sues Pfizer. http://product-liability.weil.com/uncategorized/murder-suicide-allegedly-linked-to-anti-smoking-drug-estate-sues-pfizer/. Accessed December 28, 2015.
59. Anonymous. Erdlen et al vs. Pfizer. https://dockets.justia.com/docket/pennsylvania/pawdce/2:2011cv00605/196940. Accessed December 28, 2015.
60. Carpenter DO, Nevin R. "Environmental causes of violence." *Physiol Behav.* 99 (2): 260–268.
61. Collaborative on Health and the Environment. Mental health and environmental exposures, November 2008. https://www.healthandenvironment.org/uploads-old/MentalHealth.pdf. Accessed July 24, 2021.
62. Haynes EN, Chen A, Ryan P, Succop P, Wright J, Dietrich KN. "Exposure to airborne metals and particulate metals and particulate matter and risk for youth adjudicated for criminal activity." *Environ Res.* 2011; 111 (8).
63. Spiegel AD, Suskind PB. "Chloroform-induced insanity defence confounds lawyer Lincoln." *Hist Psychiatry.* 1997; 8 (32): 487–500.
64. Senay EC, Wettstein R. "Drugs and homicide: A theory." *Drug Alcohol Depend.* 1983; 12 (2): 157–166.
65. Feix J, Wolber G. "Intoxication and settled insanity: A finding of not guilty by reason of insanity." *J Am Acad Psychiatry Law.* 2007; 35 (2): 172–182.
66. Sadoff RL. "Forensic psychiatry." In SH James, JJ Nordly, eds. *Forensic Science, 2nd ed.* New York, NY: Taylor & Francis, 2005, 593–604.
67. D'Orban PT. "Drugs and alcohol-the psychiatrist as expert witness in court." *Br J Addict.* 1986; 81 (5): 631–639.
68. Trott RJ. "Diminished responsibility and the drug scene." *Br J Addict.* 1992; 87 (2): 189–192.
69. Anonymous. Diminished capacity. Legal Information Institute. https://www.law.cornell.edu/wex/diminished_capacity. Accessed December 28, 2015.

40 Forensic Drug Testing

James J. O'Donnell III and James T. O'Donnell

The authors would like to thank Anne ImObersteg M.S., J.D., MBA, B.A. (deceased) for her contributions as a co-author of this chapter in prior editions of this book.

SYNOPSIS

DOI: 10.1201/9781003615323-44

40.1 INTRODUCTION

Drug use in the United States has increased across most generations, genders, and demographics at an alarming rate. This includes the use of prescription drugs and illicit substances alike. In 2020, over 37 million Americans, aged 12 years and older, were current illegal drug users (used within the past 30 days) and over 59 million had used illegal drugs or misused prescription drugs within the last year. In adults (18 years of age or older), 18.7% reported use of marijuana, 3.6% were users of opioids, and 3.5% were users of prescription pain medication (Figure 40.1). According to this 2020 report, 13.5% of Americans 12 and overused drugs in the last month, a 3.8% increase from 2019.[1]

The opioid epidemic contributes to staggering socioeconomic costs in the United States. Approximately 24.7% of those with drug disorders have an opioid disorder; this includes prescription pain medication and heroin. Of these opioid misusers, 7.4% abuse heroin and 4.0% use heroin and prescription medications. Hydrocodone remains the most popular prescription pain medication, with 5.1 million misusers.[2]

In June 2020, the Centers for Disease Control and Prevention (CDC) reported that 13% of Americans initiated or increased substance use as a way of coping with stress or emotions related to the COVID-19 pandemic. Drug overdoses and adverse events also increased since the onset of the pandemic.[3]

Substance	% Usership	
	Youth 12-17	Adults 18+
Marijuana	10.1%	18.7%
Opioids	1.6%	3.6%
Prescription pain medication	1.6%	3.5%
Prescription stimulants	1.2%	1.9%
LSD	0.9%	1.0%
Cocaine	0.3%	2.0%
Prescription sedatives	0.1%	2.4%
Methamphetamines	0.1%	1.0%
Heroin	*	0.4%

Substance Usership Rates, 12-Month Usage

**Insufficient data.*

FIGURE 40.1 Prevalence of Drug Use in the United States.

Drug use remains highest among individuals between the ages of 18 and 25 (39%), compared to individuals aged 26–29 (34%)—the emerging workforce in America. Based on gender, 22% of males and 17% of females used illegal drugs or misused prescription drugs within the last year.[4] These recent statistics on drug use in the United States showcase the widespread prevalence and underscore the potential impact that drug use may impose across aspects of the economy and daily living.

The impact of substance use can be measured in direct, tangible, and measurable costs, such as association with adverse health conditions and public health concerns. These direct, tangible, and measurable health costs are further increased by enormous intangible social and economic costs related to the social impact of substance abuse. These include domestic violence, child abuse, workplace, and motor vehicle accidents. Additionally, substance use contributes to other social problems with serious economic effects, including lost work productivity, decreased quality of life, and premature death.

In 2017, the cost of drug abuse in the United States was estimated at $272 billion. A total of $193 billion was incurred in overall costs for illegal drugs in addition to $78.5 billion for prescription drugs such as opioids. Healthcare costs were estimated at $11 billion related to the use of illegal drugs and $26 billion for prescription opioids. In 2016, a total of 326,000 hospitalizations occurred for nonfatal drug poisonings or overdoses. The emergency department (ED) saw 577,794 visits for nonfatal drug poisonings or overdoses with most patients experiencing opioid poisoning.[5] The current estimated economic cost of substance abuse disorder in the United States is approximately $3.73 trillion (T) annually, including $0.50 T in tangible measured costs and $3.23 T in intangible costs.[6]

The top four categories contributing to societal costs include health ($118,535 M), productivity loss ($206.753 M), crime ($97,882 M), and traffic collisions ($56,529 M). These direct costs do not reflect the intangible costs that include losses that are not commonly assessed such as the economic value assigned to loss of life, injury, and reduced quality of life. Examples of intangible costs of substance abuse disorder are those associated with the loss in quality of life of users who do not receive treatment ($0.39 T) and the emotional and physical impact of deaths, traffic deaths, and victims of violent crime associated with substance use ($2.84 T).

The corporate world incurs a large share of this cost in the form of lost productivity, untimely deaths, and illnesses

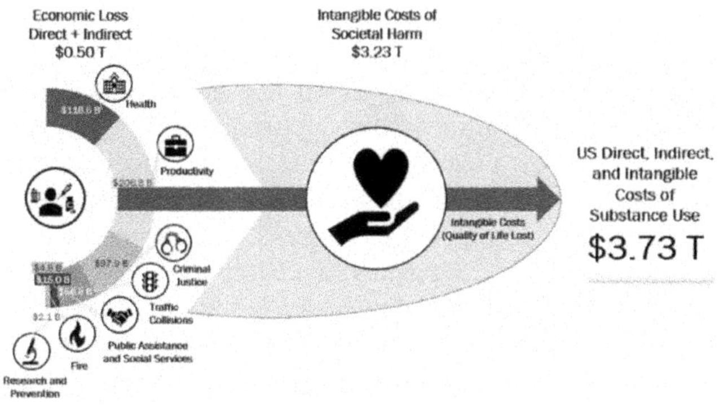

FIGURE 40.2 Economic Cost of Substance Abuse Disorder in the United States (2019).

Categories	Cost ($M)	Adj. for Double Counting[2]	%
Health	$135,457	$118,535	3.2%
Productivity Loss	$236,268	$206,753	5.5%
Crime, Law Enforcement, Criminal Justice	$111,855	$97,882	2.6%
Traffic Collisions	$64,599	$56,529	1.5%
Public Assistance and Social Services	$17,155	$15,012	0.4%
Fires	$5,106	$4,468	0.1%
Research Prevention	$2,398	$2,098	0.1%
Tangible (Direct and Indirect) Costs	$572,838	$501,277	13.4%
Death	$2,943,951	$2,576,182	69.1%
Crime Victims	$158,190	$138,428	3.7%
Quality of Life Lost	$441,078	$385,977	10.3%
Traffic Deaths	$147,181	$128,795	3.5%
Intangible Costs	$3,690,400	$3,229,382	86.6%
Total Costs	$4,263,237	$3,730,658	100.0%

FIGURE 40.3 Estimated Economic Costs Associated with Drug Use.

associated with drug use. Increased absenteeism, workplace accidents, workers' compensation claims, medical costs, and decreased productivity all negatively affect the economy and American businesses.[7]

A survey by the Hazelden Foundation determined that more than 60% of adult Americans know individuals who have gone to their place of business under the influence of either drugs or alcohol.[8] In fact, it is estimated that 70% of all illegal drug users are currently employed, affecting the efficiency of the workplace.[9] Drug-impaired employees not only are costly to the business owner and industry but also can pose a substantial safety risk to themselves, to their coworkers, and to the general public. Occupational injuries are a serious public health issue and cause significant morbidity and mortality in the United States. Occupational injuries may result in a myriad of injuries that range from minor to major and even fatal. As an apparent response to these alarming statistics, over 80% of American companies now conduct some type of workplace testing.[10] Workplace testing may take place in live specimen sampling or postmortem in cases of injuries or accidents, resulting in death.

40.2 NON-REGULATED DRUG TESTING

The interest of an employer in the productivity and welfare of their employees is not a new concept. As early as 1914, the industry attempted to regulate the "sobriety" of its employees. In the 1940s, accidents and absenteeism in the Kaiser shipyards were so prevalent that Kaiser created an in-house healthcare system, financed by payroll deductions. These early attempts at identifying drug use risk factors and drug testing by industry leaders, however, were fundamentally flawed—the plans were unregulated, lacked clear policy statements, and had no standards of performance.

40.3 REGULATED DRUG TESTING

In 1983, the Department of Transportation (DOT), in conjunction with the National Institute on Drug Abuse (NIDA), drafted a drug program for regulated testing. This program was initiated in response to the concerns of the National Traffic Safety Board over the increase in drug- and alcohol-related accidents in that industry.[11] However, it was not until 1986, when President Reagan's Commission on Organized Crime released a report connecting drug use with trafficking and organized crime that regulated testing got into full swing.[12] In the report, the commission called upon the president to issue a policy statement expressing the unacceptability of drug use among federal employees and to outline the measures necessary to achieve the commission's goals. In response, on September 15, 1986, President Reagan signed Executive Order 12564, the first step toward the ultimate goal of a "Drug-Free Federal Workplace." The order recognized the impact of drug use in the workplace and established the unprecedented rule of prohibiting federal employees from using illegal drugs on- or off-duty. The order states, in part,

> The Federal Government, as the largest employer in the Nation, can and should show the way towards achieving drug-free workplaces through a program designed to offer drug users a helping hand and, at the same time, demonstrating to drug users and potential drug users that drugs will not be tolerated in the Federal workplace.[13]

On July 11, 1987, Congress passed legislation affecting the implementation of the order. The goals of Congress were to establish uniformity among the drug testing plans of the various agencies, ensure reliable and accurate drug testing, allow employees access to drug testing records, provide confidentiality of drug testing results, and centralize oversight of the drug testing program.[14] This legislation was made under Section 503 of the Supplemental Appropriations Act of 1987.[15]

The act placed the burden of providing mandatory guidelines on the U.S. Department of Health and Human Services (HHS). The HHS was directed to establish

> "comprehensive standards for all aspects of laboratory drug-testing and laboratory procedures to be applied in carrying out Executive Order Numbered 12564, including standards which require the use of the best available technology for enduring the full reliability and accuracy of drug tests and strict procedures governing the chain of custody of specimens collected for drug-testing.[16]

The Secretary of the HHS was required to set the mandatory standards for all aspects of laboratory drug testing, including who would be tested, when the tests would be conducted, what drugs would be covered, and how the tests would be conducted. Testing was authorized for applicants, random testing of employees in designated "sensitive" positions, reasonable suspicion testing, accident or unsafe practice testing, voluntary testing, and testing as part of or as a follow-up to counseling or rehabilitation.

In 1988, the first guidelines were published by HHS in the document titled "Guidelines for Federal Workplace Drug-testing Programs." In 1994, the guidelines were revised and republished.[17] They established the testing criteria, the allowable specimen matrix, and the limited number of drugs that may be tested in the specimen.[18]

The following entities are mandated to follow the guidelines:

- Executive agencies, as defined in 5 U.S.C. § 105
- Uniformed services, as defined in 5 U.S.C. § 2101(3), except for the armed forces, as defined in 5 U.S.C. § 2101(2)
- Any other employing unit of the federal government, except for the U.S. Postal Service, the Postal Rate Commission, and employing units of the judicial and legislative branches
- Laboratories that possess or seek certification to perform urine drug testing for federal agencies under a drug testing program conducted under Executive Order 12564
- The intelligence community, as defined by Executive Order 12333, to the extent supported by the head of the affected agency

HHS established the National Laboratory Certification Program (NLCP) to certify laboratories before they are permitted to test specimens collected for federal agency drug testing programs. The DOT, the Department of Energy, and the Nuclear Regulatory Commission also require the industries they regulate to use these certified laboratories for their workplace drug testing programs. The DOT, in particular, has followed the guidelines very closely in its drug testing program. The DOT's program was codified in the Federal Register (49 C.F.R. Part 40) and became applicable nationwide with the passage of the Omnibus Transportation Employee Testing Act of 1991.[19]

40.4 VOLUNTARY PROGRAMS

Many private companies perform functions that do not require mandatory adherence to the federal HHS guidelines yet still have a regulated internal program. One such voluntary program, administered by the College of American Pathologists, is called the Forensic Urine Drug Testing Program (FUDT). The FUDT program establishes the minimum criteria for reliable urine drug testing procedures, which parallel the general consensus of the scientific community. While participation in the FUDT program is voluntary, many laboratories have an interest in being accredited by FUDT, since the program is one of the few non-governmental programs available to forensic laboratories.

The lack of formal regulation has some benefits and drawbacks. The most notable drawback is the possible development of a workplace drug testing program that lacks procedural oversight and mandatory adherence to basic forensic testing standards. Lack of adherence to scientifically accepted standards in a company's policies and procedures could increase employee-based legal challenges to any enforcement and sanctions incurred through the administration of the program. However, non-regulated testing allows employers to conduct more extensive testing of an employee's biological sample. For example, regulated testing may narrow the groups of drugs to be tested to five major drugs of abuse: cocaine, phencyclidine (PCP), opiates, amphetamines, and cannabinoids. Regulated testing often limits the sample matrix to urine and dictates the methods of testing. Non-regulated testing may allow testing for a multitude of drugs, including prescription drugs, in a variety of testing matrices such as blood, hair, sweat, urine, or saliva.

Regardless of whether the private company chooses to follow the federal program, a private program, or its own program, certain program guidelines should be followed. Only by establishing a comprehensive program can an effective program be created.

40.5 ESTABLISHMENT OF A WORKPLACE PROGRAM

The decision to develop and implement a drug-free workplace program begins with the establishment of policies guiding the program to the ultimate goal of increased safety and productivity in the workplace. Guidance for the components of a complete program can be found in Section 503 of the Supplemental Appropriations Act of 1987 (Section 503). Section 503 requires that all agencies establish a reliable workplace drug program containing five major components: a written policy statement, provision for supervisor training, provision for employee education, provision for employee assistance, and the guidelines for drug testing. All five steps are not necessary in non-regulated testing, but the establishment of all five steps makes the policy clear and may minimize legal ramifications on any employer-based action taken when an employee violates the program.

40.5.1 Written Policy

A written policy statement provides the basis for an agency or company's program. Thus, an obvious starting point for the establishment of an effective program is a written policy documenting the requirements of the employer, program adherence expectations, and ramifications of non-compliance with the policy. For federal programs, the act requires the agency to state why the drug-free program is being implemented, provide a clear description of what behaviors are prohibited, and provide a thorough explanation of the consequences of violating the policy. Regardless of whether the employer is or is not mandated to follow the steps established by the act, the following program components must be included:

- The rationale for the establishment of a policy
- A clear description of the prohibited substances and behaviors
- The type of required drug testing, and the circumstances (random, post-accident, reasonable cause, etc.) prompting drug testing
- Procedures for the determination of a policy violation
- The consequences for the violation of the policy (and any available appeals processes)
- A statement of when the policy will be enforced
- The documentation of what types of employees will be covered by the policy (safety-sensitive employees, contractors, pre-employment, all employees, and so forth)
- The treatment and rehabilitation services available to the employee
- Issues of employee confidentiality

40.5.2 Employee Assistance Programs

Employee Assistance Programs (EAPs) provide drug abuse education to company managers and counseling for employees seeking assistance for drug or alcohol abuse problems. An EAP program is a benefit to the employer, in that it allows managers to become educated in drug abuse issues while keeping them separated from the actual counseling process. An EAP is also an excellent benefit to the employee, since it often becomes an alternative to dismissal, and can provide resources for treatment facilities and counseling.

An EAP is a necessary component of any effective program and is a requirement in HHS-regulated testing. The act states that an agency must provide an EAP to help resolve poor work performance due to alcohol or drugs, as well as for personal problems. A successful EAP must provide treatment and rehabilitation to employees who have tested positive on a drug test or who have referred themselves for assistance. In addition, an EAP should disseminate knowledge on drug abuse and its effects and reinforce the impact of drug use in the workplace. Above all, any effective EAP program must assure the employee that all functions provided by the EAP, including test results and medical treatment, will be conducted with confidentiality.

40.5.3 Employee Awareness Training

Policies that are established and enforced in a draconian manner are often not financially beneficial to the employer. Legal consequences and the cost of training and hiring new employees make the establishment of an employee education program beneficial. Aside from educating the employee on the contents of the program and the new company policy, basic information on alcohol and drug abuse in the workplace is recommended. The act requires that the EAP administrator provide employee education to all federal employees. A model program under the act would include education on the types and effects of drugs, symptoms of drug use, effects of drugs on performance, the role of the EAP, treatments available, and confidentiality issues. Employee awareness programs should also include the recognition of substance abuse in the family or coworkers, the safety hazards of drug abuse in the workplace, and the available resources for addiction assistance in the company and community.

40.5.4 Supervisor Training

Supervisors provide the first line of drug detection for employees. The act requires that federal agencies provide and implement training to assist their supervisors in recognizing illegal drug use.[20] In addition, an agency must develop a training package or course covering the following issues:

- Employee problems with drugs and alcohol
- The role of EAP and the EAP supervisor
- Recognition of employees with drug or alcohol problems
- Documentation of performance or behavior problems
- Skills in confronting employees
- Agency procedures regarding referral to the EAP
- Disciplinary action and removal from safety-sensitive positions (Section 5 of the Executive Order)
- Reintegration of the employee into the workforce
- Written materials for the supervisor

Supervisors should be trained to recognize and understand drug abuse and job performance issues. The monitoring of job performance, rather than the diagnosis of drug abuse or drug abuse counseling, is the main purview of the supervisor. Documentation of performance problems will prompt the employee's referral to the available assistance. The act requires the supervisor's training to include the organization's policy, the supervisor's specific responsibilities, and how to deal with employees who have performance problems. In addition, the supervisor should be trained on how to monitor employee job performance, document performance issues, enforce the policy, and make referrals for testing based on reasonable suspicion.

40.5.5 Drug Testing

A standard drug-free workplace program must allow for drug testing, since any sanctions against an employee for mere suspicion of drug use or influence may not stand up to legal review. Drug testing may take place prior to hiring, upon reasonable suspicion, for cause, post-accident, randomly, periodically, or post-rehabilitation. Executive Order 12564 defines illegal drugs as any drug on Schedule I or II of the Controlled Substance Act. Since it is impractical to test for all the drugs listed in these schedules, the guidelines require that random drug testing programs shall test urine for marijuana and cocaine at a minimum. The agency may add to the minimum list by also testing for opiates, amphetamines, and PCP or request a waiver from the HHS to routinely test drugs other than the five listed. However, when testing for reasonable suspicion, accident, or unsafe practice testing, other drugs in Schedule I or II may be tested.[21]

In non-regulated testing, the employer and the testing laboratory have wide discretion in choosing the methods used and the drugs tested in a biological specimen. HHS restricts the matrix to urine. However, non-regulated programs may allow for the testing of an unlimited number of drugs in a variety of matrices, including sweat, saliva, and hair.

40.6 THE DRUG TESTING PROCESS

A vital part of any drug-free workplace program is the collection of the chosen biological matrix, the analytical testing of the matrix for a series of illegal drugs, and the accurate reporting of the results. Non-regulated testing laboratories are not limited to testing only urine and may use any method for testing. However, their practices may not be in accordance with the opinions and recommendations of the relevant scientific community, particularly in areas which have been updated as technology and the body of relevant knowledge progress. Regulated testing, on the other hand, may take the form of the private CAP-FUDT program or the HHS guidelines.

Federal agencies of the executive branch must comply with Executive Order 12564 (1986), which establishes the on- and off-duty abstinence from illegal drugs as a condition for employment in a federal job. Federal grantees and contractors with contracts valued at $100,000 or more must comply with the Drug-Free Workplace Act of 1988. In addition, laboratories that perform testing on federal employees must be certified by the NLCP under the HHS. In the transportation industry (DOT), employers must comply with the Omnibus Transportation Employee Testing Act of 1991 by establishing an alcohol and drug program for safety-sensitive employees. The NRC has established standards for nuclear-power producers, and employers with Department of Defense (DOD) contracts must also establish a drug-free program for employees in "sensitive" jobs.

Private programs and federal programs have some similarities—they are dedicated to maintaining a high analytical standard. All programs must require the laboratory to have in place a standard operating procedure (SOP) manual that includes a description of the laboratory's chain-of-custody procedures, analytical testing procedures, quality control and quality assurance programs, equipment and maintenance, accessioning and security, personnel qualifications and training, and reporting procedures. The laboratory must also be subject to inspections by the administering program, which must send proficiency samples to the laboratory on a regular basis.

The following drug testing guidelines contain the basic scientific concepts of the testing process and provide some examples of the basic requirements of different programs. However, the complete guidelines for the College of American Pathologists Forensic Urine Drug Testing program (CAP-FUDT), the federal program as outlined in the federal mandatory guidelines, and the DOT program will not be provided here. Drug testing programs are always subject to change with increasing needs and technology. Therefore, for a more thorough list of requirements, clarification on each activity, and new changes, the latest revision of the original documents should be consulted.

40.6.1 Specimen Collection

The collection of the specimens is a vital part of the workplace testing process. It is the foundation of the process and can affect the reliability and effectiveness of the entire program. During the entire drug testing process, the integrity and identity of the specimen must be maintained—from the collection of the specimen to the reporting of the specimen results. The manner in which the specimen is collected, the safeguards against specimen tampering during the collection of the specimen, the correct identification of the specimen, and the accompanying chain-of-custody are all factors impacting the identity and integrity of the specimen.

A chain-of-custody must be maintained to document the location of the specimen at all times. To maintain the integrity of the specimen, the chain of possession of the specimen must remain intact and must not be broken at any time. The common acceptable chain-of-custody formation is generally called the "Z" formation. A "Z" formation (representing a "Z" character when the chain-of-custody documentation form has two entries per line) takes the following form: A to B, B to C, C to D, and so on. The following represents an unacceptable chain-of-custody: A to B, C to D, and so on. In the latter example, there is no documentation of where "B" placed the specimen and from where "C" received the specimen—the chain has been broken. The HHS requires that its standardized custody control form (CCF) be used and that the control and accountability of specimens be maintained at all times. Every individual in the chain must be identified, and documentation of the individual handling the specimen—as well as the date and purpose for access to the specimen—must be contained on the chain-of-custody document.[22]

The integrity of a urine drug test hinges on the proper collection of the specimen. The DOT has set into place strict requirements for the collection of specimens. All procedures for DOT collection must be performed as per 49 C.F.R. Part 40.21. The correct collection procedure must be followed, a proper chain-of-custody form must be used at all times (CCF), the identity and integrity of the sample must always be maintained, and the collector must meet the training requirements of Section 40.33 of Part 40.

The DOT's collector training requirements are extensive and thorough. The procedures for collection of urine under these rules are very specific and must be followed whenever a DOT-required urine specimen collection is performed. As of January 2018, the collector must be trained in a series of procedures and must meet the requirements of 40.33 of Part 40. The collector must show knowledge and compliance in the following areas. To be permitted to act as a collector in the DOT drug testing program, you must meet each of the requirements of this section:

a. Basic information. You must be knowledgeable about this part, the current "DOT Urine Specimen Collection Procedures Guidelines," and DOT agency regulations applicable to the employers for whom you perform collections, and you must keep current on any changes to these materials. The DOT Urine Specimen Collection Procedures Guidelines document is available from ODAPC (DOT, 1200 New Jersey Avenue, SE, Washington DC, 20590, 202-366-3784) or on the ODAPC website (http://www.dot.gov/ost/dapc).
b. Qualification training. You must receive qualification training meeting the requirements of this paragraph. Qualification training must provide instruction on the following subjects:

    1. All steps necessary to complete a collection correctly and the proper completion and transmission of the CCF;
    2. "Problem" collections (e.g., situations like "shy bladder" and attempts to tamper with a specimen);
    3. Fatal flaws, correctable flaws, and how to correct problems in collections; and
    4. The collector's responsibility for maintaining the integrity of the collection process, ensuring the privacy of employees being tested, ensuring the security of the specimen, and avoiding conduct or statements that could be viewed as offensive or inappropriate.
c. Initial Proficiency Demonstration. Following your completion of qualification training under paragraph (b) of this section, you must demonstrate proficiency in collections under this part by completing five consecutive error-free mock collections.

    1. The five mock collections must include two uneventful collection scenarios, one insufficient quantity of urine scenario, one temperature out-of-range scenario, and one scenario in which the employee refuses to sign the CCF and initial the specimen bottle tamper-evident seal.
    2. Another person must monitor and evaluate your performance, in person or by a means that provides real-time observation and interaction between the instructor and trainee, and attest in writing that the mock collections are "error-free." This person must be a qualified collector who has demonstrated necessary knowledge, skills, and abilities by
        i. Regularly conducting DOT drug test collections for a period of at least a year;
        ii. Conducting collector training under this part for a year; or
        iii. Successfully completing a "train the trainer" course.
d. Schedule for qualification training and initial proficiency demonstration. The following is the schedule for qualification training and the initial proficiency demonstration you must meet:

    1. If you became a collector before August 1, 2001, and you have already met the requirements of paragraphs (b) and (c) of this section, you do not have to meet them again.
    2. If you became a collector before August 1, 2001, and have yet to meet the requirements of paragraphs (b) and (c) of this section, you must do so no later than January 31, 2003.
    3. If you become a collector on or after August 1, 2001, you must meet the requirements of paragraphs (b) and (c) of this section before you begin to perform collector functions.
e. Refresher Training. No less frequently than every five years from the date on which you satisfactorily complete the requirements of paragraphs (b) and (c) of this section, you must complete refresher training that meets all the requirements of paragraphs (b) and (c) of this section.
f. Error Correction Training. If you make a mistake in the collection process that causes a test to be cancelled (i.e., a fatal or uncorrected flaw), you must undergo error correction training. This training must occur within 30 days of the date you are notified of the error that led to the need for retraining.
    1. Error correction training must be provided and your proficiency documented in writing by a person who meets the requirements of paragraph (c)(2) of this section.
    2. Error correction training is required to cover only the subject matter area(s) in which the error that caused the test to be cancelled occurred.
    3. As part of the error correction training, you must demonstrate your proficiency in the collection procedures of this part by completing three consecutive error-free mock collections. The mock collections must include one uneventful scenario and two scenarios related to the area(s) in which your error(s) occurred. The person providing the training

must monitor and evaluate your performance and attest in writing that the mock collections were "error-free."

g. Documentation. You must maintain documentation showing that you currently meet all requirements of this section. You must provide this documentation on request to DOT agency representatives and to employers and C/TPAs who are using or negotiating to use your services.

[65 FR 79526, Dec 19, 2000; 66 FR 3885, Jan. 17, 2001, as amended at 66 FR 41950, Aug. 9, 2001; 73 FR 33329, June 12, 2008]

Each agency or company must have designated collection sites. These sites must be secure, accessible only to designated personnel, and have the proper procedures in place to ensure the integrity and identity of the urine specimen. Such procedures include the deterrence of possible dilution of the sample by the donor, the presentation of a photo identification card by the donor upon arrival, the removal of any clothing that may conceal adulteration materials, the washing of the donor's hands prior to urination, the elimination of access of the donor to water during the physical voiding of the bladder, and the collector's observation of the donor prior to urination. All collections must be performed in accordance with applicable regulations and must ensure the privacy of the donor by the use of a donor number rather than the donor's name.

Many programs require or allow the collection of "split specimens." Split specimens allow a portion of the collected sample to be poured into an additional container for independent testing or to preserve the specimen in the event that the original or first container becomes destroyed or contaminated. An example of a split collection procedure can be found in the DOT agency drug testing requirements. In the DOT program, all specimens must be split-specimen collections. At least 45 mL of urine must be collected; 30 mL must be poured by the collector into Bottle "A," the primary testing bottle, and at least 15 mL must be poured into Bottle "B." The donor may urinate into a specimen container or a designated Bottle "A." The collection site person then pours the urine into two specimen bottles that are labeled Bottle "A" and Bottle "B" or, if Bottle "A" was used to collect the specimen, pours an appropriate amount into Bottle "B."

During the physical collection of the specimen, the donor is given a clean specimen bottle and allowed privacy to complete the voiding of the bladder. On receiving the voided specimen from the donor, the collector must ascertain that a sufficient amount of urine has been voided. The specimen temperature should always be checked immediately. A urine temperature less than 90–100°F indicates that dilution or substitution of the specimen may have occurred. If not enough urine has been voided, and the urine temperature is within range, most programs allow the donor to drink fluids and attempt another collection in the same manner as described earlier. All specimens—even those suspected of being adulterated or diluted—are considered evidence and must be sent to the laboratory for testing.

After collection, the specimen is checked for color and any signs of contaminants. Any signs inconsistent with a valid sample must be noted on the chain-of-custody collection form. The specimen bottle is sealed with tamper-evident tape by placing the tape over the cap and down the sides of the bottle. A pre-labeled identification label containing the date, the donor's specimen number, and other identifying information (other than the donor's name) is placed on the bottle. The donor then signs the chain-of-custody form, verifying the collection process.

The privacy of the donor during collection is maintained unless certain criteria are met. Under certain circumstances, direct observation of the actual collection may be allowed. For example, employers may specify a direct collection when it is determined that there is no valid medical reason for the specimen to have been considered "invalid," when the donor's test is a return-to-duty test or a follow-up test. The collector must conduct a direct observation of urine collection if the specimen temperature is out-of-range, or if there is evidence of specimen tampering or adulteration.

40.6.2 Accessioning

The accessioning procedure is the gateway to the laboratory testing process. The biological specimen must arrive at the laboratory with the shipping package intact, a proper chain-of-custody form, and the specimen correctly identified. Broken specimen containers, seals, or gaps in the chain-of-custody all call into question the integrity of the specimen. Specimens without all the indicia of reliability should not be tested.

When the specimen is received, laboratory personnel must inspect the package for evidence of possible tampering and must compare information on specimen bottles to the information on the accompanying CCF. The CCF consists of the following five copies:

Copy 1. Test Facility Copy—accompanies the specimen to the laboratory
Copy 2. Medical Review Officer Copy—sent to the MRO
Copy 3. Collector Copy—retained by the collector
Copy 4. Employer Copy—sent to the employer
Copy 5. Employee Copy—given to the employee

Most drug testing programs have requirements in place for the acceptance or rejection of specimens during the accessioning process. Some flaws are not considered "fatal" and may be easily corrected by an affidavit from the collector. The laboratory must inspect the CCF and the specimen and note if there are "fatal" or correctable flaws. Some types of identified fatal flaws are:

- The specimen ID numbers on the specimen bottle and CCF do not match.

- The specimen Bottle "A" seal is broken or shows evidence of tampering. Exceptions are when split specimens can be redesignated as Bottle "A."
- The collector's printed name and signature are omitted from the CCF.
- Specimen bottle "A" has insufficient urine. Exceptions are when split specimens can be redesignated as Bottle "A."

Fatal flaws are not correctable, and the specimen must be rejected for testing.[23] Nonfatal flaws can be corrected within five days by affidavit.

Since the accessioning area receives and maintains the urine specimens, the area must be secure and limited to authorized individuals. Entry and exit from the area must be documented. Authorized visitors are allowed in the accessioning area but must be escorted at all times.

40.6.3 Drugs to Be Tested

Non-regulated testing has no restriction on which drugs or drug classes a laboratory may test in a specimen. Generally, in regulated testing, only five classes of drugs are covered: PCP, opiates, amphetamines, cocaine, and cannabinoids. The HHS requires that an "Agency requesting the authorization to include other drugs shall submit to the Secretary in writing the agency's proposed confirmatory test methods, testing levels, and proposed performance test program."

When performing an analysis for a particular drug or drug class, a laboratory must clearly establish the criteria for the determination of a positive or negative result, including a proper "cutoff point," below which the specimen result must be reported as "negative." In non-regulated testing, the laboratory has broad discretion in determining what cutoff level will be used and how the ultimate result will be reported. A non-regulated laboratory may allow the cutoff to be determined by the lower limit of detection (LOD) of the instruments used or may allow the reported result to be worded in vague terminology such as "possible presence" or "indicated." In regulated testing, however, cutoffs for screening and confirmation are mandatory (Table 40.1). The proper threshold to indicate a positive test is the limit of quantitation (LOQ), not the LOD. The LOD merely indicates the drug was found in the sample at the time of testing. The LOQ is the smallest value that can be reliably detected *and* quantified. Often the threshold for a positive test is established to exclude valid reasons for trace amounts of a drug in the sample. For instance, the cutoff for a positive test should be high enough that the small amount of morphine in poppy seeds would not trigger a positive test after eating a bagel with those seeds.

40.6.4 Screening Tests

Laboratory analysis of a donor's urine sample is performed in two separate stages. The first analysis is generally called an "initial test," "screening," or "presumptive" test. Non-regulated programs may allow a laboratory to use thin layer chromatography (TLC) or similar technology to screen the urine specimen. TLC is a technology which distinguishes chemical compounds based on their size and polarity. HHS and DOT guidelines mandate that immunoassay techniques be employed. Immunoassays are biochemical tests that measure the presence or concentration of a macromolecule in a solution through the use of an antibody or immunoglobulin. The molecule detected by the immunoassay is often referred to as an "analyte" and it provides selective binding of antibodies targeted against a drug or drug class. Most commercially available immunoassay kits are screening tests for the common drugs of abuse (cocaine, methamphetamine, marijuana, PCP, morphine), although some kits are available for testing other types of drugs such as benzodiazepines and phenothiazines.

TABLE 40.1
Cutoffs for Urine Screening and Confirmation Tests

Drug or Metabolite	Initial Test (ng/mL)	Confirmation Tests (ng/mL)
Marijuana metabolites	50	15
Deltra-9-tetrahydrocannabinol-9-carboxylic acid (THC-COOH)		
Cocaine metabolites	300	150
Benzoylecgonine		
Phencyclidine	25	25
Amphetamines:	100	500
Amphetamine		500
Methamphetamine		(with amphetamine present at a concentration ≥ 200)
Opiate metabolites:	2000	2000
Codeine		2000
Morphine		10
6-Acetylmorphine		(Only tested if morphine ≥ 2000 ng/mL)

The requirements do not specify which initial immunoassay product to use as long as the product meets all the requirements of the Food and Drug Administration (FDA) for commercial distribution.

Presumptive drug screening is simple to perform but difficult to interpret. Most immunoassays are called presumptive or screening tests since a positive reaction is an indication that a drug or drug class is present, yet the method does not rise to the required level of certainty. Confirmation by a second test is required. The main reason why presumptive tests are not used forensically is because there is considerable cross-reactivity with drugs other than the target drug.

There are a variety of different types of immunoassay techniques on the market. Some common technologies utilized are radioimmunoassay (RIA), enzyme immunoassay (EIA), kinetic interaction of microparticles in a solution, and fluorescence-polarization immunoassay. Some immunoassay techniques are more specific to the target drug than others. However, all immunoassay techniques use an antibody–antigen relationship to identify a drug class in a sample.

40.6.4.1 Immunoassays

Lack of specificity is a common problem with immunoassay tests. For example, an immunoassay test for "opiates" will flag positive for codeine, naloxone, morphine, heroin, hydrocodone, and hydromorphone. Thus, a presumptive "positive" opiates result may mean that an individual has taken Tylenol with codeine, Vicodin for pain relief, or heroin. In addition, depending on the kit used and the manufacturer of the kit, other drugs that are not considered an "opiate" may still cross-react. Moreover, sometimes the analysis will give a random "false positive," flagging a sample positive when there is no target drug present at all.

There are a variety of different types of immunoassay techniques on the market. Some immunoassay techniques are more specific to the target drug than others. However, all immunoassay techniques utilize an antibody–antigen relationship to identify a drug class in a sample. An antigen is a foreign substance, such as a drug, that has been introduced into a host body. This antigen will cause an immune response in the host's body, which, in turn, will prompt the host's B lymphocytes and plasma cells to create an antibody protein. This antibody will then be able to identify and bind to any similar antigen that is introduced into the host.

Commercial immunoassay kits contain a substrate with an antibody to a specific class of drugs, and also the target drug that is "labeled" with a tracer. In radioimmunoassay kits, the label is radioactive iodine or carbon. In fluorescence immunoassays, the label is a fluorochrome. In EIAs, the label is a lysozyme or other enzyme. One of the most popular EIA kits is the enzyme multiplied immunoassay test (EMIT) developed by Syva Corporation.

The EMIT utilizes a technique known as "competitive binding," which indirectly measures the concentration of analyte (drug) present in the sample. This system consists of an antibody targeting the analyte, the analyte bound to the enzyme, the enzyme substrate, and the sample containing the analyte. The first three components are provided in the kit, and the sample containing the analyte is obtained from the person whose drug levels are being measured. In immunological terms, the drug is an antigen for the antibody in the kit. The analyte (drug) bound to the enzyme competes with any drug found in the subject's sample for a limited supply of antibodies. When the enzyme-linked drug in the kit is bound with the antibody, the enzyme activity is inhibited. When a sample has a measurable amount of the target drug, antibodies will not bind to some of the enzyme-linked drugs, disinhibiting the enzyme. The enzyme, in turn, converts more of the substrate to a product. The conversion of substrate is measured and is proportional to the concentration of unlabeled drug (i.e., drug without a conjugated enzyme). Therefore, substrate conversion gives a measure of the target drug concentration in the tested sample.

More target drugs in the subject's sample means that there are fewer antibodies available to bind to the kit's enzyme-labeled analyte. By measuring the magnitude of enzymatic change on a substrate, the amount of drug present in the subject's sample can be determined. For example, a subject's sample with no target drug will enable most of the kit's enzyme-labeled drug to be bound to the antibodies and will result in an inhibition of the enzyme's activity. When the enzyme activity is inhibited, the substrate in the kit, NAD, cannot be oxidized into NADH. The result is a small absorbance change at 340 nm, measured by a spectrometer. Conversely, a large amount of drug in a subject's sample will leave few antibodies to react with the kit's enzyme-labeled drug, and many enzymes will be able to convert NAD to NADH, resulting in a large absorbency change. The amount of NAD produced and measured is inversely proportional to the amount of target drug in the sample.

40.6.4.2 Thin Layer Chromatography

In the past, TLC was occasionally used as a confirmation test. However, with the advent of more specific instruments, such as the gas chromatograph and mass spectrometer (GC/MS), TLC is now generally used as a screening test. TLC is a simple procedure that enables the chemist to determine the number and possible identity of each compound present in a mixture. This instrument allows a mixture of two or more substances in a specimen (such as urine or a pharmaceutical pill dissolved in a volatile solvent) to distribute between a stationary phase and a mobile phase. The stationary phase is a thin layer of adsorbent material (silica gel or alumina) coated on a glass, metal, or plastic plate.

The mobile phase is a solvent into which one edge of the plate is placed. A small amount of the mixture to be analyzed is spotted on the stationary phase, near the bottom of the TLC plate. The plate is then placed in a solvent in a developing chamber so that only the very bottom of the plate is in the liquid. The chamber is capped, and the solvent, by way of capillary action, is allowed to rise up the layer of silica on the plate. For each one of the mixture's components, as the solvent moves through the spot that was applied, equilibrium is established between the molecules that have adsorbed on the solid and the molecules in the solution.

Since the components in the applied mixture differ in solubility in the mobile phase and in the strength of their adsorption to the stationary phase, each component will move up the plate at a unique rate, based on its partitioning between the mobile liquid phase and the stationary phase. Highly polar organic molecules interact fairly strongly with the polar adsorbents and will tend to adsorb onto the particles of the adsorbent. In contrast, weakly polar molecules are allowed to move more freely.[24] Thus, weakly polar molecules will move through the adsorbent more rapidly than the polar species and will be seen higher up the plate than the polar molecules. In this manner, the components of a specimen are separated and may be identified by comparison to known compounds and molecular weights.

When the solvent front reaches the other edge of the stationary phase, the plate is removed from the solvent reservoir and dried. When the plate is examined, the original sample will have resolved into a row of spots running up the plate, with each spot containing one of the components of the original mixture.

Some substances are colored, which allows a simple visual comparison of the amount of movement up the plate the compound traveled. Generally, however, the spots are difficult to detect and must be visualized with an ultraviolet lamp or with staining agents. When the dried plate is placed in a chamber with iodine vapor, the iodine vapor oxidizes the substances in the various spots, making them visible to the eye. Ninhydrin (0.2% solution) is effective for visualizing amino acid spots.[25] When sprayed on the plate, amino acids display a purple coloration. In addition, visualization can be achieved through the use of an ultraviolet lamp. In this method, the adsorbent is impregnated with a fluor (zinc sulfide), which enables the plate to fluoresce everywhere except where an organic compound is present on the plate.

The amount of movement up the plate is determined by and compared against a known standard. This "retention factor," or Rf, is defined as the distance traveled by the compound divided by the distance traveled by the solvent. If the two substances have the same Rf value, they may be the same compound. If they have different Rf values, they are definitely different compounds. Since the amount of movement up the plate is also dependent on the solvent system used, the type of adsorbent, the thickness of the adsorbent, and the amount of material spotted, Rf values will change from system to system. For this reason, a known standard must be run on the same plate as the unknown specimen (so that their relative Rf values may be compared).

There are a variety of different TLC separation techniques. TLC can be automated using forced solvent flow in a vacuum-capable chamber. The ability to program the solvent delivery makes it convenient to do multiple developments in which the solvent flows for a short period of time. This method enables a higher resolution than in a single run.[26] A two-dimensional TLC process can also be applied. After running a sample in one solvent, the TLC plate is removed, dried, rotated by 90 degrees, and run in another solvent. After this process, any of the spots from the first run that contain mixtures can now be separated.

Although TLC seems like a simple procedure, there are some potential difficulties. For example, a sample that has been too heavily applied will be visualized as a streak rather than a spot. A sample possessing a strongly acidic or basic group (such as an amine) may be visualized as a smear or an upward crescent. The plate solvent front may run crookedly, which makes it harder to measure Rf values accurately. Sometimes no compound can be seen on the plate because an inadequate sample was applied, or, due to heavy sample application, components with similar Rf values may not be resolved and may appear to be one large spot.

Regardless of whether immunoassay or TLC technology is used, a legal action cannot be scientifically supported solely by a screening test, since a positive result may be due to a different substance or a random error. The laboratory must perform a "confirmation" test on an instrument—such as a GC/MS—capable of differentiating between the many drugs in a drug class and quantifying the amount of drug present in the specimen. However, a biological specimen must first be properly prepared before it can be analyzed on a GC/MS instrument.

40.6.5 Confirmation Tests

Once an initial screen indicates that the specimen may be positive for a particular drug or drug class, a confirmation test is performed. Only those specimens confirmed positive by a test utilizing an analytical technology different from the screening test may be reported as positive. In non-regulated testing, the option exists of using a variety of confirmation methods, some of which may not be considered acceptable by the majority of the scientific community. Under regulated testing, substances must be tested by laboratories with confirmation methods such as GC/MS or related technologies. Acceptable alternatives include liquid chromatography/mass spectrometry (LC/MS) or more sensitive variations of these methodologies such as GC/MS/MS or LC/MS/MS. The difference between GC and LC is the mobile phase, which is gas in the former case and liquid in the latter. However, the underlying principles are the same. Mass spectrometry (MS) is more sensitive and selective than FID and thus MS is the preferred method for confirmatory tests in general. For ethanol quantification, GC coupled with a flame ionization detector (GC-FID) is appropriate for use as the instrument for a confirmatory test, however. In this case, FID can be used as the detector because a great deal of sensitivity or selectivity is not required.[27]

There are a variety of laboratory instruments capable of identifying and quantifying the drugs that may be found in a biological specimen. Most procedures call for the use of mass spectrometry. Mass spectrometry is arguably the most versatile technology used in forensic analysis today in that it enables the analyst to determine chemical and structural information about the different types of molecules found in the specimen.

There are many techniques that combine the power of mass spectrometry with other instruments to achieve the goals of selectivity, specificity, and sensitivity. The most common—by far—are the instrument combinations described in the following text.

40.6.5.1 GC/MS

The GC/MS utilizes the GC to separate the components (drugs) of a mixture by injecting the mixture into a metal or glass column inside the instrument; the MS is used to identify these compounds by piecing together the respective structural makeup. The instrument's inner capillary column is coated with a chemical and packed with sand-like, chemical-coated particles. The column is contained in a heated oven designed to liquefy the coating. When a sample is injected into the column, the injection port is at a temperature capable of volatilizing the sample (transforming it into a gas). A carrier gas pushes the volatilized sample through the column.

The chemical makeup of each of the mixture's compounds and each component's interaction with the liquefied chemicals in the column determine how long the component will take to travel the entire length of the column. Some molecules will make a slow migration through the column, and some will travel quickly through the column relatively unhindered. This is based on the affinity of the molecule for the stationary phase. In any event, each component of the mixture will travel as a group through the column. The amount of time the compound is retained in the column is called the retention time (RT) of the compound. As each compound exits the column, a detector recognizes the passing of a compound and records the event on chart paper.

A drug may be identified in a specimen by comparing the RT of any instrumental response from the analysis of the specimen with that of a calibrator or control sample, using just a GC alone. The quantity is determined by measuring the magnitude of the response. However, with the GC/MS, the GC functions as a separating mechanism, and the identification and quantification are mainly the responsibility of the MS. The MS creates fragments of each compound in the form of gas phase ions, separates these ions in accordance with mass and charge, and measures the quantity of ions of each mass-charge ratio.

Gas phase ions can be prepared by a variety of methods. Perhaps the most common methods are chemical ionization (CI) and electron impact (EI). As each component exits the GC column, it enters the MS. In CI, molecules are ionized by a reaction between the analyte molecules and a reagent ion to form ions by proton or hydride transfer. The other method, EI, uses an electron beam to ionize gas phase molecules. CI is sometimes used instead of EI because it provides increased sensitivity and provides more specific molecular-weight information. However, the method requires a high level of technical expertise. Hardware limitations also make EI more common.

In EI, the MS bombards the drug with electrons and shatters the structure into pieces, depending on the weak points in the drug's structure and the relative stability of the resulting fragments. Theoretically, since each drug structure is different, each different drug will break at different points on the molecule and thus shatter into predictable fragments. The size and quantity of the fragments form a "fingerprint" of the drug. If one looks at all the pieces and their relative size, one can identify the drug in the sample.

The data set produced by looking at all the fragmentation pieces of the molecule is called a "scan" (see Figure 40.4). Scans are sometimes used when the identity of the molecule causing the instrument response is unknown and does not match any of the known drugs analyzed with the specimen. The fragmentation pattern of the specimen can be identified by the pattern produced, and the relative sizes of each of the fragments can be compared with one another. Identification can be performed by computation or by library match. In manual computation, the analyst must determine the chemical structure of the molecule by determining the source of the fragment. For example, a fragment with one carbon and three hydrogen atoms will have a mass of 15 (C = 12, H = 1; 12 + 3 = 15), and a fragment of 15 will be seen on the chromatogram. A trained mass spectrometrist will be able to look at an ion chromatogram, with all the ion fragments, and determine the molecular structure of the drug. An easier way, however, is to compare the pattern of the fragments with a known library match. Library databases can be purchased or created in-house. However, library matches are rarely 100% accurate, and most library programs will give the analyst the best match, leaving the decision up to the analyst of whether an 80% or 90% match constitutes an

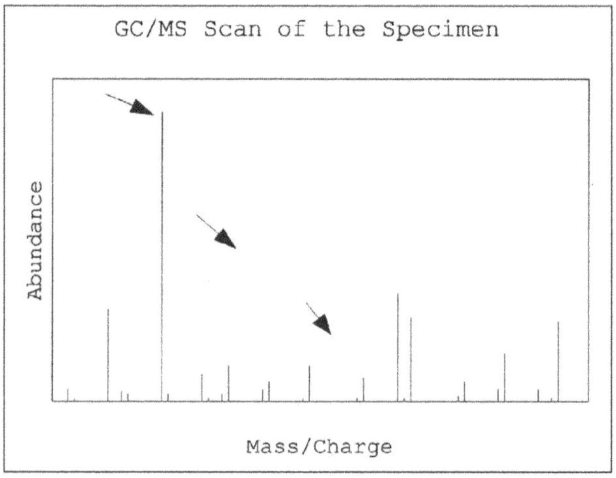

FIGURE 40.4 GC/MS Scan of the Specimen.

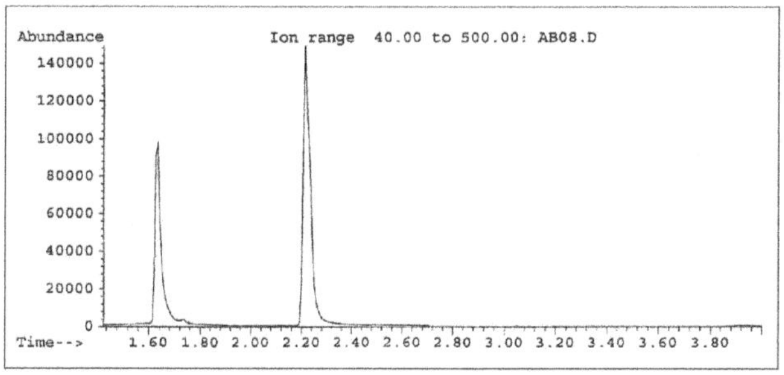

FIGURE 40.5 The Total Ion Chromatogram.

identification. Scans can be performed to identify a drug, but not to quantify the amount of drug present.

Determining the amount of drug present in the specimen is performed using selected ion monitoring (SIM). In the SIM method, the analyst selects only specific ions (rather than all the ions, as in the scan method). The benefit of using the SIM method is the greater instrument sensitivity, better chromatography, and better accuracy and precision. It is up to the laboratory method to decide which ions to use for identification, but they should be unique (to differentiate between the target drug and any similarly structured drugs).

In a typical analysis, the analyst will choose a "target" (generally the most abundant ion in the molecule) or "parent" ion for quantifying a drug and "qualifier" ions to assist in identifying the drug. These qualifier ions are two more pieces from the electron fragmentation that must be in correct proportion to the target ion for the identification to be made. (See Figure 40.5) The calibrators will establish what the proportion will be for the method. When analyzing an unknown specimen, the analyst/method allows the relative sizes of the qualifier ions to the target ion to differ by about 20%. Thus, if the qualifier ion is generally 80% as abundant as the target ion, a range of 64% to 96% is acceptable when analyzing an unknown specimen. Taken together, with the RT as recorded by the gas chromatograph and the presence of a target ion and the qualifier ions in proper proportion, these methods can identify a drug with fairly high certainty.

40.6.5.2 Quantifying a Drug Using the GC/MS

Quantifying a drug on the GC/MS is generally performed by the use of an internal standard. An internal standard aids in quantification and is used to monitor the efficiency of the extraction procedure, to ensure that the amount detected is not due to an erroneous injection, or to account for changes in signal-to-analyte-amount ratio between runs. The internal standard is usually a compound closely related in structure to the drug being sought, since it must have an RT within a few minutes of the target drug. However, the analyst must be careful and select an internal standard that will not likely be found in the sample to be analyzed. In the GC/MS, the internal standard is usually a deuterated version of the target drug.

The internal standard is typically added at the beginning of the extraction procedure. Since the internal standard is added to an aliquot of the specimen at the beginning of the analysis, there exists from the start of the analysis a relationship of the internal standard to the drug that never changes. No matter if one drop or one cup of the extracted sample is tested, the ratio of drug to internal standard will remain constant. By plotting the ratio obtained by the instrument for a suspect's sample against a variety of standards of known drug concentrations and their respective ratios, one can determine the amount of drug present in the sample.

For the specimen to be quantitated, there needs to be a relationship established between the instrument response and the concentration of the specimen. To establish this relationship, a series of samples of known concentrations, called calibrators, must be created and tested. This is performed by taking a solution of the target drug and spiking the same type of biological fluid as the specimen to be tested with the drug at various concentrations. A calibrator or control without a drug must also be tested. These calibrators are extracted in the same manner and around the same time as the specimen to be tested and have the same amount of internal standard as the test specimen.

A "target" ion is chosen to be used to quantify the drug. The more abundant the target ion, the higher the concentration of the calibrator/sample. Since an internal standard is used, the ratio of the target ion of the internal standard to the target ion of the calibrator is used to help eliminate the possibility of an incomplete or excess injection onto the GC/MS.

After the analysis of the calibrators, the relationship between the calibrator/internal standard instrument responses versus the calibrator concentration can be plotted. A straight line will be generated by the analyst or performed automatically by the computer-assisted instrument.

The line generated is tested by the use of quality control. The quality control is a sample of known concentration, which is created separately from a different solution than the calibrators. The result of the quality control, utilizing the line plotted by the calibrators, must fall within specified guidelines, generally no more than ± 20% of the true value.

Once a relationship has been created between drug concentration versus instrument response and the line is validated by the acceptability of the quality control result, the analyst can begin to analyze the specimen of unknown concentration. This analysis results in the determination of the instrument response, the abundance of target ions of the unknown specimen, and the target ions of the specimen's internal standard. Utilizing the line generated by the analysis of the calibrators, the analyst can then mathematically determine the concentration of the drug in the sample (see Figure 40.6).

40.6.5.3 GC/MS/MS

The GC/MS/MS is similar to the description for the GC/MS given previously, but a third step is added. The initial fragmentation goes through yet another fragmentation to produce daughter fragments. This method is often used for better sensitivity and specificity but is not as common as

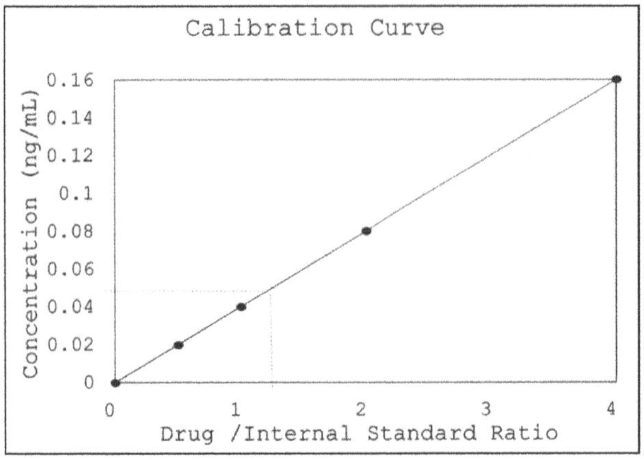

FIGURE 40.6 Calibration Curve Figure.

the GC/MS because of the cost of the instrument and the technical expertise required to operate it.

40.6.5.4 The LC/MS

LC is a separation technique whereby the test specimen is forced over a chemical system contained in a column by means of a flowing solvent stream rather than via gas (as with the GC). As with a GC, the individual compounds in the mixture travel at different rates down the column, depending on the chemical interaction of the mixture with the chemical system contained in the column.

The solvent system can have a single buffered solvent (isocratic) or a combination of several solvent systems (gradient). The benefit of a gradient system is the versatility in analyzing a wide range of compounds and the ability to produce a higher concentration of the drug. Gradient is most often used when the specimen contains unknown drugs. The isocratic method is faster and thus is more attractive to laboratories that analyze large quantities of specimens.

LC can be used alone with the traditional ultraviolet, visible, fluorescence, or electrochemical detector, or coupled with an MS. Use of LC/MS is steadily increasing in the field of toxicology, partly due to the ease in sample preparations, and partly because of the instrument's simple extractions and lack of need for derivatization. LC/MS/MS is also available, which has greater sensitivity and specificity compared to LC/MS.

40.6.5.5 GC-FID

GC-FID is a common methodology used for the quantitation of ethanol.[28] In FID, an organic sample is mixed with hydrogen and undergoes combustion in a flame. This results in ions that generate a current when an electrical potential is applied by an electrode. This current is proportional to the abundance of the molecule as well as the number of carbon atoms in the molecule. Advantages of GC-FID include simplicity, reproducibility, reliability, a wide linearity range, and ease of use. However, it is a non-selective detector, responding to all hydrocarbons. Also, the analyte must be able to be vaporized without decomposition, and the detector destroys the sample.[29] In general, GC-FID is much less sensitive and selective compared to GC/MS and related technologies such as GC/MS/MS, LC/MS, and LC/MS/MS. Blood alcohol concentration (BAC) measurements do not require much sensitivity and there are few sources of volatile, interfering agents in biological fluids, so the limitations of FID do not preclude its use in the measurement of alcohol. In fact, GC-FID in conjunction with headspace sampling is the standard for BAC measurement. In contrast, detection of trace amounts of drugs is best done with MS.

40.6.5.6 Sources of Instrumental Error

Regardless of the instrument chosen, there are many opportunities for error to be introduced into the testing process. The magnitude of the error is dependent on the type and degree of error allowed by the analyst of the method employed. Regardless of the source, appreciable error results in uncertainty of the identification and quantitation of the drug in the specimen and may directly impact litigation.

Errors can include the following:

- Improper sampling of the aliquot from the sample vial
- Error in spiking calibrators from which the instrument response line will be generated
- Improper addition of the internal standard
- Poor chromatography
- Inadequate testing of other drugs to eliminate interference or misidentification
- Improper range of calibrators
- Lack of proper controls
- Lack of linearity of the concentration/instrument response curve
- Carryover or contamination from the sample analyzed immediately preceding

Errors in sample preparation, including extraction, directly affect the resulting numerical result. Improperly prepared calibrations and changes in the amount of sample used for extraction introduce the greatest magnitude of error. For these reasons, the quality control sample must always be used to ensure that the calibrators were properly made. Likewise, the internal standard must be added as soon as possible in the preparation steps.

Errors in analysis can be introduced in many ways. One way is by the improper selection of calibrators to create the concentration/instrument response relationship. The calibration line does not always travel through zero and may not be linear at all levels. Of special concern is when the drug concentration of the unknown specimen is greater than the highest calibrator used to create the linear relationship, since the relationship can only be shown to be linear through the range of the calibrators. After the highest or lowest calibrator, the line may cease to be linear and may curve. Thus, it is important to elicit the experimental upper range of linearity from the testing laboratory. It should be noted that although the laboratory has scientifically determined this upper level in the past, only the calibrators used at the time of the test can determine the working parameters of the instrument at the time of the subject's test.

To overcome the problem of a sample being higher than the calibrators, some laboratories dilute the sample, or use less sample volume, and then multiply the calculated concentration by the dilution factor. This dilution step, unfortunately, introduces another possible source of experimental error.

Sometimes the concentration of the drug in the subject's sample is too minute for the LOD for the method and instrument used. Although the GC/MS is state of the art, there is a level of target molecule so low that the instrument cannot identify or consistently quantify the sample. These levels are, respectively, called the LOD and the LOQ.

The analyst must be careful to measure the amount of response properly so that a proper ratio can be determined. Typically, the responses should be Gaussian in shape or much like a sharp triangle. However, when the chromatography starts to deteriorate, "shoulders" and other bumps start to distort the Gaussian peak. When this happens, area is added to the peak and is erroneously attributed to the amount of drug.

40.6.6 Reporting and Storage of Samples

After analysis, the final test result must be reviewed and approved by a person authorized to review the analytical data for accuracy. In regulated programs, this duty is assigned to a "certifying scientist." The certifying scientist reviews all the data of the initial and confirmation test and chain-of-custody and determines if the result is justified. This initial review is then sent to the MRO within an average of five working days after the laboratory receives the specimen. The completed CCF is sent by fax, mail, or courier or electronically to an MRO—not to the employer. The laboratory may transmit results to the MRO by facsimile or computer, although this must be done in a manner designed to ensure confidentiality of the information.

Confidentiality of records is protected under the Privacy Act, 5 U.S.C. § 552a et. seq. and Section 503(e) of the act. Results may not be disclosed without written permission of the employee, unless the disclosure is to the MRO, the EAP administrator who is providing counseling to the employee, a supervisory or management official in the agency, or pursuant to a court order. An applicant for employment is not entitled to the results of the drug test, but an employee may obtain information by written request.

Results may not be provided verbally over the telephone. Quantitative results are not routinely sent, except when the sample is positive for morphine or codeine at a level of 15,000 ng/mL or above. This is done to ensure that additional information is provided to address the poppyseed contribution to positive opiate urine tests. All other reports for quantitation require a letter from the MRO asking for the quantitative results. All confirmed positive specimens must be maintained in long-term frozen storage for a minimum of one year. All records must be maintained for two years.

40.6.7 Prevention Against and Detection of Drug Test Cheating

A positive drug test may result in criminal prosecution or loss of employment; thus, there is considerable motivation to cheat on the drug test. Drug test cheating is prevalent. "No one knows for sure, but many drug testing experts believe that as many as 10% of all drug tests samples are adulterated, switched, or tampered with in some manner."[30]

The most common methods of cheating a urine drug test are diluting the sample, replacing the urine sample with a drug-free sample, and flushing out the sample by drinking a product which will reduce drug excretion or adulteration of the sample. Dilution of the sample may occur by simply drinking a lot of fluids or by adding water to the sample after urination.[31]

Dilution of the sample or replacing the urine sample with synthetic urine or someone else's urine sample can be prevented by close monitoring during the collection process. However, people are usually not monitored during collection in pre-employment drug screens, so in this case, the test may be circumvented. Dilution of the urine sample may be detected by aberrant creatinine concentrations, specific gravity, and pH. Synthetic urine has the same creatinine, specific gravity, and pH levels as normal urine, so in this case one would need to test for other compounds found in normal urine but not in synthetic urine, such as hormones. Another simple way to detect that the urine sample was not recently excreted is by quickly monitoring the temperature of the sample; the sample should be 90–100°F.

Adulteration by adding substances which interfere with the assay and cause false negatives is common. Pyridinium chlorochromate, nitrate-containing agents, peroxidases, and gluteraldehydes are common adulterants. Spot tests have been developed to test for these adulterants, including AdultaCheck 4, AdultaCheck 6, and Intect 7.[32] Also, as of 2010, 15 states have enacted laws to prohibit the sale or use of adulterants.[33]

40.7 ADDITIONAL PROGRAM ASPECTS

40.7.1 The Medical Review Officer

The DOT and Federal Mandatory Guidelines require that an MRO review positive results. An MRO is a licensed physician with knowledge of substance use disorders who is responsible for receiving laboratory results generated by an agency's drug testing program and is qualified to interpret and evaluate an individual's positive test. The MRO is typically a licensed physician (Doctor of Medicine or Osteopathy) who has been specially trained to review and evaluate the laboratory's implementation of the relevant program's testing of urine samples and controlled substance abuse disorders. The MRO must not have a conflict of interest with the employer's laboratory.

The DOT program requires that, when a positive result is reported, the MRO is to use due diligence to contact the employee directly and confidentially to determine whether the employee wishes to discuss the result. If the employee can present proof of a legitimate explanation for the positive test, the test will be deemed negative. After three unsuccessful attempts to contact the employee, the MRO requests that the designated employer representative (DER) contact the employee and have the employee call the MRO. Positive results can be verified without interviewing the employee if more than ten days have passed since the reported result and there has been no success in contacting the employee. Interviews are also not required when more than 72 hours have passed since the employee was told to contact the MRO or if the employee refuses to speak with the MRO.

The MRO verifies a confirmed positive test for PCP, cocaine, amphetamines, and marijuana unless a legitimate medical explanation exists for the presence of the drug in the employee's urine. However, the MRO may still raise fitness for duty issues with the employer. If the sample contained 6-acetylmorphine (6-AM), the test is verified positive for heroin. If, however, the test is negative for 6-AM, the result will still be verified positive if the morphine or codeine is at 15,000 ng/mL or above. All other opiate-positive tests must be accompanied by clinical evidence of unauthorized use of opiate or opium derivatives. Adulterated or substituted test results are treated as a verified positive if, after interviewing the employee, there is no medical reason for the result.

40.7.2 Public Interest Exclusions

To help protect the public against service agents who fail to meet the DOT regulations, the federal government has instituted a public interest exclusion (PIE) proceeding policy. PIE proceedings may be initiated against an MRO, a laboratory, a substance abuse professional (SAP), a collector, or any service agent who is non-compliant with the program's provisions. The issuing party has the burden of proving by a preponderance of the evidence that the agent was in serious non-compliance with the regulations. The duration of a PIE can last about one to five years.

40.7.3 Blind Performance Testing

Blind quality control specimens are used as a test of the entire testing process. The current guidelines require each federal agency to ensure that a minimum of 3% blind quality control samples are submitted with the donor specimens. An employer may provide blind samples to the collector, who submits the quality control sample as if it were a donor specimen. The collector will generate a fictitious social security number or employee identification number, complete a CCF, and properly label a specimen bottle. Only the MRO's copy of the CCF, copy four, will have the designation "Quality Control Sample" in the donor's name section. The MRO is to determine whether the laboratory reported the correct result when the second copy of the CCF is received from the laboratory after the laboratory's analysis. If the laboratory reports a result different from the one expected, the MRO must contact the laboratory to determine if there is a reason the laboratory did not report the correct result. The MRO may request that the laboratory retest the specimen or have an aliquot sent to another certified laboratory for confirmatory testing. If the retest result does not confirm the original result, the laboratory likely made an error.

A false-negative result is not considered as serious as a false positive. If the retest result has confirmed that a false positive was reported by the laboratory on a blind quality control sample, the employer and the regulatory office will be contacted so that an investigation can be conducted. If a specific cause for the false positive is identified, the laboratory will be required to take corrective action to prevent the recurrence of the error.

40.7.4 Alcohol Testing

Not all drug testing programs allow for the testing of ethyl alcohol. By a 1994 amendment to 49 C.F.R. Part 40, alcohol testing for the DOT is now mandated. These are separate regulations from the drug testing requirements, and an MRO review is not required. Alcohol testing may be done in four situations: post-accident, reasonable suspicion, random testing, return-to-duty, and follow-up. At this time, pre-employment testing is not required. Alcohol screening tests may be performed on breath or saliva. If the alcohol concentration result is greater than 0.02% (g/100 mL), a confirmation test must be performed on a specified breath-alcohol testing device within 30 minutes of the screening test. Specially trained screening test technicians or breath-alcohol technicians (BATs) may perform breath-alcohol testing procedures. Only a qualified BAT may conduct a confirmation test. A confirmation test device must be on the NHTSA-conforming products list (CPL) for evidential testers. The screen test may be on the CPL list for evidential and non-evidential devices.

All confirmation results must be printed in triplicate, and the printed record must include the results, date and time, a sequential test number, and the name and serial number of the evidential breath tester (EBT). Confirmation tests on an EBT must be performed after a 15-minute observation period, to ensure that alcohol in the oral cavity does not contaminate the breath test. Before beginning the test, an air blank must be conducted on the EBT.

A positive result is any confirmation test that is 0.04% or higher. Employees who have a positive test must be removed from safety-sensitive duty and referred to a SAP. A test result between 0.02% and 0.039% is considered neither positive nor negative. Employees at this level must be removed from safety-sensitive functions until they are below 0.02%, or their next duty period (at least eight hours).

A measurement equal to or below 0.019% means the test is considered negative, and the employee may return to work.

40.8 SPECIAL DRUG TESTING ISSUES

40.8.1 Type of Matrix

Determining what matrix to use to detect the use or presence of drugs depends on the concentration of the drug used, route of administration, distribution in tissues, and metabolism and excretion of the drug. Drug distribution in interstitial and cellular fluids is dependent on the physiological and physicochemical properties of the drug. For example, lipid-insoluble (lipophobic) drugs cannot permeate cell membranes easily and thus are restricted in their distribution and sites of action. Some drugs bind to plasma proteins, such as the binding of acidic drugs to plasma albumin. Lipid-soluble (lipophilic) drugs, such as cannabinoids, accumulate in tissues and fat cells, which act as a reservoir, prolonging drug action and subsequent elimination from the body. Consideration must be made to the recognized fact that chronic cannabinoid users may test positive for a month or longer after cessation of use. These factors, and many more, affect the concentration and detection levels of various drugs in different matrices.

Generally, the purpose for the testing and the information desired often dictates the type of sample preferred. If the employer wishes to test an employee "for cause" or post-accident, a blood sample is far superior to a hair or urine sample, provided the employee is available close to the time of the accident or occurrence. However, if the employer wishes to determine if the employee or hiring candidate has a long-term history of drug use, a hair sample might be the best option.

The following is an overview of the benefits and drawbacks of different sample matrices for the presence of drugs of abuse in workplace testing.

40.8.1.1 Hair Testing

Hair serves as a repository for drugs, drug metabolites, vitamins and minerals and other substances, which are delivered to the hair root by the blood supply. Most of the drug is deposited in the central part of the hair, called the cortex.[34] It takes approximately three to five days for the hair to extrude from the scalp to enable it to be cut for collection. The amount of sample required for testing varies, but generally 60 to 360 hairs are required, depending on the length of the hair and the testing technology used. Hair testing can be performed by the analysis of the whole shaft of hair or segmented to assist in the determination of the dates of ingestion. Segmentation is not very useful, since not all individuals grow hair at the same rate and not all hair on one person's head is in the growth cycle phase at the same time.

A major benefit of using hair as a drug testing sample is the ability to determine long-term drug abuse. Unlike urine or blood, hair represents a lengthier record of drug exposure. The amount of hair growth per month depends on the health and sex of the individual and the anatomical location of the hair. In general, the average rate of growth for head hair is about 1 centimeter (0.4 inch) per month.[35] For example, if a 2-inch length of hair is tested, it may represent drug use over the past five months. While it may be possible for an employee to maintain sobriety for a short period of time to test negative in an anticipated urine test, it would be more difficult for an employee to abstain for several months.

Drugs become incorporated into hair from three major sources—the blood supply, the sweat and sebum, and from passive exposure to the smoke or solid form of the drug.[36] In general, hair testing is less susceptible to intentional adulteration or substitution by the donor; the donor is always in sight of the collector. However, there have been other contentions of contamination of the hair from external sources: environmental drug contamination from exposure to methamphetamine or cocaine smoke has been shown to be present in children exposed to drug smoke in the home environment.[37]

Studies have shown that despite a washing procedure prior to testing, environmental contamination of the hair may still cause a false-positive test result.[38] Smith and Kidwell performed a study where cocaine-using adults and their non-using children were tested for drug use and exposure. Hair from the adult subjects showed cocaine in 92% of the cases and hair from the children was positive in 88% of the cases.[39] In addition, hair is continuously in contact with body sweat. Sweat also contains drugs, which may be incorporated into the hair matrix after the hair has extruded from the skin. One study demonstrated that deuterated cocaine may be found in previously drug-free hair when volunteers, who were administered deuterated cocaine, held the hair in their hands for 30 minutes.[40] This positive result persisted even after the standard pre-test washing procedure.

Other issues in the hair-testing arena are the different amounts of uptake in the hair depending on ethnicity and hair color.[41] Studies by Henderson et al. have shown a bias in ethnic hairstyles to the incorporation of cocaine vapor into the hair. The order of the degree of incorporation was largest for Asian hair, followed by African hair, and finally Caucasian hair.[42] Hair color bias was also demonstrated in a study by Reid et al., in which the binding of benzoylecgonine was different for black, brown, and blond hair types.[43]

Hair testing has enjoyed some popularity in a variety of arenas, including family law, insurance cases, custody cases, pre-employment, law enforcement, and the military. In workplace testing, hair is most often used for pre-employment testing only, since it best represents a history of drug use over a long period of time. If a company's goal is to determine long-term drug use, a hair sample may be the best matrix.

40.8.1.2 Saliva Testing

Saliva is an oral liquid composed of water (90%) and various other substances, such as mucins and enzymes. Hair testing is simple to perform and is the easiest noninvasive method available. Saliva is a substance that, compared to sweat and hair, most reliably can be correlated to blood concentrations for certain drugs.[44] Additionally, saliva differs from urine in that saliva contains higher concentrations of the parent drug than inactive metabolites. However, there are a variety of factors that affect the concentration of drugs in the saliva.

It is well-known that an increase in saliva pH can alter the partitioning of certain drugs from the blood into the saliva.[45] Many drugs are weak acids or bases. The distribution of a weak electrolyte is determined by its pKa and the pH gradient across the membrane. For drugs with a pKa less than 5.5, saliva concentrations are not pH dependent, and the concentration will correlate with the plasma portion of the blood. However, drugs with a pKa greater than 5.5 are highly pH dependent. For example, cocaine (pKa 8.6) concentration in saliva may change by a factor of 12 if the saliva pH changes from 6.5 to 7.6.[46]

Saliva is a good matrix for the determination of drug use during a 12-to-24-hour period of time.[47] Compared to hair, saliva would not be useful for the determination of a historical drug use pattern but may be useful for testing employees prior to their engagement in safety-sensitive functions.

40.8.1.3 Sweat Testing

Sweat is a body fluid that was not, until recently, fully utilized in the drug testing arena. Sweat is mainly produced by eccrine glands in the transdermal layer of the skin surface or apocrine glands in specific regional areas in the body. Sweat is about 99% water and 1% sodium chloride and other trace materials. Researchers have known since 1911 that drugs are excreted in the sweat.[48]

Over the years, there have been several devices that have been used to collect sweat. However, many of these devices consisted of a pad covered by an occlusive membrane, which would trap both water and solute. This type of patch design could not always eliminate bacterial growth under the patch or allow the skin under the patch to remain healthy for long-term application. However, more recent technological developments have enabled the invention of an absorbent pad covered by a non-occlusive membrane, which facilitates comfort to the wearer by allowing oxygen, water, and carbon dioxide to pass through the patch.[49] The invention of a "sweat patch" collection device developed by Sudormed™ and marketed by PharmChem™ Laboratories under the trade name Pharm-Chek™ is such a device. After approval by the FDA, the patch was introduced in the drug-detection and testing arena.

The Pharm-Chek patch is left on the subject for about a week, at which time it is removed. The removed patch is placed in a vial with an elution buffer to extract the drug from the patch. Testing is performed with the conventional immunoassay screening procedure, and positive results are confirmed with a GC/MS procedure. The benefits of sweat testing are that it is noninvasive and that it can detect use—even a one-time use—for a longer period of time than urine testing.[50] Other benefits include the detection of parent compounds rather than the more polar metabolites and the tamper-evident membrane that will likely tear if there is an attempt to tamper with the patch after it is applied. These facts have made the device popular in the drug treatment field as well as in custody cases, probation, parole, and the social-service arena.

While the use of sweat as a testing matrix may be suitable to guide treatment in a rehabilitation facility, the sweat patch would likely be unsuitable in "for cause" or in post-accident testing. The concentration of the drug in the sweat patches is expressed as ng/mL of buffer eluate. This convention of reporting makes it difficult to interpret or correlate the concentration with blood levels or to determine the degree of "under the influence." In addition, certain drugs tend to deposit in adipose tissue, making an issue of "recent use" more difficult to interpret.[51]

> The manufacturer claims that the patch is carefully designed so that contaminants from the environment cannot penetrate the adhesive barrier from the outside, and therefore the patch can be worn during most normal activities (bathing and swimming, for example) without affecting the integrity of the test.[52]

Several scientific articles have mirrored that opinion in stating that the molecular pore structure of the plastic membrane will exclude substances greater in molecular size than vapor-phase isopropanol.[53] However, there have been questions of contamination of the patch, during application and removal of the patch, or external contamination. Early studies indicate that the cleaning solution used (70% isopropanol) on the skin prior to the application of the patch does not adequately remove external contaminants from the skin.[54]

> Other than CFWO [external contamination of patch membrane from without] can occur and generate false positive results, one may ask whether false positive results may arise from the prior presence of drugs on the exterior of the skin, not removed by the cleaning process (external contamination from within, under the patch, CFWI). CFWI is distinct from the process where drugs permeate the skin in areas not covered by the patch, enter the blood stream, and are re-excreted in sweat into the patch. Except in extreme cases of external contamination, this is unlikely to occur because, generally speaking, drugs do not enter the bloodstream through skin in high concentrations. For CFWI to be observed, only a source of drugs, a plausible transfer mechanism to the skin, and binding of the drugs to the skin need occur. Because most individuals tested for drug use by the patch are previous drug users, their environment is more likely to be contaminated with drugs, increasing the likelihood that their skin will contact drugs from prior drug using episodes. Because the skin is "cleansed" using 70% isopropanol swabs before application of the patch, it was thought that prior drug exposures of the skin should not affect the results. Our previous research showed that 70% isopropanol does not remove all the drug deposited on the skin. Thus, the very people most likely to be tested by the sweat patch are also the most likely to be externally contaminated.[55]

40.8.1.4 Blood Testing

Blood is a valuable matrix, especially for post-accident drug use determinations. A 1985 DOT study evaluated existing data on the concentrations of a variety of drugs in drivers to assess the ability of different matrices to detect drug impairment. The study concluded that urine testing would be suitable for establishing the need to obtain and analyze blood specimens for THC (the active ingredient in marijuana) and that blood is the only body fluid that can relate drug levels to impairment albeit limitedly.[56] For practical purposes, especially in DUI and DRE (drug recognition), urine and blood samples are taken simultaneously, and if a urine-positive result is noted, the blood sample is tested for a particular drug or drugs. Typically, post-accident testing rules require urine and blood specimen collection from the involved and surviving employees and also tissue from deceased employees (these collection procedures can go well beyond the normal Part 40 procedures, e.g., Federal Railway Administration). A blood sample showing the presence of a significant concentration of a drug that impairs the safe operation of large machinery can be beneficial to the ultimate determination of impairment. Other factors that may affect the ultimate determination of impairment are whether the blood is drawn from the employee during the expected timeframe of active drug action and whether the employee exhibits consistent signs of the expected effects. Another benefit is the plethora of studies and literature delineating therapeutic versus toxic concentrations of drugs in whole blood or plasma.

The major disadvantage to blood testing is the invasiveness of the collection process, the increased hazardous exposure of the collector to possible virulent blood, and the lower concentration of drugs found in the blood compared to urine.

40.8.1.5 Urine Testing

HHS currently mandates that only urine may be tested. However, even in non-regulated testing, urine appears to be the most popular matrix. Since most workplace testing is either random testing or pre-employment, recent use (not drug impairment) is the information sought. Urine is suitable for the determination of recent use, especially during the past 72 hours. The time frame in which a drug may be detected depends on several factors, including the amount of drug initially consumed, the frequency of drug use, the lipid solubility of the drug in question, and the half-life ($t_{1/2}$) of the drug. For example, some drugs, such as cannabinoids, can be detected for over a month if the donor is a chronic user. Another benefit to using urine for drug testing is that drug concentration in urine is 10 to 100 times more concentrated than in the blood, making detection easier using conventional drug testing instruments.

In urine collection, the substitution of another substance as urine, the addition of chemicals to the urine, or the dilution of the specimen with water are common methods of tampering with the specimen during collection. Adulteration of urine samples to mask drug use or cause a false-negative result when tested can be achieved *in vivo* or *in vitro*. *In vivo* adulteration is caused by the consumption of some substance that will dilute the urine or change the amount of drug excreted into the urine of drugs. Consumption of large amounts of water or the use of diuretics will increase the amount of urine produced and will cause the drug concentration in the urine to be lowered. Consumption of a substance that makes the pH more alkaline will slow down the excretion of amphetamines and result in a lower amount in the urine per unit time. Both of these methods will effectively lower the concentration in the urine and may result in the drug concentration falling below the cutoff value of the test.

The addition of chemicals directly into a specimen may create a false negative in an otherwise positive specimen. Chemicals may interfere with the screening kit's reagents, causing the test to report the specimen as negative when it is truly positive. Some common chemicals used include detergents, vinegar, and bleach. The addition of plain water to the sample cup dilutes the specimen and lowers the concentration of the drugs in the specimen. The dilution may be so great that the specimen may test below the laboratory's cutoff concentration to determine which specimens are to be considered positive. The substitution of another substance, or another person's urine, results in the false specimen being negative for drugs.

When choosing a program or laboratory, the employer must evaluate the safeguards in place at the collection site and the testing laboratory. During the actual voiding of the specimen, the employee must not have access to water to dilute the specimen. Turning the water line to the sink off during voiding or having the employee void where no sink is accessible is necessary. The placement of the bluing agent in the toilet enables the collector to check the color of the sample to make sure the specimen was not diluted with water from the toilet. A temperature indicator on the specimen cup allows the collector to check the temperature of the specimen immediately after the voiding to ascertain if the temperature is consistent with the body temperature. The HHS guidelines call for the collector to check the temperature of the urine within four minutes of collection. The temperature of the urine must be within 90–100°F. Despite these precautions, a negative urine specimen may be heated to body temperature by the concealment on or in the donor and substituted for the donor's urine at the time of collection. The collector's evaluation of specimen temperature, color, or smell during the collection process may still not be sufficient to detect donor adulteration. The laboratory, then, has to determine the adulteration of a specimen.

In an effort to ascertain whether a specimen has been tampered with during collection, the laboratory should test the urine for creatinine levels, specific gravity, nitrites, and/or pH. If the specimen falls outside the normal ranges expected for normal urine, the integrity of the specimen might have been compromised. Unregulated laboratories often do not have criteria in place for the determination of an adulterated or dilute specimen. However, regulated programs have addressed this issue. The DOT requires specimen validity testing, and the HHS program strongly encourages the practice, through its publication of Program Document #35 for reporting urine specimen validity test results.[57] The publication discusses the issues of adulterated, diluted, and substituted urine specimens. Under the reporting guidelines, a specimen is considered "substituted" if the urine creatinine concentration is <5 mg/dL and the urine specific gravity is <1.001 or >1.020. A specimen is considered dilute if the creatinine is less than 20 mg/dL and the specific gravity is less than 1.003. A sample is considered adulterated if the pH is less than or equal to 3 or greater than or equal to 11, or if it contains exogenous substances, such as nitrites.

Natural polyuria can occur in medical conditions such as diabetes insipidus or nephrogenic diabetes.[58] However, scientific research on medical conditions resulting in severe overhydration (polyuria) and water-loading studies has indicated that guidelines can be established to enable a laboratory to detect a specimen condition that is not consistent with normal human urine. Analytical criteria for laboratories testing federal and federally regulated specimens are outlined in Program Document #37.[59] To report a specimen as "substituted," creatinine must be quantitatively measured on two different aliquots, both using a cutoff of 5 mg/dL, with the results reported to the first decimal place. Specific gravity must be determined by refractometry on at least one of these aliquots, using cutoffs of 1.001 or 1.020, and reported to the third decimal place.

Occasionally, the donor may have trouble urinating because of what is termed "shy bladder" or merely be unable to provide a sufficient amount of urine for the test. If this is the case, the specimen must be discarded, and the collector must attempt another collection. Consumption of copious amounts of water may encourage the production and collection of sufficient urine. The DOT guidelines direct the donor to consume approximately 40 ounces of fluid during a three-hour period following the unsuccessful collection. However, an employee's decision not to drink fluids in a "shy bladder" situation will not be regarded as a refusal to test. If the employee still cannot provide a specimen, the procedure is halted and the collector must make a notation on the CCF and notify the DER and MRO within 24 hours. The DER must then direct the employee to obtain a medical evaluation from a licensed physician within five days to explain the medical condition that would have precluded the employee from providing an adequate specimen. If a medical condition does exist, the MRO must determine whether there is clinical evidence that the employee is an illicit drug user. Evidence of a dilute specimen allows the employer to ask the employee to take another test immediately. Positive specimens that are determined to be dilute are treated as a valid positive test.

40.8.2 Alternate Sources of Drug Exposure

The main focus of drug testing programs is to detect illegal drug use by the employee. However, some positive urine drug tests may have their origins in the use of a legal substance rather than in the use of an illegal substance or in the unintentional exposure to substances used by another. Passive inhalation of smoked drugs, dermal absorption, foodstuff ingestion, or a laboratory's technical inability may be just a few of the other reasons for a positive urine test.[60] Thus, it is imperative that the employer or MRO be versed in the alternative explanations for positive drug test results prior to the imposition of any sanctions.

The use of certain beauty products, health oils, and food products are typical routes of drug exposure. The use of hemp products, such as hemp-seed oil or tea, has been shown to cause a positive urine test for cannabinoids.[61] In one study, a 49-year-old man consumed a total of 30 mL of cold-pressed hemp-seed oil a day for four days. Urine samples were collected periodically from the start of the first ingestion through 177 hours. Urine specimens from collections between hours 45 through 142 were determined to contain THC-COOH from 12 to 68 ng/mL.[62,]

In the 1980s, health food stores sold tea under the trade name "Health Inca Tea." Health Inca Tea, containing about 1.87 mg of cocaine per cup, was found to produce positive benzoylecgonine screening results 21 and 26 hours after ingestion.[63] This tea no longer contains cocaine, since the FDA banned the importation of any tea containing residual cocaine into the United States.

The ingestion of poppy seeds can cause a positive urine test for opiates. The type of poppy seeds used, the concentration of morphine and codeine per gram of seeds, and the amount of seeds ingested play an important role in the amount of morphine ultimately found in the urine. Numerous studies have been undertaken to determine whether poppy seeds can cause a positive urinalysis result. In one study, ingestion of three poppy seed bagels resulted in 214 ng/mL codeine and 2797 ng/mL morphine at three hours.[64] In another study, the ingestion of 25 grams of poppy seeds from four brands of poppy seeds, containing between 17 and 294 mcg of morphine per gram, resulted in serum levels of up to 131 ng/mL and urine detectability over 48 hours.[65] The vast majority of the searched literature indicates that, depending on the cutoff level utilized by the laboratory, the detection of morphine in the urine does not necessarily indicate illegal drug use.

The HHS also recognizes that a positive for codeine or morphine may be a result of the donor consuming "normal dietary amounts" of poppy seeds. The MRO is directed to report the result as negative unless clinical evidence of abuse or illegal use of opiates is verified. The guidelines state the MRO "shall determine that there is clinical evidence—in addition to the urine test—of illegal use of any opium, opiate, or opium derivative." Since 6-acetylmorphine metabolite comes only from heroin, its presence confirms the illegal use of heroin, not the legal consumption of poppy seeds. In addition, the guidelines permit an MRO to have a blanket written request on file at the laboratory to routinely receive the quantitative values associated with a positive codeine and morphine result or request quantitative information on the presence of codeine below the cutoff for specimens that have been reported positive for morphine only.

Passive inhalation or absorption of drugs can also occur. Secondary smoke contains active ingredients and pyrolysis products of the burning substance. The lungs have a large surface area and an abundant blood flow, enabling the drug to pass readily into the blood stream. Passive inhalation can occur with any smoked substance—marijuana, PCP, cocaine, methamphetamine, and so on. The level of the drug ultimately found in the bystander from the smoke depends on the proximity of the subject to the smoke, the ventilation in the confined area, the amount of smoke, the concentration of the substance smoked, and the chemical nature of the substance.

The combustion of cannabis results in the conversion of various chemical precursors to form the active constituent of marijuana, THC. Most of the dose enters the smoker's lungs during inhalation, but a small amount is released into the environmental air. The concentration of THC in the air is directly related to the THC concentration in the cigarette and the size of the room where the smoke is released. The amount of THC absorbed by the passive inhaler depends on several factors. Not only is the size of the room in which the smoke is confined important, but also the number of "joints" smoked, and the number of hours exposed to the smoke. It is shown that casual contact with marijuana smoke in a room containing approximately four smoking cigarettes may result in the passive inhaler testing positive for marijuana use by urine analysis. In a study by Cone et al., several volunteers were subjected to two differing concentrations of THC smoke in a confined room.[66] The study took place over six days, and the exposure time was limited to one hour per day. Individuals exposed to concentrations of THC smoke from 16 cigarettes reached RIA levels of up to 100 ng/mL and up to 87 ng/mL on the GC/MS. A subject confined to a medical ward tested positive for marijuana metabolites due to passive inhalation and tested positive for marijuana in the urine in concentrations up to 260 ng/mL.[67] Cannabinoids in the blood and urine were also detected by Morland et al., eliciting the conclusion that "the demonstration of cannabinoids in blood or urine is not unequivocal proof of active cannabis smoking."[68] HHS recognizes that passive inhalation of marijuana smoke does occur and can result in detectable levels of THC and its metabolites in urine. However, HHS also takes the position that it is unlikely that a nonsmoking individual could unknowingly passively inhale smoke that results in a drug concentration in urine at or over the cutoff levels used in the federal program. As such, HHS directs the MRO to report the result as "positive" for cannabinoids.

Passive exposure is not limited to the cannabinoids. There are numerous articles citing incidences of passive exposure by children and infants exposed to cocaine (crack) vapor, which resulted in a positive urine test for benzoylecgonine.[69] A study conducted at NIDA Addiction Research Center has demonstrated that individuals passively exposed to "crack" smoke did not produce a urine positive for cocaine using the guidelines' established testing levels.[70] In another unrelated study, a 73-kilogram man exposed to vapors produced by the volatilization of 200 mg of "free-base" cocaine for 30 minutes prompted the authors to conclude that "passive exposure to free-base cocaine vapor can produce low-positive results . . ." and that it was "probable that a longer exposure period, larger cocaine dose, or a more efficient (lower) vaporization temperature would lead to higher urinary benzoylecgonine concentrations."[71]

Accidental exposure of police officers to cocaine in work-related situations led the authors to conclude that "passive micro-ingestion of cocaine needs to be considered when examining persons who are in cocaine intensive environments."[72] Passive exposure of crime-lab personnel to cocaine during processing and analysis was also discovered by Le et al., prompting the authors to emphasize the use of protective equipment and short exposure times.[73]

The issue of passive exposure to PCP has not been studied extensively in the literature. However, there have been numerous laboratory studies determining the levels of animals exposed to PCP pyrolysis products. In addition, the literature cites a few instances of accidental or occupational exposure to PCP. A woman living above an illegal PCP synthesis laboratory developed psychiatric manifestations of PCP exposure and levels of PCP in her blood.[74] In another study, law enforcement personnel handling illegal PCP have been shown to have PCP in their blood and urine for at least six months after their last-known occupational exposure.[75]

It is clear that when reviewing a case for the possibility of a positive result due to passive exposure the circumstances around the exposure should be carefully evaluated. Casual contact in a social setting, or a one-time exposure, may yield only a low-positive test. However, testing individuals exposed to large amounts of smoke, smoke with a high concentration of the drug, or lower amounts on a daily basis for a long period of time may yield highly positive results. Lipid-soluble drugs pose a special problem in that daily exposure to even low amounts of smoke over a long period of time may result in the accumulation of the drug in the body and result in a high-positive test.

40.8.3 Amphetamine Testing Issues

Analysis of the phenethylamines, also called amphetamines, has always posed a challenging problem to toxicologists and drug testing personnel. A positive amphetamine test result could occur because of a medical use of amphetamines, use of a legal drug that metabolizes to an amphetamine or methamphetamine, identification of enantiomers of methamphetamine, and the conversion of ephedrine or pseudoephedrine to methamphetamine during the GC/MS testing process.

Conversion of ephedrine to methamphetamine during the testing process has been shown to occur. In 1990, a certified laboratory reported a false-positive result in the analysis of a proficiency sample. Further investigation by the HHS and the NLCP of the laboratory revealed that the misidentification was due to analytical lab error and confounding factors. Specimens reported positive by the affected laboratory were sent to other laboratories and found not to contain methamphetamine. The culprit in the false identification appeared to be the presence of high levels of ephedrine or pseudoephedrine. Other factors included the use of high injection port temperatures in the GC/MS, and the use of derivatizing agents such as 4-carbethoxyhexafluorobutyryl chloride (CB), heptafluorobutyric anhydride (HFBA), *N*-trifluoro acetcy-L-propyl chloride (TPC), or pentafluoropropionic anhydride (PFPA).

In an attempt to eliminate further similar problems, the NLCP now requires that for the laboratory to report a specimen positive for methamphetamine, the specimen must also contain the metabolite, amphetamine, at a concentration equal to or greater than 200 ng/mL. If this criterion is not met, the specimen must be reported negative for methamphetamine. Another way to virtually eliminate the problem is for the laboratory to incorporate an extraction procedure utilizing periodate. Periodate oxidizes primary amines, by reacting with -OH and -NH on adjacent carbon atoms. The result is a change in the molecule such that the ion fragments will not be similar to methamphetamine.

Once methamphetamine is identified, the structural or chiral form should be elicited. Methamphetamine and amphetamine exist in two forms known as enantiomers. Enantiomers are non-superimposable mirror images. The two isomers of each substance are designated as D- (dextro) and L- (levo), indicating the direction in which they rotate a beam of polarized light. The D-isomer of each substance has a strong central nervous system stimulant effect, while the L-isomer of each substance has primarily a peripheral action. A Vicks® Inhaler contains L-methamphetamine, affording the possibility that a laboratory-positive result could be reported for L-methamphetamine and/or L-amphetamine. Selegiline, a monoamine oxidase inhibitor used in the treatment of Parkinson's disease, is metabolized to L-methamphetamine and L-amphetamine.

HHS dictates that the MRO should request the laboratory to perform a D-, L-isomer differentiation. Following Vicks Inhaler use, there will be close to 100% L-methamphetamine, with perhaps a small amount of D-methamphetamine present as a contaminant inhaler. When isomer differentiation is conducted and there is greater than 80% L-methamphetamine, the results are considered to be consistent with Vicks Inhaler use.

40.8.4 Medical Use of Drugs

Not all drugs found in the urine are the product of illegal use. Some drugs can be directly prescribed by a medical professional (see Table 40.2) or can be present as a metabolite of a prescribed substance (see Table 40.3). In certain medical conditions, the use of drugs that are usually illegal may be permitted. Over-the-counter (OTC) preparations may contain drugs that may interfere with or be misidentified as an illegal substance. The MRO has the burden of interpreting the results found by a laboratory. As such, the MRO should request the donor to submit a copy of his medical record or evidence of medications taken during the period around the time of the drug test.

Methamphetamine is a sympathomimetic amine legally prescribed for medical conditions such as obesity, narcolepsy, and attention-deficit disorder.[76] Methamphetamine or amphetamine can be metabolically produced by the ingestion of prescribed drugs as well. Some common drugs that metabolize to amphetamine are found in Table 40.3. Some of these drugs, such as dimethylamphetamine, ethylamphetamine, and fenrthylline, are Schedule I drugs in the United

TABLE 40.2
Key Drugs Present in Drug Products

Product	Drug Present
Marinol®	**Cannabinoids**
Astramorph PF	Morphine
Duramorph	
MSIR	
MS Contin Tablets	
Roxanol	
Amogel PG	
Diabismul	
Donnagel-PG	
Infantol Pink	
Kaodene with Paregoric	
ParegoricQuiagel PG	
Actifed with Codeine Cough Syrup	Codeine
Codimal PH	
SyrupDimetane-DC Cough Syrup	
Phenaphen with Codeine	
Robitussin A-C	
Triaminic Expectorant with Codeine	
Tylenol with Codeine (#1, 2, 3, or 4)	
Kaodene with Codeine	
Desoxyn (Gradumet)	D-methamphetamine
Adderall	D-amphetamine or racemic D, L-amphetamine
Benzedrine	
Biphetamine	
Dexedrine	
Durophet	
Obetrol	
Vicks Inhaler	L-methamphetamine

Source: All products are registered.

TABLE 40.3
Prodrug Products and Associated Metabolites (Active Drugs)

Product	Metabolizes To
Amphetaminil	Amphetamine
Clobenzorex (Dinintel®, Finedal®)	
Ethylamphetamine	
Fenethylline (Captagon®)	
Fenproporex (Tegisec®)	
Mefenorex (Pondinil®)	
Mesocarb	
Prenylamine	
Benzphetamine (Didrex®)	Methamphetamine (and amphetamine)
Dimethylamphetamine	
Famprofazone	
Fencamine	
Furfenorex	
Selegiline (Deprenyl, Eldepryl®)	

States and have no recognized medical usage.[77] However, these drugs may be found in other countries.

During the analysis of a urine specimen, the main laboratory focus is to accurately identify methamphetamine or amphetamine in the specimen. However, the MRO must consider any alternative origins for these drugs. The identification of the legal parent drug, when present, will assist in the determination of the source of the illegal substance. Some of the drugs listed in Table 40.3, such as famprofazone or fenforex, undergo extensive metabolism in the body, resulting in very little, if any, parent drug found in the urine specimen. However, if the parent drug is not present, other metabolic products of the drug may be found. For example, deprenyl will metabolize to methamphetamine, amphetamine, and desmethyldeprenyl. The presence of demethyldeprenyl may indicate deprenyl as the source. Other considerations include evidence of a valid prescription by the donor and the possible concurrent use of legal drugs and illegal amphetamines.

Dronabinol is chemically synthesized delta-9-tetrahydrocannabinol (THC). It is sold under the trade name Marinol® in gelatin capsules for oral administration. Marinol is used for stimulating appetite and preventing weight loss in patients with confirmed diagnoses of AIDS, for treating nausea and vomiting associated with cancer chemotherapy, and in the management of glaucoma. The MRO should request that the donor submit a copy of her medical record or court order authorizing the legal use of Marinol or marijuana.

There is a variety of prescription and nonprescription drugs that contain morphine, codeine, or the byproducts of opium. As mentioned earlier, though, the use of heroin can be differentiated from these other drugs in that the 6-acetylmorphine metabolite comes only from heroin. Its presence in the urine confirms the illegal use of heroin.

40.9 LEGAL ASPECTS OF WORKPLACE DRUG TESTING

The implementation and enforcement of a workplace drug testing program are always subject to lawsuits by affected employees or state and federal legal guidelines. The development of a program must consider the potential legal ramifications. The legal basis for a workplace program review and criticism may come from several sources, including constitutionality issues (right to privacy, freedom from unreasonable searches, due process), negligence or libel and slander, contract law, and discrimination. Constitutional issues generally arise in the public sector but may apply to private-sector employers under specific circumstances. However, the other three areas are applicable to all employers.

40.9.1 Constitutional Issues

Opponents of workplace drug testing often argue the fundamental right to privacy and the intrusiveness of the drug collection procedure. The Fourth Amendment to the Constitution affords an individual the right to be free from an unreasonable search and seizure by the government. Any unreasonable intrusion must be justified by the law. This amendment, in addition to the Fourteenth Amendment's allowance for due process, is the two major constitutional arguments cited in workplace drug testing litigation.[78]

By implication, the Fourth Amendment affords an individual the right to privacy. The concept of an individual's right to a constitutional-based "zone of privacy" was recognized in the 1965 case *Griswold v. Connecticut* (381 U.S. 479).[79] In the *Griswold* case, citizens were accorded a "zone of privacy" free of government intrusion and recognized an individual's right to be "let alone." The U.S. Supreme Court unanimously held that mandatory drug testing is a "search," under the Fourth Amendment in the case of *Samuel K. Skinner v. Railway Labor Executives Association* (489 U.S. 602). However, the court also held that when drug testing was performed within an employment context, the intrusion was justifiable and did not unnecessarily infringe on privacy interests (*Samuel K. Skinner v. Railway Labor Executives Association*, 489 U.S. 602, p. 625). Proponents of workplace drug testing argue that this and other court rulings are not "adequate for describing the employee's claim to privacy in an essentially social and cooperative setting like the workplace."[80] To date, it appears that the prevalent view in the workforce is that workplace drug testing is not an undue intrusion of privacy rights when the standards for employment are clearly communicated to the prospective employee, and there is a subsequent contractual basis for reasonable continued performance monitoring.

The due process provision of the Fourteenth Amendment prohibits states from denying federal constitutional rights and does not generally apply to private citizens or entities.[81] The authority of Congress to enforce the Fourteenth Amendment, Section 1983 of Title 42 of the U.S. Code, prohibits interference with federal rights under color of state law. In fact, in 1966, the Supreme Court stated, "In cases under Section 1983, 'under color' of law has consistently been treated as the same thing as 'state action' required under the Fourteenth Amendment."[82] Therefore, a private employer's action of drug testing, or discharge due to a "dirty" test, can be seen as state action in some circumstances. According to case law, a private employer's action may be considered "state action" and thus regulated under the Fourteenth Amendment if any of the following four are true:[83]

- The employer derives his income from the government.
- The employer is controlled by "extensive and detailed" regulation by the state.
- The function of the employer is "traditionally the exclusive prerogative" of the state.
- There is a "symbiotic relationship" between the employer and the government.

Similarly, the Fourth Amendment applies to government actions and generally is not applicable to private-sector drug testing. A warrant is generally required for a search to be considered reasonable under the Fourth Amendment.[84] However, in regulated industries, an exception to the warrant requirement was developed for searches of premises pursuant to an administrative inspection scheme.[85] There are two requirements that justify the unwarranted administrative search exception. One is a strong state interest in conducting an unannounced search. Additionally, the pervasive regulation of the industry has reduced the justifiable privacy expectation of the subject of the search.

40.9.2 State and Federal Mandates

An employer must be aware of the myriad state and federal mandates that affect the company's workplace drug testing policy and implementation of the program. The DOT regulations and the Federal Workplace Act of 1988 have already been briefly discussed. The following are additional mandates to consider:

- The National Labor Relations Act
- Title VII of the Civil Rights Act of 1964
- The Americans with Disabilities Act of 1990
- The Rehabilitation Act of 1973
- State drug testing laws and city ordinances

Title VII of the Civil Rights Act of 1964 applies to all private-sector employees with 15 or more employees and prohibits discrimination against applicants or employees based on race, religion, sex, or national origin.[86] Disparities in sanctions, reasonable-cause testing, or a drug testing policy that unfairly impacts a protested class may prompt a Title VII charge. Thus, applying policies evenly and without bias is critical to the successful implementation of a drug-free workplace program.

State drug testing laws may also place restrictions on an employer's right to implement random drug testing or to require certain aspects of a program to be in place. For example, the California Department of Health Services prohibits drug tests performed by anyone other than a certified laboratory or licensed physician.[87] California also requires that employers with 25 or more employees must accommodate employees who wish to participate in a substance abuse treatment program, provided the accommodation does not place an undue hardship on the employer.[88] On the other hand, Rhode Island allows drug testing only when

> the employer has reasonable grounds to believe based on specific aspects of the employee's job performance and on specific contemporaneous observations, capable of being articulated, concerning the employee's appearance, behavior or speech that the employee's use of controlled substances is impairing his or her ability to perform his or her job.[89]

The confidentiality of medical records and communications in a doctor–patient relationship is generally upheld. A cause of action may be charged, and damages may be awarded when there is an improper disclosure of confidential records or information. State statutes regarding unemployment compensation should also be considered since a positive drug test may be considered "misconduct" and render a discharged employee ineligible for unemployment compensation. For these reasons, it is highly recommended that employers have a legal professional review the proposed program and policies for compliance with the relevant state and local regulations.

The Americans with Disabilities Act of 1990 (ADA) is applicable to employers with 15 or more employees.[90] Title I of the ADA prohibits employment discrimination against a "qualified individual with a disability." Among other "qualified individuals," a person who is currently not using drugs and who is participating in or has completed a supervised drug rehabilitation program may also qualify.[91] The ADA specifically permits employers to adopt drug testing policies and expressly excludes drug testing as part of the prohibition against medical inquiries of a "qualified individual's" disability. In fact, a "qualified individual" expressly does not include an individual who is currently engaged in the use of illegal drugs.[92] The Rehabilitation Act of 1973 is similar to the ADA but protests a narrower class of individuals—"handicapped" persons—from certain types of discrimination by the federal government, federal contractors, and federal grantees.[93] A "handicapped" person may include an employee who is an "addict" and who has sought treatment voluntarily.[94] However, occasional users are not considered handicapped and are therefore not protected. Here, as with the ADA of 1990, employers are not prohibited from testing employees.[95]

The 1982 National Labor Relations Act was developed to promote, among other things, the flow of commerce and establish legitimate rights for both employers and employees.[96] Employee drug testing issues were addressed in this updated version of the 1947 Labor Management Relations Act. Case law has established that drug testing of current employees, not applicants, is a mandatory subject of collective-bargaining agreements and union contracts.[97]

Employers who hire workers who belong to a union or collective-bargaining unit need to consult with union representatives or union bylaws. Incorporation of workplace drug testing policies that are acceptable to collective-bargaining agreements is the first step toward running a smooth company program.

Clinical Laboratory Improvement Amendments of 1988 (CLIA '88) was created to establish uniform testing standards in the clinical field. Laboratories that are HHS-certified under the NLCP are specifically exempt from the requirements set forth under CLIA '88. The exemption is limited to the certified laboratories' immunoassay screening and GC/MS confirmatory testing processes for the five drug classes (HHS-5) stated in the guidelines. Certified laboratories that perform tests with procedures not in accordance with the guidelines or by methods not certified by HHS are subject to the technical and regulatory requirements of CLIA '88.

40.10 DISCOVERY: THE "LITIGATION PACKAGE"

By the time cases are filed, specimens may get lost or become unsuitable for re-testing. In these instances, the litigation package—all of the documents pertaining to the case—is the only evidence that can be used to evaluate the reliability of the analysis. The litigation package must include:

1. The CCF. The Custody and Control Form (CCF) documents the circumstances around the sample collection, including the identity of the specimen, the condition of the specimen, and the chain-of-custody. On this form, as well, any irregularities surrounding the collection (for example, the need for an affidavit of correction) or discrepancies in labeling are noted.
2. The preliminary screening data. The screening data will include the results of the calibrators (low/high) and controls (blank/quality control) and the results of the cases in question. Also included should be evidence of integrity testing, such as creatinine, nitrates, or specific gravity. Also recommended are the following:
   - The SOP, including criteria for acceptance of the data for the calibrators, controls, and case, and specificity testing (evaluation of other drugs which may cause a false positive).
   - The manufacturer's assay kit insert describing the required procedure and cross-reactivities of other drugs with the assay.
3. The confirmation data. Confirmation is performed with GC/MS or related technologies such as GC/MS/MS, LC/MS, or LC/MS/MS. Data should include the spectrograms for the calibrators and controls as well as the case sample. Some laboratories use a historical (established monthly etc.) calibration curve and one calibrator and control. Also recommended for evaluation are the following:
   - The standard operating procedure (SOP), including the extraction method (chemical preparation of the specimen prior to testing on the GC/MS); criteria for acceptance of the data for the calibrators, controls, and case sample; criteria for acceptable chromatography; specificity (evaluation of other drugs which may cause a false-positive) testing; and data establishing of the LOD and limit of quantitation.
   - Maintenance and standard tune (evaluation of the working parameters of the machine for the day) data for the instrument (e.g., GC/MS).
4. Results of proficiency tests (SAMHSA and others) for two years prior to and after the case in question. This should include any reports of noncompliance or errors in identification or quantity found.

40.11 CASE REPORTS

CASE REPORT 1: POSITIVE COCAINE TESTING IN HAIR SAMPLE

Mr. R had an accident at the auto plant and had a mandatory urine test, which was positive for cocaine. According to Mr. R, he was required to go to Serenity for an outpatient drug treatment program for 21 days. While there, he tested positive again (urine test). This was May 2007. He had hair tests "every three months," and his December 2007 hair test was positive (8.3 ng/10mg cocaine; 2.9 ng/10mg benzoylecgonine—BE); a MediTest test on December 19, 2007, was negative. At this time, he was told he had one "last chance"—one more time and he is out. On March 22, 2008, he was tested for hair (positive for cocaine 24.2 ng/10 mg; BE 2.6 ng/10 mg). A urine test by MediTest was negative. On his own initiative, Mr. R had his hair sampled and tested by Acculab Laboratories on March 29, and the report came back cocaine positive 1236 pg/mg.

OPINIONS

In my opinion, the March 22, 2008, and the March 29, 2008 positives are likely due to residual cocaine in the hair, which can stay for several months. That is, these tests in March are identifying the same cocaine and metabolite found in the December 2007 test. The quantities measured are miniscule and, put in perspective, considering that billionths of a gram (pg = picogram) are being measured, do not vary substantially. Further, variance in sampling from time to time and location to location is well described. In my opinion, the "positive" tests conducted in March 2008 do not provide evidence of re-use of cocaine; thus, there is no evidence supporting a "last chance" violation.

There are many shortcomings with hair testing for drugs, one of which is the imprecision of determining when the exposure occurs, and the possibility that subsequent positives (like the March 2008 tests) are not really caused by re-use, but, rather, the cocaine staying in the hair shaft until the hair is cut off or falls off the scalp. Extensive discussions of this phenomenon, the variability between samples taken from different locations on the scalp and samples taken at different times, and the increased binding of cocaine in African American hair are discussed at length in the following text discussion.

CASE REPORT 2: ALCOHOL IMPAIRMENT DURING A VEHICLE COLLISION/DRAM SHOP

An intoxicated Mr. D collided with Ms. C's vehicle, causing serious injuries to himself, Ms. C, and her child—a passenger in her car. The collision occurred at 7:58 on June 5, 2015. Law enforcement considered Mr. D intoxicated. Serum alcohol was tested at 10:48, which showed 0.127 g/dL. While in treatment with EMS, Mr. D was administered 2 L of normal saline. While in treatment and transport by/with air evac, Mr. D was administered 3 L of normal saline. Mr. D was arrested for felony DUI, pled guilty, and was sentenced to a period of home confinement. Mr. D worked as a cook in the kitchen at a bar on the day of the accident. He left work at 4:30 pm and returned to the bar at 5:00 pm. He paid for six rum drinks with cash. The tab was paid at 7:46. The drinking started at 5:00 pm, and the last drink was served at 7:20–7:30 pm. For purposes of calculating absorption and BACs, it is assumed that the drinks were served at 5:00, 5: 30, 6:00, 6:30, 7:00, and 7:20–7:30 pm, and consumption was continuous. Mr. W served Mr. D drinks at 6:00 pm and 6:30 pm; Mr. H served the last two of the six drinks. The toxicologist calculated the amount consumed as the equivalent of nine standard drinks, 1.5-ounce 80-proof alcohol, suggesting that Mr. D was over served. The bar is being sued for serving alcohol to a person who was "visibly intoxicated," over-serving, failure to count and pace drinks, failure to mitigate, and failure to prevent a "visibly intoxicated" patron from driving a vehicle.

Bartender Mr. H testified that Mr. D was noticeably intoxicated. "He went from being fine to what I call a buzz to intoxicated pretty quickly, all of a sudden." He testified that he observed, served, and talked with him for about an hour and a half. Mr. H described Mr. D having "glassy eyes, slurred speech, overall motor skills dash poor." He testified that he later saw him leaving the back door, followed him out, and told him he couldn't drive—"I took your keys"—but apparently Mr. D had a second set of keys in this vehicle, which allowed him to drive his vehicle. He described him as "definitely not walking straight, stumbling a little bit, he had the appearance of someone that was intoxicated." He crashed approximately ten minutes later. Bartender Mr. H served Mr. D his fifth drink at approximately 7:00 pm and his last drink at approximately 7:30 PM.

DEFENSE TOXICOLOGY EXPERT OPINIONS AND BASES

1. The toxicologist opined that if only six drinks were consumed per the cash receipt, each drink must have had an additional 50% volume, 2.25 ounces instead of 1.5 ounces.
2. The toxicologist opined that retrograde extrapolation from the time of the alcohol test, 10:48 pm, could not be performed to the time the last drink was served, 7:30 pm.
3. The toxicologist calculated the BAC at the time of serving the sixth drink with the goal of determining if the calculated BAC was above or below 150 mg/dL (0.150 g/dL), a level that was reported in a 1932 publication, translated from German, that concluded that greater than 50% of subjects would be visibly intoxicated with a BAC of 0.150 g/dL. (The data for the 0150 g/dL includes subjects whose BACs ranged from 141 to 160 g/dL.) This discussion and BAC level has been repeated several times in subsequent years, including statements like "this definition is set at an alcohol concentration at which there is no doubt of obvious intoxication (excess of 50%)."
4. The toxicologist used certain parameters on serum alcohol to blood alcohol conversions, metabolic rate, and absorption rates. The toxicologist opined that since the Sprite mixer in the rum drink contains sugar, that the scientific consensus describing rapid transit time from the stomach to the small intestine (through the pyloric valve) did not apply, and that the expected rapid absorption time of an empty stomach would

not apply. The toxicologist cited two published papers evaluating the effect of sugar versus no sugar on the BAC on absorption rates. Marzynski studied 16 subjects and found breath-alcohol measures were higher in the diet drinks compared to regular sugar mixtures. Wu studied eight male subjects and concluded that the substitution of artificial sweeteners for sugars in mixed alcoholic drinks potentially has a profound impact on BACs. The implications expressed by the toxicologist in his deposition are that sugar in the mixer slows gastric emptying and thus slows the absorption rate similar to the fed state.

5. The toxicologist was asked about any dilution effect of the administration of 3 L normal saline to Mr. D during the AirEvac flight. He dismissed the potential dilution and BAC lowering effect of the three liters of normal saline and used a standard volume of distribution of 0.65 L, not the usual Widmark V_d (0.7 L/kg) applied to males.
6. The toxicologist calculated/estimated the BAC at the time of the fifth drink (~7:00 pm) as a range from 0.111 g/dL to 0.121 g/dL. The "Dram shop model" calculated Mr. D's BAC concentration at the time of the serving of his sixth (final) drink—7:20–7:30 pm, at 0.129–0.144 g/dL. The range is caused by substituting different *beta* factors (metabolic rates) 0.015–0.020, with an average of 0.017 g/dL, thus different results.
7. The toxicologist opined that "nonetheless, it is clear that when Mr. D was served his last drink at the bar, his BAC would have been lower than the level reported to consistently cause outward signs of impairment in at least 50% of the population. Even with the highly conservative calculations, his BAC was never above the point at which impairment is observed in more than 50% of the population."
8. The toxicologist opined that alcohol produces well-documented effects in humans that become more predictable as the amount of alcohol consumed rises. Also, it is unquestionable that alcohol impairs many different sensory and motor skills essential to operating any motor vehicle, and it does so in a dose-dependent fashion.
9. The toxicologist had no opinion on whether Mr. D was visibly intoxicated at the time of the serving of the sixth drink. "I don't know how to answer that question."
10. The toxicologist opined that Mr. D was solely responsible for his alcohol consumption.
11. The toxicologist testified, "There's not enough information for me to determine whether or not he is a social drinker or whether he's a binge drinker or whether he's a constant drinker."
12. The toxicologist referred to a "peer reviewed dram shop model"; he testified that he developed the model and presented it at a conference; he considered it to be "peer-reviewed" based on the fact that it was presented at a conference.
13. The toxicologist discounted any effect of marijuana on Mr. D, based on the urine toxicology screen positive.

OPINIONS OF PLAINTIFF'S PHARMACOLOGIST EXPERTS

1. Mr. D was intoxicated at the following times:
   - He was so visibly intoxicated prior to leaving the bar that the server took his keys. He was visibly intoxicated at or before the serving of the sixth drink. This is based on my review of the undisputed testimony of the server.
   - Ten minutes after he left the bar, he lost control of his vehicle and crashed into Ms. C and her six-year-old daughter. He was intoxicated based on his blood alcohol of 0.127, which was measured 2 hours and 50 minutes after the collision.
   - Serving a gentleman of the size and weight of Mr. D, it is expected that after four drinks, he would be intoxicated by well-known scientific research and literature.
   - To a reasonable prudent server of alcohol, Mr. D would have been visibly intoxicated by the ingestion of alcohol at the subject bar prior to the fifth and sixth drinks he was served.
2. Mr. D was certainly visibly intoxicated at the time the last drink was served. Mr. H described an instant change in sobriety to an intoxication state while talking with Mr. D for an hour and a half. "He went from being fine to what I call a buzz too intoxicated pretty quickly—all of a sudden—probably within the hour and a half we were talking. He had glassy eyes, slurred speech, overall motor skills were poor." Mr. H's testimony is pharmacologically impossible. Alcohol actions are dose related. The higher the dose, the higher the BAC, the more manifestations consistent with the anticipated BAC. They do not appear "all of a sudden." This is a basic concept. Based on the toxicologist's report, I assume he would agree with me. Mr. H's testimony of Mr. D's obvious, visible intoxication would have been present at the time of the serving of the sixth drink, and most likely before (the fifth drink).

3.Mr. D rarely drank alcohol, twice a year according to his deposition. He would not have developed any type of tolerance to the effects of alcohol or adjusted the effects of alcohol as suggested by the toxicologist.

Therefore, any suggestion by the toxicologist that Mr. D had tolerance or behavioral tolerance and was able to mask outward signs of alcohol intoxication is not relevant; indeed, it is scientifically inaccurate. The toxicologist testified that he had insufficient information to determine social, binge, or constant drinking status. Based on Mr. D's testimony, I consider him a "social drinker." As such, "6 drinks" over 2 hours (4 × 2.25 oz), in my opinion, would more likely than not cause "visible intoxication" in Mr. D—the serving of the fifth drink.

4. A few months earlier Mr. D was "cut off," and no more alcohol was served by "Mr. L," a bartender on duty. Same bar, same drink, same person, same amount of alcohol. Therefore, it is more likely than not that his visible intoxication at the prior "cutoff" experience would manifest at five drinks on June 5.

5. As a novice drinker, assuming that all the alcohol in the first four drinks was absorbed, it is my opinion that Mr. D would manifest visible signs of intoxication. This would be apparent at 7:00 pm (the fifth drink).
6. Mr. D was administered 2000 mL of normal saline by EMS, and 3000 mL by air evac, a total of 5000 mL fluid boluses. Physiologically, his blood had to be diluted to some extent, thus lowering the reported alcohol concentration result. Absent mass dilution, Mr. D's BAC at 10:48 pm would have been higher than the 127 mg/dL reported. For the same physiological reasons, the volume of distribution would be larger. Five liters of normal saline represents a 6% to 7% increase in the total body water (incidentally the volume of distribution of alcohol). Mr. D had a low hematocrit shortly after admission. Low hematocrits imply greater water content in the blood. Any calculations or conversions of the hospital serum tests would be affected by this artificial dilution effect.
7. The toxicologist's calculations using a delayed food effect time of one hour caused by Sprite regular are new and novel and not a consensus in the scientific community. While two studies were provided and discussed the delaying absorption effects on a total of 24 subjects, this does not change the science. The alcohol toxicology community, and consensus literature in that community, is silent on "sugared mixer" slowing gastric emptying and thus absorption. The current discussion in Garriott's *Medical Legal Aspects of Alcohol*[98] describes gastric transit time and subsequent absorption rapidly and does not differentiate based on sugar-containing beverages. An empty stomach or full stomach and the type of food are the major determinants of the rate of absorption. *Garriott* excerpts may be found on page 217 of the sixth edition. Absorption through the stomach wall is slow whereas the absolute option from the swollen testing is rapid. Therefore, anything that delays the emptying time of the stomach will slow the absorption of alcohol. The rate of flow from the stomach to the small intestine is controlled by the pyloric valve, situated at the base of the stomach, which opens and closes to control the passage of solids, semi-solids, and liquids. Food in the stomach slows stomach emptying time; hence absorption of alcohol is delayed. This applies to eating while drinking and to eating shortly before drinking; loss of blood alcohol level will have a lower peak and a lower rise to that level following a meal, compared to consumption on an empty stomach. The rate of absorption varies from person to person. Generally, most alcohol is absorbed in 30 minutes in a fasting person after a single dose; nearly 90% is absorbed within one hour when drinks are consumed successively. When several drinks are consumed in a very short period of time, maximum blood alcohol levels may be delayed until 45 minutes or longer after ingestion of the last drink to summarize factors which delay stomach emptying time such as food in the stomach or large amounts of strong or dilute drink lead to a lower BAC compared to blood levels attained from rapid absorption in the small intestine as a result of increased stomach motility absorption rate depends on the concentration composition and amount of alcohol ingested is slowing down and strong beverages is fastest for about a 20% solution the slow absorption is due to a delayed evacuation of the stomach and irritation of the gastrointestinal laws. Maximum absorption and in turn maximum blood concentrations following alcohol are taken in moderate amounts. The presence of carbon dioxide in carbonated beverages, sparkling wines, and champagne promotes evacuation of the stomach, which in turn enhances the absorption of alcohol.
8. The toxicologist's "Peer reviewed Dram Shop Model" is not "peer reviewed." A poster at a scientific meeting does not ordain "peer review."
9. The toxicologist's use of 0.65 L/kg volume of distribution is incorrect. The common "rho" factor (Vd) for alcohol for men is 0.7 L/kg. The figure is 0.6 L/kg women, owing to their high percentage of body fat, and thus less percentage of body water. Since alcohol distributes in water and not in fat, the same alcohol content given to a man and a woman of normal weight for height will result in higher BAC in the woman because the volume of distribution is smaller. The larger the volume of distribution, the lower the BAC; The smaller the Vd, the higher the BAC. Current literature recommends a body mass index (BMI) calculation be made. The mean variable is proportional to fat to lean tissue in the body, which in turn depends on age, gender, and obesity as reflected in the BMI.

10. Mr. D's calculated Vd is 0.53 L/kg, based on his height and weight (18.5% lower than the 0.65 L/kg Vd used by the toxicologist).
11. Mr. D is not normal weight. He is obese. His height and weight are calculated to a BMI equal to 32.3 (obese); thus any "peer-reviewed Dramshop calculators" will underestimate the BAC, since the volume of distribution of 0.65 used by the toxicologist is too high for Mr. D. The higher the BMI, the lower the volume of distribution: the lower the volume of distribution, the higher the BAC.
12. The 150 mg (0.150 g/dL) criteria for frank or obvious intoxication of the majority of people tested includes a range of 140–160 milligrams for that grouping. Thus, even the toxicologist's calculations are in this range (144) and therefore would meet the criteria for a greater than 50% probability of visible intoxication. Brick[99] includes a description of an alcohol concentration of 0.15 g/dL at which there is no doubt of obvious intoxication.
13. Brick and Bennett[100] published a report on alcohol calculations in emergency and forensic medicine reports subjects who were measured with a peak BAC of approximately 30 minutes post-drinking. If drinking is constant then absorption is also constant, so the peak is not always at the end of the cessation of the drink. Brick (2009) states, "It's reasonable to expect the intoxicated person would be under the influence as a result of the amount served; this means that servers need to count the drinks."
14. The bartenders failed to count drinks and anticipate intoxication based on the amount and volume and frequency of drinks served—they should have anticipated intoxication and ceased serving.
15. The positive marijuana drug screen does not support using marijuana at a particular time. There is no evidence that Mr. D smoked marijuana in the 10–12 minutes after leaving the bar and the collision with Ms. C.
16. Using the corrected Vd and absorption time of 30 and a metabolic rate of 0.015 g/dL/hour, I calculate the BAC at the time of serving the sixth drink a BAC of 0.147.5 g/dL. The metabolic rate of 0.015 g/dL/hour metabolic elimination rate is selected based on the (stated) alcohol history (social drinker) of Mr. D. The 30" absorption time is justified because of the empty stomach and type of alcoholic beverage.

Subject parameters for the BAC estimation:

Wt = 200 lb = 90.9 kg Vd = 0.5295 L/kg
Rate of elimination = 0.015 g/dL/hr
Absorption rate = 30 min; 21 g ethanol per "drink" 80 proof (40% ABV)

Mr. D himself is a good clinical model. At an earlier time—months before—Mr. D was in the bar, and the bartender stopped serving him after five drinks, ostensibly because he was visibly intoxicated. In this case, considering all the evidence, in my opinion, Mr. D would have been visibly intoxicated before the sixth drink was served. Mr. D was arrested and pled guilty to driving drunk. Mr. D left the bar at the completion of the sixth drink. Trial in this matter is scheduled for Spring of 2023.

CASE REPORT 3: POTENTIAL DRUG IMPAIRMENT DURING A TRAFFIC STOP

On June 16, 2020, at 8:07 pm, Mr. G was driving his truck and mistakenly drove through an intersection on a red light (left turn green was activated). This was witnessed by PD Officer H, who executed a traffic stop one block away. Mr. G immediately stated that he went through the intersection on a red light (paraphrased). On questioning about alcohol and drugs, Mr. G admitted consumption of one 16 oz Bud Lite beer and his usual early evening medications, duloxetine and trazodone. Mr. G also answered questions about any infirmities/health conditions. Field Sobriety Tests were administered (HGN, VGN, WNT, OLS), and Mr. G was placed under arrest, handcuffed, placed in Officer H's squad car, and taken in for booking. He was then taken to a local hospital for a blood sample for toxicology testing. The toxicology report noted trazodone 1669 ng/mL, lamotrigine 1.8 μg/mL (mcg), duloxetine 25 ng/mL, and ethanol (alcohol)—none detected.

Officer H is not a drug recognition evaluation (DRE) trained/certified officer. Specific observations/comments by Officer H include the following:

1. Eyes bloodshot and watery; speech slightly slurred; odor of alcoholic beverage emitting from his breath; (slightly) unsteady balance, slurred, thick-tongued speech, Drug Group suspected—CNS depressant. During the consent blood draw, the defendant stated he took 1 trazodone 150 mg and two (2) melatonin 5 mg at approximately 5:30 hours on the offense date (different than the narrative report and video). At the time of the chemical test, did the defendant appear to be more or less intoxicated than the roadside investigation? "About the same."

2. "Mr. G stated he consumed prescription sleep medication (Trazodone 150 mg) at approximately 5:30 hours."
3. ". . . did not feel impaired of buzzed and believed he could properly operate a motor vehicle."
4. HGN; lack of smooth pursuit in both eyes, distinct and sustained nystagmus at maximum deviation in both eyes, and onset of nystagmus prior to 45 degrees. Negative VGN.
5. WNT: Started too soon ("this is what you have to do"), miss heel to toe, step off (imaginary) line.
6. OLS: Put his leg down (after ~13 seconds) and resumed; use his arms for balance (rarely).
7. Small amount of an alcoholic beverage found in truck (other officer stated "empty").
8. Officer H noted: I believe he lost the normal use of his physical and mental faculties due to the consumption of alcoholic beverages and prescription sleep medication.
9. Taken to the hospital, a specimen of his blood was drawn by a nurse at 9:39 hours.
10. Mr. G was charged with Driving While Intoxicated W/Child under 15 YOA, Driving While intoxicated.

INTERVIEW OF MR. G

Mr. G was taking his usually prescribed medications, some of which had been changed since the arrest date. He reported drinking a 16 oz Bud-Light at home that evening (6–6:30 pm) using the same Arctic cup that he keeps in his truck for coffee. He took his trazodone at ~ 6:30 pm. He always takes the (OTC) melatonin at ~9:00 pm; "Otherwise it wears off when I need it to go to sleep." He admits that he mistakenly drove through a red-light intersection and has been confused by the left green arrow and moving traffic on prior occasions. He reports a "hereditary insomnia," "my mother has it too; I noticed it in college"; he has trouble getting to sleep (his medical records list pathophysiological insomnia). He (mistakenly) thought the trazodone was used for sleep; "because of my hereditary insomnia, I must take sleep meds in the early evening to be able to fall asleep ~ midnight." He brought the phone very close to his eyes, which appeared "red and bloodshot"; clinical description—conjunctiva injection. He also showed me several lubricating eyedrops that he uses chronically for his eyes, which apparently become red and bloodshot due to environmental pollen.

OPINIONS

1. Mr. G was not intoxicated, not under the influence, and not impaired by either alcohol or any prescription medications at the time of the traffic stop/arrest—6/16/20; 8:07 pm
2. The medications reported in the toxicology report (duloxetine, lamotrigine, trazodone) were:
   a. Legally prescribed.
   c. Detected/reported at subtherapeutic (Lamotrigine) or therapeutic (duloxetine, Trazodone) levels and therefore would not be expected to cause any significant CNS depression that would affect driving (cognition, motor function).
   d. Used chronically and monitored by his physician. On questioning, he denied any somnolence as a result of using duloxetine and trazodone early evening. He stated melatonin was used several hours later (~9:00 pm), as the effect would wear off if taken in the early evening.
   d. The prescribing physician never noted or observed any signs of drug impairment/abuse in his records and has provided a letter stating so.
3. The FSTs are "near perfect." There are no signs of impairment of balance, gait, or speech.
4. Mr. G was conversant, articulate, courteous, and cooperative demonstrated no signs of confusion and was in full control of his faculties.
5. Mr. G's speech sounded the same on the arrest videos as on the FaceTime video. His eyes were "bloodshot." Watery eyes is too non-specific to comment. Mr. G reported (and sent me a picture of various) lubricating eye drops for chronic eye irritation (red/injected/"bloodshot") eyes.
6. FSTs are not validated for any prescription medications. They are validated (NHTSA) for alcohol and potentially may be valid for marijuana. Even for alcohol, FST are clue of impairment, not evidence.
7. Mr. G has long been diagnosed with physiological insomnia (noticed in college). His mother has the same condition. This may explain the need for early evening administration of Trazodone to counteract the SSRI stimulation that contributes to insomnia.
8. Trazodone, an antidepressant, is not a sleep medication. It is prescribed commonly in patients using antidepressants (like duloxetine) that cause insomnia due to stimulant effects. Trazodone may cause drowsiness, but that effect usually dissipates with therapeutic use; otherwise it is discontinued. If taken at bedtime, any drowsiness effects are inconsequential and may not even be evident to the patient.
   a. Data from a meta-analysis of a limited number of controlled trials in patients with and without comorbid conditions (including Alzheimer's disease, depression, and opioid dependence) suggest that trazodone may be beneficial in the short-term to decrease the number of awakenings and improve sleep quality in patients with insomnia.

CASE REPORT 4: OPIATE-INDUCED HOMICIDE

Mr. H was found by his girlfriend Ms. K unresponsive at approximately 8:00 am on Sunday morning, June 9, 2019. Ms. K administered several doses of Narcan to Mr. H, as did her mother and sister and EMS. EMS was called. EMS was unable to resuscitate Mr. H. He was declared dead at the scene. An autopsy was performed by a pathologist on June 11, 2019. The immediate cause of death is listed as adverse effects of heroin, fentanyl, and acetyl fentanyl. The right and left lungs weigh 1130 and 1120 grams, respectively; the pulmonary parenchyma is purple showing severe vascular congestion and edema. The brain shows moderate edema. A history of drug (heroin and marijuana) abuse is noted. Blood, urine, and vitreous samples (were) collected at autopsy. Specimens analyzed: blood and urine. Ms. K was later arrested and charged with drug-induced homicide.

TOXICOLOGY

Axis Toxicology Labs
Peripheral Blood
7-aminodoclonazepam 37.5 ng/ml (metabolite of clonazepam)
THC (marijuana active) 1.4 ng/ml; THC-COOH (inactive metabolite) 8.7 ng/ml
Morphine 9.5 ng/ml
Fentanyl 11.2 ng/ml
Acetyl fentanyl 7,211 pg/ml; (7.21 ng/ml) "designer-synthetic" fentanyl analog
Positive for 4-ANPP (an intermediate precursor in the synthesis of fentanyl)
Urine
7-aminodoclonazepam, fentanyl, norfentanyl (metabolite of fentanyl)
Morphine (heroin converts immediately to morphine); codeine (an impurity of heroin and morphine)
6-MAM (metabolite of heroin)
Codeine
ISP Rockford Crime Lab
Six clear baggies with small basketball emblems, each containing gray/brown powder substance: fentanyl

INTERVIEW OF MS. K

The evening of Mr. H's death, Ms. K drove her car to Chicago. Mr. H was her passenger. She would not have driven to Chicago alone, especially to an area where drugs could be purchased. She described a previous experience where she had been there, someone put a gun to her head, and she feared she was being abducted. Mr. H could not drive. His car was damaged in a DUI accident; he didn't have a valid driver's license. While driving to Chicago, Mr. H used Ms. K's phone GPS and gave instructions to Ms. K. When they arrived in Westside Chicago, a male came to their car and spoke to Mr. H. That person gave Mr. H two "samples" of heroin and his phone number and asked Mr. H to call his phone then and in the future to contact him for drug purchases. That person later called Ms. K's phone and spoke to Mr. H. Mr. H gave one (sample) bag to Ms. K, and both snorted the contents of the bag. Then Mr. H left the car, went into an alley, and came back to her car. Mr. H returned from the alley and took eight or nine colored baggies out of his pocket and gave them to her. Ms. K then drove to a restaurant where Mr. H purchased ~$30.00 of food, which they ate outside the restaurant. They each snorted the contents of one bag (from their own respective supply) either at the restaurant or on the way back to her home. At no time did Ms. K see or use any "basketball" bags of drugs. Once home, they both stayed together in her room. Later that evening, each used another bag of heroin from their own respective supplies. They spent the evening watching TV and "hanging out." They went to sleep at ~ 3–3:30 am. Ms. K last saw Mr. H alive at ~ 7:00 am; they spoke, he was out of bed, standing. He then got back into bed with her. An hour later she discovered him unresponsive and unable to wake him up, "freaked out," screamed, her mother and sister came to her room, attempted CPR, called 911, and several doses of Narcan were given intramuscularly without response. EMS arrived and was also unsuccessful in reviving Mr. H. Mr. H was pronounced dead at 8:42 am on June 9, 2019.

Ms. K and Mr. H were friends and had used drugs together and with a large group of (drug using) friends since she was 13. She was not sure when they became girlfriend/boyfriend. Extensive use of alcohol, cocaine, marijuana, LSD, Ecstasy, and heroin were the drugs used; eventually, heroin became their drug of choice. Most of their drugs were purchased by Mr. H's "best friend" and neighbor, a "drug dealer" who "supplied the neighborhood" and was "known and surveilled by the Police." Heroin use was by snorting, never by needle injection or smoking. Ms. K tried to control excessive use of heroin (she tried to stop and did stop from time to time), she had very little money for it, and she wanted to be able to wake up (not sick) and go to work. She described Mr. H's drug use, including heroin, as "take as much as he got to get as high as he could." Ms. K "OD'd" once (overdose). EMS was called. Mr. H "OD'd" ten times, three of which he was resuscitated by EMS and other times by friends. Both Ms. K and Mr. H had been to several detox (detoxifications) treatments, as well as residential rehabilitation. Both were in a MAT (Medication Assisted Treatment)—methadone treatment center. Ms. K was in the MAT for ~10 months, Mr. H for a shorter period—"he was locked up."

On the day of Mr. H's death, Ms. K snorted (two bags) of heroin before the police arrived ("devastated") and four bags after the police arrived. She was concerned about a search warrant; she hoped that she would "not wake up" from the heroin herself. On that day, she was immediately admitted to a detoxification center and then transferred to a Rehab treatment center, where she stayed for 109 days. Since discharge from Rehab, she has been employed. She is on pre-trial probation, which includes weekly urine drug tests (until COVID-19); all drug tests have been negative. She has been and is currently treated by Dr. BD with Suboxone (MAT), which is helping her—it has eliminated her craving for heroin.

OPINIONS

1. Mr. H was a long-term heroin addict; each time he used heroin he risked death.
2. Only blood levels are useful in determining drug effects or intoxication. Urine levels only serve to document that a particular drug has been used within a detection period.
3. Mr. H suffered fatal fentanyl intoxication. Fentanyl was found at lethal levels. Acetylfentanyl, common contaminant of "heroin" spiked with or substituted with fentanyl, was found in very low levels.
4. Morphine was found in subtherapeutic levels, even for a naïve acute user for moderate to severe analgesia.
5. The fentanyl alone is detected at lethal levels. Death would have occurred without exposure to acetylfentanyl and/or morphine.
6. Mr. H and Ms. K used the same "heroin" source twice on the evening of the 9th. That "heroin" used did not cause or contribute to Mr. H's death. The heroin was effective. Ms. K reports it created a high, which wore off, and then another bag was used. Both were awake and functioning throughout the evening, albeit "high," communicating, watching TV, having sex, and so on. Both were awake at 7:00 am; Mr. H was up and walking and talking. Ms. K used six bags on June 9. While she was noticeably intoxicated and the police suspected she was using drugs, she did not suffer serious or fatal opiate intoxication.
7. Mr. H's "shoe stash," that is, the six bags of gray-brown fentanyl found in "basketball" baggies, contained no heroin, morphine, or codeine. This is an alternate source of the heroin used by Ms. K and Mr. H the evening prior to his death. Had Ms. K used "heroin" from the "basketball" baggies, she most likely would have died as well. Ms. K denied ever seeing any "basketball" baggies, using any drugs from any "basketball" baggies, or seeing Mr. H with any "basketball" baggies.
8. The "basketball" fentanyl is the cause of Mr. H's death. Mr. H more likely than not used "basketball" fentanyl after 7:00 am; he was unresponsive at ~8:00 am and was not revivable with Narcan. Fentanyl use after 7:00 am. caused his death.
9. Morphine in blood and morphine, codeine, and 6-MAM in urine emanate from use more than eight hours before Mr. H's death. The effects would have dissipated ("wore off"). The remaining morphine in the blood (9.5 ng/ml) would cause no additional toxicity to the fentanyl.
10. 7-amino-clonazepam is a metabolite (break-down) product of clonazepam, a benzodiazepine used for seizure control, obsessive conditions, and anxiety. The metabolite does have a drug effect. However, the measured levels (37 ng/ml) are substantially lower than levels associated with sedation (impairment, >100 ng/ml (ug/L). Therefore, in my opinion, there is insufficient clonazepam to cause any clinical impairment or contribute to fentanyl-induced respiratory depression and death.
11. Mr. H died from a self-administered fentanyl overdose from a source—"basketball" baggie—different than the heroin shared with Ms. K.
12. The presence of morphine (9.5 ng), codeine, and 6-MAM is consistent with remote heroin use. Mr. H's death one hour after being alert and oriented (and not obviously under the influence of anything) with fatal fentanyl blood levels can be only related to an acute use of fentanyl after 7:00 am.

The clinical evidence and the laboratory evidence support a lack of contribution of any of Ms. K's actions to Mr. H's death. The case was tried by a judge who found Ms. H. not guilty of the drug-induced homicide she had been charged with.

CASE REPORT 5: MARIJUANA AND OPIATE TESTING IN A CIVIL MATTER

Mr. H, (39 y/o) was killed by a tire explosion while working at a Tire Company on August 17, 2015. The explosion occurred shortly after 3:00 pm. He was taken emergently to the hospital, where he was pronounced dead at 3:59 pm after unsuccessful resuscitation attempts. An autopsy was performed the next day (August 18, 2015). The medical examiner determined that the cause of death was traumatic blunt force; the manner of death was accident. Other significant conditions: "Acute combined cannabinoid and heroin intoxication."

A subclavian blood sample at autopsy reported the following toxicology findings:

- 6-MAM < 1.0 ng/ml
- Morphine 25 ng/ml
- THC 4.2 ng/ml THC-COOH 12 ng/ml
- Amphetamine 73 ng/ml

A report by the defendant's toxicologist (HCN) lists the following opinions:

1. Mr. H had recently ingested both cannabis (marijuana—THC) and heroin.
2. Mr. H was under the influence of heroin and THC drugs at the time he sustained his fatal injury.
3. Mr. H was possibly impaired by amphetamine.
4. The finding of (delta-9 THC) this compound indicates to me that Mr. H was acutely intoxicated (marijuana) and likely suffered deficits in short-term memory, along with increased heart rates and CNS depression.
5. The presence of a detectable amount of 6-monoacetylmorphine (6-MAM) is consistent with the ingestion of heroin.
6. Mr. H was possibly impaired by amphetamine. The source and dose cannot be determined; the blood concentration (of amphetamine) at autopsy is consistent with that found in people who have taken doses of 10–30 mg.
7. The previous impairments contributed to his death through increased reaction times, lack of motor coordination, inability to sustain vigilance to danger, and slow response to stimuli.
8. HCN reports that the autopsy blood sample was taken from "peripheral blood."

A pharmacologist expert was retained by the decedent's estate and consulted/provided testimony in the case.

1. Do you have an opinion as to whether Mr. H was intoxicated at the time of the injury causing his death? Please respond and provide the factual and pharmacological basis for your opinion.
   Answer: No, Mr. H was not intoxicated at the time of the injury.
2. Do you have an opinion as to whether the toxicology findings related to Mr. H, would be a substantial factor in causing injury leading to his death?
   Answer: No, the toxicological findings do not provide evidence. The levels individually are too low, subject to post-mortem changes, and indefinite (6-MAM). The injury could and did occur absent intoxication by any substances.

OPINIONS

1. The medical examiner's report lists "subclavian blood" for toxicology. Subclavian blood is considered "central" and thus subject to greater post-mortem redistribution (PMD) than peripheral blood.
2. Post-mortem blood samples cannot be accurately related/extrapolated to ante-mortem levels.
3. Post-mortem redistribution phenomenon is reported for morphine, THC, and THC-COOH.
4. THC and THC-COOH levels may persist in chronic users; the levels detected in this case may represent remote use and thus would not cause any impairment or intoxication nor can any be reliably predicted.
5. THC level of 4.2 ng/ml (potentially elevated by PMD) is below presumptive levels of intoxication in some states that allow medical and/or recreational use. Even this level has limited relevance as a predictor of intoxication or impairment. Since this level may be a result of persistent presence from remote use (24–48 hours prior), no claims or opinions related to marijuana acute intoxication or impairment may be made in this case.
6. The morphine level reported in this case (25 ng/ml) is relatively low, even for therapeutic use, and definitely low for a heroin user. Thus, there is no evidence of any impairment or acute morphine (heroin) intoxication at the time of the fatal injury.

7. 6-MAM is detected at "<1 ng/ml." There is no lower limit or quantification. Depending on the sensitivity of the assay, the detectability may exceed the usual published time limit, thus, beyond eight hours as noted by HCN.
8. No workers at the Tire company reported any abnormal behavior or actions by Mr. H on the date of his death. He had been there for at least several hours before the fatal explosion.
9. The effect of amphetamine on Mr. H, if any, is unknown. If indeed it was having any effect, the effect is CNS stimulation, which counters any existing CNS depression. In this case, there is no evidence of any impairment from amphetamine.

Nothing in the records supports drug impairment in this case. There is no evidence/observations/reports of behavior before the time of the fatal explosion that would indicate Mr. H's conduct was a substantial factor in his death. There is no toxicology laboratory evidence supporting "acute intoxication" and impairments by marijuana and/or heroin and/or amphetamine that would support any "substantial contribution to his death." I do not dispute that Mr. H used heroin, marijuana, and amphetamine at some remote point; this is the only statement that one can state with certainty. The timing of use cannot be stated to be temporally related (proximity) to the explosion.

CASE REPORT 6: QUALITATIVE TESTING OF DRUG IN GLASS PIPE IN BEAKER OF ISOPROPYL ALCOHOL

Mr. H has been charged with Possession of 160 grams of methamphetamine and Possession with Intent to Deliver, which subjects him to enhanced sentencing, based on the weight of the substance. The Illinois State Police (isp) chemist stated that they were following protocol; "it doesn't matter what concentration of controlled substance is in the seized and tested material that tested positive (qualitative only) for methamphetamine, only the weight of the material."

The ISP documents describe Item #12 (positive methamphetamine) as ~200 ml volume liquid, which had a measured weight of 160 gm. They further described the liquid contained a glass pipe. The analytical methodology used for this qualitative test was liquid chromatography/mass spectroscopy (LC/MS).

OPINIONS

1. The liquid that measured ~200 mL and weighed 160.04 g was isopropyl alcohol. The specific gravity (the ratio of the density of a substance to the density of a standard, usually water for a liquid or solid, and air for a gas) of isopropyl alcohol is 0.79. The liquid material/alcohol weighed 160 g/200 ml, thus a specific gravity of 0.8, almost a perfect match.
2. Methamphetamine is highly soluble (dissolves completely) in alcohol (1 gm/3 ml). The pipe found in the sample liquid (alcohol) likely contained methamphetamine, which is usually smoked through a pipe. Alcohol is used to clean the pipe. Any methamphetamine in or on the pipe before the pipe is placed in the alcohol solution will be dissolved completely and will be distributed throughout the sample.
3. LC/MS identifies extremely small amounts/concentrations of analytes (drugs being tested for). Another way of expressing this concept is the LOD (level of detection)—the smallest amount (or concentration of analyte that can be detected with an acceptable SNR (signal-to-noise ratio)—typically 3). LODs as low as 1 ng/ml are reported.
   a. 1 ng/ml = 0.001 mcg/ml = 0.000001 mg/ml = 0.000000001 gm/ml
   b. 1 g contains 1,000,000,000—one billion ng
4. Used methamphetamine pipes build up a visible and sometimes invisible residue that contains measurable quantities of methamphetamine and pyrolysis products. Assume the meth pipe contains 0.100 g (100 mg), like Item #11, a sealed evidence bag containing a glass tray with (methamphetamine positive) white powder—0.114 g, just slightly above the typical dose (0.100 g) of methamphetamine smoked.
   a. 0.100 gram = 100 mg = 100,000 mcg = 100,000,000 ng.
   b. If only 1% of the residue contains methamphetamine, 1 mg = 1,000 mcg = 1,000,000 ng.
   c. To put these numbers in perspective, let's examine a teaspoon of table sugar (sucrose). A teaspoon is 5 g.
   d. 5 g = 5,000 mg = 5,000,000 mcg = 5 billion ng of sugar.
   e. Thus, even an infinitesimally small "rinse" alcohol solution from cleaning the meth pipe can result in a qualitative positive methamphetamine presence. Assuming a LOD of 1, 50, or even 100 nanogram for a ~200 ml amount of alcohol, only 200 ng, 10,000 ng, or 20,000 ng of methamphetamine IN TOTAL

need be in the alcohol solution containing the meth pipe. Comparing these numbers to a 1 mg contamination (see b. immediately preceding), it is clear that even meth vapor in the air or on one's hands has the potential to contaminate/adulterate a "wash" solution meant to clean the pipe.

f. If one were to wash/rinse/extract/test the clothes of a methamphetamine user/handler, the rinse solution would be contaminated and would test "positive." This circumstance would not be considered "possession" of a controlled substance. A recent scientific research publication concluded that wastewater contamination findings of methamphetamine and amphetamine were partly caused by human consumption (and metabolism), with elimination into sewers. Other findings suggested that pure methamphetamine was discarded into the sewers. Can you imagine if law enforcement extracted materials from a citizen's septic system, tested it, and, on finding methamphetamine, charged that citizen with "possession of a controlled substance" and based the criminal charge on the weight (a few kilograms of septic sludge)? While this is extreme, it is similar to charging a defendant with the "weight" of the alcohol "wash" liquid that contained a glass pipe, obviously contaminated with methamphetamine smoking facilitated by the pipe.
g. Neither should an infinitesimally small "positive" identified by LC/MS with a highly sensitive LOD. It is not possession; it is contamination.

The wash solution has no abuse value and no monetary value and should not be treated as "possession of a controlled substance," with the severity and gravity based on weight. To do so would make absolutely no scientific or rational sense and be an injustice to the defendant. The case was pending at press time; the outcome is not known.

CASE REPORT 7: MARIJUANA IMPAIRMENT WHILE DRIVING

EH was driving a company truck/with a trailer on Interstate 64 at 10:44 am on February 14, 2020, and lost control of the truck, resulting in the truck crossing the medium into oncoming traffic, striking and tragically killing four persons. Four oncoming vehicles were involved in the collision. EH was taken by EMS to the hospital. The EMS crew administered ketamine to EH (as documented in the EMS patient care report). EH was arrested by a State Trooper W at 11:03 am, charged with Operating a Motor Vehicle in a Careless and Imprudent Manner—Involving an Accident. While at the hospital, EH told the Trooper that he used marijuana on occasion, the last use "last night" (February 13, 2020). RH told Trooper W that he was trying to manually roll up the front passenger's window by reaching across the seat to his right, while driving, when he lost control of the Ford. A sample of EH's blood was taken at 1:10 pm. The hospital urine drug screening test reported positive opiates, oxycodone, and cannabinoids in his urine. (Oxycodone and fentanyl had been administered to EH prior to the urine drug screening test.)

On Tuesday, March 10, 2020, Troopers interviewed a co-worker of EH, who stated: "When looking at EH. I didn't notice anything out of the ordinary. His eyes were clear. He didn't smell like marijuana or alcohol at all. We exchanged small talk about work and arrived at 10:00 am. We both went separate ways." When asked how EH appeared earlier at the job site by some coworkers, my response was "he was bright eyed and bushy tailed."

A TV broadcast by a prosecutor included a statement (paraphrased) that a metabolite of marijuana was detected in EH's blood, indicating that marijuana was used hours earlier that morning. EH is being charged with driving while under the influence (intoxication) of marijuana.

INTERVIEW OF EH

EH was employed by the company and duty on the day of the accident. WH was a long-term user of marijuana from the age of 20 to 21 years old, usually in the evening after work to relax. He stated that the marijuana replaced the use of alcohol in his earlier years. His last use of marijuana was to smoke a "blunt," ~ 0.5 g the evening before, February 13, 2020, between 8:00 and 9:00 pm. He described the effect of THC was calm, relaxing, and decompressing. On that evening, he watched TV and played a game. He reported never having a "hangover" on any morning following THC use the evening before. He was "on call" on 2/14, arose at 7:30 am, had breakfast, showered, and prepared to leave for work. He arrived at work at 10:00 am, picked up a co-worker, loaded a truck, and smoked a cigarette in his truck. He denies smoking THC on the morning before the accident. He left his company for his assigned work designation and drove ~3 miles before the collision. He reached over to close the passenger window, tried to roll the window up, and, in doing so, lost control of his truck, which veered left across the center median and collided head-on with the van.

OPINIONS

1. There is no evidence, analytical toxicology or clinical, supporting THC intoxication or impairment at the time of the accident. The finding of THC or any of its metabolites, unquantified, provides no evidence or support of a close (proximate) time of use and thus of any THC intoxicating effects.
2. All three THC compounds (delta 9 THC, 11-hydroxy THC, and carboxy THC) are detectable for at least 24 hours in blood. A finding of "metabolites indicating use a few hours earlier" is scientifically wrong.
3. EH was not under the influence, not impaired, and not intoxicated by marijuana (THC) at the time of the accident. His co-worker was with EH shortly before the accident. On questioning, he told law enforcement that "he didn't notice anything out of the ordinary. His eyes were clear. He didn't smell like marijuana or alcohol at all. We exchanged small talk about work and arrived at 10:00 am. We both went separate ways." When asked how EH appeared earlier at the job site by some coworkers, my response was "he was bright eyed and bushy tailed."
4. An alternate competent proximate cause of the accident is EH reaching over to close the passenger window in his truck.
5. Therefore, no inference or conclusion of the exact time of use/exposure can be made based on the detection of the substances alone. The only conclusion that can be drawn is that EH was exposed to/used marijuana within the shortest detection period of the three substances.
6. THC use by EH the evening before did not and could not have any effect on EH 12–14 hours later. The acute effects of the drug are short-lived, a few hours. Overwhelmingly, the scientific literature describes marijuana effects gone with eight hours of use.

The laboratory tested the blood using a gas chromatography/mass spectrometry (GC/MS) analytical methodology. The following substances were detected and reported:

THC (tetrahydrocannabinol)—active marijuana
Hydroxy-THC—intermediate metabolite of THC (some drug activity)
Carboxy-THC—inactive metabolite of THC (no drug activity)

Assuming naïve/occasional use (not chronic/daily), each substance has different time periods of detection in blood/plasma. THC is present and detectable in the blood for up to 24 hours and in chronic users even longer. 11-Hydroxy THC is present and detectable for up to 72 hours, with substantial levels (~10 ng/ml) at 24 hours. A prominent NIDA scientist and renowned marijuana expert reports hydroxy THC detectable for up to 16 hours in plasma (blood). Carboxy THC is present and detectable for up to seven days. The scientific literature on this topic is clear, strong, and consistent on this issue. After intravenous administration of tritiated (radioactive tagged) hydroxy THC, plasma levels of total radioactivity and unchanged tritiated hydroxy THC declined rapidly during the first few hours. Eight hours after administration, total radioactivity in the plasma (blood) and unchanged hydroxy THC declined more slowly, with half-lives of 40 hours (range 35–56 hours) and 22 hours (range 19 to 24 hours), respectively.

Detection of the presence of any or all of the three cannabinoid substances (THC, hydroxy THC, and carboxy THC) by GC/MS simply means they were present. There is no evidence of a precise time of use. After a report by the defendant EH's pharmacologist, the prosecutor dropped the Aggravated DUI charge; reckless driving charges remained. EH pled guilty to counts of reckless driving. A judge sentenced EH to ten years in prison.

CASE REPORT 8: IMPAIRMENT FROM OXYCODONE DETECTED IN URINE

WD's semi-tractor/trailer collided with the trailer of Mr. J's truck. Both were taken to the hospital ER. EMS evaluated Mr. J and found him to have a GCS of 15, neurologically stable, eyes/pupils equally reactive to light (4 mm/4 mm). Mr. J had bilateral knee surgery in January 2015, at which time he was prescribed oxycodone 5 mg for pain.

On March 29, 2018, at some time after the MVA, urine was collected and sent to the Quest Laboratories for testing for drugs of abuse. Oxycodone 101 ng/ml (threshold for reporting is 100 ng/ml) as well as oxymorphone (a metabolite of oxycodone), 200 ng/ml (threshold for reporting is 100 ng/ml).

REPORT OF PLAINTIFF TOXICOLOGIST

1. Mr. J would have had to have taken a single 5 mg immediate-release oxycodone tablet between 10:00 pm and midnight on Wednesday, March 28, 2018. That is, he took the oxycodone between the time he awoke and was leaving for work, and not on Tuesday, March 27th between 7:00 and 8:00 pm as he stated in his deposition.

2. Mr. J was operating his semi-tractor trailer immediately prior to the crash incident (4:55 am) when the ingested oxycodone and its more potent active metabolite oxymorphone reached their peak (maximum) concentration, and thereby their well-known and documented maximum adverse effects on the skills necessary and required to safely operate a motor vehicle.
3. Mr. J was taking the long-acting centrally active antihistamine meclizine for his vertigo on the day of and prior to the crash incident . . . since 2016. This drug has documented adverse effects on the skills necessary and required to safely operate a motor vehicle.
4. Acute oxycodone ingestion is further enhanced by the presence of meclizine (a drug-drug interaction), more likely than not producing drowsiness, prolonged reaction time, impaired vigilance and attention, impaired coordination, and failure to keep in lane. Thus oxycodone impaired Mr. J's ability to safely operate his commercial motor vehicle and thereby directly and substantially contributed to his collision on March 29, 2018.

OPINIONS

1. The finding of oxycodone and oxymorphone present in urine in the extremely low amounts quantitated is consistent with remote use, as Mr. J testified in this deposition. Indeed, as stated earlier, the threshold or "cutoff" for reporting oxycodone is 100 ng/ml. 101 ng/ml was reported. Ng = nanogram = 1 billionth of a gram.
2. The oxycodone was prescribed for Mr. J by a licensed physician to relieve knee pain. Mr. J took oxycodone on March 27, 2018, to relieve knee pain.
3. There is no time limit to the validity, possession, or use of a prescribed controlled or non-controlled prescription medication. It is his property. There is no violation of any law or regulation. A patient's use of a "pain pill" in their possession for the same or similar pain is indeed a common occurrence.
4. One of the metabolites of oxycodone is oxymorphone. Both oxycodone and oxymorphone are eliminated from the body primarily via the urine. The oxymorphone content is stated to be 11%. Metabolites are not believed to contribute significantly to the pharmacological effects of oxycodone due to their lesser presence in the plasma and lower potency.
5. Oxycodone is detectable in the urine for two to four days, depending on the literature reference and the sensitivity of the assay.
6. Mr. J testified he took one oxycodone tablet (the last from his 2015 prescription) 33 hours before the collision.
7. The presence of extremely low amounts of oxycodone and metabolites in urine is reflective of an even lower amount circulating in Mr. J's blood. The half-life of oxycodone is short, three to six hours. Based on an excess of five half-lives, the oxycodone would have no effect on Mr. J's body or brain.
8. The urinary presence of oxycodone and oxymorphone had no effect on Mr. J's driving ability. These substances could not cause any impairment at such a remote exposure.
9. There was no violation of any motor vehicle laws or U.S. DOT regulations related to remote use or detection following remote use.
10. Urine levels can never be used to infer/prove impairment. Urine levels are only indicative of prior exposure to a substance.
11. The urine screening test for oxycodone is a "screening test"; it was confirmed, one billionth of a gram—(101/100 ng) over the "no report" threshold. Misinterpretation of drug tests can have serious consequences, such as unjust termination from a job, risk of a prison sentence, inappropriate exclusion from a sporting event, and possibly inappropriate medical treatment in emergencies.
12. Even a confirmed urine test can never be used to infer or confer drug effect or impairment. It is only evidence that a drug substance is present and has been used. The CDC MMWR reported the following in 1983:
    a. Only blood-sample measurements are likely to correlate with a person's degree of exposure; attempts to correlate urine concentration with impairment or time of dose are complicated by variations in individual metabolism, metabolite accumulation in the chronic user, and urine volume changes due to diet, exercise, and age. Therefore, a positive result in a urine sample indicates only the likelihood of prior use.
13. Meclizine is not a "long-acting" antihistamine. While meclizine may cause sedation and while Mr. J did have a prescription for meclizine, there is no evidence in the case (toxicology tests, sworn testimony of Mr. J) that he consumed meclizine on the day before or the morning before the accident. Indeed, he had filled a prescription as early as 2009 and filled prescriptions for 30 tablets of meclizine monthly, allowing for the use of no more than one tablet daily (if consumed every day) for a drug with instructions to take in divided doses AS NEEDED for dizziness or vertigo. Since there is no evidence of use, there can be no opinion of impairment from meclizine or any added effect of meclizine to oxycodone.

CRITIQUE/REBUTTAL OF PLAINTIFF TOXICOLOGIST REPORT

The toxicology report evaluates and interprets the urine drug tests of Mr. J for oxycodone and its active metabolite, oxymorphone. The main conclusions are that oxycodone was at or around its peak blood concentration at the time Mr. J lost control of his vehicle and that, therefore, he was impaired by oxycodone and/or its metabolite. However, this report contains several fatal flaws which undermine the validity of these conclusions.

The key erroneous inference in the report is the extrapolation of urine drug levels to make predictions on the blood concentration levels over time, which then is extended to justify the conclusion that Mr. J was impaired. Moreover, the rationale behind the toxicologist's analysis is unclear. One must assume this is based on either pharmacokinetic modeling or empiric data linking dose to urine concentration. Standard a priori pharmacokinetic modeling cannot explain his conclusions (i.e., modeling based on the dosing regimen and known pharmacokinetic parameters), and the cited references do also not justify Dr. DF's conclusions. While one small study cited by the toxicologist does report a relationship between dosing regimen and the level and temporality of urine concentrations, it would be inappropriate to generalize that these relationships hold among the wider population. In fact, the authors cautioned against such generalizing, and their stated objectives for the study were quite limited. Specific flaws, rebuttals, and objections to the DF report are enumerated in the following list.

1. Urine drug concentrations do not correlate to drug plasma concentration, recency of drug usage, or impairment from drug

   Urine drug tests, even confirmatory ones, can only detect that the substance was present in the urine and therefore in the body at some time in the past. Urine concentration does not correlate to plasma concentration, the latter of which is determinative of drug impairment. Consequently, the urine drug test cannot be used to infer clinical impairment. The urine concentration values must be disregarded outright for use in determining impairment. The literature is dogmatic and emphatic on this point. Several excerpts illustrating this point are shown in the following text.

   The most significant drawback to urine testing is that, in general, drug use testing as currently practiced, when urine is the tested biological specimen, does not provide information about past or present patterns of drug use, abuse, or drug dependence, or about drug-related mental or physical impairment, or other effects, at any time.

   Urine drug levels provide no interpretive data.

   It is for these reasons that 11 noted toxicologists, in a consensus report regarding the interpretation of urine drug testing results in a forensic context, wrote: "Testing of drugs or drug metabolites in urine is only of qualitative value in indicating some prior exposure to specific drugs. Inferences regarding the presence or systemic concentration of the drug at the time of driving or impairment from drug use are generally unwarranted."[101] This is the fatal flaw in the toxicologist's opinions.

2. Pharmacokinetic analysis of blood concentration predicts negligible levels of oxycodone at the time of the crash. A pharmacokinetic analysis of blood concentration after administration of a single 5 mg dose of immediate-release oxycodone predicts a concentration of < 0.1 ng/mL at the time of the crash, which is 33 hours after administration, according to Mr. J's sworn testimony. This is a negligible level of oxycodone and would not be expected to cause impairment. Notably, only blood levels of the drug (not urine) correlate with impairment.

   Assumptions: first-order elimination kinetics, instantaneous absorption, half-life = 2.6, volume of distribution Vd = 2.0 L/kg, bodyweight = 138 kg. Pharmacokinetic parameters used are extracted from the oxycodone monograph in *Goodman & Gilman's The Pharmacological Basis of Therapeutics*.

3. Mass balance between the drug eliminated from blood and the drug appearing in urine does not hold since oxycodone is primarily metabolized.

   Even ignoring the increase in the concentration of drugs in the urine due to the reabsorption of water, the mass of the drug eliminated (from the body) does not necessarily correlate with the mass appearing in the urine. It is not clear if DF is using this assumption to correlate the amount (mass) of drug eliminated with the amount introduced into the urine, and then using this to correlate blood and urine concentrations. In the case of oxycodone, an oxycodone molecule may be eliminated from the body through metabolism. In fact, oxycodone is primarily metabolized, so metabolism is the most likely fate of an oxycodone molecule compared to being excreted unchanged by the kidney. That is, there is no mass balance of the drug in the body and an unchanged drug in the urine if that drug is primarily metabolized.

   The fact that the drug does not pass directly from the blood to the urine compartment when eliminated is one reason that it is inappropriate to correlate blood to urine concentrations (opinion #1). There are many more scientific/physiological reasons why urine presence and concentrations can never be used to infer clinical effects.

4. Oxycodone half-lives cannot be applied to renal excretion.

   Half-lives cited in the literature for oxycodone primarily correlate to metabolism rate, not renal excretion of unchanged oxycodone. The toxicologist cites the half-life of oxycodone in his discussion of the urine concentration. Half-life ($t_{1/2}$) correlates with the rate constant of elimination (k), which in the case of oxycodone is mostly controlled by the metabolic rate constant rather than the renal rate constant (the rate constant describing the transfer of unchanged oxycodone from the blood to the urine). The overall rate constant of elimination is equal to the weighted sum of the rate constant of metabolism and the rate constant for renal excretion.

   k = (% excreted unchanged) *kr + (% metabolized)*km.

   According to *Goodman & Gilman*, "up to 19%" of an oral oxycodone dose is excreted unchanged in the urine. Thus, over 81% of oxycodone is metabolized. The bottom line is that it is inappropriate to use the overall half-life of oxycodone to model the excretion of unchanged oxycodone. If the toxicologist is using a renal half-life rather than an overall half-life, as is most often listed in literature sources, he should indicate that. Importantly, the rate constants (and thus half-lives) of oxycodone metabolites are different from oxycodone itself. These are reasons that it is inappropriate to extrapolate blood levels to urine levels (DF opinion #1).
5. Drugs are concentrated in the urine to an extent that is dependent on many variables.

   Drug concentrations are generally higher in the urine due to the reabsorption of water in the renal tubule. "Interpretation of results must take into account that urine concentrations can vary extensively with fluid intake and other biological variables." This is another reason why it is inappropriate to predict blood levels from urine levels.
6. A study relating dose to urine concentration versus time curve cannot be applied to the general population.

   The toxicologist cites a single study by Cone et al.,[102] which studies urine concentration of oxycodone (and metabolites) versus time after oral oxycodone administration. He is using this study to perform retrograde extrapolation to predict the time of drug usage based on the urine drug levels. This is an overinterpretation of this study for many reasons. The study contained only 12 subjects. This sample size is insufficient to validate the relationship between urine drug levels, the time of usage, or the time of the peak of blood concentration. The study authors noted high variability among the subjects. Sources of individual variability cited by study authors included: "amount of fluid intake and individual rates of absorption, metabolism, and excretion." They continue, "The amount of recent fluid intake has been shown to greatly influence urine drug and metabolite concentrations." The study authors note that there is variation in the enzymes that metabolize oxycodone among the general population. In particular, there are fast or slow metabolizers, which would naturally affect the elimination rate of oxycodone and the degree to which metabolites are generated. For example, in one individual a CYP2D6 enzyme could biotransform oxycodone much more slowly than in another individual. The study noted the "detection times for some analytes may be underestimated because of the study design, which allowed the discharge of subjects between 36 and 48 h with no specimen collections performed during that time." The study used a controlled-release formulation of oxycodone, not the immediate-release formulation Mr. J took. The pharmacokinetics are different for controlled compared to immediate release. The objective of the study was to increase oxycodone pharmacokinetic knowledge so that an oxycodone test may be considered as part of a federal drug testing program. Such programs only test for the presence of drugs. They do not attempt to predict the time of usage or establish the peak concentration in the blood or when it occurred. There is no indication by study authors in the Discussion section or elsewhere that this (Cone et al.) study should be used to allow retrograde extrapolation of urine concentrations to time of usage, dose, or blood concentrations.
7. Prediction of detection times is not justified with any rationale.

   The toxicologist makes the following statement, "Following a single dose of 5 mg immediate-release oxycodone, this urine level occurs between 10- and 12-hours post-dosing." No reasoning is provided for this extrapolation. There are several problems with this that are enumerated in Opinion #6.
8. Basic Pharmacokinetic term is misused in analysis.

   The toxicologist states: "Oxycodone (OC) and oxymorphone (OM) have high bioavailability such that after a single oral dose of 5,15, or 20 mg of oxycodone, OC and OM appear in the blood in less than 1 hour." Bioavailability is the fraction of the drug dose that reaches systemic circulation. It is not related to the onset of action as is suggested in the previous statement. If the rigorous definition of pharmacokinetic terms is not used in the rest of the analysis, this contributes to confusion over the analysis and rationale behind the toxicologist's claims. For instance, it is unknown whether the toxicologist is equating elimination with excretion in his analysis; if so, that would confound the critique of his analysis. It should be noted that "elimination" is not synonymous with excretion. Elimination refers to either the biotransformation of a drug or the excretion of that parent drug unchanged (usually renally). Excretion is the removal of a substance from the body.

So a drug would be eliminated as soon as it is metabolized, not when the metabolite is excreted. In at least one case, the toxicologist misuses a fundamental pharmacokinetic term (bioavailability); if elimination and excretion are similarly misused, that would contribute to the misunderstanding of his analysis.

9. Oxymorphone does not contribute significantly to the drug effect of oxycodone.

The toxicologist posits that "Mr. J's urine OM concentration at the time of the semi-trailer truck crash would have been on the rising phase of the dose-response curve . . . and thereby would exert its maximum pharmacological effects." Oxymorphone is an active metabolite of oxycodone. However, the *Baselt* Toxicology text states, "The metabolites are not believed to contribute significantly to the pharmacological effects of oxycodone due to their lesser presence in plasma." In the study *Baselt* cites, they state, "The predictions argue for a very low presence of oxycodone metabolites in the brain relative to the parent drug (i.e., at < 6%)."

The case was resolved; there was no trial in the case.

CASE REPORT 9: METHAMPHETAMINE IMPAIRMENT AND VEHICULAR MANSLAUGHTER

JP had just dropped his wife off at work and was driving home shortly after 6:00 am on July 4, 2016, when he allegedly struck a pedestrian—DK—who died six months later as a result of the injuries he sustained in the collision. JP thought he had struck a mailbox; he panicked, left the scene, and drove home. Police came to his parents' home at ~10:00 am and found his damaged vehicle, questioned JP extensively, administered field sobriety tests (11:54 am), PBT = 0.00, and arrested him at 12:01 pm. He was later administered a DRE (drug recognition evaluation) (1:40–230 pm), along with blood and urine samples for toxicology testing, blood drawn ~7.5 hours after the collision.

The DRE Officer C wrote in his report that JP was intoxicated/impaired by CNS stimulants at the time of the collision and that, at the time of the examination, JP was "on the downside of CNS stimulant impairment." Officer C and other officers described JP as giving long rambling answers, sweating profusely, appeared excited. Later, he appeared sleepy and fell asleep at various times. Officer C expressed the opinion that JP was under the influence of a CNS stimulant and that, during the DRE exam, he was on the "downside" of the stimulant.

Toxicology blood results showed methamphetamine (300 ± 60 ng/ml) and amphetamine (37 ± 8 ng/ml).

JP has been charged Manslaughter, Aggravated Assault, Leaving the Scene of an Accident, and Tampering with Evidence in connection with the incident that allegedly occurred on July 4, 2016.

Descriptions of DRE include:

A drug recognition expert (DRE) is a specialized law enforcement officer who has completed training to expertly identify individuals who are exhibiting impaired behavior caused by drugs other than, or in addition to, alcohol. DREs are commonly employed in identifying impaired drivers, but their utility extends to other areas of law enforcement as well. DREs are trained to recognize the effects of depressants, stimulants, inhalants, PCP, cannabis, hallucinogens, and narcotics. A 12-step protocol is used to examine mental, physical, and medical factors resulting in an official officer opinion on (1) subject impairment, (2) if impaired, if the impairment is drug-related, and 3) if drug-related, which drug group or combination is likely responsible for the impairment (1, 2). The 12-step process is to be documented along with the final opinion on a standardized Drug Influence Evaluation (DIE) form (2). (For a complete review of DRE, see Chapter 37 by Gengo and Mantle.)

DEFENSE PHARMACOLOGISTS REVIEW AND OPINIONS IN JP'S CASE

Officer C's ("DRE") initial report states:

> It is my opinion as a certified DRE, that JP is under the influence of CNS stimulant and is not able to operate a vehicle safely. While on scene JP was exhibiting symptoms to include sweating profusely, red, watery blood shot eyes, flush face. JP could not stand still and was very animated in his movements. JP was talking very fast and his words were mumbled and running together. Prior to the DRE evaluation (~2 hours after the arrest), JP was very lethargic and unsteady on his feet. While sitting in the chair he fell asleep several times and his eyelids were droopy. JP's speech was slow and mumbled. He concluded that JP was 'on the downside' of CNS stimulant impairment, and Officer C opined that he was impaired by a CNS stimulant at the time of the alleged motor vehicle/pedestrian accident at 6:12 that morning.

OPINIONS

1. "On the Downside" is neither a recognized nor common term in the pharmacy, pharmacology, or medical texts, journals, and other authorities to describe the effects of any drug.

2. In the context in which "On the Downside" is used in Officer C's report, as well as in the DRE Manual, the statement "When the body reacts to the presence of a drug by releasing neurotransmitters and hormones to counteract the effects of the drug consumed to return to homeostasis" is physiologically, pharmacologically, and medically incorrect—Downright Wrong! Whoever wrote this manual is obviously untrained and unfamiliar with the scientific disciplines of pharmacology and physiology.
3. Officer C's opinions contain inconsistencies, contradictions, and conclusions which are clinically incorrect or have no physiologic basis for his findings, clues, cues, and observations, which formed the basis for his opinions on drug impairment.
4. No competent evidence supports any drug impairment at the time of the collision (6:12 am).

After the pharmacologist's report, a Daubert Challenge was filed. The drugged driving charges were dropped.

CASE REPORT 10: CLAIMED PSEUDOEPHEDRINE IMPAIRMENT IN VEHICLE CRASH

A pharmacologist was retained to assess the validity of a driver charged with Aggravated DUI/death. On October 12, 2017, at 5:11 am, CP's vehicle crossed the center line and crashed into an oncoming semi-tractor trailer. The driver of the truck was fatally injured. CP received minor injuries and was taken by EMS to the hospital. CP told a Sheriff Deputy that she was coughing and blacked out, and the next thing she remembers was the airbags deploying. An eyewitness described CP's vehicle "drift" across the center line, crashing into the truck.

Blood and urine samples were taken from CP by hospital personnel at 7:40 am. Toxicology reports indicated the following:

NIRCL blood: ethanol (alcohol—BAC) 0.041 g/dL
Urine: pseudoephedrine/ephedrine
NMS blood: pseudoephedrine 370 ng/mL

Opinions provided to the driver's criminal defense attorney are as follows:

1. Since the blood was sampled 2.5 hours after the crash (0740–0511). The BAC at the time of the crash extrapolates to 0.086 g/dL
   (86 mg%) (41 + (2.5 × 18) = 86 mg% (0.086 g/dL))
2. The pseudoephedrine, a "behind the pharmacy counter," controlled sale decongestant product level is very high, higher than could be attained with recommended use. The level represents abuse/overdose of pseudoephedrine and would cause significant stimulant toxic effects in CP.
3. CP was intoxicated by alcohol (driving drunk) when she crossed the center line and crashed into the truck.
4. Her description of coughing and passing out would cause erratic, jerky vehicular movements and could result in crossing the center line. Coughing and passing out would not result in a "drift" movement of the vehicle. A "drift" movement across the center line is consistent with falling asleep at the wheel. The 5:11 time, depending on the amount of awake time since last slept, the time and amount of alcohol consumption, would all be factors in significant sleep deprivation, and resultant related impaired driving.

CASE REPORT 11: ZOLPIDEM URINE DRUG TESTING

Can a single urine drug concentration be used to determine the dosage and timing of administration of zolpidem (Ambien©)? A medical toxicologist provided the following opinions:

Based on the pharmacokinetics of zolpidem, a urine zolpidem level of 137 ng/ml is significantly higher than expected 11 hours after a single 10 mg dose. A urine zolpidem concentration of 137 ng/ml is five- to six-fold higher than expected after a single 10 mg dose of zolpidem and is consistent with recent ingestion of additional (i.e., in addition to a 10 mg dose) zolpidem.

The toxicologist based his opinions on the following:[103]

1. Villain, 2004, a "study" of three volunteers, ranges of zolpidem 5 ng/ml to ~27 ng/ml, a range of five-fold.
2. Reidy, 2011,[104] a "study" of eight subjects taking 10–12.5 mg doses of zolpidem had peak urinary zolpidem concentrations of 15–79 ng/ml, a five-fold range of concentration, with the upper limit (79) only a two-fold difference from 137 ng/ml.

OPINIONS

Three (3) subjects and/or (8) subjects do not make science. These reports (Villain and Reidy) are anecdotal and can't and shouldn't be extrapolated to base a dose/concentration relationship between urine drug concentrations. Nor did the authors make such a claim or set it as a primary or secondary aim of the "research." The pharmacokinetic literature and forensic toxicology literature are dogmatic on the limitations of interpreting urine drug presence to qualitative only; it only proves that the subject was exposed to the drug. Use of a urine drug concentration to estimate the time of exposure (other than a window), dosage amount, and time of a dose can't be done. To my knowledge, urine drug level/dosage interpretation is never used in research, clinical, or forensic settings in the manner it was used by Dr. C in this matter.

1. Urine drug concentrations do not correlate to drug plasma concentration, recency of drug usage, or impairment from the drug. Urine drug tests can never be used to infer any clinical effect, let alone impairment. The literature is dogmatic and emphatic on this point. Several excerpts illustrating this point are shown in the following text.

   The most significant drawback to urine testing is that, in general, drug use testing as currently practiced, when urine is the tested biological specimen, does not provide information about past or present patterns of drug use, abuse, or drug dependence, or about drug-related mental or physical impairment, or other effects, at any time.

   It is for these reasons that 11 noted toxicologists, in a consensus report regarding the interpretation of urine drug testing results in a forensic context, wrote:

   Testing of drugs or drug metabolites in urine is only of qualitative value in indicating some prior exposure to specific drugs. Inferences regarding the presence or systemic concentration of the drug at the time of driving or impairment from drug use are generally unwarranted.

   Even if it was the urine test was confirmed, a urine test can never be used to infer or confer drug effect or impairment. It is only evidence that a drug substance is present and has been used. The CDC MMWR reported the following in 1983:

   Only blood-sample measurements are likely to correlate with a person's degree of exposure; attempts to correlate urine concentration with impairment or time of dose are complicated by variations in individual metabolism, metabolite accumulation in the chronic user, and urine volume changes due to diet, exercise, and age.

   Therefore, a positive result in a urine sample indicates only the likelihood of prior use. In 35 years, the science has not changed!
2. Despite widespread use, the interpretation of urinalysis results is still very complex. Parent drugs are often present in urine in very low concentrations or not detected at all. Inter-subject variations in urine drug concentration, even after similar dosing, are high.
3. The daily amount and composition of urine vary widely depending on many factors, such as fluid intake, urinary voiding, diet, health, drug effects, and environmental conditions. The volume of urine produced by a healthy adult ranges from 102 liters in a 24-hour period, but normal values outside these limits are frequently reported.
4. HHS currently mandates that only urine may be tested. However, even in non-regulated testing, urine appears to be the most popular matrix. Since most workplace testing is either random testing or pre-employment, recent use (not drug impairment) is the information sought. Urine is suitable for the determination of recent use, especially during the past 72 hours. The time frame in which a drug may be detected depends on several factors, including the amount of drug initially consumed, the frequency of drug use, the lipid solubility of the drug in question, and the half-life ($T_{1/2}$) of the drug. For example, some drugs, such as cannabinoids, can be detected for over a month if the donor is a chronic user. Another benefit to using urine for drug testing is that drug concentration in urine is 10 to 100 times more concentrated than in the blood, making detection easier using conventional drug testing instruments.
5. Misinterpretation of drug tests can have serious consequences, such as unjust termination from a job, risk of a prison sentence, inappropriate exclusion from a sporting event, and possibly inappropriate medical treatment in emergencies.

Dr. C's opinion and bases do not represent a consensus of the scientific community; indeed, the opinions are opposite to those of the scientific community. His conclusion was that the 137 ng/ml in the Banner patient was five- to six-fold higher than those found (Villain and Reidy). Yet Villain and Reidy (limited number of subjects) data themselves had ranges of five to six-fold. Mr. C's methodology is invalid, his conclusions have not been subject to peer review, and his opinion is not the product of reliable principles and methods.

CASE REPORT 12: FALSE-POSITIVE OPIATE FROM PASTRY POPPY SEED CONSUMPTION

Two urine samples were taken and showed positive on preliminary screening tests by the probation department. The first test was sent to Acculab Toxicology Laboratory for confirmation testing using the sophisticated GC/MS, and the confirmation test was confirmed using a cutoff of 150 ng/ml (not quantified). The second sample had insufficient volume for Acculab to conduct a confirmation test. Since only the first test was confirmed, I will not discuss the second test.

Mr. S, a methadone maintenance patient and former heroin abuser, has tested positive for morphine in the past and admitted to "using." He adamantly denies using heroin during the time period preceding the confirmed test.

GC/MS—gas chromatography/mass spectroscopy—is the gold standard for analytical toxicology. It is extremely accurate, and besides positively identifying a drug, it also has the capacity to measure the amount of drug present—that is, quantify, quantitate—usually in a ng/ml measurement that is related to some amount beyond the cutoff (established to rule out false positives). In this test, no quantitation was conducted. Therefore, it is unknown as to how much morphine was present in the urine. The amount is important, for the consumption of common food products, specifically those containing poppy seeds, is well known to contribute to morphine-positive tests on urine, easily far exceeding the outdated and low cutoffs set for routine urine drug screens.

OPINIONS

Dr. Autry (Substance Abuse and Mental Health Services Administration) provides regulatory documentation of the level of advanced analytical toxicology science supporting higher confirmation cutoffs for opiates to rule out "poppy seed" defenses. The current understanding of the science prompted the adoption of higher cutoffs for use for federal employees and DOD personnel.

It is well known that poppy seeds contain morphine. In one study, ingestion of three poppy seed bagels resulted in 2797 ng/mL morphine at three hours.[105] In another study, the ingestion of 25 grams of poppy seeds from four brands of poppy seeds, containing between 17 and 294 mcg of morphine per gram, resulted in urine detectability over 48 hours.[106] The vast majority of the searched literature indicates that, depending on the cutoff level utilized by the laboratory, the detection of morphine in the urine does not necessarily indicate illegal drug use.

Even before the 1997 FR Notice, the federal government (Department of Health and Human Services) also recognized that a positive for morphine may be a result of the donor consuming "normal dietary amounts" of poppy seeds. The MRO, assigned to review the analytical results prior to reporting, is directed to report the result as negative unless clinical evidence of abuse or illegal use of opiates is verified. The guidelines state the MRO "shall determine that there is clinical evidence—in addition to the urine test—of illegal use of any opium, opiate, or opium derivative" prior to reporting the result as positive. One exception to this rule: if the specimen is negative for 6-monoacetlymorphine, the result may still be verified positive if the morphine is at 15,000 ng/mL or above.[107]

In this case Mr. S is charged with violating the terms of his supervised release by "using" an illegal controlled substance based on the finding of morphine in his urine. The laboratory tests that were conducted and reported can be explained by the normal consumption of poppy seeds in the routine diet (bagels, muffins). There is no proof that heroin or any opiate-controlled substance was used.

Therefore, with reasonable pharmacological certainty, there is no evidence that Mr. S used any morphine or heroin, prescription or illegal. The presence of the morphine reported in the urine screening and (unquantified) confirmation tests—if you believe Mr. S—was probably the result of dietary consumption of poppy seeds, which is certainly not a violation of anything. If you do not believe Mr. S, there is still no proof!

As a final note, this confounding interpretation would be eliminated by quantifying the confirmation test, not just reporting the tests that exceed thresholds. Levels beyond 2 to 4,000 are *not* considered to be caused by food ingestion of poppy seeds.

The urine test in question does not prove that Mr. S used heroin or any illicit opiate prior to the "morphine" positive test. Eating poppy seed bakery products will result in exactly the same imprecise finding that is the basis of the probation revocation action.

CASE REPORT 13: POSITIVE DRUG SCREENING AND VEHICLE CRASH

At approximately 3:53 pm on Saturday, September 14, 2019, Mr. H's motorcycle collided with the right rear quarter panel of TP's vehicle. Mr. H was ejected from the motorcycle and died as a result of traumatic injuries. TP was interviewed and observed for several hours at the scene and for a short period at a police station after he was taken into custody. Toxicology reports were negative for volatiles (alcohol) in blood. EMIT screening "Detected" marijuana, marijuana metabolite, cocaine, cocaine metabolite (methylecgonine), acetaminophen, and guaiphenesin in urine. SM, the ISP chemist, identified the testing as qualitative. Marijuana metabolite was the only substance confirmed in the urine. The confirmation testing was performed with GC/MS. TP was issued two traffic citations on the day of the accident. He was charged with Aggravated DUI after the toxicology reports were reviewed by the police and the State's Attorney. The Indictments state " while under the influence of any other drug or combination of drugs, at a degree that rendered him incapable of safely driving."

INTERVIEW OF TP

TP reported the following:

1. He was at home all day in bed before the accident. He had taken Dayquil that day and Mucinex on the day or two prior.
2. He smoked a "blunt"—"the same as two joints"—of marijuana at 8:30 pm the evening prior. He used marijuana in the evening only after working, as often as five to six times a week.
3. He denied any cocaine use for at least 20 years.
4. He was not intoxicated or impaired by anything at the time of the accident.
5. He was driving to a barber and then intended to work as an Uber driver when the accident occurred.
6. TP's speech patterns were the same in the scene videos as in the Zoom interview.

VIEW OF VIDEOS—CLINICAL OBSERVATIONS

1. No slurring of speech; no altered gait. Understood and answered questions.
2. Alert, responsive, aware, concerned ("worried") about the victim.
3. Extensive verbal interaction with Police Officer.
4. "I smoked marijuana last night."

OFFICER'S OBSERVATION

1. No signs of impairment or intoxication.
2. t should be noted that during the interview of TP, R/TS did not observe any signs of impairment or intoxication about the person of TP.

ISP TOXICOLOGY REPORT

1. Blood—negative volatiles (no alcohol)
2. Urine:
   a. "Detected" marijuana, marijuana metabolite, cocaine, cocaine metabolite (methylecgonine), acetaminophen, and guaifenesin. Testing methodology was EMIT—EIA.
   b. Confirmed only marijuana (THC) metabolite (GC/MS).

OPINIONS

1. TP was neither intoxicated nor impaired by marijuana (THC), cocaine, or any other substance at the time of the crash.
2. THC 19 hours before the accident would have no pharmacological or toxicological effect on TP at the time of the accident.
3. Since the only drug that was confirmed in the urine was marijuana metabolite, there is no confirmed toxicological evidence of the presence of active marijuana (THC), cocaine or cocaine metabolite, or any other drug in TP's urine sample.
4. Urine drug tests can never be used to infer clinical effects or impairment for any drug. They are evidence that the drug was introduced to the body during the window of detection-residence time of the substance) in the body.
5. Chronic daily use of THC results in frequent results in measurable THC and THC metabolites remotely, especially on the day after last use, and reported up to five days.
6. No signs or symptoms of marijuana and/or cocaine effects, toxicity, or actions are visible on the video, nor noted by the CPD officer. Indeed, the officer specifically noted no signs of drug intoxication or impairment.

7. The confirmed THC metabolite test was not quantitated. Illinois statutes related to Medical Marijuana and Recreational Marijuana 625 IlCS 5/11–501(a)(7) and 625 IlCS 5/11-501.2(a)(6) description of > 5 ng THC in blood or >10 ng THC or any THC metabolite in any body fluid or tissue as presumptive of marijuana impairment is not met by a "detected" qualitative toxicology finding alone. Thus, there should be no charge related to marijuana.

BASES FOR OPINIONS

1. TP interacted with three (3) Chicago Police Department officers. No officers observed any signs of drug impairment.
2. TP did not manifest any signs or symptoms of marijuana impairment on any of the videos that I viewed.
3. Consumption/smoking of two joints 18 hours prior to the accident is too remote for any active or residual effects, toxicity, impairment, or "hangover." Marijuana effects are generally dissipated in several hours; most literature limits any effects to no more than eight hours.
4. Chronic use (daily) of marijuana results in deposition (storage) of THC in fat[108] and other tissues, resulting in release/leaching from the tissues into the blood, resulting in positive findings of marijuana hours to days following use.
5. Urine drug concentrations do not correlate to drug plasma concentration, recency of drug usage, or impairment from the drug. Urine drug tests can never be used to infer any clinical effect, let alone impairment.[109,110,111]

The literature is dogmatic and emphatic on this point. Several excerpts illustrating this point are shown as follows.

> The most significant drawback to urine testing is that, in general, drug use testing as currently practiced, when urine is the tested biological specimen, does not provide information about past or present patterns of drug use, abuse, or drug dependence, or about drug-related mental or physical impairment, or other effects, at any time.

It is for these reasons that 11 noted toxicologists in a consensus report regarding the interpretation of urine drug testing results in a forensic context, wrote: "Testing of drugs or drug metabolites in urine is only of qualitative value in indicating some prior exposure to specific drugs. Inferences regarding the presence or systemic concentration of the drug at the time of driving or impairment from drug use are generally unwarranted (Consensus Development Panel, 1985)."

Marilyn Huestis PhD, perhaps the foremost marijuana expert in the United States, provides the following information in a National Institutes on Drug Abuse (NHTSA) position paper:[112]

> Interpretation of Urine Test Results: Detection of total THC metabolites in urine, primarily the THC-COOH-glucuronide, only indicates prior THC exposure. Detection time is well past the window of intoxication and impairment. Published excretion data from controlled clinical studies may provide reference for evaluation urine cannabinoid concentrations; however, these data are generally reflective of occasional marijuana use rather than heavy, chronic marijuana exposure. It can take as long as four hours for THC-COOH to appear in the urine at concentrations sufficient to trigger an immunoassay (at 50 ng/mL) following smoking. Positive test results generally indicate use within one to three days; however, the detection window could be significantly longer following heavy, chronic use.

The toxicology findings "detected" evidence of marijuana, cocaine, acetaminophen, and guaifenesin. "Detected" urine drug tests can't infer effect or predict when a drug was exposed. Acetaminophen and guaifenesin have no impairing effects and are OTC drugs. TP admitted to using marijuana the night before, which could not impair him at the time of the accident. The urine "detected" marijuana is not quantitated and therefore does not exceed permissible blood or urine levels, according to the Illinois statutes cited earlier. TP's occupation exposed him to large amounts of currency notes, thus exposing him to inhalation and percutaneous absorption of cocaine. GC MS methodology is an extremely sensitive analytical methodology, able to detect substantially lower concentrations than typical urine screening tests, and thus have the potential for a "false-positive" cocaine—in that there is no use, but rather exposure. The cocaine metabolites absent support that the source of cocaine that resulted in a positive test was from currency contamination rather than systemic/international use of the drug.

TP's case was tried by a judge (bench trial), who found him Not Guilty of Aggravated DUI charges.

40.12 SUMMARY AND CONCLUSIONS

Workplace drug testing programs need continual revisions to keep up with the advances in technology. Drugs outside the DHS-5 and the inclusion of matrices other than urine are likely to be adopted. New analytical methods will likely be more specific and sensitive, allowing for a more accurate and reliable testing period as the concept of workplace drug testing matures, formal policies, and the scope of programs will change. Regardless of the program implemented, voluntary or mandatory, the employer must have all of the basic aspects of a program in place including the written policy statement, provisions for supervisor training, employee education and assistance, and guidelines for drug testing. The inclusion of all these steps will increase the effectiveness of any program and help to achieve a drug-free workplace.

Interpretation of the results of forensic drug testing is dependent on the quality and quantity of the data given to the expert to review. The expert must be given all the screening and confirmation data from the specimen, as well as data from the standards and controls used in the analysis. A copy of the laboratory's SOP should be reviewed to ensure that the proper steps were taken. The laboratory's validation data should be reviewed to ensure that the method used has the necessary level of sensitivity and accuracy for the test. Finally—but perhaps most importantly—the identity and integrity of the specimen must be documented through each step.

NOTES

1 Drug Abuse and Statistics. National Center for Drug Abuse Statistics. https://drugabusestatistics.org/
2 Drug Abuse and Statistics. National Center for Drug Abuse Statistics. https://drugabusestatistics.org/
3 Czeisler MÉ, Lane RI, Petrosky E, et al. Mental Health, Substance Use, and Suicidal Ideation During the COVID-19 Pandemic: United States, June 24–30, 2020. MMWR Morb Mortal Wkly Rep. 2020;69:1049–1057.
4 Drug Abuse and Statistics. National Center for Drug Abuse Statistics. https://drugabusestatistics.org/
5 Drug Abuse and Statistics. National Center for Drug Abuse Statistics. https://drugabusestatistics.org/
6 Recovery Centers of America. Economic Cost of Substance Abuse Disorder in the United States, 2019.
7 U.S. Department of Health and Human Services. National Household Survey on Drug Abuse, August, 1998.
8 Addiction in the Workplace Survey. Center City, Minnesota: Hazelden Foundation, October 22, 1996.
9 National Institute on Drug Abuse. National Household Survey on Drug Abuse. United States Department of Health and Human Services, 1991.
10 1996 AMA Survey Workplace Drug-Testing and Drug Abuse Policies Summary of Key Findings. New York: American Management Association, 1996, 1–8.
11 Walsh, Michael J. Development and Scope of Regulated Testing. In Drug Abuse Handbook. CRC Press, 1998, 730.
12 President's Commission on Organized Crime. Report to the President-and Attorney General: America's Habit; Drug Abuse, Drug Trafficking, and Organized Crime. Washington, DC: United States Government Printing Office, 1986.
13 Executive Order 12564. Federal Register, Vol. 51, No. 180, September 15, 1986.
14 United States Department of Health and Human Services. Modal Plan for a Comprehensive Drug-Free Workplace Program. Publication No. (ADM) 90-1635, 1990.
15 Supplemental Appropriations Act of 1987, Section 503, Pub. L. 100-71, July 11, 1987, 101 Stat. 391, 468–471, codified at 5 U.S.C. Section 7301.
16 Supplemental Appropriations Act of 1987, Section 503(a)(1)(A)(ii)(I), Pub. L. 100-71, July 11, 1987. 101 Stat. 468, codified at 5 U.S.C. Section 7301.
17 Mandatory Guidelines for Federal Workplace Drug-Testing Programs. Federal Register, Vol. 59, No. 110, 29908–29931, June 9, 1994.
18 Substance Abuse and Mental Health Services Administration. Mandatory Guidelines for Federal Workplace Testing Programs. United States Department of Health and Human Services, September 1, 1994.
19 Omnibus Transportation Employee Testing Act of 1991; Public Law 102-143, Title V.
20 United States Department of Health and Human Services. Modal Plan for a Comprehensive Drug-Free Workplace Program. Publication No. (ADM) 90-1635, 1990.
21 Substance Abuse and Mental Health Services Administration. Mandatory Guidelines for Federal Workplace Testing Programs. United States Department of Health and Human Services, September 1, 1994. Subpart B, Section 2.1.
22 Substance Abuse and Mental Health Services Administration. Mandatory Guidelines for Federal Workplace Testing Programs. United States Department of Health and Human Services. Subpart B, Section 2.4.
23 Department of Transportation. Federal Register 49 C.F.R. 40, December 19, 2000.
24 Caplan, Y.A. Analytical Techniques. In Cravy, B. and Baselt, R., Eds. Introduction to Forensic Toxicology. Davis, CA: Biomedical Publications, 1981, 160.
25 Caplan, Y.H.; Levine, B. "Abbott Phencyclidine and Barbiturates Abused Drug Assays Evaluation and Comparison of ADx FPIA, TDx FPIA, EMIT, and GC/MS Methods." J. Anal. Toxicol. 13:289, 1989.
26 Chen, X.H.; Franke, J.P.; DeZeeuw, R.A. Solid Phase Extraction for Systematic Toxicological Analysis. Forensic Sci. Rev. 4:147, 1992.
27 Schug, K.A. The LCGC Blog: Forensic Drug Analysis: GC–MS VERSUS LC–MS. Chromatography Online. https://www.chromatographyonline.com/view/lcgc-blog-forensic-drug-analysis-gc-ms-versus-lc-ms. Published July 4, 2018. Accessed July 24, 2022.
28 Hage, D.S. Chromatography. In Rifai, N., Horvath, A.R. and Witter, C.T., Eds. Principles and Applications in Clinical Mass Spectrometry. Elsevier, 2018, 1–32.
29 Chaulya, S.K.; Prasad, G.M. Gas Sensors for Underground Mines and Hazardous Areas. In Chaulya,

S.K. and Prasad, G.M., Eds. Sensing and Monitoring Technologies for Hazardous Areas. Elsevier, 2016, 161–212.

30 Current, B. Beat Drug Test Cheaters at Their Own Game. Addiction Professional, 2014.

31 Cone, E.J.; Lange, R.; Darwin, W.D. In Vivo Adulteration: Excess Fluid Ingestion Cause False Negative Marijuana and Cocaine Urine Test Results. J. Anal. Toxicol. 22:460–473, 1998.

32 Dasgupta, A.; Wahed, A.; Wells, A. Rapid Spot Tests for Detecting the Presence of Adulterants in Urine Specimens Submitted for Drug Testing. Am. J. Clin. Pathol. 117(2):325–329, 2002 Feb.

33 Dasgupta, A. A Health Educator's Guide to Understanding Drugs of Abuse Testing, 1st ed. Sudbury, MA: Jones & Bartlett Publishers, 2010, 124.

34 Kintz, P., ed. Drug Testing in Hair. Boca Raton, FL: CRC Press, 1996.

35 Montagna, W.; Van Scott, E.J. The Anatomy of the Hair Follicle. In Ellis, R.A., Ed. The Biology of Hair Growth. New York: New York Academic Press, 1958, 39.

36 Montagna, W.; Van Scott, E.J. The Anatomy of the Hair Follicle. In Ellis, R.A., Ed. The Biology of Hair Growth. New York: New York Academic Press, 1958, 39.

37 Lewis, D.; et al. Determination of Drug Exposure Using Hair; Application to Child Protective Cases. Forensic Sci. Int. 84(1–3):123–128, 1997.

38 Kidwell, D.A. Analysis of Drugs of Abuse in Hair by Tandem Mass Spectrometry. Proceedings of the 36th American Society of Mass Spectrometry Conference on Mass Spectrometry and Allied Topics. American Society of Mass Spectrometry, San Francisco, 1364–1365, June 6–10, 1988. Also Kidwell, D.A.; Blank, D.L. Deposition of Drugs of Abuse in Human Hair. Society of Forensic Toxicology Conference on Hair Analysis, Washington, DC, May 26, 1990.

39 Smith, F.P.; Kidwell, D.A. Environmental Contamination Causes Positive Hair Analysis Results. The International Association of Forensic Toxicologists, XXXV Annual Meeting, 1997.

40 Henderson, G.L.; Harkey, M.R.; Jones, R. Hair Analysis for Drugs of Abuse. Final Report on Grant Number NIL 90-NIJ-CX-0012 to National Institutes of Justice, September 1993.

41 Henderson, G.L.; Harkey, M.R.; Jones, R. Hair Analysis for Drugs of Abuse. Final Report on Grant Number NIL 90-NIJ-CX-0012 to National Institutes of Justice, September 1993. Also Kidwell, D.A.; Blank, D.L. Mechanisms of Incorporation of Drugs into Hair and the Interpretation of Hair Analysis Data. In Cone, E.J. and Welch, M., eds. Research Monograph. National Institute of Drug Abuse, 1994.

42 Henderson, G.L.; Harkey, M.R.; Jones, R. Hair Analysis for Drugs of Abuse. Final Report on Grant Number NIL 90-NIJ-CX-0012 to National Institutes of Justice, September 1993.

43 Reid, W.; O'Connor, F.; Crayton, J. The In Vitro Binding of Benzoylecgonine to Pigmented Human Hair Samples. Clin. Toxicol. 32:405, 1994.

44 Cone, E.J.; et al. Correlation of Saliva Cocaine Levels With Plasma Levels and With Pharmacologic Effects After Intravenous Cocaine Administration in Human Subjects. J. Anal. Tox. 12:200–206, 1998.

45 Kato, K.; et al. Cocaine and Metabolite Excretion If Saliva Under Stimulated and Nonstimulated Conditions. J. Anal. Tox. 17:338–341, 1993.

46 Thompsom, L.K.; et al. Confirmation of Cocaine in Human Saliva After Intravenous Use. J. Anal. Tox. 11:36–38, 1987.

47 Huestis, M.; Cone, E. Alternative Testing Matrices. In Karch, S., Ed. Drug Abuse Handbook. Boca Raton, FL: CRC Press, 1998, 804.

48 Schramm, W.; et al. Drugs of Abuse in Saliva: A Review. J. Anal. Toxicol. 16:1–9, 1992.

49 Kintz, P. Drug-Testing in Addicts: A Comparison Between Urine, Sweat, and Hair. Therapeut. Drug Monit. 18:450–455, 1996.

50 Burns, M.; Baselt, R. Monitoring Drug Use With a Sweat Patch: An Experiment With Cocaine. J. Anal. Toxicol. 17:41–48, 1995.

51 Levisky, J.A.; et al. Drug Deposition in Adipose Tissue and Skin: Evidence for an Alternative Source of Positive Sweat Path Tests. Forensic Sci. Int. 110(1):3–46, 2000.

52 Fortner, N. (Vice-President, PharmChem, Inc.). Prepared Statement Before the House Committee on Government Reform and Oversight Subcommittee on National Security. International Affairs and Criminal Justice. Federal Information Systems Corporation Federal News Service, June 5, 1988.

53 Spiehler, V.; et al. Enzyme Immunoassay Validation for Qualitative Detection of Cocaine in Sweat. Clin. Chem. 42(1):34–38, 1996.

54 Kidwell, D.; Blanco, M.; Smith, F. Cocaine Detection in a University Population by Hair Analysis and Skin Swab Testing. Forensic Sci. Int. 84:65–86, 1997.

55 Kidwell, D.; Smith, F. Susceptibility of PharmChekTM Drugs of Abuse Patch to Environmental Contamination, 2002.

56 Drugs Feasibility Assessment of Chemical Testing for Drug Impairment. United States Department of Transportation. HS 806 920, September 1985.

57 Guidance for Reporting Specimen Validity Test Results. Program Document (PD) 35, September 28,1998. Notice to the National Laboratory Certification Program (NLCP) Inspectors and HHS Certified Laboratories.

58 Kern, K.B.; Meislin, H.W. Diabetes Insipidus: Occurrence After Minor Head Trauma. J. Trauma. 24:69–72, 1984. Also Buridi, A., Corman, L.; Redinger, R. Hypokalemic Nephropathy and Nephrogenic

Diabetes Insipidus Due to Excessive Consumption of a Soft Drink. S. Med. J. 91:1079–1082, 1998.
59 General Guidance/Criteria for Specimen Validity Testing. Program Document (PD) 37, July 28, 1999. Notice to the National Laboratory Certification Program (NLCP) Inspectors and HHS Certified Laboratories (Federal Register/Vol. 69, No. 71/Tuesday, April 13, 2004/Notices).
60 ElSohly, M.; Jones, A. Drug-Testing in the Workplace: Could a Positive Test for One of the Mandated Drugs Be for Reasons Other Than Illicit Use of the Drug? J. Anal. Tox. 19(6):450–458, 1995.
61 Steinagle, G.; Upfal, M. Concentration of Marijuana Metabolites in the Urine After Ingestion of Hemp Seed Tea. J. Occup. Environ. Med. 41(6):510–513, 1999.
62 Struempler, R., Nelson, G.; Urry, F. A Positive Cannabinoids Workplace Drug Test Following the Ingestion of Commercially Available Hemp Seed Oil. A. Anal. Tox. 21(4):283–285, 1997.
63 Jackson, G.; Sooday, J.; Poklis, A. Urinary Excretion of Nemzoylecgonine Following Ingestion of Health Inca Tea. F. Sci. Int. 49(1):57–64, 1991.
64 Struempler, R. Excretion of Codeine and Morphine Following Ingestion of Poppy Seeds. J. Anal. Tox. 11(3):97–99, 1987.
65 Hayes, L.; Krasselt, W.; Mueggler, P. Concentration for Morphine and Codeine in Serum and Urine After Ingestion of Poppy Seeds. Clin. Chem. 33(6):806–808, 1987.
66 Cone, E.; et al. Passive Inhalation of Marijuana Smoke: Urinalysis and Room Air Levels of Delta-9-Tetrahydrocannibinol. J. Anal. Tox. 11:89–96, 1987.
67 Zeidenberg, P.; Bourdon, R.; Nahas, G. Marijuana Intoxication by Passive Inhalation: Documentation by Detection of Urinary Metabolites. Am. J. Psychiatry 134(1):76–78, 1977.
68 Morland, J.; et al. Cannabinoids in Blood and Urine After Passive Inhalation of Cannabis Smoke. JJFSCA 30(4):997–1002, 1985.
69 Heidemann S.; Gietting, M. Passive Inhalation of Cocaine by Infants. Henry Ford Hosp. Med. J. 38(4):252–254, 1990.
70 Cone, E.J.; et al. Passive Inhalation of Cocaine. J. Anal. Toxicol. 19:399–411, 1995.
71 Baselt, R.; Yoshikawa, D.; Chang, J. Passive Inhalation of Cocaine. Clin. Chem. 37(12):2160–2161, 1991.
72 Mieczkowski, T. Distinguishing Passive Contamination From Active Cocaine Consumption: Assessing the Occupational Exposure of Narcotics Officers to Cocaine. Forensic Sci. Int. 84(1–3):87–111, 1997.
73 Le, S.; et al. Occupational Exposure to Cocaine Involving Crime Lab Personnel. J. For. Sci. 37(4):959–968, 1992.
74 Aniline, O.; et al. Incidental Intoxication With Phencylidine. J. Clin. Psychiatry 41(11):393–394, 1980.
75 Pitts, F.; et al. Occupational Intoxication and Long-Term Persistence of Phencyclidine (PCP) in Law Enforcement Personnel. Clin. Toxicol. 9:1015–1020, 1981.
76 Medical Economics Staff. Physicians Desk Reference, 55th ed. Montvale, NJ: Medical Economics Company, 2001, 438.
77 Cody, J.T. Metabolic Precursors to Amphetamine and Methamphetamine. Forensic Sci. Rev. 5:109, 1993.
78 Fogel, S.M.; et al. Survey of the Law on Employee Drug-Testing. U. Miami L. Rev. 42:553, 1988.
79 Griswold v. Connecticut, 381 U.S. 479.
80 Cranford, M. Drug-Testing and the Right to Privacy: Arguing the Ethics of Workplace Drug-Testing. J. Bus. Ethics 17:1805–1815, 1988.
81 Shelly v. Kraemer, 334 U.S. 1, 13, 1948.
82 United States v. Price, 383 U.S. 787, 794, n. 7, 1966.
83 Rendell-Baker v. Kohn, 457 U.S. 830, 1982.
84 Payton v. New York, 445 U.S. 573, 1980.
85 Donovan v. Dewey, 452 U.S. 594, 602–605, 1981.
86 Title VII of the Civil Rights Act of 1964, 42. U.S.C. § 2000c et. seq.
87 Cal. Bus. & Prof. Code § 1206, Supp. 2014. http://part40california.blogspot.com/p/cal-bus-prof-code-1206.html
88 Cal. Lab. Code § 1025 et. seq.
89 Rhode Island Chapter 136. R.I. Gen. Laws § 28-6.5-1 and § 28-6.5-2 (Supp. 1997).
90 The Americans with Disabilities Act of 1990, PL 101-336, § 108.
91 The Americans with Disabilities Act of 1990, PL 101-336, ¶ 104(a).
92 The Americans with Disabilities Act of 1990, PL 101-336, § 104 d1.
93 The Rehabilitation Act of 1973, 29 U.S.C. §§ 701–796, 1982.
94 Nispero v. Buck, 720 F. Supp. 1424, 1427, N.D. Cal 1989.
95 Heron v. McGuire, 803 F. 2d 67, 68, 2d Circuit 1986.
96 Labor Management Relations Act, 1947, 29 U.S.C § 141.
97 Johnson-Bateman Co., 295 NLRB No. 26, 1331 L.R.R.M. Cas. (BNA) 1391 (1989); Labor Management Relations Act, 1947, 29 U.S.C § 141, 8(d)).
98 Caplin, Y.; Goldberger, B., Eds. Garriott's Medicolegal Aspects of Alcohol, 6th Edition. Tucson: L&J Publishing Company, Inc., 2015.
99 Brick, J.; Erickson, C.K. Intoxication is Not Always Visible: An Unrecognized Prevention Challenge. Alcohol Clin. Exp. Res. 33(9):1489–1507, 2009.
100 Brick, J.; Bennet, W. Alcohol Calculations in Emergency and Forensic Medicine. J. Addict. Med. Ther. Sci. 3(3):24–29, 2017.
101 https://www.nhtsa.gov/sites/nhtsa.gov/files/809725-drugshumanperformfs.pdf. Accessed December 24, 2022.

102 Cone, E.J.; et al. Prescriptions Opioids. I Metabolism and Excretion Patterns of Oxycodone in Urine Following Controlled Single Dose Administration. J. Anal. Toxicol. 37(5):355–364, 2013.

103 Villain, M.; et al. Windows of Detection of Zolpidem in Urine and Hair: Application to Two Drug Facilitated Sexual Assaults. Forensic Sci. Int. 143(2–3):157–161, 2004 Jul 16.

104 Reidy, L.; et al. Zolpidem Urine Excretion Profiles and Cross-Reactivity With ELISA Kits in Subjects Using Zolpidem or Ambien CR as a Prescription Sleep Aid. J. Anal. Toxicol. 35(5):294–301, 2011 Jun.

105 Struempler, R. Excretion of Codeine and Morphine Following Ingestion of Poppy Seeds. J. Anal. Tox. 11(3):97–99, 1987.

106 Hayes, L., Krasselt, W., Mueggler, P., "Concentration of Morphine and Codeine in Serum and Urine After Ingestion of Poppy Seeds," Clin Chem, 1987, 33(6): 806-8.

107 Mandatory Guidelines for Federal Workplace Drug-testing Programs," Federal Register, Vol. 59, Number 110, pp. 29908-29931, June 9, 1994; Department of Health and Human Services, Substance Abuse and Mental Health Services Administration, "Mandatory Guidelines for Federal Workplace Testing Programs," September 1, 1994.

108 Baselt, R.C. Tetrahydrocannabinol Monograph. In Disposition of Toxic Drugs and Chemicals in Man. Seal Beach, CA: Biomedical Publications, 2014 at 1948–1941.

109 Cone, E.J. Marijuana Effects and Urinalysis After Passive Inhalation and Oral Ingestion. NIDA Res Monogr. 99:88–96, 1990.

110 Diagnostics Reagents, Inc. Cannabinoid (THC) Enzyme Immunoassay, Package Insert, Limitations of the Assay Results, August 1999.

111 Limitations of the Urine Drug Screening Assay Positive Test Results. In Leiken & Paloucek, Eds. Poisoning & Toxicology Handbook, 3rd ed. Washington, DC: APHA, 2006, 1201.

112 Huestis, M. Cannabis/Marijuana (Delta-9-Tetrahydrocannabinol, THC). Drugs and Human Performance Fact Sheets. www.nhtsa.gov/people/injury/research/job185drugsd/cannabis.htm.

41 Postmortem Redistribution and Interpretation of Drug Levels

Gourang P. Patel

SYNOPSIS

41.1 REVIEW OF A CASE FILE

The initial steps of an investigation require a careful review of the subject's case file. Prior to any interpretation of a drug level, there are several variables which need to be addressed. One such variable is the subject's medical history. The medical history can often provide vital information in regard to the patient's medication history (or evidence of prior exposure), and laboratory values, which all need to be integrated for a conclusion or opinion of the investigator to be formed.[1,2]

The concept of a patient being naïve (or non-tolerant) to a medication is often very helpful, as reaction and side effects can be quite different for a subject without previous exposure, versus one with a long history.[1] There are several types of information gathered during the investigation which can be grouped into either qualitative or quantitative data. Qualitative data can provide information about exposure; however, no further details on the extent of exposure can be gathered.[2] In the case of quantitative data, a drug level from a site in the subject's body (e.g., blood, organs) can provide additional information with regard to the degree of exposure in many cases. In both scenarios, the investigator is cautioned about false-positive and false-negative results which may alter the perception, conclusion, or opinion from a case review. The analytical procedure of choice for most substances is gas chromatography/mass spectrometry (GC/MS), which carries a minimal risk of false positives in comparison to antibody-based tests. An additional piece of information that needs to be researched is whether the measured drug concentration falls within the acceptable safe range, as given by a standard reference.[3–5] The reference text provides factual information. What it does not provide, however, is an etiology or circumstances leading up to an event, so it cannot be solely relied upon to draw legally binding conclusions. An investigator should also consider specific autopsy findings that may indicate toxicity with a certain agent. For example, pulmonary edema is usually found in conjunction with a fatal opioid overdose.

41.2 POSTMORTEM CONSIDERATIONS

The alterations and changes that occur to medication after ingestion during life are grouped under pharmacokinetics. The concept of pharmacokinetics describes the transformation of a drug via absorption, distribution, metabolism, and elimination that occurs during the process.[1,6] Postmortem redistribution (PMR) is a term used to describe the changes that may occur after death in the human body and relates it to alterations in chemistry and pharmacology which need to be considered. Changes that occur in drug levels due to redistribution after death are also termed necrokinetics. The concept of necrokinetics is critical when interpreting the postmortem drug level. PMR can be divided into categories: physiologic changes in the body after death (macro level and cellular level) and drug characteristics.[1,2] The quest for research into the drug changes which occur during PMR in humans is inherently difficult to construct and incomplete for obvious reasons; therefore, a fair amount of data is extrapolated from animal models as well.

41.2.1 Physiologic Changes in the Body After Death

At a cellular level there are several changes to incorporate into an investigation. The main variables affected after death are cell membranes, respiration, synthesis of proteins, and preservation of deoxyribonucleic acid (DNA). All of these are affected after death and need to be considered. For example, a cell's death can result in a release of its contents and/or create an environment of acidosis secondary to anaerobic metabolism that occurs. In addition, blood potassium (K) levels are increased postmortem secondary

DOI: 10.1201/9781003615323-45

to cessation of the sodium/potassium (Na/K) ATPase pump function.[7] Drugs also have the capability to diffuse from organs/tissues in the body and back into circulation, as this process is passive. In addition, body decomposition or putrefaction can create an environment in which either bacteria can facilitate further metabolism of the drug, or in some instances substances can be produced during putrefaction. For example, alcohol can be produced secondary to the process of putrefaction which begins shortly after the time of death.[8] In addition, the main substrate for ethanol production is glucose; therefore, after death, the liver, lungs, and heart can be sites where it is generated and detected. The major sites of drug deposition are the lungs, heart, liver, and gastrointestinal tract (GI). Depending on the drug characteristics, medications are able to facilitate movement from these areas and translate into either lower or higher than normal blood levels.[9] For example, alcohol has been well-known to diffuse from the GI tract into circulation after death.[10] In addition, certain organs (e.g., the lungs) facilitate the process due to their enriched blood supply, vascular access to the body, and membrane thinness. The liver appears more complicated, as the drug can diffuse via hepatic circulation and/or directly into adjacent organs. The heart is also more complex, in the respect that drugs may concentrate into the organ initially while a subject is alive; however, after death the right or left chamber can serve as a sampling site postmortem. As a result of the PMR changes, a drug sample which is evaluated for a concentration level may appear "falsely elevated" secondary to these physiologic changes.[11–15]

41.2.2 Drug Characteristics

The drug's pharmacokinetic characteristics that are involved in PMR are the following: absorption, distribution, metabolism, and elimination. Absorption can be affected by the integrity of the cell membrane and the pH of the medium in which the drug travels. The movement of the drug can also be affected by the lipophilic solubility and the ionic state (i.e., pKa) of the drug. Drugs that have lipophilic properties are able to concentrate in major organ tissues (i.e., heart, lungs, and liver).[1,6] In addition, after death the cellular medium becomes more aqueous and acidic; therefore, the movement of basic drugs becomes more likely. The distribution of drugs can also be altered after death.[12,13] In general, drugs that are more lipophilic will tend to have further redistribution after death and can translate into increased movement from tissues/organs into circulation where these are measured.[2]

The volume of distribution (Vd) refers to the total volume into which the total amount of drug would be distributed to reach the plasma. According to several experts, a Vd of greater than 3–4 L/kg can be indicative of PMR changes and increasing serum concentration after death.[2,16] However, this is not an absolute rule. Drugs which are highly protein-bound generally will not have a high or extensive Vd; however, drugs which are not heavily bound to plasma proteins are able to undergo PMR changes. For example, morphine is a drug that undergoes extensive metabolism, and its glucuronide byproducts can be detected after death. In the era of opioid abuse, heroin is another example. Heroin is metabolized to 6-acetylmorphine (6-MAM), both of which have fairly short half-lives and limited activity on the mu receptors in the brain. However, the metabolite is morphine, which has a significant impact on the mu receptors in the brain and does demonstrate PMR. Additional examples are included in Table 46.2.[18] There are also characteristics which drugs can have which would make them more likely to stay within the plasma or even increase after death. Characteristics which are notable are polar compounds and medications with a low Vd (e.g., valproic acid, antibiotics, and furosemide).[1,17] Metabolism is also affected during PMR. Metabolism can persist for several hours after death has occurred and can include the breakdown of a drug into metabolites and byproducts secondary to residual enzyme activity. Obtaining both drug and drug-metabolite levels help determine the true effect of PMR on the metabolism process. Elimination of drugs occurs mainly via the hepatic and renal routes. Both processes are affected shortly after death and can result in the accumulation of drug/metabolite(s) which may later be detected via laboratory analysis, if postmortem samples are obtained within these organ compartments by a pathologist/coroner. The main factors regarding drug characteristics which are known to affect PMR include lipophilic nature, pKa, and Vd.[14,15,17,19]

TABLE 41.1
Variables That Support PMR and Drug-Level Variance[4,16,17]

Drug characteristics (e.g., pKa, Vd, lipophilicity)
Putrefaction
Drug interactions (e.g., inhibition, induction, protein binding-displacement)
Site (e.g., arterial, venous, heart) of drug-level sample
Diffusion from the stomach to other organs
Body position and movement postmortem

41.3 ANALYSIS OF DRUG-LEVEL INFORMATION

An investigator needs to have several concepts at the base of her practice when beginning the analysis of all the information and data available. Integrating the subject's clinical scenario with past medical history, medication profile (recent and past), and laboratory information (where applicable) is the key factor. This series of steps can provide the guidance needed to formulate the appropriate conclusion or opinion. One step that would be helpful in the drug-level analysis would be the central to peripheral blood compartment ratio (C/P). The C/P ratios are generally the highest for basic compounds with a large Vd.[2,20] A caution about the C/P ratio is that there is still active research as to whether these can be correlated to therapeutic, toxic, or fatal drug levels; therefore, the interpretation and true utility of these is still debated. Scientific literature has demonstrated the general concept that concentrations obtained from the central compartment tend to be higher than the peripheral compartment. An additional factor that needs to be determined is the timing and location of the sample postmortem.[12,21,22] The drug level at the time of the autopsy will not reflect the drug level at the time of death. Autopsies may be performed after death: hours, days, weeks, or even months later. The time interval between death and autopsy can translate into changes in concentrations of a drug and/or its metabolite(s) as well. Generally, the drug is less likely to be altered in the peripheral compartment immediately after death; however, the central compartment (blood from the heart) can reflect a higher drug level secondary to diffusion and translocation of the drug from other compartments (e.g., lungs) especially those with a high Vd. In addition, several drugs have been demonstrated to have movement within the body that is dependent on the time of sampling after death. For example, due to bacterial metabolism and enzyme activity, the concentrations of certain medications can become elevated or decreased (e.g., clozapine and promethazine).[14,15,21,22]

In addition, there are inherent challenges with postmortem drug levels. Newly introduced drugs by the Food and Drug Administration often may not have therapeutically defined serum reference levels or a standard assay to which to measure them. In clinical practice, blood samples taken for drug-level analysis are typically obtained from a peripheral vein in the arm. During an autopsy, a blood sample may be obtained from the femoral artery or the heart chamber. In addition to the C/P ratio, another technique that is being utilized is to review the blood/plasma ratios. The postmortem blood/plasma ratio was introduced to attempt to more accurately describe the degree of redistribution, protein binding, and differences in acidic/basic drugs. One study reviewed over 57,000 autopsies in which the concentrations were analyzed for 129 different drugs.[23] Therefore, utilizing the blood/plasma ratio may be another method/tool to help supplement any clinical data regarding an incident in which medication concentration was thought to have a role.

Another technique when reviewing postmortem drug levels is to review the subject's medical records that note the patient's condition before death. Did the subject exhibit classical signs and symptoms of the toxicity of the suspected agent? For example, a person overdosing on bupropion would have convulsions. When the suspect is treated in a hospital, ambulance, or other clinical situation just prior to death, the relevant records should be reviewed as part of the forensic investigation. Unfortunately, a common scenario is that the decedent is found in the home after an apparent sudden death.

TABLE 41.2
Drugs and Toxins That May Undergo PMR[2,4,16]

Alprazolam
Amitriptyline
Amphetamine
Cocaine
Dextromethorphan
Diazepam
Flecanide
Gammahydroxybutarate
Haloperidol
Ketamine
Lidocaine
Morphine
Nicotine
Phencyclidine
Propafenone
Remifentanyl
Sufentanil
Venlafaxine
Zolpidem

41.4 SUMMARY AND CONCLUSIONS

An investigator has several important concepts to incorporate during the analysis of postmortem drug levels. Integrating the subject's case with past and current medical and medication history and laboratory values is vital in determining a plausible scenario. The information recorded above will allow the investigator to proceed with the next steps in determining the time and the location in the body where the postmortem drug levels were obtained. As autopsies may not be performed on the same day as a subject's death, PMR may have a significant role in drug levels, depending on the drug(s) in question. Finally, the investigator needs to concentrate on several drug properties which can alter the drug-level postmortem, which include, but are not limited to, the lipophilic nature, pKa, and Vd of the drug.[14–17] Performing a scientific conclusion also requires the utilization of a methodology which is sustainable under cross-examination. A careful analysis of the subject's case, autopsy report, and a review of the drugs' characteristics allows the investigator to form a more scientific and reliable conclusion or opinion for a forensic case involving a postmortem drug level.[21]

REFERENCES

1. Roberts DM and Buckley NA. Pharmacokinetic considerations in clinical toxicology. *Clin Pharmacokinet.* 2007;46:897–939.
2. Ferner RE. Post-mortem clinical pharmacology. *Br J Clin Pharmacol.* 2008;66:430–443.

3. Winek CL, Wahba WW, Winek CL Jr, Balzer TW. Drug and chemical blood-level data 2001. *Foren Sci Int*. 2001;122:107–123.
4. Baselt R. *Disposition of Toxic Drugs and Chemicals in Man*, 8th edition, 2008. Biomedical Publications.
5. Wennig R. Threshold values in toxicology: Useful or not? Forensic Sci Int. 2000;113:323–340.
6. Brunton LL, Chabner BA, Knollmann BC. Chapter 2: Pharmacokinetics; Buxton IL, Benet LZ. Chapter 3: Pharmacodynamics; Blumenthal DK, Garrison JC. Chapter 4: Drug toxicity and poisoning; Osterhoudt KC, Penning TM. In *Goodman and Gilmans Pharmacologic Basis of Therapeutics*, 11th edition, 2006. Biomedical Publications.
7. Pélissier-Alicot AL, Gaulier JM, Champsaur P, Marquet P. Mechanisms underlying postmortem redistribution of drugs: A review. *J Anal Toxicol*. 2003;27:533–544.
8. Robertson MD, Drummer OH. Post-mortem metabolism by bacteria. J Forensic Sci. 1995;40:382–386.
9. Pounder DJ, Adams E, Fuke C, Langford AM. Site to site variability of postmortem drug concentrations in liver and lung. J Forensic Sci. 1996;41:927–932.
10. Pounder DJ, Smith DRW. Postmortem diffusion of alcohol from the stomach. Am J Forensic Sci. 1995;16:89–96.
11. Flanagan RJ, Connally G. Interpretation of analytical toxicology results in life and at postmortem. Toxicol Rev. 2005;24:51–56.
12. Skopp G. Preanalytic aspects in postmortem toxicology. Forensic Sci Int. 2004;142:75–100.
13. Jones GR, Pounder DJ. Site dependence of drug concentrations in postmortem blood: A case study. J Anal Toxicol. 1987;11:186–190.
14. Brockbals L, Staeheli SN, Gascho D, Ebert LC, Kraemer T, Steuer AE. Time dependent postmortem redistribution of opioids in blood and alternative matrices. J Anal Toxicol. 2018;42:365–374.
15. Kennedy M. Interpreting postmortem drug analysis and redistribution in determining cause of death: A review. Pathol Lab Med Int. 2015;7:55–62.
16. Yarema MC, Becker CE. Key concepts in postmortem drug redistribution. *Clin Toxicol*. 2005;43: 235–241.
17. Leikin JB, Watson WA. Post-mortem toxicology: What the dead can and cannot tell us. Clin Toxicol. 2003;41:47–56.
18. Gerostamoulos J, Drummer OH. Postmortem redistribution of morphine and its metabolites. J Forensic Sci. 2000;45:843–845.
19. Drummer OH. Postmortem toxicology of drugs of abuse. *Forensic Sci Int*. 2004;142:101–113.
20. Kennedy MC. Post-mortem drug concentrations. *Int Med J*. 2010;40:183–187.
21. Drummer OH. Forensic toxicology. *Mol Clin Environ Toxicol*. 2010;100:579–603.
22. Maurer HH. Analytical toxicology. *Mol Clin Environ Toxicol*. 2010;100:317–337.
23. Launiainen T, Ojanpera I. Drug concentrations in post-mortem femoral blood compared with therapeutic concentrations in plasma. Drug Test Anal. 2014;6:308–316.

42 Addiction as Mitigation

Barry D. Hargan and James T. O'Donnell

SYNOPSIS

42.1 INTRODUCTION

The author (BDH) is an addictive disorders expert witness in capital murder cases who has testified as such in several states and in a variety of hearings over the years in both the guilt and penalty phases of a trial and a variety of other types of hearings and depositions.

When I am examined on the witness stand, my testimony under direct examination typically opens with a description of addiction. I have used the term "description" versus "definition" here since different experts may have different perceptions as to what addiction is based on their particular training and experience. An expert who subscribes to the learned behavior theory of addiction, for example, will define addiction from that particular perspective or paradigm while a physician may define addiction in medical terms consistent with the American Medical Association's 1956 description of alcoholism as a disease (versus a behavioral disorder). The debate rages on. I tend to take a more eclectic approach when describing addiction, since it is apparent to me that addiction is actually best described as any combination of genetics, learned behavior, and biochemical changes in the brain associated with cellular adaptation, tolerance, and the impact of a drug's half-life on brain function. Many other experts and I then tend to describe addiction in court as a brain disorder characterized by the continued use or abuse of a mood-altering substance despite known risks and prior negative consequences from the use of that drug.

42.2 CLINICAL VARIABLES WHICH CONTRIBUTE TO THE ONSET OF ADDICTION

There are several reliable clinical variables which this writer explores when conducting a substance abuse examination with an offender for court. The primary variables

DOI: 10.1201/9781003615323-46

which need to be investigated include ruling out the presence of a genetic predisposition to the development of an addictive disorder or ruling out environmental or learned behavioral considerations, psychological trauma by history, or the presence of any particular neurobiological changes in brain function as a result of addiction.

42.2.1 Genetic Predisposition

When examining a patient or offender during a substance abuse evaluation, the first thing I do is to take a family history since an offender's inherited tendency to develop an addiction can be considered mitigating evidence in the penalty phase of a criminal trial. A genetic predisposition in an alcoholic family constellation will elevate a given family member's vulnerability to the development of addiction, especially in the sons of alcoholic fathers. The Swedish geneticist Dr. Robert Cloninger is known for his landmark 1981 Stockholm Adoption Study concerning twins born to alcoholic parents but raised by adoptive parents who abstained from alcohol. His work resulted in our understanding today that alcoholism can be inherited and that alcoholism can be broken out into two separate categories referred to as Type I and Type II alcoholism. Alcoholism typing actually dates back to the work of the reputed alcoholism researcher Dr. E. M. Jellinek in the 1930s and 1940s. He reported that there were five different types of alcoholism at the time.

His typing was based on the presence, absence, or combination of the clinical variables of psychological dependence and/or physical dependence.[1]

In 1996, Dr. Cloninger published an update on his 1981 twins research in *Alcohol Health & Research World* associated with his original Stockholm Adoption Study. In that article, he noted that, of children born to alcoholic parents who were then adopted out to teetotaler adoptive parents, 14.7% of the birth parents' sons and 2.8% of their daughters developed alcoholism, while 22.4% of their sons and 3.5% of their daughters developed alcoholism when the father was alcoholic but the mother was not; 26.0% of their sons and 10.3% of their daughters developed the disorder when the father was not alcoholic but the mother was; and 33.3% of their sons and 9.1% of their daughters developed alcoholism when both birth parents were alcoholic.[2]

Type II alcoholism was also discussed in a paper presented to Congress in 1993. In the *Eighth Special Report to the U. S. Congress on Alcohol and Health*, the following description of Type II alcoholism was provided to Congress:

> A cross-fostering analysis from a large adoptee sample in Sweden demonstrated the existence of two forms of inherited vulnerability to alcohol, referred to as Type I and Type II . . . More common than Type II alcoholism, Type I alcoholism occurred in both men and women, was less severe than Type II and was associated with mild, adult onset in either biological parent . . . Type II alcoholism was characterized by a severe type of susceptibility that is significantly influenced by genetics; its expression appeared to be relatively unaffected by environmental factors. This form of alcoholism occurred only in men, and their problem drinking developed early, often during adolescence. In addition, persons classified as Type II alcoholics were characterized by aggressive behavior and involvement with the police. Similar characteristics were found in the biological fathers of these individuals. (page 63)

I have made references to the various aspects of Type II alcoholism many times over the years while on the witness stand educating the court or the jury and as to how Type II alcoholism can cause emotional and behavioral management difficulties for the alcoholic at the time of an offense and arrest.

Type II alcoholics were found by Cloninger to develop an early onset of the disease by age 25, although my experience has taught me that Type II alcoholism will frequently emerge in adolescence in the sons of alcoholic fathers. Type II alcoholics were characterized by Cloninger as having aggressive behavior and frequent contact with law enforcement. Our jails and prisons are full of Type II alcoholics. With an earlier onset than Type I alcoholism, they tend to get into trouble with law enforcement and other social institutions at an earlier age, develop tolerance at an earlier age, and die at an earlier age. Not all alcoholics develop alcoholism by inheriting it from their parents, but the more generations an investigator can uncover that seem to be evidence of the disorder, the more vulnerable the off-spring will be to developing the addiction.

Consequently, when examining an offender, I will investigate any genetic predisposition to the development of addiction and, in particular, whether there is a link between the male alcoholic's history of alcoholism and that of his father. There is then a wealth of mitigating evidence to be found in the potential genetic predisposition in addictive family systems.

The observation that sons of alcoholics tend to suffer from an alcoholic family's genetic predisposition has been shared by other genetics researchers as well. A study sponsored by the National Institute of Drug Abuse (NIDA) reported that NIDA-sponsored studies involving male and female twins showed that genetic factors for drug abuse are stronger in males than in females. Dr. Roy Pickens and Dr. Marianne van den Bree with the National Institutes of Health's Intramural Research Program studied 188 twin pairs and found that

> For females, genetic influences accounted for 47 percent of the differences between identical and fraternal twins in abuse, dependence, or both for any drug, compare with 79 percent for males. The impact of genetic factors also seems to differ for specific drugs, Dr. Van den Bree. The researchers found no evidence for genetic influence for opiate or sedative abuse, dependence, or both in females, but "in males genetic influences were generally larger than environmental influences."

Genetic influences trumped learned behavior, according to their findings.

Furthermore, NIDA-supported research showed that Drs. George Uhl and Quing-Rong Liu, who were also with the Intramural Research Program's Molecular Neurobiology Branch, found that 89 genes displayed clusters of genetic variants that are likely involved in the genetic transmission of addiction from one generation to the next and that genetics seemed to play a larger role in that transmission than environmental factors. Again, genetics trumped learned behavior in their findings as well. Finn and Justus found that researchers have been able to differentiate sons of alcoholics from sons of non-alcoholics on several measures. They found, for example, that drinking alcohol dramatically reduced sons of alcoholics' reactivity to stressful stimuli, that sons of alcoholics were less sensitive to the effect of alcohol consumption when compared with sons of non-alcoholics, and that sons of alcoholics experienced a more rewarding feeling from consuming alcohol than sons of non-alcoholics. Sons of alcoholics felt less impaired when consuming alcohol. We frequently hear this in impaired driving court cases, where the defendant claimed he did not feel as impaired as the documented blood alcohol concentration suggested he actually was.

42.2.2 Learned Behavior

There is also evidence to suggest that addictive behavior can be learned as well. Children of addicts are frequently raised in a family system whereby the primary parental focus is on obtaining and using substances or recovering from the effects of substance abuse and where parental binge drinking or heavy and compulsive drug use is seen over time by their children as normal patterns of drinking and drug using behavior. Exposure to parental substance abuse inadvertently models inappropriate behavior for their children, who will then mimic parental behavior later on in adolescence, because that is how they learned to use or abuse mood-altering substances; by watching and learning from their addicted parents. Studies have already shown that children tend to mimic their parents' drinking habits as they get older, a phenomenon which researchers and learning theorists refer to as "observational learning."

42.2.3 Psychopathological Exposure

When we are addressing the issue of psychopathological exposure as a mitigating factor in the development of an addictive disorder, we are referring, for example, to an individual's exposure to trauma such as incest, which can occur during childhood or adolescence within an addictive family, and trauma which can occur outside of the family such as assault or combat in a war zone. Examples of familial or parental pathology to which children of addicts are most often exposed include parental clinical depression or antisocial behavior, mood swings, irritability, aggression, domestic violence and frequent police contacts, parental absence, negligence, or lack of family cohesion or communication. Psychopathological experiences outside of the family can refer to an individual's exposure to war, sexual or other types of assault and violation, and other issues associated, which can result in the development of psychiatric disorders.

Regier reported on the findings of a landmark federal research project, which investigated the relationship between co-occurring psychiatric and addictive disorders in patients. He reported that 78% of male alcoholics and 86% of female alcoholics met lifetime criteria for having at least one other psychiatric disorder, that 72% of individuals with a drug addiction were also found to have a co-occurring psychiatric disorder, and that 56% of patients diagnosed with bipolar disorder were also found to have a substance abuse disorder. Furthermore, 36% of patients diagnosed with a mood disorder such as clinical depression also had met diagnostic criteria for having a substance abuse disorder while up to 50% of men and 30% of women diagnosed with posttraumatic stress disorder were also found to have a substance abuse disorder.

The reason for the elevated rate of substance abuse among individuals who have experienced psychological trauma has to do with the tendency of traumatized individuals to self-medicate those symptoms of anxiety and depression with alcohol or drugs for relief. It has been my clinical experience that individuals suffering from anxiety tend to be attracted to mood-altering substances with sedative properties (such as alcohol, marijuana, and opiates) while individuals suffering from depression tend to gravitate toward stimulants (such as amphetamines, cocaine, and methamphetamine). Abuse of any of these substances can lead to psychological or physical dependence or addiction. The traumatized individual will then have to manage both his or her psychiatric disorder and the secondary addictive disorder to prevent relapse, since relapse in one of these two types of disorders can trigger relapse in the other.

42.2.4 Substance/Medication-Induced Mental Disorder

I have also testified many times to what was previously called the substance-induced mood disorder, which was described in the previous edition of the *Diagnostic and Statistical Manual of Mental Disorders, Fourth Edition* (*DSM-IV*). The substance-induced mood disorder was described as a transient central nervous system phenomenon that could be triggered during acute intoxication or withdrawal from a given mood-altering substance. Symptoms range from dysphoria (mild depression) to violent behavior. These symptoms always subsided once the individual returned to sobriety, so this was a transient or short-term disorder, often with long-term consequences. The *Diagnostic and Statistical Manual of Mental Disorders, Fifth Edition* (*DSM-5*) now refers to this transient disorder as substance/

medication-induced mental disorder. The phenomenon refers to extreme changes in mood or behavior during bouts of acute intoxication, which seem out of character for the individual and which often results in criminal or violent behavior. I had a patient once who became acutely intoxicated and was involved in a barroom brawl. He punched a man in the face so hard that the victim fell back and hit his head on a radiator and died. Our patient woke up in jail the next morning charged with Manslaughter; he had no recollection of the tragedy because he was in an alcoholic blackout at the time.

Most of the murder cases I was involved with in Chicago and other cities in the early 2000s involved defendants who committed their crimes while coming down from crack cocaine, although the explanation for this is more biological than psychological. The mood swings, violent behavior, and psychotic episodes this writer encountered in addicts charged with capital murder seemed at times to have been associated more with the effects of the substance and/or medication-induced mental disorders than simply having a very high degree of psychopathology. They become desperate and sometimes dangerous. The shootings in those cases seemed to be at times an over-reaction to a move or comment by the victim and were not always consistent with the shooter's character or past record. The symptoms such as mood swings and violent behavior diminish once the intoxication or withdrawal syndromes have run their course, and the individual returns to their usual personality organization. The *DSM-5*, however, notes that symptoms may occur anytime within a month of abstinence, which is a recent finding, similar to the "flashbacks" that methamphetamine users experience. From my own 30 years of training and clinical experience, it would seem, however, that the majority if not all of the symptoms resolve once the intoxication or withdrawal syndromes have run their course.

42.3 FORENSIC TOXICOLOGY CASE REPORT: NEUROTOXICOLOGY EVALUATION FOR MITIGATION PURPOSES—EXCESSIVE ALCOHOL AND ANABOLIC STEROID USE IN AN ADOLESCENT MALE/DEATH PENALTY CASE

A recent consultation (by JTOD) in a death penalty case was conducted for mitigation purposes. The goal of the attorney was to determine if such an evaluation should have been offered in the case in chief and, if so, what findings would have been presented to the Court and Jury.

42.3.1 Executive Summary of Opinion

Excessive and prolonged use of alcohol and anabolic steroids damages the adolescent brain, preventing normal brain development, and substantially increases the risk of behavioral toxicity and aggressive and violent behavior.

42.3.2 Neurotoxicity Mechanisms of Alcohol and Anabolic Steroids in the Developing Brain

Adolescence is a critical developmental stage in the maturation of the human brain. The continuing growth in neural connectivity occurs throughout important cortical and subcortical brain regions and associated neural circuitry, making this time highly sensitive to environmental influence. Decades of research have demonstrated that the adolescent brain continues to undergo significant structural and functional changes, rendering the brain uniquely vulnerable to the neurotoxic effects of ingested substances such as alcohol and drugs. Exposure of the immature brain to these substances can result in acute and long-term ramifications subsequent to their neurotoxic effects. Alcohol and drug use (e.g., anabolic steroid use) can result in significant changes in structural, neurotransmitter, and hormone systems, which greatly influence the maturation of certain brain areas and neural circuitry. Healthy brain development throughout adolescence is important for optimal neurocognitive and behavioral performance. Even subtle changes in neurodevelopmental trajectories (e.g., changes in neurocircuitry, cortical thickness and volume, and myelination) can impact cognitive, emotional, behavioral, and social functioning. Heavy alcohol use during adolescence has been studied extensively and is cross-sectionally associated with impairment in many neuropsychological domains, including memory, executive functioning, visuospatial processing and skills, inhibitory functioning, and attention. Chronic alcohol use in adolescents is also correlated with psychosocial abnormalities, reduced academic success, and significant neurocognitive consequences. Heavy-drinking patterns which begin during adolescence often continue into early adulthood and significantly increase the risk for subsequent adult alcohol use disorders and related problems.[3] Altered brain development due to exposure to neurotoxins, such as alcohol and drugs, during adolescence, can significantly impact adulthood, conferring functional consequences throughout the individual's lifetime.

Adolescence is marked by an increased level of risk-taking behaviors. Evidence suggests a mismatched development in critical brain regions that drive pleasure-seeking versus executive decision-making behaviors. Executive functioning (i.e., reasoning) is not fully developed in higher cortical brain regions, leaving subcortical limbic structures (i.e., those involved in pleasure-seeking, emotion, and motivation) largely influencing behavioral choices. Brain maturation generally begins in lower-order sensorimotor regions, while brain regions associated with higher-order executive functioning (e.g., frontal-cortical brain structures) develop later in adolescence. The pre-frontal cortex is one of the last brain regions to fully mature and is responsible for driving rational and reasonable decision-making.[4] This contributes to risk-taking and novelty-seeking among adolescents who, in turn, are more likely to engage in alcohol and drug abuse during this critical time of brain maturation.

Alcohol and drug use is widespread among adolescents. In particular, binge drinking, or heavy episodic drinking, typically defined as >4 drinks/occasion for females or >5 or more drinks for males, is a prevalent occurrence among youth. Exposure to heavy alcohol is concerning as the adolescent brain undergoes extensive morphometric and functional maturation during this time period. In particular, changes in white matter (myelinated axons that serve to connect different parts of the brain) and gray matter (consisting of the brain cell bodies, dendrites, and axon terminals) of the brain are prevalent throughout the maturation process. Gray matter reductions are noted during early adolescence and are considered related to synaptic changes such as the pruning of excess neurons throughout the brain, and these processes extend into early adulthood (mid-20s). Reductions in gray matter are linked to the elimination of weak synaptic connections.[5] In parallel, white matter volumes increase throughout adolescence, attributed to synaptic changes which strengthen the formation of neural connectivity via myelin proliferation. These tandem processes are a critical element in neurocognitive and behavioral development, and, throughout these extensive maturational changes, the developing adolescent brain is highly sensitive to the detrimental effects of alcohol and drug abuse.[6]

Imaging techniques, such as structural magnetic resonance imaging (MRI), are important diagnostic tools that can assess specific metrics (i.e., tissue thickness, surface area, and volume) of the adolescent brain to determine abnormalities. Evidence from cross-sectional studies shows long-term brain structural changes following binge and heavy drinking of various lengths in adolescence. Reductions in the volume of neocortical regions, in particular, the frontal cortices, which are important regulators of executive function and cognition, are observed in addition to volume deficits in temporal and parietal cortices. Reduced gray matter has been reported in critical cortical structures such as the anterior cingulate cortex, orbitofrontal cortex, temporal gyrus, and insular cortex in adolescents who participated in heavy drinkers and were followed for ten years.[7,8]

Initiation of heavy alcohol drinking during adolescence disrupts normal, differential growth trajectories of selective cortical gray matter regions. These effects may be attributed to the acceleration of normal pruning mechanisms in brain regions with high cerebral blood flow (CBF) during alcohol exposure.[9] Reductions in hippocampal and cerebellar volumes are also observed in heavy-drinking adolescents compared to non-drinking controls.[10] A large cross-sectional study reported reductions in volumes and thinner cortical tissue in total, frontal, and temporal gray matter in addition to thinner cingulate cortex compared to normal.[11] Altogether, widespread cortical thinning, tissue volume reductions, and alterations in white/gray matter in these developing brain regions likely underlie the subsequent behavioral pathology abnormalities observed in adolescent binge drinkers.

Cognitive (thinking) functions, such as those that can be measured using spatial working memory, are also disrupted following adolescent drinking. A spatial working memory task can be used as a neurocognitive marker of alcohol's impact on the brain. These deficits may translate to behaviors such as driving safety, academic performance, and neuropsychological performance. Abnormalities in both females and male binge drinkers are seen in multiple brain regions including the bilateral frontal, anterior cingulate, temporal, and cerebellar cortices. These abnormalities were associated with changes in attention and working and spatial memory performance. This study also reports on gender-specific differences and shows that females may be more vulnerable to the neurotoxic effects of heavy alcohol use during adolescence.[12] Evidence from longitudinal studies shows reductions in spatial functioning and attention span in adolescents who initiated binge drinking at 3-year follow-up, suggesting that certain cognitive tasks may show increased vulnerability to the effects of adolescent drinking.[13] It is postulated that changes in cognitive function, at the molecular level, may relate to disruption of myelination, as white matter abnormalities have been observed among adolescent binge drinkers. Enhanced brain activity in fronto-parietal regions during working memory, verbal learning, and inhibitory control tasks are also seen in adolescent binge drinkers. In response to alcohol-related cues, binge and heavy drinkers show increased neural response in mesocorticolimbic regions, including the striatum, anterior cingulate cortex, hippocampus, and amygdala.[14]

At the molecular level, binge drinking during adolescence alters numerous aspects of synaptic transmission both directly and indirectly to alter brain function and behavior. These changes are speculated to occur through modifications at the synaptic level. Alcohol induces acute and long-term effects at the synapse. Acute exposure increases the function of ligand-gated ion channels, enhancing the activity of gamma amino benzoic acid (GABA) and glycine receptors to increase synaptic and extra-synaptic inhibition. Synaptic excitation is dampened in many brain regions, and most forms of synaptic plasticity are impaired. Long-term effects of chronic alcohol exposure include a hyperexcitable central nervous system status with enhanced function of *N*-methyl-D-aspartate (NMDA) receptors, increased glutamate release, and increased responses to other glutamate receptors. GABAergic synapses show altered efficacy of inhibitory synaptic transmission, leading to changes in synaptic tone. Synaptic proteins, such as synapsin IIa, syntaxin 4, SNAP-25, and synaptotagmin, are downregulated following alcohol exposure.[15]

42.3.3 Anabolic Steroid Effects on Brain Structure and Function

Similar to the detrimental effects that alcohol can impose on the maturing brain, the use and abuse of certain drugs can likewise cause significant impairment. The transition from adolescence to adulthood is highly dependent on gonadal sex hormones. These hormones also play a contributing role in brain maturation. These naturally occurring hormones, such as testosterone, are associated with changes in cerebral gray matter morphology during puberty.[16,17] High circulating testosterone levels have been associated with differential effects on hippocampal, amygdala, and hypothalamic volumes (gender specific). Increases in hormones and sex steroids are associated with temperamental and behavioral changes (e.g., elevated risk-taking and social and exploratory behavior).[18] Steroids are known to disrupt neural communication in brain regions that govern mood. External influence on these hormonal markers through the use of anabolic-androgenic steroids (AASs) can affect brain development, cognition, and behavior. AASs are a class of drugs that have been abused at alarming rates among adolescents, in particular, adolescent males. These drugs are commonly abused for their advantageous properties in improving strength and muscle mass. These drugs are taken chronically and are linked to significant changes in mood, anxiety, aggressiveness, and behavior.[19]

Preclinical (animal) studies indicate that adolescent anabolic steroid exposure induces structural changes in many brain regions that regulate mood and memory, including the hippocampus, amygdala, and neurotransmitter systems such as serotonin, catecholamines, vasopressin, GABA, and glutamate. Changes in the structure and neurotransmitter systems of these limbic regions impact a range of functions that include aggression, learning, and rational responses to external stimuli. Preclinical (animal) evidence confirms the association of aggressive behavior following exposure during adolescence to anabolic steroids and naturally occurring hormones, such as testosterone. Long-term behavioral and structural changes in the brain following anabolic steroid exposure were also observed. The long-term effects of adolescent anabolic steroid use in humans are largely unknown; however, aggression has been shown to remain elevated for several weeks (2–17 weeks) following the withdrawal of anabolic steroid exposure.[20] Alterations in neural connectivity through increased neuronal spine density, a measure of excitatory action in the brain, are observed in limbic brain regions following anabolic steroid withdrawal.[21] These molecular changes are in parallel with the observations of long-term aggressive behavioral effects.

42.3.4 Translational Impact—What Does This Mean to a Teenager Abusing Large Amounts of Alcohol and Steroids?

Given the clear ramifications on the brain during adolescent alcohol and drug use, it warrants investigation into the clinical and social-behavioral consequences that occur following exposure during this critical time in brain maturation. As described previously, many deficits in the development of the cortical regions of the brain are noted in adolescents who engage in drug use and heavy drinking. These deficits are of high concern as the cortex is one of the last brain regions to fully develop, and thus highly vulnerable to the neurotoxic impact of these exposures. The cortex is involved in many important functions governing behavior; however, the impact on executive control processes is of high importance when considering subsequent high-risk behaviors which may lead to adverse adult outcomes in this population. Studies indicate that an interplay exists between the rational reasoning of the frontal-cortical regions (e.g., pre-frontal cortex) and subcortical structures governing reward (e.g., ventral striatum, nucleus accumbens [NAc]). Brain regions governing reward-seeking mature earlier, thus predisposing adolescents to be more impulsive in their decision-making. It is the development of the frontal cortices throughout adolescence and young adulthood that acts to reduce these risk-taking or impulsive behaviors commonly noted in adolescents, thus promoting success in adulthood. However, detrimental effects on the development of a healthy cortical system will have long-lasting consequences on behavior into adulthood.[22]

Impulsive decision-making and drug and alcohol abuse have a complex relationship. Impulsive and risky decision-making is associated with drug and alcohol abuse, both as a contributing influence and as a consequence of exposure, eliciting a cyclical series of cause and effect that has significant consequences and long-lasting problematic influence on behavior. The acute and chronic effects of drug and alcohol abuse may increase impulsive behaviors, which may facilitate choices to engage in future use. As a determinant, the adolescent brain status predisposes this population to engage in impulsive decision-making due to immature neural maturation. Risky decision-making is a contributing factor to drug experimentation, problematic drug use, and high relapse rates. These maladaptive behaviors may be increased through the use of drugs and alcohol through both acute and long-term consequences of continued drug and alcohol use. High levels of impulsivity are observed in individuals with a history of alcohol or drug use. Many studies show deficits in reward processing that include discounting behavior. Higher discounting, that is, the preference for more immediate rewards versus larger, delayed rewards, has been observed in individuals who are current drug and alcohol users or those with a history of abuse.[23] These deficits in reward processing may underlie many of the behavioral consequences seen in this population. Prolonged exposure to alcohol and drug use may impair critical inhibitory processes due to permanent neurological sequelae of long-term exposure.[24,25]

Adolescent alcohol and drug abuse is associated with adverse outcomes affecting health and social functioning in adulthood. These negative effects include continued drug and alcohol use, enhanced risk of dependence, sexual risk-taking, criminal activity, reduced education, unemployment, homelessness, psychiatric morbidities, and social complications. Evidence collected from drinking-discordant twin pairs following the transition from adolescence to adulthood provides a compelling causal interaction between the effects of adolescent alcohol exposure and adverse adult outcomes. Outcomes assessed included truncated (interrupted) education, financial difficulties, frequent intoxication, smoking and high-density drinking, poor health, multiple sexual partners, and life dissatisfaction.[26]

Alcohol and drug use and criminal activity are correlated and commonly seen in the criminal justice system. Alcohol use is a risk factor for violent behavior and alcoholic binge drinking is found to be more prevalent in violent criminal offenders.[27] Adolescent alcohol problems are predictive of having any officially recorded criminal convictions in the subsequent 15 years.[28] Anabolic steroid use is also linked to greater involvement in violent behaviors (e.g., shooting or stabbing someone) and even homicide.[29] Systematic reports demonstrate a range of alcohol abuse and dependence (18–30% in males; 10–24% in females) and drug abuse and dependence (10–48% in males; 30–60% in females) in prison populations.[30] These reports highlight the influence that drug and alcohol use have on criminal activity. Increasing the availability of longitudinal data on the development of conduct problems and delinquency in adolescents has suggested specific developmental paths, resulting in certain types of delinquency that may be associated with substance abuse. Therefore, it is not surprising that the neural (brain) consequences experienced during adolescent exposure to drugs and alcohol can promote long-term dysfunctional behavioral outcomes which are linked to problematic or delinquent behaviors occurring later in life.[31,32,33,34]

The adolescent brain is in a critical developmental stage that renders it uniquely susceptible to the neurotoxic effects of alcohol and drug use. There is substantial evidence to demonstrate that alcohol and drug use (i.e., alcohol and anabolic androgenic steroids) during adolescence causes acute and long-term cognitive and behavioral dysfunction. Altered brain plasticity, neural structure, changes to neurotransmitter systems, and synaptic modifications following exposure to alcohol or drugs in adolescents may be related to the neurotoxic (brain damaging) effects during a highly plastic (molding/forming) neurodevelopmental period. These functional changes are correlated with impairment in many neurobehavioral domains, including memory and executive functioning—which permits an individual to inhibit their impulses and natural, habitual, or dominant behavioral responses to stimuli. These effects may impact the normal trajectory for brain development and thus predispose adolescents to potential cognitive and behavioral impairments in adulthood. These impairments may significantly alter an individual's adult success through impact on education, finances, mentality, and social and legal constructs.

42.3.5 Clinical and Practical Applications of Basic Neuroscience

The causes of violence are far from being completely understood but are multifactorial and involve biological, psychological, sociological, economic, and environmental factors. Biological causes include genetics, hormones, disease states, sleep deprivation, poor nutrition, drugs, head trauma, seizures, and tumors. Psychological causes include major mental illness and a history of abuse. Ethanol or drinking alcohol is the most common social drug, and the evidence linking alcohol to violence is overwhelming. Ethanol has a broad range of effects including incoordination, altered perceptions, sedation, and decreased inhibitions. Alcohol contributes to aggression in many ways including increased sensation-seeking and impulsive behaviors. Alcohol contributes to aggression in many ways including increased sensation-seeking and impulsive behaviors.[35]

Alcohol consumption is linked to aggressive behavior and increases the risk of being the victim (or perpetrator) of a violent act. This is more notable in heavy users. Alcohol-related aggression is caused by a decline in cognitive functioning and inaccurate expectations about the alcohol effect. Preventative efforts focused on educating college students may aid in identifying risky situations that might facilitate the expression of intoxicated aggression. These studies portray a compelling relation between alcohol and aggression, particularly on college campuses. Nevertheless, it would also be important to consider other dispositional traits that could increase the probability of exposure to such "high-risk" contexts such as problem behaviors prior to college and preexisting attitudes that promote disinhibited behavior, violence, and excessive drinking.

A large number of controlled experimental laboratory investigations have also demonstrated a strong relation between alcohol use and aggressive behavior. Experimental studies are advantageous over correlational studies in that their design structure allows for the formulation of causal inferences. Another important reason for paying attention to the results of experimental studies is that although many of these studies utilize samples of convenience, these samples tend to consist mainly of college students. Finally, Geen added that, even in a highly aroused or angered state, the expression of aggression can still be moderated by paying attention to alternative non-aggressive means of coping with the situation. However, if such attentional resources are lacking, the probability of an aggressive response will be heightened.

Approximately 40% of crimes are alcohol related. Alcohol can enhance aggressive moods that may start to appear after a person has drunk too much. Scientists have linked aggression to the consumption of too much alcohol—so it's not surprising that a person is more likely to argue after drinking.

42.3.6 Behavioral Abnormalities Associated With Anabolic Steroid Use

AASs include testosterone and its derivatives. AASs possess both anabolic steroids and have been studied as a treatment for depression in men. Toxic effects of AAS, specifically orally ingested products, include cardiovascular, hepatic (liver), endocrine, and psychiatric reactions. Cardiovascular side effects include a lowering of high-density lipoprotein cholesterol, elevations of low-density lipoprotein cholesterol, and impairing the contractile functions of the heart. Psychiatric adverse effects include distractibility, delirium, psychosis, hypomania and mania, insomnia, hostility, and mood lability.

An excerpt from Aitchison's extensive review of AASs is instructive and summarizes several published reviews and studies on behavioral abnormalities associated with AAS use.

> Individual behavioral and psychiatric responses to chronic AAS abuse are extremely variable, depending on preexisting psychiatric conditions, personality, and type and dose of AAS. Case reports and some epidemiology studies associate chronic AAS use with changes in behavior, mood, and somatic perceptions in a small subset of chronic AAS abusers.

Psychiatric complications associated with chronic AAS use include mania, aggression, and agitation, but no large-scale epidemiologic studies have confirmed a causal relationship between chronic AAS abuse and severe psychiatric complications (e.g., psychosis). Depression may occur, particularly in the immediate period after cessation of use, along with fatigue, decreased libido, insomnia, anorexia, and headaches. Studies suggest that male AAS users have more frequent and prolonged periods of anger, aggression, irritability, and hostility than non-users. Multivariate models based on data from the National Longitudinal Study of Adolescent Health indicate that young men using AASs report greater involvement in violent behaviors than non-users after controlling for the effects of key demographic variables, previous violent behavior, and polydrug use. In a study of two sets of male monozygotic twins with only one twin using AASs, the use of AASs was associated with anxiety, hostility, aggressiveness, and paranoid ideations. Behavioral abnormalities include distractibility, delirium, delusions, irritability, paranoia, impulsivity, insomnia, hostility, anxiety, agitation, aggression, violence, and mood lability. These behavioral effects are dose dependent, with effects ranging from mild effects (increased confidence, enhanced self-esteem, and euphoria) to serious behavioral abnormalities (mood swings, grandiose thinking, paranoia, impulsivity, hostility, violence, and antisocial behavior).

Abusing steroids is linked to a multitude of complications including high cholesterol and liver damage. The development of aggressive "roid rage" behavior is controversial. The term "roid rage" was first coined in the 1980s, following a series of violent crimes committed by bodybuilders. A more scientific basis for the uncontrollable, hulk-esque fury points to alterations in impulse control, increased pain thresholds, and psychosis.

42.3.7 Defendant's Alcohol and Anabolic Steroid Use

I spoke with the defendant on the telephone in late 2019, specifically to ask him what he remembered about the use, type, amounts, frequency, and effects of both alcohol and anabolic steroids.

At the time of the arrest, the defendant was 195 pounds and had 2% to 3% body fat (normal: 15–20% in adolescent athletes)—his weight did fluctuate up and down. At 14 years old he started using AAS. He was introduced to these by his football coach (who, by the way, denies this). The coach had a "connection" in Mexico. He would provide them to his athletes. The defendant put on a great deal of muscle weight. At the same time, he was constantly trying to lose weight to get under the 170 lb weight limit for the football division. He was using AAS extensively at the time of the murder.

Although he stopped playing football at 16 years old due to several concussions, he did continue as an athlete in track and pole vaulting, and he avidly pursued bodybuilding. He continued using the steroids until the time of his arrest.

Prior to taking steroids, he was a shy kid. On steroids, he was an arrogant and "cocky" athlete. He experienced frequent anger and distinct swings in mood, "like a switch going on." His friends would tell him that he had "snapped" and he would blow things out of proportion.

42.3.7.1 Alcohol

Alcohol played a big part in his life. His stepfather and mother were heavy drinkers. He learned that his biological father was an alcoholic. At 14 years old, he realized that he had a messed-up family life, and he escaped into alcohol, drinking anything he could get, including beer, vodka, whatever! Indeed, he had fake IDs as a 15-year-old and was going to clubs and drinking alcohol in clubs. When he started, he was only drinking mixed drinks on the weekends. He recalls frequent times when he was drunk and experienced blackouts.

With alcohol, he became the life of the party. He liked the feeling, but he hated being drunk. In high school sometimes he would even drink before classes in the morning. After high school graduation, he worked in a teen dance club and drank while he was working there. He kept the alcohol in his office, as the club did not serve alcohol.

On the day of the murder, he had no intention to rob the shop owner. He went to purchase jewelry that he had previously quoted a price. The price was now higher. The defendant describes that he "literally saw RED" and didn't know anything until he realized he was on top of his bloodied victim. He had a "total loss of control." He was already under the influence (of alcohol). He had been "drinking all night." That morning he "snapped-went into a rage."

42.3.8 Expert Opinions Regarding Substance-Induced Brain Damage Affecting Behavior

My opinions are expressed with reasonable pharmacological certainty.

1. The defendant heavily abused alcohol and anabolic steroids for several years as an adolescent before the murder which occurred when he was a 19-year-old. The brain is not considered to be

mature until approximately 24 years of age. He would be considered to have had alcohol use disorder and substance use disorder (SUD) from steroid abuse.
2. This excessive substance abuse is well known to cause brain damage and arrested brain development in adolescent brains and causes numerous behavioral disturbances which alter cognition (clear thinking), reasoning (deliberation—considering consequences), judgment (risk-taking), impulsivity, hyperaggression, and other specific psychopathologies.
3. The defendant was acutely intoxicated by alcohol at the time of the murder.
4. The defendant's extensive SUDs substantially increased his risk for aggressive and violent behavior and impaired his ability to think and act and deliberate his actions.

42.4 THE SIMPLIFIED VERSION OF NEUROBIOLOGY AND THE ADDICTED BRAIN

Most experts refer to addiction as a brain disorder because addiction develops within a particular neural pathway in the midbrain and because addiction alters brain biochemistry within that all-important neural pathway. As an ongoing addictions expert witness (BDH) for the Cook County Public Defenders Office's Homicide Task Force between 1999 and the abolition of the death penalty in Illinois in 2011, it was my job to investigate any connection between the capital murder and the suspect's addiction history. This was primarily during the crack cocaine epidemic in this country during the early to mid-2000s as noted earlier, and it was also during this time when I became more interested in the neurobiological aspect of addiction.

First, it should be generally noted that addiction develops within a specific neural pathway of the mesolimbic system within the midbrain. This neural pathway runs between the NAc, which terminates within the frontal cortex of the brain, and the ventral tegmental area (VTA), which is rich in dopamine, a brain neurotransmitter which activates other critical systems within the brain. The NAc is also rich in opiate receptors and includes the pleasure center of the brain, as well as the amygdala structure, which is thought to be responsible for emotional management, rage formation, and possibly the imprinting of certain emotional memories, which assist the brain in forming a fight or flight response when appropriate.

Dopamine is associated with pleasure and reward, attention, motivation, and planning. The dopaminergic system is at the basis of the pleasure or euphoria experienced in the brain with the use of certain mood-altering substances. Certain drugs of abuse activate the release of dopamine from the VTA into the terminal regions of the NAc, resulting in a sense of euphoria that addicts endlessly crave, despite known risks and prior negative consequences in the use of said drug. When elevated levels of dopamine are released in the brain by the use of cocaine or methamphetamine, for example, the addict will experience the initial sense of euphoria but will also experience a heightened degree of attention or alertness known as hypervigilance. Paranoia refers to a sense of hypervigilance. Toxic levels of dopamine released into the brain by the use of amphetamine, cocaine, or methamphetamine commonly result in panic, delusions such as ideas of reference, paranoia, psychosis, and violence. These complications most often occur not only during a state of acute stimulant intoxication but also during periods of substance withdrawal as well.

Second, there is the issue of molecular or cellular adaptation which leads to tolerance. After repeated administrations of a given mood-altering drug at the same dose, brain cells will adapt to the presence of the drug, resulting in a decreased sensitivity to the effect of the drug on mood and behavior. Cellular adaptation is thought to be the mechanism behind the development of tolerance in the addicted brain. The neurons within the mesolimbic system not only adapt to the frequent exposure to the presence of a given drug but eventually develop a dependence on the presence of that drug within the cell to function. As the blood alcohol or cocaine levels diminish following the last administration, those cells become hyperexcitable as a rebound effect which adversely affects the user. Adverse effects may include agitation and even violence, along with cravings to obtain more of the drug at any cost arising from the mesolimbic system in crack cocaine addicts. For example, while heroin addicts may experience severe withdrawal symptoms of indigestion, cramping, nausea, and vomiting, the addicted brain facing tolerance and withdrawal will often compel the addict to engage in criminal behavior in order to obtain more of the drug.

At the time of this publication, opiate addiction has surpassed cocaine addiction but not methamphetamine abuse in this country. The methamphetamine epidemic continues its march eastward from the West Coast, state by state and mainly in rural areas where mobile meth labs are harder to detect. Criminal behavior commonly associated with opiate addiction is less violent than that which was associated with crack cocaine or methamphetamine addiction but still carries with it life-threatening consequences. While crack cocaine addicts were often known to become involved with robbery, assault, burglary, and manslaughter, opiate addicts typically rely on retail theft and drug trafficking to support their habits. Sometimes, addicts will sell opiate drugs to another addict who overdoses and dies. The person who sold the deceased addict the heroin is then liable to be charged with that addict's death under the Anti-Drug Abuse Act of 1986 (H.R. 5484) or what is commonly referred to as the Len Bias Law. Other times they may resort to burglary, theft, or other property crime. Violent behavior is generally associated with stimulant abuse while property crime is generally associated with opiate abuse.

When experts refer to the way addiction alters brain biochemistry, structure, and function, they are referring to the way addiction alters the dopaminergic system within the brain, alters perception and mood, or simply contributes to the destruction of nerve cells within the brain, as demonstrated with imaging technology. The changes in brain structure and function vary depending on the type of drug abused by the addict.

It was debated for years as to whether brain damage in alcoholics was associated with alcohol's ability to dissolve the fatty myelin sheath of brain cells, thus impairing the transmission of chemical messages from one neuron to the next. Others claimed that alcoholic brain damage was caused more so by malnutrition. The usual example used to support that argument was the observation that Korsakoff Syndrome has also been diagnosed in Third World countries such as Africa where there were significantly high levels of malnutrition but where alcoholic beverages were not generally consumed by the populations sampled.

42.5 COCAINE

Cocaine is still a problem in many areas of our country, although that epidemic is receding in light of the continuing problem with methamphetamine and the growing epidemic of opiate drug abuse. However, older generations and many alcoholics still depend on the drug. Alcoholics claim they use cocaine to keep them awake long enough to continue their drinking binge. Cocaine acts on the addicted brain by stimulating the release of excessive levels of dopamine into the synapses of the frontal cortex of the brain, specifically in the area of the NAc, while simultaneously blocking uptake of the dopamine back into the neurons. The resulting excessive levels of dopamine in the synapses of the frontal cortex will result in the euphoria cocaine addicts crave but can also lead to toxic levels of dopamine in the brain, which can result in episodes of paranoia, agitation, and violence. Chronic use of cocaine will result in a depletion of dopamine in the brain, which will result in depression, agitation, violence, impulsivity, and impaired judgment and planning. Following a period of several months of abstinence and a healthy diet, however, the brain will regenerate sufficient levels of dopamine to eliminate the depletion, which gradually returns brain function back to normal. The disruption of brain function then is considered transient when compared with the effects of chronic methamphetamine abuse, as previously described.

As to opiate addiction and heroin dependence, in particular, most of the discussion as to deleterious effects on the brain has to do with the possible long-term effects of hypoxia or reduced levels of oxygen to the brain and not on long-term drug-induced brain damage per se, although research is underway looking for evidence of brain damage associated with heroin addiction. At this time, however, it is generally thought that opiate addiction does not result in chronic brain damage or long-term syndromes aside from residual effects associated with post-acute withdrawal, which can last up to several months. Likewise, sedative dependence is also not thought to result in long-term damage to brain function. Chronic inhalant abuse, however, is a matter of concern. Chronic huffing or inhaling toluene, for example, has been shown through brain imaging studies to result in a marked atrophy or shrinking of the cerebral cortex.[36]

42.6 EXPERT TESTIMONY CONCERNING ADDICTIVE DISORDERS

42.6.1 Role of the Addictions Expert

This writer is retained in cases where there is a need for an understanding of (a) the defendant's substance abuse history, (b) the impact of that defendant's substance abuse history on his cognitive abilities, and (c) how his or her cognitive impairment may have been a mitigating factor in the commission of the alleged behavior. I have testified in numerous motion-to-suppress hearings on these same issues.

When examining a defendant's substance abuse or dependence history, this writer states up front that the scope of my clinical investigation is limited to the defendant's substance abuse history and related issues. It is essential to state those parameters up front because identifying the limits of the investigation helps avoid some of the traps and pitfalls set for me by the opposing counsel on cross-examination. I then discuss the issue regarding no confidentiality in this process with the offender and that my report will be distributed to the defense attorney, the prosecution, and the judge presiding over the case. The defendant is then asked if he or she would like to proceed under those conditions. These two statements concerning lack of confidentiality and permission to proceed offer me protection.

42.6.2 Some Testimony Experiences and the Limits of Opinions

When I (BDH) am testifying and undergoing cross-examination, the prosecution will often try to set traps or detours. I have learned early to rely on an assertiveness training technique known as the "Broken Record Technique."[37] Whenever I am posed with a question from the attorney, which I know is meant to take me down a road I do not wish to go, I will state on the stand that "the scope of my investigation was limited to the alcohol and drug use habits of the defendant," assuming the question is not directly related to the substance abuse habits of the defendant. I repeat that statement, verbatim, every time I am asked a leading question on the stand, which is outside my disclosed opinions. The process allows me to remain in control of the verbal exchange and usually will lead to frustration on the part of the attorney and occasionally a slight smile on the part of the judge.

For example, I was retained by the defense in a very aggravated or "bad case" in Southern Illinois wherein the stepdaughter of the town's former police chief was found brutally stabbed in her apartment, and the defendant, in that case, had an extensive history of alcoholism. The prosecutor asked me if I was aware that the murder weapon had been found in a dumpster only a few yards away from the defendant's apartment. I responded, "The scope of my investigation was limited to the alcohol and drug use habits of the defendant." "But Mr. Hargan, the defendant's fingerprints were found on the murder weapon. What do you think of that?" I calmly replied, "The scope of my investigation was limited to the alcohol and drug abuse habits of the defendant." The prosecutor tried different ways to solicit more information from me, but I continued to repeat the same statement. That happens often.

In a murder case in Indiana in which I testified, the prosecutor showed me graphic crime scene photos of the victims and demanded to know if I thought this was the work of a madman. Again, I responded, "The scope of my investigation was limited to the alcohol and drug use habits of the defendant." If the prosecutor had asked me if the sky was indeed a pretty shade of green that day, I would have given the exact same answer. Courts have never rebuked me in any way, because I am allowed to limit my testimony to the original parameters of my examination. Otherwise, I might stray into other areas outside of my training and experience, which would diminish the credibility of my testimony. Always play to your strengths, as they say.

42.6.3 Preparation

Preparation as an expert for court involves being not only completely familiar with the details and implications of your report but also clinically up to date on the substances you identified as being a part of the defendant's history of addiction. Since the 1980s and 1990s, the evolution of imaging technology has enabled us to better understand the effect which different mood-altering drugs have on different areas of brain structure and function. Technology or related data used in the inpatient substance abuse treatment and research fields have included the use of computerized tomography (CT) scans, MRI scans, positron emission tomography (PET) scans, and CBF studies. In the late 1980s, clinicians were able to visualize significant cerebral atrophy in the brains of chronic alcoholics using CT scans. In the 1990s, PET scans enabled us to visualize different areas of the brain that were activated during undergoing acute cocaine intoxication. In the early 2000s, CBF studies showed how methamphetamine-induced brain damage reduced blood flow to the frontal lobe of the brain.

The use of technology in understanding the adverse changes in brain structure and function following years of chronic exposure to alcohol and drugs revolutionized the substance abuse treatment process. Technology can be used in explaining diminished capacity (when relevant) or changes in personality and behavior which may be relevant to explaining motivation for a particular crime. It is also helpful to know that courts prefer the hard science results of brain imaging when attempting to make a point. Courts prefer hard science (as in research findings associated with imaging studies) to soft science (such as the rambling speculation as to psychosocial functioning).

I was retained by a defense attorney in Arizona wherein a known and documented chronic methamphetamine addict in his mid-20s shot and killed a police officer who had come to his house to serve him with a warrant. I examined the defendant and found he was a chronic methamphetamine addict. I interviewed his mother, brother, and ex-wife in person and on the phone. The interview with the ex-wife hit pay dirt. She had no interest in her ex-husband since their divorce, so she was considered a credible witness. She went on at length about how paranoid and delusional the defendant had been during their marriage. He was prone to delusional thinking and auditory and visual hallucinations. He even kept a video camera running at home at all times to videotape his wife and anyone else who entered their home when he was not there. He talked about people, places, and things that were not there. He could not always distinguish right from wrong or conform his behavior to the letter of the law.

On the day that the unfortunate deputy approached the defendant in his front yard, the defendant had a gun tucked into his waistband and shot the officer dead instantly. I conducted a literature search on the most recent research findings concerning chronic methamphetamine addiction and its impact on brain structure and function. I found that there was considerable documentation describing a phenomenon referred to as methamphetamine psychosis (MAP). Despite all the documentation this writer easily uncovered on the subject and its relevance to this case, the expert for the state, a clinical psychologist, had never heard of the phenomenon. The jury voted to take death off the table and to recommend a sentence of life in prison instead.

42.7 ADDITIONAL CONSIDERATIONS CONCERNING ADDICTION MITIGATION

Acute intoxication in and of itself is generally not accepted by the courts as a mitigating circumstance since intoxication is considered a voluntary action and thus not a defense in the guilt phase of a trial or plea bargaining. Acute intoxication may be taken into account, however, during the penalty phase of a trial and also when impaired suspects are being interrogated since they may be more suggestible or vulnerable to making false confessions, thus compromising their Fifth Amendment protection against self-incrimination. I have also seen many instances in which murder suspects are interrogated by detectives while undergoing heroin withdrawal instead of interrogating them after the withdrawal syndrome has run its course. Acute heroin withdrawal typically takes up to five days to run its course, depending on the length of time the heroin was used and the quantity the addict was using on a daily basis prior to his or her arrest.

Specific instances associated with acute intoxication, however, sometimes are acceptable in court if said intoxication resulted in the defendant's inability to discern right from wrong or if he or she was unable to conform their behavior to the letter of the law. A defendant's behavior while in a substance-induced psychotic state can be considered a mitigating circumstance in the penalty phase of a trial. Psychotic states are usually associated with stimulant or hallucinogen abuse although there have been reported instances of alcoholic hallucinosis as a part of delirium tremens during alcohol withdrawal.

It has been my experience thus far that a defendant's claim of being in an alcohol-induced blackout at the time of the offense will fall on deaf ears in court. A blackout is described as an individual's failure to be able to recall specific events that occurred during a state of acute intoxication because, under blood alcohol concentrations of 0.20% or more, the brain's ability to imprint new memories can become impaired or disabled. The alcoholic will still interact with his or her environment but have no recall of doing so the next day. This is different from "passing out" wherein the alcoholic will lose consciousness altogether. To show that the defendant was indeed in a blackout, one must show documentation of the BAC at the time of the offense or at least have a BAC value at the time of the arrest which can then be retroactively computed to show what his or her BAC was at the actual time of the offense.

Delirium associated with acute intoxication during the course of intense police interrogation may be recognized by the courts however as a mitigating factor in their defense. In a May 23, 2003, issue of the *Milwaukee Journal Sentinel*, an article entitled "Suspect Delirious, So Statement Is Improper" reported that a murder suspect's statements could not be used in court because he was delirious when the police questioned him, the State Supreme court ruled. The article went on to say, "The court ruled that police used subtle interrogation tactics that were beyond Paul Hoppe's ability to resist because he was suffering from symptoms of alcohol withdrawal. The tactics rendered his statements involuntary and inadmissible," the court said "The Supreme Court's decision upheld rulings by lower courts that Hoppe's statement was not voluntary because police subtly coerced him into talking even though he was obviously impaired."[38]

This writer recalls another case involving a capital murder suspect. My medical record collection of his prior numerous hospitalizations for alcohol withdrawal documented many admissions which reported the patient's withdrawal delirium and withdrawal seizures. Prior to my examination, the suspect had been arrested and interrogated by the police approximately 24 hours after his last drinking binge. He was quite sick at the time of his interrogation to the point that the detectives decided to bring in the paramedics for a wellness check. The paramedics arrived, and the detectives asked them to give the suspect medication so they could finish interviewing him. The paramedics said they could not do this and were dismissed. The interrogation resumed. I could not simply rely on the suspect's word on this disturbing report, so I placed a call to the fire chief at the station from which the paramedics were dispatched (next door to the police station); the fire chief verified the paramedics visit to the police station and their dismissal.

Brain damage associated with chronic drug addiction certainly can serve as a mitigating factor, depending on the nature of the damage and the type of drug. For example, NIDA-sponsored researchers noted in one study that *Brain Imaging Studies Show Long-Term Damage From Methamphetamine Abuse*.[39] NIDA researchers have also found that new imaging technology confirms earlier PET Scan evidence: methamphetamine abuse linked to human brain damage.

Further research referenced earlier in this chapter showed that chronic methamphetamine addicts who experienced MAP when triggered by a given stressor while using the drug can experience a methamphetamine-induced paranoid-hallucinatory state or "flashback" and that these transient psychotic breaks or "flashbacks" can even occur up to a year after the drug was last administered.[40] In a NIDA presentation in Thailand in 2001, it was noted that "researchers have documented dose-related abnormalities that reflect neuronal damage or loss more than one year after the subjects stopped taking methamphetamine".[41] It was the latter studies that this writer used on the stand in Pinal County, AZ, to show that the murder of the deputy was in all likelihood the result of a methamphetamine paranoid-hallucinatory or "flashback" state. The penalty phase in that capital murder case resulted in a hung jury and life imprisonment instead of death.

42.7.1 Alcoholic Dementia

It is well documented through brain imaging studies using CT or PET scans that chronic alcoholics usually have some degree of brain damage ranging from mild to moderate impairments associated with what used to be referred to in psychiatry as organic brain syndrome (OBS) or organic mental disorder (OMD) to the more advanced brain damage associated with the Korsakoff Syndrome. The OBS and OMD have been largely replaced today by the term "dementia" in the *DSM-5*. I worked at the inpatient level for many years with chronic alcoholics diagnosed with OBS and noted that, after six months or so, symptoms that did not resolve upon abstinence were considered permanent cognitive impairments.

Symptoms of OMD or alcoholic dementia typically include confusion, memory impairment, delirium, impaired judgment, and agitation. These patients typically did not process information as quickly as patients not diagnosed with this disorder, and they became irritable and agitated when feeling overwhelmed or overstimulated with too much information or decision-making demands. Prior to their hospitalization, they typically self-medicated their frustration and agitation with more alcohol, which sometimes resulted in domestic violence, property damage, or other related offenses. Otherwise, while in the hospital, their personalities were generally rather flat but pleasant.

On the other end of the alcoholic brain damage spectrum is the Korsakoff Syndrome. This form of encephalopathy was first described in Russia by the researcher Sergei Korsakoff during the late 19th century. The most prominent symptoms associated with this form of brain damage include anterograde and retrograde amnesia and confabulation. Anterograde amnesia refers to the brain's inability to imprint new memories, while retrograde amnesia refers to the brain's inability to recall previously imprinted memories. Confabulation refers to a phenomenon whereby the patient absolutely believes a "memory" to be true even though evidence shows that memory to be false. It is thought that the brain's ability to properly sequence retrieved memories is permanently impaired. In my previous clinical practice, I was involved with the case management of a group of Korsakoff patients. When I asked one patient what he had for breakfast that morning, he insisted he had pancakes for breakfast, his favorite kind of breakfast. When I checked with his nurse, however, I was informed that the kitchen had prepared bacon and eggs for breakfast and pancakes had been served for breakfast two days earlier. It is all part of the global disorientation Korsakoff patients live with.

Korsakoff Syndrome patients' experience following many years of heavy drinking and malnutrition and vitamin deficiency are associated with the etiology of some forms of brain damage. I conducted a treatment group consisting only of Korsakoff patients every Thursday evening in 1977. I would welcome the group and ask them what year it was. They would reply "1964," "1969," "1974," so we would take a vote. Then I would ask them what month it was. They would look outside the windows for hints as to the season and then suggest "February," "December," and "January." When I would ask what day of the week it was, they would get upset and argue with each other as to what day it was, complaining that I was using "trick questions." Months spent in reality orientation classes helped to some degree with their orientation as to the basics concerning time, place, and so forth, but their frustrating inability to learn or retrieve memories was very difficult for these patients.

42.7.2 Neuropsychological Evaluation

To consider the possibility of impaired brain function as a mitigating factor in a given criminal case, one must retain the services of a licensed neuropsychologist, preferably one with courtroom experience, to conduct the kind of precise neuropsychological examination needed to pinpoint precise areas of impaired brain function and to determine the nature and extent of those impairments. That expert should be expected to testify as to his or her findings and recommendations following any such neuropsychological work-up.

While voluntary intoxication is not a defense, the effects of *substance withdrawal* can offer mitigation in explaining an addict's criminal behavior, especially during the penalty phase of a case. Opiate addicts are not typically violent persons except for the violence which occurs between gangs vying for control over various neighborhoods for their drug trafficking activities. In the mid- to late 2000s, my capital murder cases were typically involved with crack cocaine addicts undergoing cocaine withdrawal. However, the average heroin addict undergoing withdrawal, however, is too sick to be violent. Heroin addicts as a group are not usually violent but instead are a major nuisance to retailers who are victims of retail theft by these addicts.

Heroin intoxication and withdrawal originate within the mesolimbic system of the midbrain as discussed earlier and as such are not limited by the constraints of the cerebral cortex. The primary major symptoms of heroin withdrawal are associated with a shutdown of the digestive system resulting in cramping, nausea, vomiting, and diarrhea, along with an increased sensitivity to pain and other secondary symptoms. Additionally, there is a major escalation in craving, which also originates from the more primitive mesolimbic system. I have found that a detailed explanation of the half-life of opiate drugs, the severity of opiate withdrawal symptoms, and the creation of a timetable outlining the progression over time from the point of arrest following the last dose of heroin to the endpoint of interrogations is helpful in my preparation for court. It is easier then to explain the mitigating circumstances associated with each stage of withdrawal along with the increased vulnerability for giving a false confession to obtain relief from the pain, nausea, vomiting, chills, hot and cold flashes, and fever, which all peak during the time of these interrogations. This is useful information which can be used in motion-to-suppress hearings by defense attorneys.

42.8 SUMMARY AND CONCLUSIONS

The field of addiction provides rich mitigation evidence for use by experts. Mitigation evidence can be identified in the addict's family history, including genetic and environmental considerations. Also, self-medication behavior to alleviate symptoms associated with psychosocial trauma or psychiatric issues, extreme mood swings or behavioral changes while undergoing a state of acute intoxication or withdrawal, or even the neurobiological changes that occur within the addicted brain may impact the addict's ability to discern right from wrong or to conform his or her behavior to the law.

NOTES

1 Jellinek EM. Alcoholism, a genus and some of its species. Can Med Assoc J. 1960 Dec 24;83(26):1341–1345.
2 Cloninger CR, Sigvardsson S, Bohman M. Type I and type II alcoholism: An update. Alcohol Health Res World. 1996;20(1):18–23.
3 Cservenka A, Brumback T. The burden of binge and heavy drinking on the brain: Effects on adolescent and young adult neural structure and function. Front Psychol. 2017;8:1111.

4 Squeglia LM, Jacobus J, Tapert SF. The effect of alcohol use on human adolescent brain structures and systems. Handb Clin Neurol. 2014;125:501–510.
5 Squeglia LM, Jacobus J, Tapert SF. The effect of alcohol use on human adolescent brain structures and systems. Handb Clin Neurol. 2014;125:501–510.
6 Squeglia LM, Rinker DA, Bartsch H, Castro N, Chung Y, Dale AM, Jernigan TL, Tapert SF. Brain volume reductions in adolescent heavy drinkers. Dev Cogn Neurosci. 2014;9:117–125.
7 Squeglia LM, Rinker DA, Bartsch H, Castro N, Chung Y, Dale AM, Jernigan TL, Tapert SF. Brain volume reductions in adolescent heavy drinkers. Dev Cogn Neurosci. 2014;9:117–125.
8 Heikkinen N, Niskanen E, Könönen M, Tolmunen T, Kekkonen V, Kivimäki P, Tanila H, Laukkanen E, Vanninen R. Alcohol consumption during adolescence is associated with reduced grey matter volumes. Addiction. 2017;112(4):604–613.
9 Pfefferbaum A, Kwon D, Brumback T, Thompson WK, Cummins K, Tapert SF, Brown SA, Colrain IM, Baker FC, Prouty D, De Bellis MD. Altered brain developmental trajectories in adolescents after initiating drinking. Am J Psychiatry. 2018;175(4):370–380.
10 Squeglia LM, Rinker DA, Bartsch H, Castro N, Chung Y, Dale AM, Jernigan TL, Tapert SF. Brain volume reductions in adolescent heavy drinkers. Dev Cogn Neurosci. 2014;9:117–125.
11 Pfefferbaum A, Rohlfing T, Pohl KM, Lane B, Chu W, Kwon D, Nolan Nichols B, Brown SA, Tapert SF, Cummins K, Thompson WK. Adolescent development of cortical and white matter structure in the NCANDA sample: Role of sex, ethnicity, puberty, and alcohol drinking. Cereb Cortex. 2016;26(10):4101–4121.
12 Squeglia LM, Schweinsburg AD, Pulido C, Tapert SF. Adolescent binge drinking linked to abnormal spatial working memory brain activation: Differential gender effects. Alcohol Clin Exp Res. 2011;35(10):1831–1841.
13 McQueeny T, Schweinsburg BC, Schweinsburg AD, Jacobus J, Bava S, Frank LR, Tapert SF. Altered white matter integrity in adolescent binge drinkers. Alcohol Clin Exp Res. 2009;33(7):1278–1285.
14 McQueeny T, Schweinsburg BC, Schweinsburg AD, Jacobus J, Bava S, Frank LR, Tapert SF. Altered white matter integrity in adolescent binge drinkers. Alcohol Clin Exp Res. 2009;33(7):1278–1285.
15 Lovinger DM, Roberto M. Synaptic effects induced by alcohol. Curr Top Behav Neurosci. 2013;13:31–86.
16 Koolschijn PC, Peper JS, Crone EA. The influence of sex steroids on structural brain maturation in adolescence. PLoS One. 2014;9(1):e83929.
17 Cunningham RL, Lumia AR, McGinnis MY. Androgenic anabolic steroid exposure during adolescence: Ramifications for brain development and behavior. Horm Behav. 2013;64(2):350–356.
18 Koolschijn PC, Peper JS, Crone EA. The influence of sex steroids on structural brain maturation in adolescence. PLoS One. 2014;9(1):e83929.
19 Cunningham RL, Lumia AR, McGinnis MY. Androgenic anabolic steroid exposure during adolescence: Ramifications for brain development and behavior. Horm Behav. 2013;64(2):350–356.
20 Cunningham RL, Lumia AR, McGinnis MY. Androgenic anabolic steroid exposure during adolescence: Ramifications for brain development and behavior. Horm Behav. 2013;64(2):350–356.
21 Cunningham RL, Claiborne BJ, McGinnis MY. Pubertal exposure to anabolic androgenic steroids increases spine densities on neurons in the limbic system of male rats. Neuroscience. 2007;150(3):609–615.
22 Rose RJ, Winter T, Viken RJ, Kaprio J. Adolescent alcohol abuse and adverse adult outcomes: Evaluating confounds with drinking-discordant twins. Alcohol Clin Exp Res. 2014;38(8):2314–2321.
23 de Wit H. Impulsivity as a determinant and consequence of drug use: A review of underlying processes. Addict Biol. 2009;14(1):22–31.
24 de Wit H. Impulsivity as a determinant and consequence of drug use: A review of underlying processes. Addict Biol. 2009;14(1):22–31.
25 Jones SA, Lueras JM, Nagel BJ. Effects of binge drinking on the developing brain. Alcohol Res. 2018;39(1):87–96.
26 Rose RJ, Winter T, Viken RJ, Kaprio J. Adolescent alcohol abuse and adverse adult outcomes: Evaluating confounds with drinking-discordant twins. Alcohol Clin Exp Res. 2014;38(8):2314–2321.
27 Hakansson A, Jesionowska V. Associations between substance use and type of crime in prisoners with substance use problems: A focus on violence and fatal violence. Subst Abuse Rehabil. 2018;9:1–9.
28 McCambridge J, McAlaney J, Rowe R. Adult consequences of late adolescent alcohol consumption: A systematic review of cohort studies. PLoS Med. 2011;8(2):e1000413.
29 Beaver KM, Vaughn MG, DeLisi M, Wright JP. Anabolic-androgenic steroid use and involvement in violent behavior in a nationally representative sample of young adult males in the United States. Am J Public Health. 2008;98(12):2185–2187.
30 Hakansson A, Jesionowska V. Associations between substance use and type of crime in prisoners with substance use problems: A focus on violence and fatal violence. Subst Abuse Rehabil. 2018;9:1–9.
31 Health, N.I.O. *What Are the Risks of Anabolic Steroid Use in Teens?* Steroids and Other Appearance and Performance Enhancing Drugs (APEDs).
32 *Steroid Abuse by School Age Children: A Guide for Parents and School Officials.* US Department of Justice; Drug Enforcement Administration.

33 Lumia AR, McGinnis MY. Impact of anabolic androgenic steroids on adolescent males. Physiol Behav. 2010;100(3):199–204.
34 House JC. *After the Webinar: Policing Vulnerable Populations*. Q&A with Jason Winsky.
35 House JC. *After the Webinar: Policing Vulnerable Populations*. Q&A with Jason Winsky.
36 http://www.inhalants.org/damage.htm. Accessed December 29, 2015.
37 Harris T. *I'm OK, You're OK*. New York: Harper & Row, 1969.
38 *The Milwaukee Journal Sentinel*. Suspect delirious, so statement is improper, May 23, 2003, 6B.
39 Ernst T, Chang L, Leonido–Yee M, Speck O. Evidence for long-term neurotoxicity associated with methamphetamine abuse. Neurology. 2000;54(6):1344–1349.
40 Yui K, Ishiguro T, Goto K, Ikemoto S, Kamata Y. Spontaneous recurrence of methamphetamine psychosis: Increased sensitivity to stress associated with noradrenergic hyperactivity and dopaminergic change. Clin Neurosci. 1999;249:1–2.
41 *NIDA Invest*. Southeast Asian scientists explore methamphetamine research, Winter 2001.

Index

Note: Page numbers in *italics* indicate a figure and page numbers in **bold** indicate a table on the corresponding page.

B

C

P

Q

R

U

V

W

X

Z

For Product Safety Concerns and Information please contact our EU
representative GPSR@taylorandfrancis.com
Taylor & Francis Verlag GmbH, Kaufingerstraße 24, 80331 München, Germany

www.ingramcontent.com/pod-product-compliance
Ingram Content Group UK Ltd.
Pitfield, Milton Keynes, MK11 3LW, UK
UKHW050318071126
477531UK00012B/680

* 9 7 8 1 0 4 1 0 2 0 8 0 6 *